AF709563

Pediatric Sedation Outside of the Operating Room

Keira P. Mason
Editor

Pediatric Sedation Outside of the Operating Room

A Multispecialty International Collaboration

Second Edition

Springer

Editor
Keira P. Mason
Department of Anesthesia
Harvard Medical School
Children's Hospital Boston
Boston, MA, USA

ISBN 978-1-4939-1389-3 ISBN 978-1-4939-1390-9 (eBook)
DOI 10.1007/978-1-4939-1390-9
Springer New York Heidelberg Dordrecht London

Library of Congress Control Number: 2014950071

© Springer Science+Business Media New York 2012, 2015
This work is subject to copyright. All rights are reserved by the Publisher, whether the whole or part of the material is concerned, specifically the rights of translation, reprinting, reuse of illustrations, recitation, broadcasting, reproduction on microfilms or in any other physical way, and transmission or information storage and retrieval, electronic adaptation, computer software, or by similar or dissimilar methodology now known or hereafter developed. Exempted from this legal reservation are brief excerpts in connection with reviews or scholarly analysis or material supplied specifically for the purpose of being entered and executed on a computer system, for exclusive use by the purchaser of the work. Duplication of this publication or parts thereof is permitted only under the provisions of the Copyright Law of the Publisher's location, in its current version, and permission for use must always be obtained from Springer. Permissions for use may be obtained through RightsLink at the Copyright Clearance Center. Violations are liable to prosecution under the respective Copyright Law.
The use of general descriptive names, registered names, trademarks, service marks, etc. in this publication does not imply, even in the absence of a specific statement, that such names are exempt from the relevant protective laws and regulations and therefore free for general use.
While the advice and information in this book are believed to be true and accurate at the date of publication, neither the authors nor the editors nor the publisher can accept any legal responsibility for any errors or omissions that may be made. The publisher makes no warranty, express or implied, with respect to the material contained herein.

Printed on acid-free paper

Springer is part of Springer Science+Business Media (www.springer.com)

This book is primarily dedicated to my mother and father, whose sacrifice, love, and encouragement enabled me to pursue my goals and dreams. Leading by example, they showed me to persevere, remain positive, optimistic, and always strive to achieve my personal best.
Thank you to my husband, Ed, for continuing in my parents' footsteps of encouragement and support. Finally, thanks to God for the gift of Tyler and Colin, my sons whom I can only hope to guide, nurture, and provide for as my parents did for me.

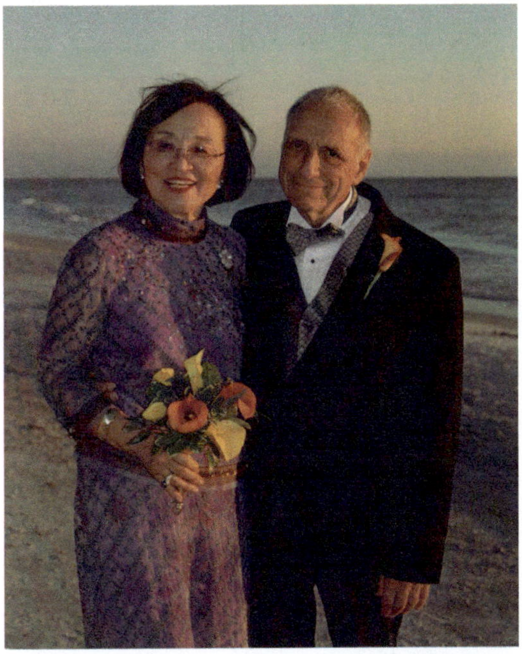

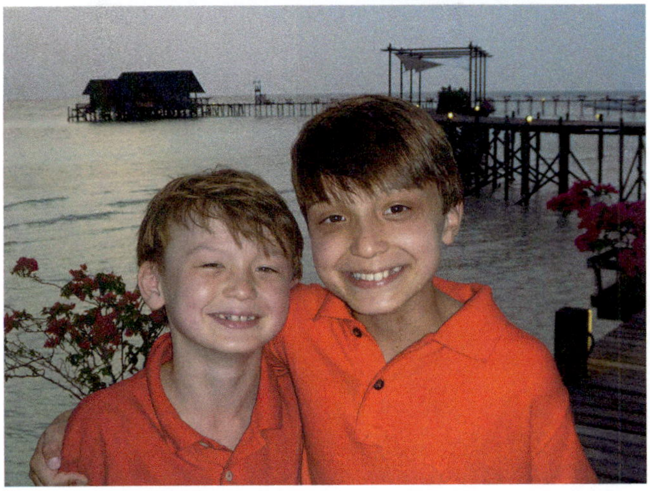

Preface

I am honored and thrilled to present within the short span of only 2 years, this updated and expanded 2nd edition. The book has doubled in size, chapters, and authorship, most notably with the significant expansion of contributions from international leaders. These authors are pioneers in their areas of expertise, both in the United States and abroad, not only in the field of sedation but also in the areas of law, ethics, child psychology, child development, pediatrics, neonatology, simulation, drug development, patient safety, and pharmacology. This book is a testimony to the passion and commitment of all the contributing authors to advance the knowledge and practice of pediatric sedation. *Pediatric Sedation Outside of the Operating Room: A Multispecialty International Collaboration* is intended to represent and be applicable to sedation providers of any specialty from around the world. Our international contributors represent Australia, Belgium, Brazil, Chile, China, Israel, the Netherlands, New Zealand, South Africa, Switzerland, and the United Kingdom. I am very appreciative of their efforts. Each chapter has been revised and edited a minimum of three times (some as many as six) and I extend a sincere "thank you" to each author.

This book is a unique and authoritative contribution to the field of pediatric sedation. As an expansion of the first book, it is directed to all specialties and specifically acknowledges and reviews the contributions and viewpoints of a broad range of international societies and specialists. Sedation has evolved to include all specialties. Although each chapter is written by a specialist in his/her particular area, it is intended to be of value to those who do not necessarily practice in that area. For example, the pediatrician in the United States will learn something in the *Pediatric Sedation: The South Pacific Approach* chapter that can be applied or considered for his own practice.

Those chapters that are clinically oriented conclude with Case Studies, which present challenging clinical scenarios. This is a unique finale as it is the author's presentation of real-life cases. The intent of these Case Studies is to guide the reader through the challenges, thought processes, and management options for each situation. Certainly there are many possible solutions to each scenario: Exploring them through the eyes of the experienced author offers a unique and valuable perspective.

This book may be read cover to cover or read a chapter at a time, out of succession. There is intentional, albeit minimal, repetition in the book. The repetition is intended not only to solidify important information for the reader but also to convey relevant information for those who may not be reading the book cover to cover. Even the "repetition" is presented in a different style by the individual authors, in most cases masking the repeated elements.

The final form of this book went to the publisher in April 2014. Every chapter was updated in these final weeks with any recently published papers. The galley proofs were reviewed and again the chapters were all updated as recently as the summer of 2014.

This book represents a global collaboration. Currently the field of sedation is being challenged by politics, differing viewpoints and our inability to reach a consensus. Our ability to come together, outside of this book, will be essential to the future of our pediatric patients who receive sedation.

There will continue to be new clinical and research studies that advance our knowledge of sedation. New sedatives, physiological monitors, and sedation delivery systems will certainly be introduced over the next decade. Regardless, the approach to sedation and the information conveyed in these chapters is intended to distinguish this book as a timeless relic that marks an important era in the field of sedation.

Boston, MA, USA
April 15, 2014

Keira P. Mason, M.D.

Acknowledgments

The most important and heartfelt acknowledgment is to my family. Thank you to my husband, Ed, and to my two sons, Colin and Tyler, for bearing with the "motherless" weekends and evenings as I worked on this book. You have all supported me not only for this book but also throughout my career: Understanding that sharing sedation experience with others to advance the practice, safety, and knowledge of sedation is my passion and has taken me away from home, even missing on occasion some of your important events. Thank you, Tyler, for sitting beside me in the early morning and late night hours to read over my shoulder, encouraging and helping me edit and revise chapters. Thank you, Colin, for your efforts in helping me organize the book and come up with new ideas for book chapters.

I would like to express my respect, gratitude, and appreciation to Shelley Reinhardt, Senior Editor in Clinical Medicine and Maureen Pierce, Developmental Editor of Springer. Their gentle prodding, attention to detail, kindness, expertise, and professionalism inspired me to meet all deadlines. Most importantly, they were committed to this project: Committed to supporting all efforts to produce *Pediatric Sedation Outside of the Operating Room* as a contribution to the field. Shelley, I am so grateful to have benefitted from your expertise, encouragement and, most importantly, your friendship. THANK YOU.

My final acknowledgment is to Ms. Amanda Buckley and Ms. Bailey Mannix. From the inception of the 1st edition of this book to the final moments of its galley proof approval, Amanda devoted even the after-hours ensuring that all references and source information were accurate, the grammar and typos corrected, the copyrights were obtained, and that everything from the table of contents to the final chapter flowed appropriately. Thank you, Bailey, for following Amanda's footsteps and for creating footsteps of your own with this 2nd edition. I have esteem for your commitment to this edition: Your organization, encouragement, tireless enthusiasm, and sleuthing skills to uncover important contributions to this book were invaluable. I will always be appreciative of you both.

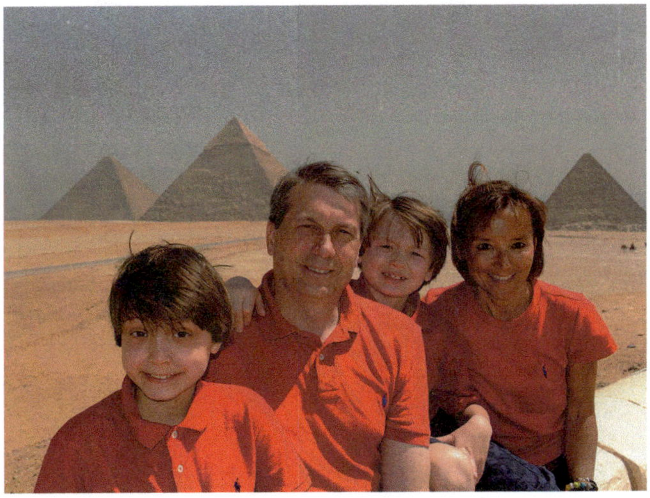

Contents

Contributors

*For more information on the credentials of each author, please see the Epilogue.

Anthony R. Absalom, MBChB, MD Department of Anesthesiology, University Medical Center Groningen, Groningen, The Netherlands

Karel Allegaert, MD, PhD Department of Growth and Regeneration, KU Leuven and Neonatal Intensive Care Unit, University Hospitals Leuven, Leuven, Belgium

Brian J. Anderson, PhD Department of Anesthesiology, University of Auckland School of Medicine, Auckland, New Zealand

Dean B. Andropoulos, MD, MHCM Department of Anesthesiology, Texas Children's Hospital, Baylor College of Medicine, Houston, TX, USA

Franz E. Babl, MD, MPH Emergency Department, Royal Children's Hospital, Melbourne, VIC, Australia

Douglas W. Carlson, MD Division of Pediatric Hospitalist Medicine, Department of Pediatrics, St. Louis Children's Hospital, Washington University, St. Louis, MO, USA

Xuan Chen, M Med Department of Anesthesia, University of Hong Kong Shenzhen Hospital, Shenzhen, Guangdong, China

Vincent W. Chiang, MD Department of Medicine, Harvard Medical School, Boston Children's Hospital, Boston, MA, USA

Stewart L. Cohen, Esq Cohen, Placitella & Roth, P.C., Philadelphia, PA, USA

Paulo Sérgio Sucasas da Costa, MS, PhD Department of Pediatrics, Federal University of Goiás, Goiania, Goias, Brazil

Joseph P. Cravero, MD Department of Anesthesiology, Perioperative, and Pain Medicine, Boston Children's Hospital, Boston, MA, USA

Stuart R. Dalziel, MBChB, FRACP, PhD Children's Emergency Department, Starship Children's Hospital, Auckland District Health Board, Auckland, New Zealand

Andrew Davidson, MBBS, MD, FANZCA Department of Anaesthesia and Pain Management, The Royal Children's Hospital, Murdoch Children's Research Institute, Melbourne, Australia

James J. Fehr, MD Department of Anesthesiology and Pediatrics, St. Louis Children's Hospital, St. Louis, MO, USA

Lynne R. Ferrari, MD Departments of Anesthesiology, Perioperative and Pain Medicine, Boston Children's Hospital, Boston, MA, USA

Daniela Hearst, BSc (Hons), M Phil Department of Pediatric Psychology, Psychosocial and Family Services, Great Ormond Street Hospital for Children NHS Foundation Trust, London, UK

Robert S. Holzman, MD, MA (Hon), FAAP Department of Anesthesiology, Perioperative and Pain Medicine, Boston Children's Hospital, Boston, MA, USA

Timothy Horeczko, MD, MSCR Department of Emergency Medicine, Harbor – UCLA Medical Center, Torrance, CA, USA

Marie Therese Hosey, DDS, MSc, BDS Department of Pediatric Dentistry, King's College Hospital, London, UK

Michael G. Irwin, MBChB, MD Department of Anesthesiology, Queen Mary Hospital, The University of Hong Kong, Hong Kong, China

Ian A. Jenkins, MBBS, FRCA Department of Pediatric Intensive Care & Anesthesiology, Bristol Royal Hospital for Children, Bristol, UK

Robert M. Kennedy, MD Department of Pediatrics, St. Louis Children's Hospital, St. Louis, MO, USA

Baruch S. Krauss, MD, Ed M, Division of Emergency Medicine, Boston Children's Hospital, Boston, MA, USA

Piet L.J.M. Leroy, MD, PhD, Division of Pediatric Critical Care, Department of Pediatrics, Pediatric Procedural Sedation Unit, Maastricht University Medical Centre, Maastricht, The Netherlands

Bi-lian Li, MD Department of Anesthesiology, Guangzhou Women and Children's Medical Centre, Guangzhou, Guangdong, China

Jenifer R. Lightdale, MD, MPH Division of Pediatric Gastroenterology and Nutrition, Department of Pediatrics, UMass Memorial Children's Medical Center, University of Massachusetts, Worcester, MA, USA

Yuan-Chi Lin, MD, MPH Department of Anesthesiology, Perioperative and Pain Medicine, Medical Acupuncture Service, Boston Children's Hospital, Harvard Medical School, Boston, MA, USA

Mohamed Mahmoud, MD Radiology Anesthesia and Sedation, Department of Anesthesia, Cincinnati Children's Hospital Medical Center, Cincinnati, OH, USA

Keira P. Mason, MD Department of Anesthesia, Harvard Medical School, Children's Hospital Boston, Boston, MA, USA

Lisa L. Mathis, MD Department of Global Regulatory Affairs and Safety, Maternal and Pediatric Safety and Regulatory, Amgen Inc., Thousand Oaks, CA, USA

Ian McKenzie, MBBS, FANZCA Department of Anaesthesia and Pain Management, The Royal Children's Hospital, Parkville, VIC, Australia

Suzanne S. Mendez, MD Department of Pediatrics, Santa Clara Valley Medical Center, San Jose, CA, USA

Alan F. Merry, FANZCA, FPMANZCA Department of Anesthesiology, University of Auckland and Auckland City Hospital, Auckland, New Zealand

James R. Miner, MD Department of Emergency Medicine, Hennepin County Medical Center, Minneapolis, MN, USA

Gail A. Van Norman, MD Department of Anesthesiology and Pain Medicine, University of Washington Medical Center, Seattle, WA, USA

Department of Biomedical Ethics, University of Washington Medical Center, Seattle, WA, USA

Itai M. Pessach, MD, PhD Israel Center for Medical Simulation (MSR), Sheba Medical Center, Tel-Hashomer, Israel

Randy P. Prescilla, MD Department of Anesthesiology, Perioperative and Pain Medicine, Boston Children's Hospital, Boston, MA, USA

Luciane Rezende Costa, DDS, MS, PhD Division of Pediatric Dentistry, Federal University of Goiás, Goiania, Goias, Brazil

Mark G. Roback, MD Department of Pediatrics, University of Minnesota Children's Hospital, Minneapolis, MN, USA

James A. Roelofse, MBChB, M Med Department of Anesthesiology, Tygerberg Hospital, Bellville, Cape Province, South Africa

Joel S. Rosen, Esq Cohen, Placitella & Roth, P.C., Philadelphia, PA, USA

Cyril Sahyoun, MD Division of Pediatric Emergency Medicine, Morgan Stanley Children's Hospital of New York, Columbia University Medical Center, New York, NY, USA

Steven M. Selbst, MD Department of Pediatrics, Nemours/Alfred I. duPont Hospital for Children and Sidney Kimmel Medical College at Thomas Jefferson University, Wilmington, DE, USA

Wang Ning ShangGuan, MD, PhD, Department of Anesthesiology, The 2nd Affiliated Hospital, Wenzhou Medical University, Wenzhou, Zhejiang, China

Devona J. Slater, CHA, CHC, CMCP Auditing for Compliance and Education, Inc. (ACE), Overland Park, KS, USA

Sulpicio G. Soriano, MD Department of Anesthesiology, Perioperative and Pain Medicine, Boston Children's Hospital, Boston, MA, USA

Michael J. Stabile, MD, MBA Department of Anesthesia, Centennial Medical Center, Nashville, TN, USA

St. Louis University School of Medicine, St. Louis, MO, USA

Michael R.J. Sury, MBBS, FRCA, PhD Department of Anaesthestics, Great Ormond Street Hospital NHS Trust, London, UK

Joss Thomas, MD, MPH, FCCP Pediatric Anesthesia, Critical Care Medicine, Department of Anesthesia, University of Iowa Children's Hospital, Iowa City, IA, USA

Joseph D. Tobias, MD Department of Anesthesiology & Pain Medicine, Nationwide Children's Hospital, Columbus, OH, USA

Johannes van den Anker, MD, PhD Department of Pediatrics, Pharmacology and Physiology, Children's National Medical Center, Washington, DC, USA

Department of Intensive Care, Erasmus Medical Center-Sophia Children's Hospital, Rotterdam, The Netherlands

Department of Pediatric Pharmacology, University Children's Hospital Basel, Basel, Switzerland

Robert A. Veselis, MD Department of Anesthesiology/CCM, Memorial Sloan Kettering Cancer Center, New York, NY, USA

Pablo Sepúlveda Voullième, Dr Med Servicio de Anestesia, Clinica Alemana Santiago Chile, Santiago, Chile

Laszlo Vutskits, MD, PhD Department of Anesthesiology, Pharmacology and Intensive Care, University Hospital of Geneva, Geneva, Switzerland

Chunyan Wang, M Med Department of Anesthesiology, University of Hong Kong Shenzhen Hospital, Shenzhen, Guangdong, China

Craig S. Webster, BSc, MSc, PhD Centre for Medical and Health Sciences Education, University of Auckland, Auckland, New Zealand

Graeme S. Wilson Department of Anesthesia, University of Cape Town, Red Cross War Memorial Children's Hospital, Rondebosch, Western Cape, South Africa

Stephen Wilson, DMD, MA, PhD Division of Pediatric Dentistry, Cincinnati Children's Hospital Medical Center, Cincinnati, OH, USA

Ying Xu, PhD, MD Department of Anesthesiology, Children's Hospital of Chongqing Medical University, Chongqing, China

Lynne P. Yao, MD Office of New Drugs, Center for Drug Evaluation and Research, US FDA, Silver Spring, MD, USA

Vivian Man-ying Yuen, MBBS Department of Anesthesiology, University of Hong Kong Shenzhen Hospital, Shenzhen, Guangdong, China

Part I

Pediatric Sedation Outside the Operating Room

The History of Sedation

1

Robert S. Holzman

Abstract

The history of induced altered states as a means of tolerating the intolerable is as old as man, and for eons has been alternately welcomed, worshipped, and vilified. As in ancient times, these three attitudes still often coexist, and our professional duty is to care for and educate our patients and public and to control the end effects to enhance safety. The history of sedation and the history of anesthesia were, and often continue to be, inseparable, particularly for children. This chapter will focus on the various modalities and practices over time, emphasizing the differences but remaining in awe of the similarities through the ages.

Keywords

History • Pediatrics • Sedation • Anesthesia • Analgesia • Opium • Narcotics • Ether • Hypnosis • Nitrous oxide • Micky Finn

Introduction

The history of induced altered states as a means of tolerating the intolerable is as old as man, and for eons has been alternately welcomed, worshipped, and vilified [1]. Ironically, as in ancient times, these three attitudes often coexist, and our professional duty is to care for and educate our patients and public, to minimize risks, and to enhance safety [2–4].

Is the history of sedation different from the history of anesthesia? They were, and often continue to be, inseparable, particularly for children,[1] so we will focus on the various modalities and practices over time, emphasizing the differences but remaining in awe of the similarities through the ages.

Inebriation, Intoxication, Hallucination, and Anesthesia

A *Forme Fruste* of the Sedation Continuum

Alcohol is a fermentation product of many fruits and cereals. Winemaking was first practiced in the Middle East about 6,000–8,000 years ago, and was already well established in

[1]The Committee on Drugs of the American Academy of Pediatrics emphasizes that "the state and risks of deep sedation may be indistinguishable from those of general anesthesia."[2] The American Dental Association Council on Education defines general anesthesia to include deep sedation.[3] The minimal distinction between deep sedation and general anesthesia has been recognized by the current author as well.[4]

R.S. Holzman, M.D., M.A. (Hon.), F.A.A.P. (✉)
Department of Anesthesiology, Perioperative and Pain Medicine, Boston Children's Hospital, Boston, MA 02115, USA
e-mail: robert.holzman@childrens.harvard.edu

K.P. Mason (ed.), *Pediatric Sedation Outside of the Operating Room: A Multispecialty International Collaboration*, DOI 10.1007/978-1-4939-1390-9_1, © Springer Science+Business Media New York 2015

ancient Egypt. Wine production was not well developed in ancient Greece, but wine was imported from other countries and often used for medicinal purposes. Benefitting from the breadth of their empire, the Romans developed the art of winemaking.

Winemaking was ubiquitous in the ancient world—the Moors prepared date wines, the Japanese rice wines, the Indians (Mexico) made *pulque* from agave, the Vikings fermented honey to make *mead*, and the Incas made *chicha* from maize. Modern beer making (yeast—*Saccharomyces cerevisiae*) probably had its origin in Babylon as long ago as 5,000–6,000 BCE. The addition of hops is a much more recent modification. Beer drinking and drunkenness was common in ancient Egyptian life; the Greeks learned their brewing skills from the Egyptians. Britons and Hiberni[2] drank *courni* made from fermented barley.

Wine remained an inebriant and intoxicant, however, until distillation technology was developed in the tenth century. Distillation exploits the fact that alcohol has a lower boiling point than water and therefore can be boiled out of an aqueous solution and condensed, approaching (but never achieving) purity—although 95 % by volume is achievable. *Liquors* (such as rum or whisky) involve fermentation of sugar cane or barley, respectively, than distillation. *Liqueurs* are usually produced by steeping fruits and/or herbs in brandy or vodka, with subsequent filtration to remove the vegetable residues. In this regard, absinthe, prepared from *wormwood* (*Artemisia absinthium*, *A. maritime*, or *A. pontica*), *anise* (*Pimpinella anisum*), and *fennel* (*Foeniculum vulgare*), plus nutmeg, juniper, and various other herbals, added to 85 % alcohol, is then filtered and diluted to 75 % alcohol by volume. Wormwood was the most important ingredient because of its psychotropic properties, recognized by ancient and medieval herbalists (Ebers Papyrus, Hippocrates, Dioscorides, John Gerard).

The dose–response of alcohol is interesting as a proxy for the continuum of sedation and general anesthesia. Mild intoxication occurs with a blood concentration of 30–50 mg/dL (0.03–0.05 %), and mild euphoria is achieved. Once the concentration has reached 100 mg/dL (0.10 %), more serious neurological disturbances result in slurred speech and a staggering gait. At concentrations of 200 mg/dL (0.20 %), vision and movement are impaired, and coma results at twice that concentration.

Ancient History

Much of what we know in the twenty-first century about attempts to provide analgesia and sleep is derived from the written records of ancient civilizations in widely separated areas: China, India, Sumeria, and Egypt, for example. The recorded knowledge began approximately in the fourth millennium BCE, codifying oral drug lore that had undoubtedly preceded such codification by centuries. In rough chronological order of the records (but not by the use of the drugs themselves), we can begin with China.

[2]Hibernia is the Latin name for Ireland; its people were the Hiberni.

Chinese Drug Lore

The *Pen Tsao* (the symbols of which represent the compilation of medicinal herbs) was said to have been authored by Emperor Shen-nung in approximately 2700 BCE. As the father of agriculture (the "Divine Husbandman"), he was said to have tasted all herbs in order to become familiar with their usefulness. Likewise, the *Nei-Ching* was said to have been written by Emperor Hant-Ti (about 2700 BCE). Although these texts describe the effects of naturally occurring herbs, the preparation of medicinals from herbs was attributed to I-Yin, a prime minister of the Shang Dynasty (1767–1123 BCE). The details of these preparations were recorded by making knots in strings, arranged vertically on a narrow bamboo surface. The ideograms utilized were uncannily similar to those chosen by Egyptian physicians in their hieroglyphs.[3] As recording transitioned from string knots on bamboo to pen and paper, clinical cases and treatment recommendations were more easily recorded, initially by Chang Chung-Ching and the surgeon Hua Tuo (c. 140–208), who probably used *Cannabis indica* (*mafeisan*[4]) for anesthesia (Fig. 1.1). This was probably no accident, as there is ample suggestion that Hua Tuo may have developed many of his medical ideas from Ayurvedic practices in an area of China richly influenced by Buddhist missionaries [5].

Hindu Drugs

Brahman priests and scholars were the medical leaders in the earliest recorded histories, three of which are of primary importance:

- *Charaka Samhita* (second century CE, but copied from an earlier work)
- *Susruta* (fifth century CE)
- *Vagbhata* (seventh century CE)

[3]The ideogram for "physician" (pronounced i) contained an arrow or a lancet in the upper half and a drug—or bleeding glass—in the lower half.

[4]The name *mafeisan* combines *ma* ("cannabis; hemp; numbed"), *fei* ("boiling; bubbling"), and *san* ("break up; scatter; medicine in powder form"). *Ma* can mean "cannabis, hemp" and "numbed, tingling." Other historians have postulated that mandrake or datura was used rather than cannabis, along with the wine. Still others have suggested hashish (bhang) or opium.

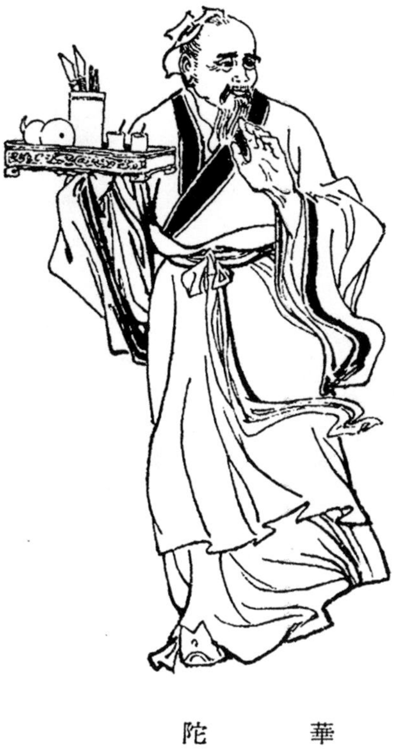

Fig. 1.1 Hua Tuo (c. 140–208 CE). The ancient texts *Records of the Three Kingdoms* and *Book of the Later Han* record Hua as the first person in China to use anesthesia during surgery, referring specifically to mafeisan. The illustration portrays Hua Tuo's surgical and medicinal abilities as well as his use of moxibustion

The *Susruta* detailed more than 700 medicinal plants, the most common of which were condiments such as sugar, cinnamon, pepper, and various other spices. Included among them were descriptions of the depressant effects of *Hyoscyamus* and *Cannabis indica*. The eponymously named text (Susruta, c. 700–600 BCE) described Susruta's use of wine to the point of inebriation as well as fumitory cannabis in preparation for surgical procedures. Part of the difficulty with so many drugs was that they were not well codified and were prescribed in casual ways by numerous practitioners, who relied on (clinical) observation of effects [6].

Sumerian Drugs

Agriculture developed in the area between the Tigris and Euphrates rivers, and a sophisticated cultivation of plant materials useful for the alleviation of symptomatic disease was not only practiced, but also recorded. Nearly 30,000 clay tablets from the era of Ashurbanipal of Assyria (568–626 BCE) were discovered in the mid-nineteenth century near the site of Nineveh, capital of the neo-Assyrian Empire, with numerous references to plant remedies. Beers were especially well developed in ancient Babylon. *Cannabis indica* was known for producing intoxication, ecstasy, and hallucinations, when reinforced with hemp. This was all under the supervision of the priesthood. In addition, hallucinogenic mushrooms were employed in ancient Sumeria. Poppies were used mainly as a condiment in Sumerian life. Although there is no drug activity in the poppy leaves, fruit, or root, if the unripe seed capsule is opened, the white juice resulting from that is (raw) opium, the dried "latex" of which forms alkaloids as it dries. However, opium was not described (as far as we know) in the Ashurbanipal tablets.

Table 1.1 List of Egyptian medical records

Document	Date	Comment
Kahun Papyrus	1900 BCE	Primarily veterinary medicine
Edwin Smith Papyrus	1600 BCE	Consists of 48 case histories; a well-organized surgical text
Ebers Medical Papyrus	1550 BCE	Deals with medical rather than surgical conditions; emphasizes recipes
Hearst Medical Papyrus	1550 BCE	Poorly organized; a practicing physician's formulary
The Erman Document	1550 BCE	Deals largely with childbirth and diseases of children
The London Papyrus	1350 BCE	Poorly organized; a practicing physician's formulary
The Berlin Papyrus	1350 BCE	Poorly organized; a practicing physician's formulary
The Chester Beatty Papyrus	1200 BCE	Formulary for anal diseases; one case report

Jewish Medicine

Jewish medicine received significant contributions from the Babylonians during the Babylonian captivity (597–538 BCE) as well as from the Egyptians during the Egyptian Captivity (a date which is much less clear, based on 430 years of captivity prior to the Exodus, accepted as 1313 BCE in rabbinic literature [7]). Jewish potions were prepared by the priesthood for pain relief and the imparting of sleep during surgical procedures, venesection, and leeching; *Samme de shinda* was probably a hemp potion, but probably not an opium derivative [8].

Egyptian Medicine

The major influence on the emerging Greek world of medicine came from Egypt. Our knowledge of their codification is relatively robust because of the medical papyri, most of which were hieratic (hieroglyphics or ideographs), compiled from around 2000–1200 BCE (Table 1.1). They themselves were probably copied from older originals, as evidenced by the use of archaic terminology within the medical papyri, more characteristic of language from around 3,000 BCE.

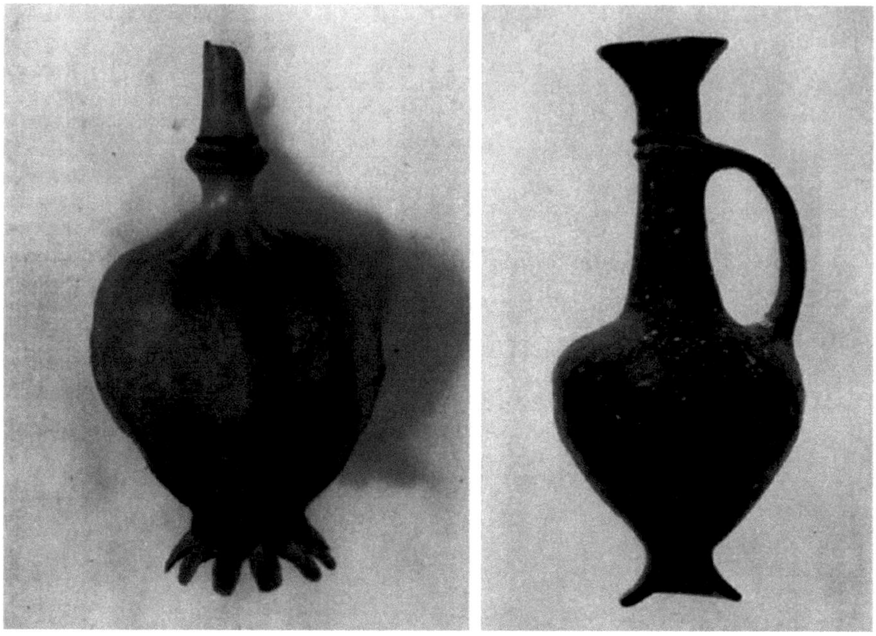

Fig. 1.2 Comparison of an opium poppy capsule and a base ring juglet. An inverted opium poppy capsule on the *left*, and a base ring juglet from the Bronze Age (dated to Egypt's 18th Dynasty). Note that the solid pottery base ring takes the place of the serrated upper portion of the capsule, but the flaring angle is almost identical. Overall, the outline of the body of the juglet almost parallels that of the poppy head, and its tall slender neck corresponds to the poppy's thin stalk

It is ironic, and somewhat puzzling, that despite the richness of ancient documentation from the aforementioned artifacts, there is a paucity of information about narcotics and sedatives in ancient Egypt. Most of the suggestions about the use of such medications are by inference. For example, Ebers 782 cites "*shepnen* of *shepen*" (poppy seeds of poppy) to settle crying children. Interestingly, the poppy seed contains relatively little morphine; it is the latex produced from the incision of the seed pod that actually contains the active ingredient. Another suggestion, by inference, is that base ring juglets were used to import opium from Cyprus in about 1500 BCE, because of the resemblance of these juglets, when inverted, to a poppy head [9] (Fig. 1.2) and the reported finding of morphine in an Egyptian juglet from the tomb of Kha (19th Dynasty), although this has been disputed [10]. Cannabis (*C. sativa*) was prescribed by mouth, rectum, vagina, and delivered transdermally and by fumigation, yet central nervous system effects were not described. The London and Ebers papyri refer to *mantraguru*, an obvious common origin with mandrake, or *Mandragora*. Some species of lotus (*Nymphaea caerulea* and *N. lotos*) are native to Egypt and contain several narcotic alkaloids that can be extracted in alcohol, leading to a logical hypothesis that lotus-containing wine might have additional narcotic effects. Ebers 209 and 479 both refer to preparations for the relief of right-sided abdominal pain and jaundice (respectively) containing lotus flower as an ingredient, but directing that the lotus flower has to "spend the night" with wine and beer—conditions that would likely permit alkaloid extraction. It is therefore interesting that depictions of the lotus flower being sniffed are the only artifactual suggestion of the possible medical use of lotus (Fig. 1.3).

All over the world, indigenous people have learned the medicinal properties of plants in their environments and have applied them to medical use. The remarkable acquisition of a sufficient amount of experience to provide the basis for a systematic analysis and an accumulated fund of knowledge, probably transmitted initially through oral tradition and along specific lines of professional authority (physicians, priesthood, specialized castes of drug-gatherers and preparers), undoubtedly took a long time. It is extraordinary, moreover, for its survival and consistency through the ages, laying the groundwork for Classical civilization and beyond.

Classical History

Greek Medicine

Chaldo-Egyptian magic, lore, and medicine were transferred to the coasts of Crete and Greece by migrating Semitic Phoenicians or Jews and the stage was then set for incorporating ancient Egyptian drug lore into Greek medicine. Two prominent medical groups developed on the mainland of Asia Minor: the group on Cnidos, which was the first, and then the group on Kos, of which Hippocrates (460–380 BCE) was one member. While they were accomplished surgeons, they generally eschewed drugs, believing that most sick people get well regardless of treatment. Although Hippocrates did not gather his herbal remedies, he did prescribe plant drugs, and a cult of root diggers (*rhizotomoi*) developed, as did a group of drug merchants (*pharmacopuloi*). In Greece, plants were used not only for healing but also as a means of inducing death, either through suicide or execution; perhaps

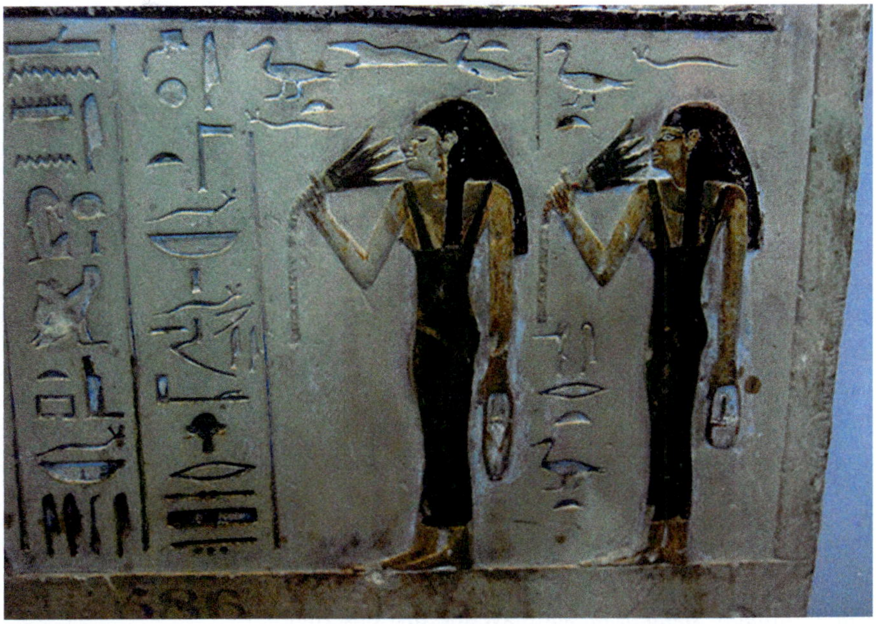

Fig. 1.3 Stela of Ity (from the British Museum EA 586). Painted limestone Stela of Ity, dated to the 12th Dynasty, c. 1942 BCE. Ity's many titles and the names of his mother, wife, sons, and daughters are listed. Note the illustration of the lotus flower being sniffed

the best example was the death of Socrates. Later, Theophrastus (380–287 BC), a pupil of Aristotle (384–322 BCE), classified plants and noted their medicinal properties. This was a departure from previous recordings, as Theophrastus analyzed remedies on the basis of their *individual* characteristics, rather than a codification of combinations as in Egyptian formularies. He provided the earliest reference in Greek literature to mandragora [11].

The father of history, Herodotus (484–425 BCE) (Fig. 1.4), left a detailed description of the mass inhalation of cannabis in the Scythian baths [12]:

> The Scythians, as I said, take some of this hemp-seed, and, creeping under the felt coverings, throw it upon the red-hot stones; immediately it smokes, and gives out such a vapour as no Grecian vapour-bath can exceed; the Scyths, delighted, shout for joy, and this vapour serves them instead of a water-bath; for they never by any chance wash their bodies with water.

Compression of the great vessels of the neck was also recognized as a form of inducing unconsciousness. It was recognized that compression of the carotid[5] arteries would result in unconsciousness and insensibility, as would pressure on the jugular veins. Aristotle recognized this, saying of jugular vein compression, "if these veins are pressed externally, men, though not actually choked, become insensible, shut their eyes, and fall flat on the ground" [13].

The poets Virgil and Ovid described the soporific effects of opium. Virgil (70–19 BCE) described the power of the poppy through the personification "Lethaeo perfusa papavera somno" ("poppies steeped in Lethe's slumber"),[6] while Ovid (43 BCE–17/18 BCE) also invoked the personification of Lethe by stating, "There are drugs which induce deep slumber, and steep the vanquished eyes in Lethean night."[7]

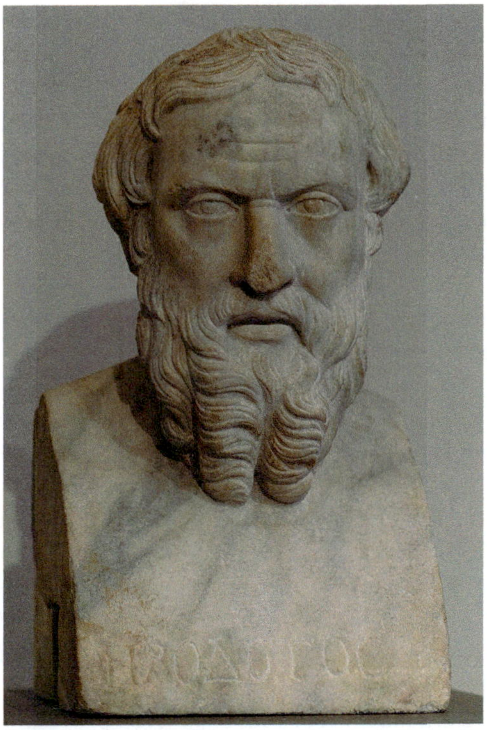

Fig. 1.4 Herodotus (484–425 BCE). *Source*: Marie-Lan Nguyen (2011)/ Wikimedia Commons

[5]The Greek word *carotid* means drowsiness, stupor, or soporific—hence the carotid artery is the artery of sleep. Galen incorporated its use as an adjective when he stated, "I abhor more than anybody carotic drugs."

[6]Virgil, Georgics 1. 78

[7]As recorded in Fasti, a Roman calendar, 4:661

Roman Medicine

After the decline of the Greek empire following the death of Alexander the Great (323 BCE), Greek medicine was widely disseminated throughout the Roman Empire by Greek physicians, who often were slaves. Dioscorides (c. 40–90 CE) described some 600 plants and non-plant materials including metals. His description of mandragora is famous—the root of which he indicates may be made into a preparation that can be administered by various routes and will cause some degree of sleepiness and relief of pain [14]. Pliny the Elder (23–79 CE) described the anesthetic efficacy of mandragora in the following manner [15]:

> …(mandragora is) given for injuries inflicted by serpents and before incisions or punctures are made in the body, in order to insure insensibility to pain. Indeed for this last purpose, for some persons the odor is quite sufficient to induce sleep.

In the first century, Scribonius Largus compiled *Compositiones Medicorum* and gave the first description of opium in Western medicine, describing the way the juice exudes from the unripe seed capsule and how it is gathered for use after it is dried. It was suggested by the author that it be given in a water emulsion for the purpose of producing sleep and relieving pain [16]. Galen (129–199 CE), another Greek, in *De Simplicibus* (about 180 AD), described plant, animal, and mineral materials in a systematic and rational manner. His prescriptions suggested medicinal uses for opium and hyoscyamus, among others; his formulations became known as galenicals.

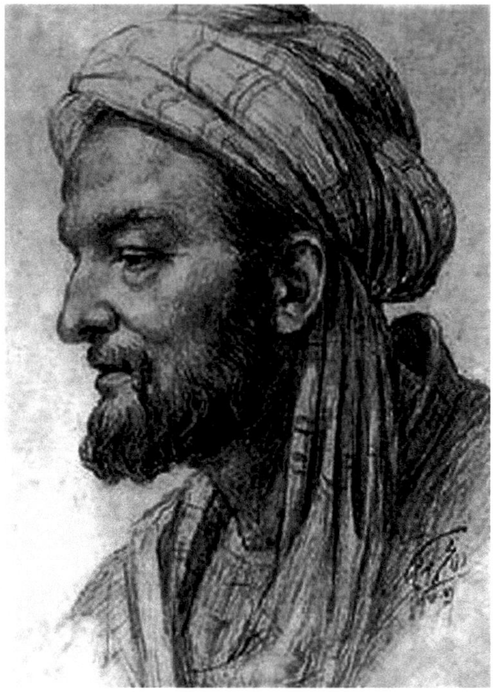

Fig. 1.5 Avicenna (930–1036 CE). "If it is desirable to get a person unconscious quickly, without his being harmed, add sweet-smelling moss or aloes-wood to the wine. If it is desirable to procure a deeply unconscious state, so as to enable the pain to be borne, which is involved in painful application to a member, place darnel-water into the wine, or administer fumitory opium, hyoscyamus (half dram dose of each); nutmeg, crude aloes-wood (four grains of each). Add this to the wine, and take as much as is necessary for the purpose. Or boil black hyoscyamus in water, with mandragora bark, until it becomes red, and then add this to the wine" [17]

Islamic Medicine

In 640 CE, the Saracens conquered Alexandria, Egypt's seat of ancient Greek culture, and by 711 CE they were patrons of learning, collecting medical knowledge along the way. Unlike the Christians, who believed that one must suffer as part of the cure, the Saracens tried to ease the discomfort of the sick. They flavored bitter drugs with orange peels and sweets, coated unpleasant pills with sugar, and studied the lore of Hippocrates and Galen. Persian physicians became the major medical teachers after the rise of the Baghdad Caliphate around 749 CE, with some even penetrating as far east as India and China. By 887 there was a medical training center with a hospital in Kairouan in Northern Africa.

The most prominent of the Arab writers on medicine and pharmacy were Rhazes (865–925 CE) and Avicenna (930–1036 CE), whose main work was *A Canon on Medicine*. The significance of this thread of ancient medical philosophy was that during the eleventh and twelfth centuries this preserved knowledge was transmitted back to Christian Europe during the Crusades. Avicenna noted the special analgesic and soporific properties of opium, henbane, and mandrake [17] (Fig. 1.5).

Medieval Medicine

The first Christian early medieval reference to anesthesia is found in the fourth century in the writings of Hilary, the bishop of Poitiers [18]. In his treatise on the Trinity, Hilary distinguished between anesthesia due to disease and "intentional" anesthesia resulting from drugs. While St. Hilary does not describe the drugs that lulled the soul to sleep, at this time (and for the following few centuries) the emphasis remained on mandragora.

From 500 to 1400 CE, the church was the dominant institution in all walks of life, and medicine, like other learned disciplines, survived in Western Europe between the seventh or eighth and eleventh centuries mainly in a clerical environment. However, monks did not copy or read medical books merely as an academic exercise; Cassiodorus (c. 485 CE–c. 585 CE), in his efforts to bring Greek learning to Latin readers and preserve sacred and secular texts, recommended books by Hippocrates, Galen, and Dioscorides while linking the purpose of medical reading with charity care and help.

Conventional Greco-Roman drug tradition, organized and preserved by the Muslims, returned to Europe chiefly through Salerno, an important trade center on the southwest coast of

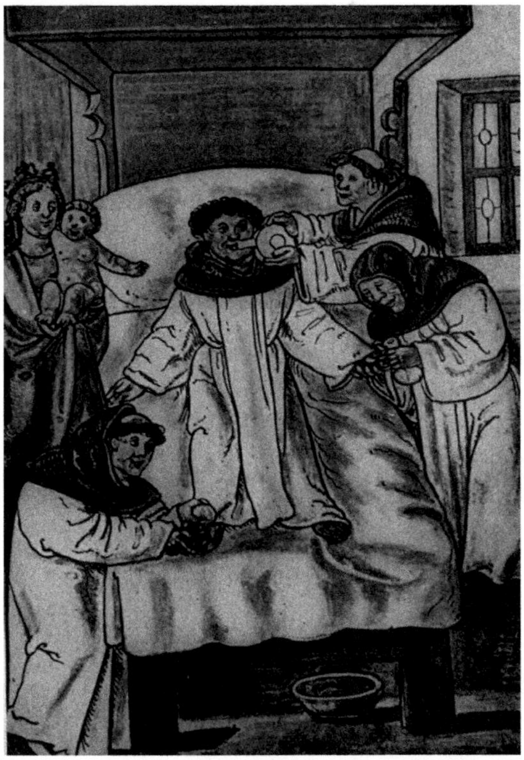

Fig. 1.6 The Alcohol Sponge [46]. "Take of opium, of the juice of the unripe mulberry, of hyoscyamus, of the juice of hemlock, of the juice of the leaves of mandragora, of the juice of the wood-ivy, of the juice of the forest mulberry, of the seeds of lettuce, of the seeds of the dock, which has large round apples, and of the water hemlock—each an ounce; mix all these in a brazen vessel, and then place in it a new sponge; let the whole boil, as long as the sun lasts on the dog-days, until the sponge consumes it all, and it is boiled away in it. As oft as there shall be need of it, place this sponge in hot water for an hour, and let it be applied to the nostrils of him who is to be operated on, until he has fallen asleep, and so let the surgery be performed. This being finished, in order to awaken him, apply another sponge, dipped in vinegar, frequently to the nose, or throw the juice of the root of fenugreek into the nostrils; shortly he awakes" [47]

Italy in the mid 900s. One of the more impressive practices documented at Salerno was intentional surgical anesthesia, described in *Practica Chirugiae* in 1170 by the surgeon Roger Frugardi (Roger of Salerno, 1140–1195), in which he mentions a sponge soaked in "narcotics" and held to the patient's nose. Hugh of Lucca (ca. 1160–1252) prepared such a sleeping sponge according to a prescription later described by Theodoric of Cervia (ca. 1205–1296). As an added precaution, Theodoric bound his patients prior to incision. The description of the soporific sponge of Theodoric survived through the Renaissance largely because of Guy de Chauliac's (1300–1367) *The Grand Surgery* and the clinical practices of Hans von Gersdorff (c. 1519) and Giambattista della Porta (1535–1615), who used essentially the same formula of opium, unripe mulberry, hyoscyamus, hemlock, mandragora, wood-ivy, forest mulberry, seeds of lettuce, and water hemlock (Fig. 1.6).

Ether

Ether was discovered in 1275 CE by the Spanish chemist Raymundus Lullus (c. 1232–1315). This new discovery was given the name "sweet vitriol." In 1540 CE, the synthesis of ether was described by the German scientist Valerius Cordus (1514–1544 CE) who carefully specified the materials to be used, the apparatus, and the procedure to be followed in order to distill "strong biting wine" (alcohol) with "sour oil of vitriol" (sulfuric acid). He recommended it for the relief of cough and pneumonia [19]. Paracelsus (1493–1541), a contemporary of Cordus, came surprisingly close to the recognition of ether as an anesthetic [20]. Later, in 1730, German scientist W. G. Frobenius changed the name of sweet vitriol to ether.

Varied Preparations of Varying Potencies

If the constituents of the plants were combined with fats or oils, they would penetrate through the skin or could be easily absorbed via the sweat ducts in the axillae or body orifices such as the vagina or rectum. This would allow the psychoactive tropane alkaloids, especially hyoscine, access to the blood and brain without passage through the gut, thus avoiding the risk of poisoning. A few prominent surgeons offered statements about the mode of application of such salves or "oyntments." John Arderne (1307–1380) (Fig. 1.7), known for his success-curing fistula in ano, and Andres De Laguna (1499–1560) (Fig. 1.8), physician to Emperor Charles V and Philip II, provided unambiguous descriptions of soporifics.

The uncertainty of the potency and action of the narcotic drugs rendered their application dangerous and by the end of the sixteenth century such anesthetics had largely fallen into disrepute and disuse. Indeed, even if physicians tried to use "narcotic" herbals in the middle of the seventeenth century, they were condemned, arrested, and fined or tried for practicing witchcraft [21]. Many of the early books were herbals, and Gerard (1545–1612) warned of the alkaloids "...this kind of Nightshade causeth sleepe...it bringeth such as have eaten thereof into a ded sleepe wherein many have died" [22].

The Scientific or Modern Epoch

The divergence of herbalism (botany) and medicine began in the seventeenth century as part of the larger movement known alternatively as natural philosophy, scientific deism, and the scientific revolution. An attempt to develop quantitative methodology characterized science, and at the forefront of these attempts was the chemical analysis of the active ingredients in medicinal plants.

Following his clinical observation of poisoning in children who had mistaken water hemlock for parsnip root, Johann

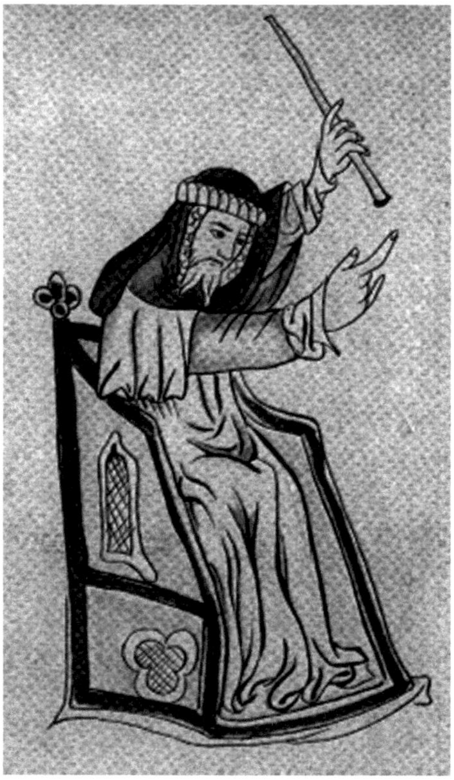

Fig. 1.7 John Arderne (1307–1380). "An ointment with which if any man be anointed he shall suffer cutting in any part of his body without feeling or aching. Take the juice of henbane, mandragora, hemlock, lettuce, black and white poppy, and the seeds of all these aforesaid herbs, if they may be had, in equal quantities; of Theban poppies and of poppy meconium one or two drachms with sufficient lard. Braise them all together and thoroughly in a mortar and afterwards boil them well and let them cool. And if the ointment be not thick enough add a little white wax and then preserve it for use. And when you wish to use it anoint the forehead, the pulses, the temples, the armpits, the palms of the hands and the soles of the feet and immediately the patient will sleep so soundly that he will not feel any cutting" [48, 49]

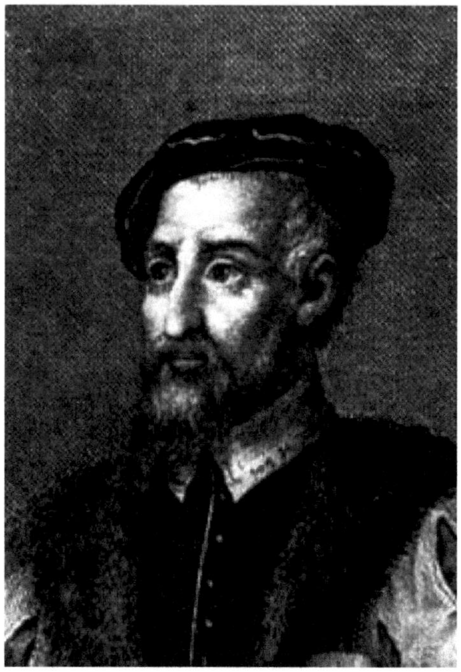

Fig. 1.8 Andres de Laguna (1499–1560 CE). "...a pot full of a certain green ointment...with which they were annointing themselves...was composed of herbs...such as hemlock, nightshade, henbane, and mandrake...I had the wife of the public executioner anointed with it from head to foot...she...had completely lost power of sleep...no sooner did I annoint her than she opened her eyes, wide like a rabbit, and soon they looked like those of a cooked hare when she fell into such a profound sleep that I thought I should never be able to awake her...after a lapse of thirty-six hours, I restored her to her senses and sanity" [50]

Jakob Wepfer (1620–1695) demonstrated dose-dependent toxic effects in dogs of the alkaloids eventually isolated as strychnine, nicotine, and conine [23, 24]. Thus, this early quantitative approach gave rise to the development of modern chemistry and pharmacology. This was first successfully applied to anesthetic pharmacology by Friedrich Wilhelm Adam Serturner (1783–1841) who, in 1805, described the isolation of meconic acid from the crude extract of opium and in 1806, extracted opium. He further experimented with this crystal on dogs, finding that it caused sleep and indifference to pain and called this new substance morphine, in honor of the Greek god of dreams, Morpheus. This science of pharmacology—the interaction of chemistry with living matter—thus began to replace the ancient and descriptive materia medica of herbalism, and set the stage for the advances of the second half of the nineteenth century, which included modern surgical anesthesia.

The introduction of these drugs directly into the vascular system was developed by (Sir) Christopher Wren (1632–1723) at Oxford in 1656 when he convinced his friend Robert Boyle (1627–1691) to experiment with a quill attached to a syringe through which opium was injected into a dog. What they found was that the opium made the dog stuporous, but did not kill him. Not long thereafter, in 1665, Johann Sigismund Elsholtz (1623–1688) administered opiates intravenously to humans in order to achieve unconsciousness, as described in his 1667 work *Clysmatica nova* [25] (Fig. 1.9). He performed early research into blood transfusions and infusion therapy, and speculated that a husband with a "melancholic nature" could be re-vitalized by the blood of his "vibrant wife," leading to a harmonious marriage. Direct transfusion of blood between animals was accomplished later that same year, and human transfusion followed 2 years later. Lamb's blood was usually used, until James Blundell (1791–1878) transfused human blood into humans.

By the 1830s, physiologists and elite doctors envisioned a level of unconscious life separable from the higher functions and the mind, including suffering. Advances in surgical thought, including more conservative and slower surgery, intensified the problem of pain for both patient and surgeon.

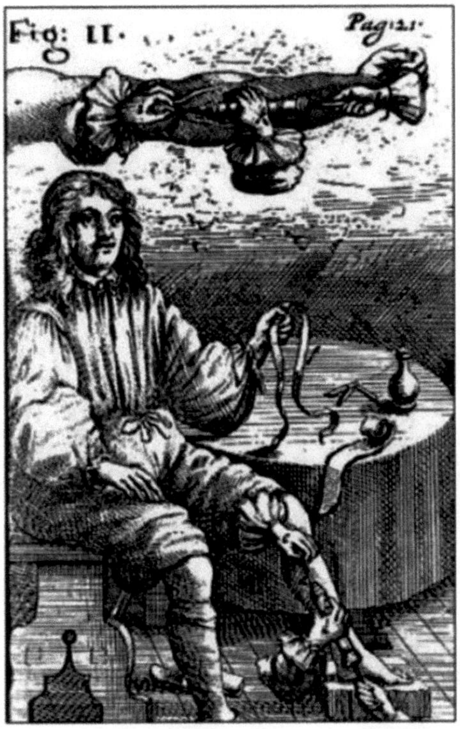

Fig. 1.9 Illustration of venous injection, from *Clysmatica nova* (1667). Note the disembodied hands delineating the vascular anatomy and illustrating the technique

By the mid 1840s, pain no longer seemed physiologically necessary or socially acceptable, but the intensive use of drugs known to diminish surgical pain was dangerous, and non-pharmacological alternatives such as Mesmerism were highly contentious and controversial.

Mesmerism, the predecessor of hypnosis, was based on Franz Anton Mesmer's (1734–1815) belief that a magnetic field existed around people and could be controlled for health purposes to heal the sick. Mesmer's strategy was to induce a trancelike state [26], rendering his patients hyperalert while asleep, a state referred to as "artificial somnambulism" by the Marquis de Puysegur (1751–1825), which eventually became known as "hypnosis" (de Cuvillers, in 1820) (Fig. 1.10). Hypnosis was used as an adjunct to surgery in the 1830s by Cloquet (mastectomy) and Elliotson, and ironically (in 1846) Esdaile (1808–1859) reported on the use of hypnoanesthesia in approximately 300 surgical patients in India [27]. Because the public demonstration of ether was virtually simultaneous, medical applications of hypnosis rapidly fell into disuse, and intriguingly, it was relegated to entertainment—much like nitrous oxide before the "acceptance" of chemically induced anesthesia. Turnabout was fair play. Hypnosis is making a comeback for sedation, especially with children [28–30], and has been shown to reduce required amounts of propofol and lidocaine, with accompanying reductions in pain, nausea, fatigue, discomfort, and emotional upset. It has also been shown to reduce the cost per patient by more than $750, mainly due to a shorter time in the operating room [31, 32].

The time was thus ripe for the integration of science and medicine, and the introduction of pneumatic medicine by Thomas Beddoes (1803–1849). He was committed to the notion that chemistry, especially the use of medicinal gases, could transform medicine and was convinced that the newly discovered respirable gases nitrogen, hydrogen, and oxygen could be therapeutic for various lung conditions, such as tuberculosis [33]. It was his employee Humphrey Davy's experiments with nitrous oxide that fueled the therapeutic use of gases, including his experiments with nitrous oxide's ability to be breathed longer than any of his other experimental gases (except air and oxygen) with animals showing an initial period of excitement, followed by exhaustion. Furthermore, he noted that even if the animal stopped breathing gas before complete exhaustion was reached, it was still possible to restore "healthy living action" by letting the animal breathe atmospheric air. The "peculiar changes" in the blood and organs were therefore reversible. This concept of death as a process, a continuum, rather than an absolute, was evolutionary and revolutionary.

Pari passu, Henry Hill Hickman (1800–1830) was born in the year Humphrey Davy suggested that nitrous oxide might be used for pain relief during surgery. Hickman, a country doctor, conceived, promoted, and attempted to practice "pain-free surgery," a novel concept at the time. Hickman experimented at a time when understandings of asphyxia were changing and death began to be conceived as a *process*. Medical research began to focus on resuscitation and the various techniques that could restore life in a body lacking a pulse or respiration. Thus Hickman understood suspended animation as a form of asphyxia; a state in which respiration had been suspended but life still existed—hence his use of bellows during a 17-min amputation of the leg of a dog. It is clear too that Hickman was incorporating a new understanding of the nervous system from the work of Charles Bell (1774–1842) in Britain and François Magendie (1783–1855) in France in the 1810s, supporting the separation of mind and body. Hickman based his experiments on the belief that if applied to humans, the key benefit would be the suspension of the mind of the patient and thus the absence of anticipation of suffering, as well as the relief of physical pain. Hickman advocated what he called "suspended animation" (general anesthesia) for surgery on humans as well. He had the right idea about inhalation anesthesia but unfortunately, in selecting carbon dioxide, picked the wrong agent. Carbon dioxide can indeed induce unconsciousness, but the gas also often results in panic attacks. In larger quantities, it is lethal.

In a scathing letter to the editor in 1826, Hickman's work was brutally criticized in an article in *The Lancet* entitled "Surgical Humbug" [34]. In his attempt to seek support abroad, Hickman decided to try his luck in Paris in 1828 and presented a paper to King Charles X. The paper was forwarded

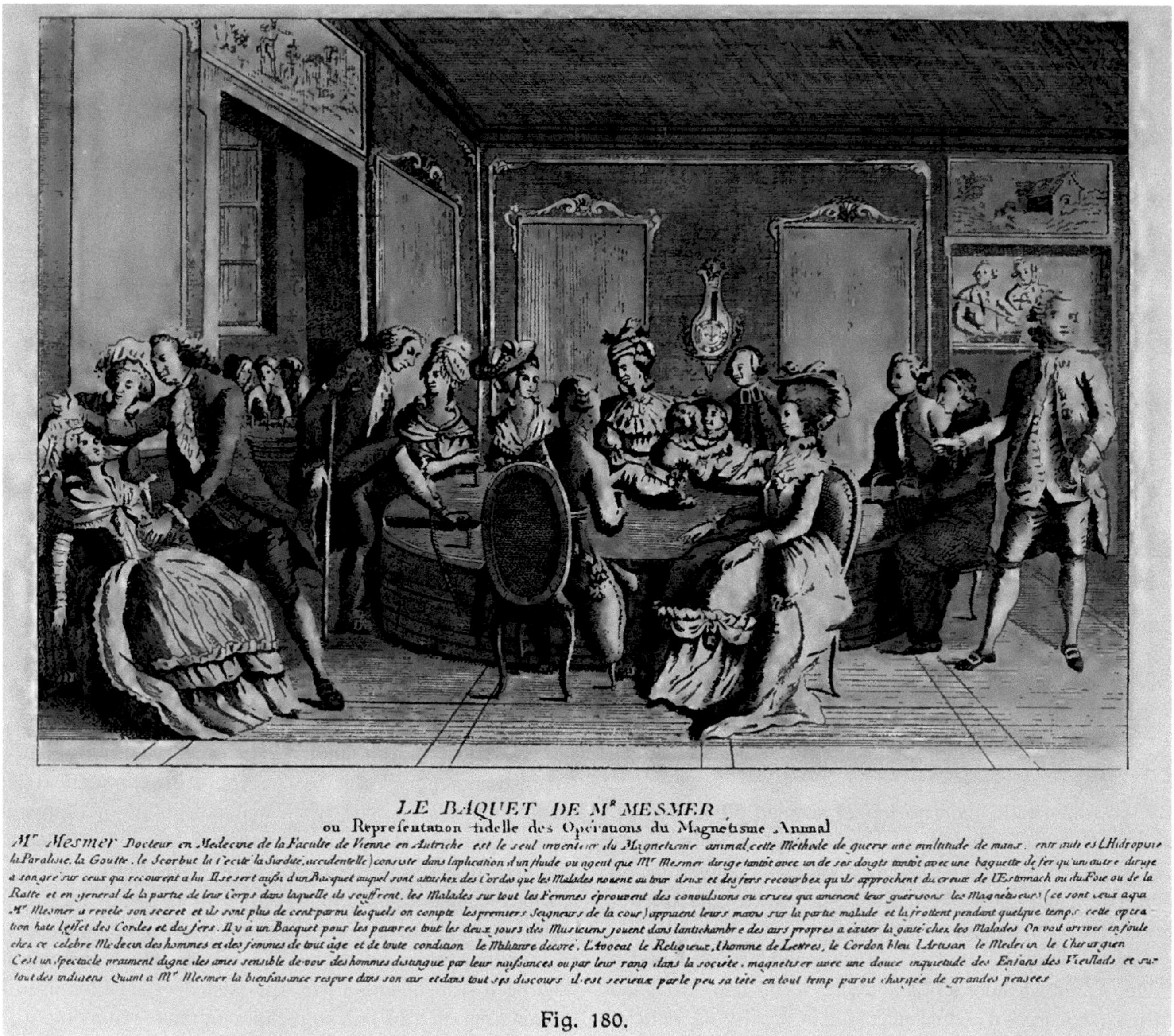

Fig. 1.10 Mesmer practicing animal magnetism, from Hollander's *Die Karikatur und Satire in der Medizin*, 1921. The title "Le Baquet de M. Mesmer" refers to Mesmer's "tub" or cabinet, around which a group of patients would sit in order to press their afflicted body areas against the tub's emerging metal rods. The patients would link their fingers to complete an "electric" circuit. The milieu was equally dramatic—an incense-filled room, haunting background music, mirrors, heavy drapes, and astrological symbols. There was a tremendous popular interest in medical applications of electricity, and serendipitously, Benjamin Franklin was the United States ambassador to France

to the Academie Royale de Medecine. A committee was set up to investigate Hickman's proposal for painless surgical operations on humans but was unsupported by French scientists. He went back to England to live out his remaining years and work hard in his poor practice, dying of tuberculosis 2 years later at 30 years of age.

Interest in the intravenous methods persisted as well, and Pierre-Cyprien Oré injected chloral hydrate in 1872 in order to produce an anesthetic state in humans (following animal experimentation). Again, unfortunately, an incorrect drug was chosen, because intravenous chloral hydrate has a very narrow therapeutic margin. Emil Fischer (1852–1919) synthesized barbital in 1902, and although it was ineffective as an intravenous anesthetic because its onset and termination was too slow, hexobarbital (Evipal) followed 30 years later and was first reported for anesthetic use in 1932. Sodium thiopental followed in 1943.

The Modern Story of Anesthesia

The modern story of anesthesia began with the reaction in Philadelphia to Humphrey Davy's (1778–1829) account of nitrous oxide and its biological effects. In 1808, William P. C.

Barton (1786–1856) emphasized the brain disorientation caused by inhaling nitrous oxide, and cited Davy. Meanwhile, an anonymous note, often ascribed to Michael Faraday, indicated that the inhalation of ether would produce effects similar to those of nitrous oxide [35].

In 1839, William E. Clarke (1818–1878) in Rochester, New York, began the fad of ether frolics among young people. He is said to have given ether for extraction of a tooth in 1842. In Jefferson, Georgia, Crawford W. Long (1815–1878) noted that one of the participants in an ether frolic fell heavily, but seemed to lack pain. On March 30, 1842, Long gave ether by inhalation to a patient for removal of a neck tumor; there was no evidence of pain. Unfortunately, he failed to report his anesthetic success for several years. William T. G. Morton (1819–1868), a student at Harvard Medical School, learned of sulfuric ether, and practiced anesthetizing various small animals at his home. He tried to perfect an inhaling device, and a demonstration was arranged at the Massachusetts General Hospital on October 16, 1846, a turning point in the history of medicine. Gardner Quincy Colton (1814–1898) first gave nitrous oxide for anesthetic purposes to Horace Wells in 1844 and revived its use in dentistry for dental extractions in 1863. Colton and Smith established the Colton Dental Institute in New York in 1864, and over a period of 30 years treated 186,500 patients without "a single accident from the gas" [36]. In England, Alfred Coleman (1828–1902) became the chief advocate for the use of nitrous oxide in dentistry. Clinical administration, of course, was not without its risks. In the latter half of the nineteenth century, before co-administration with oxygen, 100 % nitrous was administered, in the sitting position (with the head flexed in order to prevent the tongue from falling backward onto the hard palate):

> until breathing was rapid, the face was (at first) pale, then cyanotic…The aspect of the patient is at this time ghastly in the extreme, there being every physical indication of impending asphyxia…These appearances are coincident with anesthesia sufficiently profound for the needs of minor surgery and the inhaler must be withdrawn and the operation swiftly performed. [37]

Supplemental oxygen was introduced by Hewitt at the turn of the century [38]. The presumptive risks of hypoxia associated with nitrous oxide (especially the technique of "secondary saturation" practiced by clinicians since the late nineteenth century) were finally proven by C. B. Courville (a neuropathologist) in 1939 [39], although the concepts did not enter into clinical practice until after World War II. The principal advance, however, was the reformulation of the goals of nitrous oxide administration—for its sedative rather than anesthetic or analgesic properties. With patients never reaching the excitement stage, nitrous oxide was used to produce sedation, and local anesthesia to control pain. The formation of the American Dental Society of Anesthesiology in 1953 furthered this concept.

There were additional "sleep-producing" agents available in the second half of the nineteenth century. For example, it was recognized by Robert Glover that potassium bromide would cause drowsiness in animals and by Charles Locock that it would effectively treat epileptic seizures in obstetrical patients being treated for dysmenorrhea. Behrend reported its use for the treatment of insomnia, nervous excitement, and irritability. This led to the therapeutic use of "bromides" (of lithium, sodium, and potassium) as anticonvulsants. It was only a short time later that chloral hydrate was introduced by Liebreich as a soporific for medical purposes [40] as well as more nefarious purposes (it was the chief ingredient in the "Micky Finn" cocktail, for which the bartender, Michael Finn, was tried in 1903 in Chicago). Additional soporifics were paraldehyde, ethanol, sulfonal, diethyl-malonyl-urea (Veronal or barbital), and phenyl-ethyl-malonylurea (Luminal or phenobarbital).

"Modern" Sedation and Analgesia Services

There is an inseparable continuum, particularly in pediatrics, between general anesthesia and sedation and analgesia. Not surprisingly, it was the early efforts of dental surgeons at the beginning of the twentieth century that spearheaded ambulatory anesthesia, much as early general anesthesia was associated with dental procedures. Many dentists produced, purified, and stored their own nitrous oxide. The first Day Surgery began at the Royal Hospital for Sick Children in Glasgow with pediatric surgeon James Nicholl, who began to operate on children as outpatients. In 1909 he reported a 10-year history of almost 9,000 operations on children as outpatients; unfortunately, there is no mention of anesthesia [41]. In 1916, Ralph Waters (1883–1979) opened the Downtown Anesthesia Clinic in Sioux City, Iowa, caring for dental and minor surgery patients, but avoiding ether in favor of nitrous oxide along with the selection of appropriately short surgical procedures such as dental extractions, circumcisions, simple fractures, or incision and drainage of abscesses [42]. Intermittently, pediatric anesthesiologists filled the role of sedation experts in order for children to tolerate unpleasant diagnostic procedures (Fig. 1.11).

"Twilight Sleep" was also introduced in the early part of the twentieth century; it is a term that persists to this day, perhaps because of its colorful name, which originated from the German *Dammerschlaf*, introduced by Gauss in 1906 to describe the state of clouded consciousness produced by a combination of scopolamine and morphine. The technique had actually been introduced several years earlier, but Gauss (and obstetrician Bernhard Kronig) broadened its use in hundreds of patients at the Frauenklinik of the State University of Freiburg and reported their results in 500 patients [43]. The impact, particularly among women, in the early twentieth century was astounding—reporters from the *Ladies' Home Journal*, the *Women's Home Companion*, and *McClure's* journeyed to Germany to investigate the heralding of a new age in obstetrical analgesia. Popular favorable

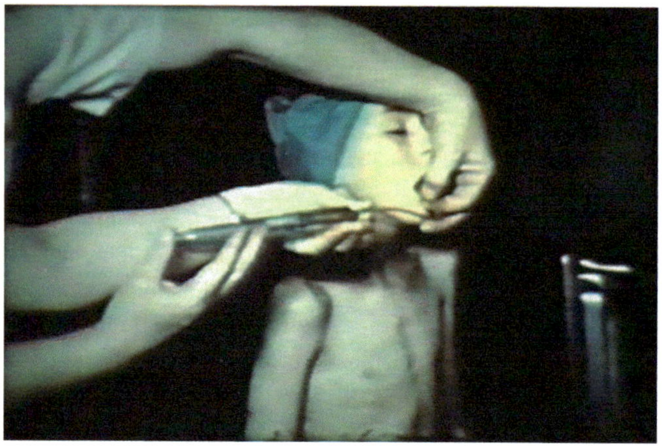

Fig. 1.11 A cachectic child undergoing intrapulmonary contrast injection via an intratracheal catheter for radiographic evaluation of tuberculosis. The tracheobronchial tree was topically anesthetized with local anesthetic, and intermittent sedation was provided by the inhalation of nitrous oxide (From a pediatric anesthesia training film made by Dr. M. Digby-Leigh in 1947)

reports rapidly followed, galvanizing a political movement for obstetrical pain relief largely advanced by women. In a rallying statement, the *Ladies' Home Journal* correspondent who eventually wrote *Truth About Twilight Sleep* stated [44]:

> I now make my last appeal to every woman who has read this book to take up the battle for painless childbirth where I left off…Fight not only for yourself, but for your sisters, your sex, the cradle of the human race…Through Twilight Sleep a new era has dawned for woman and through her for the whole human race.

The technique was not perfect. There was wide variation in the response to the drug combination, from incomplete analgesia to incomplete erasure of memory. Patients continued to groan and scream in agony, they just could not remember afterwards. Kronig would therefore not allow the presence of any family members—nor reporters or professional observers—to directly verify the efficacy of the technique. The end result, however, was that the majority of patients would not recall anything about the birth, and would awaken after delivery and state that they hoped the labor would begin soon, which then gave rise to the debate about whether there is pain if there is no memory of pain.

It further highlighted a problem that Gauss faced every day—his attempts to standardize the dose were difficult at best. He expressed it clearly, "If you could trust to having an average women, you could use an average dose; but the dose is easier to standardize than the woman." Competing institutions adopted Gauss' recommendations, with results ranging from praise to condemnation. In America, similar ambivalence was encountered. Twilight Sleep was adopted wholeheartedly and enthusiastically at Long Island College Hospital in Brooklyn (by patient request) but was abandoned at Johns Hopkins. This controversy reflected the narrow therapeutic range of the technique, again summarized succinctly by Gauss: "Twilight Sleep is a narcotic condition of extremely narrow breadth, like a narrow mountain crest. To the left of it lie the dangers of too deep action, with narcosis and absence of birthpains; to the right, the danger of shallow action, with retention of consciousness and sensibility of pain." The tensions developed between the medical profession, the medical press, and the public are outlined very thoughtfully by Caton in *What a Blessing She Had Chloroform* (1999).

Waters' prescience was followed by a long gap, until the 1960s, when increasing interest in employing shorter-acting anesthetic strategies with more rapid return to "street-fitness" predated the explosion onto the medical diagnostic scene of computed tomography (1974), magnetic resonance imaging (1977), interventional radiology procedures, cardiac catheterization (diagnostic and interventional), and various other imaging modalities. In addition, further miniaturization and engineering improvements continued for both gastrointestinal and pulmonary endoscopy and the use of radiation therapy as an adjunct to surgical and medical treatment of cancer patients. All of these took place in nontraditional anesthetizing locations, popularly known as "outfield" anesthesia [45].

The Future of Sedation

As an increasing number of procedures are developed that are accessible by percutaneous, intravascular, or natural orifice routes, they will be less painful in both the awake and asleep state. However, the need for motionlessness for children as well as adults will remain, especially as these imaging techniques and procedures are likely to be longer and require increasingly sophisticated instrumentation. At the same time, progress will inevitably continue in understanding the neurophysiology of pain mechanisms as well as consciousness, and we are perhaps not that far removed from the "tricorder" settings in *Star Trek* to noninvasively control mediators of pain, attention, and neuromuscular competence, all in scalable fashions. (Refer to Chaps. 31 and 38.)

References

1. Holzman R. Uncertainty by choice: anesthesia and the children of night. J Clin Anesth. 2002;14:46–51.
2. Committee on Drugs, American Academy of Pediatrics. Guidelines for monitoring and management of pediatric patients during and after sedation for diagnostic and therapeutic procedures. Pediatrics. 1992;89:29–34.
3. Holzman R, Cullen D, Eichhorn J, Philip J. Guidelines for sedation by nonanesthesiologists during diagnostic and therapeutic procedures. J Clin Anesth. 1994;6:265–76.
4. Kallar S, Dunwiddie W. Conscious sedation. In: Wetchler B, editor. Outpatient anesthesia. Philadelphia: Lippincott; 1988. p. 93–100.

5. Mair V. The biography of Hua-t'o. In: Mair V, editor. History of the three kingdoms. New York: Columbia University Press; 1994. p. 688–96.
6. Chopra R. Indigenous drugs of India: their medical and economic aspects. Calcutta: Art Press; 1933.
7. Finegan J. Handbook of biblical chronology: principles of time reckoning in the ancient world and problems of chronology in the Bible. Peabody, MA: Hendrickson Publishers; 1998.
8. Friedenwald H. The Jews and medicine; essays by Harry Friedenwald. Baltimore: The Johns Hopkins Press; 1944.
9. Merrillees R. Opium trade in the Bronze Age Levant. Antiquity. 1962;36:287–92.
10. Nunn J. Ancient Egyptian medicine. London: University of Oklahoma Press; 1996.
11. Holzman R. The legacy of Atropos, the fate who cut the thread of life. Anesthesiology. 1998;89:241–9.
12. Herodotus. The histories. New York: Everyman's Library/Knopf; Random House; 1997. (Translated by: Rawlinson G. 440 BCE).
13. Aristotle. The history of animals, Book III, Part 3; 1907. (Translated by D'Arcy Wentworth Thompson.
14. Dioscorides Pedanius of Anazarbus. The Greek herbal of Dioscorides (Illustrated by a Byzantine A.D. 512, Englished by John Goodyer A.D. 1655). Oxford: Oxford University Press; 1933.
15. Pliny the Elder. The natural history (c.77 AD). London: Taylor and Francis; 1855. (Translated "with copious notes and illustrations" by John Bostock and H. T. Riley. London. H. G. Bohn).
16. Leake C. An historical account of pharmacology to the 20th century. Springfield, IL: Charles C. Thomas; 1975.
17. Avicenna. Qanun dar tibb (Canon of Medicine). Tehran: Surush; 1987. (Translated by: Hazhar).
18. Humphrey J, Oleson J, Sherwood A. Greek and Roman technology: a sourcebook: annotated translations of Greek and Latin texts and documents. London: Routledge; 1998.
19. Cordus V. Annotationes in Pedacii Dioscorides Anazarbei de materia medica. Strassburg. Argentorati: Excudebat Iosias Rihelius, MDLXI 1561.
20. Temkin O, Rosen G, Zilboorg G, Sigerist H. Defensiones, in four treatises of Theophrastus von Hohenheim called Paracelsus. Boston: Johns Hopkins Press; 1941.
21. Summers M. The history of Witchcraft and demonology. New York: Knopf; 1926.
22. Gerard J. The Herball, or Generall Historie of Plantes. London: Adam Islip, Joice Norton & Richard Whitakers; 1633.
23. Eichenberger P. Autobiographic material on Johann Jakob Wepfer (1620-1695) in correspondence with Johann Conrad Brotbeck (1620-1677). Gesnerus. 1967;24:1–23.
24. Maehle AH. Scientific and moral justification of toxicologic animal trials in the 17th century. Johann Jakob Wepfer and Johann Jakob Harder. Gesnerus. 1986;43:213–21.
25. Gladstone E. Clysmatic Nova (1665): Elsholtz' Neglected Work on Intravenous Injection. Cal West Med. 1933;39:119–23.
26. Holländer E. Die Karikatur und Satire in der Medizin: medikokunsthistorisches Studie. Stuttgart: Verlag von Ferdinand Enke; 1921.
27. Esdaile J. Mesmerism in India, and its practical application in surgery and medicine. New York: Arno Press; 1976.
28. Butler L, Symons B, Henderson S, Shortliffe L, Spiegel D. Hypnosis reduces distress and duration of an invasive medical procedure for children. Pediatrics. 2005;115:e77–85.
29. Calipel S, Lucas-Polomeni M, Wodey E, Ecoffey C. Premedication in children: hypnosis versus midazolam. Pediatr Anesth. 2005; 15:275–81.
30. Saadat H, Drummond-Lewis J, Maranets I, Kaplan D, Saadat A, Wang S, Kain Z. Hypnosis reduces preoperative anxiety in adult patients. Anesth Analg. 2006;102:1394–6.
31. Montgomery G, Bovbjerg D, Schnur J, David D, Goldfarb A, Weltz C, Schechter C, Graff-Zivin J, Tatrow K, Price D, Silverstein J. A randomized clinical trial of a brief hypnosis intervention to control side effects in breast surgery patients. J Natl Cancer Inst. 2007;99:1304–12.
32. Spiegel D. The mind prepared: hypnosis in surgery. J Natl Cancer Inst. 2007;99:1280–1.
33. Snow S. Operations without pain: the practice and science of anaesthesia in Victorian Britain. Hampshire, UK: Palgrave Macmillan; 2006.
34. Antiquack. Surgical humbug. Lancet. 1826;5:646–7.
35. Anonymous. Effects of inhaling the vapour of sulphuric Ether. Q J Sci. 1818;4:158–9.
36. Mead S. Anesthesia in dental surgery. St. Louis: C.V. Mosby; 1935.
37. Litch W. Anaesthesia and anaesthetics. In: Litch W, editor. The American system of dentistry. Philadelphia: Lea Brothers; 1887. p. 144–98.
38. Smith W. A history of nitrous oxide and oxygen anaesthesia. XI: the use of Hewitt's "mixture" and the development of nasal administration. Br J Anaesth. 1972;44:106–14.
39. Courville C. Untoward effects of nitrous oxide anesthesia. Mountain View, CA: Pacific Press Publishing; 1939.
40. Liebreich O. Das Chloralhydrat: Ein neue Hypnoticum und Anaestheticum. Arch Deutsch Ges Psychiat. 1869;16:237.
41. Nicoll J. The surgery of infancy. Br Med J. 1909;2:753–4.
42. Waters R. The down-town anesthesia clinic. Am J Surg (Suppl). 1919;33:71–3.
43. Gauss C. Births in artificial Dammerschlaf: Translated from Archiv Für Gynäkologie. 1906;78:579–631. Berlin. 1914. http://books.google.com/books?id=rEXdNwAACAAJ
44. Rion H. The truth about twilight sleep. New York: McBride, Nast & Co.; 1915.
45. Hui-Lin L. The origin and use of Cannabis in Eastern Asia: linguistic-cultural implications. Econ Bot. 1973;28:293–301.
46. Schilling D. Diebold Schillings Spiezer Bilderchronik: kommentar zur Faksimile-Ausgabe der Handschrift Mss. hist. helv. I. 16 der Burgerbibliothek Bern/herausgegeben von Hans Haeberli und Christoph von Steiger; mit Beiträgen von Vinzenz Bartlome. Luzern: Faksimile Verlag; 1513. (Translated by: Haeberli H, Steiger C, Bartlome V, Zahnd M).
47. Borgognoni T. The surgery of Theodoric. Tr. from the Latin. New York: Appleton-Century; 1995. (Translated by: Campbell E, Colton J).
48. Fraenkel W. Uber Narkosen und Weckmittel des John Arderne, Schmerz-Narkose-Anesthesie. Leipzig; 1937.
49. Piomelli D, Pollio A. A study in Renaissance psychotropic plant ointments. Hist Philos Life Sci. 1994;16:241–73.
50. Rothman T. De Laguna's commentaries on hallucinogenic drugs and witchcraft in Dioscorides' Materia Medica. Bull Hist Med. 1972;46:562–7.

Sedation Policies, Recommendations, and Guidelines Across the Specialties and Continents

2

Joseph P. Cravero

Abstract

The provision of sedation for children undergoing tests or procedures outside of the operating room has evolved significantly over the last 40 years. Professional societies around the globe have helped make this area of care safer by providing recommendations or guidelines for practitioners. Some organizations, such as the American Academy of Pediatrics (AAP), have published a series of these guidelines over the years that have adopted the most relevant information and newest technologies as they have developed. Most of the guidelines share common elements. They are intended to maximize the safety and effectiveness of sedation by defining the appropriate evaluation of patients, recommending strategies for sedation, outlining appropriate monitors for patients during sedation, and defining discharge criteria after the procedure/sedation is completed. In this chapter there is a detailed discussion of several of the historically most cited sedation guidelines for children and a brief review of a number of other organizational guidelines from around the world.

Keywords

Sedation • Children • Guidelines • International • Monitoring • Recommendations • American Academy of Pediatrics (AAP) • American Academy of Pediatric Dentistry (AAPD) • American Society of Anesthesiologists (ASA) • American College of Emergency Physicians (ACEP) • Joint Commission • Deep sedation • Monitored Anesthesia Care (MAC) • Center for Medicare and Medicaid Services (CMS) • American Dental Association (ADA) • American Society of Gastroenterologists (ASG) • Scottish Intercollegiate Guidelines Networks (SIGN) • Society for the Advancement of Anesthesia in Dentistry (SAAD) • South African Society of Anesthesiologists (SASA)

Introduction

The practice of pediatric sedation involves a wide variety of sedation providers and pediatric medical subspecialists. There are no "universally" applicable and acceptable guidelines that apply to all the physicians and nurses who are taking part in sedating children. A number of guidelines, policies, and recommendations for sedation care have been promulgated by different subspecialty societies over the last 30 years. This chapter will consider the evolution of North American and international guidelines, and put them into context and perspective.

The common dictionary definition of "guideline" is "general rule, principle, piece of advice." With this definition in mind, this chapter will consider several forms of guidelines—including those that come in the form of "Statements," "Practice Advisories," "Clinical Policies," or "Recommendations." These documents range from those that contain broad descriptions of appropriate monitoring and treatment to those

J.P. Cravero, M.D. (✉)
Department of Anesthesiology, Perioperative, and Pain Medicine, Boston Children's Hospital,
300 Longwood Avenue, Boston, MA 02115, USA
e-mail: Joseph.Cravero@childrens.harvard.edu

K.P. Mason (ed.), *Pediatric Sedation Outside of the Operating Room: A Multispecialty International Collaboration*,
DOI 10.1007/978-1-4939-1390-9_2, © Springer Science+Business Media New York 2015

offering specific guidelines on the use of particular drugs or nil per os (NPO) intervals. There is variability in the manner in which different pediatric subspecialties (and different countries) have addressed the specifics of sedation care, but the common elements and considerations largely outweigh the differences.

It should be noted that the methodologies used to produce these guidelines vary from organization to organization. For example, the American Academy of Pediatrics (AAP), guidelines were put together by a workgroup on sedation from the Committee on Drugs [1–3]. While these guidelines were based on a careful consideration of the available literature, the exact nature of how studies were "weighted" and how conclusions were drawn is not explicitly described. The most recent guidelines of the American Society of Anesthesiologists (ASA) [4] and American College of Emergency Physicians (ACEP) [5–8] are founded on an evidence-based review of pediatric sedation literature and the methodologies are quite explicit. Even in these cases, however, the lack of definitive or comparative data on outcomes from sedation encounters necessitates that many of the guidelines are based on "consensus" rather than evidence.

This chapter will review the most recently published sedation guidelines of the various specialties in the United States and will then present the guidelines of some international specialties in order to provide comparison and contrast.

American Academy of Pediatrics Guidelines

In the United States, the AAP's guidelines for monitoring and management of pediatric patients during and after sedation for diagnostic and therapeutic procedures [9] are the most widely applied guidelines with respect to pediatric sedation. While other statements from the AAP have expanded on the importance of the use of sedation and analgesia for children [10, 11], these guidelines remain of primary importance and have influenced the creation of safe sedation systems around the United States and internationally. Much of their lexicon and recommendations have been largely adopted by the Joint Commission and regulatory bodies in Europe and Australia in evaluating institutional compliance for safe sedation standards.

The first AAP guideline for pediatric sedation was written in response to three dental deaths in 1983 (published in 1985) [1] on behalf of the AAP Section on Anesthesiology. Written in collaboration with the American Academy of Pediatric Dentistry (AAPD) and the ASA, the purpose was to develop a framework from which improved safety could be developed for children requiring sedation in order to perform a needed procedure. This initial guideline emphasized standardization on issues such as the need for informed consent, appropriate fasting prior to sedation, frequent measurement and charting of vital signs, the availability of age- and size-appropriate equipment, the use of physiologic monitoring, the need for basic life support skills, and proper recovery and discharge procedures. The concept of an independent observer whose only responsibility is to monitor the patient was introduced for deeply sedated pediatric patients. Advanced airway and resuscitation skills were encouraged but not specifically required for deep sedation providers. These original guidelines defined three terms for depth of sedation: conscious sedation, deep sedation, and general anesthesia. The descriptive term "conscious sedation" was defined as "A medically controlled state of depressed consciousness that allows the protective reflexes to be maintained; retains the patient's ability to maintain a patent airway independently and continuously; and permits an appropriate response by the patient to physical stimulation or verbal command, e.g., "open your eyes"" [1].

In 1992 the Committee on Drugs of the AAP revised the 1985 guideline [2]. The new iteration recognized that a patient could readily progress from one level of sedation to another and that the practitioner should be prepared to increase vigilance and monitoring as indicated. Pulse oximetry was recommended for all patients undergoing sedation. This new guideline also discouraged the practice of administering sedation at home by parents—a practice that was not infrequent in dental and radiologic sedation at that time. An addendum to the guideline was produced by the same Committee on Drugs of the AAP 2002 [9] ending the use of the term "conscious sedation" and clarifying the fact that these guidelines apply to any location where children are sedated—in or out of the hospital. This set of guidelines use the terminology of "minimal sedation, moderate sedation, deep sedation, and anesthesia." These descriptions of sedation levels have been adopted by the ASA, the Joint Commission, and multiple international organizations (see later). The addendum emphasized that sedatives should only be administered by those skilled in airway management and cardiopulmonary resuscitation [9].

The most current iteration of the AAP sedation guidelines was published in Pediatrics in December 2006 [3]. This document represents a significant landmark for the field of pediatric sedation. For the first time, the Joint Commission, ASA, AAP, and the AAPD officially adopted common language to define sedation categories (minimal, moderate, deep, and anesthesia) and the expected physiologic responses for each category. The authors emphasize the idea that sedation is a continuum and that the sedation provider must be capable of rescuing a patient for a level of sedation one step deeper than that which is intended. They recommend "ongoing maintenance of critical skills for airway rescue" and reference some resources, but stop short of specific directions for how best to teach or maintain critical competencies.

The authors contend that deep sedation requires special expertise and personnel resources.

Credentials required to administer deep sedation [3]:

1. There must be one person available whose sole responsibility is to constantly observe the patient's vital signs, airway patency, and adequacy of ventilation and to either administer drugs or direct their administration.
2. At least one individual, trained and competent to provide advanced pediatric life support, airway management, and cardiopulmonary resuscitation, must be present [3].

This iteration of the guidelines emphasizes that plans for rescue by Emergency Medical Systems (EMS) must be put in place for settings such as a free-standing clinic or office.

The guidelines also include an interesting section on drug interactions and cautions on alternative medications such as St. John's wort, kava, and echinacea and their possible impact on sedation provision. In regard to propofol, they do not make any statement or recommendation on its administration, either by anesthesiologists or nonanesthesiologists.

Monitoring requirements are based on the depth and setting of sedation. Pulse oximetry, heart rate, and intermittent blood pressure should be followed during moderate sedation. For deep sedation, "precordial stethoscope or capnography should be implemented for patients who are difficult to observe (i.e., magnetic resonance imaging (MRI)) to aid in monitoring adequacy of ventilation" [3]. Capnography is "encouraged" but not required, particularly in situations where other means of assessing ventilation are limited.

These guidelines suggest that predicting the exact depth of sedation (other than minimal sedation) that will result from the administration of a sedative drug is impossible. In light of this fact, the authors make recommendations on fasting (NPO) status, which assume airway protective reflexes could be lost at any time during a moderate or deep sedation and therefore mirror the recommendations made for patients undergoing anesthesia.

NPO Guidelines

- Clear liquids: 2 h; include water, fruit juices without pulp, carbonated beverages, clear tea, black coffee
- Breast milk: 4 h
- Infant formula, nonhuman milk
- Light meal and solid food: 6 h

Note: These guidelines state that in urgent/emergent sedation situations, the benefit of waiting for appropriate NPO intervals must be weighed against the necessity of the procedure [3].

Finally, recovery criteria and considerations are enumerated, including a suggestion for the use of (new) simple "wakefulness" measures as part of the discharge criteria (where a child is simply observed for his/her ability to remain awake for a specified period of time [15–20 min] prior to discharge).

American Society of Anesthesiologists Policies and Recommendations

While the ASA has not produced a document specific for pediatric sedation, issues relating to pediatric patients are mentioned in almost all of the sedation-related publications it has produced. The ASA has many statements and guidelines that address sedation by non-anesthesia providers including:

- "Practice Guidelines for Sedation and Analgesia by Nonanesthesiologists" [4]
- "Continuum of Depth of Sedation—Definition of General Anesthesia and Levels of Sedation/Analgesia"
- "Statement on Granting Privileges for Administration of Moderate Sedation to Practitioners Who Are Not Anesthesia Professionals"
- "Practice Guidelines for Preoperative Fasting and the Use of Pharmacologic Agents to Reduce the Risk of Pulmonary Aspiration—Application to Healthy Patients Undergoing Elective Procedures"
- "Statement on Safe Use of Propofol"
- "Standards for Basic Anesthesia Monitoring"
- "Statement on Granting Privileges to Nonanesthesiologist Practitioners for Personally Administering Deep Sedation or Supervising Deep Sedation by Individuals Who Are Not Anesthesia Professionals"[1]

The "Practice Guidelines for Sedation and Analgesia by Nonanesthesiologists" [4] is probably the most widely quoted document concerning sedation the ASA has produced. The latest iteration of this document was published in 2002 [4] as an update/revision of the original 1996 guidelines [12]. The stated purpose of the guideline is to "allow clinicians to provide their patients with the benefits of sedation/analgesia while minimizing the associated risks." These guidelines were developed by a task force using an evidence-based "strength of the evidence" methodology.

The ASA guidelines are consistent with the AAP in many respects. They describe the sedation levels identical to the AAP and the Joint Commission guidelines. They require that the sedation provider be able to rescue patients from a level deeper than intended. The authors also apply the current ASA recommendations on NPO times (2 h for clear fluids, 4 h for breast milk, 6 h for light meals and formula, 8 h for full meals) to elective sedation. The ASA guidelines are similar to those of AAP in their recommendation for electrocardiogram (ECG), blood pressure, and pulse oximetry for all deep sedation patients. In contrast to the AAP, the ASA places more emphasis on capnography, stating that capnography should be considered, but is not required, for all patients receiving deep sedation and for patients whose

[1] All statements and other documents available at: http://www.asahq.org/publicationsAndServices/sgstoc.htm.

ventilation cannot be directly observed during moderate sedation. Continual monitoring of sedation depth through stimulation/response analysis is also recommended.

In 2005 the ASA published the "Statement on Granting Privileges for Administration of Moderate Sedation to Practitioners Who Are Not Anesthesia Professionals." This is a detailed statement that defines the different groups/qualifications of sedation providers:

1. Anesthesia Professional—anesthesiologist, certified registered nurse anesthetist (CRNA), anesthesiologist assistant (AA)
2. Nonanesthesiologist Sedation Practitioner—other physicians, dentists, podiatrists
3. Supervised Sedation Professional—licensed registered nurse, advanced practice nurse, etc.

This grouping has raised some controversy, as the term "nonanesthesiologist" can represent physicians of various levels of skill, training, and experience [13].

The ASA defines the rescue capabilities that are required for sedation providers at each level of sedation. In 2006 they deviated from the AAP in that they advocated the limitation of the administration of deep sedation to those practitioners with anesthesia training: Specifically they state that this practice should be limited to those practitioners who are qualified to administer general anesthesia or to appropriately supervise anesthesia professionals [14]. This individual should have no other responsibilities except to deliver sedation and monitor the patient throughout. The "Statement on granting privileges to non-anesthesiologist practitioners for personally administering deep sedation or supervising deep sedation by individuals who are not anesthesia professionals" was supplanted on October 20, 2010 by the ASA advisory on "Granting Privileges for Deep Sedation to Non-Anesthesiologist Sedation Practitioners" [15]. It recommends that the nonanesthesiologist be able to bag-valve-mask ventilate, insert an oropharyngeal airway and laryngeal mask airway, and perform an endotracheal intubation. The advisory states that training for these individuals should include a minimum of 35 patients, inclusive of simulator experience. Practitioners should be familiar with the use and interpretation of capnography. Finally, this document recommends that deep sedation of children requires Pediatric Advanced Life Support (PALS) and Advanced Cardiac Life Support (ACLS) certification as well as separate education training and credentialing in sedation.

Most recently, in October of 2012, the ASA passed an amendment of its original (2006) advisory on deep sedation by nonanesthesiologists. In this iteration the statement is worded "Because of the significant risk that patients who receive deep sedation may enter a state of general anesthesia, privileges for deep sedation should be granted only to non-anesthesiologist physicians who are qualified and trained in the medical practice of deep sedation and the recognition of and rescue from general anesthesia" [16]. This guideline goes on to advise against nonanesthesiologists delegating or supervising the administration of sedation by individuals who are not similarly qualified [16].

In 2011, the ASA amended the Standards for Basic Anesthesia Monitoring (first published in 1986) to specify that during moderate and deep sedation, ventilation should be followed by clinical observation and capnography [17]. Exceptions to capnography would be situations whereby patient, procedure, or equipment precludes or invalidates the monitoring.

The ASA recognizes the Center for Medicare and Medicaid Services (CMS) as defining those qualified to administer deep sedation. The Hospital Anesthesia Services Condition of Participation 42 CFR 482.52 (a) of 2010 [18] limits deep sedation to be delivered only by an anesthesiologist, nonanesthesiologist MD or DO, dentist, oral surgeon, podiatrist, CRNA, or anesthesia assistant [18, 19].

The CMS guidelines regarding nonanesthesiologist providers of sedation were revised in January 2011 in the PUB 100-07 State Operations Provider Certification, which revises Appendix A for various provisions of 42 CFR 482.52 concerning anesthesia services. These revisions were made in response to feedback from practitioners. Important changes in these guidelines stem from the CMS acknowledgement that the individual hospitals may establish their own policies and procedures with respect to the qualifications of analgesia providers and the clinical situations that distinguish anesthesia from analgesia. The policies must follow nationally recognized guidelines and can include guidelines of one or more specialty societies.

The ASA "Statement on Safe Use of Propofol" first published in 2004 and amended in 2009, advises "the involvement of an anesthesiologist in the care of every patient undergoing anesthesia is optimal. However, when this is not possible, non-anesthesia personnel who administer propofol should be qualified to rescue patients whose level of sedation becomes deeper than initially intended and who enter, if briefly, a state of general anesthesia" [20].

The distinction between sedation, deep sedation, and monitored anesthesia care (MAC) is frequently misunderstood. To clarify these definitions, the ASA in 2009, amended the document entitled "Distinguishing Monitored Anesthesia Care ('MAC') from Moderate Sedation/Analgesia (Conscious Sedation)" to differentiate between the two levels of care [21]. Important distinctions were that MAC entails an anesthesia assessment and the delivery of sedation by a provider who is prepared and qualified to assess and manage physiological or medical issues as well as to convert to a general anesthetic. This is distinguished from those who administer moderate sedation where one would not expect progression to a condition in which the patient could not maintain his own airway [21].

The Joint Commission: Where We Stand Now

Issues relating to sedation (in general) and pediatric sedation (specifically) are found in a variety of locations in the Joint Commission Handbook and website.[2] The JCAHO 2004 Comprehensive Accreditation Manual for Hospitals was intended to set the standards for sedation and anesthesia care for patients in any setting [22].

The Joint Commission recommendations are important when considering the credentialing and privileging of sedation providers. The Joint Commission requires that hospitals define the scope of practice for practitioners. It is important to distinguish the term "credentialing" from "privileging." Credentialing is the process whereby designated hospital appointees assure that physicians who work in the hospital have the appropriate education, training, and licensure to practice in the institution. Privileging specifically gives permission to staff to provide care in various clinical settings or perform particular procedures in a given institution. With regard to sedation privileging, each healthcare facility is mandated by the Joint Commission to approve a plan to provide sedation and anesthesia care. Each institution must outline the criteria for determining which practitioners are qualified to provide the service.

It is important to recognize the evolution of the role of the Anesthesiology Department in the delivery of sedation as outlined by the Joint Commission. Earlier Joint Commission publications placed responsibility for sedation oversight on the Department of Anesthesiology and its Chairman [22]. Subsequent revisions of this document have revised the language: The Anesthesiology Department plays an important advisory role but is not directly responsible for sedation care, privileging, or quality assurance.

In the current 2007 Joint Commission manual there are recommendations for the training that may be provided for other sedation providers: "Individuals administering moderate or deep sedation and anesthesia are qualified and have the appropriate credentials to manage patients at whatever level of sedation or anesthesia is achieved, either intentionally or unintentionally" [23]. Referring specifically to deep sedation it states, "individuals must be qualified to rescue patients from general anesthesia and are competent to manage an unstable cardiovascular system as well as a compromised airway and inadequate oxygenation and ventilation" [23]. It goes on to specify, "Each organization is free to define how it will determine that the individuals are able to perform the required types of rescue. Acceptable examples include, but are not limited to, ACLS certification, a satisfactory score on a written examination developed in concert with the Department of Anesthesiology, a mock rescue exercise evaluated by an anesthesiologist" [23].

Although the Joint Commission still believes that anesthesiology departments should play a role in the development of training and privileging programs for sedation, they no longer hold the central role of being "in charge" of sedation services. Key roles in sedation oversight may be filled by qualified specialists of many different subspecialties.

American College of Emergency Physicians Guidelines

The American College of Emergency Medicine (ACEP) has put forward a wide range of statements, clinical practice advisories, and clinical policy statements concerning sedation. The 2008 American College of Emergency Physicians Policy Compendium includes a statement "Procedural Sedation in the Emergency Department" [24]. This statement begins with a strongly worded sentence: "Emergency physicians and nurses under their supervision are qualified to provide procedural sedation/analgesia in the emergency department, and ACEP is the authoritative body for the establishment of guidelines for procedural sedation and analgesia by emergency physicians."

In 1998 and 2005 the ACEP published "Clinical Policy: Procedural Sedation and Analgesia in the Emergency Department" [7]. Similar to the ASA guidelines, the ACEP guidelines apply to all patients—adults and children—who receive sedation. They recognize that sedation is a continuum and maintain that practitioners should possess competence in cardiovascular resuscitation and airway management that should include a patient who has achieved general anesthesia. The ACEP considers these skills, including the administration of deep sedation, to be a fundamental part of the emergency medicine training curriculum of all board-certified emergency physicians [7, 25].

The ACEP guidelines deviate from those of the AAP and ASA with respect to NPO guidelines. Both the AAP and ASA recommend fasting intervals for elective cases similar to those required for general anesthesia—specifically 2 h for clear liquids, 4 h for breast milk, 6 h for formula, and 8 h for full meals. These guidelines do not make recommendations for the nonelective sedation case. The ASA guidelines state "Patients undergoing sedation/analgesia for elective procedures should not drink fluids or eat solid foods for a sufficient period of time to allow for gastric emptying before their procedure. In urgent, emergent, or other situations in which gastric emptying is impaired, the potential for pulmonary aspiration of gastric contents must be considered in determining (1) the target level of sedation, (2) whether the procedure should be delayed, or (3) whether the trachea should be protected by intubation." The AAP guidelines are

[2]http://www.jointcommission.org

a bit less specific, stating only "for emergency procedures the risks of sedation and the possibility of aspiration must be weighed against the benefits of performing the procedure promptly."

By the very nature of their work, emergency medicine sedation providers must cope with patients who do not meet appropriate NPO criteria and are not having "elective" procedures. In the last 10 years there have been several studies in the emergency medicine literature that have reported very low rates of aspiration or pulmonary complications in patients who were sedated without meeting the NPO recommendations from the AAP or ASA [26, 27]. Previous publications from the ACEP have concluded that there is insufficient evidence to conclude that fasting actually changes outcome for sedation (see previous) [28].

In 2006, ACEP produced a document on fasting prior to sedation [29]. This clinical practice advisory is titled "Fasting and Emergency Department Procedural Sedation and Analgesia: A Consensus-Based Clinical Practice Advisory." The paper begins with an extensive review of the guidelines that have been set forth by the ACEP, AAP, and ASA concerning NPO status, and considers them in the context of the emergency department setting. This consensus-based clinical advisory concludes that there is actually scarce literature to document the perceived risk that various NPO times pose with respect to sedation complications. The authors suggest that the issue of NPO interval needs to be considered in the context of the urgency and duration of the procedure as well as the risk stratification of the patient, nature of food intake, and depth/type of sedation targeted. The result is a somewhat complex strategy that weighs NPO time versus emergent/urgent/semiurgent nature of the case versus duration of the procedure.

Table 2.1 schematically describes the recommendations that result from these guidelines [29]. It is important to note the guidelines for nonelective sedation of patients who are not considered NPO by ASA or AAP standards. The guidelines state that although "recent food intake is not a contraindication for administering procedural sedation and analgesia, the emergency physician must weigh the risk of pulmonary aspiration and the benefits of providing procedural sedation and analgesia in accordance with the needs of each individual patient" [7, 29].

In 2004 and 2008, the ACEP published evidence-based guidelines on the use of specific medications for use in pediatric sedation: "Clinical policy: evidence-based approach to pharmacologic agents used in pediatric sedation and analgesia in the emergency department" [5] and "Clinical policy: Critical issues in the sedation of pediatric patients in the emergency department" [28]. The "Critical Issues" statement supported earlier recommendations on NPO status and reviewed the use of sedatives including nitrous oxide, chloral hydrate, and sucrose. Their recommendations have been accepted by a wide range of surgical and nursing organizations and have been published in corresponding journals [30, 31].

Other ACEP publications include a clinical practice advisory on propofol use in the emergency department [25], and a clinical practice guideline on ketamine use in the emergency department [6]. Both of these documents support the use of these drugs for sedation in the emergency department, expanding on the evidence-based guideline recommendations from the clinical policy on pharmacological agents mentioned previously [5]. The ACEP recommendations for physiological monitoring also differ from the ASA and AAP with respect to pulse oximetry application: Pulse oximetry is not mandatory. The guidelines advise that pulse oximetry may not be necessary when the patient's level of consciousness is minimally depressed and verbal communication can be continually monitored. Pulse oximetry is recommended, however, when there is an increased risk of developing hypoxemia, such as when high doses of drugs or multiple drugs are used, or when treating patients with significant comorbidity. Capnography, although not required, is acknowledged to be a monitor that may allow more rapid identification of hypoventilation than pulse oximetry alone [32].

In February 2014, the ACEP released the most recent clinical policy to date. Entitled "Clinical Policy: Procedural Sedation and Analgesia in the Emergency Department," it updates the 2005 policy [33]. This paper highlights the value of designing studies to specifically examine patient-specific outcomes. It also recognizes that unique patient-care environments and high-risk patient populations may pose unique challenges which may require modification of the clinical policy. Reviewing the literature, the College of Emergency Physicians Clinical Policies Committee made evidence-based recommendations for important clinical questions. The following questions were addressed [33]:

1. Is preprocedural (nil per os/NPO) fasting necessary to decrease risk of emesis and aspiration during sedation in the emergency department?
2. Does capnography decrease risk of adverse events?
3. How many personnel are necessary to manage sedation-related complications?
4. Are ketamine, propofol, etomidate, dexmedetomidine, alfentanil, and remifentanil appropriate sedatives for the emergency department?

The clinical policy was based on literature review, with recommendations identified as levels A, B, and C. The levels were determined from the degree of clinical certainty after review of the literature. High certainty, moderate certainty, and inadequate/absence evidence corresponded to levels A, B, and C recommendations, respectively. The importance of NPO was a level B recommendation, advising that there was no evidence to support preprocedural fasting of children for procedural sedation in the emergency department. The routine use of capnography was assigned a level B recommendation,

Table 2.1 ACEP NPO considerations and aspiration risk (adapted from [28])

STANDARD RISK				
ORAL INTAKE IN THE PRIOR 3 HOURS	**Urgency of the Procedure**			
	Emergent	***Urgent***	***Semi-Urgent***	***Non-Urgent***
Nothing	All levels of sedation	All levels of sedation	All levels of sedation	All levels of sedation
Clear liquids only	All levels of sedation	All levels of sedation	Up to and including brief deep sedation	Up to and including extended moderate sedation
Light snack	All levels of sedation	Up to and including brief deep sedation	Up to and including dissociative sedation; non-extended moderate sedation	Minimal sedation only
Heavy snack or meal	All levels of sedation	Up to and including extended moderate sedation	Minimal sedation only	Minimal sedation only

HIGHER RISK				
ORAL INTAKE IN THE PRIOR 3 HOURS	**Procedural Urgency**			
	Emergent Procedure	***Urgent Procedure***	***Semi-Urgent Procedure***	***Non-Urgent Procedure***
Nothing	All levels of sedation	All levels of sedation	All levels of sedation	All levels of sedation
Clear liquids only	All levels of sedation	Up to and including brief deep sedation	Up to and including extended moderate sedation	Minimal sedation only
Light snack	All levels of sedation	Up to and including dissociative sedation; non-extended moderate sedation	Minimal sedation only	Minimal sedation only
Heavy snack or meal	All levels of sedation	Up to and including dissociative sedation; non-extended moderate sedation	Minimal sedation only	Minimal sedation only

↓ Increasing Potential Aspiration Risk ↓	**Procedural Sedation and Analgesia Targeted Depth and Duration**
	Minimal sedation only
	Dissociative sedation; brief or intermediate-length moderate sedation
	Extended moderate sedation
	Brief deep sedation
	Intermediate or extended-length deep sedation

Brief: <10 min
Intermediate: 10–20 min
Extended: >20 min

recognizing that as an adjunct to pulse oximetry, it may detect hypoventilation and apnea earlier than pulse oximetry or clinical assessment. The recommendation for the number of personnel necessary to manage sedation-related complications was a level C—without supporting evidence, the recommendation was that in addition to the provider performing the procedure, a nurse or other qualified individual needed to be continuously present. The final recommendations with respect to sedatives were levels A, B, and C. Ketamine and propofol were considered level A recommendations, deemed safe for pediatric sedation in the emergency department. Etomidate for children was considered level C, supported with expert consensus, despite absent/inadequate supporting published literature. The combination of ketamine and propofol was considered level B for safe pediatric sedation in the emergency department. No recommendations could be made for dexmedetomidine, as there is only one case report of its use in the emergency department.

American Dental Association Sedation Guidelines

The American Dental Association (ADA) guidelines regarding sedation are posted on its website [34]. The guideline acknowledges the depths of sedation consistent with that described by the AAP and the ASA. It contains descriptions of routes of administration for sedative medications, ASA classification for sedation patients, and monitoring guidelines for sedated patients. There is a very specific outline of the training required for dentists regarding various levels of sedation, including specific educational programs and life support training. In this regard, the guidelines are more detailed than those provided by other organizations. Deep sedation requires the presence of a minimum of three individuals: one dentist who is credentialed to administer deep sedation or anesthesia and two additional personnel who have current certification of successfully completing a Basic Life Support (BLS) Course for the Healthcare Provider. There are two requirements to qualify for deep sedation certification: (1) completion of an advanced education program on the administration and management of deep sedation or anesthesia, which must be accredited by the ADA Commission on Dental Accreditation, and (2) a current certification in both BLS for Healthcare Providers and ACLS or an appropriate dental sedation/anesthesia emergency management course. The dentist administering deep sedation or general anesthesia must remain within the facility until the patient meets discharge criteria (or is discharged) and must monitor the patient continuously until the patient meets the criteria for recovery. Those who provide pediatric sedation must have PALS in addition to directed pediatric training and education [35, 36].

The guidelines are presented in sections, each of which relates to a sedation level: minimal, moderate, and deep sedation. Specific recommendations are given for training of sedation providers, preoperative preparation of patients, monitoring and documentation, recover and discharge criteria, and personnel/equipment requirements. For children 12 years of age and under, the ADA refers to the AAP/American Academy of Pediatric Dentists (AAPD) Guidelines for Monitoring and Management of Pediatric Patients During and After Sedation for Diagnostic and Therapeutic Procedures that was discussed earlier in the AAP section [3, 37]. These guidelines address some issues unique to the office-based dental practice and to the special needs child. If the dental patient is mentally and/or physically challenged, it may not be possible to have a comprehensive physical examination or appropriate laboratory tests prior to administering care. In these situations, the dentist responsible for administering the deep sedation should document the reasons preventing the recommended preoperative assessment prior to administering sedation [3]. In addition, recognizing the long history of nitrous oxide use in dentistry, this document specifically mentions it as an acceptable sedative, alone or in combination with other sedatives [3].

In 2012, AAPD published a revision of its "Guideline on Use of Anesthesia Personnel in the Administration of Office-based Deep Sedation/General Anesthesia to the Pediatric Dental Patient" [38]. This document reaffirms the fact that there are several categories of pediatric patients, such as those with developmental delays and autism, who require deep sedation for dental interventions. It further recognizes that when this care is provided in the dental office, it is much more cost effective and convenient to schedule than when it is delivered in a large hospital setting. The authors are careful to define the aspects of training that are required in order to deliver this care. Specifically, the provider must have completed a 1- or 2-year dental anesthesia residency approved by the ADA or a medical anesthesia residency as approved by the AMA. This provider must be licensed in the state where the care is provided. Emergency preparedness must be updated and practiced on a regular basis and recovery must be monitored by an experienced provider at all times until the patient has met discharge criteria. There is a directive that the facility must meet the standards for anesthesia delivery as set by state or local codes and the "Guidelines on Monitoring and Management of Pediatric Patients During and after sedation for Diagnostic and Therapeutic Procedures." The new document concludes by reinforcing the need for appropriate pre-, intra-, and postoperative documentation as well as ongoing quality assurance standards.

American Society of Gastroenterologists

The Standards of Practice Committee of the American Society for Gastrointestinal Endoscopy has recently published guidelines for deep sedation, the administration of propofol by nonanesthesiologists, and pediatric sedation for gastrointestinal procedures and endoscopy [39]. All of these guidelines were written after a review of the MEDLINE and PubMed database. The recommendations are rated "A," "B," or "C" based on the weight of the evidence available. A level identifies statements supported by prospective randomized trials and C level identifies expert opinion in the absence of peer-reviewed evidence. The chronological history leading up to these 2009 guidelines will be detailed as follows.

The first guideline was published in 2002 and entitled "Guidelines for the Use of Deep Sedation and Anesthesia for GI Endoscopy" [40]. This guideline reviews the levels of sedation and the importance of presedation assessment in order to customize sedation for the needs of the patient. Planning is identified as particularly important for those with specific emotional issues, drug use history, and those who are undergoing extensive procedures. There are no specific references to or recommendations for the pediatric population.

Pharmacologic agents are reviewed including guidelines for the indications and use of droperidol (in addition to midazolam and fentanyl) and propofol for deep sedation during endoscopy. This guideline is unique in its recommendation for droperidol as a third drug if needed. There is an accompanying warning about cardiac issues related to droperidol and the need for extended ECG monitoring when it is utilized.

The majority of this guideline is devoted to the role of propofol and the relative risks versus benefits of its use in endoscopy. Personnel preparation and monitoring requirements for propofol sedation are carefully delineated [40]:

1. At least one person who is qualified in both basic and advanced life support skills (i.e., tracheal intubation, defibrillation, use of resuscitation medications).
2. Physiologic monitoring should include pulse oximetry, electrocardiography, and automated blood pressure measurement. Monitoring oxygenation by pulse oximetry is not a substitute for monitoring ventilatory function.
3. Equipment for airway management and resuscitation.
4. Trained personnel dedicated to the continuous and uninterrupted monitoring of the patient's physiologic parameters and administration of propofol.
5. Extended monitoring with capnography should be considered as it may decrease the risks during deep sedation.

Published in 2002, it concludes that although propofol does not appear to offer a significant advantage over standard benzodiazepine/opiate techniques for routine endoscopy procedure, it does confer significant advantages for longer and more complicated procedures (level "A" recommendation). The authors also discuss the provision of propofol sedation by nonanesthesiologists including other physicians and registered nurses. Anesthesiology assistance is recommended for specific situations including: prolonged or therapeutic endoscopic procedure requiring deep sedation, anticipated intolerance to standard sedatives, increased risk for complication because of severe comorbidity (ASA class III or greater), increased risk for airway obstruction because of anatomic variant. These final recommendations are included at a "C" level.

A second publication, "Guidelines for Conscious Sedation and Monitoring during Gastrointestinal Endoscopy," was published in 2003 in the journal *Gastrointestinal Endoscopy* [41]. It refers to "conscious sedation" as a level of equivalence to "moderate sedation." These guidelines review the data on endoscopy-related complications—noting that over 50 % of complications are related to cardiopulmonary side effects with the majority relating to aspiration, oversedation, hypoventilation, vasovagal episodes, and airway obstruction. The authors note that the risk of cardiovascular complications is dependent on the patient's underlying medical condition and the procedure to be performed—high-risk patients and high-risk procedures at highest risk.

These guidelines support the monitoring recommendations of the ASA and AAP. Required monitoring during sedation for endoscopy includes recording of the heart rate, blood pressure, respiratory rate, and oxygen saturation. Capnography is advised for prolonged cases.

Several drugs are mentioned for conscious sedation during endoscopy. Benzodiazepines and opiates (along with reversal agents) are reviewed along with droperidol and promethazine. Unique to this set of guidelines, "pharyngeal" anesthesia is reviewed. Specific mention is made of the risk of methemoglobinemia when excessive benzocaine is administered to the mucosa. In reference to deep sedation, the authors suggest that propofol is superior to standard benzodiazepine/opiate sedation for complex procedures. On the other hand, the authors recognize that its use in routine upper and lower endoscopic procedures is controversial with little proven benefit over standard moderate sedation [41].

The most recent and pertinent publication regarding sedation specifically for pediatric endoscopy was published in 2008 as "Modifications in Endoscopic Practice for Pediatric Patients" [42]. This document addresses many issues relating to sedation in children and for pediatric endoscopy. For example, the authors review indications and contraindications for endoscopy in children, the appropriateness of pediatric versus adult endoscopists for various procedures in children, and the appropriate preparation of patients for these studies. They include discussions of the proper equipment to use for pediatric endoscopy and the indications for antibiotic prophylaxis.

Important cautions are included, such as the fact that airway obstruction is more common in children and (because of higher oxygen consumption) can lead to the rapid onset of hypoxia in the face of apnea. Therefore the routine use of oxygen is recommended during endoscopic sedation in this age group. The authors note that general anesthesia is often used for pediatric endoscopy and that the number of centers using propofol sedation or general anesthesia for endoscopy appears to be increasing [42, 43]. One study from 1995 cites equivalent safety and efficacy when using a standardized procedural sedation protocol (opiate plus benzodiazepine) when compared to general (potent inhalation) anesthesia [44]. The authors also note that when propofol is compared to "general anesthesia" it has been found to result in less total time for anesthesia and equal safety [45].

In 2009, the American Society of Gastroenterologists (ASG) published their position statement for nonanesthesiologist administration of propofol for GI endoscopy [39]. The guidelines state that clinically important benefits of propofol in average-risk patients undergoing upper endoscopy and colonoscopy have not been consistently demonstrated with regard to patient satisfaction and safety. It supports that propofol can be safely and effectively given by nonanesthesiologist physicians and nurses provided they have undergone appropriate training and credentialing in administration and rescue from potential pulmonary and cardiovascular complications. The summary section makes specific recommendations for sedation for pediatric endoscopy. They generally follow AAP and ASA standards [39]:

1. All sedation pediatric patients should receive routine oxygen administration and should be monitored with a minimum of pulse oximetry and heart rate monitoring.
2. In deeply sedated patients, one individual having no other responsibilities should be assigned to monitor the patient's cardiac and respiratory status and to record vital signs.
3. The presence of personnel trained specifically in pediatric life support and airway management during procedures requiring sedation is strongly recommended.

International Guidelines

A wide variety of sedation guidelines specific to pediatrics, or with application to pediatrics, have been published by various specialty societies and international organizations. Most of these guidelines are consistent with the recommendations from the AAP and ASA, others are not. Of particular interest are the recommendations on effective and safe sedation of children and young people undergoing common diagnostic and therapeutic procedures from the National Institute of Health and Clinical Excellence (NICE) in the United Kingdom (2011) [46]. This document was written after a comprehensive review of the best available evidence and expert opinion. The recommendations are wide ranging and include the mandate for a full presedation evaluation that incorporates medical condition, current medications, airway assessment, ASA physical status, and an evaluation of the psychosocial makeup of the child. In addition, there is a clear outline of indications for seeking advice from a specialist before undertaking sedation based on the presedation assessment. These referral indications include ASA status 3 or greater, airway difficulties, and *all* infants and newborns. Notably, these recommendations include an extensive description of available sedation techniques. The authors include a section that recommends specific drugs and drug combinations for sedation encounters based on the targeted level of sedation, the procedure, and patient/family preference. Contraindications for sedatives are also covered. Recommendations concerning other elements of sedation practice, such as choosing appropriate resuscitation equipment, personnel, and informed consent, follow closely with the guidelines put forward by the AAP and ASA.

Chapters 18 and 25 detail the most recent sedation guidelines from the Dutch Institute of Healthcare Improvement in the Netherlands (2011) [47], the Endoscopy Section of the German Society for Digestive and Metabolic Diseases (2009) [48] and the adult and pediatric guidelines of the South African Society of Anesthesiologists (2010 and 2011) [49, 50].

Notable sedation statements and guidelines published worldwide include:

Scottish Intercollegiate Guidelines Network. "SIGN Guideline 58: safe sedation of children undergoing diagnostic and therapeutic procedures" [51]

This is a comprehensive, evidence-based sedation review that includes discussions of appropriate evaluation of pediatric patients as well as recommendations for equipment, environment, recovery, parental information, and quality improvement. There are specific sections addressing the needs of medical pediatrics versus dentistry versus radiology versus emergency medicine. There is also a section on sedation techniques that recommends various drugs for certain situations and specifically reserves potent medications such as propofol and short-acting opiates for use by anesthesiologists.

Australasian College for Emergency Medicine, Australian and New Zealand College of Anesthetists. "Statement on clinical principles for procedural sedation" [52]

A very brief statement of basic principles of sedation (preparation, staffing, facilities, medication, recovery) that is in line with recommendations from British and American organizations. Source material is not referenced.

Canadian Consensus Guidelines. Canadian Association of Emergency Physicians "Procedural sedation and analgesia in the emergency department" [53]

This is a slightly dated consensus statement conceived in conjunction with the Canadian Association of Anesthesiologists. It outlines general principles of safe sedation care in line with those mentioned previously, including assessment of the patient, facility preparation, training of providers, fasting status, and recovery. This document also includes an example of a sedation record, which is somewhat unique. While no specific sedation regimens are recommended, there are useful links to other publications that involve sedation recommendations.

British Society of Gastroenterology "Recommendations for standards of sedation and patient monitoring during gastrointestinal endoscopy" [54]

An older set of recommendations for sedation that is intended for a general population, not strictly for children. This document is focused primarily on basic safety issues including the use of appropriate monitoring, record keeping, equipment, and personnel. There is a specific recommendation to evaluate patients for "risk factors" and the authors include a helpful checklist to aid in this assessment. Strategies for sedation are not outlined, although there are general statements that the dosage of all drugs should be kept to the "minimum necessary" and antagonists (for benzodiazepines and opiates) should be available.

Society for the Advancement of Anesthesia in Dentistry (SAAD) Standards in Conscious Sedation for Dentistry [55]

This is a set of general standards that were written for adult and pediatric patients care. The standards are meant to apply to any setting in which "conscious" sedation is being provided for dental patients. The authors define conscious sedation as "A technique in which the use of a drug or drugs produces a state of depression of the central nervous system enabling treatment to be carried out, but during which verbal contact with the patient is maintained throughout the period of sedation. The level of sedation must be such that the patient remains conscious, retains protective reflexes, and is able to understand and respond to verbal commands." The standards do not define other levels of sedation except to point out that "Any technique resulting in the loss of consciousness or abolition of protective reflexes is defined as General Anesthesia."

General guidelines for education and training of providers include the need for "practical training in the use of drugs and equipment." There is also a mandate for training in the management of conscious sedation-related complications, although no guidance is given as to how or what situations should be tested. All members of the sedation team are recommended to have basic life support training. Supervised, hands on experience must be acquired by the sedation providers and their assistants in each of the conscious sedation techniques used. The setting, timing, and number of these experiences will vary with local circumstances but the authors advise that the experience should be commensurate with those specified by "appropriate authorities."

These standards also contain general recommendations for specific equipment—such as the inhalation relative analgesia machines and intravenous equipment that could be used for sedation. The authors of these standards go further to state that a clinical assessment of the patient is required and should result in an ASA classification as well as consideration of any "absolute contraindications" for sedation, although these are not defined. Consent for sedation is outlined along with a detailed description of the need for supervision and transportation requirements after sedation.

A sizable portion of these standards is left to a discussion of techniques for sedation, which include oral, inhalation, or intravenous sedation. Inhalation sedation is limited to titrated doses of nitrous oxide. Intravenous sedation is described as a dose of benzodiazepine, however the authors mention that propofol infusion "has become popular in recent years." (No warnings about this practice or special requirements are included.) Oral/intranasal/transmucosal sedation is mentioned, and midazolam and temazepam are cited as drugs that produce sedation by this route.

Monitoring is mentioned in general terms. Clinical monitoring of "color, pulse, and respiration is of particular importance." No electromechanical devices are required for this purpose for inhalation induction—few other details are offered.

For the purposes of this document, "children" are considered as any patient under the age of 16. There is very little detail offered concerning special requirements for the care of children except the warning that children have different responses to sedation and teams that deliver sedation to children should be trained and have experience in this age group.

Neuroanesthesia and Neurointensive Study Group of the Italian Society of Anesthesia "SIAARTI-SARNePI Guidelines for sedation in pediatric neuroradiology" [56]

These guidelines are based on a literature review and graded on the basis of the evidence in the literature to support them. In spite of their origins from an Italian professional society, these guidelines use the AAP terminology for levels of sedation. As with the other guidelines reviewed here, there is a detailed discussion of the need for an appropriate presedation evaluation. NPO recommendations and monitoring guidelines follow closely with the AAP and ASA. This guideline cites the use of the Pediatric

Coma Scale and the Ramsay Scale for monitoring of depth of sedation during procedures performed on children. Capnography is recommended, although the authors recognize the lack of clear evidence for outcome improvement with this monitor. There are extensive reviews of emergency equipment required for sedation sites and drug choices/combinations for sedation. Finally, the authors include some helpful thoughts on "special situations" including angiography, endovascular treatment, computed tomography (CT) scans, and MRI.

The Working Group on Endoscopy, Austrian Society of Gastroenterology, and Hepatology. "Austrian Society of Gastroenterology and Hepatology (OGGH)—guidelines on sedation and monitoring during gastrointestinal endoscopy" [57]

This is a very brief guideline of sedation specific to the gastroenterology field. There are many references, but the methodology involved in coming up with specific statements is not explained. The authors include a brief discussion of risk factors for patients (and those that might be designated "difficult") and a review of the specific procedures and terminology that is involved in gastroenterology. The authors include a significant section on the use of propofol and cite several studies that support the use of propofol by nonanesthesiologists (including trained nurses) for endoscopic procedures. The document concludes with some specific comments on the need to assure full recovery prior to discharge.

South African Society of Anesthesiologists "Guidelines for the safe use of procedural sedation and analgesia for diagnostic and therapeutic procedures in children: 2010" [58]

This is a comprehensive document that reviews multiple aspects of the provision of sedation of children. It represents the most complete guidelines/review of pediatric sedation produced by any national organization or policy-making entity. The introduction of the document clearly identifies those responsible for authoring the guidelines, but there is no description of the manner in which evidence was used to formulate the recommendations. The authors do not reference the document in a way that would allow one to check or review the sources of their recommendations.

These guidelines begin with an interesting listing of the defined levels of sedation that is a blending of the AAP and ACEP levels of sedation. The list includes the various levels defined by the AAP and ASA, but adds the level of "dissociative sedation" which is aimed at the sedation provided by ketamine. The state is defined as one where spontaneous breathing and cardiovascular stability are maintained. The section includes the statement that this anesthetic state "does not operate on the sedation continuum." The statement goes on to define "simple sedation" as that provided by single oral or transmucosal medications and contrasts this to "advanced sedation," which includes sedation with multiple medications or that given by the intravenous or inhalational route. "Failed sedation" is also defined and includes sedation that fails to achieve the desired level of sedation and results in the procedure being abandoned. The guidelines go on to specifically define patients that require a presedation evaluation by an anesthesiologist or a "highly experienced sedation practitioner." These patients include those of young age <1 year, as well as those with specific comorbidities such as congenital syndromes or congenital heart disease. The balance of the document includes an extensive section on the presedation patient assessment, NPO guidelines (same as AAP), and a detailed description of a wide variety of sedation medications—ranging from minimal sedation with oral midazolam to deep sedation/anesthesia (propofol). There is a review of the key elements of the sedation environment—which are independent of the setting (office versus hospital)—and monitoring requirements. The authors advise that even patients who are under simple sedation require someone other than the procedure operator to monitor the patient and those undergoing advanced sedation should have a separate individual who is responsible for the administration, monitoring, and rescue of the patient. This individual is recommended to be a medical practitioner. Discharge criteria are described. These are the most safety oriented and conservative of any guidelines currently published. They include the recommendation of the use of maintenance of wakefulness criteria such as the ability to keep eyes open for at least 20 min. The authors include a unique and thought-provoking discussion of the various adverse events associated with the sedation of children and subdivide these events into those attributable to the procedure, the skills of the sedation provider, and the environment. The final portion of the document includes a discussion of strategies for sedation aimed at specific procedures or tests.

Sedation Guidelines for Gastrointestinal Endoscopy (2008) of German Society for Digestive and Metabolic Diseases [59]

This is a very detailed document available only in German. The authors begin with a discussion of all safety-related issues such as patient evaluation, monitoring, and resuscitation concepts. The majority of these guidelines involve a detailed discussion of the use of various drugs and combinations for sedation. Propofol is featured with a significant section to the literature supporting nurse-delivered propofol sedation as well as a review of literature comparing propofol to other sedatives for endoscopic procedures. There is further discussion of propofol target-controlled infusions for endoscopic sedation as well as propofol computer-assisted personalized sedation. Later sections review the use of benzodiazepines and opiates alone or in combination with other medications. The guidelines conclude with a discussion of complications of sedation for endoscopy and treatment of complications. The authors include 232 references.

"European Society of Gastrointestinal Endoscopy, European Society of Gastroenterology and Endoscopy Nurses and Associates, and the European Society of Anesthesiology Guideline: Non-Anesthesiologist Administration of Propofol for GI Endoscopy" [60]

This guideline represents the combined effort of a number of European societies involved with gastrointestinal endoscopy. The authors have undertaken an evidence- and consensus-based guideline on the use of propofol for non-anesthesiologists for GI endoscopy. Recommendations are graded based on the evidence. The guideline concludes that propofol sedation has similar rates of adverse events as more traditional sedation regimens. There is a strong recommendation for appropriate training for propofol sedation. Physicians and registered nurses are considered appropriate candidates for propofol sedation training and practice. Human patient simulation is recommended as an enhancement of the training for propofol sedation. High-risk patient groups are noted, including those with high ASA status, risks for airway obstruction, patients who take potent pain medications, and those undergoing prolonged procedures. The combination of propofol with other drugs is neither advised nor discouraged. Monitoring with full ASA monitors and regular assessment of the level of sedation is recommended. Discharge using standardized discharge scoring system is recommended.

Lago P, Garetti E, Merazzi D, Pieragostini L, Ancora G, Pirelli A. "Guidelines for procedural pain in the newborn" [61]

These guidelines were written with the intent of informing the Italian neonatology community about the most up-to-date, evidence-based information on the management on neonatal patients who are undergoing procedures. While not strictly sedation related, the guidelines do address the management of procedural stress and pain—and some sedatives are described. The authors outline a very careful review of the current literature at the time of publication and their methodology for "weighting" the evidence. They outline sensible "principles" for management of neonates during procedures—such as optimizing the environment, use of sucrose, and distraction techniques. Finally, they advise waiting for a baseline state of quiet restfulness prior to beginning a procedure and limiting the number of sequential procedures that a neonatal patient experiences in any one time period. The bulk of these guidelines describe optimal management of one procedure at a time starting with heel lancing, venipuncture, central venous catheter insertion, tracheal intubation, lumbar puncture, chest tube insertion, and ending with screening examinations for ROP. In each case, the pertinent literature on environmental, behavioral, and pharmacologic interventions are cited and rated according to significance. There is a sensible emphasis on the use of local anesthetics and titration of pharmacological agents as needed.

In an era where the appropriate treatment for pain in this age group is uncertain, these guidelines offer a well-researched and reasonable approach to management.

Consideration of these various guidelines leads to the inevitable conclusion that there is more agreement than disparity among the opinions and recommendations that are presented internationally. Almost all of the guidelines focus on careful assessment and risk stratification of patients. All are careful to advise appropriate monitoring, rescue systems, and recovery when sedating children. The primary area where there is lack of agreement lies in the use of specific medications for sedation—and in particular with deep sedation involving potent opioids and propofol. As an example, we can consider the Scottish National Guidelines of 2004, which were written only for minimal and moderate sedation, as anything beyond this (deep sedation included) is recommended for an anesthesiologist and is treated as a general anesthetic [51]. On the other hand, guidelines from the Austrian Society of Gastroenterology and the German Society for Digestive and Metabolic Diseases [57] point specifically to literature that supports the use of propofol by nonanesthesiologists for endoscopic procedures and recommends the practice.

Conclusion

The delivery of sedation for children has advanced considerably over the last 40 years. Similarly, sedation guidelines have evolved, with new editions, updates, and addendums in order to reflect the change in practice and the published literature. As outlined in this chapter, there are a large number of guidelines that address pediatric sedation. Most agree on the important aspects of sedation safety and monitoring. On the other hand, there is a lack of consensus on the duration of NPO status for sedation and whether nonanesthesiologists should administer deep sedation with propofol. Future efforts should be aimed at designing clinical studies with defined endpoints and outcomes. Worldwide participation in these studies, involving all specialties, could establish safety data that would allow the creation of more unified sedation guidelines. Unified recommendations from the AAP, ASA, AAPD,

ADA, the Joint Commission, ACEP, and American Society of Gastroenterologist, together with the different specialty societies worldwide, would offer a landmark first step in the advancement of pediatric sedation.

References

1. [no authors listed] Guidelines for the elective use of conscious sedation, deep sedation, and general anesthesia in pediatric patients. Committee on Drugs, American Academy of Pediatrics. Section on Anesthesiology. Pediatrics. 1985;76:317–21.
2. [no authors listed] American Academy of Pediatrics Committee on Drugs: Guidelines for monitoring and management of pediatric patients during and after sedation for diagnostic and therapeutic procedures. Pediatrics. 1992;89(6 Pt 1):1110–5.
3. Cote CJ, Wilson S. Guidelines for monitoring and management of pediatric patients during and after sedation for diagnostic and therapeutic procedures: an update. Pediatrics. 2006;118(6):2587–602.
4. [no authors listed] American Society of Anesthesiologists Task Force on Sedation and Analgesia by Non Anesthesiologists. Practice guidelines for sedation and analgesia by non-anesthesiologists. Anesthesiology. 2002;96(4):1004–17.
5. Mace SE, Barata IA, Cravero JP, Dalsey WC, Godwin SA, Kennedy RM, et al. Clinical policy: evidence-based approach to pharmacologic agents used in pediatric sedation and analgesia in the emergency department. Ann Emerg Med. 2004;44(4):342–77.
6. Green SM, Krauss B. Clinical practice guideline for emergency department ketamine dissociative sedation in children. Ann Emerg Med. 2004;44(5):460–71.
7. Godwin SA, Caro DA, Wolf SJ, Jagoda AS, Charles R, Marett BE, et al.; American College of Emergency Physicians. Clinical policy: procedural sedation and analgesia in the emergency department. Ann Emerg Med. 2005;45(2):177–96.
8. Zempsky WT, Cravero JP. Relief of pain and anxiety in pediatric patients in emergency medical systems. Pediatrics. 2004;114(5):1348–56.
9. [no authors listed] Committee on Drugs. American Academy of Pediatrics. Guidelines for monitoring and management of pediatric patients during and after sedation for diagnostic and therapeutic procedures: addendum. Pediatrics. 2002;110(4):836–8.
10. American Academy of Pediatrics Committee on Fetus and Newborn; American Academy of Pediatrics Section on Surgery; Canadian Paediatric Society Fetus and Newborn Committee, Batton DG, Barrington KJ, Wallman C. Prevention and management of pain in the neonate: an update. Pediatrics. 2006;118:2231–41.
11. [no authors listed] American Academy of Pediatrics. Committee on Psychosocial Aspects of Child and Family Health; Task Force on Pain in Infants, Children, and Adolescents. The assessment and management of acute pain in infants, children, and adolescents. Pediatrics. 2001;108:793–7.
12. [no authors listed] Practice guidelines for sedation and analgesia by non-anesthesiologists. A report by the American Society of Anesthesiologists Task Force on Sedation and Analgesia by Non-Anesthesiologists. Anesthesiology. 1996;84(2):459–71.
13. Green SM, Krauss B. Replacing the outmoded term "nonanesthesiologist". Anesth Analg. 2005;100:1862.
14. http://www.asahq.org/For-Healthcare-Professionals/Standards-Guidelines-and-Statements.aspx. Accessed 16 Dec 2013.
15. Granting privileges for deep sedation to non-anesthesiologist sedation practitioners. (Approved by the ASA House of Delegates on October 20, 2010). Available at: http://www.asahq.org/publications AndServices/sgstoc.htm. Accessed 16 Dec 2013.
16. http://www.asahq.org/For-Members/Standards-Guidelines-and-Statements.aspx. Accessed 16 Dec 2013.
17. American Society of Anesthesiologists. Standards for basic anesthetic monitoring. 2010. http://www.asahq.org/For-Members/~/media/ ForMembers/documents/Standards Guidelines Stmts/Basic Anesthetic Monitoring 2011.ashx. Accessed 4 Feb 2014.
18. Department of Health & Human Services. Centers for Medicare & Medicaid Services Revised Hospital Anesthesia Services Interpretive guidelines—state operations manual (SOM) Appendix A Ref: S&C-10-09-Hospital. Revised 2-05-2010. Available at: https://www.cms.gov/SurveyCertificationGenInfo/downloads/SCLetter10_09.pdf. Accessed 6 Dec 2013.
19. Department of Health & Human Services. Centers for Medicare & Medicaid Services. CMS Manual System. Pub. 100-07 State Operations Provider Certification. Transmittal 59. Clarification of the Interpretive Guidelines for the Anesthesia Services Condition of Participation. 2010. Available at: https://www.cms.gov/transmittals/downloads/R59SOMA.pdf. Accessed 20 Jan 2011.
20. Statement on safe use of propofol. (Approved by the ASA House of Delegates on October 27, 2004, and amended on October 21, 2009). Available at: http://www.asahq.org/publicationsAndServices/sgstoc.htm. Accessed 16 Dec 2013.
21. Distinguishing Monitored Anesthesia Care ("MAC") From Moderate Sedation/Analgesia (Conscious Sedation). (Approved by the ASA House of Delegates on October 27, 2004 and last amended on October 21, 2009). Available at: http://www.asahq.org/publications AndServices/sgstoc.htm. Accessed 16 Dec 2013.
22. Joint Commission on Accreditation of Healthcare Organizations (JCAHO). Comprehensive accreditation manual for hospitals: the official handbook. Oakbrook Terrace, IL: Joint Commission on Accreditation of Healthcare Organizations; 2004.
23. Joint Commission for Accreditation of Hospitals. Operative or other high-risk procedures and/or the administration of moderate or deep sedation or anesthesia. The comprehensive accreditation manual for hospitals: official handbook. Oakbrook Terrace, IL: Joint Commission on Accreditation of Healthcare Organizations; 2007. PC-41.
24. American College of Emergency Physicians Policy Compendium. Procedural sedation in the emergency department. 2008. http://www.acep.org/practres.aspx?id=29644. Accessed 16 Dec 2013.
25. Miner JR, Burton JH. Clinical practice advisory: emergency department procedural sedation with propofol. Ann Emerg Med. 2007;50(2):182–7, 187.e1.
26. Roback MG, Bajaj L, Wathen JE, Bothner J. Preprocedural fasting and adverse events in procedural sedation and analgesia in a pediatric emergency department: are they related? Ann Emerg Med. 2004;44(5):454–9.
27. Agrawal D, Manzi SF, Gupta R, Krauss B. Preprocedural fasting state and adverse events in children undergoing procedural sedation and analgesia in a pediatric emergency department. Ann Emerg Med. 2003;42(5):636–46.
28. Mace SE, Brown LA, Francis L, Godwin SA, Hahn SA, Howard PK, et al.; EMSC Panel (Writing Committee) on Critical Issues in the Sedation of Pediatric Patients in the Emergency. Clinical policy: critical issues in the sedation of pediatric patients in the emergency department. Ann Emerg Med. 2008;51(4):378–99, 399.e1–57.
29. Green SM, Roback MG, Miner JR, Burton JH, Krauss B. Fasting and emergency department procedural sedation and analgesia: a consensus-based clinical practice advisory. Ann Emerg Med. 2007;49(4):454–61.
30. Mace SE, Barata IA, Cravero JP, Dalsey WC, Godwin SA, Kennedy RM, et al.; EMSC Grant Panel on Pharmacologic Agents Used in Pediatric Sedation and Analgesia in the Emergency Department. Clinical policy: evidence-based approach to pharmacologic agents used in pediatric sedation and analgesia in the emergency department. J Emerg Nurs. 2004;30(5):447–61.
31. Mace SE, Barata IA, Cravero JP, Dalsey WC, Godwin SA, Kennedy RM, et al.; EMSC Grant Panel (Writing Committee) on Pharmacologic Agents Used in Pediatric Sedation and Analgesia in

the Emergency Department; American Academy of Pediatrics; American Pediatric Surgical Association; Emergency Nurses Association. Clinical policy: evidence-based approach to pharmacologic agents used in pediatric sedation and analgesia in the emergency department. J Pediatr Surg. 2004;39(10):1472–84.
32. Miner JR, Heegaard W, Plummer D. End-tidal carbon dioxide monitoring during procedural sedation. Acad Emerg Med. 2002;9(4): 275–80.
33. Clinical policy: procedural sedation and analgesia in the emergency department. Ann Emerg Med. 2014;63(2):247–58.e18.
34. http://www.ada.org/prof/resources/positions/statements/anesthesia_guidelines.pdf. Accessed 16 Dec 2013.
35. The American Dental Association. Guidelines for the Use of sedation and general anesthesia by dentists: as adopted by the October 2007 ADA House of Delegates. http://www.ada.org/sections/about/pdfs/anesthesia_guidelines.pdf. Accessed 16 Dec 2013.
36. The American Dental Association. Guidelines for teaching pain control and sedation to dentists and dental students: as adopted by the October 2007 ADA House of Delegates. http://www.ada.org/sections/professionalResources/pdfs/anxiety_guidelines.pdf. Accessed 16 Dec 2013.
37. American Academy of Pediatrics and the American Academy of Pediatric Dentistry. Guideline for monitoring and management of pediatric patients during and after sedation for diagnostic and therapeutic procedures. http://www.aapd.org/media/Policies_Guidelines/ G_Sedation.pdf. Accessed 16 Dec 2013.
38. [no authors listed] American Academy of Pediatric Dentistry. Clinical Affairs Committee Sedation and General Anesthesia Subcommittee. Guideline on use of anesthesia personnel in the administration of office-based deep sedation/general anesthesia to the pediatric patient. Pediatr Dent. 2012;34(5):170-2
39. Vargo JJ, Cohen LB, Rex DK, Kwo PY. Position statement: non-anesthesiologist administration of propofol for GI endoscopy. Hepatology. 2009;50(6):1683–9.
40. Faigel DO, Baron TH, Goldstein JL, Hirota WK, Jacobson BC, Johanson JF, et al.; Standards Practice Committee, American Society for Gastrointestinal Endoscopy. Guidelines for the use of deep sedation and anesthesia for GI endoscopy. Gastrointest Endosc. 2002;56(5):613–7.
41. Waring JP, Baron TH, Hirota WK, Goldstein JL, Jacobson BC, Leighton JA, et al.; American Society for Gastrointestinal Endoscopy, Standards of Practice Committee. Guidelines for conscious sedation and monitoring during gastrointestinal endoscopy. Gastrointest Endosc. 2003;58(3):317–22.
42. ASGE Standards Of Practice Committee, Lee KK, Anderson MA, Baron TH, Banerjee S, Cash BD, Dominitz JA, et al. Modifications in endoscopic practice for pediatric patients. Gastrointest Endosc. 2008;67(1):1–9.
43. Koh JL, Black DD, Leatherman IK, Harrison RD, Schmitz ML. Experience with an anesthesiologist interventional model for endoscopy in a pediatric hospital. J Pediatr Gastroenterol Nutr. 2001;33(3):314–8.
44. Squires Jr RH, Morriss F, Schluterman S, Drews B, Galyen L, Brown KO. Efficacy, safety, and cost of intravenous sedation versus general anesthesia in children undergoing endoscopic procedures. Gastrointest Endosc. 1995;41(2):99–104.
45. Kaddu R, Bhattacharya D, Metriyakool K, Thomas R, Tolia V. Propofol compared with general anesthesia for pediatric GI endoscopy: is propofol better? Gastrointest Endosc. 2002;55(1): 27–32.
46. Sury M, Bullock I, Rabar S, Demott K. Sedation for diagnostic and therapeutic procedures in children and young people: summary of NICE guidance. BMJ. 2010;341:c6819.
47. Summary of draft guidelines on sedation and/or analgesia (PSA) at locations outside the operating theatre. Part III: in children. Initiators: Netherlands Society of Anesthesiologists and Dutch Society of Pediatrics. Organization. Utrecht: Dutch Institute for Healthcare Improvement (Central Accompaniment Organization (CBO)); 2011.
48. Riphaus A, Wehrmann T, Weber B, Arnold J, Beilenhoff U, Bitter H, et al. S3 guideline: sedation for gastrointestinal endoscopy 2008. Endoscopy. 2009;41(9):787–815.
49. Reed A, Thomas J, Roelofse JA, Gray R, de Kock M, Piercy J. Paediatric Procedural Sedation and Analgesia (PSA) guidelines; S Afr J Anaesthesiol Analg 2010:16(5) (Supplement 1):S1–S37.
50. SASA Guidelines. Paediatric procedural analgesia and sedation guidelines. S Afr J Anaesthesiol Analg. 2010;16(5):1612.
51. [no authors listed] Scottish Intercollegiate Guidelines Network. SIGN guideline 58: safe sedation of children undergoing diagnostic and therapeutic procedures. Paediatr Anaesth. 2008;18(1): 11–12.
52. [no authors listed] Australasian College for Emergency Medicine, Australian and New Zealand College of Anaesthetists; Faculty of Pain Medicine and Joint Faculty of Intensive Care Medicine. Statement on clinical principles for procedural sedation. Emerg Med (Fremantle). 2003;15(2):205–6.
53. Innes G, Murphy M, Nijssen-Jordan C, Ducharme J, Drummond A. Procedural sedation and analgesia in the emergency department. Canadian consensus guidelines. J Emerg Med. 1999;17(1): 145–56.
54. Bell GD, McCloy RF, Charlton JE, Campbell D, Dent NA, Gear MW, et al. Recommendations for standards of sedation and patient monitoring during gastrointestinal endoscopy. Gut. 1991;32(7): 823–7.
55. The Society for the Advancement of Anaesthesia in Dentistry (SAAD). Standards in conscious sedation for dentistry. Report of an independent working group. 2000.
56. Levati A, Paccagnella F, Pietrini D, Buscalferri A, Calamandrei M, Grossetti R, et al. SIAARTI-SARNePI guidelines for sedation in pediatric neuroradiology. Minerva Anestesiol. 2004;70(10):675–97; 698–715.
57. Schreiber F. Austrian Society of Gastroenterology and Hepatology (OGGH)–guidelines on sedation and monitoring during gastrointestinal endoscopy. Endoscopy. 2007;39(3):259–62.
58. Guidelines for the safe use of procedural sedation and analgesia for diagnostic and therapeutic procedures in children: 2010. S Afr J Anaesthesiol Analg. 2010:16(5 Suppl. 1):S1–37.
59. Riphaus A, Wehrmann T, Weber B, Arnold J, S3-guidelines—sedation in gastrointestinal endoscopy. Z Gastroenterol. 2008; 46(11):1298–330.
60. Dumonceau JM, Riphaus A, Aparicio JR, Beilenhoff U, Knape JT, Ortmann M, et al. European Society of Gastrointestinal Endoscopy, European Society of Gastroenterology and Endoscopy Nurses and Associates, and the European Society of Anaesthesiology Guideline: non-anesthesiologist administration of propofol for GI endoscopy. Endoscopy. 2010;42(11):960–74.
61. Lago P, Garetti E, Merazzi D, Pieragostini L, Ancora G, Pirelli A. Guidelines for procedural pain in the newborn. Acta Paediatr. 2009;98(6):932–9.

Procedural Sedation: Let's Review the Basics

3

Vincent W. Chiang

Abstract

In a pediatrician's practice, there are a number of indications for the provision of procedural sedation. This chapter aims to provide a framework for procedural sedation from a pediatrician's point of view, including understanding of the practice setting, the patients, and the procedures themselves. Although written from a pediatrician's perspective, this chapter is designed to apply to all sedation providers across specialties. Additionally, in trying to create an approach to procedural sedation, it is equally important to consider when the risks of the sedation outweigh the benefits that may be achieved by the procedure.

Keywords

Sedation • Analgesia • Anxiolysis • Risk • Benefits • Cognitive development • Patient age • American Academy of Pediatrics (AAP) • Basic life support (BLS) • Pediatric advanced life support (PALS) • Emergency medical service (EMS)

For the welfare of children

—Motto, American Academy of Pediatrics

Introduction

Pediatricians, by their very nature, are patient advocates. As such, it is no wonder that pediatricians have taken a leadership role in trying to define standards around the management of pain, anxiety, and motion in children undergoing medical procedures. In 1985, the American Academy of Pediatrics (AAP) published its first set of guidelines for the elective use of conscious sedation. These guidelines have continued to evolve over the last 20 plus years [1]. In this time, our understanding of pediatric pain experiences as an interplay of genetic, experiential, and developmental factors has grown considerably [2, 3]. Simultaneously, the widespread availability of noninvasive monitoring, short-acting opioids and sedatives, and specific opioid and benzodiazepine antagonists has greatly increased our ability to provide procedural sedation in a wide array of practice settings [4].

The practice of procedural sedation, however, is not simply the administration of pharmacologic agents to remove all pain. In every clinical setting, pediatricians must weigh the balance of all the risks and benefits of their potential treatment. Virtually every agent in the procedural sedation armamentarium can have negative effects on a patient's cardiovascular and/or respiratory status and the physician providing sedation must be prepared to handle these potential adverse effects. Furthermore, there are a number of adverse reactions, such as nausea and vomiting, that may also result from the provision of procedural sedation. As much as pediatricians serve as the advocates for their patients to minimize pain and anxiety, they are also their patient's advocates with regard to their safety. For example, it is unlikely that procedural sedation would ever be routinely used for procedures such as venipuncture or vaccine administration [3].

In a pediatrician's practice, there are a number of indications for the provision of procedural sedation. This chapter aims to provide a framework for procedural sedation from a pediatrician's

V.W. Chiang, M.D. (✉)
Department of Medicine, Harvard Medical School, Boston Children's Hospital, Boston, MA, USA
e-mail: vincent.chiang@childrens.harvard.edu

K.P. Mason (ed.), *Pediatric Sedation Outside of the Operating Room: A Multispecialty International Collaboration*, DOI 10.1007/978-1-4939-1390-9_3, © Springer Science+Business Media New York 2015

point of view, including understanding of the practice setting, the patients, and the procedures themselves. This chapter is designed to apply to all sedation providers across specialties. Additionally, in trying to create an approach to procedural sedation, it is equally important to consider when the risks of the sedation outweigh the benefits that may be achieved by the procedure.

Questions to Be Asked

Prior to the initiation of any procedural sedation, the following questions need to be considered:

1. What are the goals of the procedural sedation? Eliminating or reducing pain (analgesia)? Alleviating or reducing anxiety (anxiolysis)? Maintaining motionlessness for an imaging procedure?
2. Do I have the appropriate personnel to provide the therapy, both with regard to knowledge and experience? The proper equipment? The time to do the procedure and to monitor the patient during the recovery period?
3. Does the patient have an underlying medical condition that may complicate the provision of procedural sedation?
4. Am I prepared to handle an adverse reaction or unanticipated complication of the procedural sedation?

This chapter will attempt to provide a framework for these questions and will lay the foundation for future chapters.

Setting

First and foremost, the provision of sedation in a safe manner requires a setting that has immediately available personnel, equipment, monitoring, and protocols to manage emergency and rescue situations [5]. In particular, practitioners providing sedation must be prepared to handle the patient who has a compromise of the airway or depressed respiratory effort, both of which can result in airway obstruction, hypoventilation, hypoxemia, apnea and, at worst, frank respiratory arrest. Fortunately, most severe outcomes are extremely rare. One large study found that even in centers with dedicated and specialized sedation services, one in every 200 sedations outside of the operating room required airway and ventilation intervention and one in every 400 procedures is associated with stridor, laryngospasm, wheezing, or apnea [6]. While it is difficult to predict when and for whom adverse events will occur, advanced preparation may be the most critical factor in minimizing an adverse outcome [7, 8].

Personnel

Properly trained personnel are of the utmost importance in the provision of procedural sedation and there should be, at a minimum, two trained professionals present at each sedation.

The primary caregiver is the one who is responsible for providing the sedation itself. This person must be credentialed to provide sedation and should have current training in both basic (e.g., BLS) and advanced (e.g., PALS) life support. Simple certification, however, is not enough. This primary practitioner needs to be able to recognize all potential complications of the sedation, especially the earliest signs of airway difficulties, and to manage them accordingly [9]. According to the Joint Commission, this level of competence requires not only training and education, but experience as well [10].

The secondary provider's primary responsibilities are to monitor the patient during the procedure and to inform the primary provider of any changes in the patient's cardiovascular or respiratory status. Most, if not all, healthcare facilities require that all providers be properly trained and educated as well as take part in a minimum number of sedations annually in order to ensure competence and maintain sedation privileges.

Equipment

The space where the procedural sedation takes place must have the proper equipment to minimize any adverse consequences. Table 3.1 lists the minimum equipment that must be available to provide sedation and rescue a sedated patient [5, 11].

Monitoring

A number of physiologic parameters should be monitored to ensure the safety of the patient. The most recent guidelines from the AAP state that there should be a "functioning pulse oximeter with size-appropriate oximeter probes and other monitors as appropriate for the procedure (e.g., noninvasive blood pressure, respiratory rate, heart rate, electrocardiogram [ECG], capnography and a precordial stethoscope is encouraged in those circumstances in which the patient is not easily visible)" [5]. In July 2011, the American Society of Anesthesiologists updated the Standards for Basic Anesthetic Monitoring. These standards specify that "during moderate or deep sedation the adequacy of ventilation shall be evaluated by continual observation of qualitative clinical signs and monitoring for the presence of exhaled carbon dioxide unless precluded or invalidated by the nature of the patient, procedure or equipment" [12].

Protocols

Protocols or algorithms for how to activate back-up emergency services are essential for every setting where procedural sedation is practiced [5]. For nonhospital facilities, this includes the activation of the Emergency Medical Service (EMS) system and ambulance/transport services to the

Table 3.1 Equipment required for procedural sedation

Code cart Defibrillator Emergency airway equipment • Face masks • Self-inflating bag-valve-mask setup • Oro- and nasopharyngeal airways • Laryngeal mask airways (LMAs) • Laryngoscope handles and blades • Endotracheal tubes and stylettes
Oxygen source May be from wall or oxygen tank, but should be able to provide positive pressure for at least 60 min or the minimum time required to be able to continuously support a patient during transfer to another medical facility or another area within the medical facility
Suction (both Yankauer-type and suction catheters for endotracheal tubes)
Vascular access equipment Intravenous catheters Intraosseous needle Equipment to place, secure, and use the catheters (i.e., tubing, tape, arm boards, alcohol wipes, tourniquets, syringes, etc.)
Reversal agents Naloxone or nalmefene for opioid reversal Flumazenil for benzodiazepine reversal
Monitoring equipment Pulse oximetry Three-lead electrocardiogram Noninvasive blood pressure monitoring End-tidal CO_2 monitoring
Means of two-way communication
Adequate lighting, electricity, and space
Medical record for documentation

Source: Data from Henderson and Womack [11] and from Cote et al. [5]

Table 3.2 Preprocedure health assessment

Age of the patient
Weight of the patient
Health history • Allergies and previous adverse drug reactions • Medication history • Relevant medical diseases, physical anomalies, or neurologic impairment that might increase the potential of airway obstruction • Pregnancy status • Relevant past hospitalizations and surgeries • History of sedation or anesthesia, especially with regard to complications or adverse outcomes • Relevant family history, especially with regard to anesthesia
Review of systems focusing on cardiac, pulmonary, renal, and hepatic function that might alter the patient's response to the medications used in the procedure
Vital signs
Physical examination, including a focused evaluation of the airway
Physical status evaluation (i.e., ASA classification)
Name and contact information of the patient's medical home

Source: Data from Cote et al. [5]

receiving hospital. It is implicit that the availability of EMS services does not obviate the practitioner's responsibility in providing initial management and rescue of the potential complications of the sedation.

There need to be written guidelines and protocols for the preprocedure assessment as well as for the monitoring of the patient during and following the procedure. Table 3.2 lists the information that should be obtained in a preprocedure assessment [5]. Documentation during the procedure should be a time-based record of the monitored physiologic parameters and the timing, dosage, and effect of the administered drugs. This should start with the "time out," during which time the patient's name, procedure to be performed, and the site of the procedure are confirmed [10]. All complications, unanticipated patient reactions, and ensuing treatment should be documented. Finally, there must be instructions for patients and families for care of the patient postprocedure and following discharge, including contact information should there be a concern after the patient is discharged.

Patients

The practice of pediatrics is dependent on having an understanding of how patients change over time. From infancy to adolescence, children undergo tremendous physical, cognitive, and mental development. Where a patient is in his/her development will alter how we as physicians interact with our patients. An understanding of the child's cognitive development is paramount to effectively manage a patient who is about to undergo a medical procedure.

While the pain from a medical procedure may be short-lived, there is recent data to suggest that there are long-term detrimental effects on neuronal development, pain threshold and sensitivity, coping strategies, and pain perception [13]. While procedural sedation may remove the acute pain, the anxiety surrounding the procedure may actually heighten the pain experience or the patient's response to pain [13]. As such, how we prepare a patient for a medical procedure may have tremendous subsequent impact [14]. Recommendations regarding preparation for the procedure can be partitioned into timing, format, and content.

Timing refers to when one informs a patient about the procedure that is going to happen. Data suggest that information provided too far in advance of a procedure may serve to increase anxiety: Children may dwell on or exaggerate the anticipated pain or forget the pertinent information completely [13]. On the other hand, inadequate time to process the information about a procedure may heighten stress. Patients undergoing a major medical procedure (e.g., surgery) will need more advanced timing as compared to something more routine, such as the administration of a vaccine.

Table 3.3 Childhood developmental considerations for preprocedure preparation

Age (years)	Characteristics	Strategy for preprocedure preparation
1–4	Understanding of world through sensory experiences	Use real objects to help child master the situation
	Egocentric	Reinforce good behavior
	Trusts primary caregiver	Keep parent with child as much as possible
	Animism	
	Understanding > verbal ability	
4–10	Development of reasoning	Allow time for questioning
	Elimination of egocentrism	Provide detail
	Improved verbal communication	Use concrete teaching materials and simple medical terms
10+	Can think abstractly	Involve patient in decision-making
	Future thinking	Provide information in advance
	Heightened self-consciousness	Support need for self-control and independence
		Offer explanations in clear, technical terms
		Respect privacy and self-image concerns

Adapted from [15]

The timing will also be influenced by the developmental stage of the patient. In general, children who cannot reason or think abstractly will benefit less from early advanced information.

Format refers to how information about a procedure is conveyed. Examples of various formats include models, puppets, schematic drawings, etc. The appropriate format to be used depends greatly on one's cognitive development. For instance, young children who are at an egocentric phase of their development may not have the cognitive maturity to understand role playing with a puppet or doll.

The *content* about a procedure should relay information about the procedure itself and what the patient can expect. Accurate expectations will allow a patient to gain a sense of self-control and better cope with what is about to happen. As with timing and format, the content is greatly influenced by the developmental stage of the patient. Table 3.3 presents the sequential stages of cognitive development and the accompanying strategies to prepare a patient for a medical procedure [15].

The language we choose to explain a given procedure may also have an impact on how an upcoming procedure is perceived [16]. Dialogue that is negative, vague, or critical can increase anxiety and stress. For instance, warning that something will "hurt" or "burn" creates a negative focus. On the other hand, language that allows for distraction or provides a positive focus can attenuate anxiety and stress. For example, stating "this may feel like a pinch" or "some children say this feels warm and tingly" gives children a sensory as opposed to negative focus. Positive reinforcement such as "you are being brave" or "you did a good job of holding still" is a nice way of providing encouragement or praise. Finally, children are often very concrete thinkers. Stating that "the nurse is going to draw your blood" is too vague for most children to understand. Rather, describing the procedure in a stepwise fashion (e.g., "the nurse is going to clean your arm, you will feel a cold pad to wash your skin, we will use this tourniquet to give your arm a hug, etc.") provides both sensory and detailed information that allow the children a greater sense of control [13].

Procedures

A pediatrician will encounter many different common procedures that may require procedural sedation. Depending on the procedure, a patient may require analgesia or sedation/anxiolysis or both. For instance, an infant who needs a head MRI will likely require a sedative agent, while a cooperative adolescent may only require pain medication for a lumbar puncture. On the other hand, a child with an angulated forearm fracture will need both analgesia and sedation for the reduction. It is difficult to characterize procedures to predict the medication requirement. The temperament, cognitive development, and patient's past experience will alter what is needed for any given procedure. Table 3.4 lists the most commonly encountered procedures that may require procedural sedation. This list is not intended to be inclusive nor exhaustive. For instance, some very common procedures may require procedural sedation in a minority of patients (e.g., venipuncture). Additionally, there are some procedures on the list (e.g., endotracheal intubation, thoracentesis) that most general pediatricians will not perform once they have completed residency training.

While the choice of agents is covered in great detail in other chapters, there are a few points that bear repeating. It should be noted that while opioids do have some sedative effects, sedation often enhances analgesic efficacy. In a patient who is anxious or stressed, concomitant treatment

Table 3.4 Procedures that may require procedural sedation

Procedures
Radiologic imaging procedures (e.g., CT scan, MRI, ultrasound)
Laceration repair
Lumbar puncture
Foreign body removal
Abscess management (e.g., incision, drainage, and packing)
Burn or wound debridement
Relocation of a dislocated joint
Fracture reduction
Joint aspiration
Prepubescent gynecologic examination
Hernia reduction
Peripherally inserted central catheter (PICC) placement
Bone marrow aspiration
Central line placement
Thoracentesis
Chest tube placement
Cardioversion
Endotracheal intubation

CT computed tomography, *MRI* magnetic resonance imaging

with a sedative may reduce the needed dose of narcotic. Furthermore, the use of local and regional anesthetics (e.g., nerve blocks) may reduce the total dose of sedatives and analgesics required.

Other Considerations

Given the large number of resources required to safely perform procedural sedation, only primary care pediatricians in a hospital or medical center setting will likely be able to perform procedural sedation for their patients. However, this does not mean that pediatricians outside of these settings cannot assist and advise in the sedation of their patients. Our understanding of these patients and the process will allow us to play an integral role in the planning and implementation of the sedation.

As previously stated, it would be extremely unlikely that procedural sedation becomes common for, painful procedures such as phlebotomy or IV placement. Local anesthetics, however, can dramatically lessen the pain associated with procedures that require penetration of the skin [13]. In general, there are three processes by which the local anesthetic is delivered to the skin. The anesthetic can be injected locally via a small-gauge needle; it can diffuse passively through the skin via a cream or gel or be administered by a needleless system that enhances passage of the local anesthetic through the skin (e.g., heat-enhanced diffusion, iontophoresis, sonophoresis, laser-assisted passage, or pressurized gas delivery) [17]. Another topical treatment to reduce pain is the use of a vapocoolant spray. By rapidly cooling the skin, it is thought that initiation and conduction of nerve impulses are reduced and the refractoriness is increased [18]. A differentiating feature of these different methodologies is the timing and onset of anesthesia. Finally, less invasive routes, such as intranasal administration, allow for the delivery of both analgesics and anxiolytics without the need for intravenous access [19, 20].

There have been a number of studies that have demonstrated the effectiveness of distraction as a technique to minimize pain and anxiety around painful medical procedures [13]. (Refer to Chap. 34.) While there are several postulated theories as to how distraction works to reduce pain, there is much anecdotal evidence to suggest that it is an excellent pain-management intervention. Child life therapists are another excellent resource to assist in pain management, both with regard to preparing for a procedure and providing distraction during a procedure [21]. Even proper positioning can assist in making a painful procedure less traumatic [13]. Depending on the procedure, sitting on a parent's lap or allowing a child to hold a parent's hand can help reduce procedure-related anxiety. For young infants, skin-to-skin contact, nonnutritive sucking, and sucrose water have been demonstrated to be helpful in reducing perceived pain and should be considered for certain procedures when medically allowable.

Future Directions

One of the most recent advances in our understanding of adverse reactions due to medication use lies in our increasing knowledge of pharmacogenetics. The observed differences in response between patients to the same dose of the same drug likely are attributed to how a given individual metabolizes a given agent. For instance, differences in the level of cytochrome P-450-dependent monooxygenase activity may result in differences in both efficacy and toxicity of certain agents [22]. As an example, variants in the genotype CYP2D6 likely explain different responses to codeine, including potentially life-threatening toxicity as the result of accumulation of active metabolites of the drug [22]. In the future, our understanding of pharmacogenetics will likely be integrated into the decision-making process as we choose agents to provide procedural sedation in the safest manner possible.

Conclusion

In summary, it is the responsibility of the sedation provider to advocate for his/her own patients, especially with regard to pain, fear, and anxiety that may accompany a medical procedure. Being an advocate, however, does not mean that all patients should be sedated for every painful procedure. In reality, the provider must balance the pain associated with the procedure with what is safest for the patient. In essence, the approach to procedural sedation is as much about choosing when not to sedate as it is to tailoring the sedation to the patient and procedure.

Case Studies

Case 1

You are in your office when a father brings his son in for evaluation. He is a healthy 14-year-old with no significant past medical history who accidentally slammed his finger in a door. You obtain X-rays, which are negative. However, he has a large subungual hematoma that is moderately painful to touch. What would be your approach to managing pain for the treatment of the hematoma?

Considerations: The treatment for a subungual hematoma involves draining the hematoma by placing a hole in the nail itself (trephination). Since the nail is not innervated, this is a relatively painless procedure and in general, does not require any analgesia. However, there are still patients who may be quite anxious. Most 14-year-olds can be reasoned with, for example, pointing out that it does not hurt when one clips one's nails. One can also position one's body between the patient and the affected finger during the procedure so as to "prevent" the patient from seeing the procedure itself. In extreme cases, the use of a short-acting anxiolytic may be warranted.

Case 2

You and a nurse are together seeing urgent patients for your clinic. A mother brings her 2-year-old son in for blood work. She is here because she herself is quite needle phobic and thinks that her son is as well. She would like her son to be sedated for the blood draw and the local lab said that they do not sedate patients for phlebotomy. What would your approach be to this patient?

Considerations: Whenever a patient undergoes procedural sedation, one has to weigh the risks and benefits. In general, phlebotomy is not considered a typical procedure for which procedural sedation is used. That being said, it does not mean one should not try to minimize the discomfort associated with the procedure. For 2-year-olds, depending on the urgency, one could consider the use of a topical anesthetic prior to a blood draw. Also, this is a great age where distraction techniques may help as well.

Case 3

Your office is in a small medical center that shares a procedure room where you can provide procedural sedation. The procedure room is well stocked, including having a pediatric code cart that is kept up to date. You and your nurses have done a number of procedures there and in general you feel quite comfortable providing procedural sedation. One of your 2-year-old patients is brought in after a fall through a glass coffee table. The patient has multiple deep lacerations to both forearms, which will require significant repair. Of note, the patient has trisomy 21. What would your approach be to this patient?

Considerations: The provision of procedural sedation is not simply about providing the medications, but also managing the potential complications that may occur. While this patient may tolerate sedation without any difficulty, there are other factors to consider. Patients with trisomy 21 often have macroglossia and hypotonia, which can increase the difficulty of managing the patient's airway should hypoventilation or apnea occur. Additionally, patients with trisomy 21 can also have complex congenital heart disease, which can affect which agents are chosen for the procedural sedation. At the very least, consultation with an expert in procedural sedation, if not transfer to a facility with even more resources should be considered.

References

1. American Academy of Pediatrics Committee on Drugs. Section on anesthesiology: guidelines for the elective use of conscious sedation, deep sedation, and general anesthesia in pediatric patients. Pediatrics. 1985;76:317–21.
2. Walco GA. Needle pain in children: contextual factors. Pediatrics. 2008;122 Suppl 3:S125–9.
3. Kennedy RM, Luhmann J, Zempsky WT. Clinical implications of unmanaged needle-insertion pain and distress in children. Pediatrics. 2008;122 Suppl 3:S130–3.
4. Krauss B, Green SM. Sedation and analgesia for procedures in children. N Engl J Med. 2000;342:938–45.
5. Cote CJ, Wilson S, The Work Group on Sedation. Guidelines for monitoring and management of pediatric patients during and after sedation for diagnostic and therapeutic procedures: an update. Pediatrics. 2006;118:2587–602.

6. Cravero JP, Blike GT, Beach M, et al. Incidence and nature of adverse events during pediatric sedation/anesthesia for procedures outside the operating room: report from the pediatric sedation research consortium. Pediatrics. 2006;118:1087–96.
7. Cote CJ, Karl HW, Notterman DA, et al. Adverse sedation events in pediatrics: analysis of medications used for sedation. Pediatrics. 2000;106:633–44.
8. Cote CJ, Notterman DA, Karl HW, et al. Adverse sedation events in pediatrics: a critical incident analysis of contributing factors. Pediatrics. 2000;105:805–14.
9. Flood RG, Krauss B. Procedural sedation and analgesia for children in the emergency department. Emerg Med Clin North Am. 2003; 21:121–39.
10. Joint Commission on Accreditation of Healthcare Organizations. Comprehensive accreditation manual for hospitals: the official handbook by the JCAHO. Oakbrook Terrace, IL: Joint Commission on Accreditation of Healthcare Organizations; 2005.
11. Henderson K, Womack W. Noninvasive monitoring for procedural sedation. In: Krauss B, Brustowicz RM, editors. Pediatric procedural sedation and analgesia. Philadelphia, PA: Lippincott, Williams & Wilkins; 1999.
12. Standards for Basic Anesthetic Monitoring. Committee of Origin: standards and practice parameters (Approved by the ASA House of Delegates on October 21, 1986, and last amended on October 20, 2010 with an effective date of July 1, 2011). http://www.asahq.org/ForHealthcare-Professionals/Standards-Guidelines-and-Statements.aspx.
13. Cohen LL. Behavioral approached to anxiety and pain management for pediatric venous access. Pediatrics. 2008;122 Suppl 3:S134–9.
14. Jaanist T, Hayes B, von Bayer CL. Providing children with information about forthcoming medical procedure: a review and synthesis. Clin Psychol Sci Pract. 2007;14:124–43.
15. Moynihan R, Kurker C. The perioperative environment and the pediatric patient. In: Ferrari LR, editor. Anesthesia and pain management for the pediatrician. Baltimore, MD: The Johns Hopkins University Press; 1999.
16. McMurty CM, McGrath PJ, Fortson BL, et al. Reassurance can hurt: parental behavior and painful medical procedures. J Pediatr. 2006;148:560–1.
17. Zempsky WT. Pharmacologic approaches for reducing venous access pain in children. Pediatrics. 2008;122 Suppl 3:S140–53.
18. Burke D, Mogyoros I, Vagg R, Kiernan MC. Temperature dependence of excitability indices of human cutaneous afferents. Muscle Nerve. 1999;22:51–60.
19. Grassin-Delyle S, Buenestado A, Naline E, Faisy C, Blouquit-Laye S, Couderc LJ, Le Guen M, Fischler M, Devillier P. Intranasal drug delivery: an efficient and non-invasive route for systemic administration: focus on opioids. Pharmacol Ther. 2012;134(3): 366–79.
20. Wolfe TR, Braude DA. Intranasal medication delivery for children: a brief review and update. Pediatrics. 2010;126(3):532–7.
21. Leahy S, Kennedy RM, Hesselgrave J, et al. On the front lines: lessons learned in implementing multidisciplinary peripheral venous access pain-management programs in pediatric hospitals. Pediatrics. 2008;122 Suppl 3:S161–70.
22. Gasche Y, Daali Y, Fathi M, Chiappe A, Cootini S, Dayer P, et al. Codeine intoxication associated with ultrarapid CYP2D6 metabolism. N Engl J Med. 2004;351:2827–31.

The Pre-sedation Assessment and Implications on Management

4

Timothy Horeczko and Mohamed Mahmoud

Abstract

In this chapter we will present the essentials of pre-sedation screening and risk stratification, discuss fasting guidelines, and review the most commonly encountered scenarios and comorbidities that impact sedation management and outcomes. Today's practice of pediatric sedation (PS) involves ever more complex patients whose care is coordinated with multidisciplinary teams. Technological advances have allowed for the development of various invasive and noninvasive pediatric procedures and imaging modalities, resulting in a tremendous demand for and growth in PS in children. Despite the increasing complexity and patient volume, sedation providers generally meet the child and his family only minutes before the scheduled (or unscheduled) procedure. The provider must assess the situation quickly and accurately to ensure safety and optimal effectiveness. Important data from all available resources should be gathered and synthesized before the procedure to formulate a successful sedation plan within the context of the urgency of the procedure.

Keywords

Pediatric sedation • Pre-sedation • Screening • History • Physical exam • Fasting guidelines • Asthma • Reactive airway disease • Autism spectrum disorders (ASD) • Developmental delay • Intellectual disability • Bronchopulmonary dysplasia (BPD) • Cerebral palsy • Congenital heart disease • Cystic fibrosis • Diabetes mellitus • Endocrinopathies • Mitochondrial disease • Allergies • Muscular dystrophy • Musculoskeletal disorders • Obstructive sleep apnea • Pregnancy • Premature infant • Psychiatric disorders • Behavioral disorders • Sickle cell disease • Syndromes • Trauma • Tuberous sclerosis • Upper respiratory tract infection • Food and Drug Administration (FDA) • Cyanotic heart disease • New York Heart Association classification (NYHA) • Congestive heart failure (CHF)

Introduction

In this chapter we will present the essentials of pre-sedation screening and risk stratification, discuss fasting guidelines, and review the most commonly encountered scenarios and comorbidities that impact sedation management and outcomes.

Today's practice of pediatric sedation (PS) involves ever more complex patients whose care is coordinated with multidisciplinary teams. Technological advances have allowed for the development of various invasive and noninvasive pediatric procedures and imaging modalities, resulting in a

T. Horeczko, M.D., M.S.C.R.
Department of Emergency Medicine, Harbor—UCLA Medical Center, Torrance, CA, USA

M. Mahmoud, M.D. (✉)
Radiology Anesthesia and Sedation, Department of Anesthesia, Cincinnati Children's Hospital Medical Center, Cincinnati, OH, USA
e-mail: mohamed.mahmoud@cchmc.org

K.P. Mason (ed.), *Pediatric Sedation Outside of the Operating Room: A Multispecialty International Collaboration*, DOI 10.1007/978-1-4939-1390-9_4, © Springer Science+Business Media New York 2015

tremendous demand for and growth in PS in children. Despite the increasing complexity and patient volume, sedation providers generally meet the child and his family only minutes before the scheduled (or unscheduled) procedure. The provider must assess the situation quickly and accurately to ensure safety and optimal effectiveness. Important data from all available resources should be gathered and synthesized before the procedure to formulate a successful sedation plan within the context of the urgency of the procedure.

The saying "an ounce of prevention is worth a pound of cure" encapsulates the pre-sedation mindset. The main objective for the sedation provider during pre-procedural assessment is to answer the question: **Is this child optimized for the procedure or not?**

Components of a successful sedation plan include readily accessible medical records, a thorough medical history with review of systems and careful attention to red flags, pre-sedation tests, or consultation if indicated, a targeted physical exam, and a complete understanding of the procedure and its potential physiologic effects on the patient.

Pre-sedation Screening

All children scheduled for elective sedation should receive a prescreen telephone call before the scheduled invasive or noninvasive procedure. Last-minute cancellation due to new information surfacing on the day of the procedure can result in delay of care and economic loss for the parents and the institution. The telephone screening allows for review of the medical history, gives the opportunity to determine if there is some underlying medical issue that requires further investigation, confirms that the child has not been recently ill, and reinforces *nil per os* (NPO) instructions. Pertinent data points should be clearly documented and attached to a standardized, hospital-approved sedation assessment form.

Once the screening process is complete, an established triage system can help to determine whether the procedure is appropriate for non-anesthesiologist sedation or whether the expertise of an anesthesiologist is needed. In many centers there is a "point person" to whom non-anesthesiologists may direct questions regarding patient management issues in off-site venues. This coordinator should be familiar with the requirements, challenges, and needs of the individual specialists. In the case of an urgent or emergent (non-elective) procedure, the same logic applies: **Gather as much information as possible and reasonable for your setting to make the most informed decision regarding the timing and approach to the procedure**.

History

The process of constructing a successful sedation plan starts with a careful, targeted history focusing on a few critical domains. Ask about past problems or known abnormalities of the respiratory, cardiovascular, neurologic, gastrointestinal, and endocrine systems. Some parents may not be familiar with medical terminology or may assume that you are aware of the child's history; the provider can work around this by describing common problems and/or procedures, pursuing anything that "sounds familiar." Review any available medical records and contact the primary care provider if possible. Examine previous records in regard to previous problems with airway management, obtaining intravenous access, or prior adverse events related to sedatives-anesthetics.

Antenatal history should be reviewed, as maternal medical conditions or complications may affect the neonate adversely. Determine gestational age and conceptional age—premature infants may have pulmonary, cardiovascular, neurologic, gastrointestinal, and hematologic conditions that may lead to decompensation during sedation.

Elicit a history of prior sedation-anesthesia and any known adverse reactions, such as marked nausea, vomiting, increased or decreased sensitivity to sedatives or analgesics, and/or prior need for intervention during sedation or unexpected hospitalization after procedures. The complete list of current medications and allergies should be carefully documented.

Confirming NPO status is important: Children can never be trusted to have fasted. The child and parent should be carefully questioned about any recent intake by mouth, however trivial it may seem.

Physical Examination

The initial physical examination provides the sedation practitioner with an opportunity to become familiar with the patient's baseline physiologic status. **Perform a targeted physical examination, including airway assessment, respiratory status, and volume status**. Some children will present with a syndrome that the parents do not disclose, either because they assume you are aware or for personal reasons; in these cases, tactfully ask about any special needs. Specific syndromes may be recognized by unusual features, many of which appear as a constellation of associated findings. Inquire as to what extent the child is affected by the syndrome and his current functional status.

Fasting Guidelines and Sedation

Although the presence of gastric contents theoretically increases the risk of aspiration pneumonia, **there is no known gastric fluid volume (GFV) that places a particular patient at clinically relevant risk or that eliminates all risk** [1]. The traditional teaching is that the risk of aspiration increases with gastric acid volume greater than 0.4 mL/kg and a pH of less than 2.5 [2]. However, if these threshold values were applied, a great number of appropriately fasted patients would be classified as at risk for aspiration. **That is, the stomach is rarely completely empty**—even in the fasted state—given ongoing salivary (1 mL/kg/h) and gastric (0.6 mL/kg/h) secretions [3]. The provider may expect GFV to be minimal in most fasting patients, but some patients may have large residual GFV despite having followed traditional fasting guidelines (Fig. 4.1). Prolonged fasting in children is not entirely benign: The fasting child is always at risk for hypoglycemia and/or hypovolemia. Optimize your patient's volume and metabolic status before the procedure with the appropriate intravenous fluids if needed. Due to high metabolic needs, an infant should be offered clear fluids until 2 h before sedation.

There is a presumption that the relative risk of aspiration is lower during sedation than under general anesthesia, and that protective airway reflexes are retained fully during sedation. It is important to note that the progression from mild sedation or analgesia to general anesthesia represents a continuum not easily divided into discrete stages [4]. **Anyone receiving moderate or deep sedation should be treated similarly to those receiving general anesthesia because the sedation level can change rapidly and deepen subtly with subsequent impairment of airway reflexes.**

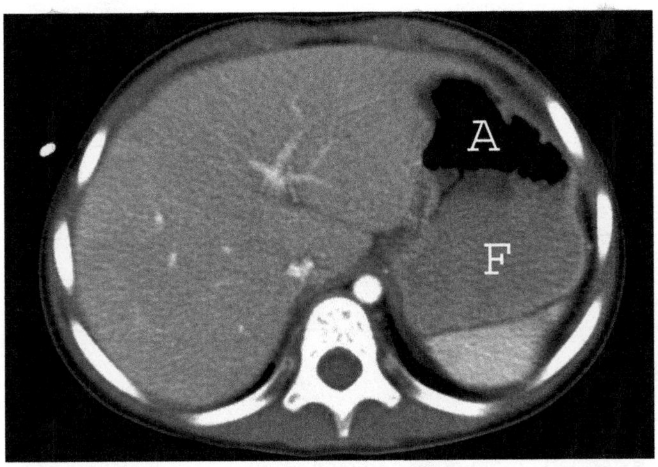

Fig. 4.1 CT of the abdomen without administration of oral contrast in a fasting 2-year-old child in supine position. CT shown in axial (A) plane. Note fluid (labeled "F") and air (Labeled "A") in distended stomach. Measured volume of fluid in stomach was 41.8 mL (3.3 mL/kg). Courtesy of Mohamed Mahmoud, MD

Although aspiration is a widely feared complication of general anesthesia, fortunately clinically relevant aspiration in modern anesthesia practice is exceptionally rare in pediatrics. The incidence is estimated to be 1 in 10,000 to 10 in 10,000, with the wide reported range likely due to variation in research methodologies, definitions, and reporting sensitivities [5]. In those undergoing general anesthesia, approximately two-thirds of aspiration occurs during manipulation of the airway (endotracheal tube placement and removal) [6]. The multicenter Pediatric Sedation Research Consortium collected data on 49,836 propofol sedations in children: Aspiration during sedation occurred four times (0.04 %) [7]. A retrospective study by Sanborn et al. of 16,467 sedations during imaging procedures in children using chloral hydrate, midazolam, fentanyl, or pentobarbital found 70 (0.4 %) respiratory incidents; only two patients of 16,467 aspirated (0.012 %) [8].

The low incidence of aspiration pneumonia with sedation and anesthesia may be attributed to the fact that the stomach is very distensible and can accommodate a large volume before resting intragastric pressure rises [9]. Intragastric pressure must exceed the barrier pressure of the lower esophageal sphincter (LES) for regurgitation to occur. The barrier pressure of the LES does not appear to be as easily overcome under general anesthesia as is widely believed [9].

The **American Society of Anesthesiology's (ASA) Task Force on Fasting** has published consensus guidelines for elective anesthesia: clear fluids, 2 h; breast milk, 4 h; formula, 6 h; and solids, 8 h [10]. These guidelines are intended for healthy patients of all ages undergoing elective procedures; they are not intended for patients with coexisting diseases or conditions that may delay gastric emptying such as diabetes, hiatal hernia, gastroesophageal reflux, or bowel obstruction. The ASA acknowledges that there is insufficient evidence to codify preoperative fasting times. In addition, the task force does not offer specific guidance for fasting times for emergency procedures.

When practitioners formulate a plan for sedation for emergency procedures in children who have not fasted, the risks of sedation and the possibility of aspiration must be balanced against the benefits of performing the procedure emergently. **The American College of Emergency Physicians (ACEP)** Clinical Policy on Sedation assesses risk based on the nature of last oral intake and the urgency of the procedure (Table 4.1) [11]. In this setting, aspiration has been found to be very rare among patients sedated in an emergency room setting for procedures, regardless of fasting status [12].

There is an ongoing debate regarding the **administration of oral contrast for Computerized Tomography (CT) prior to sedation**. The administration of oral contrast less

Table 4.1 Prudent limits of targeted depth of ED procedural sedation

STANDARD RISK				
ORAL INTAKE IN THE PRIOR 3 HOURS	Urgency of the Procedure			
	Emergent	*Urgent*	*Semi-Urgent*	*Non-Urgent*
Nothing	All levels of sedation	All levels of sedation	All levels of sedation	All levels of sedation
Clear liquids only	All levels of sedation	All levels of sedation	Up to and including brief deep sedation	Up to and including extended moderate sedation
Light snack	All levels of sedation	Up to and including brief deep sedation	Up to and including dissociative sedation; non-extended moderate sedation	Minimal sedation only
Heavy snack or meal	All levels of sedation	Up to and including extended moderate sedation	Minimal sedation only	Minimal sedation only
HIGHER RISK				
ORAL INTAKE IN THE PRIOR 3 HOURS	Procedural Urgency			
	Emergent Procedure	*Urgent Procedure*	*Semi-Urgent Procedure*	*Non-Urgent Procedure*
Nothing	All levels of sedation	All levels of sedation	All levels of sedation	All levels of sedation
Clear liquids only	All levels of sedation	Up to and including brief deep sedation	Up to and including extended moderate sedation	Minimal sedation only
Light snack	All levels of sedation	Up to and including dissociative sedation; non-extended moderate sedation	Minimal sedation only	Minimal sedation only
Heavy snack or meal	All levels of sedation	Up to and including dissociative sedation; non-extended moderate sedation	Minimal sedation only	Minimal sedation only

↓ Increasing Potential Aspiration Risk ↓	Procedural Sedation and Analgesia Targeted Depth and Duration
	Minimal sedation only
	Dissociative sedation; brief or intermediate-length moderate sedation
	Extended moderate sedation
	Brief deep sedation
	Intermediate or extended-length deep sedation

Modified with permission from Green SM, Roback MG, Miner JR, Burton JH, Krauss B. Fasting and Emergency Department Procedural Sedation and Analgesia: A Consensus-Based Clinical Practice Advisory. Ann Emerg Med. 2007; 49(4): 454–461

Brief: <10 min

Intermediate: 10–20 min

Extended: >20 min

than 2 h before sedation-anesthesia is at odds with elective NPO guidelines, and in theory would increase the risk of aspiration pneumonia. Sedation practitioners are asked to make an exception to the fasting guidelines and permit the use of enteric contrast material with CT in order to obtain an accurate study. There does not appear to be a perfect resolution to this issue, since waiting several hours after administration of contrast often results in inadequate opacification of the small bowel and a poor study [13].

Small bowel transit time can be as rapid as 15 min and on average is 1 h 24 min [14]. In one study, in 83 % of cases small bowel transit time was less than 2 h [14]. Inadequate opacification of the small bowel can lead to lack of distinction between small bowel loops and fluid collections or masses [13].

At one author's institution, administration of contrast begins 2 h before and ends 1 h prior to anesthesia-sedation. The challenge lies in balancing technical factors governing the image quality of the study with safety concerns related to sedating a child with a potentially full stomach for an elective CT. A recent retrospective chart review concluded that administering oral contrast material within 2 h of propofol sedation for abdominal CT in children appears to be relatively safe. The data sample, however, was small relative to the reported incidence of aspiration in the literature [15]. Currently we are not aware of any clear consensus among institutions that care for these patients. Some clinicians may choose to perform rapid sequence induction of general anesthesia with endotracheal intubation while others may choose deep sedation without definitive airway protection. Others may negotiate with radiologists to have the oral contrast given 2 h before the study or administered through an oral gastric tube after placement of an endotracheal tube [16, 17].

When Not to Proceed

Barring emergent or life-threatening circumstances, situations arise in which—despite pressure from consultants, providers, and/or families—the practitioner should forgo sedation outside of the operating room for a more opportune time, setting, or facility. Proper monitoring, rescue equipment, and sufficient staff should be in place. The provider should use sound clinical judgment before proceeding, informed by the patient's risk for complications and the urgency of the procedure, as well as practical concerns such as the ability to dedicate the necessary time, attention, and human resources to the endeavor. The following section is a broad overview that will address specific safety considerations and focused assessments in important special populations.

Preparation for and Considerations in Special Populations

Asthma and Reactive Airway Disease

The child who wheezes presents a common challenge to the sedation practitioner. *Transient wheezers* are infants whose symptoms are provoked by an active viral respiratory infection. These children typically "outgrow" their reactivity within the first few years of life. After the toddler and preschool period, *non-atopic wheezers* continue to experience wheezing with active viral illnesses, but are not likely to develop lifelong symptoms. Both transient and non-atopic wheezers tend to have mild reactions to the inciting event. *Atopic wheezers* are equally sensitive to viral illnesses, but often also suffer from allergy, allergic rhinitis, and atopic dermatitis. These children are at highest risk for severe and persistent symptoms exacerbated by a variety of infectious and/or environmental factors [18].

The diagnosis of asthma is difficult to make under the age of 6, since there is significant overlap with reactive airway disease and pulmonary function tests are problematic in young children. In those with an established diagnosis of asthma, the assessment of symptoms follows a step-wise approach (Table 4.2).

In addition to the assessment of severity of symptoms, confirm the overall control of symptoms and what level of therapy the child is currently receiving. It is also helpful to ascertain the responsiveness that the child has shown to previous exacerbations [19]. This is especially important in the planning of procedures that involve airway stimulation or those that would require frequent suctioning.

Children with a history of either reactive airway disease or diagnosed asthma are at risk for **bronchial hyperreactivity** (40 % of school-aged children with asthma) [20]. Bronchial hyperreactivity may persist for weeks after an exacerbation. For this reason, a careful history of recent illness, changes in medication, and history of hospitalization are important in all children with a history of wheezing. In general in children with stable and controlled asthma or reactive airway disease, the peri-procedural risk for bronchospasm is low and is not associated with a significant morbidity [21].

A recent prospective study found that patient factors (readily known on pre-procedural assessment) such as active respiratory symptoms, eczema, family history of asthma, rhinitis, or exposure to tobacco smoke were associated with an increased relative risk of peri-procedural respiratory adverse events such as airway obstruction, oxygen desaturation (<95 %), and severe or sustained cough [22]. In patients with active symptoms, the practitioner should determine the *severity of illness* and weigh this with *the urgency and importance* of

Table 4.2 Asthma severity assessment in children older than 5 years of age

Clinical features	Mild intermittent asthma	Mild persistent asthma	Moderate persistent asthma	Severe persistent asthma
A. Symptoms: wheezing, coughing, chest tightness	Symptoms ≤2 times/week	Symptoms >2 times/week but <1 time/day	Daily symptoms	Continual symptoms
	Asymptomatic between brief exacerbations		Exacerbations 2 or more time/week; may last days	Frequent exacerbations
B. Activity limitations	No activity limitations	Activity may cause exacerbations	Activity causes exacerbations	Limited physical activity
C. Nocturnal symptoms	≤2 times/month	>2 times/month	>1 time/week	Frequent nighttime symptoms
D. Lung function	PEF or $FEV_1 \geq 80$ % of predicted or personal best	PEF or $FEV_1 \geq 80$ % of predicted or personal best	PEF or $FEV_1 > 60$ % and <80 % of predicted or personal best	PEF or $FEV_1 \leq 60$ % of predicted or personal best

Modified from: National Heart, Lung, and Blood Institute: National Asthma Education and Prevention Program. *Expert Panel Report 3: Guidelines for the Diagnosis and Management of Asthma*. 2007

the procedure. The actively wheezing patient should have his current illness addressed immediately, and if the procedure is to go forward, a plan for pre-, intra-, and post-procedure treatment should be formulated to anticipate and manage potential complications such as bronchospasm.

Autism, Developmental Delay, and Intellectual Disability

Autism spectrum disorders (ASD) are characterized by neurodevelopmental impairments in three major domains: **behavior, communication, and socialization** [23]. Although the rate of diagnosis of ASD has markedly increased recently, its pathogenesis is incompletely understood; the current consensus is that autism has a genetic basis with possible contributing environmental factors. Approximately 40–62 % of children with ASD demonstrate some learning disability [24].

Children with intellectual disability, developmental delay, or ASDs require a holistic view in preparation for sedation. Caretakers are typically very helpful in sharing the child's past reactions to the procedure, and may be vocal in their preferences in the timing, type, and route of administration of sedatives. The practitioner would do well to consider the caregivers' experience with their child and weigh this with the practicalities and requirements of the procedure at hand.

These children may exhibit challenging behavior, especially when anxious or stressed, such as punching/slapping/pulling (50 %) or kicking (24 %) [25]. Boys and adolescent males form the majority (66 %) of children with challenging behavior [26]. These behaviors may be exacerbated by frequent and sometimes unpleasant interactions with the health care system. **Observing the child while non-stressed during the pre-sedation assessment may help to reveal caregiver-patient dynamics as well as to inform the clinician of how best to keep him calm and cooperative.** Non-pharmacologic methods such as distraction, storytelling, watching videos, or playing games are particularly helpful in this setting and during the induction/pre-procedural period. (Refer to Chap. 34.)

Intellectual, developmental, and learning disabilities are not a specific medical condition, but rather manifestations of neurologic disease. It is important to note that **comorbidities are common**, such as epilepsy (44 %), psychiatric disorders (50 %), and gastroesophageal reflux (49 %) [24]. The pre-procedural assessment should include a review of medical conditions, frequency and control of symptoms, and current medications.

A small observational study found that as a group, children with developmental delay (given the prevalence of substantial neurologic comorbidities) may have a smaller airway diameter at the level of the soft palate when sedated for magnetic resonance imaging (MRI). The authors' findings were thought to be multifactorial: anatomic (different airway shape), physiologic (abnormal airway tone), and pharmacologic (increased susceptibility to sedative) [27]. In this light, concurrent illness such as viral respiratory symptoms should be considered carefully in these patients.

If the child requires pretreatment, one may start with noninvasive approaches such as the oral route for pre-sedation, the intranasal route to facilitate IV access if needed, and the intramuscular route if necessary. Nitrous oxide, if available, may be a good choice if the child sees the device as a novelty or game, rather than as a restraint. Close attention to risk factors for pre-procedural anxiety or behavioral challenges is important, as these are associated with post-procedural delirium and maladaptive behaviors, which complicate the feasibility of a successful outpatient visit [28].

Anticipating behavioral disruptions and having a ready plan for escalation of treatment are essential. Discussion with the caregiver before the procedure may help to decrease his or her anxiety, allowing for a capable, present, and calm ally in the endeavor. This includes the timing and threshold for physical restraint if needed, based on the urgency and nature of the procedure. A brief pre-sedation "team huddle" with caregivers and staff to review the sedation plan may promote a smooth procedure and help to avoid injury to the patient, parents, practitioner, or staff.

Bronchopulmonary Dysplasia

Bronchopulmonary dysplasia (BPD) is the most common cause of chronic lung disease in infants. It affects premature infants who survive the acute phase of respiratory distress syndrome and is characterized by the need for supplemental oxygen beyond 4 weeks of life. BPD is thought to develop after prolonged periods of mechanical ventilation and exposure to high concentrations of inspired oxygen. Other proposed pathophysiologic mechanisms include initial volume overload, increased pulmonary blood flow, and generalized inflammation. These patients typically have decreased lung compliance, airway hyperactivity, lung hyperinflation, rapid respiration, wheezing, cough, and frequent episodes of fever, desaturation, hypercarbia, abnormal functional airway growth, and increased risk for bradycardia and congestive heart failure (CHF) [29].

Implications of BPD in sedation-anesthesia include tracheomalacia, tracheal granuloma, subglottic stenosis, increased airway reactivity and bronchospasm, and diuretic-induced electrolyte disorders. **Adequate pre-procedure preparation should focus on optimizing oxygenation, reducing airway hyperactivity, and correcting electrolyte abnormalities.** These children require special attention to fluid balance with careful titration of fluids during the procedure. A laryngeal mask airway (LMA) is less irritating to both the upper and lower airways; it may offer some advantage in reducing the incidence of post-procedural coughing, wheezing, and hoarseness compared to endotracheal intubation in these patients.

Cerebral Palsy

Cerebral palsy (CP), a nonprogressive, permanent disorder of motor function and posture, is the most common physical disability in childhood, occurring in 2–2.5 in 1,000 births [30]. The majority of cases are of unknown etiology. Known associations are multifactorial: prematurity (78 %), intrauterine growth restriction (34 %), intrauterine infection (28 %), antepartum hemorrhage (27 %), and maternal alcohol use (threefold increased risk) [31, 32]. One in four have epilepsy and one in five have a sleep disorder [33].

The spectrum of disease varies from mild focal weakness with normal intelligence to total body spasticity and severe intellectual disability. CP may be classified by the predominant motor component: **spasticity, ataxia, or dyskinesia** [34]. Medical therapy emphasizes control of spasticity with medications, injections, or surgery. In the pre-sedation assessment, the type, dosage, and route of medications are important especially if there will be prolonged fasting. The clinician should determine the presence (and recent setting changes) of an intrathecal pump. Although rarely an issue, children with recent Botulinum toxin type A injection (for local control of spasticity) if unwittingly overdosed may later experience relative respiratory muscle weakness, which may be exacerbated during sedation [35].

Common comorbidities such as scoliosis, gastroesophageal reflux, decubitus ulcers, and skin infections should be assessed for control of disease. This will help in planning for successful positioning (to optimize ventilation and comfort), IV access, and ready access to the airway if advanced measures are needed during the procedure. Children with CP often have considerable drooling due to difficulty in swallowing secretions; **plan for frequent suctioning**. Atropine or glycopyrrolate may be considered for their antisialagogue effect, but they may also thicken lung secretions and potentially increase the risk of lung infection in CP patients [34].

Part of the pre-sedation assessment is anticipating and avoiding pitfalls in the care of children with CP. **Chronic low fluid intake and relative malnutrition put the child at risk for pre-renal failure and the development of pressure ulcers**. Careful attention to fluid replacement (especially during prolonged fasting periods) and proper positioning of the patient during the procedure will help to attenuate these risks. Other common challenges are the presence of extremity casts that may obscure blood loss (from trauma or the procedure itself) or developing compartment syndrome from malpositioning.

Pain control in intellectually disabled children is an important issue. Clinician understanding of the analgesic needs of these children is changing, and there is evidence to suggest that they may, in fact, be more sensitive to pain than non-disabled children [36]. Unfortunately, these vulnerable children are often undertreated due to barriers in communication or misinterpretation of behaviors [37]. Children on chronic opioids may have 30–100 % higher dosage requirements than opioid-naïve children [38]. Control of symptoms should begin early in the visit to promote a successful procedure and post-procedure course.

Congenital Heart Disease

Congenital heart disease (CHD) occurs in approximately 8 in 1,000 live births [39]. The most common acyanotic

Table 4.3 Classification systems of heart failure [45, 46]

Class	NYHA classification	Ross classification
I	No symptoms	No limitations or symptoms
II	Symptoms with moderate exertion	Mild tachypnea or diaphoresis with feeding in infants; dyspnea on exertion in older children
III	Symptoms with mild exertion	Marked tachypnea or diaphoresis with feeding or exertion
IV	Symptoms at rest	Symptomatic at rest with tachypnea, retractions, grunting, or diaphoresis

Table 4.4 Heart failure staging for infants and children [43]

Stage	Interpretation
A	Increased risk of developing heart failure, but with normal cardiac function and size
B	Abnormal cardiac morphology or function, with no heart failure symptoms or history of symptoms in the past
C	Underlying structural or functional heart disease and heart failure symptoms past or present
D	End-stage heart failure

Table 4.5 Cardiac conditions associated with the highest risk of adverse outcome from endocarditis for which prophylaxis with dental procedures is reasonable [48]

Prosthetic cardiac valve or prosthetic material used for cardiac valve repair
Previous infectious endocarditis
Unrepaired cyanotic CHD, including palliative shunts and conduits
Completely repaired congenital heart defect with prosthetic material or device, whether placed by surgery or by catheter intervention, during the first 6 months after the procedure
Repaired CHD with residual defects at the site or adjacent to the site of a prosthetic patch or prosthetic device (which inhibit endothelialization)
Cardiac transplantation recipients who develop cardiac valvulopathy

lesion is a ventricular septal defect; the most common cyanotic lesion is the tetralogy of Fallot. Although lesions may be classified as acyanotic or cyanotic and/or ductal dependent or not, the clinician may risk stratify based on whether the child has been fully repaired or whether his lesion involves palliation. That is, a child with a repaired ventricular septal defect and normal baseline oxygenation may have no long-term sequelae relevant to sedation while a child with single ventricle pathology, a palliative shunt (e.g., hypoplastic left heart syndrome status-post Fontan procedure), or baseline low oxygen saturation requires a more judicious approach.

Children with cyanotic disease with or without palliative surgery are very sensitive to changes in volume status, as many are pre-load dependent. In addition, certain lesions are more prone to dysrhythmias [40]. Their low baseline oxygen saturations offer little to no reserve in times of stress. For this reason and in general, **children with cyanotic heart disease are poor non-emergent outpatient candidates for sedation beyond mild anxiolysis** [40–42].

Although each lesion has a unique set of considerations in the pre-sedation assessment, current functional status is most informative of appropriateness for sedation outside of the operating room. Children with CHD (both cyanotic and acyanotic lesions) often develop some degree of CHF. The New York Heart Association (NYHA) classification was originally designed for adults, and is often applied to children (Table 4.3) [41]. The Ross classification was designed specifically for children and mirrors the NYHA classification [43]; recently a detailed age-specific modification to the Ross classification has been proposed [44].

Both the NYHA and the Ross classifications assess current symptoms; neither discriminates well in the early stages of disease. Since overt heart failure symptoms are a late sign in children (due to compensatory mechanisms), and the sedating clinician is interested in detecting subtle risk factors, an updated heart failure staging classification has been proposed (Table 4.4).

Stages A and B correspond to NYHA I, and stage C corresponds to NYHA II and III. Stage D patients typically require inotropic and/or ventilator support. In addition to the above, the assessment should include the child's general health and change in behavior, oral intake, or urine output. A recent cough or taking longer to feed may be subtle alerts to hypervolemia and poor control of CHF. On examination, infants may be in mild to moderate respiratory distress and/or have evidence of hepatic engorgement, a sign of right-sided heart failure (*N.B.* peripheral edema as seen in adults in CHF is rare in children).

Recent illnesses, especially upper respiratory tract infections (URIs), are especially important to note in these children, as airway reactivity and changes in pulmonary vascular resistance are not well tolerated in children with CHD. A thorough review of previous surgeries and complications, current medications, and drug allergies is required. Anticoagulants may need to be held for the procedure in consultation with the child's cardiologist. The presence of an implantable cardiac defibrillator or pacer should be determined and recent changes or complications noted [47].

Prophylaxis for bacterial endocarditis is recommended for all dental procedures only in children with high-risk historical features (Table 4.5). In eligible children, it is reasonable to give prophylaxis for procedures on the respiratory tract, infected skin, or musculoskeletal tissue. Prophylaxis is no longer recommended for gastrointestinal or genitourinary procedures.

Cystic Fibrosis

Cystic fibrosis (CF) is the most common fatal inherited disease in Caucasians, and exists in smaller frequencies in other racial groups [49]. The basis of its pathophysiology is a mutation in the cystic fibrosis transmembrane conductance regulator (CFTR) protein, a chloride channel found in all exocrine tissues. As such, **CF is a multi-organ system disease**, involving impaired lung function, pancreatic insufficiency and diabetes mellitus, hepatobiliary disease and cirrhosis, bone disease, and genitourinary disease. Pulmonary complications account for over 90 % of the morbidity and mortality in CF patients [50].

CF demonstrates a spectrum not only in terms of organ systems involved but also in severity of disease burden in the individual patent [51]. For this reason, the pre-sedation assessment should include pointed questioning about the child's frequency of illness, strength of cough, amount of sputum produced, airway reactivity, and history of recovery from procedures and illnesses. A thorough review of current therapies and recent acceleration of treatment may reveal the child's current trajectory of disease.

Younger children with CF have more reactive airways, which may respond to β(beta)-agonists. **It is important to note, however, that older children may have worsening expiratory airflow with the use of bronchodilators**. This is due to progressive damage to cartilaginous support in the lower airways; bronchial muscle hypertrophy may in fact help to "stent" the airways open [52]. In these patients, bronchodilators may result in "floppy" lower airways, and impaired gas exchange. A careful history regarding response to β(beta)-agonists is important to anticipate and avoid intra-procedure complications.

In addition to acute exacerbations and worsening lung infections, children with CF are at risk for apical blebs (up to 3.4 %) that may cause spontaneous pneumothorax [50]. Planning for sedation of a child with CF should include preparation for the management of this complication, such as oxygen therapy, IV catheters for decompressive thoracostomy, and a plan for emergent definitive chest tube thoracostomy. Chronic lung disease may manifest in chronic hypoxia and hypercarbia with resulting increases in pulmonary vascular resistance and pulmonary hypertension. An electrocardiogram (ECG) with evidence of *cor pulmonale* is an ominous sign [53].

Control of diabetes mellitus, if present, should be addressed. The presence of liver disease should be noted, as hepatic clearance of medications may be enhanced in early disease and impaired with the onset of cirrhosis; liver function tests are unreliable in this context [54]. Older CF patients may develop distal intestinal obstruction syndrome (DIOS) in the colon and ileum, mimicking medical and surgical causes of nausea, vomiting, abdominal pain, and distention [55]. Volume depletion, chronic narcotics, and medication nonadherence put the patient at higher risk [50].

If possible, a review of the medications given during previous procedures may be helpful in planning for sedation. Patients with CF may have higher opioid and benzodiazepine requirements than patients without CF [56]. Plan to balance titrating to effect with possible impairment of overall oxygenation and ventilation during the procedure.

Diabetes Mellitus

Type 1 (insulin-dependent) diabetes mellitus (DM) accounts for over 90 % of DM cases in children [57]. Early onset of type 2 (non-insulin-dependent) DM is rising with obesity rates in children [57]. Other less common causes of DM in children include maturity onset diabetes of youth (MODY), insulin resistance syndromes (idiopathic), genetic syndromes (chromosomal abnormalities, congenital disorders of the pancreas), and secondary diabetes (e.g., drugs such as corticosteroids) [58].

The clinician should gain a general view of the patient's overall diabetes control and any recent change in regimen. A thorough account of the child's medications (e.g., insulin, oral hypoglycemic sulfonylureas, oral biguanide) and timing of the last dose should be reviewed. Patients may have taken a recent dose of medication, only to be unexpectedly fasting during the visit. Physical exam should pay close attention to volume status, as these children are at risk for hypovolemia. If an insulin pump is found, the silastic catheter may be removed before the procedure to ensure that ongoing insulin is not administered to the fasting child. A baseline fingerstick blood glucose will be helpful in the initial assessment.

Regardless of the type or current control of the patient's diabetes, **the overall goal during sedation is to avoid hypoglycemia and excessive hyperglycemia** [58, 59]. When appropriate, IV fluids may be given, and if the procedure is prolonged, supplemental glucose with frequent fingerstick blood glucose monitoring. Case reports demonstrate the importance of glucose monitoring in DM patients undergoing sedation: hypoglycemic coma may be confused for deep or prolonged sedation [60].

Endocrinopathies

Knowledge of the normal anatomy and physiology of the endocrine glands is essential in understanding their potential pathophysiologic effects relevant to procedural sedation. In this section we will outline the considerations for sedating a child with adrenal insufficiency, hypothyroidism, hyperthyroidism, or diabetes insipidus (DI).

The adrenal cortex synthesizes and secretes steroid hormones (glucocorticoids, mineralocorticoids, and sex steroids) that are essential to life. Glucocorticoids (especially cortisol) play a critical role in the body's response to stress and play an important role in maintaining vascular tone.

Causes of adrenal insufficiency can be classified as primary (adrenal gland dysfunction), secondary (the pituitary gland dysfunction), or tertiary (hypothalamic dysfunction). The most common cause of adrenal insufficiency is long-term administration of exogenous glucocorticoids via oral, intravenous, inhaled, intranasal, or topical routes. Even a short course (5 days) of prednisone mildly suppresses the hypothalamic–pituitary–adrenal axis for 5 days after discontinuation (usually without clinical sequelae in the healthy patient). Long-term glucocorticoid use produces adrenal cortical atrophy as a result of chronic suppression of ACTH production, requiring variable recovery times of up to 1 year [61].

The practice of providing perioperative glucocorticoid replacement therapy to patients with adrenal insufficiency is well established. Insufficient levels of cortisol can be produced in response to stress in these patients, posing the risk of acute adrenal crisis with hypotension and cardiovascular collapse.

Peri-procedural stress dosing depends on the duration and invasiveness of the procedure. Most elective minor procedures and noninvasive diagnostic studies do not warrant supplementation with additional glucocorticoids. A continuation of the current dose of corticosteroids is sufficient to maintain cardiovascular function in patients who receive long-term administration of exogenous glucocorticoids [62]. It is extremely important to note that **primary hypopituitarism is a condition that always requires peri-procedure steroid supplementation** regardless of the daily dose taken. Parenteral cortisol (e.g., Solu-Cortef) at a dose of 0.5–1 mg/kg every 6 h is recommended for perioperative, intensive care, or emergency department indications for up to 72 h [63].

Thyroid hormones are integral to the normal physiology of every organ system of the human body, playing a crucial role in regulating myocardial function, pulmonary ventilation, energy homeostasis, vascular tone, water and electrolyte balance, and normal function of the central nervous system. **The most important adverse effects of hypothyroidism include impaired cardiac contractility with decreased cardiac output, increased peripheral vascular resistance, and decreased blood volume and peripheral oxygen consumption.**

A detailed history should be obtained from the patient or the family about prior thyroid disease, thyroid surgery, radiation therapy (radioactive iodine or neck irradiation), treatment with any thyroid medications, or family history of thyroid disease. Physical examination is equally important. Dry skin, a slowed deep tendon reflex relaxation phase, bradycardia, and hypothermia are all signs of clinical hypothyroidism. Children with known hypothyroidism have increased sensitivity to anesthetic-sedative agents; these children should have documented normal thyroid function tests before elective procedures.

Hyperthyroidism is less common in children than hypothyroidism and is most commonly caused by Graves disease. The classical features of thyrotoxicosis include hyperactivity, weight loss, tremor, heat intolerance, dyspnea, insomnia, diarrhea, and nervousness. Cardiovascular effects of hyperthyroidism include palpitations, tachycardia, atrial fibrillation, and congestive cardiac failure. **Thyroid storm can be lethal.** Fortunately, it is rarely seen due to widespread use of antithyroid drugs. In an attempt to prevent this catastrophic complication, **these children should be euthyroid before the procedure**. Thyroid storm responds to symptomatic treatment including parenteral β(beta)-blockers and propylthiouracil.

The clearance and distribution volume of propofol are increased in hyperthyroid patients. When total intravenous anesthesia is used, propofol infusion rates should be increased to reach anesthetic blood concentrations [64].

Optimal anesthetic-sedative care of patients with history of DI requires an understanding of the complex pathophysiology of this disease. Arginine vasopressin (AVP) is produced within the hypothalamus, and it is normally stored for release in the posterior pituitary gland. After its release, AVP acts on V2 receptors in the collecting tubules of the nephron in order to allow for effective urine concentration.

DI is a syndrome manifested by high output urine, low urine specific gravity (<1.005), high plasma osmolality (>200 mOsm/L), and high plasma sodium (>150 mEq/L). **Nephrogenic DI** occurs when the kidney is unable to control plasma osmolality due to a defect in the action of AVP. Medications such as demeclocycline, lithium, amphotericin B, and fluoride [5], and electrolyte abnormalities such as hypokalemia and hypercalcemia [6] are known to cause or precipitate nephrogenic DI. **Central DI** occurs due to destruction of the posterior pituitary and eventually lack of AVP production or release. Without treatment, intravascular volume depletion occurs, cardiac stroke volume decreases, and eventually heart rate increases. These patients will have orthostatic hypotension, weak pulses, rapid breathing, and decreased level of consciousness. They may present with seizures if significant hypernatremia is present.

A child undergoing procedural sedation should receive his usual morning dose of desmopressin. The sedation provider should pay attention to fluid management in the patient on desmopressin therapy, as some degree of fluid restriction is required. Intravenous fluids (use 5 % dextrose-0.9 % saline) should total 1 L/m^2/24 h to approximate insensible losses and obligate urine output. Oral fluids may be offered once the child is awake.

Mitochondrial Disease

Mitochondrial disease (MD) is a group of disorders that arise from defects in the oxidative phosphorylation or electron transport chain involved in generation of ATP [65]. Primary mitochondrial disorder is caused by deletions in nuclear DNA or mitochondrial DNA. Secondary disorders are due to mitochondria dysfunction caused by various drugs and by free radicals.

The ten most common syndromes associated with MD are: Kearns-Sayre syndrome; Leigh syndrome; mitochondrial DNA depletion syndrome; mitochondrial encephalomyopathy, lactic acidosis and stroke-like episodes (MELAS); myoclonic epilepsy with ragged red fibers; neurogastrointestinal encephalomyopathy, neuropathy, ataxia and retinitis pigmentosa (NARP); and external ophthalmoplegia. There is no definitive treatment for MD, although some patients improve with specific therapies such as coenzyme Q10; those with seizures may respond to a ketogenic diet.

MD may present with any symptom in any organ at any age, but some symptoms and signs are more suggestive of a mitochondrial disorder than others. These red-flag features require the initiation of a diagnostic evaluation for mitochondrial disease (Table 4.6).

Sedating-anesthetizing children with MD may perplex many practitioners. Currently there is no clear evidence-based guidance in the literature regarding the anesthetic-sedative management of these patients. Complicating matters further is the risk of clinical deterioration related to the stress of the procedure itself, unrelated to nature of the anesthetic-sedative agents used. It is well known that **children with mitochondrial defects (MD) may have an increased risk for cardiorespiratory and neurological and metabolic complications from anesthesia-sedation**. Any organ may be affected in MD: meticulous individualized pre-sedation assessment is essential. Sedation providers should review and consider obtaining complete blood count, basic metabolic panel, liver function tests, thyroid function tests, sleep studies, and ECG and/or echocardiogram as indicated by the patient's condition and the associated syndrome.

Patients with MD often develop hypoglycemia and lactic acidosis, which can be exacerbated by the stress of the procedure. Hypoglycemia is common: diseased mitochondria cannot keep up with the body's energy requirements via fatty acid oxidation during stress, which leads to drawing on and rapid depletion of carbohydrate stores. Minimizing periods of fasting and routine use of lactate-free intravenous fluids (such as 5 % dextrose-0.9 % saline) in all patients with MD undergoing sedation-anesthesia is recommended. Prolonged procedure time requires lactate and blood glucose monitoring. This is especially important for infants, as glucose is the major energy supply to the myocardium, and hypoglycemia may contribute to myocardial depression.

The prevalence of cardiomyopathy in children with MD is reported to be 20 % [66, 67]. The severity of MD correlates with the severity of impairment of cardiac function. Cardiac impairment occurs in Barth syndrome, Kearns-Sayre syndrome, ocular myopathy, and MELAS. *A pre-procedure baseline ECG is strongly recommended* and can be extremely valuable; red flags in the ECG include any form of heart block or prolonged QT. If the screening ECG is abnormal, a cardiology consult is recommended before proceeding with elective sedation-anesthesia in these patients. For those with cardiomyopathy, an echocardiogram within the past year is recommended.

Table 4.6 Factors that warrant initiation of a diagnostic evaluation in mitochondrial disease

Possible indicators of mitochondrial disease
Neurologic
• Nonvascular pattern for cerebral stroke-like lesions
• Basal ganglia diseases
• Encephalopathy—either recurrent or induced by low or moderate dosing of valproate
• Neurodegeneration
• Epilepsia partialis continua (Kojevnikov's epilepsia)
• Myoclonus
• Ataxia
• Magnetic resonance imaging consistent with Leigh disease
• Characteristic magnetic resonance spectroscopy peaks:
– Lactate peak at 1.3 ppm TE (echo time) at 35 and 135 ms
– Succinate peak at 2.4 ppm
Cardiovascular
• Hypertrophic cardiomyopathy with rhythm disturbance
• In a child: unexplained heart block
• Cardiomyopathy combined with lactic acidosis (>5 mM)
• Dilated cardiomyopathy combined with muscle weakness
• Wolff-Parkinson-White arrhythmia
Ophthalmologic
• Retinal degeneration. May include:
– Decreased visual acuity
– Night blindness
– Deficits in color vision
– Pigmentary retinopathy
• Ophthalmoplegia/paresis
• Disconjugate movement of eyes
• Ptosis
• Sudden-onset or insidious-onset optic neuropathy or atrophy
Gastroenterologic
• Liver failure: unexplained or valproate-induced
• Severe dysmotility
• Pseudo-obstructive episodes
Other red flags
• Newborn, infant, or young child experiencing:
– Unexplained hypotonia
– Weakness
– Failure to thrive
– Metabolic acidosis (particularly lactic acidosis)
• Exercise intolerance disproportionate to weakness
• Hypersensitivity to general anesthesia
• Acute rhabdomyolysis

Adapted from [166]

There is no absolute contraindication to any particular anesthetic-sedative agent for patients with MD. Many anesthetic agents adversely affect mitochondrial function in vitro but adverse events in vivo are only sparsely reported. Furthermore, the anesthetic agents implicated in these cases have been used without incident in many other reports. Opioids, ketamine, midazolam, and dexmedetomidine do not appear to inhibit mitochondrial function. At the present time there is no need to avoid volatile agents in patients with MD; **inhalational anesthetics have been used without ill effects in these children.** Keep in mind that patients with MD may have impaired upper airway and respiratory response to hypoxia and hypercarbia. Sedative agents should be titrated carefully in order to avoid respiratory depression.

Patients with MD may be more susceptible to the effects of lipophilic agents such as propofol. Propofol uncouples oxidative phosphorylation in mitochondria and suppresses ATP production by interfering with the electron transport chain [68]. There are cases in which short-term use of propofol has resulted in propofol infusion syndrome (acute bradycardia resistant to treatment and progressing to asystole). These patients may have subclinical forms of mitochondrial disease that are uncovered by the infusion of propofol. Single dose propofol has been used safely in many patients, but the true risk associated with this practice and the safe total dose and duration of infusion is not established. **Since there are many sedative-anesthetic alternatives, it is reasonable to avoid the use of propofol infusion in these patients.**

As in any child with a known myopathy, children with MD are at risk at baseline for rhabdomyolysis. Further, due to abnormal neuromuscular endplates with the subsequent risk of hyperkalemia, a **depolarizing agent such as succinylcholine is contraindicated.** Note also that patients with MD also exhibit variable sensitivity to the non-depolarizing neuromuscular blocking agents. Many report mitochondrial patients' experiencing prolonged neuromuscular block with non-depolarizing neuromuscular blocking agents. Careful titration of neuromuscular blocking agents by twitch monitoring and consideration of administration of reversal agents are recommended.

To summarize, the most important anesthetic-sedative considerations in these patient are: **to maintain normoglycemia and normothermia, to avoid any period of hypoxia, to maintain normovolemia, and to avoid metabolic stresses that can lead to or worsen lactic acidosis.**

Multiple Allergies

The term "drug allergy" is often misused by clinicians and patients to describe any reaction (proven or perceived) to a medication. The preferred general term is *adverse drug reaction*, which encompasses the important subcategories. Three clinically relevant subcategories are: **drug allergy** (reaction resulting from an immunologic mechanism), **drug intolerance** (reaction resulting from non-immunologic and/or unknown reasons), and **pseudo-allergy** (reaction resembling allergy, but with a multifactorial, unknown, or idiosyncratic cause) [69].

It may not be feasible to differentiate the above in the pre-sedation assessment [70]. Allergists suggest referring to these events as **predictable reactions** (drug overdose, side effects, drug–drug interactions) and **unpredictable reactions** (allergy, intolerance, pseudo allergy). Predictable reactions are often benign, and account for approximately 80 % of adverse drug reactions. Unpredictable reactions account for the remaining 20 %, with allergic or pseudo-allergic reactions comprising 5–10 % of adverse drug reactions [69].

Confirming the diagnosis of a drug allergy is not the goal of the pre-sedation assessment; drug provocation testing performed in other settings remains the criterion standard. However, it is important to note that drug allergy is over-diagnosed in children [71]. Although it is prudent to avoid drugs that may have provoked some reaction in the past, when few alternatives remain the clinician should focus on determining the risk and potential severity of unpredictable reactions during sedation. **Type I** allergic reactions are immediate and due to drug-specific antibodies; they require prior exposure and sensitization to the drug. Clinical manifestations include urticaria, angioedema, bronchospasm, and/or anaphylaxis. **Type II** reactions (anti-tissue cytotoxic, e.g., hemolytic anemia or thrombocytopenia) and **Type III** reactions (immune complex, e.g., serum sickness) are readily identified by a history of severe illness or hospitalization. **Type IV** reactions (the most common) are delayed hypersensitivity reactions evolving over hours to days, and often present with maculopapular exanthems (but may also manifest as eczematous, pustular, or bullous lesions) [69].

Documenting the timing, course of the reaction, and likely inciting drug may help the clinician to understand the safety of the use of the proposed medication during the procedure. Electronic medical records may be a good source of information, as many include entries on when the drug was given and the nature of the reaction [72].

Multiple drug allergy syndrome (MDAS) describes a condition in which the patient experiences allergic or pseudo-allergic reactions to related and non-related drugs [73]. Most cases involve urticarial and/or angioedema; however, Stevens-Johnson syndrome and anaphylaxis have been reported. Interestingly, **skin testing in these patients may be negative, even after significant clinical manifestations have been documented**. These patients typically are older, most are adults, and many have multiple comorbidities and a long past medical history (with many opportunities to become sensitized to many different types of drugs). Information about the pathophysiology of MDAS remains limited, as there is no criterion standard for diagnosis and prospective studies are lacking [70].

Multiple drug intolerance syndrome (MDIS) may be a separate entity from that which is described above. MDIS is defined as a hypersensitivity to three or more drugs that are "chemically, pharmacologically, and immunogenically unrelated, taken on three different occasions, and with negative allergy skin tests" [74, 75]. MDIS patients are also typically older, have anxiety, depressive and/or somatoform symptoms, and are typically convinced that they are allergic to all drugs. These patients often require allergy and psychiatric consultations as an outpatient [76].

In summary, the pre-sedation assessment should focus on true allergic or pseudo-allergic signs or symptoms associated with a particular drug and the severity of the presentation. When in doubt and feasible, the clinician in this setting may avoid the drug altogether. If there is a conflict or no acceptable alternative, a frank discussion about the risks, benefits, and other possible alternatives is needed.

Muscular Dystrophies

The muscular dystrophies (MD) are a group of progressive myopathic disorders characterized by muscle wasting and weakness. The most common are Duchenne and Becker MDs; other types present at different stages in life, with varying degrees of severity and involving different muscle groups: fascioscapulohumeral, limb-girdle, distal, oculopharyngeal, and Emery-Dreifuss [77]. The morbidity of the most common, Duchenne and Becker MDs, involves progressive respiratory failure with recurrent lung infections.

The disease is characterized by severe proximal muscle weakness, progressive degeneration, and fatty infiltration of the muscles. Symptoms typically appear at the age of 2–6 years; delayed walking beyond 15 months of age is a common initial sign. Affected children never run properly and have difficulty climbing stairs; only approximately 10 % manage to jump with both feet together. Many children require the use of a wheelchair by age 12, and may not live past their 20s [77]. **Most MDs involve some degree of cardiomyopathy and all are at risk for heart failure** [78]. Other manifestations include pseudohypertrophy of the calves and markedly elevated creatine kinase levels. The progressive nature of the disorder results in restrictive pulmonary disease, multiple contractures, and scoliosis. Due to advances in medical management, many of these patients may now be expected to live into adulthood.

The pre-procedure assessment should focus on the child's overall function (ambulatory or wheelchair) with careful attention to respiratory toilet. The child with disturbed sleep, nightmares, daytime drowsiness, or early morning headaches may have unrecognized nocturnal hypoventilation. This may be a clue to a recent worsening trajectory of illness and make the child more likely to benefit from noninvasive positive pressure ventilation during sleep or sedation. Worsening respiratory symptoms may preclude outpatient sedation.

Symptoms of dizziness, chest pain, intermittent increased shortness of breath, nausea, and decreased oral intake may be consistent with developing (or worsening) cardiomyopathy. A thorough cardiovascular exam with careful attention to signs of heart failure (hepatic congestion in infants and toddlers, facial and extremity edema in older children; presence of an S3 or precordial heave) is warranted. One-third of these patients have dilated cardiomyopathy by age 14, with nearly all patients developing some degree of cardiomyopathy by age 18. Due to the prevalence of cardiac disorders in these patients, the American Academy of Pediatrics recommends that children with DMD should undergo cardiac evaluation and optimization of cardiovascular status prior to elective anesthesia [79].

While it is important to investigate and optimize cardiovascular status before the elective procedure, these patients can develop complications despite the presence of reassuring pre-procedure tests. Unexplained tachycardia should raise the suspicion of cardiomyopathy. *A pre-procedure baseline ECG* and potentially an echocardiographic assessment (within a year from the date of the procedure) are recommended to optimize cardiac function and avoid a dysrhythmia. A child with **a pre-procedure echocardiogram showing good left ventricular function may not respond adequately to myocardial stress during the procedure**. Some children with particular MDs are at higher risk for dysrhythmias, and require a prophylactic implantable defibrillator [80]. **The severity and progression of skeletal muscular disease may be outpaced by worsening cardiac muscular disease, such as non-ischemic cardiomyopathy** [81].

Another important concern in these patients is careful evaluation of the airway and respiratory apparatus. These patients may have a difficult airway due to a combination of macroglossia, weak upper respiratory muscles, limited cervical spine mobility, and limited mandibular mobility. DMD is characterized by weakness of the diaphragm, intercostal muscles, and the accessory muscles of respiration, resulting in restrictive pulmonary impairment and a progressive decrease in total lung capacity and vital capacity. For patients with declining respiratory function, it may be necessary to prepare for noninvasive ventilation prior to the procedure.

During sedation, patients with MD are at risk for rhabdomyolysis, with subsequent acute renal failure or hyperkalemia. A careful review of the child's past procedures and outcomes is recommended. Ideally the child is euvolemic prior to the procedure; care should be taken for proper positioning and potentially adjusting positions during long procedures to discourage the development of rhabdomyolysis. Keep in mind that **children with MDs are often sensitive to small doses of opioids and sedatives, which may cause a sudden and prolonged apnea** [82]. Plan for minimum presedation and small titratable aliquots.

Controversy exists concerning the role of inhalational anesthetics and succinylcholine in "triggering" rhabdomyolysis or malignant hyperthermia [78, 83–85]. Some experts recommend against their use based on case reports. Many clinicians avoid their use altogether in children with MD. Propofol, dexmedetomidine, and ketamine (among others) have all been used with success in intravenous sedation in these children [78, 86–88]. Nitrous oxide may be considered in children with MD without significant cardiomyopathy or cardiac dysfunction [66].

Musculoskeletal Disorders

Children with musculoskeletal disorders may present repeatedly for diagnostic procedures. These children should be managed with sensitivity. Positioning for the procedure can be challenging, especially in those with limb deformities and contractures. Whenever possible, offer the child a position of comfort and minimize focal pressure during sedation.

Achondroplasia is the most common nonlethal skeletal dysplasia. There are two causes for this disorder: the child has either a de novo mutation of the fibroblast growth factor receptor 3 gene or inherits the disorder from his parents. These patients have midface hypoplasia, a depressed nasal base, small nasal airways, narrow oropharynx, and upper airway muscle hypotonia, which predispose them to development of obstructive sleep apnea (OSA) [89]. They tend to have a large head, a bell-shaped chest, cupping of the ribs, and short arms and legs.

Sedative-anesthetic risks in these patients include a challenging airway and increased sensitivity to sedative-anesthetic agents. Patients with severe kyphoscoliosis and restrictive lung disease may have baseline hypoxemia and low lung volumes, predisposing them to hypoxemia during sedation. Review of CT scans and MRI of the spine is helpful before sedating these children. Hyperextension of the neck should be avoided and special consideration should be taken before manipulating the neck due to the possibility of cervical cord compression [90].

The sedation practitioner must be aware of potential complications when sedating a patient with history of significant scoliosis. The primary aim of pre-procedure evaluation is to detect the presence and extent of cardiac or pulmonary compromise. The earlier the age of onset and the more immature the bone growth at the time the process begins, the worse the disease burden. Children with *idiopathic scoliosis* tend to have less pulmonary embarrassment than children with *neuromuscular scoliosis*, who may have abnormalities in the central control of breathing and impaired airway reflexes. Poor coordination of laryngeal and pharyngeal muscles may result in abnormal control of secretions and inadequate cough, increasing the risk of aspiration.

Respiratory function should be assessed by a thorough history, focusing on functional impairment (exercise tolerance). Physical examination should include a good understanding of vital capacity (review any pulmonary function tests that may be available). If pre-procedure vital capacity is less than 30–35 % of predicted, post-procedure ventilation is likely to be required. Cardiac dysfunction may occur in scoliosis from distortion of the mediastinum; patients may develop cor pulmonale from chronic hypoxemia and pulmonary hypertension. Cardiac studies (ECG, echocardiogram) may be performed as indicated.

Osteogenesis imperfecta (OI) is an inherited disorder of the connective tissue whose primary manifestation is an increased susceptibility to fractures. Patients usually present with growth retardation, multiple fractures, progressive kyphoscoliosis, vertebral compression, megalocephaly, macroglossia, blue sclera, dentinogenesis imperfecta, bleeding diathesis, and temperature dysregulation. Anesthetic-sedative challenges in OI include airway anomalies, chronic lung disease (due to kyphoscoliosis, rib fractures, intrinsic pulmonary hypoplasia, and defective lung collagen), coagulation dysfunction, hyperthyroidism, and an increased tendency to develop peri-procedure hyperthermia [91, 92]. Fractures occur from minor trauma and result in severe deformity of the extremities complicating intravenous access and blood pressure cuff placement [91, 92].

Obstructive Sleep Apnea

OSA is an increasingly recognized disorder in children that can present unique challenges to the sedationist and pose substantial morbidity to the patient. It belongs to the spectrum of anomalies known as sleep-related breathing disorders in which the airway may become completely (as in apnea) or partially (as in hypopnea) occluded despite respiratory effort. These abnormalities lead to abnormal gas exchange resulting in increasing hypoxemia, hypercapnia, and sleep fragmentation. Common clinical manifestations include snoring (pauses and gasps), disrupted sleep, daytime somnolence, and behavioral problems. Systemic manifestations in the cardiovascular, pulmonary, metabolic, and neurologic systems

Table 4.7 STOP-BANG scoring model[a]

S	Snoring: Do you snore loudly (louder than talking or loud enough to be heard through closed doors)?	Yes	No
T	Tired: Do you often feel tired, fatigued, or sleepy during the daytime?	Yes	No
O	Observed: Has anyone observed you stop breathing during your sleep?	Yes	No
P	Blood pressure: Do you have or are you being treated for high blood pressure?	Yes	No
B	BMI: BMI more than 35 kg/m^2	Yes	No
A	Age: Age over 50 years	Yes	No
N	Neck circumference: Neck circumference greater than 40 cm	Yes	No
G	Gender: Male	Yes	No

Reprinted with permission from Mehta PP, Kochhar G, Kalra S, Maurer W, Tetzlaff J, Singh G, et al. Can a validated sleep apnea scoring system predict cardiopulmonary events using propofol sedation for routine EGD or colonoscopy? A prospective cohort study. Gastrointest Endosc. 2013 Nov 9. pii: S0016-5107(13)02407-3

[a]High risk of obstructive sleep apnea: yes to ≥3 questions; low risk of obstructive sleep apnea: yes to <3 questions

occur secondary to recurrent hypoxemia, activation of the sympathetic nervous system, and sleep disruption. There is an **increased incidence of OSA among children with syndromes affecting the upper airway** such as Down syndrome, Treacher Collins syndrome, and Pierre Robin sequence.

A description of symptoms related to OSA, their severity, and provocative and palliative factors should be sought from the parents or caregiver. Ask about a history of snoring, as this is common in children with OSA. Further questioning for paradoxical breathing, episodes of apnea, mouth breathing, behavioral disturbances, and restless sleep alert the clinician to undiagnosed OSA. Observe for failure to thrive, obesity, micrognathia, midface hypoplasia, retrognathia, and macroglossia, all of which are associated with OSA. Interventions during sleep, such as supplemental oxygen, bilevel positive airway pressure (BiPAP), and special positioning aids should be noted. It is important to realize that tonsil size does not predict the presence or severity of OSA [93].

In cases of severe OSA, pulmonary hypertension can develop secondary to pulmonary vasoconstriction with subsequent right ventricular failure and cor pulmonale; fortunately this presentation in children is uncommon. High-risk features for cor pulmonale include signs of right ventricular failure and the presence of severe OSA: patients may experience episodes of desaturation to less than 70 %. These children should have an ECG, echocardiogram, and an evaluation by a cardiologist [94]. A complete metabolic panel helps to determine the degree of chronic hypercarbia, which manifests as a compensatory metabolic alkalosis.

Polysomnography (PSG) is the criterion ("gold") standard for diagnosis and quantification of OSA. PSG includes electroencephalography (EEG), electrooculography, chin-leg electromyography, transthoracic impedance, video recording, oral-nasal thermal sensors, nasal airflow pressure transducer, chest/abdomen plethysmography monitors, pulse oximeter, end tidal or transcutaneous CO_2, and snore microphone. OSA should be differentiated from primary snoring (snoring without hypopnea or apnea). **Central sleep apnea** is characterized by the absence of both airway flow and respiratory effort. Some patients, especially those with neuromuscular conditions, may display mixed sleep apnea (central and obstructive sleep apnea).

The sedation provider must identify which patients are most at risk and who can be managed as an outpatient. PSG provides clues to the severity of the airway obstruction during sleep by noting the lowest oxygen saturation observed, as well as the types of apnea (obstructive, central, or mixed) experienced and the frequency of apnea events. The apnea-hypopnea index (AHI) measures the number of hypopnea/apnea episodes per hour of sleep (the AHI does not take into account duration of the obstructive events). The American Society of Anesthesiologists Task Force on Perioperative Management of Patients with Obstructive Sleep Apnea defines OSA as: mild, with an AHI of 1–5; moderate, with an AHI of 5–10; and severe, with an AHI > 10 [95]. The respiratory disturbance index (RDI) is calculated from all respiratory events (including central apnea) occurring in 1 h. AHI and RDI are sometimes used interchangeably but the bottom line is that they may be used to risk-stratify OSA. Nocturnal oximetry assesses the severity of OSA. Isolated severe desaturation (<80 %) or clusters of desaturation (more than three desaturations <90 %) are considered abnormal.

In 2008, the STOP-BANG questionnaire was introduced and validated as a screening tool to identify OSA in adults (Table 4.7) [96]. This questionnaire consists of eight questions (yes/no answers) that together can total a score from 0 to 8. Chung et al. found that in adults, a high STOP-BANG score (5–8) was predictive of moderate and severe OSA [97]. Cote et al. found that in adults high STOP-BANG scores (3 or greater) were predictive of the need for airway intervention (chin lift, mask ventilation, nasal airway, endotracheal intubation) and oxygen desaturation to <90 % with propofol sedation [98]. This scoring tool has not been validated in children. Although one question pertains mostly to adults (neck circumference greater than 40 cm), this screening tool may be relevant to predict OSA and sedation-related complications in children. Future studies are needed in order to determine whether there is a predictive application of this questionnaire to extrapolate outcomes and the presence of OSA in children.

Children with OSA are sensitive to respiratory depression by opioids, sedatives, and hypnotics; they are especially vulnerable to the development of upper airway obstruction during sedation-anesthesia [99]. Investigations on the effect of these drugs on airway morphology indicate the pharynx to be a primary site of obstruction during anesthesia [100]. Changes in airway patency in sedation and anesthesia mirror those associated with sleep disordered breathing: increased airway collapsibility due to an increase in closing pressure [101], loss of tonic activity in pharyngeal muscles [102], and failure of coordination of phasic activation of upper airway muscles with diaphragmatic activity [103]. Residual effects of sedatives/anesthetics can lead to similar changes in airway dynamics resulting in significant post-procedure airway obstruction. Recurrent episodes of apnea, hypopnea, desaturation, and hypercarbia that occur during the pre-procedure sleep state are expected to occur in the recovery room, on the ward, and at home.

Sedatives (such as diazepam and midazolam) relax the pharyngeal musculature, causing a reduction of the pharyngeal space [104]. Propofol, barbiturates, opioid analgesics, and sub-anesthetic concentrations of inhalational agents similarly exacerbate upper airway obstruction and increase the risk of respiratory depression and/or apnea [99]. In contrast to other sedatives, dexmedetomidine induces a state that mimics non-rapid eye movement sleep, without significant respiratory depression. These properties make dexmedetomidine an attractive agent for noninvasive procedural sedation in children with OSA [105]. Increasing doses of dexmedetomidine in children without OSA have minimal effect on the upper airway and are not associated with clinical signs of airway obstruction. However, the effect of high doses of dexmedetomidine in children with OSA is unknown [106]. Ketamine is a good alternative: it has been shown to preserve hypopharyngeal caliber in adults [107].

Examination of patterns of dynamic airway collapse in patients with OSA during sleep permits identification of anatomic causes of airway obstruction and facilitates planning for treatments required to relieve airway obstruction. MRI sleep studies demonstrate airway motion abnormalities that are related to OSA [108]. The most common challenge faced during sleep MR airway imaging studies is the inability of the child breathing via the native airway to tolerate an adequate level of sedation or anesthesia without experiencing significant oxygen desaturation. There is no strict consensus among sedation providers as to when to interrupt airway imaging for interventions to improve oxygenation. Absolute lower limits of oxygen saturation below which artificial airway adjuncts are required may differ from patient to patient depending on the benefits to be gained from the imaging study and the severity of the patient's condition. It is helpful to review overnight PSG reports, noting in particular the severity of oxygen desaturations during natural sleep, as a guide to acceptable minimal arterial oxygen saturations for a particular patient. Dexmedetomidine provides an acceptable level of sedation-anesthesia for MRI sleep studies in children with OSA and makes it possible to complete the study successfully in the majority of children without resorting to the use of artificial airways [109].

A recent study using an electronic survey of national and international members of the Society of Pediatric Anesthesia and a closed claims database (from 1990 to 2011) focused on OSA and reported all deaths and neurologic injury in relation to apnea. Closed claims involving death or neurologic injury after tonsillectomy due to apparent apnea in children suggest that at least 16 children out of 86 may have been rescued had respiratory monitoring been continued throughout first- and second-stage recovery, as well as on the ward during the first postoperative night. The authors recommended a validated pediatric-specific risk assessment scoring system to identify children at risk for OSA [110]. Another recent review of the LexisNexis "MEGATM Jury Verdicts and Settlements" database reported that sleep apnea was inculpated in 17 fatal malpractice claims related to post-tonsillectomy management [111].

An essential duty of the sedationist is to determine which patients are at risk for post-procedure respiratory adverse events and which can be managed as an outpatient. Currently we are not aware of any consensus among institutions that care for these patients as to clear post-procedure discharge criteria. The most recent literature is insufficient to offer definitive guidance regarding which patients with OSA can be safely managed as an outpatient, who should be admitted, and the appropriate time for discharge of these patients from the facility [112].

The ASA's Practice Guidelines for the Perioperative Management of Patients with Obstructive Sleep Apnea recommend **the following factors to be considered in determining whether outpatient care is appropriate** or not. These factors include: (1) sleep apnea status, (2) anatomical and physiologic abnormalities, (3) status of coexisting diseases, (4) nature of the surgery, (5) type of anesthesia, (6) need for postoperative opioids, (7) patient age, (8) adequacy of post-discharge observation, and (9) capabilities of the outpatient facility [112].

The authors approach these patients in the following way: at the end of the pre-procedure evaluation, we perform a risk assessment based on the presence and severity of symptoms, invasiveness of the procedure, associated comorbidities, physical examination, and, if available, the results of PSG. We have a very low threshold to admit children with OSA after procedural sedation who have any of the following comorbidities: craniofacial anomalies, obesity, history of prematurity, neuromuscular diseases, cardiac manifestations of OSA (e.g., right ventricular hypertrophy), Down syndrome, chronic lung disease, and sickle cell anemia. The decision to admit the child with whose OSA severity is yet undetermined is more challenging. If the patient develops significant episodes of obstruction during the procedure, we admit overnight with continuous monitoring for observation. OSA patients who are on home apnea monitoring or receive CPAP or BiPAP should be closely monitored in the hospital setting after the procedure to minimize respiratory complications. Patients with severe OSA undergoing lengthy procedures associated with the use of high doses of opioids require admission to the ICU.

Pregnancy

Although teenage pregnancy rates are currently in a steady decline, the pregnant teenager presenting with the need for an urgent or emergent procedure is not uncommon [108, 109, 113]. Girls of child-bearing age should have a screening pregnancy test done before procedural sedation. **Any elective procedure involving sedation-anesthesia in pregnancy is best postponed until after delivery**. In the urgent or emergent setting, the clinician must stratify risk and minimize harm to the mother and fetus.

The pregnant woman or girl experiences anatomic and physiologic changes throughout the pregnancy, many of which are important considerations in the pre-sedation assessment (Table 4.8) [114]. In general, there is increased oxygen consumption, decreased vascular resistance, increased edema of the upper airway, decreased vital lung capacity, decreased gastroesophageal motility, and decreased lower esophageal tone. Individually and in combination, these normal findings in pregnancy increase the risk of an adverse event during sedation. Screen for symptoms of heart failure, uncontrolled gastroesophageal reflux, frequent or painful uterine contractions, and vaginal bleeding.

It is important to verify the relative safety of the planned agents (and alternatives) prior to starting the procedure. In the United States, the Food and Drug Administration (FDA) has classified the relative risks of medications to the fetus into five categories (Table 4.9) [115, 116].

The clinician should always consult the most recent references for a given drug. It is important to note that sources may vary in classification of risk in pregnancy; **the timing, context, and chronicity of administration will affect the category** [117, 118]. Know and follow your institutional protocols and guidelines.

Premature Infant

Neonates are at high risk for the development of postoperative apnea after sedation-anesthesia. Infants at highest risk are those born prematurely (before the 37th week of gestation), or those with multiple congenital anomalies, a history of apnea and bradycardia, or chronic lung disease. Apneas occur postoperatively at rates of 5–49 % with spinal and general anesthesia [119]. The large variation is mainly due to the use of variable anesthetic and monitoring techniques as well as to the different study populations. The most significant risk factor of apnea in premature infants is conceptional age; the lower the conceptional age, the greater the risk of delayed apnea, with the incidence of postoperative apnea in the micropremie greater than 50 %. The frequency and duration of apnea decrease between 1 and 20 weeks postnatal age [120].

The etiology of apnea is likely multifactorial. Premature infants have decreased ventilatory control and response to hypoxia and hypercarbia—chemoreceptor responses are blunted in these babies. The normal response to hypoxemia (hyperventilation, followed by hypoventilation or apnea) is replaced by apnea only. This lack of physiologic response

Table 4.8 Anatomic and physiologic changes in pregnancy [114]

System	Anatomy	Physiology
Cardiovascular	Uterine obstruction of inferior vena cava → supine hypotensive syndrome	↑ Plasma volume ↑ Cardiac output ↓ SVR
Respiratory	Elevation of diaphragm Airway edema ↓ Upper airway caliber	↑ Minute volume ↑ Oxygen consumption ↓ $PaCO_2$
CNS		↓ Effective distribution of sedatives and hypnotics
Gastrointestinal	↓ Lower esophageal sphincter tone	↑ Gastric volume and acidity Delayed gastric motility
Hematologic		↑ Activity of coagulation factors

Table 4.9 United States FDA pharmaceutical pregnancy categories [115, 116]

Pregnancy Category A	Controlled studies in women fail to demonstrate a risk to the fetus in the first trimester (and there is no evidence of a risk in later trimesters), and the possibility of fetal harm appears remote
Pregnancy Category B	Either animal reproduction studies have not demonstrated fetal risk (but no controlled studies in pregnant women have been reported), or animal reproduction studies have shown an adverse effect (other than a decrease in fertility) that was not confirmed in controlled studies in women in the first trimester (and there is no evidence of risk in later trimesters)
Pregnancy Category C	Either studies in animals have revealed adverse effects on the fetus (teratogenic, embryocidal, or other) but no controlled studies in women have been reported, or studies in women and animals are not available. Drugs should be given only if the potential benefit justifies the potential risk to the fetus
Pregnancy Category D	Positive evidence of human fetal risk exists, but the benefits from use in pregnant women may be acceptable despite the risk (e.g., if the drug is needed for a life-threatening condition or for a serious disease for which safer drugs cannot be used or are ineffective).
Pregnancy Category X	Studies in animals or human beings have demonstrated fetal abnormalities or evidence exists of fetal risk based on human experience, or both, and the risk in pregnant women clearly outweighs any possible benefit. The drug is contraindicated in women who are or may become pregnant

may be worsened by sedative agents. Postoperative apnea can occur after surgery with inhalational-based anesthetics or even after surgery for which a regional anesthetic was used and no anesthetic drugs were utilized [121]. Apneas are frequent in the first 12 h and can continue until 48–72 h.

Kurth et al. studied the breathing patterns of 47 preterm infants less than 60 weeks postconception with pneumocardiograms before and after general inhalational anesthesia. The study found that 18 infants (37 %) had prolonged apnea (>15 s) and an additional 7 infants (14 %) had short apnea (6–15 s) postoperatively [122]. **The authors conclude that preterm infants younger than 60 postconceptional weeks of age should be monitored continuously for at least 12 h postoperatively in order to prevent apnea-related complications.**

The best evidence basis is found in a 1995 meta-analysis of eight prospective studies examining 254 premature infants undergoing general anesthesia for inguinal hernia repair; apnea was strongly inversely related to both gestational age and conceptional age [123]. Anemia (<10 g/dL) and apnea at home were also risk factors. Based on this data, many institutions adopted the study's **recommendation that all infants born <37 weeks gestational age and less than 60 weeks conceptional age be monitored for postoperative apnea for a minimum of an overnight stay in an ICU setting**.

The appropriate discharge time frame of these patients remains controversial. The cutoff for outpatient surgery in infants born before 37 weeks may be 50–52 weeks conceptional age, provided there is no anemia, prior apnea, or coexisting disease. **The most conservative approach is to admit all premature infants (for monitored 24-h observation) younger than 60 weeks conceptional age, regardless of the anesthetic used** [122]. Certainly this should be the case for any high-risk infant, such as those using a home apnea monitor or taking methylxanthine drugs.

There is considerable institutional variability in practice and hospitals have different age-based guidelines for admission. Some institutions feel comfortable performing elective outpatient procedures if the infant is born full term. Other centers prefer to wait until the infant is 2–4 weeks of age to ensure the resolution of physiologic jaundice, decreased pulmonary vascular resistance, and to give sufficient time for the ductus arteriosus to close. Still in other settings, such as the emergency department, full-term infants less than 3 months of age undergoing significant sedation for an emergent procedure are rarely discharged home on the same day. Options are limited in this high-risk population, as otherwise "safe" agents such as ketamine are contraindicated in these very young infants (<3 months of age in a full-term infant).

Regardless of the timing or setting, premature infants should have both pulse oximetry and apnea monitoring, since standard impedance pneumatography can fail to detect episodes that result in serious desaturation [123]. Although there is limited evidence that prophylactic caffeine or theophylline reduces the rate of post-procedure apnea, if the infant experiences any irregular breathing after the procedure, caffeine should be given without delay.

In-depth understanding of the preterm neonatal physiology is vital to the sedation provider. For example, in patients who have a patent ductus arteriosus, one pulse oximetry probe should be placed on the right hand (pre-ductal) and the other on a lower limb (post-ductal). In the premature infant, fetal hemoglobin persists. For example, a premature infant at first glance may have a reassuring hemoglobin concentration of 13–15 g/dL; however, 70–80 % may be fetal Hb, which is known to have a reduced ability to release oxygen to the tissues.

Another important concern in these babies is the immaturity of the renal and hepatic systems. **Preterm infants do not maintain fluids and electrolyte balance well, requiring**

care in the administration of the IV fluids and electrolytes. Liver immaturity (both in synthetic and metabolic capacity) may lead to longer duration of action of sedative agents.

Sedation providers should make every effort to **avoid hypothermia during the procedure**. Preterm infants have a high surface-area-to-body-weight ratio and decreased brown fat stores, rendering them very susceptible to heat loss. Heat loss is a major potential stress in premature babies and hypothermia-induced stress can lead to hypoglycemia, apnea, and metabolic acidosis.

In summary, sedating-anesthetizing a preterm neonate requires in-depth understanding of neonatal physiology, constant vigilance, rapid recognition of any adverse event, and rapid intervention.

Psychiatric and Behavioral Disorders

It is estimated that one in ten children meets criteria for a serious emotional disturbance, defined as "a mental health problem that has drastic impact on the child's ability to function socially, academically, and emotionally" [124, 125]. Due to changing diagnostic criteria ("diagnosis shifting") and worldwide variation, exact estimates of the prevalence of individual disorders are problematic; nonetheless, increased awareness and diagnosis are commonly seen in practice [126].

Mood disorders in children include anxiety disorders (8 %), major depression (4 %), and bipolar disorder (1 %) [125]. The pre-procedural assessment in these children should include a brief review of the child's general health, control of mood disorder, recent additions or changes to medications, and history of previous procedures and adverse drug reactions (especially to psychotropic medications). These children are at risk for eating disorders and substance abuse, and may present with hypothermia, hypokalemia, hypomagnesemia, and/or hypokalemia [127]. If an eating disorder such as anorexia or bulimia is suspected, a screening ECG or chemistry profile should be performed prior to sedation [128, 129].

Behavior disorders are multifactorial in nature, and rates vary greatly by criteria used, population studied, and survey conducted. Attention deficit hyperactivity disorder (ADHD) involves inattention, impulsivity, and hyperactivity. The National Health and Nutrition Examination Survey reveals an overall prevalence of ADHD in children 8–15 to be 8.7 % [130]. Conduct disorder (CD) and oppositional defiant disorder (ODD) are characterized by a pattern of disobedient, hostile, and defiant behavior toward authority figures [131]. As a group, rates of CD and ODD are reported to be as high as 5.5 % in recent US studies, but the rate varies greatly by country and subpopulation [125, 132]. Children with behavior disorders are often prescribed stimulant or other psychotropic medications; they may have an altered reaction to premedication (such as decreased response to benzodiazepines), increased risk of post-procedure nausea and vomiting, and a decreased seizure threshold [133]. Although the literature is inconclusive regarding the need for a special approach to the sedation of these children, the clinician may use this information especially when considering pre-procedural fasting requirements.

Substance abuse disorders in older children and adolescents are estimated to have a prevalence of approximately 5 %, with a wide range of 1–24 % [125]. **There is a significant overlap in behavior and mood disorders in this population.** Although the long-term effects of substance abuse (cardiac, pulmonary, hepatic, renal, immune) may not be evident in children, a good general history and physical examination should reveal red flags in the pre-sedation assessment. *Marijuana* use may cause relaxation and a decreased sedation requirement; however, patients may also present with tachycardia and anxiety from recent use. A mild abstinence syndrome has been reported; conversely, overuse can result in intractable nausea, as in *cannabinoid hyperemesis syndrome*. *Cocaine* is highly addictive and may cause dysrhythmias, ischemia, and heart failure. These patients often have altered pain perception. Concomitant cocaine use and β(beta)-blocker administration may precipitate hypertensive crisis, due to unopposed α(alpha)-adrenergic stimulation. *Opioid abuse* may present with altered pain tolerance, increased requirements during sedation, and acute withdrawal, depending on the timing of last ingestion. *Alcohol abuse* may present with increased sedative requirements [134].

Designer drugs (also called "club" or "party" drugs) include 3,4-methylene-dioxymethamphetamine (MDMA) or "ecstasy," phencyclidine (PCP), ketamine, inhalants, rohypnol, γ(gamma)-hydroxybutyrate, and bath salts, among others. The clinician will undoubtedly recognize an acutely intoxicated child or adolescent on presentation. However, the non-intoxicated patient with regular use of these substances may not be apparent without a focused history; many have considerable anxiety in the pre-procedure assessment. During sedation, these patients are at risk for **autonomic dysregulation with wide swings in blood pressure and heart rate**, with case reports of non-hemorrhagic cerebral vascular accidents and myocardial ischemia and infarction [135].

During the pre-sedation assessment, the clinician should screen for risk factors for pre- and post-procedural combativeness, such as previous negative experiences with procedures, sedation, or anesthesia; preoperative anxiety; parental anxiety; and other baseline emotional problems [136–138]. In children at risk for combativeness or lack of cooperation, early involvement of supportive family members, play therapists, and/or nursing staff with distraction techniques may be helpful, as well as the use of noninvasive oral premedication [139].

Sickle Cell Disease

The term sickle cell disease (SCD) includes all hemoglobinopathies that result in sickling of red blood cells (HbSS, HbSC, sickle-cell thalassemias, and other variants). SCD is characterized by hemolytic anemia and vaso-occlusive phenomena, causing painful episodes and a variety of crises affecting virtually every organ system. Although the sickle cell trait originated in West Africa, it is now estimated that more than 250,000 children worldwide are born each year with SCD [140].

Sickling occurs due to deoxygenation stress on HbS polymers, resulting in a process called *gelation*—red blood cells subsequently become less able to deform normally as they pass through capillary beds, which may result in vaso-occlusion and infarction [141]. Even fully oxygenated blood in a child in SCD is more viscous than in non-affected individuals. Volume depletion or dehydration accentuates their baseline hyperviscosity and promotes vascular stasis. For this reason, the pre-sedation assessment should carefully consider the child's volume status. Recent intake, number of wet diapers or frequency of urination, and recent illness should be assessed.

Take a careful history of past sickle-cell crises (e.g., acute chest syndrome, splenic sequestration, hemolytic crises, stroke, priapism, cardiomyopathy, renal disease, avascular necrosis of bones) and the severity of the course of illness. It is important to note whether the child is currently controlled with medications or requires intensive treatment such as red blood cell exchange transfusions [142]. Common medications in SCD include penicillin prophylaxis, hydroxyurea, and folic acid. Transfusion therapy lowers the percentage of HbS in the blood and is used to treat vaso-occlusive crises acutely or to prevent stroke or pain crisis [143]. It is helpful to know the child's recent hematocrit; if there is history of recent illness or complaint consistent with a hemolytic crisis, obtain a CBC and reticulocyte count and address the patient's current complaint and volume status before sedation.

Ask about recent illness, including any fever or atypical pain. If possible, ascertain what medications have helped to relieve pain in the past. Children with SCD typically have high opioid requirements, thought to be due to a variety of reasons, including severe pain, tolerance, and altered plasma clearance of opioids [144]. Certain medications should be avoided in the sedation or analgesia of SCD children, such as meperidine. Multiple doses of meperidine may cause an accumulation of its metabolite, associated with central toxicity such as myoclonus and seizures [145]. Expert opinion varies on the use of nitrous oxide in children with SCD, but it is generally considered safe [146–148].

When possible and appropriate, **consider liberal use of intranasal, oral, and intramuscular medications if intravenous access is not otherwise required**. Children with SCD often have limited reliable vascular access due to frequent venipuncture; be judicious with their remaining usable peripheral veins if feasible.

Syndromes

There is a vast array of pediatric genetic syndromes, each with its particular considerations and challenges in general and acute care. Syndromes may be classified by morphology into four broad categories: **malformation** (poor formation of tissue), **deformation** (unusual forces on normal tissue), **disruption** (breakdown of normal tissue), or **dysplasia** (abnormal organization of tissues). Keep in mind the variance of expression in most syndromes—some children may be mildly affected while others may be severely affected [149].

The pre-sedation assessment should focus on children with abnormal airway anatomy, as airway reflexes may be affected during sedation, and a contingency plan for airway rescue must be ready before the procedure. Ask about previous procedures, previous or current tracheostomies, problems with oral intake or reflux, snoring, or easy choking or fatigue. Some syndromes are associated with specific metabolic issues, such as frequent hypoglycemia (e.g., Beckwith-Wiedemann, pituitary dwarfism). Perform a careful review of the child's medications and ask how the child responds to and recovers from illness and stress (i.e., history of decompensation or requiring medication supplementation). Perform a careful assessment of the size and shape of the mouth and tongue, the ability to open the mouth wide, and identify the Mallampati classification of pharyngeal structures (Fig. 4.2, Table 4.10) [149–153]. **It is important to palpate the distance from the anterior ramus of the mandible to the hyoid bone**. In infants, it should measure at least one finger breadth (of the adult examiner); in children at least two finger breadths; and in adolescents at least three finger breadths. **A decreased distance correlates with a more difficult rescue airway** [150].

Down syndrome is the most common chromosomal abnormality, with an overall incidence of as high as 1 in 700 live births, varying by region and maternal age. The sedation practitioner must be familiar with its associated multisystem abnormalities including OSA, CHD (endocardial cushion defect, VSD), atlantoaxial instability, obesity, and subglottic stenosis.

Predisposing factors for OSA in these children include midfacial and mandibular hypoplasia, glossoptosis, adenoidal encroachment, increased secretions, and an increased

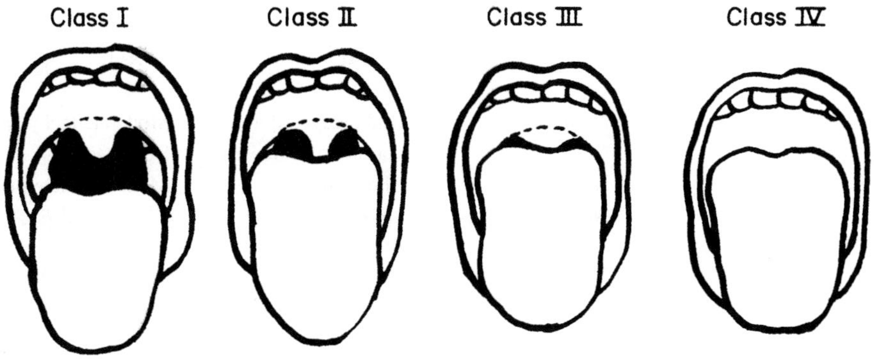

Fig. 4.2 Mallampati classification of pharyngeal structures. Reprinted with permission from Samsoon GL, Young JRB. Difficult tracheal intubation: a retrospective study. Anaesthesia. 1987;42:487–90

Table 4.10 Anatomic considerations in common syndromes [149–153]

Anatomic consideration		Associated syndromes
Alanto-occipital joint abnormalities	• Short neck	***Down syndrome*** (Trisomy 21)
	• Limited mobility	***Goldenhar syndrome*** (incomplete development of the ear, nose, palate, and mandible)
	• Instability	***Juvenile Rheumatoid Arthritis*** (JRA)
		Klippel-Feil syndrome (short neck, restricted upper spine mobility)
Abnormal airway anatomy	• Mandibular hypoplasia	***Airway mass/tumor***
	• High arched/narrow palate	***Arteriovenous malformation*** (AVM)
	• Macroglossia	***Arthrogryposis*** (congenital multiple contractures)
		Beckwith-Wiedemann syndrome (exomphalos, macroglossia, gigantism)
		Cornelia de Lange syndrome (microcephaly, dwarfism, cleft palate)
		Cri du chat (microcephaly, clinodactyly)
		Crouzon syndrome (cranial synostosis, hypotelorism, hypoplastic maxilla)
		DiGeorge syndrome (velo-pharyngeal insufficiency, hypothyroidism)
		Dwarfism (various)
		Goldenhar syndrome (incomplete development of the ear, nose, palate, and mandible)
		Mucopolysaccharidosis (various)
		Pierre Robin sequence (micrognathia, upper airway obstruction)
		Treacher Collins syndrome (micrognathia, hearing loss)
		Trisomies (especially 18, 21, 22)
Midface abnormalities	• Maxillary hypoplasia	***Apert syndrome*** (hypertelorism, craniosynostosis, hydrocephalus)
	• Nasal or choanal stenosis	***Down syndrome*** (Trisomy 21)

incidence of lower respiratory tract anomalies, obesity, and generalized hypotonia. **These children are sensitive to respiratory depression by opioids, sedatives, and hypnotics**; they are especially vulnerable to the development of upper airway obstruction during sedation-anesthesia. A smaller than normal endotracheal tube should be placed if indicated and the head should remain in neutral position during intubation.

The most common sedation-anesthesia-related complication in these patients is **bradycardia**, especially during induction. This may occur even in the absence of heart disease. Borland et al. reported the incidence of severe bradycardia associated with inhaled anesthetic induction (halothane or isoflurane) in children with Down syndrome to be 3.7 % [154]. Recently Kraemer et al. examined the incidence of bradycardia in 209 children with Down syndrome and 268 healthy control patients who had inhaled induction of anesthesia with sevoflurane over an 8-year period. On univariate analysis Down syndrome, low ASA physical status, CHD, and mean sevoflurane concentrations were factors associated with bradycardia. However, multivariate analysis showed that only Down syndrome and low ASA physical status remained as independent factors associated with bradycardia [155].

Table 4.11 ATLS hemorrhagic shock classification [156]

	Class I	Class II	Class III	Class IV
Percent blood loss (%)	Up to 15 %	15–30	30–40	>40
Heart rate	Normal	Mild tachycardia	Moderate tachycardia	Severe tachycardia
Blood pressure	Normal	Normal to decreased	Decreased	Decreased
Respiratory Rate	Normal	Mild tachypnea	Moderate tachypnea	Severe tachypnea
Urine Output	Normal	0.5–1 mL/kg/h (minimum goal)	0.25–0.5 mL/kg/h (markedly decreased)	Negligible
Mental status	Slightly anxious	Mildly anxious	Anxious/confused	Confused/lethargic
Fluid replacement	Crystalloid	Crystalloid	Crystalloid and blood	Crystalloid and blood

Cardiac output is dependent on heart rate, especially in neonates and infants, and bradycardia can have a significant effect on the patient's hemodynamic stability. Some practitioners routinely use intramuscular prophylactic atropine to prevent bradycardia before anesthesia induction. It is important to recognize that atropine will not prevent or reverse the negative inotropic effect of an inhalational anesthetic, but it may maintain heart rate. Gradual titration of the volatile agent concentration and close monitoring of blood pressure and heart rate are recommended during inhalational induction of patients with Down syndrome. If bradycardia occurs and an IV is not in place, intramuscular atropine should be administered if there is sustained bradycardia or if hemodynamic instability develops.

Trauma

The acutely injured child poses a particular challenge to the clinician performing sedation. The child may present immediately after trauma or subacutely. Only after primary and secondary advanced trauma life support (ATLS) surveys are completed and injuries addressed and stabilized is the child a candidate for sedation outside of the operating room.

In addition to the injury-specific brief history and physical examination, the pre-sedation assessment will include last intake by mouth, allergies, medications, and prior sedation or anesthesia. The urgency of procedural sedation will match the urgency of the presenting condition, such as neurovascular compromise; this will affect the clinician's decision in the amount of fasting time allowed (Table 4.1).

Keep in mind that a child with one injury is at risk for other obvious or occult injuries, due to the pliable thorax and underdeveloped musculature of the pediatric abdomen. ATLS describes four classes of hemorrhagic shock, initially developed for adults (Table 4.11) [156]. Children will compensate well with tachycardia (compensated shock) until a precipitous fall in blood pressure is noted (decompensated shock), and ominous sign [157].

Medication given during sedation may affect vital signs that would otherwise serve as an early warning sign of ongoing occult hemorrhage. For example, ketamine administered for orthopedic reduction invariably causes an increase in heart rate, which makes the recognition of compensated shock difficult. Similarly, propofol, opioids, and benzodiazepines may cause a small drop in blood pressure that may mask an underlying decompensated shock. Meticulous history and physical examination to screen for occult injuries is imperative before the urgent or elective sedation. During sedation, consideration of developing shock should always be at the forefront of the clinician's mind. Consider strategies such as peripheral nerve blocks and mild anxiolysis in these patients.

Tuberous Sclerosis

Tuberous sclerosis (TS) is one of the commonest autosomal dominant genetic disorders, displaying high genetic penetrance in affected families. TS is a neurocutaneous disorder characterized by a classic triad of epilepsy, fibroangiomas, and mental retardation. TS causes hamartomas in multiple organs, including the brain, skin, heart, kidneys, lungs, and liver. Awareness of the signs, symptoms, and organs affected is critical to reduce the risk of a life-threatening complication.

A **baseline cardiac evaluation** (regardless of presence or absence of symptoms) is an essential part of the pre-procedure work-up to determine whether the procedure is appropriate for non-anesthesiologist sedation or whether the expertise of an anesthesiologist is needed. Cardiovascular manifestations, seen in more than 50 % of affected individuals, can have major anesthetic-sedative implications. Rhabdomyomas are the most common benign cardiac tumors associated with tuberous sclerosis [158]. They tend to regress spontaneously and are not usually excised unless they become obstructive or cause severe arrhythmias. A pre-procedure ECG is recommended to exclude dysrhythmia or conduction defects. Abdominal aortic aneurysms have been reported as well as narrowing of major arteries in patients with TS.

Airway management can be challenging in these patients due to the presence of oropharyngeal or laryngeal tumors, fibromata, or papillomata. Pulmonary involvement is rare (<1 %). However, hamartomatous growths may involve the lungs or pleura and there have been a number of reports of spontaneous pneumothorax in patients with undiagnosed pulmonary manifestations of the disease. A **pre-procedure chest radiograph (X-ray)** is recommended to exclude silent pulmonary or mediastinal masses.

Renal function should also be assessed before the procedure because renal angiomyolipomas are present in 50–80 % of affected individuals [159]. Although possibly initially clinically silent, these patients are known to progress to renal failure. Anticonvulsants should be optimized and continued until the morning of surgery and should be resumed as soon as possible in order to prevent seizures [160].

Upper Respiratory Tract Infection

There is no consensus regarding the optimal management of children with URI who require sedation for an elective procedure. The economic and emotional consequences of cancelling a procedure are significant for the family and the institution. Studies showed that anywhere from 3 to 33 % of children coming for anesthesia and surgery present with an active URI [161]. Children with URIs who present for procedural sedation pose a perplexing clinical dilemma for sedation providers. Currently there is little agreement between individual providers and institutions on which children with respiratory tract infections (RTIs) should be sedated-anesthetized and under what circumstances. **Inflammation from a URI may persist for up to 6 weeks after apparent resolution of symptoms**.

An active URI may put the child at risk for laryngospasm, bronchospasm, severe coughing, major oxygen desaturations (<90 %) airway obstruction, pneumonia, and unanticipated admission. These complications are disturbing, but fortunately can be addressed with medications that should be readily available during any procedure, such as inhaled β(beta)-agonists for bronchospasm, succinylcholine followed by advanced airway management for sustained laryngospasm not amenable to positive-pressure ventilation, and supplemental oxygen for desaturation [162].

Sedation practitioners need to differentiate allergic rhinitis from URI and uncomplicated URIs from other illnesses. Typical symptoms of uncomplicated URI include low-grade fever, rhinorrhea, congestion, sneezing, sore throat, and laryngitis. If the child has a disproportionally high fever or shows signs of lower respiratory tract symptoms such as increased work of breathing, wheezing, or mucopurulent secretions, the pathology may have extended beyond the upper respiratory tract.

Many children with recurrent URIs have a very small window of opportunity to provide sedation in the symptom-free period. It is inevitable that the sedation provider will need to look to decision tools to help to disentangle this dilemma. Parnis et al. used logistic regression to determine which variables were predictors of perioperative anesthetic adverse events in 2,051 children. The analysis showed that 22.3 % of children had symptoms of an RTI on the day of surgery, and 45.8 % had a "cold" in the preceding 6 weeks [163]. Important independent preoperative predictors of anesthetic adverse events were: parental report of the child's having a "cold" on the day of surgery, nasal congestion, history of snoring, history of second-hand smoking, and cough productive of sputum. The study concluded that surgery requiring endotracheal intubation increases the probability of anesthetic complications, but when the airway is managed with a laryngeal mask or face mask the probability of complications is decreased. An interesting finding worth noting was that the identification of a viral pathogen did not help to identify individuals at risk for adverse events.

The never-ending question of what to do with a child with a URI will always be with us. In the absence of evidence-based clear criteria, the sedation practitioner should be especially aware of active signs and symptoms. A clinical algorithm has been proposed (Fig. 4.3) to guide the assessment and management of these children [164]. Most practitioners would agree that children with mild uncomplicated URIs undergoing procedures that do not involve airway manipulation can be safely anesthetized-sedated without any increase in risk [165].

Conclusion

The prepared provider should be as informed about the patient as he is about the procedure to be performed. Eliciting red flags in history and physical examination is the basis for safe sedation practice. When faced with a less-than-ideally prepared patient or situation, the provider should work to optimize the patient's status and anticipate complications before the procedure takes place.

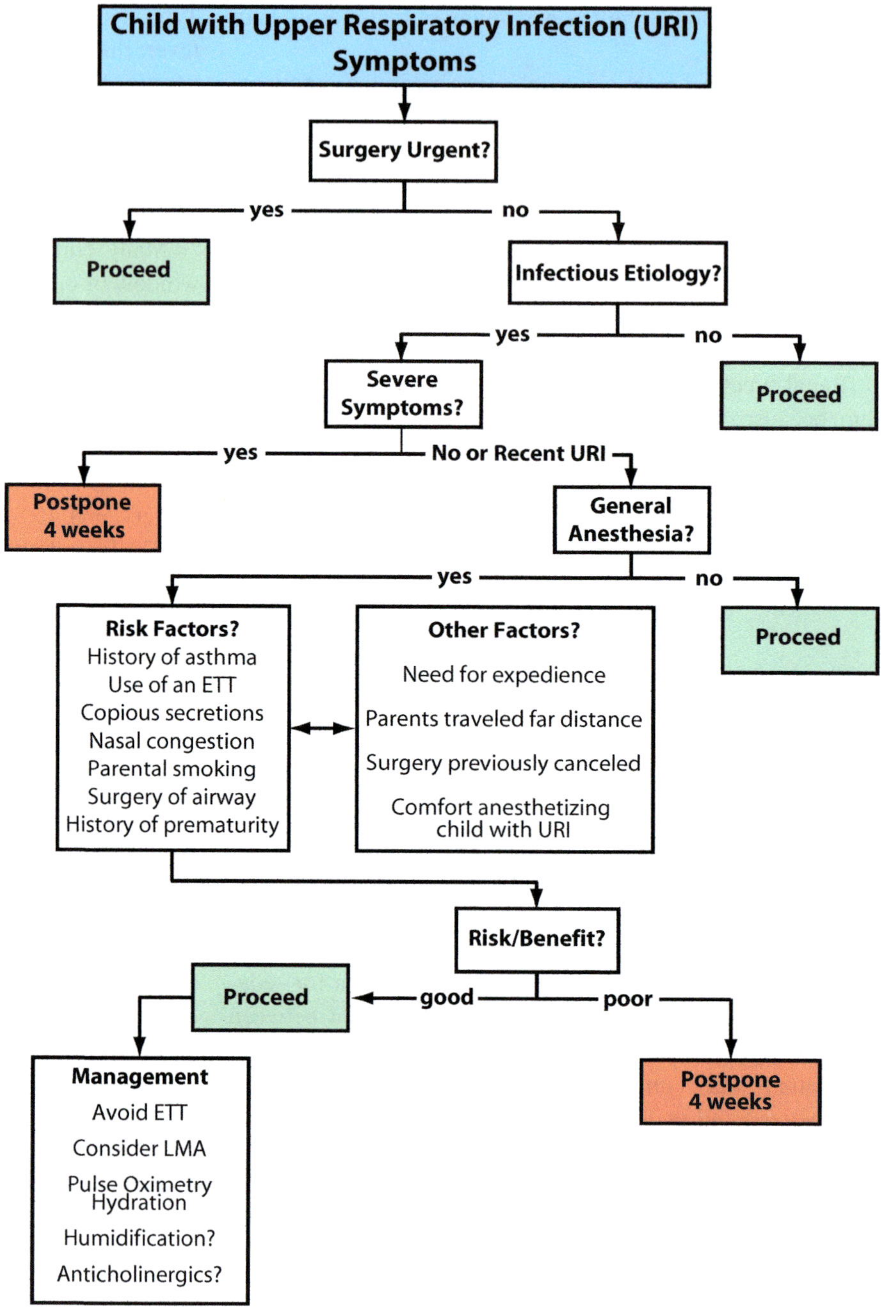

Fig. 4.3 Suggested algorithm and management of a child with upper respiratory infection. Modified with permission from Tait ATR, Malviya S. Anesthesia for the child with an upper respiratory tract infection: still a dilemma? Anesth Analg 2005;100:59–65

Case Studies in Pre-sedation Assessment

Case 1: Just Another URI?

A 4-year-old girl with a history of seizures is scheduled for magnetoencephalography (MEG) scan. She has a 4-day history of isolated clear rhinorrhea. Her lungs are clear to auscultation and she is afebrile. Her mother reported that her activity level and appetite have been unchanged since onset of rhinorrhea.

The main considerations for this child will be the pre-procedure URI and understanding the needs and requirements for MEG scan. This child appears to have an uncomplicated URI. Based on the information provided in this clinical scenario, proceeding with the scan is the most appropriate decision. Understanding the nature and demands of MEG is important to decide on the appropriate sedative agent. MEG scan records

(continued)

magnetic fields induced by the brain's electrical activity and recently is increasingly used in presurgical evaluation of epileptic children. Compared with the standard electroencephalogram (EEG), the MEG allows for a better spatial resolution in the localization of epileptogenic foci. MEG exams are conducted in magnetically shielded chambers to minimize interference of magnetic fields induced by other electric and electronic appliances. Our experience with dexmedetomidine-based technique (2 μg/kg loading dose followed by 2 μg/kg/h infusion) provides adequate depth of sedation required to prevent motion artifacts. Compared with propofol at higher doses dexmedetomidine does not appear to negatively affect inter-ictal activity and thereby does not interfere with spike identification.

Case 2: Snoring Away

A 2-year-old 16 kg boy born at 33 weeks gestation is scheduled for high resolution CT. The CT is being done as part of the work-up for recurrent aspiration pneumonias. On pre-imaging evaluation, the child's exam reveals micrognathia and a cleft palate. His mother reports that he "snores a lot" and seems to obstruct his upper airway at night. A look through the medical records shows that the patient recently underwent an overnight sleep study (PSG) that demonstrated a moderate degree of OSA with a minimum oxygen saturation of 86 %.

The considerations in this case are: difficult airway, OSA, and an imaging study requires controlled ventilation in off-site environment. A thoughtful, carefully implemented plan is essential to ensure safety and high-quality imaging study for this patient. In an ideal world this family should have been contacted prior to scheduling to ensure a proper consultation with an anesthesiologist who can guide the safest plan for sedating this infant.

It is important to evaluate the airway carefully prior to beginning anesthesia or sedation. Evaluation of the pediatric airway can be challenging as the patient may be uncooperative and the history given by parents may be misleading. The overnight PSG provides clues to the severity of the airway obstruction during sleep by providing the lowest oxygen saturation observed, as well as the types of apnea (obstructive, central, or mixed) and the frequency of apnea events. The combination of micrognathia and significant OSA in an off-site location would contraindicate non-anesthesiologist delivered sedation. This patient should be managed by an anesthesiologist who is trained in and prepared for the difficult airway. The anesthetic management is detailed below.

Before inducing this infant, the authors would manage this case as follows:

1. Discuss the benefits and risks of the study with the family and ordering physician and make arrangements for post-procedure admission if required.
2. Review previous anesthetic/sedative records and documentations for previous airway management.
3. Confirm that advanced airway management instruments are available including different sizes of face masks, endotracheal tubes, laryngoscope blades and handles, appropriate size LMA fiberoptic equipment, video laryngoscope, and the difficult airway cart.
4. Proceed with an inhalational induction with sevoflurane with maintenance of spontaneous ventilation followed by placement of LMA when it is established that the patient can be ventilated.

Help in the case of an emergency may be less readily available than in the operating room environment. A more conservative approach in this clinical scenario is to start the anesthetic in the more controlled environment of the operating room, secure the airway with an endotracheal tube, and then transport the patient to radiology. The operating room provides a safe, secure, and familiar environment in which the anesthesiologist has access to emergency airway equipment and assistance from colleagues who can assist with airway management.

Case 3: It's All in Your Head

A 5-year-old boy with developmental delay and autism is hit by a baseball on the left temporal aspect of his head. His GCS is 14, and he has a large scalp hematoma. The decision is made to perform a CT of his head. He is intermittently sleepy and agitated, but consolable by his mother.

The main questions for this potentially uncooperative patient are: (1) Is the procedure painful? (2) How long will the procedure take? (3) Will non-pharmacologic methods be appropriate?

This is an emergent study, but the provider has time to review any medical comorbidities, as well as any history of previous sedation and the outcome. In the proper context, with a calm and reassuring caregiver, a tablet computer or smart phone may be employed to distract the child for the very brief study.

(continued)

This would avoid any complication of sedation, allow the provider to watch his mental status more closely, and potentially ensure a more expedient discharge if the work-up is negative.

If this child is to be sedated, the less invasive the technique the better: Intranasal medications, such as combined midazolam and fentanyl, may give just enough sedation to accomplish this non-painful, non-distressing procedure. If this fails, the intravenous route offers a wide array of options. Rarely in children does the provider have to intubate and sedate in order to obtain advanced emergent imaging.

Case 4: Broken Heart, Broken Bone

A 7-year-old boy with hypoplastic left heart syndrome who is doing well as an outpatient falls off a slide and sustains a right femur fracture. His vital signs are his normal baseline, and he has no other evidence of trauma. On radiograph, his right femur shows a mid-shaft fracture with shortening of the thigh; he is neurovascularly intact distally. He requires emergent placement of a Steinmann pin and traction in anticipation for the operating room when it becomes available.

The urgency of this boy's condition requires action. Take a brief, focused history of previous cardiac surgeries, complications, and other comorbidities. Obtain a cardiology consultation with a pediatric cardiologist, if available, to discuss the patient's physiology and management option and concerns. Collaborate with or transfer this patient's care to an anesthesiologist, if possible. This child has had palliative surgery for his cyanotic heart disease; he has undergone a Fontan procedure, and therefore his cardiac output is pre-load dependent. His volume status should be optimized prior to the procedure. Small boluses of 10 mL/kg of normal saline may be given carefully to ensure euvolemia (with careful attention not to cause volume overload). Prior to proceeding, emergency medications and vasopressors should be immediately available for administration.

This child may be best served with a femoral nerve or fascia iliaca block, to avoid the potential problems with volume and oxygenation status. If this is not possible, a medication that preserves systemic vascular resistance, such as ketamine, would be a good option. Although short acting, a medication such as propofol would not be ideal in this child; propofol is a myocardial depressant and causes transient hypotension. In the otherwise healthy child, this is not an issue. In this child with CHD and low reserve, it is best avoided.

References

1. Splinter WM, Schreiner MS. Preoperative fasting in children. Anesth Analg. 1999;89(1):80–9.
2. Roberts RB, Shirley MA. Reducing the risk of acid aspiration during cesarean section. Anesth Analg. 1974;53(6):859–68.
3. Nordgren B. The rate of secretion and electrolyte content of normal gastric juice. Acta Physiol Scand Suppl. 1963;58(202):1–83.
4. Krauss B, Green SM. Sedation and analgesia for procedures in children. N Engl J Med. 2000;342(13):938–45.
5. Warner MA, Warner ME, Warner DO, Warner LO, Warner EJ. Perioperative pulmonary aspiration in infants and children. Anesthesiology. 1999;90(1):66–71.
6. Warner MA, Warner ME, Weber JG. Clinical significance of pulmonary aspiration during the perioperative period. Anesthesiology. 1993;78(1):56–62.
7. Cravero JP, Beach ML, Blike GT, Gallagher SM, Hertzog JH. The incidence and nature of adverse events during pediatric sedation/anesthesia with propofol for procedures outside the operating room: a report from the Pediatric Sedation Research Consortium. Anesth Analg. 2009;108(3):795–804.
8. Sanborn PA, Michna E, Zurakowski D, Burrows PE, Fontaine PJ, Connor L, et al. Adverse cardiovascular and respiratory events during sedation of pediatric patients for imaging examinations. Radiology. 2005;237(1):288–94.
9. Jones MJ, Mitchell RW, Hindocha N. Effect of increased intra-abdominal pressure during laparoscopy on the lower esophageal sphincter. Anesth Analg. 1989;68(1):63–5.
10. Anonymous. Practice guidelines for preoperative fasting and the use of pharmacologic agents to reduce the risk of pulmonary aspiration: application to healthy patients undergoing elective procedures: a report by the American Society of Anesthesiologist Task Force on Preoperative Fasting. Anesthesiology. 1999;90(3):896–905.
11. Green SM, Roback MG, Miner JR, Burton JH, Krauss B. Fasting and emergency department procedural sedation and analgesia: a consensus-based clinical practice advisory. Ann Emerg Med. 2007;49(4):454–61.
12. Agrawal D, Manzi SF, Gupta R, Krauss B. Preprocedural fasting state and adverse events in children undergoing procedural sedation and analgesia in a pediatric emergency department. Ann Emerg Med. 2003;42(5):636–46.
13. Kaufman RA. Technical aspects of abdominal ct in infants and children. AJR Am J Roentgenol. 1989;153(3):549–54.
14. Kim SK. Small intestine transit time in the normal small bowel study. Am J Roentgenol Radium Ther Nucl Med. 1968;104(3):522–4.
15. Kharazmi SA, Kamat PP, Simoneaux SF, Simon HK. Violating traditional NPO guidelines with PO contrast before sedation for computed tomography. Pediatr Emerg Care. 2013;29(9):979–81.
16. Mahmoud M, McAuliffe J, Kim HY, Mishra P, Salisbury S, Schnell B, et al. Oral contrast for abdominal computed tomography in children: the effects on gastric fluid volume. Anesth Analg. 2010;111(5):1252–8.
17. Mahmoud M, McAuliffe J, Donnelly LF. Administration of enteric contrast material before abdominal ct in children: current practices and controversies. Pediatr Radiol. 2011;41(4):409–12.
18. Doherty GM, Chisakuta A, Crean P, Shields MD. Anesthesia and the child with asthma. Pediatr Anesth. 2005;2005(15):446–54.
19. National Heart Lung, and Blood Institute. Expert panel report 3: guidelines for the diagnosis and management of asthma. National Asthma Education and Prevention Program; 2007.
20. Von Ungern-Sternberg B, Habre W. Pediatric anesthesia—potential risks and their assessment: part I. Pediatr Anesth. 2007;17:206–15.

21. Rock P, Passannante A. Preoperative assessment: pulmonary. Anesthesiol Clin North Am. 2004;22:77–91.
22. von Ungern-Sternberg BS, Boda K, Chambers NA, Rebman C, Johnson C, Sly PD, et al. Risk assessment for respiratory complications in paediatric anaesthesia: a prospective cohort study. Lancet. 2010;376:773–83.
23. Tchaconas A, Adesman A. Autism spectrum disorders: a pediatric overview and update. Curr Opin Pediatr. 2013;25(1):130–44.
24. Courtman SP, Mumby D. Children with learning disabilities. Pediatr Anesth. 2008;18:198–207.
25. Harris P. The nature and extent of aggressive behavior amongst people with learning difficulties (mental handicap) in a single health district. J Intellect Disabil Res. 1993;39:221–42.
26. Emerson E, Bromley J. The form and function of challenging behaviours. J Intellect Disabil Res. 1995;3:388–98.
27. Elwood T, Hansen LD, Seely JM. Oropharyngeal airway diameter during sedation in children with and without developmental delay. J Clin Anesth. 2001;13:482–5.
28. Lewis I, Burke C, Voepel-Lewis T, Tait AR. Children who refuse anesthesia or sedation: a survey of anesthesiologists. Pediatr Anesth. 2007;17:1134–42.
29. Goodman G, Perkin RM, Anas NG, Sperling DR, Hicks DA, Rowen M. Pulmonary hypertension in infants with bronchopulmonary dysplasia. J Pediatr. 1988;112(1):67–72.
30. Stanley F, Blair E, Alberman E. Cerebral palsies: epidemiology and causal pathways. London: Mac Keith Press; 2000.
31. Nelson KB. Can we prevent cerebral palsy? N Engl J Med. 2003;349(18):1765–9.
32. Strijbis EM, Oudman I, van Essen P, MacLennan AH. Cerebral palsy and the application of the international criteria for acute intrapartum hypoxia. Obstet Gynecol. 2006;107(6):1357–65.
33. Novak I, Hines M, Goldsmith S, Barclay R. Clinical prognostic messages from a systematic review on cerebral palsy. Pediatrics. 2012;130(5):e1285–312.
34. Wongprasartsuk P, Stevens J. Cerebral palsy and anaesthesia. Paediatr Anaesth. 2002;12(4):296–303.
35. Collier J. The management of spasticity. Drug Ther Bull. 2000; 38(6):44–6.
36. Valkenburg AJ, van der Kreeft SM, de Leeuw TG, Stolker RJ, Tibboel D, van Dijk M. Pain management in intellectually disabled children: a survey of perceptions and current practices among Dutch anesthesiologists. Paediatr Anaesth. 2012;22(7):682–9.
37. Malviya S, Voepel-Lewis T, Merkel S, Tait AR. Difficult pain assessment and lack of clinician knowledge are ongoing barriers to effective pain management in children with cognitive impairment. Acute Pain. 2005;7(1):27–32.
38. Geary T, Negus A, Anderson BJ, Zernikow B. Perioperative management of the child on long-term opioids. Paediatr Anaesth. 2012;22(3):189–202.
39. Reller MD, Strickland MJ, Riehle-Colarusso T, Mahle WT, Correa A. Prevalence of congenital heart defects in metropolitan Atlanta, 1998–2005. J Pediatr. 2008;153(6):807–13.
40. White MC. Approach to managing children with heart disease for noncardiac surgery. Pediatr Anesth. 2011;21(5):522–9.
41. Rosenthal DN, Hammer GB. Cardiomyopathy and heart failure in children: anesthetic implications. Paediatr Anaesth. 2011;21(5): 577–84.
42. Diaz LK, Jones L. Sedating the child with congenital heart disease. Anesthesiol Clin. 2009;27(2):301–19.
43. Rosenthal D, Chrisant MR, Edens E, Mahony L, Canter C, Colan S, et al. International society for heart and lung transplantation: practice guidelines for management of heart failure in children. J Heart Lung Transplant. 2004;23(12):1313–33.
44. Ross RD. The Ross classification for heart failure in children after 25 years: a review and an age-stratified revision. Pediatr Cardiol. 2012;33(8):1295–300.
45. Jessup M, Abraham WT, Casey DE, Feldman AM, Francis GS, Ganiats TG, et al. 2009 focused update: ACCF/AHA guidelines for the diagnosis and management of heart failure in adults: a report of the American College of Cardiology Foundation/American Heart Association Task Force on practice guidelines developed in collaboration with the International Society for Heart and Lung Transplantation. J Am Coll Cardiol. 2009;53(15):1343–82.
46. Ross RD, Bollinger RO, Pinsky WW. Grading the severity of congestive heart failure in infants. Pediatr Cardiol. 1992;13(2):72–5.
47. Navaratnam M, Dubin A. Pediatric pacemakers and ICDs: how to optimize perioperative care. Paediatr Anaesth. 2011;21(5): 512–21.
48. Wilson W, Taubert KA, Gewitz M, Lockhart PB, Baddour LM, Levison M, et al. Prevention of infective endocarditis: guidelines from the American Heart Association: a guideline from the American Heart Association Rheumatic Fever, Endocarditis, and Kawasaki Disease Committee, Council on Cardiovascular Disease in the Young, and the Council on Clinical Cardiology, Council on Cardiovascular Surgery and Anesthesia, and the Quality of Care and Outcomes Research Interdisciplinary Working Group. Circulation. 2007;116(15):1736–54.
49. Ratjen F, Doring G. Cystic fibrosis. Lancet. 2003;361(9358): 681–9.
50. Huffmyer JL, Littlewood KE, Nemergut EC. Perioperative management of the adult with cystic fibrosis. Anesth Analg. 2009;109(6):1949–61.
51. Fitzgerald M, Ryan D. Cystic fibrosis and anaesthesia. Contin Educ Anaesth Crit Care Pain. 2011;11(6):204–9.
52. Gibson RL, Burns JL, Ramsey BW. Pathophysiology and management of pulmonary infections in cystic fibrosis. Am J Respir Crit Care Med. 2003;168(8):918–51.
53. Fraser KL, Tullis DE, Sasson Z, Hyland RH, Thornley KS, Hanly PJ. Pulmonary hypertension and cardiac function in adult cystic fibrosis: role of hypoxemia. Chest. 1999;115(5):1321–8.
54. Kearns GL, Mallory Jr GB, Crom WR, Evans WE. Enhanced hepatic drug clearance in patients with cystic fibrosis. J Pediatr. 1990;117(6):972–9.
55. Dray X, Bienvenu T, Desmazes-Dufeu N, Dusser D, Marteau P, Hubert D. Distal intestinal obstruction syndrome in adults with cystic fibrosis. Clin Gastroenterol Hepatol. 2004;2(6):498–503.
56. Chhajed PN, Aboyoun C, Chhajed TP, Malouf MA, Harrison GA, Tamm M, et al. Sedative drug requirements during bronchoscopy are higher in cystic fibrosis after lung transplantation. Transplantation. 2005;80(8):1081–5.
57. American Diabetes Association. Diagnosis and classification of diabetes mellitus. Diabetes Care. 2011;34:S62–9.
58. Chadwick V, Wilkinson KA. Diabetes mellitus and the pediatric anesthetist. Paediatr Anaesth. 2004;14(9):716–23.
59. Gavin LA. Perioperative management of the diabetic patient. Endocrinol Metab Clin North Am. 1992;21(2):457–75.
60. Wu CC, Lin CS, Mok MS. Bispectral index monitoring during hypoglycemic coma. J Clin Anesth. 2002;14(4):305–6.
61. Lamberts SW, Bruining HA, de Jong FH. Corticosteroid therapy in severe illness. N Engl J Med. 1997;337(18):1285–92.
62. Glowniak JV, Loriaux DL. A double-blind study of perioperative steroid requirements in secondary adrenal insufficiency. Surgery. 1997;121(2):123–9.
63. Jacobi J. Corticosteroid replacement in critically ill patients. Crit Care Clin. 2006;22(2):245–53; vi.
64. Tsubokawa T, Yamamoto K, Kobayashi T. Propofol clearance and distribution volume increase in patients with hyperthyroidism. Anesth Analg. 1998;87(1):195–9.
65. Driessen J, Willems S, Dercksen S, Giele J, van der Staak F, Smeitink J. Anesthesia-related morbidity and mortality after surgery for muscle biopsy in children with mitochondrial defects. Paediatr Anaesth. 2007;17(1):16–21.

66. Lerman J. Perioperative management of the paediatric patient with coexisting neuromuscular disease. Br J Anaesth. 2011;107 Suppl 1:i79–89.
67. McFarland R, Taylor RW, Turnbull DM. A neurological perspective on mitochondrial disease. Lancet Neurol. 2010;9(8):829–40.
68. Kam PC, Cardone D. Propofol infusion syndrome. Anaesthesia. 2007;62(7):690–701.
69. Anderson J. Allergic and allergic-like reactions to drugs and other therapeutic agents. In: Lieberman P, Anderson J, editors. Allergic diseases. Totowa, NJ: Humana Press; 2007. p. 295–318.
70. Khan DA. Treating patients with multiple drug allergies. Ann Allergy Asthma Immunol. 2013;110(1):2–6.
71. Caubet JC, Eigenmann PA. Diagnostic issues in pediatric drug allergy. Curr Opin Allergy Clin Immunol. 2012;12(4):341–7.
72. Gonzalez-Gregori R, Dolores Hernandez Fernandez De Rojas M, Lopez-Salgueiro R, Diaz-Palacios M, Garcia AN. Allergy alerts in electronic health records for hospitalized patients. Ann Allergy Asthma Immunol. 2012;109(2):137–40.
73. Asero R. Multiple drug allergy syndrome: a distinct clinical entity. Curr Allergy Asthma Rep. 2001;1(1):18–22.
74. Patriarca G, Schiavino D, Nucera E, Colamonico P, Montesarchio G, Saraceni C. Multiple drug intolerance: allergological and psychological findings. J Investig Allergol Clin Immunol. 1991;1(2): 138–44.
75. Schiavino D, Nucera E, Roncallo C, Pollastrini E, De Pasquale T, Lombardo C, et al. Multiple-drug intolerance syndrome: clinical findings and usefulness of challenge tests. Ann Allergy Asthma Immunol. 2007;99(2):136–42.
76. De Pasquale T, Nucera E, Boccascino R, Romeo P, Biagini G, Buonomo A, et al. Allergy and psychologic evaluations of patients with multiple drug intolerance syndrome. Intern Emerg Med. 2012;7(1):41–7.
77. Emery AE. The muscular dystrophies. Lancet. 2002;359(9307): 687–95.
78. Hayes J, Veyckemans F, Bissonnette B. Duchenne muscular dystrophy: an old anesthesia problem revisited. Paediatr Anaesth. 2008;18(2):100–6.
79. Anonymous. American Academy of Pediatrics Section on Cardiology and Cardiac Surgery. Cardiovascular health supervision for individuals affected by Duchenne or Becker muscular dystrophy. Pediatrics. 2005;116:1569–73.
80. Groh WJ. Arrhythmias in the muscular dystrophies. Heart Rhythm. 2012;9(11):1890–5.
81. Romfh A, McNally EM. Cardiac assessment in Duchenne and Becker muscular dystrophies. Curr Heart Fail Rep. 2010;7(4): 212–8.
82. Morgan GE, Mikhail MS, Murray MJ. (eds) Anesthesia for patients with neuromuscular disease. In: Clinical anesthesiology. 4th ed. New York: McGraw-Hill Medical; 2005.
83. Driessen J, Snoeck M. Duchenne muscular dystrophy: which is the best anesthetic agent? Paediatr Anaesth. 2008;18(10):1007–8.
84. Berry FA. Succinylcholine: a premature death knell? Pediatr Anesth. 1994;4(4):205.
85. Veyckemans F. Can inhalation agents be used in the presence of a child with myopathy? Curr Opin Anaesthesiol. 2010;23(3): 348–55.
86. Raman V, Yacob D, Tobias JD. Dexmedetomidine-ketamine sedation during upper gastrointestinal endoscopy and biopsy in a patient with Duchenne muscular dystrophy and egg allergy. Int J Crit Illn Inj Sci. 2012;2(1):40–3.
87. Ross AK. Muscular dystrophy versus mitochondrial myopathy: the dilemma of the undiagnosed hypotonic child. Paediatr Anaesth. 2007;17(1):1–6.
88. Phan H, Nahata MC. Clinical uses of dexmedetomidine in pediatric patients. Paediatr Drugs. 2008;10(1):49–69.
89. Zucconi M, Weber G, Castronovo V, Ferini-Strambi L, Russo F, Chiumello G, et al. Sleep and upper airway obstruction in children with achondroplasia. J Pediatr. 1996;129(5):743–9.
90. Nelson FW, Hecht JT, Horton WA, Butler IJ, Goldie WD, Miner M. Neurological basis of respiratory complications in achondroplasia. Ann Neurol. 1988;24(1):89–93.
91. Stynowick G, Tobias J. Perioperative care of the patient with osteogenesis imperfecta. Orthopedics. 2007;30(12):1043–9.
92. Widmann R, Bitan F, Laplaza F, Burke S, DiMaio M, Schneider R. Spinal deformity, pulmonary compromise, and quality of life in osteogenesis imperfecta. Spine. 1999;24(16):1673–8.
93. Fernbach SK, Brouillette RT, Riggs TW, Hunt CE. Radiologic evaluation of adenoids and tonsils in children with obstructive sleep apnea: plain films and fluoroscopy. Pediatr Radiol. 1983; 13(5):258–65.
94. Schwengel DA, Sterni LM, Tunkel DE, Heitmiller ES. Perioperative management of children with obstructive sleep apnea. Anesth Analg. 2009;109(1):60–75.
95. Gross JB, Bachenberg KL, Benumof JL, Caplan RA, Connis RT, Cote CJ, et al. Practice guidelines for the perioperative management of patients with obstructive sleep apnea: a report by the American Society of Anesthesiologists task force on perioperative management of patients with obstructive sleep apnea. Anesthesiology. 2006;104(5):1081–93; quiz 1117–8.
96. Chung F, Yegneswaran B, Liao P, Chung S, Vairavanathan S, Islam S, et al. STOP questionnaire: a tool to screen patients for obstructive sleep apnea. Anesthesiology. 2008;108(5):812–21.
97. Chung F, Subramanyam R, Liao P, Sasaki E, Shapiro C, Sun Y. High STOP-Bang score indicates a high probability of obstructive sleep apnoea. Br J Anaesth. 2012;108(5):768–75.
98. Coté GA, Hovis CE, Hovis RM, Waldbaum L, Early DS, Edmundowicz SA, et al. A screening instrument for sleep apnea predicts airway maneuvers in patients undergoing advanced endoscopic procedures. Clin Gastroenterol Hepatol. 2010;8(8):660–5.
99. Connolly LA. Anesthetic management of obstructive sleep apnea patients. J Clin Anesth. 1991;3(6):461–9.
100. Shorten GD, Opie NJ, Graziotti P, Morris I, Khangure M. Assessment of upper airway anatomy in awake, sedated and anaesthetised patients using magnetic resonance imaging. Anaesth Intensive Care. 1994;22(2):165–9.
101. Eastwood PR, Platt PR, Shepherd K, Maddison K, Hillman DR. Collapsibility of the upper airway at different concentrations of propofol anesthesia. Anesthesiology. 2005;103(3):470–7.
102. Dhonneur G, Combes X, Leroux B, Duvaldestin P. Postoperative obstructive apnea. Anesth Analg. 1999;89(3):762–7.
103. Brouillette RT, Thach BT. A neuromuscular mechanism maintaining extrathoracic airway patency. J Appl Physiol. 1979;46(4): 772–9.
104. den Herder C, Schmeck J, Appelboom DJK, de Vries N. Risks of general anaesthesia in people with obstructive sleep apnoea. BMJ. 2004;329(7472):955–9.
105. Mahmoud M, Gunter J, Donnelly LF, Wang Y, Nick TG, Sadhasivam S. A comparison of dexmedetomidine with propofol for magnetic resonance imaging sleep studies in children. Anesth Analg. 2009;109(3):745–53.
106. Mahmoud M, Radhakrishman R, Gunter J, Sadhasivam S, Schapiro A, McAuliffe J, et al. Effect of increasing depth of dexmedetomidine anesthesia on upper airway morphology in children. Paediatr Anaesth. 2010;20(6):506–15.
107. Drummond GB. Comparison of sedation with midazolam and ketamine: effects on airway muscle activity. Br J Anaesth. 1996;76(5): 663–7.
108. Hamilton BE, Ventura SJ. Birth rates for U.S. teenagers reach historic lows for all age and ethnic groups. NCHS data brief, no. 89. Hyattsville, MD: National Center for Health Statistics; 2012.

109. Acquavella AP, Braverman P. Adolescent gynecology in the office setting. Pediatr Clin North Am. 1999;46(3):489–503.
110. Coté CJ, Posner KL, Domino KB. Death or neurologic injury after tonsillectomy in children with a focus on obstructive sleep apnea: Houston, we have a problem! Anesth Analg. 2014;118:1276–83.
111. Subramanyam R, Varughese A, Willging JP, Sadhasivam S. Future of pediatric tonsillectomy and perioperative outcomes. Int J Pediatr Otorhinolaryngol. 2013;77(2):194–9.
112. Gross JB, Bachenberg KL, Benumof JL, Caplan RA, Connis RT, Coté CJ, et al. American Society of Anesthesiologists Task Force on Perioperative Management. Practice Guidelines for the Perioperative Management of Patients with Obstructive Sleep Apnea. A Report by the American Society of Anesthesiologists Task Force on Perioperative Management of Patients with Obstructive Sleep Apnea. Anesthesiology. 2006;104(5):1081–93.
113. Givens TG, Jackson CL, Kulick RM. Recognition and management of pregnant adolescents in the pediatric emergency department. Pediatr Emerg Care. 1994;10(5):253–5.
114. Walton NKD, Melachuri VK. Anaesthesia for non-obstetric surgery during pregnancy. Contin Educ Anaesth Crit Care Pain. 2006;6(2):83–5.
115. Centers for Disease Control and Prevention. Pregnancy and medicines. Washington, DC: US Department of Health and Human Services, Office on Women's Health; 2010.
116. American College of Obstetricians and Gynecologists. ACOG educational bulletin. Teratology. Number 236, April 1997 (replaces no. 233, February 1997). American College of Obstetricians and Gynecologists. Int J Gynaecol Obstet. 1997;57(3):319–26.
117. Addis A, Sharabi S, Bonati M. Risk classification systems for drug use during pregnancy: are they a reliable source of information? Drug Saf. 2000;23(3):245–53.
118. Rathmell JP, Viscomi CM, Ashburn MA. Management of nonobstetric pain during pregnancy and lactation. Anesth Analg. 1997;85(5):1074–87.
119. Welborn LG, Rice LJ, Hannallah RS, Broadman LM, Ruttimann UE, Fink R. Postoperative apnea in former preterm infants: prospective comparison of spinal and general anesthesia. Anesthesiology. 1990;72(5):838–42.
120. Miller MJ, Martin RJ. Apnea of prematurity. Clin Perinatol. 1992;19(4):789–808.
121. Webster AC, McKishnie JD, Watson JT, Reid WD. Lumbar epidural anaesthesia for inguinal hernia repair in low birth weight infants. Can J Anaesth. 1993;40(7):670–5.
122. Kurth CD, Spitzer AR, Broennle AM, Downes JJ. Postoperative apnea in preterm infants. Anesthesiology. 1987;66(4):483–8.
123. Poets CF, Stebbens VA, Richard D, Southall DP. Prolonged episodes of hypoxemia in preterm infants undetectable by cardiorespiratory monitors. Pediatrics. 1995;95(6):860–3.
124. U.S. Department of Health and Human Services. Mental health: a report of the surgeon general. Rockville, MD: U.S. Department of Health and Human Services; 2000.
125. Merikangas KR, Nakamura EF, Kessler RC. Epidemiology of mental disorders in children and adolescents. Dialogues Clin Neurosci. 2009;11(1):7–20.
126. Belfer ML. Child and adolescent mental disorders: the magnitude of the problem across the globe. J Child Psychol Psychiatry. 2008;49(3):226–36.
127. Palla B, Litt IF. Medical complications of eating disorders in adolescents. Pediatrics. 1988;81(5):613–23.
128. Takimoto Y, Yoshiuchi K, Kumano H, Yamanaka G, Sasaki T, Suematsu H, et al. Qt interval and qt dispersion in eating disorders. Psychother Psychosom. 2004;73(5):324–8.
129. Khan MU, Patel AG, Wilbur SL, Khan IA. Electrocardiographic changes in combined electrolyte depletion. Int J Cardiol. 2007;116(2):276–8.
130. Froehlich TE, Lanphear BP, Epstein JN, Barbaresi WJ, Katusic SK, Kahn RS. Prevalence, recognition, and treatment of attention-deficit/hyperactivity disorder in a national sample of us children. Arch Pediatr Adolesc Med. 2007;161(9):857–64.
131. Steiner H, Remsing L. Practice parameter for the assessment and treatment of children and adolescents with oppositional defiant disorder. J Am Acad Child Adolesc Psychiatry. 2007;46(1):126–41.
132. Roberts RE, Roberts CR, Xing Y. Rates of DSM-IV psychiatric disorders among adolescents in a large metropolitan area. J Psychiatr Res. 2007;41(11):959–67.
133. Forsyth IAN, Bergesio R, Chambers NA. Attention-deficit hyperactivity disorder and anesthesia. Pediatr Anesth. 2006;16(4):371–3.
134. Hernandez M, Birnbach DJ, Van Zundert AA. Anesthetic management of the illicit-substance-using patient. Curr Opin Anaesthesiol. 2005;18(3):315–24.
135. Steadman JL, Birnbach DJ. Patients on party drugs undergoing anesthesia. Curr Opin Anaesthesiol. 2003;16(2):147–52.
136. Kayaalp L, Bozkurt P, Odabasi G, Dogangun B, Cavusoglu P, Bolat N, et al. Psychological effects of repeated general anesthesia in children. Paediatr Anaesth. 2006;16(8):822–7.
137. Watson AT, Visram A. Children's preoperative anxiety and postoperative behaviour. Paediatr Anaesth. 2003;13(3):188–204.
138. Fortier MA, Del Rosario AM, Rosenbaum A, Kain ZN. Beyond pain: predictors of postoperative maladaptive behavior change in children. Paediatr Anaesth. 2010;20(5):445–53.
139. Christiansen E, Chambers N. Induction of anesthesia in a combative child; management and issues. Pediatr Anesth. 2005;15:421–5.
140. Marchant WA, Walker I. Anaesthetic management of the child with sickle cell disease. Paediatr Anaesth. 2003;13(6):473–89.
141. Eaton WA, Hofrichter J. Hemoglobin s gelation and sickle cell disease. Blood. 1987;70(5):1245–66.
142. Swerdlow PS. Red cell exchange in sickle cell disease. ASH Educ Program Book. 2006;2006(1):48–53.
143. Wayne AS, Kevy SV, Nathan DG. Transfusion management of sickle cell disease. Blood. 1993;81(5):1109–23.
144. Crawford MW, Galton S, Naser B. Postoperative morphine consumption in children with sickle-cell disease. Paediatr Anaesth. 2006;16(2):152–7.
145. Ballas SK. Current issues in sickle cell pain and its management. ASH Educ Program Book. 2007;2007(1):97–105.
146. Ogundipe O, Walker M, Pearson TC, Slater NGP, Adepegba T, Westerdale N. Sickle cell disease and nitrous oxide-induced neuropathy. Clin Lab Haematol. 1999;21(6):409–12.
147. Carbajal R, Hubert P, Treluyer JM, Jouvet P, Olivier-Martin M. Nitrous oxide and morphine in children with sickle cell crisis. Lancet. 1996;347(9015):1621.
148. McGarry P, Duncan C. Anesthetic risks in sickle cell trait. Pediatrics. 1973;51(3):507–12.
149. Jones KL. Smith's recognizable patterns of human malformation. Philadelphia, PA: Elsevier; 2006.
150. Frei FJ, Ummenhofer W. Difficult intubation in paediatrics. Paediatr Anaesth. 1996;6(4):251–63.
151. Nargozian C. The airway in patients with craniofacial abnormalities. Paediatr Anaesth. 2004;14(1):53–9.
152. Mitchell V, Howard R, Facer E. Down's syndrome and anaesthesia. Paediatr Anaesth. 1995;5(6):379–84.
153. Barnett S, Moloney C, Bingham R. Perioperative complications in children with Apert syndrome: a review of 509 anesthetics. Paediatr Anaesth. 2011;21(1):72–7.
154. Borland LM, Colligan J, Brandom BW. Frequency of anesthesia-related complications in children with Down syndrome under general anesthesia for noncardiac procedures. Paediatr Anaesth. 2004;14(9):733–8.
155. Kraemer FW, Stricker PA, Gurnaney HG, McClung H, Meador MR, Sussman E, et al. Bradycardia during induction of anesthesia with sevoflurane in children with Down syndrome. Anesth Analg. 2010;111(5):1259–63.

156. American College of Surgeons. ATLS: Advanced Trauma Life Support program for doctors. 9th ed. Chicago, IL: American College of Surgeons; 2012.
157. Kleinman ME, Chameides L, Schexnayder SM, Samson RA, Hazinski MF, Atkins DL, et al. Pediatric advanced life support: 2010 American Heart Association guidelines for cardiopulmonary resuscitation and emergency cardiovascular care. Pediatrics. 2010;126(5):e1361–99.
158. Benyounes N, Fohlen M, Devys JM, Delalande O, Moures JM, Cohen A. Cardiac rhabdomyomas in tuberous sclerosis patients: a case report and review of the literature. Arch Cardiovasc Dis. 2012;105(8–9):442–5.
159. Lee JJ, Imrie M, Taylor V. Anaesthesia and tuberous sclerosis. Br J Anaesth. 1994;73(3):421–5.
160. Septer S, Thompson ES, Willemsen-Dunlap A. Anesthesia concerns for children with tuberous sclerosis. AANA J. 2006;74(3):219–25.
161. Elwood T, Bailey K. The pediatric patient and upper respiratory infections. Best Pract Res Clin Anaesthesiol. 2005;19(1):35–46.
162. Schreiner MS, O'Hara I, Markakis DA, Politis GD. Do children who experience laryngospasm have an increased risk of upper respiratory tract infection? Anesthesiology. 1996;85(3):475–80.
163. Parnis SJ, Barker DS, Van Der Walt JH. Clinical predictors of anaesthetic complications in children with respiratory tract infections. Paediatr Anaesth. 2001;11(1):29–40.
164. Tait AR, Malviya S. Anesthesia for the child with an upper respiratory tract infection: still a dilemma? Anesth Analg. 2005;100(1):59–65.
165. Cote CJ. The upper respiratory tract infection (URI) dilemma: fear of a complication or litigation? Anesthesiology. 2001;95(2):283–5.
166. Haas RH, Parikh S, Falk MJ, Saneto RP, Wolf NI, Darin N, Cohen BH. Mitochondrial disease: a practical approach for primary care physicians. Pediatrics. 2007;120(6):1326–33.

Sedation Scales and Discharge Criteria: How Do They Differ? Which One to Choose? Do They Really Apply to Sedation?

5

Dean B. Andropoulos

Abstract

Assessing the depth of sedation in children is critically important to determine whether the goals of sedation are met without exposing the patient to the risk of adverse outcomes. In Cravero's model of pediatric sedation, the patient's state ranges from fully awake undergoing a painful procedure without sedation or analgesia to apnea, hypoxia, and death from oversedation. Clearly, having the sedated child's state in the goal zone is important, and objective tools to assess sedation depth are necessary to standardize depth of sedation. Additionally, having objective assessment scales available to rate a child's readiness for discharge from a sedation recovery area is also important, as premature discharge may lead to adverse events and even death. This chapter will review commonly used pediatric sedation scales, focusing on procedural sedation. Then methods of sedation assessment using processed EEG will be reviewed and compared to pediatric sedation scales.

Keywords

Pediatric • Sedation scales • Ramsay Sedation Scale (RSS) • Observer's Assessment of Alertness/Sedation Scale (OAA/S) • Modified Observer Assessment Sedation Score (MOAA/S) • COMFORT Scale • University of Michigan Sedation Scale (UMSS) • Dartmouth Operative Conditions Scale • Modified Aldrete Score • Bispectral index (BIS) • Aldrete Score • Maintenance of Wakefulness Test • Modified Maintenance of Wakefulness Test (MMWT) • Auditory evoked potentials (AEP)

Introduction

Assessing the depth of sedation in children is critically important to determine whether the goals of sedation are met without exposing the patient to the risk of adverse outcomes. In Cravero's model of pediatric sedation [1], the patient's state ranges from fully awake undergoing a painful procedure without sedation or analgesia to apnea, hypoxia, and death from oversedation (Figure 5.1). Clearly, having the sedated child's state in the goal zone is important, and objective tools to assess sedation depth are necessary to standardize depth of sedation. Additionally, having objective assessment scales available to rate a child's readiness for discharge from a sedation recovery area is also important, as premature discharge may lead to adverse events and even death [2–4]. This chapter will review commonly used pediatric sedation scales, focusing on procedural sedation. Then methods of sedation assessment using processed electroencephalography (EEG) will be reviewed and compared to pediatric sedation scales. Finally, commonly used scales to assess recovery from sedation and readiness for discharge from sedation will be discussed.

D.B. Andropoulos, M.D., M.H.C.M. (✉)
Department of Anesthesiology, Texas Children's Hospital, Baylor College of Medicine, 6621 Fannin, WT 17417, Houston, TX 77030, USA
e-mail: dbandrop@texaschildrens.org; dra@bcm.tmc.edu

K.P. Mason (ed.), *Pediatric Sedation Outside of the Operating Room: A Multispecialty International Collaboration*, DOI 10.1007/978-1-4939-1390-9_5, © Springer Science+Business Media New York 2015

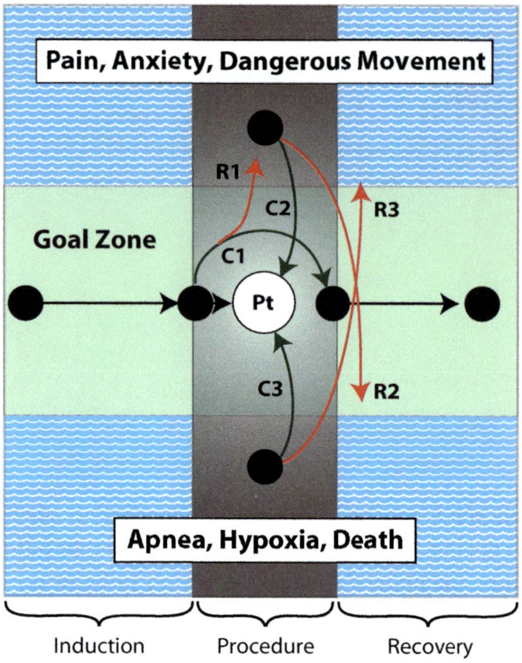

Fig. 5.1 A working model of pediatric sedation. The *x*-axis is the time of phase of sedation. The *y*-axis is the depth of sedation, ranging from inadequate to oversedation. A sedation scale should be able to accurately assess the depth of sedation and maximize the chance that the patient is in the goal zone. The *black dots* are the patient at a single point in time, ranging from preprocedure, through intra- and postprocedure. C designates the work done by the provider to counteract the adverse effects of sedation or accomplish a task. C1 is the procedure control loop, C2 the procedural pain and anxiety control loop, and C3 the sedation-related respiratory depression control loop. R1 is the undesired side effects of therapeutic action: R1 undersedation and pain, R2 oversedation, and R3 rescue from oversedation (Adapted from Cravero JP, Blike GT, Surgenor SD, Jensen J. Development and validation of the Dartmouth Operative Conditions Scale. Anesth Analg. 2005;100:1614–21, with permission from Lippincott Williams & Wilkins)

Table 5.1 American Academy of Pediatrics/Joint Commission/American Society of Anesthesiologists Definitions of Levels of Sedation

Minimal sedation (*anxiolysis*)	A drug-induced state during which patients respond normally to verbal commands
	Although cognitive function and coordination may be impaired, ventilatory and cardiovascular functions are unaffected
Moderate sedation (previously called conscious sedation or sedation/ analgesia)	A drug-induced depression of consciousness during which patients respond purposefully to verbal commands either alone or accompanied by light tactile stimulation
	No interventions are required to maintain a patent airway, and spontaneous ventilation is adequate
	Cardiovascular function is usually maintained
Deep sedation	A drug-induced depression of consciousness during which patients cannot be easily aroused but respond purposefully after repeated or painful stimulation. (*Note*: reflex withdrawal from a painful stimulus is not considered a purposeful response)
	The ability to independently maintain ventilatory function may be impaired
	Patients may require assistance in maintaining a patent airway and spontaneous ventilation may be inadequate
	Cardiovascular function is usually maintained
General anesthesia	A drug-induced loss of consciousness during which patients are not arousable, even to painful stimulation
	The ability to independently maintain ventilatory function is often impaired
	Patients often require assistance in maintaining a patent airway, and positive pressure ventilation may be required because of depressed spontaneous ventilation or drug-induced depression of neuromuscular function
	Cardiovascular function may be impaired

Source: Data from American Society of Anesthesiologists. ASA Standards, Guidelines and Statements, October

Sedation Scales

The Joint Commission, the American Academy of Pediatrics, and the American Society of Anesthesiologists have recently revised their definitions of the levels of pediatric sedation [5, 6] (Table 5.1, Figure 5.2). The four levels of sedation are now minimal, moderate, deep, and general anesthesia. The previously used term "conscious sedation" has been eliminated because it was misleading, and particularly in pediatric patients, they can change rapidly from minimal to deep levels of sedation. Any assessment of levels of sedation needs to take these basic considerations into account.

Sedation scales are indeed necessary for pediatric procedural sedation, particularly when practiced by nonanesthesiologists. For example, Reeves et al. [7] studied 16 children undergoing propofol sedation for bone marrow aspiration by nonanesthesiologists, and found that for all children, their level of consciousness, motor activity score, and bispectral index score was consistent with either deep sedation or general anesthesia at some point during the procedure. In the largest pediatric procedural cohort reported to date, Cravero et al. assessed 49,836 propofol sedations. Complications were noted in 5.92 % of patients, including an airway or pulmonary complication in 1.17 %, yet there was no assessment of depth of sedation reported [8]. Sedation scales are essential to minimize complications from sedation by providing early warning of sedation that is deeper than intended, to allow the practitioner to intervene proactively, instead of having to rescue the patient from an episode of hypoxemia from airway obstruction or apnea. The ideal sedation scale would be applicable to children of all ages, easy and rapid to administer to allow repeated objective assessment, and correlate both with depth of sedation necessary for successful completion of the procedure and with adverse effects of sedation, i.e., airway obstruction, hypoxemia, hypotension,

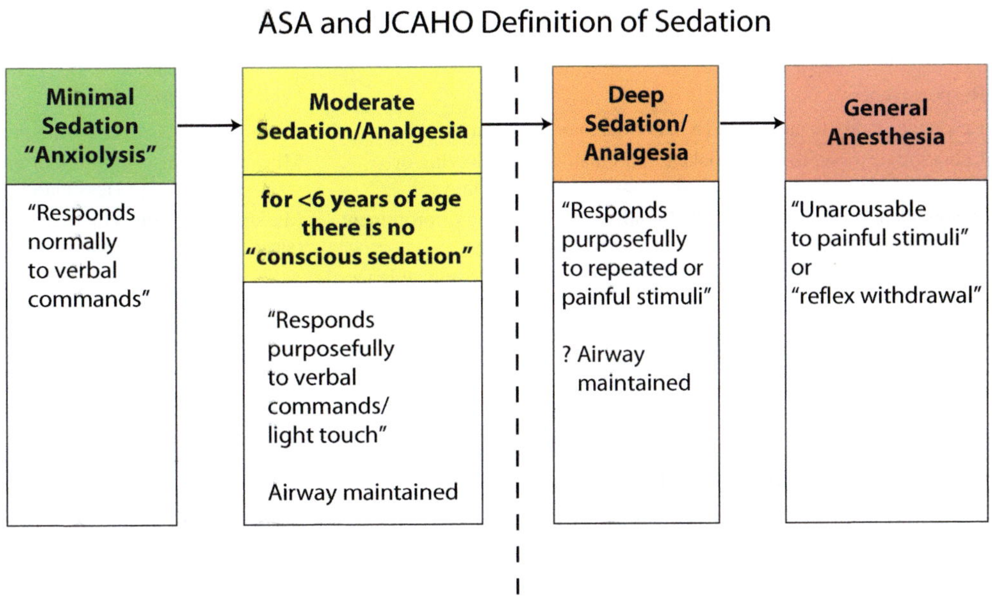

Fig. 5.2 The sedation continuum. A patient may readily pass from a light level of sedation to deep sedation or general anesthesia. Healthcare providers must be prepared to increase vigilance and intensity of monitoring consistent with the depth of sedation. One should consider all children younger than the age of 6 years as deeply sedated because "conscious sedation" in this age group for most children is an oxymoron (*ASA, American Society of Anesthesiologists; JCAHO, Joint Commission on Accreditation of Healthcare Organizations*) (Adapted from [6].)

Table 5.2 Ramsay Scale

Level	Characteristics
1	Patient awake, anxious, agitated, or restless
2	Patient awake, cooperative, orientated, and tranquil
3	Patient drowsy, with response to commands
4	Patient asleep, brisk response to glabellar tap or loud auditory stimulus
5	Patient asleep, sluggish response to stimulus
6	Patient has no response to firm nail-bed pressure or other noxious stimuli

Source: Data from Ramsay et al. [9]

and bradycardia. It would be validated against other accepted scales, and also an objective method of assessment such as a processed EEG technique. And, it would be further validated in very large numbers of patients to determine that the scale did correlate with outcomes. Unfortunately, no such ideal sedation scale exists. However, there are a number of objective and semiobjective methods, some validated, to assess depth of sedation.

Table 5.3 Modified Ramsay Sedation Scale with American Academy of Pediatrics/Joint Commission/American Society of Anesthesiologists designation

Score	Characteristics
1	Awake and alert, minimal or no cognitive impairment
2[a]	Awake but tranquil, purposeful responses to verbal commands at conversation level
3[a]	Appears asleep, purposeful responses to verbal commands at conversation level
4[b]	Appears asleep, purposeful responses to verbal commands but at louder than usual conversation level or requiring light glabellar tap
5[b]	Asleep, sluggish purposeful responses only to loud verbal commands or strong glabellar tap
6[c]	Asleep, sluggish purposeful responses only to painful stimuli
7[d]	Asleep, reflex withdrawal to painful stimuli only (no purposeful responses)
8[d]	Unresponsive to external stimuli, including pain

Source: Data from Ramsay et al. [9]
GA general anesthesia
[a] Minimal
[b] Moderate
[c] Deep
[d] GA

The Ramsay Scale

The Ramsay Sedation Scale (RSS) was described by Ramsay and colleagues in 1974 for the purpose of monitoring sedation with alphaxalone/alphadolone [9] (Table 5.2). It has been validated by several methods including a modified Glasgow Coma Scale and the Sedation-Agitation Scale [10]. The Ramsay Scale was one of the earliest sedation scales, and although not strictly validated in children, it is one of the most widely used scales for assessing and monitoring pediatric sedation in daily practice, as well as in clinical research. It spans the continuum of sedation but does not clearly separate purposeful from nonpurposeful responses.

A later modification of the Ramsey scale more clearly coincides with the AAP and Joint Commission guidelines (Table 5.3) [6]. A score of 2–3 is anxiolysis, 4–5 is moderate sedation, 6 is deep sedation, and 7–8 is general anesthesia.

Table 5.4 The Observer's Assessment of Alertness/Sedation Scale

Assessment categories				
Responsiveness	Speech	Facial expression	Eyes	Composite score level
Responds readily to name spoken in normal tone	Normal	Normal	Clear, no ptosis	5 (alert)
Lethargic response to name spoken in normal tone	Mild slowing or thickening	Mild relaxation	Glazed or mild ptosis (less than half the eye)	4
Responds only after name is called loudly and/or repeatedly	Slurring or prominent slowing	Marked relaxation (slack jaw)	Glazed and marked ptosis (half the eye or more)	3
Responds only after mild prodding or shaking	Few recognizable words	–	–	2
Does not respond to mild prodding or shaking	–	–	–	1 (deep sleep)

Source: Data from Chernik et al. [11]

The Observer's Assessment of Alertness/Sedation Scale and Modified Observer's Assessment of Alertness/Sedation Scale

The Observer's Assessment of Alertness/Sedation Scale (OAA/S) [11] was developed to measure the alertness of adult subjects who are sedated with benzodiazepines. It assesses consciousness level in four areas: responsiveness, speech, facial expression, and eyes (Table 5.4). The OAA/S was validated in 18 healthy males 19–44 years of age, who received intravenous midazolam, initial dose 0.035 mg/kg, followed by additional doses of 0.015 mg/kg every 60–90 s until one of two levels of sedation was reached: light or heavy. A placebo group was also used, and two raters determined the depth of sedation using the OAA/S and 100 mm visual analog scale (VAS) rating patients from 0 (very sedated) to 100 (completely alert). Each subject was tested three separate times in a crossover design to assess the OAA/S reliability, criterion, and construct validity. The scale was found to be reliable with high correlations between raters, to have strong criterion and behavioral validity with consistently decreasing scores for placebo, light, and heavy sedation. The construct validity among the four components was also strong, as was the validity for subsequent administration to the same subject in the crossover phase. Finally, the investigators also used two performance tests—the Digit Symbol Substitution Test and the Serial Sevens Subtraction Test—to compare to OAA/S scores and again found strong correlation.

Despite this thorough validation of the OAA/S in adult patients, and its use in several sedation research studies in children [12, 13], the OAA/S has not been separately validated in children. The OAA/S has been used in the validation of the University of Michigan Sedation Scale [14], and in assessments of the reliability of the bispectral index monitor in children [15].

The Modified Observer Assessment Sedation Score (MOAA/S) uses only the responsiveness category of the OAA/S. This category was separately validated in the original study [11] but, as with the OAA/S, has not been separately validated in children.

The COMFORT Scale

The COMFORT Scale is a physiologically based scale that was originated and validated in children receiving intensive care, and as such is not completely applicable to the procedural sedation environment [16] (Table 5.5). It was tested and validated in 37 ventilated pediatric patients, and interrater agreement and internal consistency were very strong. Criterion validity, assessed by comparison with concurrent global ratings of pediatric intensive care unit (PICU) nurses, was also high. It is included here as an example of such a physiologically based scale. An added dimension is the assessment of pain or discomfort. Generally, a COMFORT score between 18 and 26, with each area scored as 2–3, is desirable to signify appropriate levels of sedation in the ICU setting. It is clear that this scale is complex and will require several minutes to assess, and as such is appropriate for ICU care where the scale is performed no more frequently than every hour. In the context of most procedural sedation, this scale will be inappropriate.

The University of Michigan Sedation Scale

The University of Michigan Sedation Scale (UMSS) is an assessment tool that has been shown to be valid when compared to the OAA/S Scale and other scales of sedation (Table 5.6) [14]. It is a level of consciousness tool that readily separates patients into the sedation categories defined by the AAP, ASA, and Joint Commission. It does not explicitly rate pain, and does not include an assessment of vital signs. In a study of 32 children aged 4 months to 5 years undergoing computed tomography (CT) scanning with oral chloral hydrate, 50–75 mg/kg, Malviya et al. [14] validated the UMSS by comparing the scores assessed every 10 min before, during, and after the procedure by the clinical sedation nurse, with assessments made by trained, blinded observers of the videotaped assessments, which were edited and viewed in random order. UMSS was compared to a 10-point VAS and the OAA/S. One hundred sixty-four observations

Table 5.5 The COMFORT Score

Domain	Characteristics	Score
Alertness	Deeply asleep	1
	Lightly asleep	2
	Drowsy	3
	Fully awake and alert	4
	Hyperalert	5
Calmness/agitation	Calm	1
	Slightly anxious	2
	Anxious	3
	Very anxious	4
	Panicky	5
Respiratory response	No coughing and no spontaneous respiration	1
	Spontaneous respiration with little or no response to ventilation	2
	Occasional cough or resistance to ventilator	3
	Actively breathes against ventilator or coughs regularly	4
	Fights ventilator; coughing or choking	5
Physical movement	No movement	1
	Occasional slight movement	2
	Frequent slight movement	3
	Vigorous movement limited to extremities	4
	Vigorous movement including torso and head	5
Blood pressure	Blood pressure below baseline	1
	Blood pressure consistently at baseline	2
	Infrequent elevations of 15 % or more (1–3 observations)	3
	Frequent elevations of 15 % or more (more than three episodes)	4
	Sustained elevation of >15 %	5
Heart rate	Heart rate below baseline	1
	Heart rate consistently at baseline	2
	Infrequent elevations of 15 % or more (1–3 observations)	3
	Frequent elevations of 15 % or more (more than three episodes)	4
	Sustained elevation of >15 %	5
Muscle tone	Muscle totally relaxed	1
	Reduced muscle tone	2
	Normal muscle tone	3
	Increased muscle tone and flexion of fingers and toes	4
	Extreme muscle rigidity and flexion of fingers and toes	5
Facial tension	Facial muscles totally relaxed	1
	Facial muscle tone normal; no facial muscle tension evident	2
	Tension evident in some facial muscles	3
	Tension evident throughout facial muscles	4
	Facial muscles contorted and grimacing	5

were made, and the UMSS showed an excellent correlation with VAS ($r=0.955$) and OAA/S ($r=0.929$), $p<0.0001$ for both. There was excellent inter-rater agreement between sedation nurse and trained observers at UMSS 0 and 1, and good agreement at UMSS 3 and 4, as well as excellent agreement in a test–retest scenario where 75 videotaped observations were rescored at a later date. Thus it would appear that the UMSS meets several of the requirements for the ideal sedation scale, in that it is validated, rapid to administer, and allows repeated observations. A problem shared with other scales is the need to arouse the patient to make an assessment; this is not possible during a procedure such as a magnetic resonance imaging (MRI) scanning sequence, and may be undesirable if the patient remains aroused, interfering with the procedure.

Table 5.6 University of Michigan Sedation Scale (UMSS)

Score	Characteristics
0	Awake and alert
1	Minimally sedated: tired/sleepy, appropriate response to verbal conversation and/or sound
2	Moderately sedated: somnolent/sleeping, easily aroused with light tactile stimulation or a simple verbal command
3	Deeply sedated: deep sleep, arousable only with significant physical stimulation
4	Unarousable

Dartmouth Operative Conditions Scale

The Dartmouth Operative Conditions Scale [1] was designed by three experienced pediatrician/anesthesiologists, and then refined by videotaping 12 common procedures including MRI, CT scan, voiding cystourethrogram, cardiac catheterization, fracture reduction, and bone marrow biopsy (Table 5.7). Then the Dartmouth scale was validated by videotaping 95 procedures with sedation provided by a variety of providers including radiology nurses, pediatricians, pediatric residents, cardiologists, oncologists, and anesthesiologists. The scale allows quantification of children based on observable behavior. It rates level of sedation in four areas: pain or stress, movement, consciousness, and sedation side effects. In this manner the completeness of the quality of sedation can be assessed comprehensively. Inter- and intra-rater reliability, construct validity, and criterion validity were all excellent. Thus the Dartmouth scale is a well-validated tool, best suited for research because of its comprehensive nature but nonetheless applicable to routine use for procedural sedation. Assessment of this scale at frequent intervals allows for careful tracking of state of sedation, effectiveness of sedation, uncontrolled side effects, and the timing of induction of sedation and recovery. These data can be helpful in quantifying the quality of sedation and best practices. The Dartmouth scale was validated against the COMFORT score (see above), a previously well-validated scale of pain and sedation in pediatric intensive care patients. Scores range from 5 (inadequate sedation with high levels of pain, stress,

Table 5.7 The Dartmouth Operative Conditions Scale

Patient state	Observed behaviors/points			
Pain/stress	Eyes closed or calm expression: 0	Grimace or frown: 1	Crying, sobbing, or screaming: 2	–
Movement	Still: 0	Random little movement: 1	Major purposeful movement: 2	Thrashing, kicking, or biting: 3
Consciousness	Eyes open: 0	Ptosis, uncoordinated, or "drowsy": −1	Eyes closed: −2	–
Sedation side effects	SpO_2 <92 %: −1	Noise with respiration: −1	Respiratory pauses: >10 s: −1	BP decrease of >50 % from baseline: −1

Source: Data from Cravero et al. [1]

and undesired movement) to −4 (dangerously oversedated). Scores in the +2 to −2 range are desired, with more negative scores associated with deeper levels of sedation needed for more painful procedures. These scores correlate with the goal zone desired during sedation (Figure 5.1).

Modified Aldrete Score as a Sedation Scale

The modified Aldrete score has been in widespread use as a postanesthesia recovery score for many years (see below). Because of its near universal use for this purpose it is familiar to many sedation practitioners, and although not designed specifically for this purpose, it is also in wide use as both a sedation scale during the procedure itself, and as a recovery and discharge scale for procedural sedation in children. This score has not been independently validated either in children or for procedural sedation.

Processed EEG Monitors: The Bispectral Index

Several investigators have studied whether the Bispectral Index (BIS, Aspect Corporation, Newton, MA), a single-lead processed EEG that uses a proprietary algorithm to assign a number from 100 (completely awake) to 0 (isoelectric EEG), is meant to objectively assess the depth of sedation or anesthesia (Figure 5.3). The appeal of processed EEG methods is that they are continuous, objective, and do not require awakening of the patient for assessment. Problems with BIS include that the sensor, when applied to the forehead, must be secured with firm pressure to yield a valid signal, and this in itself may awaken the patient. And, its ferromagnetic electrode array is not compatible with MRI magnetic fields. Malviya et al. [17] pooled data from four studies comparing UMSS to BIS values for 3,373 observations for 248 children aged 1 month to 18 years. The patients underwent a variety of diagnostic and therapeutic procedures, with a number of different agents including chloral hydrate, midazolam, pentobarbital, propofol, ketamine, and opioids. There was a moderate inverse correlation between BIS and UMSS in all age groups; however, there was not a difference between BIS values and UMSS 3 and 4 (moderate and deep sedation) in all age groups, and UMSS 0 and 1 (awake versus light sedation) in infants. Furthermore, there was a poor correlation between BIS and UMSS with ketamine or opioid use. The authors concluded that BIS values must be interpreted with caution during procedural sedation in infants and children, with particular attention needed to the age of patient and agents used.

Haberland et al. [18] also compared BIS values and UMSS scores in 35 pediatric dental patients undergoing sedation with nasal mask nitrous oxide in addition to various other regimens, including oral hydroxyzine or chloral hydrate, transmucosal fentanyl, or intravenous (IV) meperidine or midazolam. Mean age of patients was 4.2 years, and duration of sedation was 2.5 h. BIS and UMSS values were recorded every 5 min during sedation, and during the 1-h recovery they were assessed every 15 min, resulting in 455 paired observations. There was a significant decline in BIS and UMSS from baseline to start of the dental procedure, and increase after the procedure, ($p<0.0001$), and moderate kappa coefficient of the percentage agreement between BIS values and UMSS scores 0, 1, 2, and 3–4 (0.26, 95 % confidence interval 0.21–0.20, $p<0.0001$). However, there was no difference in BIS values between UMSS 2 and 3, 2 and 4, or 3 and 4. Therefore, as in the Malviya study [17] cited previously, the authors concluded that BIS did not distinguish between moderate and deep sedation, and was best utilized to distinguish between mild and moderate sedation.

Mason et al. [19] compared BIS values immediately after an MRI or CT scan in 86 children greater than 1 year of age undergoing sedation with pentobarbital as a sole agent, who had achieved Ramsay scores of 4 or 5 (moderate or deep sedation). There was no significant difference between the sedation scores and BIS values (63 ± 12 and 64 ± 15 for RSS 4 and 5, respectively, $p=0.64$). There was a wide variation in BIS values of 31–90. The authors concluded that the BIS had limited ability to distinguish moderate from deep sedation levels.

These studies and other data suggest that BIS has limited utility in assessing sedation level in children [20].

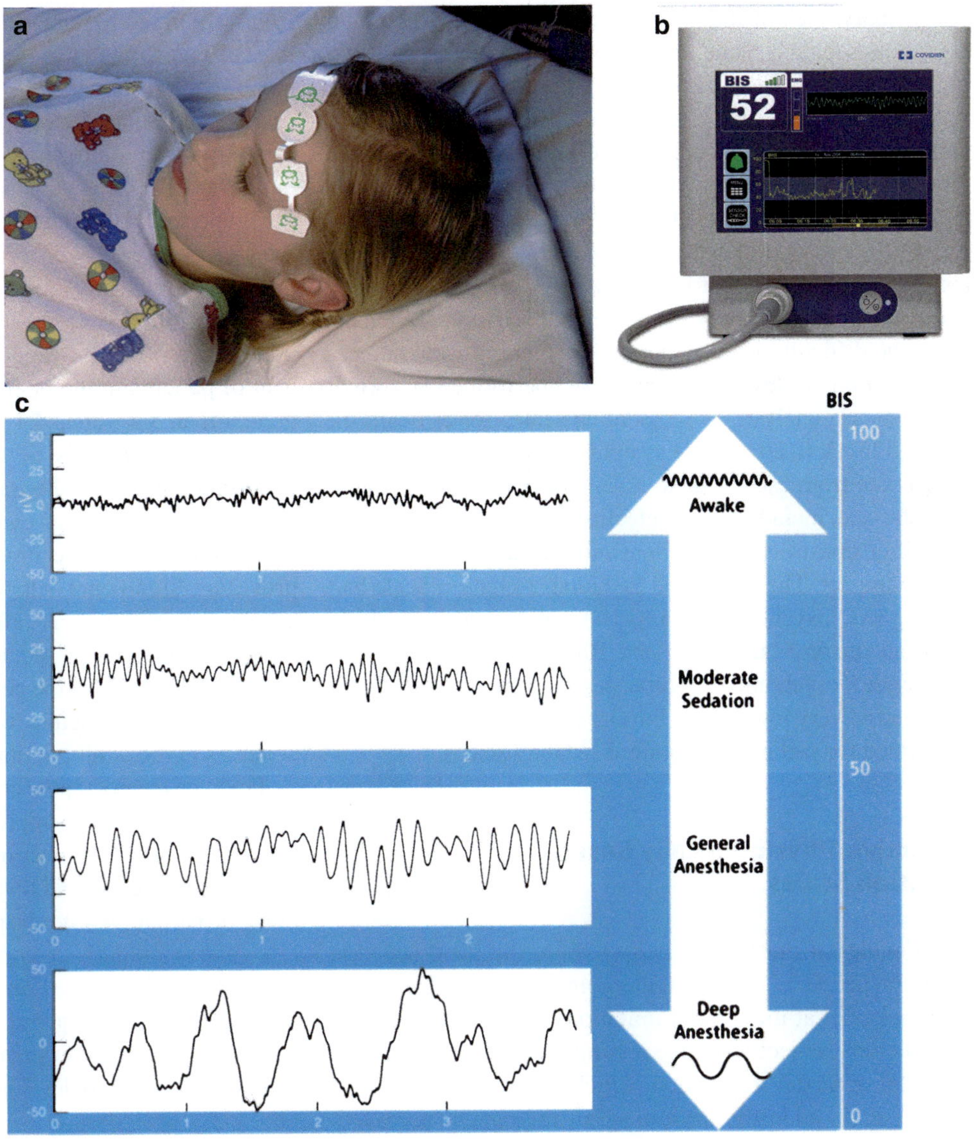

Fig. 5.3 (**a**) The bispectral index® (BIS™) pediatric sensor. A one-channel EEG monitor with reference electrode applied to the forehead. (**b**) The BIS™ monitor displays a single processed EEG number from 0 to 100, as well as the raw EEG waveform, and signal strength indicator. (**c**) The sedation continuum using the BIS algorithm. See text for details (Copyright ©2013 Covidien. All rights reserved. Used with the permission of Covidien)

This is due to several factors, including the age-related developmental differences in the EEG between infants, children, and adults; and the different values achieved with similar levels of sedation with different agents [21].

Auditory Evoked Potentials

Auditory evoked potentials (AEP) demonstrate a correlation with depth of hypnosis in adult patients, and these monitors are becoming available for clinical use. In a study of 75 children aged 1–16 years undergoing urologic surgery with propofol-remifentanil anesthesia, Chueng et al. measured mid-latency AEP produced by a 90 dB click delivered through headphones at a frequency of 6.9 Hz [22]. They compared AEP to BIS during anesthesia, and to the UMSS during emergence. Propofol target-controlled infusion levels were tested, and the BIS demonstrated a stronger correlation than AEP with predicted propofol plasma levels during the intraoperative period (BIS 0.36, AEP 0.21, $p=0.010$). The BIS and AEP performed similarly in predicting UMSS ≤ 1 (sedated versus awake) during emergence from anesthesia. However, the AEP was inferior to BIS at UMSS 2, 3, or 4 (distinguishing light, moderate, or deep sedation). Additional study of this modality in sedated children is necessary to determine its utility for procedural sedation.

Other Sedation Scales

There are a number of additional sedation scales, such as the Harris, modified Glasgow Coma Scale, Cambridge,

Bloomsbury, Neurobehavioral Assessment Scale, Richmond Agitation-Sedation Scale, PRST (pressure, rate, sweat, tearing), Vancouver Sedative Recovery Scale, Motor Activity Assessment Scale, and many others [10]. These scales are largely not applicable to pediatric procedural sedation because they were designed either for adult or for pediatric ICU care, and many have not been validated. None were designed primarily for procedural sedation. Most also measure physiologic variables as part of the assessment, and thus are long and cumbersome to apply for procedural sedation. To underscore the difficulty in selecting and employing valid subjective sedation scales, Robinson et al. performed a formal psychometric analysis of 11 sedation scales for critically ill adults. [23] A 0–20 scoring system was applied using published data from each scale to assess quality of development of each scale, including item selection and content validation, reliability, construct validity, feasibility of use, and scale relevance/impact. The Richmond Sedation–Agitation Scale had "very good" psychometric properties, with a score of 19.5. The Vancouver Scale (14.3) and Ramsay Scale (13.2) had "moderate" psychometric properties, and the OAA/S Scale (3.7) had a "very low" score. Similar assessment has not been performed for pediatric procedural sedation scales.

Objective, Physiologically Based Sedation Scales

As is evident from the prior discussion, the ideal sedation scale for pediatric patients undergoing procedural sedation does not exist at this time. Limitations of all scales include the inherent subjectivity in assessing the patient's response to verbal or tactile stimulation, which is included in most of the scales. In addition, the arousal of the patient necessary for assessment can interfere with both the sedation level itself, and interrupt the procedure. Also, many scales have not been validated, and interobserver reliability is thus in question. Finally, the ability to discriminate safe from dangerous levels of sedation (i.e., deep sedation from general anesthesia) is limited and has not been demonstrated for most of the scales, or for processed EEG monitoring, and thus the goal of preventing airway and cardiovascular complications is also problematic using current schema. Recently, Green and Mason [24] have advocated a reformulation of the sedation continuum. Instead of basing the scale on subjective or semiobjective criteria, scales based on objective physiologic monitoring would be devised (Table 5.8). Because most sedation-related adverse events begin with airway and ventilatory problems, capnography would be able to detect abnormalities (i.e., upper airway obstruction from lax pharyngeal muscle tone and tongue resulting in cessation of airflow) at its earliest occurrence (Figure 5.4). This is substantially before arterial desaturation is detected by pulse oximetry, or bradycardia or hypotension from prolonged hypoxia. Portable capnographic monitoring is easily performed via widely available divided nasal cannulae made in infant, pediatric, and adult sizes, and can be used in all situations, including the MRI suite [25]. Indeed, capnography monitoring for procedural sedation has been demonstrated to improve safety in children. Lightdale et al. [26] reported 174 moderate sedations in children for gastrointestinal endoscopy procedures, with half receiving capnographic monitoring and an intervention protocol and the other half blinded capnography with only rescue intervention, in a prospective randomized study design. Eleven percent of patients in the intervention arm had $SpO_2 < 95$ % for greater than 5 s, versus 24 % in the control arm ($p < 0.03$).

In a meta-analysis of five randomized trials in adults undergoing procedural sedation in 332 patients, Waugh et al. [27] found that respiratory depression events were 6.5–17.6 times more likely to occur without capnographic monitoring, providing significant support for the concept that capnographic monitoring is effective at detecting dangerous increases in depth of sedation. Additional controlled study would be desirable in the pediatric population, but it is highly likely that this principle would have the same strong evidence as in the adult population.

Potential capnographic criteria for increasing levels of sedation would include age-appropriate respiratory rate determined by the capnograph (slower means deeper sedation), significant decreases in end-tidal CO_2 values (signifying smaller tidal volumes or partial airway obstruction, or in worst case scenario low cardiac output), or complete absence of end-tidal CO_2, associated with complete airway obstruction. Specific, focused research would be required to stratify levels of risk based on capnographic and other parameters. A multidisciplinary effort would be required to develop updated guidelines.

Recovery and Discharge Scales

The concept of postanesthesia recovery after a surgical procedure has been expanded to procedural sedation, and scales originally designed to assess anesthesia recovery readiness for discharge to a hospital ward (Aldrete, Steward—see later) have also been expanded to include recovery from sedation, and readiness for discharge to home after procedural sedation without a painful operative procedure, e.g., an outpatient brain MRI for assessment of seizure disorder or developmental delay. Obviously the requirements for discharge can be very different in these two circumstances. The outpatient should be able to resume quiet "normal" activities before discharge from sedation, i.e., spontaneous wakefulness, eating, voiding, drinking, and ambulating with assistance. The inpatient may not need to meet all these requirements. This raises the question of whether these types of recovery scales have ever been validated for the purpose of discharge readiness, and in the case of the postanesthesia

Table 5.8 Preliminary sample schematic for an Objective Risk Assessment Tool for Sedation (ORATS). The choice of four levels here is arbitrary and for illustration purposes only; the final tool would contain the minimum number of discrete levels with independent predictive value

New levels (as yet unnamed)	Escalating risk of serious adverse event	Physiological monitoring parameters (singular or combination)[a]	Recommended sedationist skill set	Recommended resources[b]
1	≤1:10,000	Consistent with normal awake pattern and frequency	Ability to observe and interpret the agreed-upon physiological monitoring parameters	Appropriate for risk level
2	1:1,000	← Objective monitoring predicts this level of risk	Skills appropriate for maintaining sedation at this risk level and for rescuing from the subsequent level	Appropriate for risk level
3	1:100	← Objective monitoring predicts this level of risk	Skills appropriate for maintaining sedation at this risk level and for rescuing from the subsequent level	Appropriate for risk level
4	≥1:10	← Objective monitoring predicts this level of risk	Skills appropriate for maintaining a patient at this risk level	Appropriate for risk level

[a]Focused research would be required to validate the specific variables, parameters, and thresholds that predict the progressive levels of serious adverse event risk. Evaluation of capnography, for example, could include but not be limited to evaluation of waveform, frequency, pattern, and/or numerical value on inspiration or expiration

[b]To be determined at each level by consensus panel and would include but not be limited to recommendations on adjuvant personnel, intravenous access, availability of rescue medications, and airway equipment

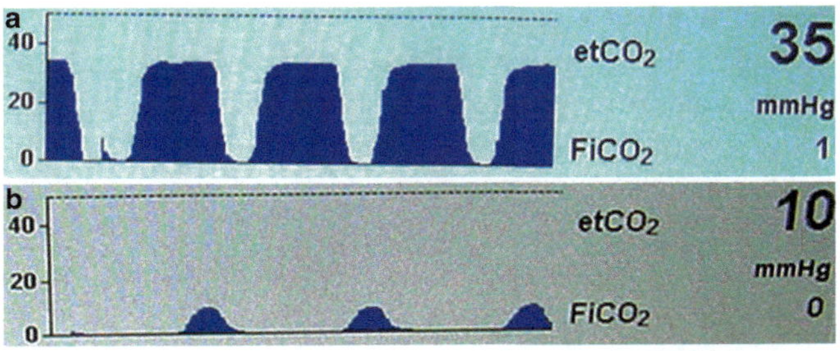

Fig. 5.4 (**a**) Normal capnograph in a sedated patient, obtained with divided nasal cannula. Respiratory rate of 16, and end-tidal CO_2 of 35 mmHg with full "area under the curve" waveform with long plateau signifies unobstructed airway and adequate tidal volumes in this patient. (**b**) Capnograph from a patient with significant respiratory depression. Respiratory rate is 10 per minute, and end-tidal CO_2 is only 10 mmHg, likely signifying small tidal volumes

recovery scales, they have not. Besides assessing readiness to resume "normal" activities, the purpose of discharge and recovery scales is to prevent adverse events. Respiratory and cardiac events, including death, have occurred after premature discharge following procedural sedation [2]. These events have mostly occurred when a long-lasting (long half-life) sedative such as chloral hydrate has been given. This can result in the child being unable to spontaneously unobstruct his or her airway.

The Aldrete score was introduced in 1970 [28], validated in adults, and quickly became the standard for PACU discharge from surgery for both adults and children. It rates five domains: activity, respiration, circulation, consciousness, and color. A point score of 0, 1, or 2 is given in each domain for a maximum score of 10 (Table 5.9). With the introduction of pulse oximetry, the score was modified to include SpO_2 instead of color [29]. Because of its familiarity, it has been used as a score for discharge from sedation as well. A score of 9 or 10 is standard to determine readiness for discharge.

The Maintenance of Wakefulness Test was devised to assess daytime somnolence in patients with sleep disorders. Polysomnography is used to measure the time taken for an adult patient to fall asleep in a dark, quiet room, after they have been instructed to stay awake [30]. The Modified Maintenance of Wakefulness Test (MMWT) is a new modification of the original test, which was devised to help

Table 5.9 The modified Aldrete Scale

Domain	Response	Points
Activity	Able to move four extremities voluntarily or on command	2
	Able to move two extremities voluntarily or on command	1
	Unable to move extremities voluntarily or on command	0
Respiration	Able to breathe deeply and cough freely	2
	Dyspnea or limited breathing	1
	Apneic	0
Circulation	BP ± 20 % of preanesthetic level	2
	BP ± 20–49 % of preanesthetic level	1
	BP ± 50 % of preanesthetic level	0
Consciousness	Fully awake	2
	Arousable on calling	1
	Not responding	0
O_2 saturation	Able to maintain $SpO_2 > 92$ % on room air	2
	Needs O_2 inhalation to maintain $SpO_2 > 90$ %	1
	$SpO_2 < 90$ % even with O_2 supplement	0
Total		

determine discharge readiness in children. In this score, the patient has to maintain a state of wakefulness or alertness in a quiet room for a minimum of 20 min after last being awakened. Malviya et al. studied 29 infants receiving either chloral hydrate or midazolam/diphenhydramine oral sedation for echocardiogram. The modified wakefulness test was combined with the UMSS sedation scale (see above) to devise new, modified discharge criteria, which were compared with the standard hospital sedation discharge criteria. A UMSS of 0 or 1 (awake or minimally sedated), combined with a modified wakefulness test of 20 min, was required to meet these criteria. These data were compared with the bispectral index, with a value of 90 or higher signifying adequate wakefulness for discharge. Standard discharge criteria were stable vital signs, oxygen saturation, and level of consciousness compared to presedation baseline. Also, the patient must maintain a patent air way, manage oral secretions independently, or demonstrate the ability to swallow or demonstrate a gag reflex. In addition, the patient should be able to move or ambulate safely consistent with their presedation baseline. Combining the MMWT and UMSS criteria correctly identified infants with BIS values >90.88 % of the time, compared with only 55 % of children assessed as "street ready" according to usual hospital discharge criteria [30]. In addition, time in recovery to discharge was only 16 ± 13 min using the standard discharge criteria versus 75 ± 76 min ($p \leq 0.007$) using the revised criteria. This very interesting study reveals that many children discharged using standard criteria may indeed not truly be back to their baseline status, and thus be potentially at risk for delayed complications. These more objective discharge criteria would need to be studied in a much larger group of patients to determine whether late complications were truly reduced.

Table 5.10 The Steward simplified postanesthetic recovery score

Domain	Level	Points
Consciousness	Awake	2
	Responding to stimuli	1
	Not responding	0
Airway	Coughing on command or crying	2
	Maintaining good airway	1
	Airway requires maintenance	0
Movement	Moving limbs purposefully	2
	Nonpurposeful movements	1
	Not moving	0
Total		

Source: Reprinted from Steward DJ. A simplified scoring system for the postoperative recovery room. Can Anaesth Soc J. 1975;22:111–3, with kind permission of Springer Science + Business Media

Steward [31], citing the difficulty of assessing patient color (pulse oximetry was not available at the time), and the sometimes inconsistent relationship of blood pressure to recovery from anesthesia, proposed a simplified score (Table 5.10). The original publication was a short description of the scale, and its rationale, but there was no actual patient data attempting to validate it as had been done in the original Aldrete score paper. Despite its use in a number of pediatric studies [32, 33] it has not been independently validated.

In a recent comprehensive review of assessment of recovery from anesthesia or sedation in infants, Sury et al. [34] cited all of the above-noted recovery scales, and several others including the Behavioral Arousal Threshold Scale, Children's Hospital of Wisconsin Sedation Scale, and Simple Pediatric Analog Sedation Score. They concluded that besides the UMSS and MMWT, none of the many other recovery/discharge scales were specifically validated in infants. Additional research to develop criteria for awakening from anesthesia and sedation specific to infants is needed.

Table 5.11 summarizes the sedation, recovery, and discharge scales reviewed above including parameters assessed, utility in various phases of the sedation process, and strengths and limitations.

A Practical Approach to Sedation Scales and Discharge Scores

Synthesizing the concepts presented in this chapter, and considering the demands of a busy sedation service that must be efficient as well as safe, I propose a practical approach to sedation scales and recovery and discharge scores. If moderate or deep sedation by a nonanesthesiologist is planned (the vast majority of pediatric sedations, as only older children undergoing non-painful procedures, will undergo light sedation), one suggested approach is to use a validated simple level of consciousness scale (Ramsay, UMSS, or Aldrete), at least every 15 min or when a change in level of sedation occurs, i.e., after an additional dose of sedative. In addition

Table 5.11 Characteristics of sedation and recovery/discharge scales

Scale	Parameters measured	Sedation, recovery, or discharge scale	Strengths	Limitations	Validated?	References
Ramsay Sedation Scale	Level of consciousness	S, R, D	Simple	No physiologic parameters, must awaken patient	Adults	[6, 9, 10]
OAA/S	Responsiveness, speech, facial expression, eyes	S, R, D	Well validated, relatively simple	No physiologic parameters, must awaken patient	Adults	[11–13]
Modified OAA/S	Responsiveness only	S, R, D	Simple	No physiologic parameters, must awaken patient	Adults	[11]
COMFORT	Alertness, agitation, and multiple physiologic parameters	S	Comprehensive, well validated	Very complex, time consuming, not appropriate for routine procedural sedation	Children	[16]
UMSS	Level of consciousness	S, R, D	Relatively simple	Does not rate pain or physiologic parameters, must arouse patient	Children	[14]
Dartmouth	Pain, movement, consciousness, physiologic parameters	S	Comprehensive, rates pain and movement	Relatively complex	Children	[1]
Modified Aldrete	Activity, respiration, circulation, consciousness, oxygen saturation	S, R, D	Widespread use and familiarity	Not designed as a sedation scale	Adults	[26, 27]
Modified Maintenance of Wakefulness	Maintenance of alertness	R, D	Simple	Requires at least 20 min to administer	Children	[28]
Steward	Consciousness, airway, movement	S, R, D	Simple	No assessment of oxygen saturation	No	[29]
Bispectral Index®	Processed electroencephalogram	S, R, D	Semiobjective; one simple number reported	Continuous, no need to awaken patient	Adults, incomplete validation in young children; not compatible with MRI	[17–20]
Capnography based	End-tidal CO_2	S, R	Objective; sensitive indicator of respiratory depression/obstruction	Many artifacts; equipment not always available	Adults and children, as monitor	[22–24]

S sedation phase, *R* recovery phase, *D* discharge phase, *OAA/S* Observer's Assessment of Alertness/Sedation Scale, *UMSS* University of Michigan Sedation Scale

to standard monitoring with continuous ECG and SpO_2, automated oscillometric blood pressure measurement at least every 5 min, the use of end-tidal CO_2 monitoring via a divided nasal cannula is encouraged. The sedation scale is not assessed if it would arouse the patient such that it would interrupt the procedure (i.e., MRI sequence) and the patient has not exhibited any signs of oversedation (i.e., hypotension or respiratory depression). In this way, the frequent physiologic monitoring is used instead of a more extensive and difficult to administer scale that scores the vital signs, i.e., COMFORT scale. A recovery and discharge score is also used—a modified Aldrete score of 9 or 10, a UMSS of 0 or 1, or a modified wakefulness test of 20 min. It may be simplest to use the same scale for both the sedation and the recovery phases, i.e., the Ramsey, UMSS, or modified Aldrete could be used throughout. The exact tests and scales are determined by institutional preferences. The sedation and recovery personnel must also be familiar with the patient's baseline heart rate, blood pressure, respiratory rate, and oxygen saturation, as well as the age-related normal ranges. Whatever scales are decided upon, they are not a substitute for well-trained sedation practitioners' exercising skill and vigilance, combined with continuous physiological monitoring to ensure the best outcomes.

Conclusion

Regular use of a sedation, recovery, and discharge scales for pediatric procedural sedation is essential, given the wide variety of practitioners involved, as well as the variety of procedures and agents used. Uniform assessment will minimize oversedation and complications, but also ensure that adequate levels of sedation and analgesia are achieved. In addition, only by more objective measurement of sedation will hospitals and departments have accurate data to improve the quality and outcomes of their programs. In the future, more objective physiologically based scales, utilizing capnography, should be devised. Any research on new agents or approaches must be validated using sedation scores that are objective and allow scientific comparison of different methods.

References

1. Cravero JP, Blike GT, Surgenor SD, Jensen J. Development and validation of the Dartmouth Operative Conditions Scale. Anesth Analg. 2005;100:1614–21.
2. Cote CJ, Karl HW, Notterman DA, et al. Adverse sedation events in pediatrics: analysis of medications used for sedation. Pediatrics. 2000;106:633–44.
3. Malviya S, Voepel-Lewis T, Prochaska G, Tait AR. Prolonged recovery and delayed side effects of sedation for diagnostic imaging studies in children. Pediatrics. 2000;105(3):e42.
4. Malviya S, Voepel-Lewis T, Tait AR. Adverse events and risk factors associated with sedation of children by non-anesthesiologists. Anesth Analg. 1997;85:1207–13.
5. Cote CJ, Wilson S; the Work Group on Sedation. Guidelines for monitoring and management of pediatric patients during and after sedation for diagnostic and therapeutic procedures: an update. Pediatrics. 2006;118:2587–602.
6. Kaplan RF, Cravero JP, Yaster M, Cote C. Sedation for diagnostic and therapeutic procedures outside the operating room, Chap. 48. In: Cote CJ, Lerman J, Todres ID, editors. A practice of anesthesia for infants and children. Philadelphia: Saunders Elsevier; 2009. p. 1023–48.
7. Reeves ST, Havidich JE, Tobin DP. Conscious sedation of children with propofol is anything but conscious. Pediatrics. 2004;114:e74–6.
8. Cravero JP, Beach ML, Blike GT, et al. The incidence and nature of adverse events during pediatric sedation/anesthesia with propofol for procedures outside the operating room: a report from the Pediatric Sedation Research Consortium. Anesth Analg. 2009;108: 795–804.
9. Ramsay MA, Savege TM, Simpson BR, Goodwin R. Controlled sedation with alphaxalone-alphadolone. BMJ. 1974;2:656–9.
10. De Jonghe B, Cook D, Appere-De-Vecchi C, et al. Using and understanding sedation scoring systems: a systematic review. Intensive Care Med. 2000;26(3):275–85.
11. Chernik DA, Gillings D, Laine H, et al. Validity and reliability of the observer's assessment of alertness/sedation scale: study with intravenous midazolam. J Clin Psychopharmacol. 1990;10:244–51.
12. Shannon M, Albers G, Burkhart K, et al. Safety and efficacy of flumazenil in the reversal of benzodiazepine-induced conscious sedation. J Pediatr. 1997;131:582–6.
13. Madan R, Kapoor I, Balachander S, et al. Propofol as a sole agent for pediatric day care diagnostic ophthalmic procedures: comparison with halothane anesthesia. Paediatr Anaesth. 2001;11:671–7.
14. Malviya S, Voepel-Lewis T, Tait AR, et al. Depth of sedation in children undergoing computed tomography: validity and reliability of the University of Michigan Sedation Scale (UMSS). Br J Anaesth. 2002;88:241–5.
15. Sadhasivam S, Ganesh A, Robison A, et al. Validation of the bispectral index monitor for measuring the depth of sedation in children. Anesth Analg. 2006;102:383–8.
16. Ambuel B, Hamlett KW, Marx CM, Blumer JL. Assessing distress in pediatric intensive care environments: the COMFORT scale. J Pediatr Psychol. 1992;17:95–109.
17. Malviya S, Voepel-Lewis T, Tait AR, Watcha MF, Sadhasivam S, Friesen RH. Effect of age and sedative agent on the accuracy of bispectral index in detecting depth of sedation in children. Pediatrics. 2007;120:e461–70.
18. Haberland CM, Baker S, Liu H. Bispectral index monitoring of sedation depth in pediatric dental patients. Anesth Prog. 2011;58: 66–72.
19. Mason KP, Michna E, Zurakowski D, et al. Value of bispectral index monitor in differentiating between moderate and deep Ramsay Sedation Scores in children. Paediatr Anaesth. 2006;16:1226–31.
20. Malviya S, Voepel-Lewis T, Tait AR. A comparison of observational and objective measures to differentiate depth of sedation in children from birth to 18 years of age. Anesth Analg. 2006;102:389–94.
21. Davidson AJ. Monitoring the anaesthetic depth in children—an update. Curr Opin Anaesthesiol. 2007;20:236–43.
22. Cheung YM, Scoones GP, Hoeks SE, et al. Evaluation of the aepEX™ monitor of hypnotic depth in pediatric patients receiving propofol-remifentanil anesthesia. Paediatr Anaesth. 2013;23:891–7.
23. Robinson BR, Berube M, Barr J, et al. Psychometric analysis of subjective sedation scales in critically ill adults. Crit Care Med. 2013;41(9 Suppl 1):S16–29.
24. Green SM, Mason KP. Reformulation of the sedation continuum. JAMA. 2010;303:876–7.
25. Mason KP, Burrows PE, Dorsey MM, et al. Accuracy of capnography with a 30 foot nasal cannula for monitoring respiratory rate and end-tidal CO2 in children. J Clin Monit Comput. 2000;16:259–62.
26. Lightdale JR, Goldmann DA, Feldman HA, et al. Microstream capnography improves patient monitoring during moderate sedation: a randomized, controlled trial. Pediatrics. 2006;117:e1170–8.
27. Waugh JB, Epps CA, Khodneva YA. Capnography enhances surveillance of respiratory events during procedural sedation: a meta-analysis. J Clin Anesth. 2011;23:189–96.
28. Aldrete JA, Kroulik D. A postanesthetic recovery score. Anesth Analg. 1970;49:924–34.
29. Aldrete JA. The post-anesthesia recovery score revisited. J Clin Anesth. 1995;7:89–91.
30. Malviya S, Voepel-Lewis T, Ludomirsky A, et al. Can we improve the assessment of discharge readiness?: a comparative study of observational and objective measures of depth of sedation in children. Anesthesiology. 2004;100:218–24.
31. Steward DJ. A simplified scoring system for the postoperative recovery room. Can Anaesth Soc J. 1975;22:111–3.
32. Finkel JC, Cohen IT, Hannallah RS, et al. The effect of intranasal fentanyl on the emergence characteristics after sevoflurane anesthesia in children undergoing surgery for bilateral myringotomy tube placement. Anesth Analg. 2001;92:1164–8.
33. Bevan JC, Veall GR, Macnab AJ, et al. Midazolam premedication delays recovery after propofol without modifying involuntary movements. Anesth Analg. 1997;85:50–4.
34. Sury MR, Bould MD. Defining awakening from anesthesia in infants: a narrative review of published descriptions and scales of behavior. Paediatr Anaesth. 2011;21:364–72.

Physiological Monitoring for Procedural Sedation: The Routine and Beyond

6

Cyril Sahyoun and Baruch S. Krauss

Abstract

Physiological monitoring of vital signs is essential for the safe practice of procedural sedation and analgesia. Oxygenation, ventilation, cortical activity, and hemodynamics can all be monitored noninvasively in spontaneously breathing patients. This chapter discusses the current guidelines and standards for patient monitoring, the essential monitoring modalities for procedural sedation and analgesia in children, and future directions in the field of monitoring.

Keywords

Physiologic monitoring • Procedural sedation • Oxygenation monitoring • Ventilation monitoring • Hemodynamic monitoring • Capnography • Depth of sedation • Bispectral index (BIS) • Cerebral oximetry • Noninvasive cardiovascular monitoring • American Academy of Pediatrics (AAP) • American Society of Anesthesiologists (ASA) • Joint Commission • American College of Emergency Physicians (ACEP) • Electroencephalogram (EEG) • Ramsay Sedation Scale (RSS) • Observer's Assessment of Alertness/Sedation Scale (OAA/S) • University of Michigan Sedation Scale (UMSS)

Introduction

Physiological monitoring of vital signs is essential for the safe practice of procedural sedation and analgesia. Oxygenation, ventilation, cortical activity, and hemodynamics can all be monitored noninvasively in spontaneously breathing patients. This chapter discusses the current guidelines and standards for patient monitoring, the essential monitoring modalities for procedural sedation and analgesia in children, and future directions in the field of monitoring.

C. Sahyoun, M.D. (✉)
Division of Pediatric Emergency Medicine, Morgan Stanley Children's Hospital of New York, Columbia University Medical Center, 3959 Broadway, CHN-1-116, New York, NY 10032, USA
e-mail: cs2476@columbia.edu

B.S. Krauss, M.D., Ed.M.
Division of Emergency Medicine, Boston Children's Hospital, 300 Longwood Avenue, Boston, MA 02115, USA
e-mail: baruch.krauss@childrens.harvard.edu

Current Guidelines and Standards

In the United States, there are numerous procedural sedation and analgesia guidelines that have been created by specialty societies to standardize procedural sedation and analgesia practice in order to optimize patient safety (Table 6.1) [1]. Worldwide, specialty societies have also contributed and championed sedation guidelines and recommendations. (Refer to Chap. 2.) The most widely disseminated guidelines in the United States are from the American Academy of Pediatrics [2], the American Society of Anesthesiologists [3], and the American College of Emergency Physicians [4]. In the early 1990s, the Joint Commission took a special interest in procedural sedation and analgesia, and in 2001 released standards for pain management, sedation, and anesthesia care, with the central theme that sedation care should be comparable throughout a given hospital [5]. Patients sedated in settings outside the operating room should not receive a significantly different level of attention or monitoring than

K.P. Mason (ed.), *Pediatric Sedation Outside of the Operating Room: A Multispecialty International Collaboration*, DOI 10.1007/978-1-4939-1390-9_6, © Springer Science+Business Media New York 2015

those sedated for a similar procedure in the operating room. To ensure this, the Joint Commission requires specific procedural sedation and analgesia protocols that apply consistently throughout each institution. These hospital-wide sedation policies vary from site to site based upon the specific needs and resources available within each institution.

At each hospital accreditation survey, the Joint Commission will evaluate whether clinicians practice procedural sedation and analgesia consistent with their hospital-wide sedation policy, and whether they provide sufficient documentation for such compliance. Physicians must be familiar with their hospital's sedation policies, and should work with their medical staff to ensure that such policies are suitably detailed. Most hospitals pattern their sedation policies after the Joint Commission standards and definitions.

The Joint Commission requires that practitioners who are permitted to administer deep sedation must be qualified to rescue patients from general anesthesia. Moderate sedation suffices for the majority of procedures in cooperative children, although it will not be adequate for extremely painful procedures, or in uncooperative patients. Deep sedation can facilitate these, but at greater risk of cardiorespiratory depression than moderate sedation [3, 5] (Table 6.2).

Table 6.1 Specialty societies with published sedation guidelines [1]

American Academy of Pediatrics
American Academy of Pediatric Dentistry
American Academy of Periodontology
American Association of Critical-Care Nurses
American College of Critical Care Medicine
American College of Emergency Physicians
American Nurses Association
American Society for Gastrointestinal Endoscopy
American Society of Anesthesiologists
American Society of Plastic and Reconstructive Surgeons
Association of Operating Room Nurses
Emergency Nurses Association
Joint Commission on Accreditation of Healthcare Organizations
National Institutes of Health
Society of Gastroenterology Nurses and Associates
Society of Nuclear Medicine

Observational Monitoring

Physiological monitoring has two components: observational monitoring by a designated clinician and electronic monitoring with mechanical monitoring devices. The most important element of procedural sedation and analgesia monitoring is close and continuous patient observation by an individual capable of recognizing adverse events. This person must be able to continuously observe the patient's face, mouth, and chest wall motion, and equipment or sterile drapes must not interfere with such visualization. This careful observation will allow prompt detection of adverse events such as respiratory depression, apnea, airway obstruction, emesis, and hypersalivation [6]. An individual with advanced life-support skills should be immediately available in all settings where deep sedation is performed.

Table 6.2 Levels of sedation (modified from [1])

Minimal sedation (anxiolysis) [7]	A drug-induced state during which patients respond normally to verbal commands
	Although cognitive function and coordination may be impaired, ventilatory and cardiovascular functions are unaffected
Moderate sedation (formerly "conscious sedation") [7]	A drug-induced depression of consciousness during which patients respond purposefully to verbal commands, either alone or accompanied by light tactile stimulation
	Reflex withdrawal from a painful stimulus is not considered a purposeful response
	No interventions are required to maintain a patent airway, and spontaneous ventilation is adequate
	Cardiovascular function is usually maintained
Dissociative sedation [57, 58]	A trance-like cataleptic state induced by the dissociative agent ketamine characterized by profound analgesia and amnesia, with retention of protective airway reflexes, spontaneous respirations, and cardiopulmonary stability
Deep sedation [7]	A drug-induced depression of consciousness, during which patients cannot be easily aroused but respond purposefully following repeated or painful stimulation
	The ability to independently maintain ventilatory function may be impaired
	Patients may require maintaining a patent airway and spontaneous ventilation may be inadequate
	Cardiovascular function is usually maintained
General anesthesia [7]	A drug-induced loss of consciousness during which patients are not arousable, even by painful stimulation
	The ability to independently maintain ventilatory function is often impaired
	Patients often require assistance in maintaining a patent airway. Positive pressure ventilation may be required because of depressed spontaneous ventilation or drug-induced depression of neuromuscular function
	Cardiovascular function may be impaired

During deep sedation, the individual dedicated to patient monitoring should be experienced with this depth of sedation and have no other responsibilities that would interfere with the required advanced level of monitoring and documentation. Individual hospital-wide sedation policies may have additional requirements for how and when deep sedation is administered based on their specific needs and available resources.

Vital signs should be measured at individualized intervals including at baseline, after drug administration, on completion of the procedure, during early recovery, and at completion of recovery. During deep sedation, vital signs should be assessed every 5 min. In addition to recording vital signs at set intervals, clinicians must be especially vigilant during key phases of the sedation. Patients are usually at highest risk of complications 5–10 min following administration of IV medications and during the immediate post-procedure period when external stimuli are discontinued.

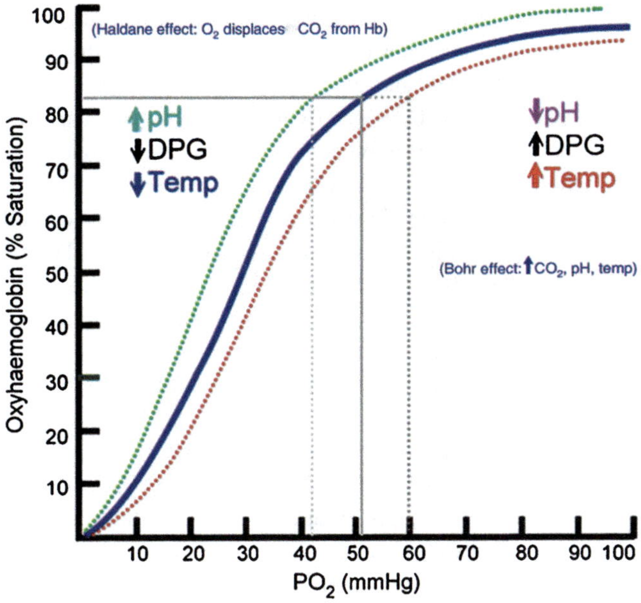

Fig. 6.1 Oxyhemoglobin dissociation curve

Electronic Monitoring

The use of electronic monitoring has greatly enhanced the safety of procedural sedation and analgesia. Continuous oxygenation (pulse oximetry with an audible signal), ventilation (capnography), and hemodynamics (blood pressure and electrocardiogram [ECG]) can all be monitored noninvasively in spontaneously breathing patients.

Oxygenation Monitoring

Pulse oximetry is the noninvasive measurement of the percent of hemoglobin bound to oxygen providing a continuous means of estimating in real time the arterial oxygen saturation. The underlying principles of oximetry were developed in 1932 based on the Beer–Lambert law (the concentration of an unknown solute dissolved in a solvent can be determined by light absorption). Modern pulse oximetry technology, using optical plethysmography and spectrophotometry, was invented in 1974 and completed in 1980 with the addition of a probe and a miniaturized computer in the monitor [7]. The probe, consisting of red and infrared (IR) light sources and a photoelectric detector, is positioned across a pulsatile vascular bed such as the finger, the foot, or the ear lobe [7, 8].

The most common type of oximetry (i.e., transmission oximetry) places the light sources on one side of the tissue bed and the photodetector on the opposite side. The pulsatile variation of the emitted red and IR light transmitted through the tissue bed is accessed by the oximeter, which divides the signal into an arterial blood pulsatile component and a non-pulsatile component (venous and capillary blood). Data averaged over several arterial pulse cycles are represented as the oxygen saturation (SpO_2) [7–9]. There is a tight correlation between the arterial hemoglobin oxygen saturation (PaO_2) and the SpO_2 in a nonlinear fashion as described by the oxyhemoglobin dissociation curve (Fig. 6.1) [8–10]. The shape of the curve has important clinical implications. In the hypoxic patient, small changes in SpO_2 on the steep part of the curve result in large changes in the PaO_2, while SpO_2 values at high levels of oxygenation (on the plateau of the curve) are relatively insensitive at detecting significant changes in PaO_2.

Patients with normal lung function and adequate gas exchange have an SpO_2 between 97 and 100 %. Pulse oximeters are accurate for saturations >70 % [10]. When SaO_2 falls below 95 %, hypoxia may be present, although patients with obstructive lung disease may live in this range [8, 9]. Oxygen saturations below 90 % represent significant hypoxia. At 75 % saturation, oximetry bias is uniformly scattered (7 % underestimation and 7 % overestimation).

The finger is the most common probe site used for pulse oximetry. If the finger is inaccessible or unsuitable, other probe sites, such as the ear lobe or the bridge of the nose, may be used. In neonates and infants, probe sites include the great toe, the heel, the sole, and the lateral aspect of the foot.

There are a number of important limitations to the accuracy of pulse oximetry: poor perfusion secondary to severe vasoconstriction (e.g., low perfusion states, shock, hypothermia), artifact from excessive patient motion, severe anemia, high-intensity ambient light, abnormal hemoglobins, venous pulsations, synthetic fingernails and nail polish, or intravenous dyes [8, 10]. Recent advances in motion control technology have made pulse oximetry more reliable during patient motion. Carboxyhemoglobin (COHb) and methemoglobin

(MetHb) contribute to light absorption and cause errors in saturation readings. The oximeter sees COHb as though it were mostly OxyHb and gives a false high reading. In the presence of high levels of MetHb, the SpO_2 is erroneously low when the arterial saturation is above 85 % and erroneously high when the arterial saturation is below 85 %. MetHb produces a large pulsatile absorbance signal at both the red and IR wavelengths. This forces the absorbance ratio toward unity, which corresponds to an SpO_2 of 85 %. Further, in dark-skinned patients, false high readings and a higher incidence of failure of signal detection have been reported [8–10].

Pulse oximetry is not a substitute for ventilation monitoring, as there is a lag time—the extent of the lag depending on the age and physical status of the patient—between the onset of hypoventilation or apnea and a change in oxygen saturation. Therefore, during procedural sedation, ventilation monitoring should always accompany oxygenation monitoring. Hypoventilation and resultant hypercapnia may precede a decrease in hemoglobin O_2 saturation by minutes [11]. Further, supplemental O_2 may mask hypoventilation by delaying the eventual O_2 desaturation for which pulse oximetry monitoring is designed to recognize [12].

Ventilation Monitoring

Capnography is the noninvasive measurement of the partial pressure of carbon dioxide in exhaled breath represented as a numerical value (end-tidal CO_2) and a waveform. The CO_2 waveform or capnogram represents changes in the CO_2 concentration over the time of one respiratory cycle (Fig. 6.2) [13]. Changes in the shape of the waveform are diagnostic of disease conditions, while changes in end-tidal CO_2 ($EtCO_2$—the maximum CO_2 concentration at the end of each tidal breath) can be used to assess disease severity and response to treatment [14].

Modern capnography was developed in the 1940s and commercialized in the 1960s and 1970s with the development of mass spectroscopy. Capnography became a routine part of anesthesia practice in Europe in the 1970s and in the United States in the 1980s [13]. Most capnography technology is built on infrared (IR) radiation techniques and based on the fact that CO_2 molecules absorb IR radiation at a specific wavelength, with the amount of radiation absorbed having a close to exponential relation to the CO_2 concentration present in the breath sample. Detecting changes in IR radiation levels with photodetectors allows for the calculation of the CO_2 concentration in the gas sample.

Carbon dioxide monitors measure gas concentration or partial pressure using one of two configurations: mainstream or sidestream. Mainstream devices measure CO_2 directly from the airway, with the sensor located on the endotracheal tube. Sidestream devices measure CO_2 by aspirating a small sample from the exhaled breath through tubing to a sensor located inside the monitor. Mainstream systems, as the sensor is located on the endotracheal tube, are configured for intubated patients. Sidestream systems, as the sensor is located inside the monitor, are configured for both intubated and non-intubated patients. The airway interface for intubated patients is an airway adapter placed on the hub of the endotracheal tube; and, for spontaneously breathing patients, a nasal–oral cannula that allows concomitant CO_2 sampling and low-flow oxygen delivery.

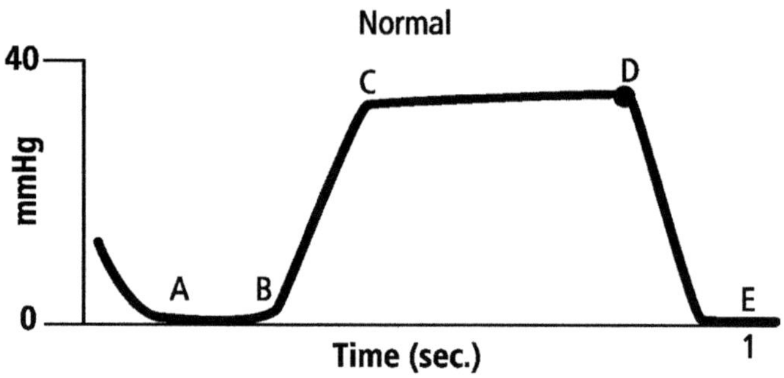

Fig. 6.2 Normal CO_2 waveform

Sidestream systems can be either high flow (with 150 cc/min as the amount of CO_2 in the breath sample required to obtain an accurate reading) or low flow (50 cc/min). Low-flow sidestream systems have a lower occlusion rate (from moisture or patient secretions) and are more accurate in patients with low tidal volumes (neonates, infants, and patients with hypoventilation and low tidal volume breathing) [15]. In high flow systems, when the tidal volume of the patient drops below 150 cc (i.e., the flow rate of the system), the monitor will entrain room air to compensate, falsely diluting the $EtCO_2$ [16–18].

The CO_2 waveform, corresponding to a single breath, consists of four phases [2, 15]. Phase 1 (dead space ventilation, A–B) represents the beginning of exhalation where the dead space is cleared from the upper airway. Phase 2 (ascending phase, B–C) represents the rapid rise in CO_2 concentration in the breath stream as the CO_2 from the alveoli reaches the upper airway. Phase 3 (alveolar plateau, C–D) represents the CO_2 concentration reaching a uniform level in the entire breath stream and concludes with a point of maximum CO_2 concentration ($EtCO_2$). Phase 4 (D–E) represents the inspiratory cycle where the CO_2 concentration drops to zero as atmospheric air enters the airway (Fig. 6.2). A normal waveform is characterized by four distinct phases, a CO_2 concentration that starts at zero and returns to zero (i.e., there is no rebreathing of CO_2), and a maximum CO_2 concentration reached with each breath (i.e., $EtCO_2$).

Patients with normal lung function have a characteristic rectangular-shaped waveform and a narrow $EtCO_2$–pCO_2 gradient (0–5 mmHg), with the $EtCO_2$ accurately reflecting the $PaCO_2$ [14, 19]. Patients with obstructive lung disease

a

Diagnosis	Waveform	Features	Intervention
Normal	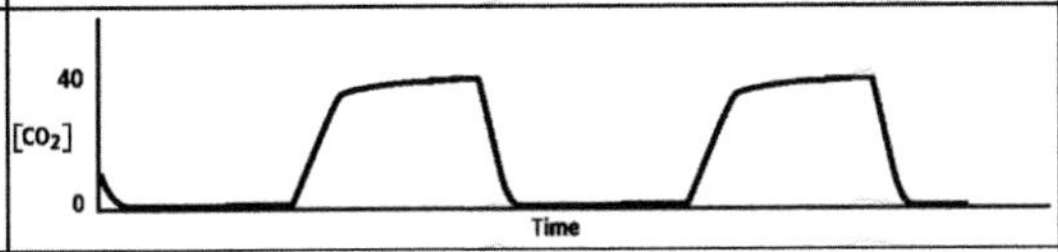	SpO_2 Normal $EtCO_2$ Normal Waveform Normal RR Normal	• No intervention required • Continue sedation
Hyperventilation	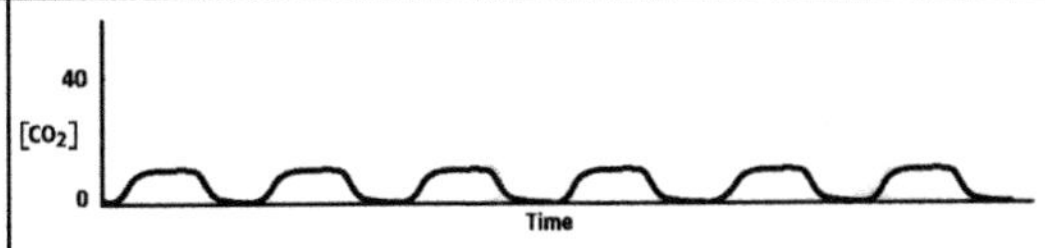	SpO_2 Normal $EtCO_2$ ↓ Waveform Decreased amplitude and width RR ↑	
Bradypneic hypoventilation (Type 1)	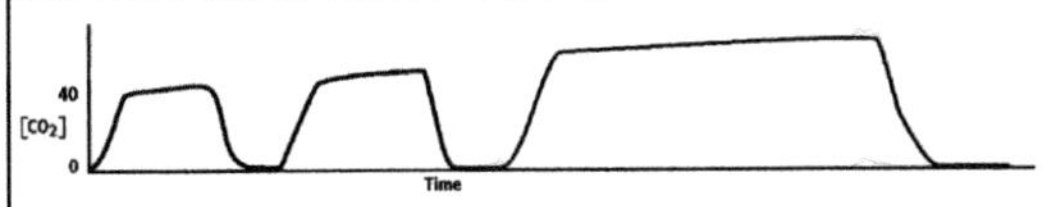	SpO_2 Normal $EtCO_2$ ↑ Waveform Increased amplitude and width RR ↓↓↓	• Reassess patient • Continue sedation
		SpO_2 ↓ $EtCO_2$ ↑ Waveform Increased amplitude and width RR ↓↓↓	• Reassess patient • Assess for airway obstruction • Supplemental oxygen • Cease drug administration or reduce dosing
Hypopneic hypoventilation (Type 2)	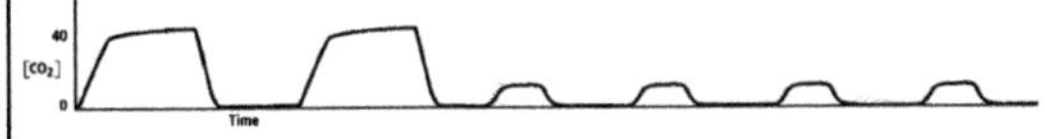	SpO_2 Normal $EtCO_2$ ↓ Waveform Decreased amplitude RR ↓	• Reassess patient • Continue sedation
		SpO_2 ↓ $EtCO_2$ ↓ Waveform Decreased amplitude RR ↓	• Reassess patient • Assess for airway obstruction • Supplemental oxygen • Cease drug administration or reduce dosing
Hyponeic hypoventilation with periodic breathing	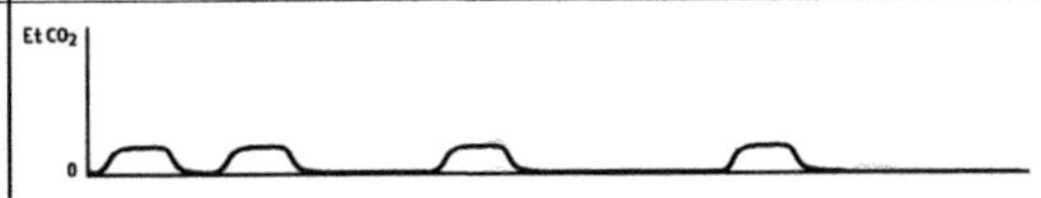	SpO_2 Normal or ↓ $EtCO_2$ ↓ Waveform Decreased amplitude RR ↓ Other Apneic pauses	

Fig. 6.3 (**a**, **b**) Capnographic airway assessment for procedural sedation and analgesia. *Source*: Krauss and Hess [24]. [a]Varying waveform amplitude and width. [b]Depending on duration and severity of bronchospasm. [c]Depending on duration of episode

will have a more rounded ascending phase and an upward slope in the alveolar plateau (Fig. 6.3) [20]. In patients with abnormal lung function secondary to ventilation–perfusion (V–Q) mismatch, the gradient will widen, depending on the severity of the lung disease [21–23].

The shape of the waveform is affected by the $EtCO_2$ and the expiratory time. The amplitude of the waveform is determined by the $EtCO_2$ value and the width is determined by the expiratory time. Hyperventilation (increased respiratory rate, decreased $EtCO_2$) results in a low-amplitude and narrow waveform, while classical hypoventilation (decreased respiratory rate, increased $EtCO_2$) results in a high-amplitude and wide waveform (Fig. 6.3). Acute bronchospasm results in a waveform with a curved ascending phase and upsloping alveolar plateau (Fig. 6.3). An $EtCO_2 > 70$ mmHg, in patients without chronic hypoventilation, indicates respiratory failure.

Capnography provides a continuous, breath-by-breath measure of respiratory rate and CO_2 exchange and can detect the common adverse airway and respiratory events associated with procedural sedation and analgesia [24]. Capnography is the earliest indicator of airway or respiratory compromise and will manifest an abnormally high or low $EtCO_2$ well before pulse oximetry detects a falling oxyhemoglobin saturation, especially in patients receiving supplemental oxygen. Early detection of respiratory compromise is especially important in infants and toddlers who have smaller functional residual capacity and greater oxygen consumption relative to older children and adults. Capnography provides a non-impedance respiratory rate directly from the airway (via oral–nasal cannula) that is more accurate than impedance-based respiratory monitoring. In patients with obstructive apnea, impedance-based monitoring will interpret chest wall movement without ventilation as a valid breath.

Both central and obstructive apnea can be rapidly detected by capnography (Fig. 6.3). Loss of the waveform, in conjunction with no chest wall movement and no breath sounds confirms the diagnosis of central apnea. Obstructive apnea is characterized by loss of the waveform, chest wall

b

Diagnosis	Waveform	Features	Intervention
Physiological variability	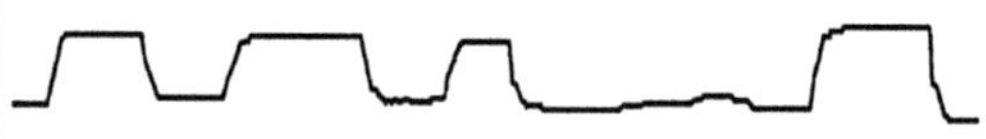	SpO_2 Normal $EtCO_2$ Normal Waveform Varying[a] RR Normal	• No intervention required • Continue sedation
Bronchospasm	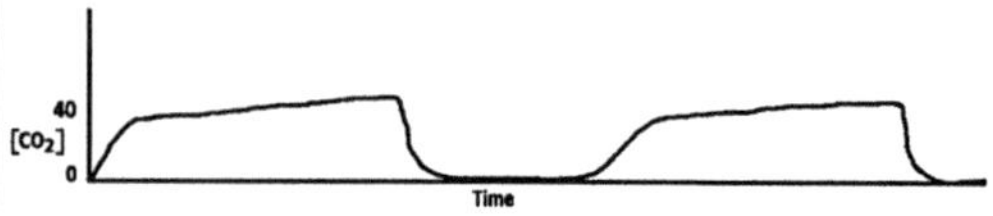	SpO_2 Normal or ↓ $EtCO_2$ Normal, ↑, or ↓[b] Waveform Curved RR Normal, ↑, or ↓[b] Other Wheezing	• Reassess patient • Bronchodilator therapy • Cease drug administration
Partial airway obstruction	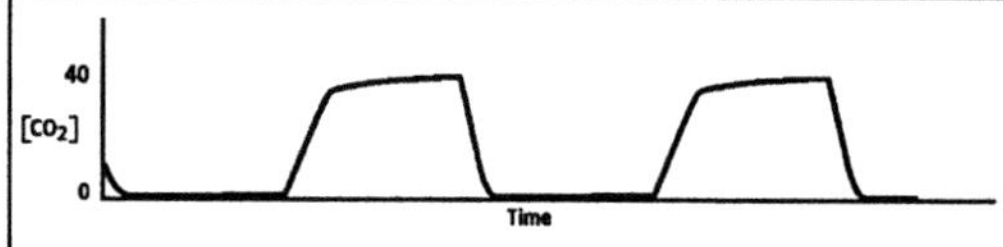	SpO_2 Normal or ↓ $EtCO_2$ Normal Waveform Normal RR Variable Other Noisy breathing and/or inspiratory stridor	• Full airway patency restored with airway alignment • Noisy breathing & stridor resolve • Reassess patient • Establish IV access • Supplemental O_2 (as needed) • Cease drug administration
Partial laryngospasm			• Airway not fully patent with airway alignment • Noisy breathing & stridor persist • Reassess patient • Establish IV access • Supplemental O_2 (as needed) • Cease drug administration
Apnea Complete airway obstruction	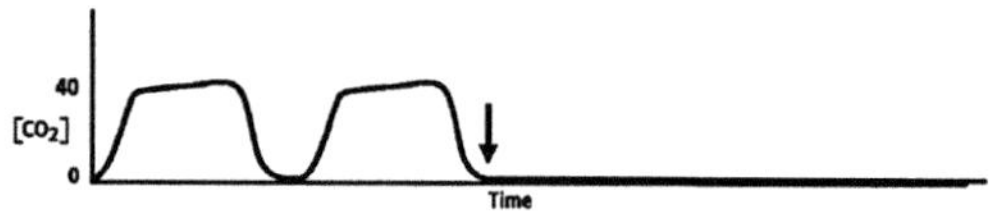	SpO_2 Normal or ↓[c] $EtCO_2$ Zero Waveform Absent RR Zero Other No chest wall movement or breath sounds	• Reassess patient • Stimulation • Bag mask ventilation • Reversal agents (where appropriate) • Cease drug administration
Complete laryngospasm		SpO_2 Normal or ↓[c] $EtCO_2$ Zero Waveform Absent RR Zero Other Chest wall movement and breath sounds present	• Airway patency restored with airway alignment • Waveform present • Airway not patent with airway alignment • No waveform — Positive pressure ventilation

Fig. 6.3 (continued)

movement, and absent breath sounds. The absence of the waveform in association with the presence or absence of chest wall movement distinguishes apnea from upper airway obstruction and laryngospasm. Response to airway alignment maneuvers can further distinguish upper airway obstruction from laryngospasm.

There are two types of drug-induced hypoventilation that occur during procedural sedation and analgesia (Fig. 6.3) [24]. Bradypneic hypoventilation, commonly seen with opioids, is characterized by an increased $EtCO_2$ and an increased $PaCO_2$. Respiratory rate is depressed proportionally greater than tidal volume resulting in bradypnea, an increase in expiratory time, and a rise in $EtCO_2$, graphically represented by a high-amplitude and wide waveform (Fig. 6.3). Bradypneic hypoventilation follows a predictable course with $EtCO_2$ increasing progressively until respiratory failure and apnea occur. Although there is no absolute threshold at which apnea occurs, patients without chronic hypoventilation with $EtCO_2 > 70$ mmHg are at significant risk.

Hypopneic hypoventilation, commonly seen with sedative–hypnotic drugs, is characterized by a normal or decreased $EtCO_2$ and an increased $PaCO_2$ as airway dead space remains constant and tidal volume is decreasing (Fig. 6.3). Tidal volume is depressed proportionally greater than respiratory rate, resulting in low tidal volume breathing that leads to an increase in airway dead space fraction (dead space volume/tidal volume). As tidal volume decreases, airway dead space fraction increases which in turn results in an increase in the $PaCO_2$–$EtCO_2$ gradient. Even though $PaCO_2$ is increasing, $EtCO_2$ may remain normal or may be decreasing, graphically represented by a low-amplitude waveform (Fig. 6.3). Hypopneic hypoventilation follows a variable course and may remain stable with low tidal volume breathing resolving over time as CNS drug levels decrease and redistribution to the periphery occurs, progress to periodic breathing with intermittent apneic pauses (which may resolve spontaneously or progress to central apnea), or progress directly to central apnea.

The low tidal volume breathing that characterizes hypopneic hypoventilation increases dead space ventilation when normal compensatory mechanisms are inhibited by drug effects. Minute ventilation, which normally increases to compensate for an increase in dead space, does not change or may decrease [25]. As minute ventilation decreases, PaO_2 decreases. If minute ventilation decreases further, oxygenation is further impaired [26, 27]. However, $EtCO_2$ may initially be high (bradypneic hypoventilation) or low (hypopneic hypoventilation) without significant changes in oxygenation, particularly if supplemental oxygen is given. Therefore, a drug-induced increase or decrease in $EtCO_2$ does not necessarily lead to oxygen desaturation and may not require intervention.

Technical problems with capnography have limited its effectiveness and restricted its clinical applications. These problems include: interference with the sensor by condensed water and patient secretions, cross sensitivity with anesthetic gases in conventional CO_2 sensors, lack of ruggedness for intra- and interhospital transport, and power consumption issues related to portable battery operation time. These issues have been resolved in the newer generation capnography monitors. Early capnography airway interfaces (i.e., nasal cannula) had difficulty providing consistent measurements in mouth-breathing patients and patients who alternated between mouth and nose breathing. The newer oral–nasal interfaces do not have these problems. Recently, an entropy monitor has been evaluated to determine whether tracheal sounds can detect obstruction or apnea [28]. Tracheal sounds reflect vibrations of the tracheal wall and surrounding soft tissue [8]. These sounds may be monitored with a microphone placed over the trachea, a means of estimating respiratory flow in awake and sleeping patients [9–14]. Entropy reflects the tracheal sounds and can provide an estimate of respiratory flow [10–12]. (See Fig. 6.4) Recent evidence suggests that in healthy adult volunteers, the entropy of the acoustic signals measured over the trachea may be a better indicator of impending apnea or obstruction than is capnography [28]. The entropy of the acoustic signals over the trachea was able to detect apnea in sedated volunteers with a sensitivity and specificity of 95 % and 92 %, respectively. Future studies will need to be done to determine whether entropy will be applicable to the pediatric population and whether it can be incorporated into a physiological monitor that will follow entropy signals as a continuous, easily interpretable variable.

Hemodynamic Monitoring

Noninvasive blood pressure (NIBP) measurement is an automated method of repetitively determining blood pressure that is accurate in both adults and children. Blood pressure can be obtained manually (only when the operator pushes a button) or automatically cycled at preset intervals with the cuff inflated to specific levels. NIBP provides a display of the heart rate, systolic, diastolic, and mean blood pressures by electronically determining the pulse amplitude. During deflation, the cuff determines the amplitude of the pulsations transmitted by movement of arterial wall under the cuff. A sudden rise in the magnitude of the pulsations accompanies the artery opening and represents the systolic pressure. The magnitude of the pulsations increases to a peak and then falls rapidly. The diastolic pressure is determined at the point where there are no further alterations in the magnitude of the pulsations. The accuracy of NIBP depends on utilizing the correct cuff size (especially important in children and obese patients) and on minimizing patient motion during measurement.

Continuous ECG monitoring is useful for the rapid detection of rhythm disturbances or ischemia. Continuous ECG monitoring for procedural sedation and analgesia is neither mandatory nor standard of care in patients without a cardiovascular disease. However, such monitoring is simple, inexpensive, and readily available and is frequently used during procedural sedation and analgesia in children.

Depth of Sedation Monitoring

Monitoring modalities that measure the brain's response to anesthetic agents have recently been studied for use in procedural sedation and analgesia [29–31]. Although these technologies have been used to monitor depth of sedation/anesthesia in the operating room, in 2006 the American Society of Anesthesiologists concluded that the clinical applicability in the operating room "has not been established" [32]. Further, the predictive value of this type of monitoring for the moderate and deep sedation outside the operating room remains unclear.

Bispectral Index

The most studied of these technologies is the bispectral index (BIS), that uses a processed electroencephalogram (EEG) signal to quantify sedation depth. A BIS value of 100 is considered complete alertness, a range of 40–60 consistent with general anesthesia, and zero is no cortical activity [33].

Several studies have shown a reasonable correlation between BIS and standard observational sedation score in children older than 6 months (i.e., University of Michigan Sedation Scale [UMSS], Observer's Assessment of Alertness/Sedation [OAA/S], Ramsay Sedation Scale) for commonly used sedatives such as midazolam, pentobarbital, chloral hydrate, and propofol. (Refer to Chap. 5.) However, other studies have failed to consistently validate a tight correlation between BIS values and specific levels of sedation as measured by standard observational sedation scores.

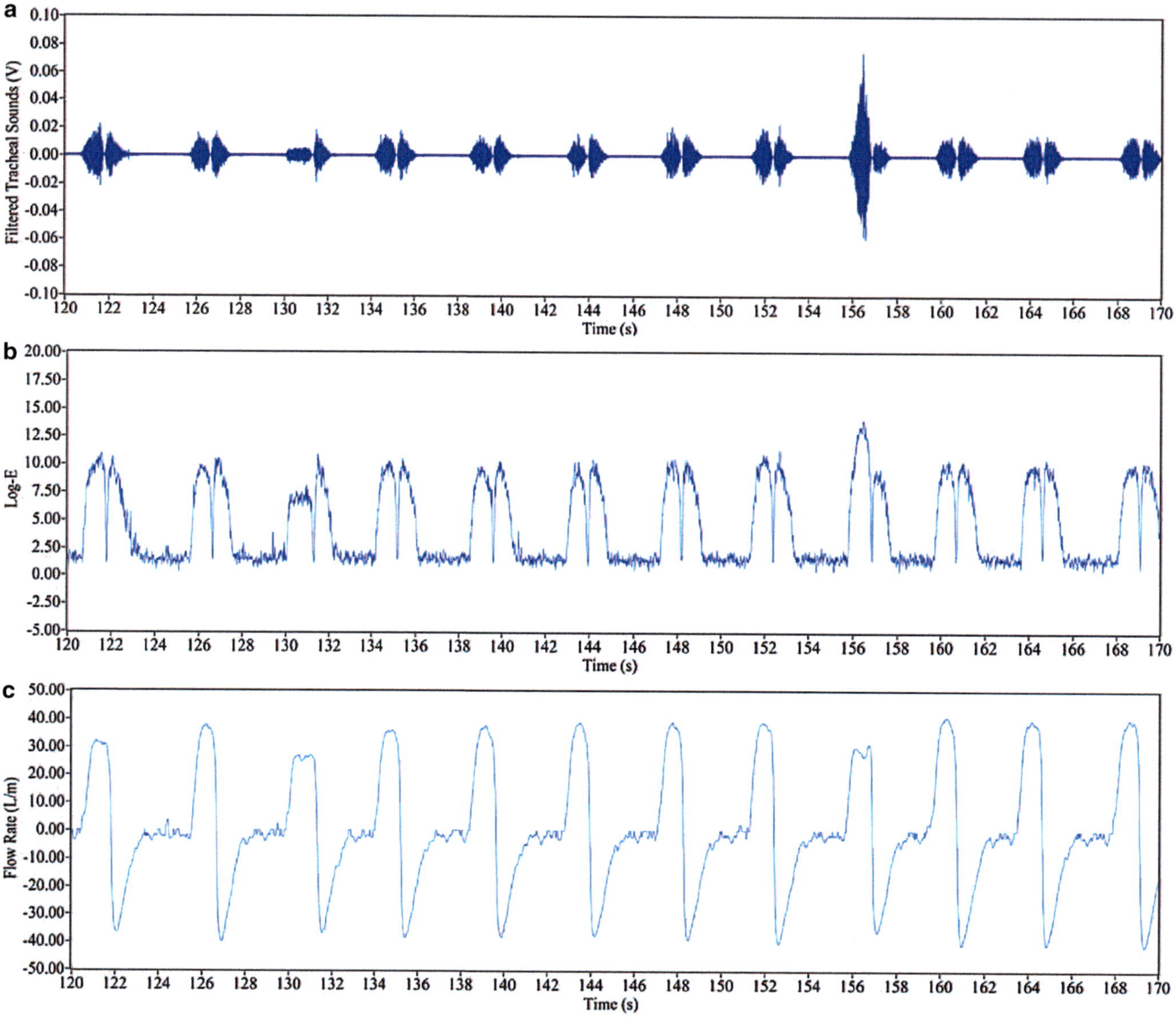

Fig. 6.4 (**a**) An example of the filtered tracheal signal from the microphone, (**b**) the processed signal, the logarithm of the tracheal sound entropy (Log-E), and (**c**) the associated airway flow signal from the pneumotachometer [28]

A 2007 study of 248 children (1 month to 18 years), using pooled raw data from four independently conducted studies, found a moderate correlation between BIS and UMSS with the use of chloral hydrate, pentobarbital, propofol, and midazolam, but poor correlation with ketamine and with opioids. BIS values were significantly lower for a same observed level of sedation with propofol and pentobarbital when compared to midazolam and chloral hydrate, making BIS an unreliable method for targeting a desired level of sedation [34]. The poor correlation observed with opioids is thought to be secondary to opioids providing sedation without hypnosis [34, 35]. Hence, it has been argued that BIS reflects cortical activity rather than level of consciousness [36].

Overly et al., in a study of 47 patients treated either with ketamine/midazolam, methohexital, propofol, or midazolam and a narcotic found a good correlation between BIS and OAA/S scale for non-dissociative agents, but not with ketamine [37]. Ketamine sedation, in multiple studies, has shown an unreliable correlation between BIS and standard sedation scoring, with persistence of high BIS or even an increase in BIS despite achieving deeper levels of sedation [34, 35, 37].

Dexmedetomidine, a selective alpha-2 adrenergic agonist that provides sedation without respiratory depression, has shown to correlate well with standard observational sedation scores. In a study of 11 mechanically ventilated children in an intensive care unit setting sedated with dexmedetomidine, significant correlations between Richmond agitation sedation scale and BIS values were found [38].

A 2009 crossover study of nine adult volunteers receiving propofol or dexmedetomidine followed by the alternate drug 7 days later also showed good correlation between BIS and OAA/S. However, for a same OAA/S score, BIS values were significantly lower in patients sedated with dexmedetomidine, suggesting that the BIS score is drug-specific with different scores signifying different levels of sedation for different sedation agents [39].

BIS scores in infants less than 6 months of age have been noted to be unreliable during general anesthesia and procedural sedation, likely secondary to the fact that the BIS algorithm was developed using adult EEG data [35, 40].

In summary, procedural sedation studies using BIS monitoring have found wide ranges of BIS values at various depths of sedation that do not correlate with standard sedation scores (e.g., UMMS, OAA/s, or Ramsey score) [29–31]. BIS scores appear to be drug specific and cannot reliably be used with common sedating agents such as ketamine. The utility of BIS monitoring to assess depth of sedation during procedural sedation remains unproven.

Cerebral Oximetry

Another new technology with potential application to procedural sedation is cerebral oximetry. Through near-infrared spectroscopy, cerebral tissue oxygenation (i.e., regional oxygen saturation, rSO_2) is measured by monitoring the nonpulsatile signal component reflecting tissue circulation of arterioles, capillaries, and venules. Unlike conventional pulse oximetry, which monitors the pulsatile signal component reflecting arterial circulation, cerebral oximetry is reliable in low perfusion states, shock, and cardiac arrest. Cerebral oximetry represents a "weighted average" of the tissue circulation and reflects a potentially more accurate measurement of oxygen consumption, similar to and correlating with mixed venous saturations [41, 42].

Cerebral oximetry has been primarily studied in the operating room, except for a recent ED procedural sedation study, which demonstrated poor correlation between cerebral oximetry, pulse oximetry, and capnography [43]. In this study, 100 children of ages 9 months to 18 years were sedated with various agents (ketamine, fentanyl, pentobarbital, dexmedetomidine, or propofol). Changes in rSO_2 occurred in 2.1 % of patients and were associated with changes in SpO_2 23 % of the time and changes in end-tidal CO_2 29 % of the time. Only a minority of hypoxic episodes resulted in a decrease in rSO_2, while the majority of changes in rSO_2 occurred in the absence of changes in cardiorespiratory parameters.

Although rSO_2 appears to be a more sensitive measure of cerebral oxygenation than pulse oximetry, isolated decreases in rSO_2 do not appear to correlate well with short- or long-term neurological outcome, as illustrated in a small study of adult patients undergoing carotid endarterectomy. Importantly, there is no clear rSO_2 threshold under which clinically significant brain hypoxia occurs [44].

Noninvasive Cardiovascular Monitoring

Methods for advanced noninvasive cardiovascular monitoring continue to be refined. Through thoracic electrical bioimpedance, and similar to impedance cardiography, electrical cardiometry (or electrical velocimetry) enables the measurement of various cardiac parameters including cardiac output, cardiac index, stroke volume, systemic vascular resistance, and index of contractility. Such methods rely on the interpretation of a signal from sensors placed on the neck and chest, which quantify changes in conductivity of the blood in the aorta during the cardiac cycle [45–47].

Electrical velocimetry measurements have been shown to correlate with measurements derived from the Fick principle applied to blood sampled invasively in pediatric patients with congenital heart disease undergoing left heart catheterization [48], and to transesophageal echocardiography in ventilated children following cardiac surgery—although electrical velocimetry appeared to underestimate cardiac output in terms of absolute values [49]. Impedance cardiography has shown good correlation with standard pulmonary artery thermodilution methods during cardiac surgery [50].

The applicability and clinical relevance of advanced noninvasive cardiovascular monitoring to pediatric procedural sedation appear promising. A recent study used noninvasive cardiovascular monitoring during procedural sedation in children to examine the effects of high-dose dexmedetomidine sedation on heart rate, cardiac index, stroke index, and systemic vascular resistance. It was found that during dexmedetomidine sedations of less than 10 min, heart rate and cardiac index decreased transiently before returning to baseline during recovery. In dexmedetomidine sedations greater than 10 min, the heart rate and cardiac index remained decreased during recovery, with an associated increase in systemic vascular resistance that preserved the noninvasive blood pressure [51].

Conclusion

There have been significant advances in noninvasive physiological monitoring of ventilation, oxygenation, and hemodynamics for procedural sedation in children with the advent of improved motion control in pulse oximetry, low-flow capnography systems, and the potential of cerebral (regional) oximetry and entropy depth of sedation monitoring. These systems bring enhanced safety and efficiency to pediatric procedural sedation. Surprisingly, and despite the added safety of monitoring, a recent report of the Pediatric Sedation Research Consortium found that adherence to guidelines set forth by multiple professional organizations was highly variable [52]. In the words of a 2012 editorial in *JAMA Pediatrics*, "this lack of adherence to sedation guidelines is akin to driving a car at night with no headlights and no speedometer; at some point a disaster will happen" [53].

Future directions in pediatric procedural sedation will include the monitoring of drug-specific parameters of cerebral activity. In a recent small study of anesthetized children by Kuhnle et al., plasma propofol concentrations correlated with mid-latency auditory-evoked potentials (MLAEP) in a dose-dependent manner, hence making MLAEP a potential useful tool for assessing the depth of sedation in children undergoing propofol sedation [54]. Another study by Cheung et al. evaluated the performance of aepEX™, an auditory-evoked potential monitor, during propofol–remifentanil anesthesia, and found it comparable to BIS for differentiating between consciousness and unconsciousness but less useful in distinguishing different depths of sedation [55]. In addition, a recent study by Purdon et al. investigated the EEG signature of unconsciousness in patients undergoing propofol sedation [56]. Other sophisticated methods (for data display, interpretive algorithms, composite indices based on integration of physiological parameters) and new technology to monitor blood pressure, vascular tone, cardiac output, ventilation, and oxygenation will likely be part of the growing sedation monitoring landscape; Yu et al., in a 2013 study, placed a microphone over the trachea of propofol- and remifentanil-sedated patients to demonstrate that the entropy of the acoustic signal may provide an early warning to the onset of obstructive and central apnea [28].

In addition to the development and validation of new technological advances, updating guidelines and monitoring adherence will continue to be paramount to the ongoing establishment of a culture of safety in pediatric procedural sedation.

References

1. Krauss B, Green SM. Procedural sedation and analgesia in children. Lancet. 2006;367(9512):766–80.
2. American Academy of Pediatrics, American Academy of Pediatric Dentistry. Guidelines for monitoring and management of pediatric patients during and after sedation for diagnostic and therapeutic procedures: an update. Pediatrics. 2006;118:2587–602.
3. American Society of Anesthesiologists. Practice guidelines for sedation and analgesia by non-anesthesiologists. Anesthesiology. 2002;96:1004–17.
4. American College of Emergency Physicians. Clinical policy: procedural sedation and analgesia in the emergency department. Ann Emerg Med. 2005;45:177–96.
5. Sedation and Anesthesia Care standards. Oakbrook Terrace: Joint Commission on Accreditation of Healthcare Organizations. http://www.jcaho.org
6. Krauss B, Green SM. Procedural sedation and analgesia in children. N Engl J Med. 2000;342:948–56.
7. New W. Pulse oximetry. J Clin Monit. 1985;1:126.
8. Alexander CM, Teller LE, Gross JB. Principles of pulse oximetry: theoretical and practical considerations. Anesth Analg. 1989; 68:368–76.
9. Tremper KK, Barker SJ. Pulse oximetry. Anesthesiology. 1989;70:98–108.
10. Sinex JE. Pulse oximetry: principles and limitations. Am J Emerg Med. 1999;17:59–67.
11. Burton JH, Harrah JD, Germann CA, Dillon DC. Does end-tidal carbon dioxide monitoring detect respiratory events prior to current sedation monitoring practices? Acad Emerg Med. 2006; 13:500–4.
12. Fu ES, Downs JB, Schweiger JW, Miguel RV, Smith RA. Supplemental oxygen impairs detection of hypoventilation by pulse oximetry. Chest. 2004;126:1552–8.
13. Swedlow DB. Capnometry and capnography: the anesthesia disaster early warning system. Semin Anesth. 1986;3:194–205.
14. Smalhout B, Kalenda Z. An atlas of capnography. Kerckebusch Zeist: Utrecht; 1975.
15. Colman Y, Krauss B. Microstream capnography technology: a new approach to an old problem. J Clin Monit. 1999;15:403–9.
16. Friesen RH, Alswang M. End-tidal PCO_2 monitoring via nasal cannulae in pediatric patients: accuracy and sources of error. J Clin Monit. 1996;12(2):155–9.
17. Gravenstein N. Capnometry in infants should not be done at lower sampling flow rates. J Clin Monit. 1989;5:63–4.
18. Sasse FJ. Can we trust end-tidal carbon dioxide measurements in infants? J Clin Monit. 1985;1:147–8.
19. Berengo A, Cutillo A. Single-breath analysis of carbon dioxide concentration records. J Appl Physiol. 1961;16:522–30.
20. Krauss B, Deykin A, Lam A, Ryoo JJ, Hampton DR, Schmitt PW, et al. Capnogram shape in obstructive lung disease. Anesth Analg. 2005;100:884–8.
21. Hoffbrand BI. The expiratory capnogram: a measure of ventilation-perfusion inequalities. Thorax. 1966;21:518–23.
22. Yamanaka MK, Sue DY. Comparison of arterial-end-tidal PCO_2 difference and dead space/tidal volume ratio in respiratory failure. Chest. 1987;92:832–5.
23. Hardman JG, Aitkenhead AR. Estimating alveolar dead space from the arterial to end-tidal CO_2 gradient: a modeling analysis. Anesth Analg. 2003;97:1846–51.
24. Krauss B, Hess DR. Capnography for procedural sedation and analgesia in the emergency department. Ann Emerg Med. 2007; 50:172–81.
25. Lumb AB, editor. Respiratory system resistance. In: Nunn's applied respiratory physiology. 6th ed. Oxford: Butterworth-Heinemann; 2005.
26. Wilson WC, Shapiro B. Perioperative hypoxia: the clinical spectrum and current oxygen monitoring methodology. Anesthesiol Clin North Am. 2001;19:769–812.
27. West JB. Respiratory physiology, the essentials. 6th ed. Philadelphia: Lippincott Williams & Wilkins; 2000.
28. Yu L, Ting C-K, Hill BE, Orr JA, Brewer LM, Johnson KB, et al. Using the entropy of tracheal sounds to detect apnea during sedation in healthy nonobese volunteers. Anesthesiology. 2013; 118(6):1341–9.

29. Agrawal D, Feldman HA, Krauss B, Waltzman ML. Can bispectral index monitoring quantify depth of sedation during procedural sedation and analgesia in the pediatric emergency department? Ann Emerg Med. 2004;43:247–55.
30. Gill M, Green SM, Krauss B. A study of the bispectral index monitor during procedural sedation and analgesia in the emergency department. Ann Emerg Med. 2003;41:234–41.
31. Miner JR, Biros M, Heegaard W, Plummer D. Bispectral EEG analysis of patients undergoing procedural sedation in the emergency department. Acad Emerg Med. 2003;10:638–43.
32. American Society of Anesthesiologists. Practice advisory for intraoperative awareness and brain function monitoring. Anesthesiology. 2006;104:847–64.
33. Rosow C, Manberg PJ. Bispectral index monitoring. Anesthesiol Clin North Am. 2001;19:947–66.
34. Malviya S, Voepel-Lewis T, Tait AR, Watcha MF, Sadhasivam S, Friesen RH. Effect of age and sedative agent on the accuracy of bispectral index in detecting depth of sedation in children. Pediatrics. 2007;120(3):e461–70.
35. McDermott NB, VanSickle T, Motas D, Friesen RH. Validation of the bispectral index monitor during conscious and deep sedation in children. Anesth Analg. 2003;97(1):39–43.
36. Hans P, Dewandre P-Y, Brichant JF, Bonhomme V. Comparative effects of ketamine on bispectral index and spectral entropy of the electroencephalogram under sevoflurane anaesthesia. Br J Anaesth. 2005;94(3):336–40.
37. Overly FL, Wright RO, Connor FA, Fontaine B, Jay G, Linakis JG. Bispectral analysis during pediatric procedural sedation. Pediatr Emerg Care. 2005;21(1):6–11.
38. Turkmen A, Altan A, Turgut N, Vatansever S, Gokkaya S. The correlation between the Richmond agitation-sedation scale and bispectral index during dexmedetomidine sedation. Eur J Anaesthesiol. 2006;23(4):300–4.
39. Kasuya Y, Govinda R, Rauch S, Mascha EJ, Sessler DI, Turan A. The correlation between bispectral index and observational sedation scale in volunteers sedated with dexmedetomidine and propofol. Anesth Analg. 2009;109(6):1811–5.
40. Rampil IJ. A primer for EEG signal processing in anesthesia. Anesthesiology. 1998;89(4):980–1002.
41. Tortoriello TA, Stayer SA, Mott AR, McKenzie ED, Fraser CD, Andropoulos DB, et al. A noninvasive estimation of mixed venous oxygen saturation using near-infrared spectroscopy by cerebral oximetry in pediatric cardiac surgery patients. Paediatr Anaesth. 2005;15(6):495–503.
42. Watzman HM, Kurth CD, Montenegro LM, Rome J, Steven JM, Nicolson SC. Arterial and venous contributions to near-infrared cerebral oximetry. Anesthesiology. 2000;93(4):947–53.
43. Padmanabhan P, Berkenbosch JW, Lorenz D, Pierce MC. Evaluation of cerebral oxygenation during procedural sedation in children using near infrared spectroscopy. Ann Emerg Med. 2009; 54(2):205–13.
44. Carlin RE, McGraw DJ, Calimlim JR, Mascia MF. The use of near-infrared cerebral oximetry in awake carotid endarterectomy. J Clin Anesth. 1998;10(2):109–13.
45. Absi MA, Lutterman J, Wetzel GT. Noninvasive cardiac output monitoring in the pediatric cardiac intensive care unit. Curr Opin Cardiol. 2010;25(2):77–9.
46. Kubicek WG, Karnegis JN, Patterson RP, Witsoe DA, Mattson RH. Development and evaluation of an impedance cardiac output system. Aerosp Med. 1966;37(12):1208–12.
47. Schmidt C, Theilmeier G, Van Aken H, Korsmeier P, Wirtz SP, Berendes E, et al. Comparison of electrical velocimetry and transoesophageal Doppler echocardiography for measuring stroke volume and cardiac output. Br J Anaesth. 2005;95(5):603–10.
48. Norozi K, Beck C, Osthaus WA, Wille I, Wessel A, Bertram H. Electrical velocimetry for measuring cardiac output in children with congenital heart disease. Br J Anaesth. 2008;100(1):88–94.
49. Schubert S, Schmitz T, Weiss M, Nagdyman N, Huebler M, Alexi-Meskishvili V, et al. Continuous, non-invasive techniques to determine cardiac output in children after cardiac surgery: evaluation of transesophageal Doppler and electric velocimetry. J Clin Monit Comput. 2008;22(4):299–307.
50. Suttner S, Schöllhorn T, Boldt J, Mayer J, Röhm KD, Lang K, et al. Noninvasive assessment of cardiac output using thoracic electrical bioimpedance in hemodynamically stable and unstable patients after cardiac surgery: a comparison with pulmonary artery thermodilution. Intensive Care Med. 2006;32(12):2053–8.
51. Wong J, Steil GM, Curtis M, Papas A, Zurakowski D, Mason KP. Cardiovascular effects of dexmedetomidine sedation in children. Anesth Analg. 2012;114(1):193–9.
52. Langhan ML, Mallory M, Hertzog J, Lowrie L, Cravero J, Pediatric Sedation Research Consortium. Physiologic monitoring practices during pediatric procedural sedation: a report from the Pediatric Sedation Research Consortium. Arch Pediatr Adolesc Med. 2012;166(11):990–8.
53. Coté CJ. American Academy of Pediatrics sedation guidelines: are we there yet? Arch Pediatr Adolesc Med. 2012;166(11):1067–9.
54. Kuhnle GE, Hornuss C, Lenk M, Salam AP, Wiepcke D, Edelmann-Gahr V, et al. Impact of propofol on mid-latency auditory-evoked potentials in children. Br J Anaesth. 2013;110(6):1001–9.
55. Cheung YM, Scoones GP, Hoeks SE, Stolker RJ, Weber F. Evaluation of the aepEX™ monitor of hypnotic depth in pediatric patients receiving propofol-remifentanil anesthesia. Paediatr Anaesth. 2013;23(10):891–7.
56. Purdon PL, Pierce ET, Mukamel EA, Prerau MJ, Walsh JL, Wong KF, et al. Electroencephalogram signatures of loss and recovery of consciousness from propofol. Proc Natl Acad Sci U S A. 2013;110(12):E1142–51.
57. Green SM, Krauss B. The semantics of ketamine. Ann Emerg Med. 2000;36:480–2.
58. Green SM, Krauss B. Clinical practice guideline for emergency department ketamine dissociative sedation in children. Ann Emerg Med. 2004;44(5):460–71. Review.

The Pediatric Airway: Anatomy, Challenges, and Solutions

7

Lynne R. Ferrari

Abstract

Sedation may alter laryngeal anatomy, function, and respiratory mechanics; therefore, it is essential that the practitioner has a thorough understanding of the pediatric airway. Physical examination reveals the general condition of a patient and the degree of the airway compromise. During sedation, adequate oxygenation and ventilation must be maintained despite a relative decrease in rate and depth of respiration. Conditions that interfere with the integrity of the laryngeal inlet or upper larynx may impair effective ventilation as a result of partial or complete airway obstruction. Sleep-disordered breathing (SDB) is a spectrum of disorders ranging from primary snoring to obstructive sleep apnea syndrome (OSAS). When sedation without a secured airway is planned it is imperative that the level of consciousness, adequacy of ventilation, and oxygenation be continuously monitored and the risk of apnea be evaluated. When a child is sedated, the best prevention is to insure that the position provides the best anatomic orientation for airway patency.

Keywords

Sleep-disordered breathing (SDB) • Obstructive sleep apnea (OSA) • Airway obstruction • Upper respiratory infection (URI) • Pharyngeal anatomy • Laryngomalacia • Anterior mediastinal mass • Obstructive sleep apnea syndrome (OSAS) • Laryngeal mask airway (LMA) • Pediatric advanced life support (PALS) • American Heart Association (AHA)

One of the most important aspects of planning sedation is consideration of the airway of each individual patient. Sedation may alter laryngeal anatomy, function, and respiratory mechanics; therefore, it is essential that the practitioner has a thorough understanding of the pediatric airway.

L.R. Ferrari, M.D. (✉)
Department of Anesthesiology, Perioperative and Pain Medicine, Boston Children's Hospital, 300 Longwood Avenue, Boston, MA 02115, USA
e-mail: lynne.ferrari@childrens.harvard.edu

Anatomy of the Pediatric Airway

Airway compromise in the infant or child may result from abnormalities in the nasal cavities, nasopharynx, oral cavity, pharynx, and neck. The airway is comprised of the larynx, trachea, bronchi, and alveoli. The trachea in the infant is smaller than that of the adult and since the function of the trachea is passive during respiration, anatomic differences in the infant and adult trachea are not as apparent as they are in the larynx [1]. The infant larynx is not a miniature version of the adult larynx and there are essential differences between these two organs. The differences are related to size, location, and configuration, and must be considered since the primary function of the larynx is to protect the lower airway and regulate airflow during respiration by controlling the resistance

K.P. Mason (ed.), *Pediatric Sedation Outside of the Operating Room: A Multispecialty International Collaboration*, DOI 10.1007/978-1-4939-1390-9_7, © Springer Science+Business Media New York 2015

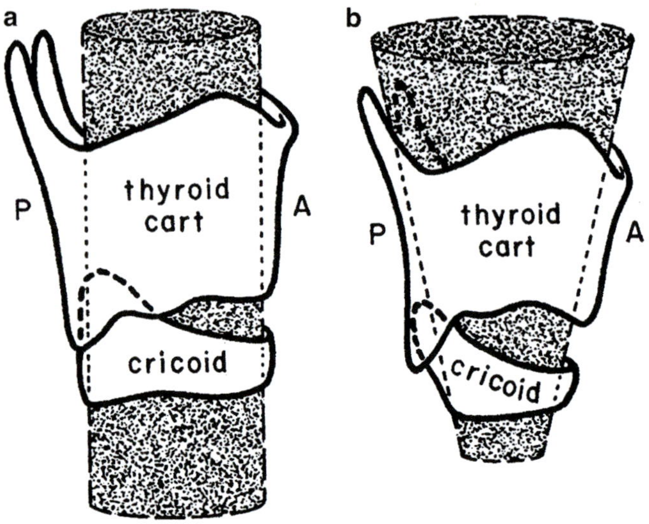

Fig. 7.1 Configuration of (**a**) the adult larynx and (**b**) infant larynx (Reprinted with permission from Wheeler M, Coté CJ, Todres D. The Pediatric Airway. Chapter 5. In: Coté CJ, Todres ID, Goudsouzian NG, Ryan JF (editors). A Practice of Anesthesia for Infants and Children, 3rd edition. Philadelphia, PA: W. B. Saunders Company. 2001)

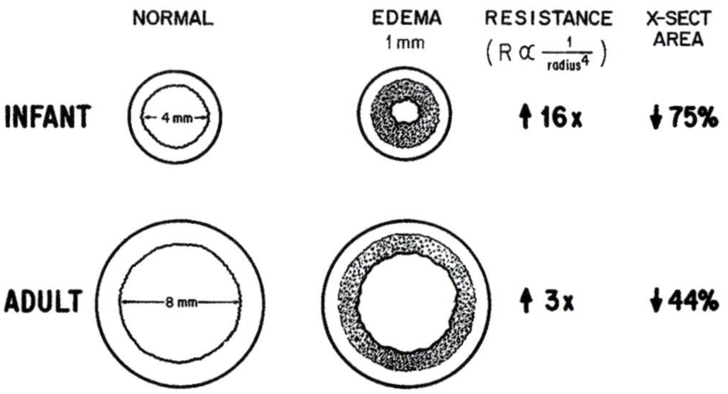

Fig. 7.2 Relative effect of circumferential edema on the infant and adult airway (Reprinted with permission from Wheeler M, Coté CJ, Todres D. The Pediatric Airway. Chapter 5. In: Coté CJ, Todres ID, Goudsouzian NG, Ryan JF (editors). A Practice of Anesthesia for Infants and Children, 3rd edition. Philadelphia, PA: W. B. Saunders Company. 2001)

during inspiration and exhalation. The cricoid ring is the narrowest portion of the infant larynx. Although this has recently been questioned, there are insufficient data to refute the validity of this anatomic finding [2]. In the infant and child, the cricoid cartilage is a non-expansile complete ring whereas, this cartilage is open at the posterior aspect in the adult patients [3, 4] (Fig. 7.1). In the adult patient the vocal cords are the narrowest part of the airway, providing the cylindrical shape of the adult larynx in contrast to the cone shape of the pediatric larynx. This is an important distinction to make since the resistance to airflow is inversely proportional to the fourth power of the radius ($R = 1/\text{radius}^4$ [5]). One cen-

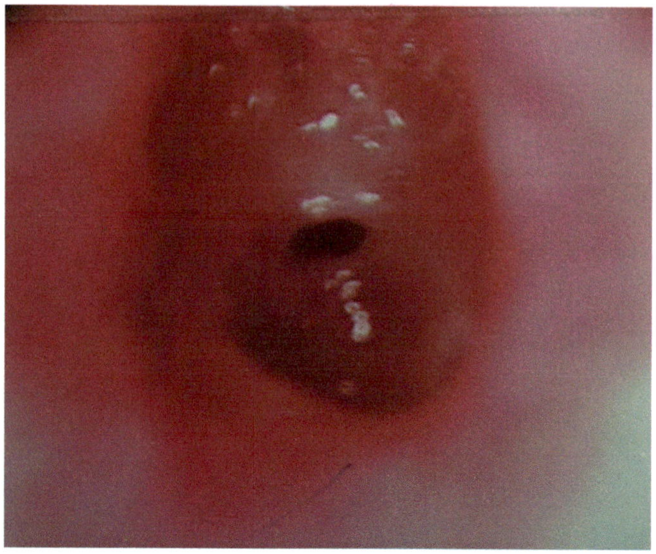

Fig. 7.3 Child with post-intubation subglottic stenosis (Photo courtesy of Reza Rahbar, DMD, MD, Children's Hospital Boston)

timeter of circumferential edema in the infant larynx will decrease the cross-sectional area by 75 % and increase the resistance by 16-fold as compared to the same one centimeter of edema in the adult larynx, which will result in a decrease in the cross-sectional area of only 44 % and threefold increase in resistance (Fig. 7.2). This becomes relevant when sedating a child with either a history of prolonged intubation in which the tracheal lumen may be narrowed, or a child with a recent upper respiratory infection or croup, which also may result in a circumferentially narrow airway (Figs. 7.3 and 7.4).

The larynx of the infant and young child is higher than in the adult patient. The adult larynx is located at C6–7, whereas it is at C4 in the infant and descends to the adult location as growth occurs during childhood. The cephalad location of the infant larynx makes oral ventilation difficult, and as a result the infant is an obligate nasal breather for the first year of life [5]. The epiglottis projects vertically in the adult, but posteriorly in the infant. The infant epiglottis is also narrower and omega shaped, which makes it more prone to obstructing the laryngeal inlet [6] (Fig. 7.5). In the setting of nasal congestion, effective ventilation may be compromised in the unaltered state and worsened after sedation.

The tongue of the infant is larger in relation to the oral cavity than that of the older child and adult. In neonates, the tongue is more anterior than the larynx so that the epiglottis can contact the soft palate and allow respirations and sucking simultaneously. This does, however, predispose the infant to airway obstruction more readily than the older child. At birth, the base of the tongue resides in the oral cavity and gradually descends with the larynx to a more caudad position

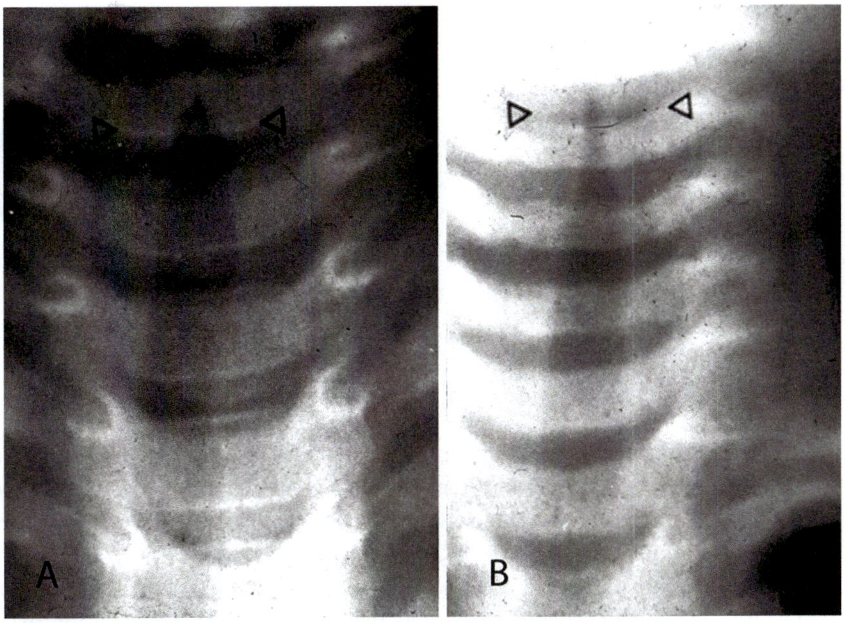

Fig. 7.4 Plain X-ray of the airway of a child with (**a**) severe croup and (**b**) mild croup. Note the subglottic narrowing and appearance of the characteristic "Chrysler Building" sign (Photo courtesy of Reza Rahbar, DMD, MD, Children's Hospital Boston)

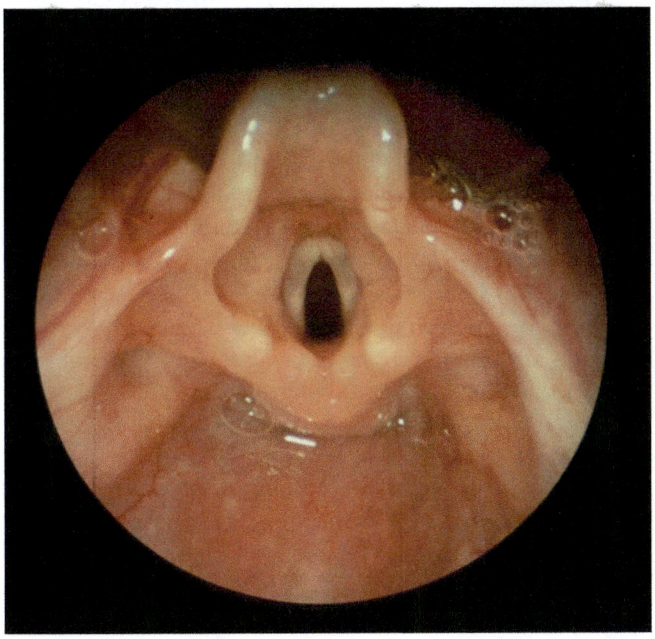

Fig. 7.5 Normal infant larynx. Note the omega-shaped epiglottis (Photo courtesy of Reza Rahbar, DMD, MD, Children's Hospital Boston)

by the fourth year of life. The ratio of soft tissue to bony structures is higher in the infant and thus predisposes this group of patients to a greater risk of mechanical oropharyngeal obstruction. The combination of small nares, large tongue, small mandible, excess soft tissue, and short neck also increases the infant's susceptibility to airway obstruction [7]. The ribs of the infant and small child are more horizontal in orientation than those of the older child and adult, and more flexible, which therefore predisposes the child to ventilatory compromise. As previously noted, since the metabolic rate and oxygen consumption of infants is double than that of the adult and the functional residual capacity is smaller, the rapidity of desaturation in the infant and child is much greater. For this reason optimal surveillance of the airway and respiratory mechanics is essential if hypoxia is to be avoided [8].

Normal spontaneous breathing is accomplished by minimal work, and obstruction of either the upper or lower airway will result in increased work of breathing. To avoid this it is essential that airway obstruction and compromises in ventilation be recognized and corrected early. Infants and children may rapidly progress from normal breathing to obstruction, and compromised respiration to respiratory distress, and eventual cardiac arrest. Since oxygen consumption is higher in infants, decreases in oxygen delivery will result in more rapid compromise than is observed in older patient populations. The presence of apnea leading to inadequate alveolar ventilation may rapidly progress to hypoxemia, hypercarbia, and eventual tissue hypoxia.

Assessment of the Pediatric Airway for Sedation

Physical examination reveals the general condition of a patient and the degree of the airway compromise. Laboratory examination may include assessment of hemoglobin, a chest

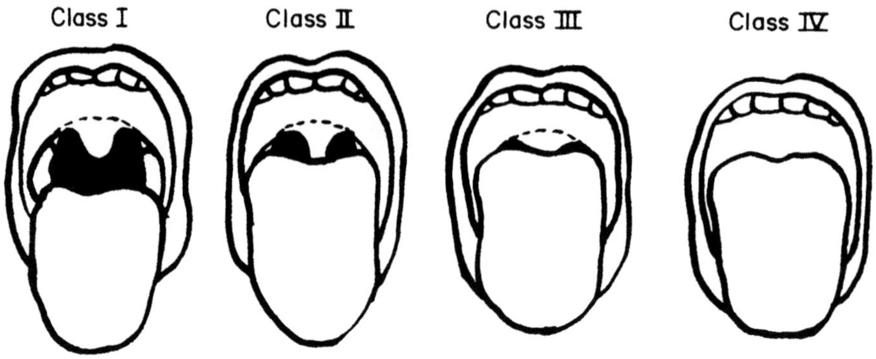

Fig. 7.6 Mallampati classification of pharyngeal structures (Reprinted with permission from Samsoon GL, Young JR. Difficult tracheal intubation: A retrospective study. Anaesthesia. 1987 May;42(5):487–490)

radiograph, and barium swallow, which can aid in identifying lesions that may be compressing the trachea. Other radiologic examinations such as magnetic resonance imaging (MRI) and computed tomography (CT) scan may be indicated in isolated instances but are not routinely ordered.

The physical examination of the airway in children begins with simple observation, since approaching an anxious child may cause inconsolable crying and distortion of the physical examination. Observation of the general appearance, noting color of the skin and the presence of pallor, cyanosis, rash, jaundice, unusual markings, birthmarks, and scars from previous operations should be documented.

The degree of mouth opening should be noted and full examination of the oropharyngeal area should be completed. The distance from the temporomandibular joint to the angle of the ramus is helpful in the assessment of the adequacy of the mouth opening. The distance between the angle of the ramus and the mentum is a good predictor of the ability of the mandibular bony structure to accommodate the oropharyngeal soft tissue. The presence of loose teeth should be documented. Special attention should be paid to the condition of the soft and hard palates, the dentition, and the size of the tongue. The relation of the tongue to the other oropharyngeal structures should be noted. For instance, a large thick tongue may pose minimal increased risk for airway obstruction in a child with an otherwise normal oropharynx but may cause severe risk in the child with a narrow oropharynx or a high arched palate (as may be present in children with craniofacial abnormalities and syndromes) where the tongue occupies a greater proportion of the bony structure volume. The amount of the posterior pharynx that can be visualized is important and correlates with the difficulty of intubation, and in sedated patients would correlate with the potential for airway obstruction. The Mallampati classification (Class I–IV) is based on the structures visualized with maximal mouth opening and tongue protrusion in the sitting position (Fig. 7.6) [9, 10]. The soft palate, fauces, uvula, and pillars are visualized in patients with a Class I airway. The soft palate, fauces, and portion of the uvula but no pillars are visualized in Class II. The soft palate and base of uvula are visualized in Class III and only the hard palate is visualized in Class IV [10]. Tonsil size should be evaluated since the tonsils of pediatric patients are frequently enlarged and may be the source of upper airway obstruction. A standardized system for evaluation of tonsils exists and is based on the percentage of pharyngeal area that is occupied by hypertrophied tonsils. Class 0 tonsils are completely limited to the tonsillar fossa. Class +1 tonsils take up less than 25 %, Class +2 tonsils take up between 25 and 50 %, and Class +3 tonsils take up 50–75 % of the pharyngeal area. Class +4 tonsils take up greater than 75 % of the oropharynx and are commonly referred to as "kissing tonsils" [11] (Fig. 7.7). Tonsillar hyperplasia may increase the risk of airway obstruction in the sedated patient when the tonsils occupy the oropharyngeal space outside of the tonsillar fossa as in Class +3 and Class +4 anatomy. Conversely, lesser degrees of hyperplasia as seen in Class +1 and Class +2 may result in airway obstruction in the sedated patient with craniofacial abnormalities such as Down syndrome.

Abnormal facies might be an indication of a syndrome or constellation of congenital abnormalities. One congenital anomaly often is associated with others. The neck should be examined primarily to determine if the trachea is midline and to evaluate tracheal length and soft tissue volume. In the child with a short neck and abundant soft tissue, the potential for oropharyngeal airway obstruction is greater.

The rate, depth, and quality of respirations should be evaluated. The pattern of breathing should be noted as well as the rate and depth of respiration. Use of accessory muscles may indicate an increased work of breathing due to an effort to overcome upper or lower airway obstruction. Nasal or upper respiratory obstruction is indicated by noisy or labored breathing. The color, viscosity, and quantity of nasal discharge should be documented. If the child is coughing, the origin of the cough (upper versus lower airway) and the quality (dry or wet) can be evaluated even before auscultation of the lungs. The presence of wheezing, audible stridor, or retractions should be noted. The airway should be evaluated for ease of intubation in the case of urgent intervention.

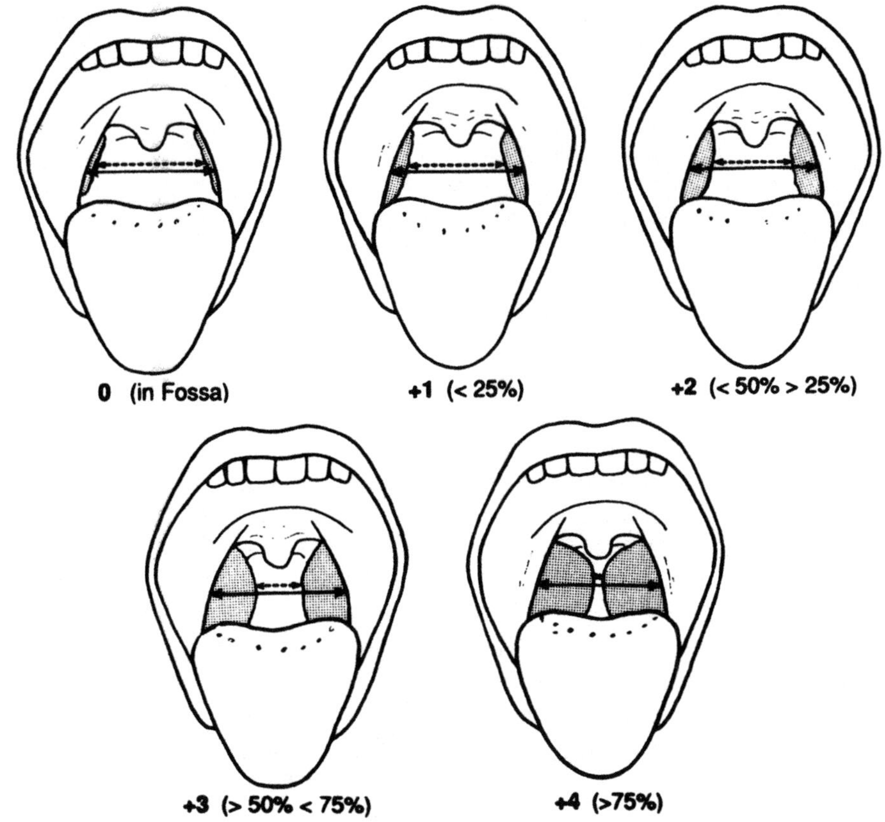

Fig. 7.7 Classification of tonsillar hypertrophy (Reprinted with permission from Brodsky L. Modern assessment of tonsils and adenoids. Pediatr Clin North Am. 1989;36: 1551–1569. WB Saunders)

If the child will not open his or her mouth, a manual estimation of the thyrohyoid distance should be made. Children with micrognathia, as in Pierre Robin syndrome or Goldenhar syndrome, may be especially difficult to intubate, especially in an unanticipated situation.

Risk Factors for Airway Compromise or Depression

During sedation, adequate oxygenation and ventilation must be maintained despite a relative decrease in rate and depth of respiration. Any condition that causes airway compromise should be thoroughly evaluated prior to administration of sedation agents to determine if alteration in respiratory parameters will result in impaired ventilation.

During normal breathing the flow of air is laminar. As previously mentioned the resistance is inversely proportional to the fourth power of the radius. Increased airway resistance occurs when the diameter of an airway is decreased under constant pressure. The radius of an airway may be decreased by circumferential edema, external compression, mucous, secretions, or bronchoconstriction. The work of breathing increases in patients with upper or lower airway disease. Increased airway resistance, decreased lung compliance, and altered central control of respiration will all affect the adequacy of respiration.

Adequacy of respiration may be based on respiratory rate, respiratory effort, tidal volume, chest auscultation, and pulse oximetry. The normal respiratory rate in infants under 1 year of age is up to 30 breaths per minute. The respiratory rate declines to 20 breaths per minute by age 8 years and equals the adult rate of 16–17 breaths per minute by age 18. Alterations in the respiratory rate can indicate underlying comorbidity such as fever, pain, acidosis, and sepsis in tachypneic patients and impending cardiovascular collapse in the bradypneic patient. Increased respiratory effort as recognized by nasal flaring, chest retractions, and uncoordinated chest excursions should alert the clinician that an increased work of breathing may increase if excessive sedation is administered.

Noisy breathing due to obstructed airflow is known as *stridor*. Inspiratory stridor results from upper airway obstruction; expiratory stridor results from lower airway obstruction; and biphasic stridor is present with midtracheal lesions. The evaluation of a patient with stridor begins with a thorough history. The age of onset suggests a cause since laryngotracheomalacia and vocal cord paralysis are usually present at or shortly after birth, whereas cysts or mass lesions develop later in life. Information indicating positions that make the stridor better or worse should be obtained, and placing a patient in a position that allows gravity to aid in reducing obstruction can be of benefit during anesthetic induction.

Patients at risk for airway compromise may have either anatomic or physiologic abnormalities that may predispose them. Anatomic abnormalities may cause the oropharyngeal or tracheobronchial airway to be compromised and ventilation to be impaired by small changes in position. The anatomic imbalance between the upper airway soft tissue volume and the craniofacial size contributes to pharyngeal airway obstruction. Pharyngeal size is determined by the soft tissue volume inside the bony enclosure of the mandible. The magnitude of pharyngeal muscle contraction is controlled by neural mechanisms and the interaction between the anatomical balance and neural mechanisms, which are suppressed in sedated patients, determines pharyngeal airway size and patient ability to maintain a patent airway. An anatomic imbalance between the upper airway soft tissue volume and craniofacial size will result in obstruction. Anatomic imbalance may be compensated for by enhanced neural mechanisms that regulate pharyngeal dilator muscles in patients during wakefulness. When neural mechanisms are suppressed during sleep or sedation, relaxation of pharyngeal dilator muscles occurs and the pharyngeal airway severely narrows [12]. Small changes in function in the setting of normal anatomy may similarly cause inadequate oxygenation. Increasing the distance between the mentum and cervical column will transiently relieve the obstruction. This is achieved by positioning the patient in the sniffing position. Similarly, the sitting position displaces excessive soft tissue outside the bony enclosure through the submandibular space.

Laryngomalacia is the most common cause of stridor in infants and is usually benign and self-limited. It occurs during inspiration and is most often due to a long epiglottis that prolapses posteriorly and prominent arytenoid cartilages with redundant aryepiglottic folds that fall into the glottis and obstruct the glottic opening during inspiration (Fig. 7.8). There is little obstruction during exhalation since the supraglottic structures are pushed out of the way during expiration. Intermittent low-pitched inspiratory stridor is the hallmark symptom, which appears during the first 2 weeks of life. Symptoms peak at 6 months of age when they are at their worst, then gradually resolve. Although most children are symptom-free by 18–24 months, the stridor can persist for years. The definitive diagnosis is obtained by direct laryngoscopy and rigid or flexible bronchoscopy. Preliminary examination is usually carried out in the surgeon's office. A small, flexible fiberoptic bronchoscope is inserted through the nares into the oropharynx, and the movement of the vocal cords is observed [13]. Other etiologies include foreign body aspiration, infection such as croup or laryngotracheobronchitis, edema, or mass lesions such as cyst or tumor.

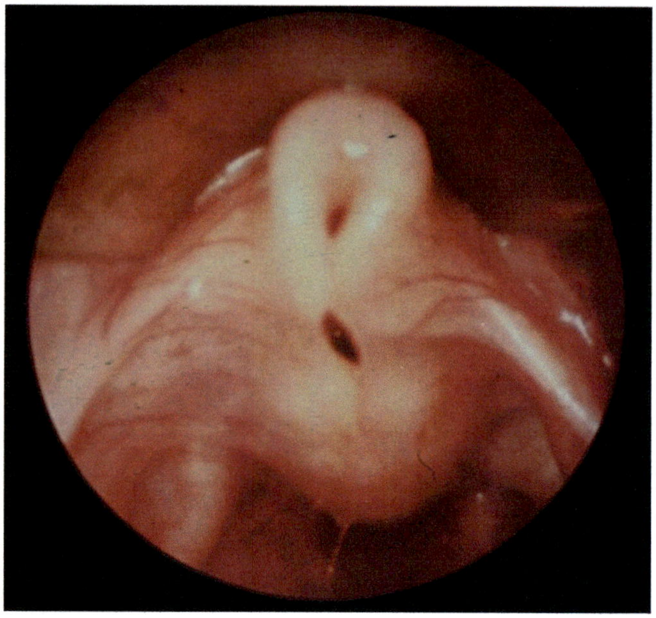

Fig. 7.8 Larynx of an infant with laryngomalacia (Photo courtesy of Reza Rahbar, DMD, MD, Children's Hospital Boston)

Grunting is a low-pitched sound that results when a patient exhales against a closed glottis and is heard on exhalation. Infants and children often grunt to keep the small airways and alveoli open in an attempt to optimize ventilation and oxygenation. The presence of grunting may be a sign of severe respiratory distress and impending respiratory failure. Underlying causes include pneumonia, acute respiratory distress syndrome, pulmonary edema, congestive heart failure, and abdominal splinting.

Wheezing during inspiration or exhalation, or both, indicates intrathoracic obstruction of small airways. It may be a result of intrinsic reactive airways, bronchospasm, or foreign body aspiration. Hypoxemia that is present in the wheezing patient may worsen during administration of sedation.

One of the most challenging decisions in caring for children is establishing criteria for cancelation of a procedure in the presence of an upper or lower respiratory infection. Children presenting with symptoms of uncomplicated upper respiratory infection who are afebrile, with clear secretions, and appear otherwise healthy should be able to safely undergo sedation. A history of nocturnal dry cough, wheezing during exercise, and wheezing more than three times in the recent 12 months, or a history of present or past eczema may be associated with an increased risk for bronchospasm, desaturation, or airway obstruction [14]. Nasal congestion, purulent sputum production, and a history of reactive airway disease are predictors of adverse respiratory events, and children with these advanced symptoms of upper and potential lower respiratory disease should not undergo sedation [15].

There are many syndromes that have anatomic components related to the airway. A large tongue is associated with Down, Hunter, Hurler, and Beckwith-Wiedemann syndromes. Congenital hypothyroidism and Pompe disease are also associated with a large tongue. Patients with Pierre Robin, Treacher Collins, and Goldenhar syndromes, as well as children with congenital hemifacial microsomia, have micrognathia, high arched palate, and a potential to have early airway obstruction when sedated. Children with tonsillar hypertrophy are at risk for mechanical airway obstruction due to large tonsils occupying a greater portion of the oropharyngeal airway than normal-sized tonsils.

Former premature infants are at risk for untoward respiratory events during sedation. There is a more gradual slope of the CO_2 response curve in the preterm infant, which predisposes this group of patients to apnea. All neonates exhibit periodic breathing, which is manifested as interrupted ventilation by self-corrected short periods of apnea without desaturation or bradycardia [16]. This tendency diminishes by 45 weeks postconceptual age. Apnea of prematurity and postanesthetic apnea are predominantly central in origin, with about 10 % due to mechanical obstruction. The response to airway obstruction with apnea is common in infants with periodic breathing and decreases with increasing postnatal age. In the sedated neonate and former premature infant, benign periodic breathing may evolve into frank apnea, which must be managed by stimulation or assisted ventilation. To detect postanesthetic or post-sedation apneic events, it is suggested that infants whose age is under 56 weeks postconception be monitored for 24 h after the procedure [17].

Conditions that interfere with the integrity of the laryngeal inlet or upper larynx may impair effective ventilation as a result of partial or complete airway obstruction. Upper respiratory infections cause increased secretions, which may occlude the larynx in addition to the inflammatory response that can compromise the internal diameter of the laryngeal inlet. Laryngotracheobronchitis or croup also decreases the internal laryngeal diameter and produces the same clinical outcome. The incidence of epiglottitis has decreased dramatically in the past decade but may still be encountered. These patients have not only inflammation of the epiglottis but edema of the surrounding structures, which severely restricts the size of the larynx and encroaches on the area for ventilation to occur.

Patients who have sustained airway trauma or thermal injury should be considered in this category as well. Children who have experienced prolonged intubation may have decreased laryngeal inlet diameter as a result of fibrosis from congenital or acquired subglottic stenosis (Figs. 7.9 and 7.10). Any agent that will decrease the pharyngeal muscle tone and rate and depth of respiration in this setting should be given with extreme caution and warrants vigilance.

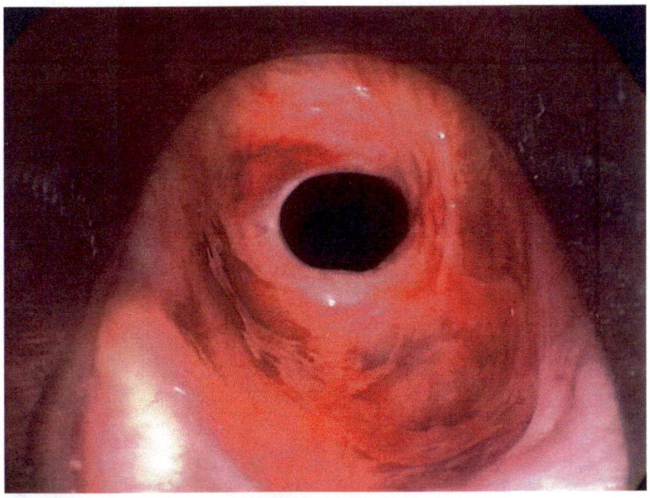

Fig. 7.9 Larynx of an infant with congenital subglottic stenosis (Photo courtesy of Reza Rahbar, DMD, MD, Children's Hospital Boston)

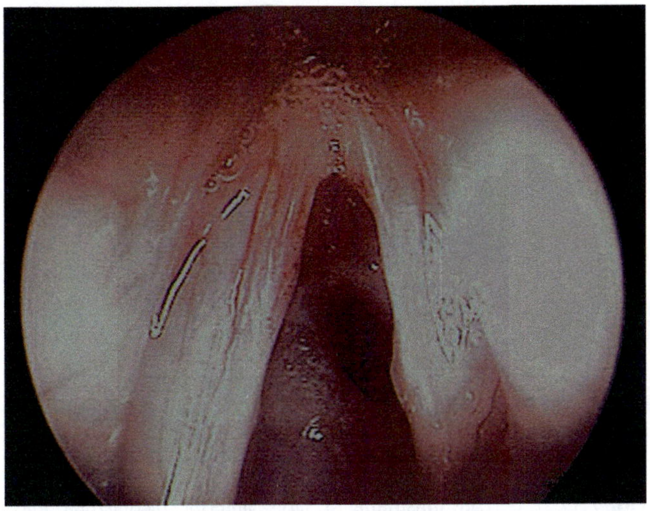

Fig. 7.10 Larynx of an infant with acquired post-intubation subglottic stenosis. (Photo courtesy of Reza Rahbar, DMD, MD, Children's Hospital Boston)

Other conditions that restrict the laryngeal inlet are subglottic stenosis, laryngeal cysts, and papillomatosis.

There is a similar concern for narrowing and compromise of the larynx from external factors. Goiter or other tumors of the neck that are extrinsic to the larynx may cause compression and functional restriction to ventilation. Children with arthrogryposis or congenital abnormalities in which the neck is fused may have difficulty with positioning and subsequent ventilation when airway function is depressed during sedation.

Children with an anterior mediastinal mass are at significant risk for airway compromise during sedation due to compression of the intrathoracic larynx (Figs. 7.11 and 7.12).

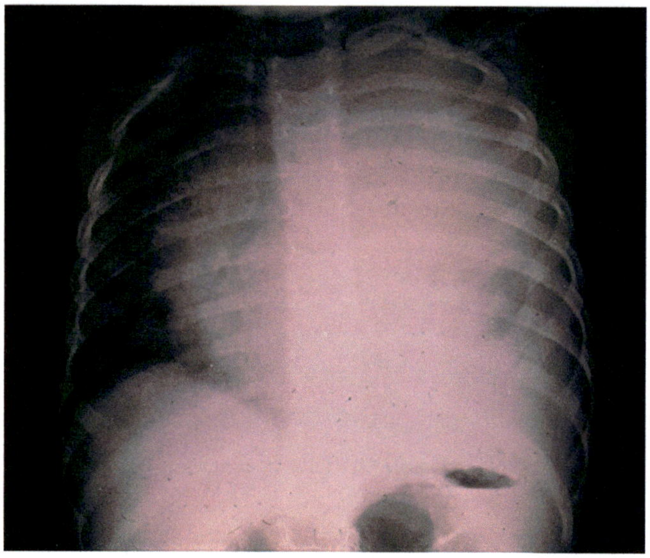

Fig. 7.11 A 20-month-old male with a large anterior mediastinal mass

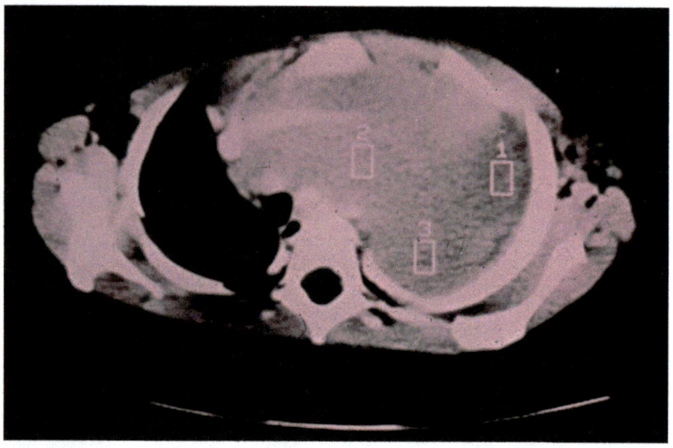

Fig. 7.12 CT scan illustrating a large anterior mediastinal mass compressing the lung and causing tracheal deviation

Although lymphomas constitute the largest group of masses that arise in the anterior mediastinum, other masses that may present in this location include teratomas, cystic hygromas, thymomas, hemangiomas, sarcomas, desmoid tumors, pericardial cysts, and diaphragmatic hernias of the Morgagni type.

To understand the pathophysiology of the anterior mediastinum, it is important to be familiar with the anatomy. The mediastinum is defined as the extrapleural space in the thorax that is bounded anteriorly by the sternum, posteriorly by the thoracic vertebrae, superiorly by the thoracic inlet, and inferiorly by the diaphragm. Structures contained within the mediastinum that may undergo compression from an enlarging mass are the trachea and the main stem bronchi, superior vena cava, aortic arch, main pulmonary artery, and a portion of the heart itself.

Patients with anterior mediastinal masses may present with varied signs and symptoms referable to both the cardiovascular and respiratory systems and are directly related to the location and size of the mass, as well as the degree of compression of surrounding structures. The most commonly observed respiratory symptom is cough, especially in the supine position, which results from anterior compression of the trachea. Infants younger than 2 years of age are more likely to experience wheezing as a sign of tracheal compression, whereas children older than 2 years of age usually present with malaise, cough, fever, and neck mass. Other respiratory findings in patients of all ages include tachypnea, dyspnea, stridor, retractions, decreased breath sounds, and cyanosis on crying, all of which should alert the practitioner to some degree of airway compromise that may worsen when positive intrathoracic pressure is generated.

Cardiovascular symptoms result from compression of the aortic and pulmonary vessels, as well as the right atrium and right ventricle. This can lead to both hypotension secondary to inadequate cardiac filling and restricted pulmonary blood flow resulting in poor oxygenation despite adequate ventilation. Findings referable to the cardiovascular system include fatigue, headache, hypotension or pallor in the supine position, a feeling of light-headedness, superior vena cava syndrome (facial edema, cyanosis, jugular venous distension), and the appearance of a new murmur, especially in the area of the pulmonary valve. It is essential that the practitioner search for these signs and symptoms when interviewing and examining patients with mediastinal masses in an attempt to ascertain the degree of respiratory and cardiovascular compromise present. Patients with minimal symptoms can have catastrophic events if subtle indicators are overlooked. Improvement of these physiologic changes is often quickly achieved by moving the patient into a sitting or left lateral position.

Sleep-Disordered Breathing

Sleep-disordered breathing (SDB) is a spectrum of disorders ranging from primary snoring to obstructive sleep apnea syndrome (OSAS). The mildest form of SDB is primary snoring, which is noisy breathing without clinical manifestations and occurs in 20 % of normal children [18]. Although SDB affects 10 % of the population, only 1–4 % will progress to OSAS. OSAS is characterized by periodic, partial, or complete obstruction of the upper airway during sleep. Airway obstruction is characterized by an anatomic imbalance between the upper airway soft tissue volume and craniofacial size. Suppression of pharyngeal dilator muscles during sleep and anesthesia occurs in the patient with obstructive sleep apnea, as opposed to patients who are just noisy breathers or have mild to moderate snoring.

Repetitive arousal from sleep to restore airway patency is a common feature as are episodic sleep-associated oxygen desaturation, hypercarbia, and cardiac dysfunction as a result of airway obstruction. Individuals who experience obstruction during sleep may have snoring loud enough to be heard through closed doors or observed pauses in breathing during sleep. They may awaken from sleep with a choking sensation. Parents report restless sleep in affected children and frequent somnolence or fatigue while awake despite adequate sleep hours. These children fall asleep easily in nonstimulating environments and are difficult to arouse at their usual awakening time. Type 1 OSAS is characterized by lymphoid hyperplasia without obesity, whereas type 2 OSAS patients are obese with minimal lymphoid hyperplasia. Approximately, 10 % of OSAS is present in preschool and school-aged children and is thought to decline after 9 years of age [4].

Obesity changes craniofacial anthropometric characteristics, therefore body mass index of 95 % for age or greater is a predisposing physical characteristic that increases the risk of developing OSAS. Children with craniofacial abnormalities including a small maxilla and mandible, large tongue for given mandibular size, and thick neck have a similar increased risk. Many of these children have syndromes that are associated with additional comorbidities. Anatomic nasal obstruction and Class IV touching tonsils reduce oropharyngeal cross-sectional area, which constitutes an additional risk. Pharyngeal size is determined by the soft tissue volume inside the bony enclosure of the mandible, and an anatomic imbalance between the upper airway soft tissue volume and craniofacial size will result in obstruction.

The magnitude of pharyngeal muscle contraction is controlled by neural mechanisms and the interaction between the anatomical balance and neural mechanisms determines pharyngeal airway size. Increased neural mechanisms can compensate for the anatomical imbalance in obstructive sleep apnea patients during wakefulness. When the neural mechanisms controlling pharyngeal dilator muscles are suppressed during sleep or anesthesia (as is present in non-OSAS patients), the pharyngeal airway severely narrows because of the anatomical imbalance. There is additional decrease in ventilator response and impairment of the arousal response. Craniofacial morphology may influence the severity of obstruction in boys more than girls [19]. Increasing bony enclosure size will provide relief of airway obstruction. This is only accomplished surgically by mandibular advancement. Increasing the distance between the mentum and cervical column by positioning will transiently relieve the obstruction as long as the sniffing position is maintained. Similarly, the sitting position displaces excessive soft tissue outside the bony enclosure through the submandibular space.

The long-term effects of OSAS are not limited to the airway. These children have other systemic comorbidities. Increased body mass index and obesity may lead to increased cognitive vulnerability as illustrated by the increased frequency of hyperactivity and increased levels of C-reactive protein. The duration of OSA has no relation to reversibility of neurobehavioral impairment since many believe that episodic hypoxia alters the neurochemical substrate of the prefrontal cortex causing neuronal cell loss. Metabolic syndrome consists of insulin resistance, dyslipidemia, and hypertension. It is felt that OSAS is a risk factor for metabolic syndrome in obese children but not in nonobese patients. Cardiovascular and hemodynamic comorbidities are more common in OSAS patients. These consist of altered regulation of blood pressure as well as alterations in sympathetic activity and reactivity. Also present are endothelial dysfunction and initiation and propagation of inflammatory response facilitated by increases in levels of C-reactive protein [20, 21]. Systemic inflammation using interleukins as a marker is a component of OSAS in both obese and nonobese children and is reversed after tonsillectomy. Systemic hypertension, changes in left ventricular geometry, and intermittent hypoxia leading to pulmonary artery hypertension are well-described comorbidities present in patients with OSAS.

The mainstay of OSAS management is surgical removal of tonsils and adenoids, which carries an 85 % success rate in resolving OSAS. Recurrence may occur in children with craniofacial abnormalities and in others, and if surgical intervention does not resolve the problem, continuous positive airway pressure (CPAP) at night is the next treatment modality. Many of these children, however, may present for imaging or require sedation prior to removal of the tonsils or adenoids.

For patients undergoing sedation, the preoperative evaluation begins with the history. (Refer to Chap. 4.) Questions to ask parents include the presence of difficulty breathing during sleep, snoring, gasping, retractions, apnea during sleep, sweating during sleep, restless sleep or behavioral problems, and/or somnolence during the day [22, 23]. A positive finding of any of the aforementioned characteristics should alert the practitioner to the possibility of some degree of OSAS [24]. Specific attention should be paid to the frequency of tonsillar infection, recent upper respiratory infections, SDB, and cardiovascular abnormalities. The physical exam should include observation of audible respiration, mouth breathing, nasal quality of speech, chest retractions, long facies, retrognathic mandible, and inspection of tonsillar size. Auscultation should be specifically directed to detect wheezing and stridor. Polysomnography (PSG), otherwise known as the sleep study, is the gold standard for diagnosis of OSAS. A sleep study is suggested to direct the postoperative or postprocedural disposition. It is essential in patients with comorbidities and high-risk features such as morbid obesity, craniofacial abnormalities, neuromuscular disorders, cor pulmonale, systemic hypertension, difficulty breathing during sleep, growth impairment due to chronic obstructed breathing, and a history of severe prematurity [25]. Obesity changes craniofacial anthropometric characteristics and a body mass index of 95 % for age or greater is a risk factor for OSA, which should be quantified by PSG. Craniofacial abnormalities that specifically include small maxilla and mandible, large tongue for given mandible size, and thick neck similarly should be evaluated by sleep study. Despite this, most patients do not have this examination prior to surgery. It is expensive, time consuming, and unavailable in some medical centers. The nadir of oxygen saturation and respiratory disturbance index (RDI), which is the number of apneic episodes per hour, are measured during PSG. Apnea is defined as decreases in airflow greater than 90 % for two breaths or more. Hypopnea is defined as decreases in airflow greater than 50 % coupled with 3 % decrease in oxygen saturation or electroencephalogram (EEG) arousal. An RDI of two or more is necessary for the diagnosis of OSAS. Mild OSAS is defined as RDI of 5–10 events, moderate 10–20 events, and severe 20–30 events. The STOP-BANG questionnaire has been in use in the adult population since 2009 to predict the presence of OSA in the absence of a sleep study [24]. It is comprised of eight questions designed to predict moderate to severe OSA. Although it has good predictive value for alerting practitioners to adults with OSA, it is not a good predictor of sedation-related adverse events (SRAE) in children [26]. Although the presence of OSA does not seem to be a risk factor for hypoxia in adults undergoing moderate sedation, this has not been demonstrated in the pediatric population [27].

When sedation without a secured airway is planned, it is imperative that the level of consciousness, adequacy of ventilation, and oxygenation be continuously monitored and the risk of apnea be evaluated. Patients exposed to recurrent hypoxia exhibit an altered response to narcotics, which is manifested by decreases in minute ventilation, respiratory frequency, and tidal volume. It is therefore suggested that no sedative premedication be administered to OSAS patients prior to a general anesthetic and narcotics be administered in incremental doses, beginning with one-half the recommended dose, until adequacy of ventilation and respiration is determined. Patients with OSAS who are given the same dose of narcotic as non-OSAS patients have a very high risk of serious respiratory compromise [28, 29]. Similarly, patients should not be discharged until fully awake and breathing at a baseline rate and depth. The supraglottic obstruction secondary to decreased muscle tone may contribute to desaturation. Children who have increased severity of OSAS, low weight, and age under 3 years exhibit a higher rate of complications [30]. They are more likely to require supplemental oxygen, the use of an oral airway, and require assisted ventilation. Slow return of upper airway tone may lead to desaturation and laryngospasm on emergence, especially in those patients who are known to have an RDI greater than 30.

There is no agreement on the specific criteria that preselect an elective OSAS patient for admission and monitoring postprocedure [31].

Inclusive characteristics may include the following: PSG-proven OSAS with RDI >40, RDI >20 plus either desaturation <70 % or age less than 3 years, or weight <3 % for age. Children with craniofacial syndromes or neuromuscular disease are included as children with complex or cyanotic cardiac disease. Additional indications include morbid obesity, known cor pulmonary and pulmonary hypertension and preexisting asthma or other unrelated respiratory comorbidities.

Identification and Treatment of Airway-Related Adverse Events

The best way to minimize airway and respiratory compromise is to optimize the situation and prevent it. When a child is sedated, the best prevention is to ensure that the position provides the best anatomic orientation for airway patency. The patient should be in the supine position with the head in a sniffing position and shoulders slightly elevated. This requires that the protrusion of the occiput is balanced by slight shoulder elevation to prevent neck flexion and airway compromise (Fig. 7.13). Supplemental oxygen should be administered by nasal prongs, mask, or blow-by to keep oxygen saturation above 95 %.

If, despite proper positioning, the airway becomes obstructed and ventilation is compromised, an oropharyngeal or nasopharyngeal airway may be placed. Both of these devices improve ventilation by maximizing the space for gas entry between the tongue and posterior pharynx. The appropriate size must be chosen to prevent worsening of the obstruction or irritation of the larynx resulting in laryngospasm (Fig. 7.14). The appropriate oropharyngeal airway size may be determined by measuring the distance between the lips and the angle of the mandible. If the airway is too large, the tip may rest on the epiglottis and cause laryngeal irritation and spasm. If the airway is too small it may compress the tongue and cause it to move posteriorly, thus causing worsening of the oropharyngeal obstruction. The proper nasopharyngeal size may be estimated by measuring the distance between the nares and the angle of the mandible. Extreme caution must be used when placing a nasopharyngeal airway in a toddler or young child due to the presence of hypertrophied adenoid tissue, which can bleed profusely when dislodged [32]. If airway patency is not restored with repositioning of the head and shoulders despite the use of an artificial airway, the jaw thrust may be useful. This maneuver increases the distance between the base of the tongue and the vocal cords and helps to provide the maximum area for air exchange. In addition, positioning the patient on his/her side with the mouth opened may also relieve obstruction.

If it is determined that ventilation must be assisted to maintain oxygenation, then bag-mask ventilation may be instituted. The laryngeal mask airway (LMA) may also be a

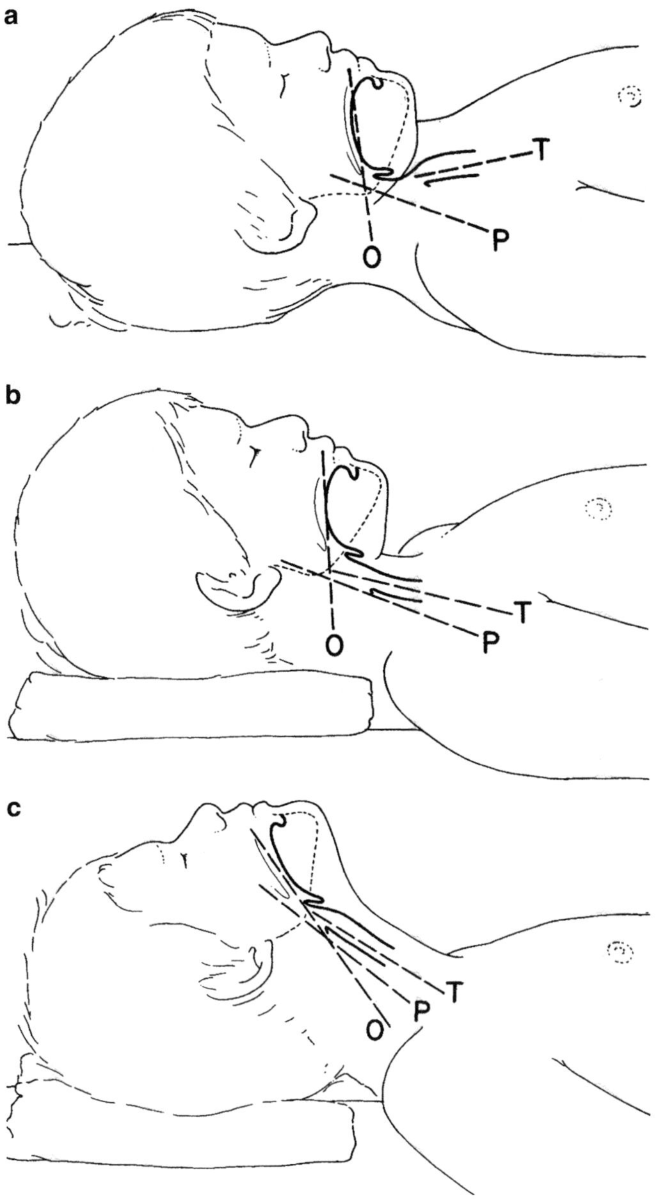

Fig. 7.13 Alignment of oral, pharyngeal, and tracheal axis variation with head position (Reprinted with permission from Wheeler M, Coté CJ, Todres D. The Pediatric Airway. Chapter 5. In: Coté CJ, Todres ID, Goudsouzian NG, Ryan JF (editors). A Practice of Anesthesia for Infants and Children, 3rd edition. Philadelphia, PA: W. B. Saunders Company. 2001)

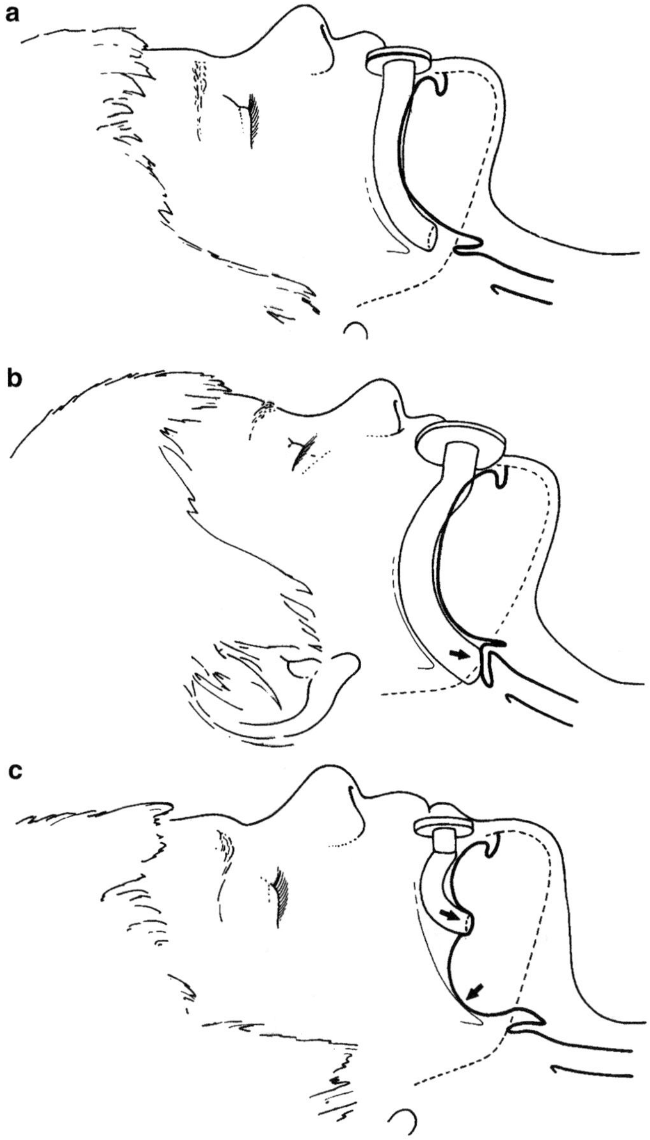

Fig. 7.14 Effects of different sizes of oropharyngeal airway placement (Reprinted with permission from Wheeler M, Coté CJ, Todres D. The Pediatric Airway. Chapter 5. In: Coté CJ, Todres ID, Goudsouzian NG, Ryan JF (editors). A Practice of Anesthesia for Infants and Children, 3rd edition. Philadelphia, PA: W. B. Saunders Company. 2001)

useful adjunct if the patient has progressed beyond spontaneous ventilation and requires assisted or controlled ventilation. The LMA is an appropriate intermediate step to maintain an airway that does not require endotracheal intubation and is a part of the Pediatric Advanced Life Support (PALS) algorithms of the American Heart Association.[1] The LMA is inserted without the need to visualize the vocal cords and forms an airtight seal around the glottis rather than plugging the pharynx. This positioning provides both a patent path for gas entry during positive pressure ventilation and simultaneously prevents the supralaryngeal structures from encroaching on the glottis. The vocal cords move freely during respiration and are not manipulated, thus avoiding a potent stimulus for laryngospasm. The ideal patient position for insertion is the supine sniffing position, but it can be inserted in the neutral position as well. In infants and young children, the epiglottis is prominent and may provide a mechanical barrier to successful placement. To overcome this, it is recommended that the LMA be

[1] http://www.heart.org/HEARTORG/

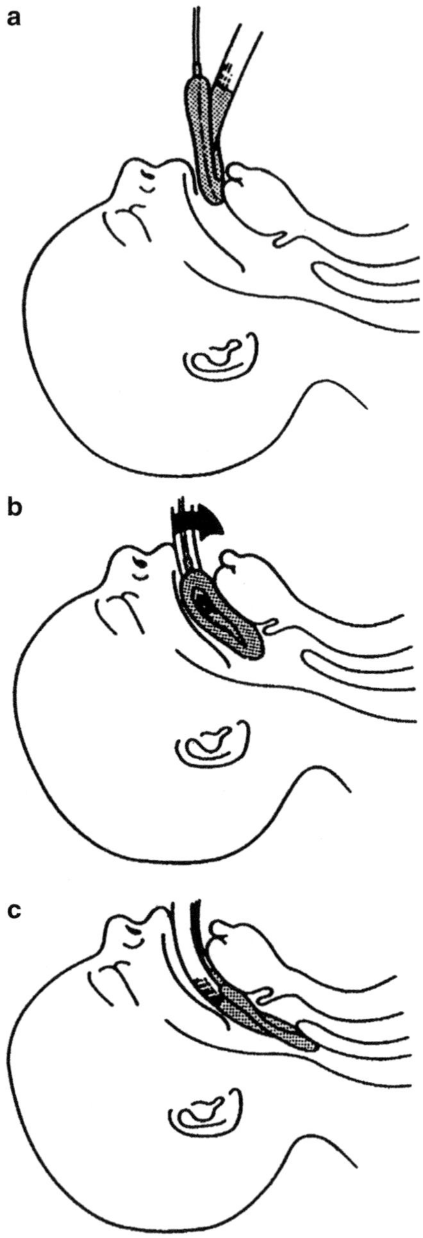

Fig. 7.15 Technique of laryngeal mask insertion in infants and children (Reprinted with permission from Haynes SR, Morton NS. The laryngeal mask airway: A review of its use in paediatric anaesthesia. Paediatr Anaesth. 1993;3:65. Blackwell Publishing)

place with the vented side facing the palate and advanced while turning in an attempt to flick the epiglottis out of the way (Fig. 7.15) [33]. Assisted spontaneous ventilation may be carried out in this manner. If undisturbed, the LMA provokes very little stimulus and can be left in place until the patient's protective reflexes have returned and respirations resume spontaneously. If ventilation cannot be achieved, endotracheal intubation with controlled ventilation may have to be instituted.

Conclusion

Sedation of children for diagnostic or therapeutic procedures is often an alternative to general anesthesia due to the common belief that it carries less risk and requires fewer resources. Although this is not a completely erroneous perspective, sedation is not without risks. A thorough understanding of the pediatric airway anatomy at each developmental stage is essential as well as the physiologic consequences that occur when consciousness is altered. Appropriate monitoring must be utilized and personnel who are knowledgeable with regard to the potential adverse events and skills to treat them must be immediately available. When these conditions are met, sedation of infants and children is a reasonable and safe practice.

Case Studies

Case 1: Obstructive Sleep Apnea

A 5-year-old boy with osteomyelitis Class 4 tonsillar hyperplasia presents to the interventional radiology suite for insertion of a peripherally inserted central catheter (PICC) for antibiotic administration. Attempts at PICC insertion were unsuccessful due to patient movement and difficulty in locating an appropriate vessel. The mother reports that the child is otherwise healthy, except that he seems to choke when he is asleep and sometimes awakens startled in the middle of the night. He is overweight for his age and has some difficulty concentrating and sitting still in school. His physical exam reveals him to be a moderately overweight boy with a short neck and nasal breathing. His oropharyngeal examination is positive for Class 4 kissing tonsils, which occupy greater that 75 % of the oropharyngeal volume and a Mallampati Class 3 classification for intubation. He is taking no medications and has not had a sleep study.

The considerations for this child would be appropriateness for sedation, choice of monitoring required, and postprocedural disposition. This is a child in whom a sleep study would be desirable, but in the absence of this information it may be assumed that he is at risk for OSAS based on his weight, short neck, and large tonsils. He may undergo sedation, but is at risk for airway obstruction and desaturation, thus he must be monitored in the presence of a practitioner who has airway management skills should this occur. Monitors should include electrocardiograph (EKG), pulse oximeter, capnography, and blood pressure measurements. Supplemental oxygen should be administered by nasal

(continued)

cannula. Some head-up position should be maintained as much as possible to facilitate diaphragmatic excursion. Agents that maintain spontaneous respirations and do not produce significant respiratory depression should be considered. Due to the probability of OSAS, this patient should be admitted to the hospital overnight for observation. The inclusion criteria for overnight admission include obesity, Class 4 tonsils, as well as a history consistent with significant SDB and probable OSAS. Alternatively, if the child underwent tonsillectomy and adenoidectomy in advance of sedation, the radiologic study could be scheduled 2–3 weeks postoperatively. Waiting this amount of time ensures that the hypopharynx would be well healed. In this case, if a repeat sleep study was repeated and improved, the post-sedation admission might be eliminated; however, in the absence of a repeat sleep study, the overnight post-sedation admission still is required.

Case 2: Anterior Mediastinal Mass

An otherwise healthy 14-year-old male presented to his pediatrician with a history of new-onset cough and difficulty sleeping. The only significant findings on physical exam were shortness of breath when lying down, some jugular venous distention in the supine position, and a single enlarged cervical lymph node. Breath sounds were diminished bilaterally but more on the left side. The child was sent to the hospital for a chest X-ray and a large anterior mediastinal mass was noted. An MRI for further classification was requested.

Patients with an anterior mediastinal mass may present with varied signs and symptoms referable to both the cardiovascular and respiratory systems. Symptoms are directly related to the location and size of the mass, as well as the degree of compression of surrounding structures. The most commonly observed respiratory symptom is cough, especially in the supine position, which results from anterior compression of the trachea by a mass located in the anterior mediastinum. Infants younger than 2 years of age are more likely to experience wheezing as a sign of tracheal compression, whereas children older than 2 years of age usually present with malaise, cough, fever, and a neck mass. Other respiratory findings in patients of all ages include tachypnea, dyspnea, stridor, retractions, decreased breath sounds, and cyanosis on crying, all of which should alert the anesthesiologist to some degree of airway compromise that may worsen when positive intrathoracic pressure is generated.

Cardiovascular symptoms result from compression of the aortic and pulmonary vessels, as well as the right atrium and right ventricle. This can lead to both hypotension secondary to inadequate cardiac filling and restricted pulmonary blood flow, resulting in poor oxygenation despite adequate ventilation. Findings referable to the cardiovascular system include fatigue, headache, hypotension or pallor in the supine position, a feeling of light-headedness, superior vena cava syndrome (facial edema, cyanosis, jugular venous distension), and the appearance of a new murmur, especially in the area of the pulmonary valve. It is essential that the clinician search for these signs and symptoms when interviewing and examining patients with mediastinal masses in an attempt to ascertain the degree of respiratory and cardiovascular compromise present. Patients with minimal symptoms can have catastrophic events when sedated if subtle indicators are overlooked.

Sedation is best accomplished with the child in the semi-Fowler or full sitting position, since the supine position leads to decreased expansion of the rib cage and cephalad displacement of the diaphragm. Patients who are asymptomatic while awake may exhibit airway obstruction during sedation in the supine position, which is explained by a reduction in the dimensions of the thorax that limits the available space for the trachea relative to the tumor. The increase in central blood volume that accompanies the supine position can also lead to increased tumor volume and size, thus contributing to the potential for airway obstruction. The patient should breathe spontaneously and a small dose of sedative agents may be administered as the patient is lowered into position. Agents that suppress respirations should be avoided. The adequacy of ventilation and blood pressure should be checked at frequent intervals until the optimum surgical position has been achieved. If at any time a decrease in blood pressure occurs and causes an inability to oxygenate despite adequate ventilation or if an inability to provide adequate ventilation is encountered, the patient should be returned to the upright or lateral position. This will generally relieve airway obstruction caused by the tumor mass.

Case 3: The Child with a "Cold"

A 4-year-old child presents for sedation for a brain MRI. He was born at 36 weeks gestation and his mother had an uncomplicated delivery. He was slightly

(continued)

hypotonic at birth and has not reached his expected milestones. He walks but still exhibits some weakness in both extremities. His pediatrician is concerned and wishes to make certain that there is no intracranial lesion or other central nervous system pathology. He has a history of reactive airway disease and uses a bronchodilator, but has not had to use it in the recent 6 months.

His mother reports that he had a "cold" 10 days ago but is "fine" now. His symptoms initially included fever to 101 ° F, purulent nasal discharge, and cough. He is now sneezing and has an occasional cough and clear runny nose, especially in the morning, and has been afebrile for 5 days. He has not been given any acetaminophen in 5 days. His lungs are clear on auscultation and he does not have wheezing, rales, or rhonchi.

When considering whether or not to proceed with the requested study in this patient, the first step is to determine the urgency of the procedure and if the result will change therapy or inform a diagnosis. Each case is unique and must be determined on the individual risk/benefit basis. Acute symptoms of an upper respiratory infection (URI) should be differentiated from the same symptoms demonstrated in noninfectious chronic conditions. For instance, sneezing and clear runny nose are present in allergic rhinitis, which does not carry the same risk for the patient as a URI. Identification of a mild URI, severe URI, or lower respiratory infection must be made since the implications are different with regard to risk and potential cancelation. Mild URI consists of minimal cough, no fever, clear runny nose, sneezing, a nontoxic appearance, normal activity level, and clear lung fields on auscultation. A severe URI is accompanied by symptoms of malaise, fever greater than 38.3 °C, sneezing, productive cough, toxic appearance, and upper airway congestion. A child with a lower respiratory infection usually has a severe productive cough with purulent sputum, wheezing, fever, rales, rhonchi, toxic appearance, and tachypnea with or without respiratory distress.

Children under the age of 5 years usually experience 4–6 URIs each year, especially during the winter season, and the inflammatory response and increased reactivity of the lower airway may persist for up to 6 weeks after a viral infection. If a child's procedure is canceled for 6 weeks, he/she is usually into the next URI, so the most prudent recommendation is to wait until the acute symptoms have resolved and then reschedule 2 weeks after that. Children with known URI may experience an increase in respiratory events when intubated or the airway is instrumented; however, there is no increase in laryngospasm or bronchospasm when there is a natural airway. There is, however, a significant risk of oxygen desaturation and hypoxemia even with the use of supplemental oxygen.

Considerations for proceeding in this child include the following: This is not an urgent procedure so the procedure may be rescheduled. This child has a resolving URI and demonstrates only mild symptoms without lower respiratory involvement. The reactive airway disease is not an active problem and not a cause of increased risk. Since there still is a risk of hypoxemia and increased oxygen requirement if the study proceeds, he should have full monitoring and supplemental oxygen administered. He should also demonstrate that he can lie flat without coughing prior to the start of the case. If he cannot, and the case is postponed, the end point should be no coughing and reschedule 2 weeks after all symptoms have resolved.

References

1. O'Connor D. Development anatomy of the larynx and trachea. In: Myer C, Cotton R, Shott S, editors. The pediatric airway an interdisciplinary approch. Philadelphia, PA: JB Lippincott. 1995:1–23.
2. Litman R, Weissend E, Shibata D, Westesson P. Developmental changes of laryngeal dimensions in unparalyzed sedated children. Anesthesiology. 2003;98(1):41–5.
3. Eckenhoff JE. Some anatomic considerations of the infant larynx influencing endotracheal anesthesia. Anesthesiology. 1951;12(4):401–10.
4. Plante J, Turgeon AF, Zarychanski R, Lauzier F, Vigneault L, Moore L, et al. Effect of systemic steroids on post-tonsillectomy bleeding and reinterventions: Systematic review and meta-analysis of randomised controlled trials. BMJ. 2012;345:e5389.
5. McGoldrick K. The larynx: normal development and congenital abnormalities in anesthesia for ophthalmic and otolaryngologic surgery. Philadelphia: WB Saunders Co.; 1992.
6. Holinger L, Lusk R, Green C, editors. Anatomy in pediatric laryngology & bronchoesophagology. Philadelphia: Lippincott-Raven; 1997.
7. Katz ES, Mitchell RB, D'Ambrosio CM. Obstructive sleep apnea in infants. Am J Respir Crit Care Med. 2012;185(8):805–16.
8. Hall S. Anesthesia for the neonate. In: Badgewell J, editor. Clinical pediatric anesthesia. Philadelphia: Lippincott-Raven; 1997. p. 163–93.
9. Samsoon GL, Young JR. Difficult tracheal intubation: a retrospective study. Anaesthesia. 1987;42(5):487–90.
10. Mallampati SR, Gatt SP, Gugino LD, Desai SP, Waraksa B, Freiberger D, et al. A clinical sign to predict difficult tracheal intubation: a prospective study. Can Anaesth Soc J. 1985;32(4):429–34.
11. Brodsky L. Modern assessment of tonsils and adenoids. Pediatr Clin North Am. 1989;36:1551–69.
12. Tsuiki S, Isono S, Ishikawa T, Yamashiro Y, Tatsumi K, Nishino T. Anatomical balance of the upper airway and obstructive sleep apnea. Anesthesiology. 2008;108(6):1009–15.
13. Zalzal GH. Stridor and airway compromise. Pediatr Clin North Am. 1989;36:1389–402.
14. von Ungern-Sternberg BS, Boda K, Chambers NA, Rebmann C, Johnson C, Sly PD, et al. Risk assessment for respiratory complica-

tions in paediatric anaesthesia: a prospective cohort study. Lancet. 2010;376(9743):773–83.
15. Tait A, Malviva S. Anesthesia for the child with an upper respiratory tract infection is still a dilemma. Anesth Analg. 2005;100:59–65.
16. Steward DJ. Postoperative apnea syndrome in premature infants. West J Med. 1992;157(5):567.
17. Cote CJ, Zaslavsky A, Downes JJ, Kurth CD, Welborn LG, Warner LO, et al. Postoperative apnea in former preterm infants after inguinal herniorrhaphy. A combined analysis. Anesthesiology. 1995; 82(4):809–22.
18. Martin LD. Anesthetic implications of an upper respiratory infection in children. Pediatr Clin North Am. 1994;41(1):121–30.
19. Di Francesco R, Monteiro R, Paulo ML, Buranello F, Imamura R. Craniofacial morphology and sleep apnea in children with obstructed upper airways: differences between genders. Sleep Med. 2012;13(6):616–20.
20. Gozal D, Kheirandish-Gozal L, Bhattacharjee R, Kim J. C-reactive protein and obstructive sleep apnea syndrome in children. Front Biosci (Elite Ed). 2012;4:2410–22.
21. Lazaratou H, Soldatou A, Dikeos D. Medical comorbidity of sleep disorders in children and adolescents. Curr Opin Psychiatry. 2012; 25(5):391–7.
22. Goldstein NA, Stefanov DG, Graw-Panzer KD, Fahmy SA, Fishkin S, Jackson A, et al. Validation of a clinical assessment score for pediatric sleep-disordered breathing. Laryngoscope. 2012;122(9):2096–104.
23. Gasparini G, Saponaro G, Rinaldo FM, Boniello R, Marianetti TM, Torroni A, et al. Clinical evaluation of obstructive sleep apnea in children. J Craniofac Surg. 2012;23(2):387–91.
24. Chung F, Elsaid H. Screening for obstructive sleep apnea before surgery: why is it important? Curr Opin Anaesthesiol. 2009;22(3): 405–11.
25. Schwengel DA, Sterni LM, Tunkel DE, Heitmiller ES. Perioperative management of children with obstructive sleep apnea. Anesth Analg. 2009;109(1):60–75.
26. Mehta PP, Kochhar G, Kalra S, Maurer W, Tetzlaff J, Singh G, et al. Can a validated sleep apnea scoring system predict cardiopulmonary events using propofol sedation for routine EGD or colonoscopy? A prospective cohort study. Gastrointest Endosc. 2014;79(3):436–44.
27. Cha JM, Jeun JW, Pack KM, Lee JI, Joo KR, Shin HP, et al. Risk of sedation for diagnostic esophagogastroduodenoscopy in obstructive sleep apnea patients. World J Gastroenterol. 2013; 19(29):4745–51.
28. Brown KA, Laferriere A, Lakheeram I, Moss IR. Recurrent hypoxemia in children is associated with increased analgesic sensitivity to opiates. Anesthesiology. 2006;105(4):665–9.
29. Moss IR, Brown KA, Laferriere A. Recurrent hypoxia in rats during development increases subsequent respiratory sensitivity to fentanyl. Anesthesiology. 2006;105(4):715–8.
30. Hanna AH, Mason LJ. Challenges in paediatric ambulatory anesthesia. Curr Opin Anaesthesiol. 2012;25(3):315–20.
31. Gross JB, Bachenberg KL, Benumof JL, Caplan RA, Connis RT, Cote CJ, et al. Practice guidelines for the perioperative management of patients with obstructive sleep apnea: a report by the american society of anesthesiologists task force on perioperative management of patients with obstructive sleep apnea. Anesthesiology. 2006;104(5):1081–93. quiz 1117–1088.
32. Wheeler M. Management strategies for the difficult pediatric airway. Anesthesiol Clin North America. 1998;16(4):743–61.
33. Haynes SR, Morton NS. The laryngeal mask airway: a review of its use in paediatric anaesthesia. Paediatr Anaesth. 1993;3:65.

Pediatric Physiology: How Does It Differ from Adults?

8

Dean B. Andropoulos

Abstract

Safe sedation of pediatric patients requires a thorough understanding of the physiological differences between infants, children, adolescents, and adults. Especially in small infants, there is much less margin for any errors in diagnosis and treatment of respiratory or cardiovascular depression during sedation procedures. This chapter will review developmental aspects of respiratory, cardiovascular, central nervous system, renal, hepatic, hematologic, and temperature homeostatic systems, highlighting the differences between children and adults and emphasizing their relevance to sedation procedures in children.

Keywords

Pediatric • Physiology • Anatomy • Airway • Lungs • Functional residual capacity (FRC) respiratory • Cardiovascular • Central nervous system (CNS) • Renal • Hepatic • Hematologic • Homeostatic • Hypothermia • Pulse oximetry • Upper respiratory infection (URI) • Functional residual capacity (FRC) • Bronchopulmonary dysplasia (BPD) • Cystic fibrosis • Nil per os (NPO) • American Society of Anesthesiologists (ASA)

Introduction

Safe sedation of pediatric patients requires a thorough understanding of the physiological differences between infants, children, adolescents, and adults. Especially in small infants, there is much less margin for any errors in diagnosis and treatment of respiratory or cardiovascular depression during sedation procedures. This chapter will review developmental aspects of respiratory, cardiovascular, central nervous system (CNS), renal, hepatic, hematologic, and temperature homeostatic systems, highlighting the differences between children and adults and emphasizing their relevance to sedation procedures in children.

D.B. Andropoulos, M.D., M.H.C.M. (✉)
Department of Anesthesiology, Texas Children's Hospital, Baylor College of Medicine, Houston, TX, USA
e-mail: dbandrop@texaschildrens.org; dra@bcm.tmc.edu

Respiratory Physiology

Many physiologic differences in respiratory physiology between children and adults can be understood by anatomical differences in the airway and lungs [1]. The major anatomical airway differences include the tongue, where the infant's tongue is relatively large compared to the adult, and more prone to airway obstruction. The larynx of the infant is more cephalad, lying at the C3–4 level, versus the adult position of C4–5. The infant epiglottis is narrow and omega shaped, versus the flat, broad, U-shaped epiglottis of the adult. The cricoid ring is the narrowest portion of the infant and child up to about 4–6 years of age; thereafter the glottic opening itself is the narrowest portion of the airway. In terms of the intrathoracic airways, they are fully formed, including the terminal bronchioles, relatively early in gestation. However, alveolar number and development are incomplete at birth, with the full-term infant having 20–50 million terminal airspaces, which are immature alveoli. Lung development occurs rapidly with nearly the adult number of 300

K.P. Mason (ed.), *Pediatric Sedation Outside of the Operating Room: A Multispecialty International Collaboration*,
DOI 10.1007/978-1-4939-1390-9_8, © Springer Science+Business Media New York 2015

million or more alveoli reached by 3 years of age [2]. Early in postnatal life the lung volume of the neonate and young infant is disproportionately small in relation to body size; the functional residual capacity (FRC) is only about 25 mL/kg in contrast to 40–50 mL/kg in the older child and adolescent. In addition, metabolic rate and therefore oxygen requirement in mL/kg/min are 2–3 times higher in the neonate compared to the adult.

Lung and chest wall mechanics are very different in the neonate and young infant, compared to the older child and adult [2, 3]. The soft and compliant thoracic cage means that the outward recoil of the thorax is very low in the neonate, and this means that resting negative thoracic pressure in infants is low. Neonates depend on the diaphragm for the power to produce lung expansion to a much greater degree than the older child. In addition, since airway resistance is proportional to the inverse of the fourth power of the radius of the airway, the much smaller airways of infants and young children experience a significant increase in resistance when partially obstructed by edema, inflammation, bronchospasm, or secretions. The low FRC, small airways, and poor elastic recoil of the thorax in neonates make the small airways vulnerable to airway closure, and thus hypoventilation and hypoxemia can occur quickly in the sedated infant who is not crying or taking deep breaths [4]. Figure 8.1 displays the difference in lung volumes between the neonate and adult [5], and Table 8.1 summarizes the developmental changes in respiratory physiology from birth through adulthood.

Fetal hemoglobin predominates in the neonate and young infant, and this causes another important difference in respiratory physiology from the older child and adult. The oxyhemoglobin dissociation curve is shifted to the left in neonates because of fetal hemoglobin, meaning that the partial pressure of oxygen necessary to produce an oxyhemoglobin saturation of 50 % (the P_{50}) is only 19 mmHg, versus 27 mmHg with mature adult hemoglobin A [6] (Fig. 8.2). This is an adaptation to fetal life, where oxygen tensions are low, and with hemoglobin F loading the hemoglobin with oxygen molecules is facilitated; however, unloading of oxygen to the tissues is more difficult with a left-shifted curve. Therefore in the neonate and young infant, a given oxygen tension will produce a higher oxygen saturation, but this extra reserve is required to provide additional oxygen to unload to the tissues. Adult hemoglobin A predominates by 6 months of age.

Pulse oximetry is the standard for monitoring of oxygenation during all sedation procedures. (Refer to Chaps. 2 and 6.) Pulse oximeter arterial saturation (SpO_2) is a very useful monitor, generally accurate to ±2 % when compared to arterial blood oxygen saturation measured by co-oximetry. In a child without cardiac or pulmonary disease, normal SpO_2 is 96–100 % on room air and unsedated. Sedative medications often cause a degree of hypoventilation, both in slowing respiratory rate, and decreasing tidal volumes and FRC. Upper airway obstruction is also common, which may interfere with oxygenation. These factors make it necessary to deliver supplemental oxygen to virtually all patients undergoing sedation procedures, either by nasal cannula or face mask, to enable SpO_2 to remain in the normal 96–100 % range. A decrease of 5 % or less from baseline, as long as the patient is otherwise stable without significant respiratory depression or upper airway obstruction, is common and can usually be treated with increased supplemental oxygen. A decrease of 10 % or more from baseline is cause for urgent intervention to detect and treat upper airway obstruction or hypoventilation—the two most common causes of arterial desaturation during sedation. Children with cyanotic congenital heart disease may have resting awake SpO_2 ranging from 70 to 95 %, and it is important to understand the anatomy, pathophysiology, and normal baseline saturations before proceeding with sedation in these patients. The general guidelines of a 5 % decrease from baseline being common and treated with additional supplemental oxygen, and a 10 % decrease, a cause for urgent intervention, are applicable to this population as well. Other patients with chronic lung diseases—i.e., bronchopulmonary dysplasia (BPD) or cystic fibrosis—may also have decreased baseline SpO_2, often ranging from 85 to 95 %.

Monitoring of respiration also often includes end-tidal CO_2, which can easily be monitored using a special or modified nasal cannula. Although dilution of the exhaled gas with inspired oxygen, poor fit of nasal cannula, increased dead space ventilation, or right to left intracardiac shunting often increases the gap between arterial blood $PaCO_2$ and end-tidal CO_2, it is a very sensitive monitor of airway obstruction, and an accurate method to measure respiratory rate. In addition, low cardiac output states or cardiac arrest is accompanied by a sudden decrease or absence of end-tidal CO_2.

Common conditions in pediatric patients that reduce respiratory reserve even further include BPD in former premature infants who suffered from respiratory distress syndrome (RDS) [7]. BPD is defined as a chronic condition of fibrosis and loss of alveoli in the lung following RDS with a requirement for supplemental oxygen beyond 30 days of life. These infants may present for sedation months or years later, and even though they have apparently recovered, pulmonary reserve is often considerably limited. Other common chronic conditions include asthma or reactive airway disease, affecting an estimated six million children in the USA [8]. Presedation assessment must always include questioning about asthma and a thorough airway and pulmonary examination; elective sedation in the face of an asthma exacerbation is contraindicated.

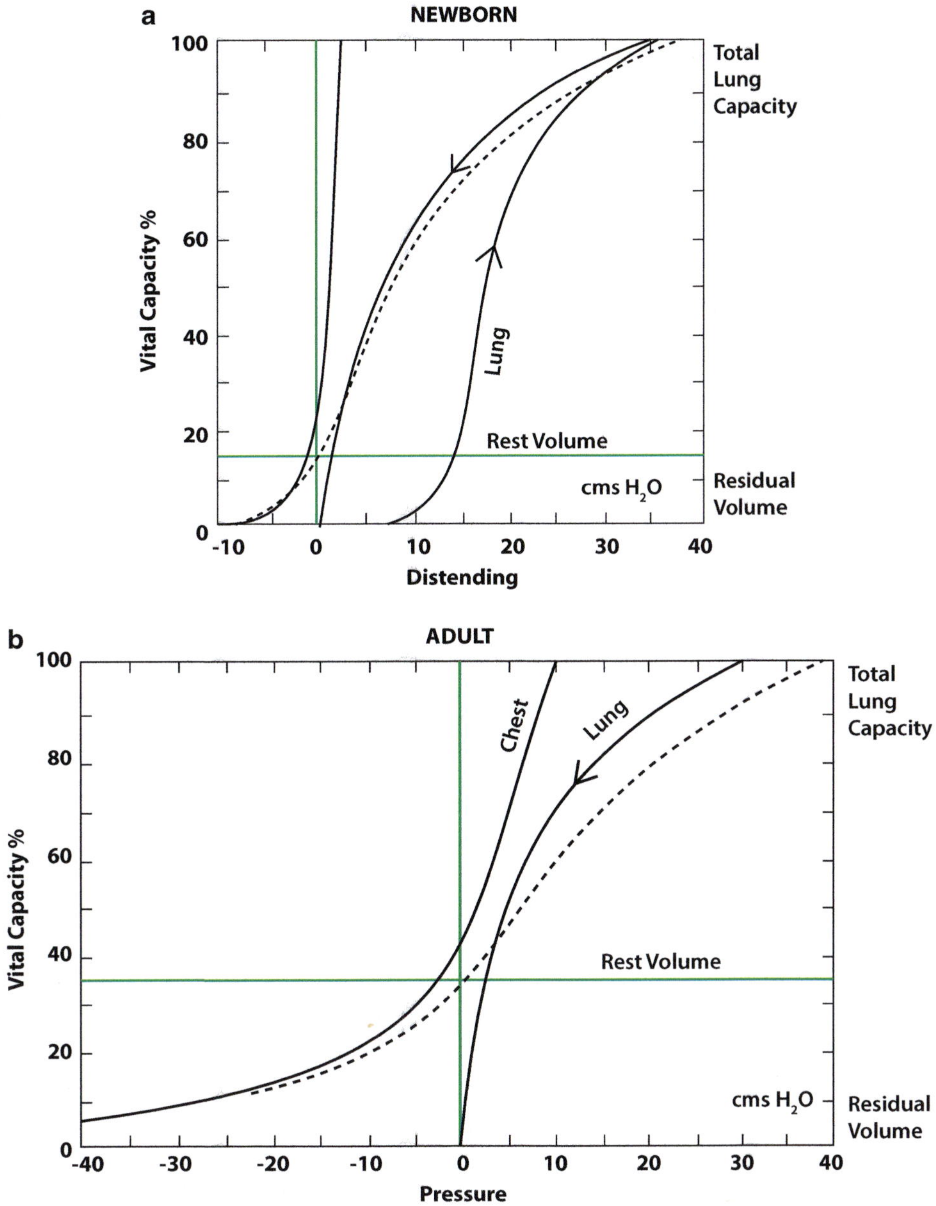

Fig. 8.1 Pressure–volume curves of the (**a**) infant and (**b**) adult respiratory systems. The rest volume is the volume at zero intrathoracic pressure, where the outward recoil of the chest wall is equal to the inward elastic recoil of the lungs. (**a**) In the neonate, this volume is very low (10–15 % of total lung capacity) compared to the adult, and is just above the FRC and often below the closing volume of the small airways. (**b**) In the adult, this value is much higher at 30–35 % of the total lung capacity. During sedation, where quiet breathing or respiratory depression may occur, the neonate and small infant are much more prone to airway closure, resulting in intrapulmonary shunting and hypoxemia (Adapted from Agostoni E, Mead J: Statics of the respiratory system. In Fenn WO, Rahn H. (eds): Handbook of Physiology. Section 3: Respiration, vol 1. Washington, DC: American Physiological Society, 1964. 387–409)

Children also have frequent upper respiratory infections (URIs), which predispose them to increased airway complications during a sedation procedure. Elective sedation procedures should be performed in children with URIs only after a thorough risk–benefit assessment.

All of the factors reviewed earlier make the small infant in particular vulnerable to rapid onset of hypoxemia and hypercarbia if sedated too deeply, and the practitioner must be vigilant especially when sedating infants. Supplemental oxygen should be used in almost every setting in which infants and children are sedated, the only exceptions being in premature neonates where retinopathy of prematurity may be a risk, and in relatively uncommon congenital heart defects in neonates with a single functional ventricle, such as hypoplastic left heart syndrome.

Table 8.1 Age-dependent respiratory variables

Variable	Units	Neonate	6 months	12 months	3 years	5 years	9 years	12 years	Adult
Approx. weight	kg	3	7	10	15	19	30	50	70
Respiratory rate	Breaths/min	50 ± 10	30 ± 5	24 ± 6	24 ± 6	23 ± 5	20 ± 5	18 ± 5	12 ± 3
Tidal volume	mL	21	45	78	112	170	230	480	575
	mL/kg	6–8	6–8	6–8	6–8	7–8	7–8	7–8	6–7
Minute ventilation	mL/min	1,050	1,350	1,780	2,460	4,000		6,200	6,400
	mL/kg/min	350	193	178	164	210		124	91
Alveolar ventilation	mL/min	665		1,245	1760	1,800		3,000	3,100
	mL/kg/min	222		125	117	95		60	44
Dead space/tidal volume ratio		0.3	0.3	0.3	0.3	0.3	0.3	0.3	0.3
Oxygen consumption	mL/kg/min	6–8							3–4
Vital capacity	mL	120			870	1,160		3,100	4,000
	mL/kg	40			58	61		62	57
Functional residual capacity	mL	80			490	680		1,970	3,000
	mL/kg	27			33	36		39	43
Total lung capacity	mL	160			1,100	1,500		4,000	6,000
	mL/kg	53			73	79		80	86
Closing volume as a % of vital capacity	%					20		8	4
No. of alveoli	Saccules × 10^6	30	112	129	257	280			300
Specific compliance	C_L/FRC:mL/cm H_2O/L	0.04	0.038			0.06			0.05
Specific conductance of small airways	Ml/s/cm H_2O/g	0.02		3.1	1.7	1.2		8.2	13.4
Hematocrit	%	55 ± 7	37 ± 3	35 ± 2.5	40 ± 3	40 ± 2	40 ± 2	42 ± 2	43–48
Arterial pH	pH units	7.30–7.40		7.35–7.45					7.35–7.45
$PaCO_2$	mmHg	30–35		30–40					30–40
PaO_2	mmHg	60–90		80–100					80–100

Adapted from [2]

Cardiovascular Physiology

Development from Neonate to Older Infant and Child

At birth the neonatal heart must suddenly change from a parallel circulation to a series circulation, and the left ventricle in particular must adapt immediately to dramatically increased preload from blood returning from the lungs, and increased afterload as the placental circulation is removed. The very high oxygen consumption of the newborn necessitates a high cardiac output for the first few months of life. However, animal models have demonstrated that the fetal and newborn myocardium develops less tension in response to increasing preload (sarcomere length), and that cardiac output increases less to the same degree of volume loading [9, 10]. Resting tension, however, is greater in the newborn compared to the mature heart. This information suggests that the newborn heart is operating near the top of its Frank–Starling curve, and that there is less reserve in response to both increased afterload and preload. The newborn myocardium also has only a limited ability to increase its inotropic state in response to exogenous catecholamines, and is much more dependent on heart rate to maintain cardiac output than the mature heart. One reason for this is the high levels of circulating endogenous catecholamines that appear after birth, necessary to make the transition to extrauterine life [11]. As these levels decrease in the weeks after birth, contractile reserve increases.

The neonatal myocardium is less compliant than the mature myocardium, with increased resting tension as noted previously, and a significant greater increase in ventricular pressure with volume loading [12]. This implies that diastolic function of the neonatal heart is also impaired compared to the mature heart [13]. The myofibrils of the newborn heart also appear to have a greater sensitivity to calcium, developing a greater tension than adult myofibrils when exposed to the same free Ca^{++} concentration in vitro [14]. Table 8.2 summarizes the major physiological differences between the neonatal and mature hearts [15]. With increased metabolic needs, including oxygen consumption and glucose for metabolic substrate, cardiac output indexed to weight in the neonate is double that of the adult [16] (Fig. 8.3).

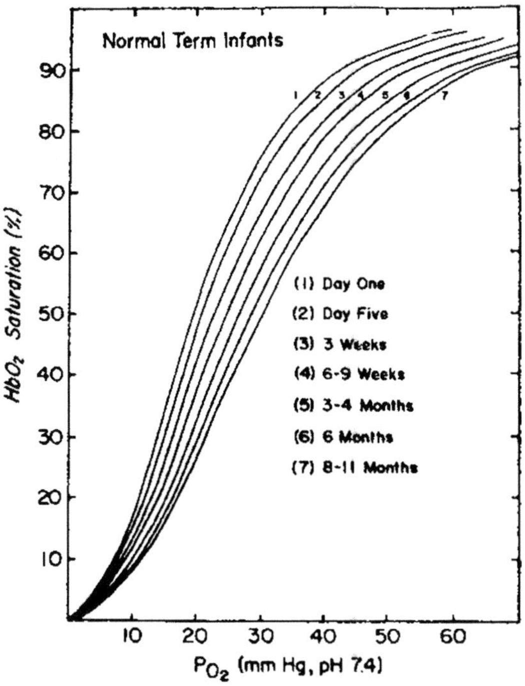

Fig. 8.2 Comparison of oxyhemoglobin dissociation curves from blood of infants at different ages. At birth the P50 is 19 mmHg, and by 8 months of age has shifted to the right and is 27 mmHg, a result of the change from predominately fetal hemoglobin F to adult hemoglobin A (Reproduced with permission from Delivoria-Papadopoulos M, Ronceric NP, Oski FA. Postnatal changes in oxygen transport of term, premature and sick infants: the role of red cell 2,3 diphosphoglycerate and adult hemoglobin. Pediatr Res. 1971;5(6):235–40.)

Innervation of the Heart

Clinical observations in newborn infants have led to the hypothesis that the sympathetic innervation and control of the cardiovascular system is incomplete in the newborn infant compared to older children and adults, and that the parasympathetic innervation is intact [17]. Examples of this include the frequency of bradycardia in the newborn in response to a number of stimuli, including vagal, and vagotonic agents, and the relative lack of sensitivity in the newborn to sympathomimetic agents. Histologic studies in animal models have demonstrated incomplete sympathetic innervation in the neonatal heart when compared to the adult, but no differences in the number or density of parasympathetic nerves [18, 19].

Autonomic cardiovascular control of cardiac activity can be evaluated by measuring heart rate variability in response to both respiration, and to beat-to-beat variability in systolic blood pressure [20]. The sympathetic and parasympathetic inputs into sinoatrial node activity contribute to heart rate variability changes with greater heart rate variability resulting from greater parasympathetic input into sinoatrial node activity [21]. Studies using these methodologies for normal infants during sleep suggest that the parasympathetic predominance gradually diminishes until approximately 6 months of age, coinciding with greater sympathetic innervation of the heart similar to adult levels [22].

Table 8.2 Summary of major differences between neonatal and mature hearts

	Neonatal	Mature
Physiology		
Contractility	Limited	Normal
Heart rate dependence	High	Low
Contractile reserve	Low	High
Afterload tolerance	Low	Higher
Preload tolerance	Limited	Better
Ventricular interdependence	Significant	Less
Ca^{++} cycling		
Predominant site of Ca^{++} flux	Sarcolemma	Sarcoplasmic reticulum
Dependence on normal iCa^{++}	High	Lower
Circulating catecholamines	High	Lower
Adrenergic receptors	Downregulated, insensitive	Normal
	β2, α1 predominant	β1 predominant Complete
Innervation	Parasympathetic predominates; sympathetic incomplete	Complete
Cytoskeleton	High collagen and water content	Lower collagen/H_2O
Cellular elements	Incomplete SR, disorganized myofibrils	Mature SR, organized myofibrils

Reprinted with permission from Andropoulos DB, Ogletree ML. Ch 3. Physiology and molecular biology of the developing circulation. In: Andropoulos DB, Stayer SA, Russell IA, editors. Anesthesia for congenital heart disease. Malden, MA: Blackwell-Futura; 2005. p. 30–47

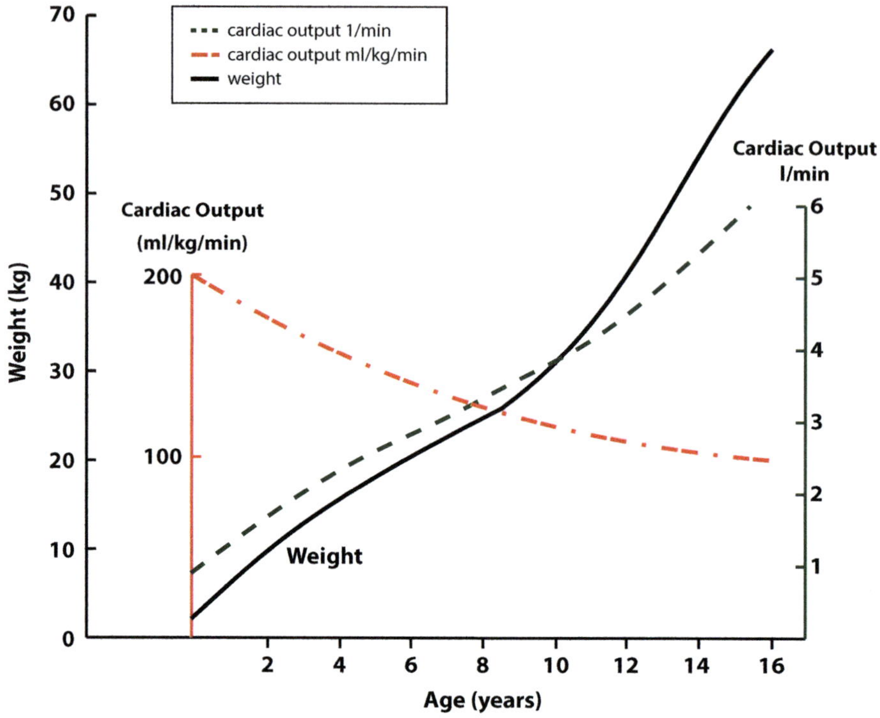

Fig. 8.3 The relationship between body weight, age, and cardiac output. Note that cardiac output in mL/min, when indexed to body weight, decreases by 50 % from birth to adolescence (Adapted with permission from Rudolph AM, editor. Changes in the circulation after birth. In: Congenital diseases of the heart. Chicago, IL: Year Book Medical; 1974)

Development from Child to Adult

Beyond the transition period from fetal to newborn life and into the first few months of postnatal life, there is not much human or animal information concerning the exact nature and extent of cardiac development at the cellular level. Most studies compare newborn or fetal to adult animals [23]. Cardiac chamber development is assumed to be influenced by blood flow [24]. Increases in myocardial mass with normal growth, as well as in ventricular outflow obstruction, are mainly due to hypertrophy of myocytes. Late gestational increases in blood cortisol are responsible for this growth pattern, and there is concern that antenatal glucocorticoids to induce lung maturity may inhibit cardiac myocyte proliferation. In the human infant, it is assumed that the cellular elements of the cardiac myocyte—i.e., adrenergic receptors, intracellular receptors and signaling, calcium cycling and regulation, and interaction of the contractile proteins—are similar to the adult by approximately 6 months of age. Similarly, cardiac depression by volatile agents is greater in the newborn, changing to adult levels by approximately 6 months of age [25].

Normal Heart Rate and Blood Pressure Ranges at Different Ages

Heart rate must be monitored continuously by 3- or 5-lead electrocardiogram (ECG) during all phases of a sedation procedure, because of the frequent effects of sedative and analgesic drugs on heart rate, and the added importance of maintaining acceptable heart rates to maintain cardiac output, especially in young infants. An understanding of the patient's baseline heart rates is important, and generally a decrease or increase of 20 % or less is well tolerated and will maintain adequate cardiac output [26]. Maintaining normal sinus rhythm is obviously important, and any non-sinus rhythm needs to be diagnosed, its effect on blood pressure and cardiac output assessed, and treated if necessary. The most common arrhythmias are sinus bradycardia caused by decreased CNS sympathetic outflow from many sedatives and sinus tachycardia caused by sympathomimetic effects of drugs. Slow junctional rhythms or supraventricular tachycardias are also seen during sedation procedures. It is important to understand the patient's baseline cardiac status, and rhythm, as many patients with preexisting arrhythmias will continue to experience them with sedation and no ill effects.

Blood pressure must be measured at least every 5 min during sedation procedures, and often more frequently (i.e., every 1–3 min) during the induction phase, or after a bolus of medication to deepen the level of sedation. Blood pressure is not equivalent to cardiac output, but perfusion to vital organs, especially myocardium and brain, needs to be preserved during sedation procedures and thus blood pressure should be maintained within acceptable limits, usually ±20 % of the baseline blood pressure, again taking into account the patient's baseline state, and pathophysiology of any disease states.

Table 8.3 Normal heart rates and systolic blood pressure as a function of age

Age	Range of normal heart rates (beats per minute)	Range of normal systolic blood pressures, measured by oscillometric blood pressure device (mmHg)
Neonate (<30 days)	120–160	60–75
1–6 months	110–140	65–85
6–12 months	100–140	70–90
1–2 years	90–130	75–95
3–5 years	80–120	80–100
6–8 years	75–115	85–105
9–12 years	70–110	90–115
13–16 years	60–110	95–120
>16 years	60–100	100–125

Blood pressure is usually measured with an automated oscillometric blood pressure device, and the cuff must be the proper size for the patient, according to the manufacturer's instructions. A cuff that is too small for the patient will read out a blood pressure that is falsely elevated, and a cuff that is too large will display a pressure that is spuriously low. Under normal circumstances, a cuff on the right or left upper arm is standard, although a properly sized blood pressure cuff on the lower leg will also provide accurate measurements. The measured systolic pressure and mean pressure are very accurate with the oscillometric devices, with the diastolic pressure being subject to increased measurement errors. Since the systolic blood pressure is most commonly used to determine high or low measurements, Table 8.3 includes this parameter for normal values.

Systolic blood pressures more than 20 % below baseline values, if accompanied by acceptable heart rate, oxygen saturation, and end-tidal CO_2, should be investigated and treatment such as fluid administration to increase cardiac preload and stroke volume, or decreasing the depth of sedation, should be instituted. If heart rate, SpO_2, or end-tidal CO_2 has also changed, very urgent diagnosis and treatment must be instituted, as this heralds a low cardiac output state, and possible impending cardiac arrest. Discontinuing sedation, administering fluid boluses and a vagolytic agent such as atropine or sympathomimetic agent such as ephedrine or epinephrine may be indicated. Elevated blood pressures may, of course, be due to inadequate sedation or analgesia, but often can be due to the drugs themselves, especially ketamine. In the latter case, the dose of ketamine should be reduced, or if sedation and analgesia judged to be inadequate, additional drugs other than ketamine should be used. Table 8.3 displays normal heart rate and systolic blood pressure for different ages.

CNS Physiology

Brain growth and development are very rapid during infancy, with the brain weight at birth about 20 % of adult weight, but by 2 years of age, the brain has attained 75 % of adult weight [27]. The brain in the infant and young child receives a correspondingly higher percentage of the cardiac output than in the older child and adult. In addition, rapid proliferation and migration of neurons to their cortical and subcortical zones are taking place in early infancy, as are myelination and synaptogenesis [28] (Fig. 8.4). The neurotransmitters gamma-aminobutyric acid, and glutamate, and their corresponding receptors, play a crucial role in synaptogenesis, and also in the natural death of some neurons during the rapid proliferation phase (apoptosis). Most sedative agents, including benzodiazepines, barbiturates, chloral hydrate, propofol (GABA), and ketamine (NMDA) interact with these receptors, giving rise to the concerns that sedative agents may increase apoptosis and potentially have adverse long-term neurodevelopmental effects [29]. Because of the relatively larger brain size and blood volume/flow, the dose per kilogram requirement for sedative agents is usually higher in the young infant to produce the desired effects than it is in the older child and adult. The exception to this is the neonate, where the tight junctions of the basement membranes of the intracerebral capillaries are not fully formed, meaning the blood–brain barrier is not as fully intact, allowing passage of higher drug concentrations into neurons, causing an exaggerated effect of most drugs in this very young age group.

Cerebral autoregulation is normally intact in the full-term neonate and older patient, albeit at lower blood pressures than in the adult patient. Responsiveness of the cerebral circulation to carbon dioxide tension is also intact, with significant hypercarbia causing maximal cerebral vasodilation.

Maturation of the EEG during infancy and childhood has important implications for any technology proposing to measure depth of sedation using EEG parameters. (Refer to Chap. 6.) All current depth of sedation monitors using processed EEG parameters are based on the adult EEG, and application of these monitors in infants and young children especially is unreliable. Infants and younger children have markedly different EEG profiles for both frequency and amplitude of EEG waveforms emanating from different regions of the brain. Older children (i.e., 8–10 years of age or older) have EEG characteristics much more similar to the adult and thus these monitors can be more reliable [30].

Developmental changes in motor, language, and behavior milestones are crucial to understand when sedating pediatric patients. Table 8.4 presents some of the important milestones

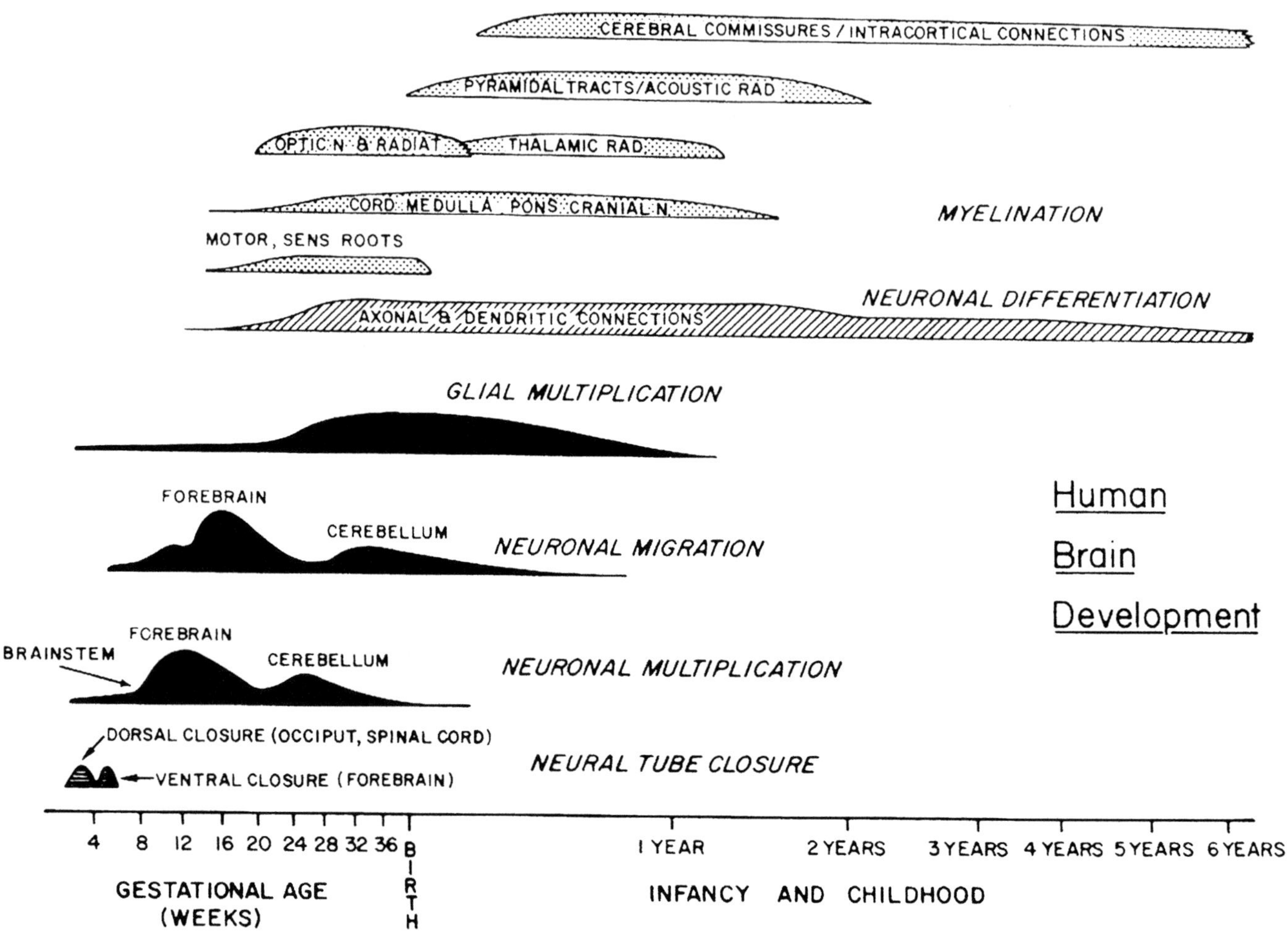

Fig. 8.4 Brain growth and development from conception to age 6 years. Note the very rapid brain growth and complexity of development from birth to age 2 years, when the majority of postnatal brain development occurs. This period of rapid development gives rise to the recent concerns that sedative agents interacting with gamma-aminobutyric acid and *n*-methyl-D-aspartate receptors could have long-term effects on the developing brain. See text for details (Reproduced with permission from Kandt RS, Johnston MV, Goldstein GW. The central nervous system: basic concepts. In: Gregory GA, editor. Pediatric anesthesia. 2nd ed. New York, NY: Churchill-Livingstone; 1989. p. 161–199)

in these areas [31]. In approaching the infant patient, with normal children of age 6–12 months, they will not experience stranger anxiety and thus will go with practitioners for sedation procedures with little to no protest. Extensive study and clinical experience demonstrate that infants from the premature neonate onward experience pain in the same manner as older children, and so will react accordingly to painful procedures such as IV catheter insertion. In the infant up to age 6 months, 24 % sucrose, 0.2 mL placed on a pacifier and given 5–10 min before a painful procedure, will alleviate pain from venipuncture and heelsticks [32]. The mechanism of action is proposed to be endorphin release. Infants from age 6 to 12 months, toddlers, and preschool children up to age 5 can be expected to be quite fearful and resistant when separated from parents or familiar caregivers, and the process of separation must be planned to ameliorate this psychological discomfort as much as possible with distraction, familiar toys, or objects, or having the parent present during initiation of sedation, if appropriate. School-aged children of 5 or 6 years or older generally can accept simple explanations of medical procedures and will often separate from parents more easily. The patient aged 8–12 years is often the easiest to approach for sedation procedures and often has a very concrete understanding of explanations and instructions. The adolescent often has great concern about body image, and respecting this is very important. The child of any age who has been hospitalized frequently or has had prior painful or stressful experiences may be very upset at the prospect of separation from parents and sedation procedures.

Table 8.4 Age-specific anxieties of pediatric patients

Age	Specific type of perioperative anxiety
0–6 months	Maximum stress for parent
	Minimum stress for infants—not old enough to be frightened of strangers
6 months–4 years	Maximum fear of separation
	Not able to understand processes and explanations
	Significant postoperative emotional upset and behavior regression
	Begins to have magical thinking
	Cognitive development and increased temper tantrums
4–8 years	Begins to understand processes and explanations
	Fear of separation remains
	Concerned about body integrity
8 years–adolescence	Tolerates separation well
	Understands processes and explanations
	May interpret everything literally
	May fear waking up during surgery or not waking up at all
Adolescence	Independent
	Issues regarding self-esteem and body image
	Developing sexual characteristics and fear loss of dignity
	Fear of unknown

Reproduced with permission from Ghazal EA, Mason LJ, Cote CJ. Ch 4. Preoperative evaluation, premedication, and induction of anesthesia. In: Cote CJ, Lerman J, Todres ID, editors. A practice of anesthesia for infants and children, 4th edition. Philadelphia, PA: Saunders-Elsevier; 2009. p. 37–69

Hematologic System Development

The neonate has a normal hemoglobin of 15–20 g/dL, and hematocrit of 45–60 %, most all consisting of hemoglobin F, as noted earlier. Over the first 6 months of life, predominate hemoglobin species changes to adult hemoglobin A, and there is a decline to a physiologic nadir of about 11–12 g/dL of hemoglobin by 2–6 months of age. These values are maintained until about age 2 years, at which time they gradually increase in boys and girls to 12–14 g/dL by about age 12. With the onset of menstruation, hemoglobin remains at this level in girls until adulthood. In boys, hemoglobin levels continue to increase gradually to adult levels of 15–18 g/dL by age 18 [33].

The concept of a physiologic nadir of hemoglobin at 2–6 months of age is important, because this is an age when oxygen consumption is still twice that of the adult, yet oxygen carrying capacity is low, with the result that there is even less oxygen reserve in these young infants.

The blood volume of the neonate is approximately 90 mL/kg body weight, and this decreases to about 85 mL/kg by 6 months, 80 mL/kg at 1 year, and 75 mL/kg until age 2 years, after which the blood volume assumes the adult value of approximately 70 mL/kg.

Table 8.5 Maintenance intravenous fluid requirements

Weight	Maintenance fluid, mL/kg/24 h	Maintenance fluid, mL/kg/h
<10 kg	100	4.16
10–20 kg	50	2.08
Each 10 kg increment above 20 kg	20	0.83

Renal Physiology, and Fluid and Electrolytes

At birth the neonate has an expansion of total body water and the extracellular water space, combined with renal function that is decreased, with glomerular filtration rate only 15–30 % of adult values. Renal function matures fairly rapidly, achieving levels of 50 % of the adult by 2 weeks of life, and then gradually increasing to adult levels by 12 months of age [3]. Total body water also decreases to adult levels by about 12 months of age. However, fluid requirements remain high throughout the first 3–4 years of life, because of the increased body surface-to-weight ratio present in young children, which results in increased insensible fluid loss. Table 8.5 displays the approximate daily and hourly maintenance fluid and requirements for normal children at various weights and ages [3]. In children with normal renal function, intravenous fluids of one-quarter normal saline (38 meq NaCl/L) and 20 meq/L KCL will provide maintenance of sodium and potassium, and 5 % dextrose for maintenance of glucose requirements. In actual practice, healthy infants and children over age 6 months will do well with a standard intravenous solution such as lactated Ringer's solution during sedation procedures. This solution, which does not contain dextrose but has a sodium concentration of 130 meq/L and osmolarity similar to plasma, will allow a fluid bolus to be administered without producing hyperglycemia.

In general, modern nil per os (NPO) guidelines allowing clear liquid intake until 2 h before a sedation procedure will prevent significant fluid deficits, but frequently there are situations where the patient has been NPO for long periods of time.

If NPO for greater than 6 h, many practitioners would calculate the fluid deficit accumulated during those 6 h, administer half the deficit during the first hour of the procedure, and one-quarter of the deficit in each of the next 3 h [31]. These fasting guidelines were published in 1999, approved by the American Society of Anesthesiologists (ASA) and represent a recommendation based on the review of clinical studies between 1966 and 1996, over 1,100 citations. They were updated in 2011, after further literature review and recommendations of experts in pediatric anesthesia. They were intended for healthy patients undergoing elective surgery [34] (Table 8.6). The guidelines were not intended nor

Table 8.6 American Society of Anesthesiologists' summary of fasting recommendations to reduce the risk of pulmonary aspiration[a]

Ingested material	Minimum fasting period[b] (hours)
Clear liquids[c]	2
Breast milk	4
Infant formula	6
Nonhuman milk[d]	6
Light meal[e]	6

Reprinted with permission from the American Society of Anesthesiologists Task Force on Preoperative Fasting. Practice guidelines for preoperative fasting and the use of pharmacologic agents to reduce the risk of pulmonary aspiration: application to healthy patients undergoing elective procedures. Anesthesiology. 1999;90:896–905

[a]These recommendations apply to healthy patients who are undergoing elective procedures. They are not intended for women in labor. Following the guidelines does not guarantee complete gastric emptying

[b]Fasting times apply to all ages

[c]Examples: water, fruit juice without pulp, carbonated beverages, clear tea, and black coffee

[d]Since nonhuman milk is similar to solids in gastric emptying time, the amount ingested must be considered when determining an appropriate fasting period

[e]A light meal typically consists of toast and clear liquids. Meals that include fried or fatty foods or meat may prolong gastric emptying time. Both the amount and type of foods ingested must be considered when determining an appropriate fasting period

considered for sedation purposes, although they have been so adopted by many.

Glucose requirement is predictably high in the neonate and young infant, being 5–7 mg/kg/min in the neonate, which is 2–3 times that of the adult. The neonate and young infant less than 3–6 months of age are also prone to hypoglycemia because of a paucity of glycogen stores, compared to the older child and adult, thus it is especially important in this age group to encourage ingestion of clear glucose-containing fluids until 2 h before a sedation procedure. And, young infants should have infusion of dextrose-containing intravenous fluids during and after the sedation procedure, until they are recovered and can ingest dextrose-containing fluids again.

Hepatic/Gastrointestinal Physiology

Liver function, both synthetic and metabolic, is immature at birth, with only about 30 % of the functional capacity of the adult [3]. Hepatic function also matures relatively rapidly, with normal function achieved by about 3 months of life. This means that drugs that depend on hepatic metabolism for clearance, especially the cytochrome P450 system, will often have prolonged effects in the very young infant once therapeutic plasma levels are reached. In addition, coagulation factor levels are low in the neonate because of this hepatic immaturity, so that normal partial thromboplastin time, which measures coagulation function in the extrinsic coagulation system and depends on proteins synthesized in the liver, is elevated at birth to as high as 60 s. Despite this, the protein factors that inhibit coagulation are also reduced in concentration, and neonates and young infants are not more prone to clinical bleeding than older patients.

As with other systems, the brush border of the neonatal small bowel is not mature, and is more prone to insults such as infections and ischemia, particularly in the premature infant, which predisposes them to necrotizing enterocolitis. The risk of this disease diminishes greatly toward term, but the ability of the full-term neonate's intestine to absorb high osmolar loads is limited. With normal intake such as breast milk or infant formulas, however, gastric emptying is rapid. This normal gastric emptying has given rise to the standard recommendation in most institutions that in patients of all ages—who do not have bowel obstruction or other condition known to delay gastric emptying—ingestion of solid food, milk, or formula until 6 h prior to a sedation procedure is acceptable. Breast milk ingestion until 4 h before sedation, and clear liquids until 2 h before, has also been shown to result in complete gastric emptying.

Temperature Regulation

Maintenance of temperature homeostasis during sedation procedures is an important goal, and the young child in particular is prone to hypothermia during prolonged sedation. Heat loss (or gain) into or from the environment is via four basic routes [35, 36]:

1. Radiation—from difference in temperature between the patient and the surrounding environment, e.g., a cold room
2. Conduction—heat transfer between two surfaces in direct contact, i.e., a cold irrigating solution
3. Convection—transfer of heat to moving molecules such as air or liquid, i.e., a cold drafty MRI scanning room
4. Evaporation—loss of heat from vaporization of water from the skin or mucosal surface

Under normal circumstances, the older infant, child, or adult will sense temperature of the blood in the anterior hypothalamus, the thermostat for the body, and use various mechanisms to keep body temperature within 0.5 of 37 °C [35]. In response to mild hypothermia, the CNS via α(alpha)-adrenergic sympathetic activation will cause cutaneous blood vessels to constrict, especially in the extremities, reducing blood flow and thus conserving heat by shunting warmed blood flow to deeper structures not vulnerable to radiation heat loss. With moderate hypothermia shivering occurs, which through muscle aerobic metabolism will generate additional heat and help return body temperature toward normal. With hyperthermia, initially blood flow to the extremities will remain at normal levels, but with further warming vasodilation will occur, and heat loss from

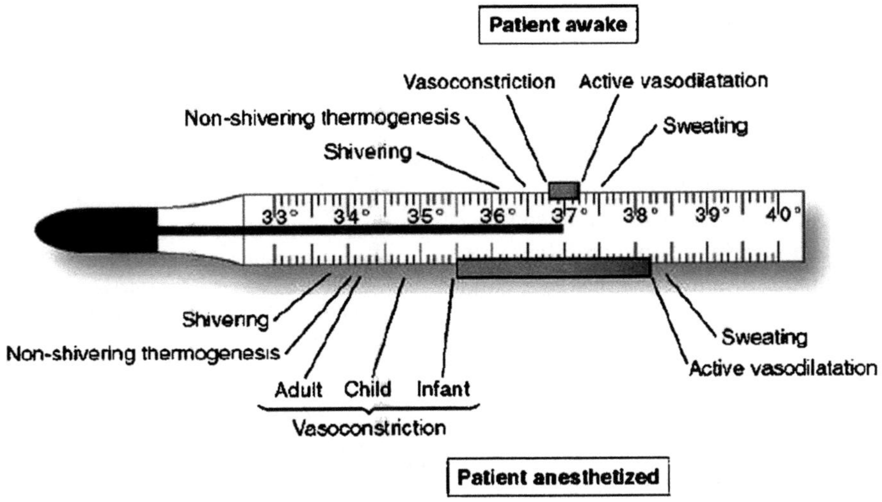

Fig. 8.5 Illustration of the thermoregulatory thresholds and gains for awake and anesthetized (sedated) infants, children, and adults in relation to the central (core) temperature. The distance between the edge of the thermometer and each effector response represents the maximal intensity of each response. The slopes of the lines (positive values for awake and negative values for anesthetized) between the thermometer and the response represent the gains of the responses. The threshold is defined as the corresponding core temperature that triggers a response. The sensitivity of the thermoregulatory system describes the range between the first cold response (vasoconstriction) and the first warm response (sweating), which is known as the interthreshold range. Sedation with agents such as propofol and dexmedetomidine produces the same dose-dependent changes in thermoregulation as general anesthesia (Reproduced with permission from Luginbuehl I, Bissonnette B. Ch 25. Thermal regulation. In: Cote CJ, Lerman J, Todres ID, editors. A practice of anesthesia for infants and children. Philadelphia, PA: Saunders-Elsevier; 2009. p. 557–567)

radiation, convection, and conduction all increase. The next response is sweating, with the evaporation of sweat resulting in significant heat loss.

Commonly used sedative agents, including propofol and dexmedetomidine, affect the thermoregulatory thresholds [35]. In general, the higher the dose of these agents, the wider the range of "normal" temperatures tolerated by the hypothalamus before the compensatory mechanisms described earlier occur, meaning that temperatures will need to decrease by 1.5–2.5 °C before vasoconstriction and shivering will begin, rather than 0.5 °C in the awake patient (Fig. 8.5).

Adverse effects of significant hypothermia include enhanced effects of intravenous sedative medication and a lower dose requirement for sedation, as well as slowed metabolism and organ function, resulting in delayed metabolism of drugs by kidney and liver. This can result in prolonged awakening from sedation. Significant hypothermia accompanied by shivering can result in metabolic acidosis from anaerobic muscle metabolism. Significant hypothermia and shivering are also profoundly uncomfortable for the patient, often resulting in an unsatisfactory sedation experience in the case of older children, or agitation and crying behaviors in the younger children.

The neonate is a special case, as in most other organ systems, in that with significant hypothermia the neonate cannot shiver, but rather starts to metabolize special brown fat cells, mostly located between the scapulae, and in the mediastinum and perirenal areas, in order to generate heat to raise body temperature, in a process termed nonshivering thermogenesis [35]. This is accompanied by a significant catecholamine discharge and anaerobic metabolism, resulting in lactic acidosis, which can have profound secondary effects on other organ systems (i.e., the heart and circulation) resulting in hemodynamic instability. Nonshivering thermogenesis is either nonexistent or insignificant after the neonatal period.

Because of the high body surface area-to-weight ratio of neonates, which decreases to adult levels by 8–9 years of age, the young child is susceptible to hypothermia by radiation. Thus, an infant or young child who is uncovered and exposed to cool ambient temperatures, especially with a draft or in a room cooled because of medical equipment (e.g., MRI scanners) will cool rapidly.

Preventing hypothermia is a crucial task for every sedation procedure in children, and often the simplest method is to cover or wrap the child in warm blankets to prevent heat loss by convection. Warming the room and employing forced air warming devices where possible are other important measures to prevent hypothermia. Continuous temperature measurement during sedation procedures in patients at risk for hypothermia should be practiced, especially during lengthy procedures such as MRI scans in infants. In these patients, temperature should be monitored along with other routine vital signs in the recovery area.

Drug Pharmacokinetics and Pharmacodynamics

All of the differences in organ system physiology discussed previously, especially cardiovascular, CNS, hepatic, renal, and body fluid composition, mean that response to sedative drugs, and initial dosage and interval dosing, are often very different especially in the infant, compared to the older child and adult.

Conclusion

Children, particularly the neonate and infant, have very substantial differences in physiology in all systems compared to the adult. The increased metabolic requirements for the rapidly growing young patient result in higher demand for oxygen and glucose, the major metabolic fuels. This translates into a much smaller margin of error during sedation procedures especially in patients less than 1 year of age, but to some extent in all growing children, and the sedation practitioner must be well aware of these physiologic differences for the safe and effective sedation procedure.

References

1. Shaffer TH, Wolfson MR, Panitch HB. Airway structure, function and development in health and disease. Paediatr Anaesth. 2004; 14(1):3–14.
2. O'Rourke PP, Crone RK. The respiratory system. In: Gregory GA, editor. Gregory's pediatric anesthesia. 2nd ed. New York: Churchill Livingstone; 1989. p. 63–91.
3. McClain CD, McManus ML. Fluid management. In: Cote CJ, Lerman J, Anderson BJ, editors. Cote and Lerman's a practice of anesthesia for infants and children. 5th ed. Philadelphia: Elsevier; 2013. p. 161–77.
4. Sly PD, Collins RA. Physiological basis of respiratory signs and symptoms. Paediatr Respir Rev. 2006;7:84–8.
5. Smith CA, Nelson NM, editors. The physiology of the newborn infant. 4th ed. Springfield: Charles C. Thomas; 1976, p. 205.
6. Delivoria-Papadopoulos M, Ronceric NP, Oski FA. Postnatal changes in oxygen transport of premature and sick infants: the role of red cell 2,3 diphosphoglycerate and adult hemoglobin. Pediatr Res. 1971;5:235–40.
7. Moss TJ. Respiratory consequences of preterm birth. Clin Exp Pharmacol Physiol. 2006;33:280–4.
8. Firth PG, Haver KE. Essentials of pulmonology. In: Cote CJ, Lerman J, Todres ID, editors. A practice of anesthesia for infants and children. Philadelphia: Saunders-Elsevier; 2009. p. 221–36.
9. Friedman WF. The intrinsic physiologic properties of the developing heart. Prog Cardiovasc Dis. 1972;15:87–111.
10. Friedman WF, George BL. Treatment of congestive heart failure by altering loading conditions of the heart. J Pediatr. 1985;106: 697–706.
11. Eliot RJ, Lam R, Leake RD, et al. Plasma catecholamine concentrations in infants at birth and during the first 48 hours of life. J Pediatr. 1980;96:311.
12. Romero T, Covell U, Friedman WF. A comparison of pressure-volume relations of the fetal, newborn, and adult heart. Am J Physiol. 1972;222:1285.
13. Teitel DF, Sisd D, Chin T, et al. Developmental changes in myocardial contractile reserve in the lamb. Pediatr Res. 1985;19:948.
14. Nassar R, Malouf NN, Kelly MB, et al. Force-pCa relation and troponin T isoforms of rabbit myocardium. Circ Res. 1991;69: 1470–5.
15. Andropoulos DB. Physiology and molecular biology of the developing circulation. In: Andropoulos DB, Stayer SA, Russell IA, Mossad EB, editors. Anesthesia for congenital heart disease. 2nd ed. Oxford: Wiley-Blackwell; 2010. p. 55075.
16. Rudolph AM, editor. Changes in the circulation after birth. In: Congenital diseases of the heart. Chicago, IL: Year Book Medical; 1974, p. 9.
17. Baum VC, Palmisano BW. The immature heart and anesthesia. Anesthesiology. 1997;87:1529–48.
18. Friedman WF, Pool PE, Jacobowitz D, et al. Sympathetic innervation of the developing rabbit heart. Biochemical and histochemical comparisons of fetal, neonatal, and adult myocardium. Circ Res. 1968;23:25–32.
19. Jacobowitz D, Koelle GB. Histochemical correlations of acetylcholinesterase and catecholamines in post-ganglionic autonomic nerves of the cat, rabbit and guinea pig. J Pharmacol Exp Ther. 1965;148:225–37.
20. Pagani M, Montano N, Porta A, et al. Relationship between spectral components of cardiovascular variabilities and direct measures of sympathetic nerve activity in humans. Circulation. 1997;95: 1441–8.
21. Constant I, Dubois M, Piat V, Moutard M, et al. Changes in electroencephalogram and autonomic cardiovascular activity during induction of anesthesia with sevoflurane compared with halothane in children. Anesthesiology. 1999;91:1604–15.
22. Katona PG, Frasz A, Egbert J. Maturation of cardiac control in full-term and preterm infants during sleep. Early Hum Dev. 1980; 4:145–59.
23. Fabiato A, Fabiato F. Calcium induced release of calcium from the sarcoplasmic reticulum of skinned cells from adult human, dog, cat, rabbit, rat, and frog hearts and from fetal and newborn rat ventricles. Ann N Y Acad Sci. 1978;307:491–9.
24. Rudolph AM. Myocardial growth before and after birth: clinical implications. Acta Paediatr. 2000;89:129–33.
25. Friesen RH, Wurl JL, Charlton GA. Haemodynamic depression by halothane is age-related in paediatric patients. Paediatr Anaesth. 2000;10:267–72.
26. Davignon A. ECG standards for children. Pediatr Cardiol. 1980; 1:133–52.
27. Kandt RS, Johnston MV, Goldstein GW. The central nervous system: basic concepts. In: Gregory GA, editor. Pediatric anesthesia. 2nd ed. New York: Churchill-Livingstone; 1989. p. 161–99.
28. Dobbing J, Sands J. Comparative aspects of the brain growth spurt. Early Hum Dev. 1979;3:79–83.
29. Loepke AW, Soriano SG. An assessment of the effects of general anesthetics on developing brain structure and neurocognitive function. Anesth Analg. 2008;106:1681–707.
30. Davidson AJ. Monitoring the anaesthetic depth in children: an update. Curr Opin Anaesthesiol. 2007;20:236–43.
31. Ghazal EA, Mason LJ, Cote CJ. Preoperative evaluation, premedication, and induction of anesthesia. In: Cote CJ, Lerman J, Anderson BJ, editors. Cote and Lerman's a practice of anesthesia for infants and children. 5th ed. Philadelphia: Elsevier; 2013. p. 31–63.
32. Stevens B, Yamada J, Ohlsson A. Sucrose for analgesia in newborn infants undergoing painful procedures. Cochrane Database Syst Rev. 2001(4):CD001069. Review. Update in: Cochrane Database Syst Rev. 2004;(3):CD001069.

33. Dallman PR, Shannon K. Developmental changes in red blood cell production and function. In: Rudolph AM, Hoffman JIE, Rudolph CD, editors. Rudolph's pediatrics. 20th ed. Stamford: Appleton & Lange; 1996. p. 1167–70.
34. American Society of Anesthesiologists Committee on Standards and Practice Parameters. Practice guidelines for preoperative fasting and the use of pharmacologic agents to reduce the risk of pulmonary aspiration: application to healthy patients undergoing elective procedures: an updated report by the American Society of Anesthesiologists Committee on Standards and Practice Parameters. Anesthesiology. 2011;114:495–511.
35. Flick R. Clinical complications in pediatric anesthesia. In: Gregory GA, Andropoulos DB, editors. Gregory's pediatric anesthesia. 5th ed. Oxford: Wiley-Blackwell; 2012. p. 1152–82.
36. Luginbuehl I, Bissonnette B. Thermal regulation. In: Cote CJ, Lerman J, Todres ID, editors. A practice of anesthesia for infants and children. Philadelphia: Saunders-Elsevier; 2009. p. 557–67.

The Pharmacology and Clinical Application of Sedatives, Analgesics, and Adjuncts

9

Randy P. Prescilla

Abstract

The overall objective in sedation outside the operating room is to provide effective and safe sedation. The American Academy of Pediatrics (AAP) provides five specific goals: "(1) to guard the patient's safety and welfare, (2) to minimize physical discomfort and pain, (3) to control anxiety, minimize psychological trauma, and maximize the potential for amnesia, (4) control behavior and/or movement to allow the safe completion of the procedure, and (5) return the patient to a state in which safe discharge is possible."

In order to achieve effective and safe sedation, it is imperative that sedation providers possess a clear understanding of the pharmacology of the drugs that will be administered. Knowledge of each drug's time of onset, peak response, and duration of action is critical. The American Society of Anesthesiologists (ASA) also mandates that the curriculum for a formal training program in sedation for nonanesthesiologists should include, among others, "the pharmacology of all anesthetic drugs…of moderate sedation."

Keywords

Pharmacology • Sedatives • Analgesics • Adjuncts • Reversal agents • Pharmacokinetics • Contraindications • Route of administration • Clinical application • Adverse events • American Academy of Pediatrics (AAP) • American Society of Anesthesiologists (ASA) • Food and Drug Administration (FDA) • Off-label • Best Pharmaceuticals for Children Act (BPCA) • Pediatric Research Equity Act (PREA) • Alfentanil • Chloral hydrate • Codeine • Dexmedetomidine • Opiod • Diazepam • Etomidate • Fentanyl • Fospropofol • Ketamine • Ketofol • Lorazepam • Meperidine (Demerol) • Methohexital (Brevital) • Midazolam (Versed) • Morphine • Nitrous oxide • Pentobarbital (Nembutal) • Propofol • Remifentanil • S-ketamine • Sufentanil • Flumazenil • Naloxone (Narcan) • Lidocaine • Ondansetron (Zofran) • Metoclopramide (Reglan) • Scopolamine • Diphenhydramine (Benadryl) • Dexamethasone (Decadron)

Introduction

The overall objective in sedation outside the operating room is to provide effective and safe sedation.

The American Academy of Pediatrics (AAP) provides five specific goals: "(1) to guard the patient's safety and welfare, (2) to minimize physical discomfort and pain, (3) to control anxiety, minimize psychological trauma, and maximize the potential for amnesia, (4) control behavior and/or

R.P. Prescilla, M.D. (✉)
Department of Anesthesiology, Perioperative and Pain Medicine, Boston Children's Hospital, 300 Longwood Avenue, Boston, MA 02115, USA
e-mail: randy.prescilla@childrens.harvard.edu

K.P. Mason (ed.), *Pediatric Sedation Outside of the Operating Room: A Multispecialty International Collaboration*, DOI 10.1007/978-1-4939-1390-9_9, © Springer Science+Business Media New York 2015

movement to allow the safe completion of the procedure, and (5) return the patient to a state in which safe discharge is possible" [1].

In order to achieve effective and safe sedation, it is imperative that sedation providers possess a clear understanding of the pharmacology of the drugs that will be administered. Knowledge of each drug's time of onset, peak response, and duration of action is critical [1]. The American Society of Anesthesiologists (ASA) also mandates that the curriculum for a formal training program in sedation for nonanesthesiologists should include, among others, "the pharmacology of all anesthetic drugs…of moderate sedation" [2].

Drug Selection and Administration

The AAP states that the goals of sedation can best be achieved by selecting the lowest dose required, and selecting the drug(s) with the highest therapeutic index for the procedure. It is essential that in the selection process of which drug to use, the practitioner should choose the least number of drugs, while matching the drug(s) to the type and goal of the procedure that is being planned. For example, analgesic medications such as opioids are indicated for painful procedures, while for nonpainful procedures, sedatives/hypnotics may suffice. Since children younger than 6 years and those with developmental delay generally require deep levels of sedation, the need for deep sedation should be anticipated [1]. Anxiolysis or mild sedation may be occasionally sufficient for computerized tomography (CT), but is often not enough in procedures such as magnetic resonance (MR) or nuclear medicine imaging.

Selection of medications and dosages should be guided by the desired key effect(s). An ideal regimen would provide acceptable analgesia, sedation, and amnesia for residual awareness of procedure-related pain or anxiety. It would cause minimal adverse effects and work reliably with a wide therapeutic index; i.e., small differences in doses would not cause oversedation or adverse events, have rapid onset and recovery, and be easy to titrate to effect. No single agent or combination of agents fully achieves these goals. Selection of procedural sedation medications therefore is based upon balancing desired effects with the potential for adverse effects. For procedures that are very painful (e.g., fracture reduction), control of the pain will be paramount. For procedures that require the child to be motionless (e.g., CT or MRI scans) immobility may be most important. Most procedures in children require some combination of analgesia and immobility along with anxiolysis; therefore, sedation planning should consider all these parameters.

Because increasing depth of sedation is associated with increasing frequency of adverse events [3, 4], use of the lightest effective sedation is usually preferred. However, frequently the depth of sedation required for a particular procedure cannot be accurately predicted in a specific patient [3]. Underappreciated anxiety and a lack of comprehension in younger children and those with developmental delay often elicit a need for deeper-than-anticipated sedation. For intensely painful procedures, deep sedation is typically required. Sedation practitioners, therefore, should be trained and prepared to administer increasingly deeper sedation as guided by the patient's response to the procedure.

Careful intravenous "titration" of medications uses repeatedly administered small doses to achieve the desired clinical effect. Titration enables the practitioner to use the smallest effective dose and reduce the risk of oversedation with its accompanying risks of respiratory depression and aspiration [3, 5–7]. Individual variation in sensitivity to the medication can also be detected, thus a smaller-than-expected dose may be found adequate for a given individual.

Knowledge of the time to peak effect of the specific medication is necessary to avoid "stacking" of doses when first gaining experience with titration. "Stacking" can occur after a subsequent dose is administered before the peak effect of the preceding dose has occurred. In these situations, deeper-than-intended sedation can easily occur. For example, morphine has a peak effect at approximately 10 min. If an additional dose of morphine is administered after 5 min because the patient is still in significant pain, by 15 min after the original dose—when both the first and second doses are near peak effects—the patient may have significant respiratory depression due to an excessive accumulative dose. For this reason, titration is difficult with drugs that have longer than 1–3 min to peak effect time.

When a "typical" total dose for a specific procedure is known, that total dose may be divided and the increments administered at intervals shorter than "the time to peak effect" without likely overshoot. This strategy of repeated administration of fractional doses for fixed dose protocols—e.g., half of the anticipated total dose administered twice with administration separated by a short interval—reduces the risk for significant respiratory depression induced by some agents, such as the combined technique using fentanyl and midazolam. This approach is suggested for practitioners as they acquire experience with a specific medication.

Use of Multiple Drugs for Sedation

A strong knowledge of pharmacology is essential when administration of several sedating agents is considered. Drugs with long durations of action must be allowed to manifest their pharmacologic actions and peak effects before additional doses are considered. The practitioner must know whether the previous dose of any drug has taken full effect before administering additional medications [1].

If the mechanisms of action of concomitant medications are similar, synergistic effects may be potentiated, and the risk of adverse events is magnified. Respiratory depression is a common pathway of adverse events, and may result unexpectedly and quickly. A study in 2000 showed that potential for adverse events may be increased when three or more medications are administered for sedation [8].

Practitioners must also be cognizant that drug interactions may occur. Drugs such as erythromycin, cimetidine, and others inhibit the cytochrome P450 system and concomitant use of these medications can result in prolonged sedation with midazolam and other medications that compete for the same enzyme systems. Even herbal medications such as St. John's wort or echinacea can affect drug pharmacokinetics resulting from altered cytochrome P450 effects.

Additional Pharmacologic Effects

One benefit that some sedatives provide is analgesia. This is critical not only for patients who are in pain at the onset of sedation but also for patients who will become uncomfortable or experience pain during the diagnostic study. Patient as well as procedural factors can amplify the pain response, for example, a child with scoliosis who may be required to lay flat on an MRI table for an hour, or a child whose elbow will need to remain flexed at a certain angle during a radiologic imaging study. By their nature as opioids, fentanyl, sufentanil, remifentanil, and alfentanil are known to produce analgesia. Dexmedetomidine has also been reported to provide analgesic effects.

An additional effect that some sedatives provide is relative amnesia. This effect is helpful for young children whose previous visit(s) may be marred by traumatic memory. An amnesic effect is also most helpful in children who will need additional sedation or procedures in the future. Drugs that have been reported to produce amnesia include propofol [9–12], fentanyl [9], ketamine [12, 13] and S-ketamine [14], and the benzodiazepines midazolam [15, 16] and lorazepam [17]. Ideally, the patient will be unable to recall procedure-related pain despite occasional moans or crying out during intensely painful parts of the procedure [18]. It is unwise to promise complete amnesia during the informed consent process.

Off-Label Use

Unfortunately, most drugs used for sedation in children do not carry pediatric information that has been reviewed and approved by the Food and Drug Administration (FDA) and as such, these drugs are used "off-label." Out of 106 drugs administered during anesthesia to pediatric patients from the operating room pharmacy, drugs were administered off-label in about 73 % of cases [19]. Implementation of legislation such as the Best Pharmaceuticals for Children Act and the Pediatric Research Equity Act has led to the addition of specific pediatric information in more than 500 product labels from 1997 to 2013 [20].)

Readers are reminded that the current FDA guidelines on off-label use state that "if physicians use a product for an indication not in the approved labeling, they have the responsibility to be well informed about the product, to base its use on firm scientific rationale and on sound medical evidence, and to maintain records of the product's use and effects" [21].

In general, the off-label use of a marketed product for the "practice of medicine" does not require the submission of an Investigational New Drug Application from the FDA [21]. However, the institution at which the product will be used may, under its own authority, require Institutional Review Board (IRB) review or other institutional oversight. The reader is advised to consult the IRB in his or her institution for specific guidelines.

Alternate Sites of Administration

Off-label use in pediatrics includes the use of routes of administration that are not contained in current FDA-approved drug information. Pediatric practitioners try to be innovative in order to decrease pain and discomfort in children through a variety of ways. These include drug administration via nasal, transdermal, oral, sublingual, and oral and rectal routes. The American Academy of Pediatrics, Committee on Drugs cautions that although new routes of administration offer advantages, controlled laboratory and clinical trials are necessary to determine safe use. When new methods or routes of drug administration are introduced, the Committee further recommends that the practitioner understand the pharmacologic actions of the drug, as well as the pharmacokinetic and pharmacodynamic implications that may be unique for pediatric patients [22].

In March 2014, the AAP and its Committee on Drugs published a policy statement on off-label drugs in children. The policy concluded that "evidence, not label indication, remains the gold standard from which practitioners should draw when making therapeutic decisions for their patients." The statement made recommendations for off-label drug administration and the advocating of off-label drug research and publication. Finally, the policy statement recommended, "institutions and payers should not use labeling status as the sole criterion that determines the availability on formulary or reimbursement status for medications in children. Similarly, less expensive therapeutic alternatives considered appropriate for adults should not automatically be considered appropriate first-line treatment in children. Finally, off-label uses of drugs should be considered when addressing various drug-related concerns, such as drug shortages" [23].

Reversal Agents

The knowledge of pharmacology should also extend to that of drugs that may be needed to "rescue" a sedated patient. Currently, pharmacologic antagonists exist only for opiates and benzodiazepines. This includes reversal agents such as flumazenil and naloxone. Drugs that are not reversal agents per se such as albuterol, ammonia spirits, atropine, diphenhydramine, diazepam, epinephrine, glucose, lidocaine, methylprednisolone, fosphenytoin, rocuronium, sodium bicarbonate, and succinylcholine may also be required in specific cases [1]. As the need for resuscitation can occur unexpectedly, the practitioner should familiarize him or herself with dosing and drug administration.

The Effects of Psychotropic Drugs on the Developing Brain

There is growing concern about the neurotoxic effects of anesthetics in the human developing brain. To date, there is no direct evidence in humans of neurotoxicity. (Refer to Chap. 27 [24].)

Formulary

The most common medications currently used in sedation in children are presented in the next section. A brief description of the pharmacologic nature of each drug is provided, along with any available pediatric pharmacokinetic data, followed by a brief discussion on the clinical applications in children and common adverse events.

As the data indicate, there are limited published pediatric data on most of these medications. The sedation practitioner is encouraged to consult the latest appropriate formulary in their institution, particularly for pediatric dosage and restrictions of use, if any. Pediatric sedation practitioners are also encouraged to conduct formal clinical studies to add to the literature in pediatric sedation.

This chapter is not intended to list which drugs are appropriate for which particular procedure.

The reader is advised to refer to the individual chapters that discuss specific sedatives in the appropriate clinical context, for indications and dosages.

Lastly, inclusion of a drug in this chapter does not imply endorsement of an off-label use.

Sedatives and Analgesics

Alfentanil (Alfenta, Rapifen)

Drug class: Opioid.

Route of administration: Primarily intravenous, although intranasal administration in children has been reported [25, 26].

The pharmacokinetics of alfentanil can be described as a three-compartment model. The liver is the major site of biotransformation; urinary excretion is the major route of elimination of metabolites [27].

The pharmacokinetics of alfentanil in children has been described [26, 28–38].

Contraindications: Alfentanil is contraindicated in patients with known hypersensitivity to the drug or known intolerance to other opioid agonists.

Clinical application: Alfentanil is an opioid analgesic with a rapid onset of action. As such it is used in sedation as an analgesic adjunct in anesthesia or monitored anesthesia care.

Alfentanil is seldom used now [39].

Common adverse events [27] include respiratory depression and skeletal muscle rigidity, particularly of the truncal muscles. Alfentanil may produce muscular rigidity that involves the skeletal muscles of the neck and extremities.

Respiratory events reported during monitored anesthesia care (MAC) included hypoxia, apnea and bradypnea, nausea, hypotension, vomiting, pruritus, confusion, somnolence, and agitation.

The incidence of certain side effects is influenced by the type of use (e.g., chest wall rigidity has a higher reported incidence in clinical trials of alfentanil induction) and by the type of surgery (e.g., nausea and vomiting have a higher reported incidence in patients undergoing gynecologic surgery). The overall reports of nausea and vomiting with alfentanil were comparable to fentanyl.

Chloral Hydrate

Drug class: Chloral derivative.

Chloral hydrate is rapidly reduced to the active compound trichloroethanol, which exerts barbiturate-like effects on GABA-receptor [40].

Route of administration: Primarily oral, but rectal administration for sedation in children has been reported [41–44].

Chloral hydrate is extensively metabolized in the liver by alcohol dehydrogenases and by erythrocytes to its major metabolite, trichloroethanol [45]. Less than 10 % of chloral hydrate is excreted in the urine.

The pharmacokinetics of chloral hydrate in children has been described [46, 47].

Approved indications: Sedative, hypnotic. (+) Pediatric labeling.

Contraindications: Chloral hydrate is contraindicated in patients with marked hepatic or renal impairment and in patients who have previously demonstrated hypersensitivity or an idiosyncratic reaction to the drug.

Clinical application: Chloral hydrate continues to be used for moderate sedation in children. The advantages and disadvantages of chloral hydrate have been reviewed [48]. Disadvantages include the long half-life: up to 48 h in children [46]. TCE has also been found to be carcinogenic in mice [48, 49].

In 1993, the AAP issued a statement on the use of chloral hydrate for sedation in children [49]. In it, the Academy states that it is an effective sedative when administered in the recommended dosage. However, repetitive dosing of chloral hydrate is of concern, as well as theoretical long-term risk of carcinogenicity. The need for additional studies was raised.

Common adverse events include prolonged sedation, respiratory depression, nausea/vomiting, gastric and esophageal irritation, diarrhea, headache, disorientation, dysphoria, dizziness, rash, and hypotension (especially in neonates).

Codeine

Drug class: Opioid.

Codeine is mentioned in this formulary only to emphasize that it is an unreliable analgesic because it is a prodrug of morphine, and the enzyme (CYP2D6) that converts codeine to morphine has many different genetic variants. This results in some patients getting little to no analgesia from codeine (poor metabolizers) and other patients overdosing because of overactive metabolism (ultrarapid metabolizers). There have been many deaths in pediatrics associated with codeine use due to overactive metabolism [50].

The FDA issued the following Drug Safety Communication in August 2012 [50] and later, a communication update in February 2013 and eventually, issued a Black Box Warning for use of codeine and contraindication on use after tonsillectomy and/or adenoidectomy [51].

Dexmedetomidine (Precedex, Dexdor)

Drug class: Alpha2 receptor agonist.

Route of administration: Intravenous [52], although buccal [53–56], intranasal [57–59], and intramuscular [60, 61] administration in children have been reported.

Dexmedetomidine undergoes almost complete biotransformation with very little unchanged dexmedetomidine excreted in the urine and feces. Biotransformation involves both direct glucuronidation and cytochrome P450-mediated metabolism. About 95 % of the drug is recovered in the urine and 4 % in the feces.

The pharmacokinetics of dexmedetomidine in children has been described [62–66].

Approved indications: Sedation.

Contraindication: None.

Clinical application: Dexmedetomidine was originally indicated for sedation of initially intubated and mechanically ventilated adult patients during treatment in an intensive care setting. It has recently been approved for sedation of non-intubated adults prior to and/or during surgical and other procedures.

Dexmedetomidine offers the advantage of providing sedation and analgesia with little respiratory depression and in most a tolerable decrease in blood pressure and heart rate [67].

Adverse events [52] include serious adverse reactions such as hypotension, bradycardia, sinus arrest, and transient hypertension in both Intensive Care Unit and procedural sedation studies.

Hypotension and bradycardia were the most common adverse reactions associated with the use of dexmedetomidine during post-approval use.

Diazepam (Valium, Antenex)

Drug class: Benzodiazepine.

Route of administration: Rectal, intravenous, oral.

After oral administration >90 % of diazepam is absorbed and the average time to achieve peak plasma concentrations is 1–1.5 h. Absorption is delayed and decreased when administered with a moderate fat meal.

Diazepam is N-demethylated to the active metabolite N-desmethyldiazepam, and is hydroxylated to the active metabolite temazepam. N-desmethyldiazepam and temazepam are both further metabolized to oxazepam. Temazepam and oxazepam are largely eliminated by glucuronidation and are excreted mainly in the urine, predominantly as their glucuronide conjugates [68].

The clinical pharmacology of diazepam in children has been reviewed [69].

Approved indications: Sedation. (+) Pediatric labeling.

Contraindications: Diazepam injection is contraindicated in patients with a known hypersensitivity to this drug, in acute narrow-angle glaucoma, and in open-angle glaucoma unless patients are receiving appropriate therapy.

Clinical application: Diazepam is administered to provide anxiolysis, with accompanying mild sedation. This state usually suffices for short diagnostic procedures.

Common adverse events include drowsiness, fatigue, and ataxia; venous thrombosis and phlebitis at the site of injection [68].

Etomidate (Amidate)

Drug class: Carboxylated imidazole.

Route of administration: Intravenous.

Etomidate is rapidly metabolized in the liver.

Approximately 75 % of the administered dose is excreted in the urine during the first day after injection. The chief metabolite is produced from hydrolysis of, and accounts for about 80 % of the urinary excretion [70].

The pharmacokinetics of etomidate in children has been described [71].

Contraindication: Etomidate is contraindicated in patients who have shown hypersensitivity to it.

Clinical application: Etomidate was more effective and efficient than pentobarbital in CT sedation in the emergency department, with rare adverse events [72]. The use of etomidate for sedation has also been compared to midazolam [73] and pentobarbital [74].

Common adverse events [70] include transient venous pain on injection and transient skeletal muscle movements, including myoclonus, hyperventilation, hypoventilation, apnea of short duration, laryngospasm, hiccup, and snoring suggestive of partial upper airway obstruction; all have been observed in some patients; hypertension, hypotension, tachycardia, bradycardia, and other arrhythmias have occasionally been observed during induction; and maintenance of anesthesia, nausea, and/or vomiting following induction of anesthesia. One case of anaphylactoid reaction (severe hypotension and tachycardia) has been reported.

Etomidate Analogs

Two derivatives of etomidate are in development. MOC-etomidate is an analog that retains the important favorable pharmacological properties of etomidate, such as rapid onset of action, high hypnotic potency, and hemodynamic stability. In addition, it is rapidly metabolized, ultra-short-acting, and does not produce prolonged adrenocortical suppression after bolus administration [75]. Carboetomidate represents an etomidate analog that contains a five-membered pyrrole ring instead of an imidazole. The loss of the free imidazole nitrogen eliminates coordination interactions with heme irons, thereby reducing adrenal suppression [76].

Fentanyl (Fentanil, Sublimaze, Actiq, Durogesic, Duragesic, Fentora, Onsolis, Instanyl, Abstral)

Drug class: A synthetic opioid related to the phenylpiperidines [77].

Route of administration: Primarily intravenous, epidural, and intrathecally. Transdermal [78–84], intranasal [85–98], and transmucosal administration [99–125] in children have been reported.

Fentanyl is primarily transformed in the liver, and is excreted mainly through the kidneys.

The pharmacokinetics of fentanyl in children has been described [126–128].

Contraindication: Fentanyl is contraindicated in patients with known intolerance to the drug.

Clinical application: Fentanyl remains a popular drug for sedation because of its relatively shorter time to peak effect, rapid termination of effect after small bolus doses, and relative cardiovascular stability. Its intravenous use has been effective but limited by clinical concerns about muscle rigidity [39], although no cases of rigid chest syndrome have been reported in the procedural sedation literature [129].

Common adverse events include respiratory depression, apnea, rigidity, and bradycardia. Other adverse reactions that have been reported are hypertension, hypotension, dizziness, blurred vision, nausea, emesis, laryngospasm, and diaphoresis. Secondary rebound respiratory depression may occasionally occur postoperatively [77].

When a tranquilizer such as droperidol is used with fentanyl citrate, chills and/or shivering, restlessness, and postoperative hallucinatory episodes (sometimes associated with transient periods of mental depression) can occur. Extrapyramidal symptoms (dystonia, akathisia, and oculogyric crisis) have been observed up to 24 h postoperatively [77].

Fospropofol (Lusedra)

Drug class: Alkylphenol derivative.

Route of administration: Intravenous.

Fospropofol is a water-soluble prodrug of propofol (see below). Since it is water soluble, fospropofol eliminates some of the known lipid emulsion-associated disadvantages of propofol such as pain on injection, narrow therapeutic window with the potential to cause deep sedation, high lipid intake during long-term sedation, and risk of infection resulting from bacterial contamination [130].

Fospropofol is metabolized in vivo to produce liberated propofol (producing the sedative effect), phosphate, and formaldehyde [131].

The use and the pharmacokinetics of fospropofol in children have not been described.

Clinical application: Monitored anesthesia care sedation in adult patients undergoing diagnostic or therapeutic procedures.

Contraindications: None.

Clinical application: The pharmacokinetic and pharmacodynamic profiles of fospropofol make it an attractive agent for sedation for procedures of short duration.

Common adverse events include paresthesia, pruritus, and cough. Serious adverse reactions include respiratory depression, hypoxemia, loss of purposeful responsiveness, and hypotension [132].

Ketamine (Ketanest, Ketaset, Ketalar)

Drug class: Phencyclidine derivative.

Route of administration: Intravenous and intramuscular.

Ketamine is rapidly absorbed following parenteral administration and rapidly distributed into body tissues [133].

The pharmacokinetics of ketamine in children has been described [134–138].

Contraindications: Ketamine is contraindicated in those in whom a significant elevation of blood pressure would constitute a serious hazard and in those who have shown hypersensitivity to the drug.

Clinical application: Ketamine is a rapid-acting dissociative agent that produces an anesthetic (dissociative anesthesia) state characterized by profound analgesia, normal pharyngeal–laryngeal reflexes, normal or slightly enhanced skeletal muscle tone, cardiovascular and respiratory stimulation, and occasionally a transient and minimal respiratory depression.

Ketamine is used for premedication, sedation, and induction and maintenance of general anesthesia. Ketamine and its S(+)-isomer are ideal anesthetic agents for trauma victims, patients with hypovolemic and septic shock, and patients with pulmonary diseases. Even subanesthetic doses have analgesic effects, so ketamine is also recommended for postoperative analgesia and sedation. The combination of ketamine with midazolam or propofol can be extremely useful and safe for sedation and pain relief in intensive care patients, especially during sepsis and cardiovascular instability [139].

The evolution of the applications of ketamine in children has been reviewed recently [140].

Common adverse events include the following [133]:

Cardiovascular: Hypertension and tachycardia are common, although hypotension and bradycardia have been observed. Arrhythmia has also occurred.

Respiration: Although respiration is frequently stimulated, severe depression of respiration or apnea may occur following rapid intravenous administration of high doses of ketamine. Laryngospasms and other forms of airway obstruction have occurred.

Eye: Diplopia and nystagmus have been noted. Ketamine may also cause a slight elevation in intraocular pressure measurement.

Psychological: Emergence reactions have been reported.

Neurological: In some patients, enhanced skeletal muscle tone may be manifested by tonic and clonic movements sometimes resembling seizures.

Gastrointestinal: Mild to moderate anorexia, nausea, and vomiting have been observed.

General: Anaphylaxis, local pain, and exanthema at the injection site have infrequently been reported. Transient erythema and/or morbilliform rash have also been reported.

Ketofol (Ketamine + Propofol)

Ketamine (see previous) was approved by the FDA in 1970. Propofol (see later) was approved by the FDA in 1989 and remains labeled as an anesthetic agent. Both ketamine and propofol are now available in generic form in the United States.

The combination of ketamine and propofol has been used successfully in anesthesiology for many years. In recent years, this combination has become more popular in procedural sedation and analgesia. The sedative effects of the two drugs are additive, thus allowing the use of lower doses of each drug. The other effects of propofol and ketamine appear to be complementary: ketamine adds an analgesic effect, unlike propofol, which in turn blunts the emetogenic and psycho-cognitive effects of ketamine. The adverse effects of ketamine and propofol tend to offset each other, with less pain on injection and evidence of reduced effect on cardiac and respiratory suppression [141, 142]. Ketofol is usually constituted as a 1:1 mixture. There is no premixed formulation approved, available, or pending. There are no published pharmacokinetic data on this empirical mixture.

In a large double-blind study in the emergency department, there was no difference in adverse respiratory events with ketofol versus propofol, 30 % versus 32 %, respectively. Ketofol, however, reduced the need for supplemental sedation to achieve Ramsay Sedation Score of 4 or greater (46 % vs. 65 %) but did not offer an advantage on the incidence of adverse respiratory events [143]. The advantage of ketofol in procedural anesthesia for children has been a reduction in narcotic and overall propofol requirement with favorable hemodynamics [144]. The pros and cons on the use of ketofol in pediatric procedural sedation have been reviewed [145].

Lorazepam (Ativan, Temesta)

Drug class: 3-hydroxyl benzodiazepine.

Route of administration: Oral, intravenous, intramuscular.

Lorazepam is extensively conjugated in the liver and is known to undergo enterohepatic recirculation. The inactive metabolite is eliminated mainly by the kidneys [146].

The pharmacokinetics of lorazepam in pediatrics has been described [147, 148].

Contraindications: Lorazepam injection is contraindicated in patients with a known sensitivity to benzodiazepines or its vehicle (polyethylene glycol, propylene glycol, and benzyl alcohol), in patients with acute narrow-angle glaucoma, or in patients with sleep apnea syndrome. It is also contraindicated in patients with severe respiratory insufficiency, except in those patients requiring relief of anxiety and/or diminished recall of events while being mechanically ventilated. The use of lorazepam injection intra-arterially is contraindicated because it may produce arteriospasm resulting in gangrene, which may require amputation.

Clinical application: Lorazepam has been used to provide anxiolysis as well as preanesthetic medication. Compared to midazolam, lorazepam has a less rapid onset of action and a longer duration of action.

Common adverse events [146] include depression of the central nervous system such as excessive sleepiness and drowsiness. Other symptoms include restlessness, confusion, depression, crying, sobbing, and delirium. Visual hallucinations were present in about 1 % and were self-limiting. Hypertension and hypotension have occasionally been observed.

As with all benzodiazepines, paradoxical reactions such as stimulation, mania, irritability, restlessness, agitation, aggression, psychosis, hostility, rage, or hallucinations may occur in rare instances and in an unpredictable fashion.

Fatalities also have been reported—usually in patients on concomitant medications (e.g., respiratory depressants) and/or with other medical conditions (e.g., obstructive sleep apnea).

Meperidine (Demerol, Isonipecaine, Lidol, Pethanol, Piridosal, Algil, Alodan, Centralgin, Dispadol, Dolantin, Mialgin, Petidin Dolargan, Dolestine, Dolosal, Dolsin, Mefedina)

Drug class: Opioid.

Route of administration: Intramuscular, subcutaneous, and slow intravenous.

The onset of action is slightly more rapid than with morphine, and the duration of action is slightly shorter. Meperidine is significantly less effective by the oral than by the parenteral route, but the exact ratio of oral to parenteral effectiveness is unknown.

Meperidine is metabolized chiefly in the liver, and extensively excreted by the kidney [149].

The pharmacokinetics of meperidine in pediatrics has been described [150].

Contraindications: Meperidine is contraindicated in patients who have shown hypersensitivity to it and in patients who are receiving monoamine oxidase (MAO) inhibitors. Therapeutic doses of meperidine have occasionally precipitated unpredictable, severe, and occasionally fatal reactions in patients who have received such agents within 14 days. The mechanism of these reactions is unclear, but may be related to a preexisting hyperphenylalaninemia. Some have been characterized by coma, severe respiratory depression, cyanosis, and hypotension and have resembled the syndrome of acute narcotic overdose. In other reactions, the predominant manifestations have been hyperexcitability, convulsions, tachycardia, hyperpyrexia, and hypertension.

Although it is not known that other narcotics are free of the risk of such reactions, virtually all of the reported reactions have occurred with meperidine.

Clinical application: Meperidine, in 60–80 mg parenteral doses, is equivalent in analgesic effect to about 10 mg of morphine. It has been used to provide analgesia and sedation in children over the past several decades.

Common adverse events: The most frequently observed adverse reactions include light-headedness, dizziness, sedation, nausea, vomiting, sweating, respiratory depression and, to a lesser degree, circulatory depression; respiratory arrest, shock, and cardiac arrest have occurred [149].

Methohexital (Methohexitone, Brevital)

Drug class: Barbiturate.

Route of administration: Intravenous, rectal.

Unlike thiopental and thiamylal, methohexital has a much more rapid clearance and therefore accumulates less during prolonged infusions. All three are primarily eliminated by hepatic metabolism and renal excretion of inactive metabolites [67, 151].

The pharmacokinetics of methohexital in pediatrics has been described [152–159].

Contraindications: Methohexital is contraindicated in patients in whom general anesthesia is contraindicated, in those with latent or manifest porphyria, or in patients with a known hypersensitivity to barbiturates.

Clinical application: Methohexital is labeled for use in pediatric patients older than 1 month: (1) for rectal or intramuscular induction of anesthesia prior to the use of other general anesthetic agents, (2) for rectal or intramuscular induction of anesthesia and as an adjunct to subpotent inhalational anesthetic agents for short surgical procedures, and (3) as rectal or intramuscular anesthesia for short surgical, diagnostic, or therapeutic procedures associated with minimal painful stimuli.

Methohexital is threefold more potent than thiopental and thiamylal.

Common adverse events include extensions of pharmacologic effects such as:

Cardiovascular: Circulatory depression, thrombophlebitis, hypotension, tachycardia, peripheral vascular collapse and convulsions in association with cardiorespiratory arrest.

Respiratory: Respiratory depression (including apnea), cardiorespiratory arrest, laryngospasm, bronchospasm, hiccups, and dyspnea.

Neurologic: Skeletal muscle hyperactivity (twitching), injury to nerves adjacent to injection site, and seizures.

Psychiatric: Emergence delirium, restlessness, and anxiety may occur, especially in the presence of postoperative pain.

Gastrointestinal: Nausea, emesis, abdominal pain, and liver function tests abnormal.

Allergic: Erythema, pruritus, urticaria, and cases of anaphylaxis have been reported rarely.

Other adverse reactions include pain at injection site, salivation, headache, and rhinitis.

Midazolam (Versed, Dormicum, Hypnovel)

Drug class: Benzodiazepine.

Route of administration: Intravenous, intramuscular and oral.

The absolute bioavailability of the midazolam administered through the intramuscular route was greater than 90 %. Midazolam is approximately 97 % bound to plasma protein, principally albumin. Elimination is mediated by cytochrome P450-3A4 to hydroxylated metabolites that are conjugated and excreted in the urine [160].

The pharmacokinetics of midazolam in pediatrics has been described [69, 161–179].

Approved indications: Sedation, induction of anesthesia, component of balanced anesthesia. (+) Pediatric labeling.

Contraindications: Midazolam is contraindicated in patients with a known hypersensitivity to the drug. Midazolam, like other benzodiazepines, is contraindicated in patients with acute narrow-angle glaucoma. It may be used in patients with open-angle glaucoma only if they are receiving appropriate therapy.

Clinical application: Midazolam is usually administered to provide anxiolysis, with accompanying mild sedation. This state usually suffices for short diagnostic procedures.

For children who do not require placement of an intravenous line, the parenteral formulation of midazolam may be orally administered 15–30 min before the procedure.

Common adverse events in pediatrics include desaturation, apnea, hypotension, paradoxical reactions, hiccough, seizure-like activity, and nystagmus. The majority of airway-related events occurred in patients receiving other CNS-depressing medications and in patients where midazolam was not used as a single sedating agent.

Morphine (MS Contin, MSIR, Avinza, Kadian, Oramorph, Roxanol, Kapanol)

Drug class: Opioid.

Route of administration: Intravenous, intramuscular, rectal.

Morphine is conjugated with glucuronic acid to form two major metabolites: morphine-6-glucuronide and morphine-3-glucuronide. The former has similar pharmacological actions compared to morphine. Both metabolites are excreted by the kidney [180].

The pharmacokinetics of morphine in pediatrics has been well described [181–200].

Contraindications: Morphine is contraindicated in those medical conditions that would preclude the administration of opioids by the intravenous route: allergy to morphine or other opiates, acute bronchial asthma, and upper airway obstruction. Morphine, like all opioid analgesics, may cause severe hypotension in an individual whose ability to maintain blood pressure has already been compromised by a depleted blood volume or a concurrent administration of drugs, such as phenothiazines or general anesthetics.

Clinical application: Morphine and other opioid agonists exert a wide range of physiological effects. In sedation, the most pertinent effects are analgesia, drowsiness, changes in mood, and mental clouding. At therapeutic levels, patients report that the pain is less intense, less discomforting, or entirely gone; drowsiness commonly follows [39].

Common adverse events include respiratory depression and/or respiratory arrest. This depression and/or respiratory arrest may be severe and could require intervention. Because of delay in maximum CNS effect with intravenously administered drug (30 min), rapid administration may result in overdosing. Single-dose neuraxial administration may result in acute or delayed respiratory depression for periods at least as long as 24 h [180].

In general, side effects are amenable to reversal by narcotic antagonists.

Nitrous Oxide

Route of administration: Inhaled.

Nitrous oxide (N_2O) is a colorless, odorless, tasteless gas that produces dissociative euphoria, drowsiness, and a "floating sensation" with anxiolysis and mild to moderate amnesia and analgesia.

The pharmacokinetics of nitrous oxide in children has been described [201, 202].

Contraindications: Nitrous oxide should not be used with any condition where air is entrapped within a body and where its expansion might be dangerous—artificial, traumatic or spontaneous pneumothorax, air embolism, decompression sickness, following a recent dive, following air encephalography, severe bullous emphysema, use during myringoplasty, and gross abdominal distension.

Clinical application: Nitrous oxide is used primarily for anxiolysis, mild analgesia, and amnesia during brief procedures, especially in conjunction with local anesthesia, e.g., laceration repair, abscess incision and drainage, lumbar puncture, intravenous line placement, and some fracture reductions. Its advantages include rapid onset of action (within 5 min), and N_2O does not require vascular access or painful administration. Recovery from N_2O sedation typically is very rapid, with the child able to sit alone within 5 min and ready for discharge within 15 min [203].

The use of nitrous oxide in children for sedation has been reported [203–222]. The applications of nitrous oxide for procedural sedation in pediatrics have been reviewed recently [223].

Common adverse events include vomiting, nausea, inadequate sedation, agitation/delirium, low oxygen saturation, unresponsive episode with low oxygen saturation, stridor, seizure, diaphoresis, burpy/hiccupy, gaggy, expectorated large amount of clear phlegm, and screaming [224].

Pentobarbital (Nembutal)

Drug class: Barbiturate.

Route of administration: Primarily intravenous, although oral administration has been reported in children [225].

Barbiturates are absorbed and rapidly distributed to all tissues and fluids with high concentrations in the brain, liver, and kidneys. Pentobarbital is metabolized primarily by the hepatic microsomal enzyme system, and the metabolic products are excreted in the urine, and less commonly, in the feces [226].

The pharmacokinetics of pentobarbital in children has been described [227, 228].

Approved indications: Sedative-hypnotic, induction of anesthesia. (+) Pediatric labeling.

Contraindications: Pentobarbital is contraindicated in patients with known barbiturate sensitivity. It is also contraindicated in patients with a history of manifest or latent porphyria.

Clinical application: Pentobarbital is a widely used barbiturate used for sedation of children. However, its delayed onset of action and prolonged sedation has led to the use of other medications for sedation. The occurrence of paradoxical hyperactivity reactions has also contributed to the decline in its use.

Common adverse events: Somnolence is the most common adverse event. Other adverse events include agitation, confusion, hyperkinesia, ataxia, CNS depression, nightmares, nervousness, psychiatric disturbance, hallucinations, insomnia, anxiety, dizziness, and thinking abnormality.

Respiratory effects include hypoventilation and apnea.

Cardiovascular system: Bradycardia, hypotension, and syncope.

Digestive system: Nausea, vomiting, and constipation.

Other reported reactions include headache, injection site reactions, hypersensitivity reactions (angioedema, skin rashes, exfoliative dermatitis), fever, liver damage, and megaloblastic anemia following chronic phenobarbital use [226].

Propofol (Diprivan)

Drug class: Alkylphenol derivative.

Route of administration: Intravenous.

Propofol promotes unconsciousness, in part, by $GABA_A$-mediated inhibition of release of the arousal-promoting neurotransmitter histamine in the cortex from the tuberomammillary nucleus in the hypothalamus [229]. Propofol is extensively distributed and rapidly cleared from the body. Clearance occurs by metabolic processes, mainly in the liver, to form inactive conjugates of propofol and its corresponding quinol, which are excreted in the urine [230].

The pharmacokinetics of propofol in children has been described [231–249].

Approved indications: Initiation of monitored anesthesia care sedation, combined sedation and regional anesthesia, induction and maintenance of general anesthesia, and Intensive Care Unit (ICU) sedation of intubated, mechanically ventilated patients. (+) Pediatric labeling (induction and maintenance of general anesthesia).

Contraindications: Propofol injectable emulsion is contraindicated in patients with a known hypersensitivity to propofol injectable emulsion or any of its components. It is contraindicated in patients with allergies to eggs, egg products, soybeans, or soy products [250].

Older studies have shown severe reactions to propofol [251–254]. Some more recent studies show otherwise. In a retrospective case review over an 11-year period in Australia, propofol was frequently administered to egg-allergic children and it was concluded that propofol was likely to be safe in the majority of egg-allergic children who do not have a history of egg anaphylaxis [255]. Another study questioned this contraindication; there was no confirmed report of propofol-induced anaphylaxis by allergy testing, in egg-allergic patients [256].

Clinical application: Propofol is a rapidly acting anesthetic used in the induction and maintenance of general anesthesia, as well as in sedation. Propofol sedation is of a similar quality to that produced by midazolam. Emergence from sedation occurs quickly due to its rapid clearance.

The use of propofol by nonanesthesiologists was discussed in several chapters.

The use of propofol in children for sedation has been recently compared to midazolam [257], midazolam and fentanyl [258], pentobarbital [259], midazolam + pentobarbital + fentanyl [260], ketamine [261], midazolam + ketamine [262], and dexmedetomidine [263, 264].

Propofol (and thiopental sodium) have also been found to be effective in the treatment of uncontrolled seizure activity such as refractory status epilepticus. Coma is induced with anesthetic drugs to achieve complete control of seizure activity [265].

The adverse events in 49,836 pediatric sedations with propofol in 37 centers were recently reviewed [266].

Common adverse events include apnea in pediatric patients. Adverse events in adults include bradycardia, arrhythmia, tachycardia nodal, hypotension, decreased cardiac output, hypertension, hypotension, burning/stinging or pain at the site of injection, hyperlipidemia, apnea, respiratory acidosis, rash, and pruritus.

A rare complication, propofol infusion syndrome (PRIS), has been described, and recently reviewed [267]. Initially reported in children and in traumatic brain injury, PRIS typically presents as severe rhabdomyolysis, acute kidney injury, hyperkalemia, metabolic acidosis, and hepatomegaly. Myocardial injury may occur in several forms. Occurrence of the syndrome, as well as its severity, appears to be dose dependent, most cases occurring in patients who received doses in excess of 5 mg/kg/h (80 μg/kg/min) for at least 48 h. However, the syndrome has been described with short-term high doses and long-term small doses. Additional well-recognized risk factors for its development include the coadministration of catecholamines or corticosteroids. PRIS has not yet been reported in procedural sedation [129].

Remifentanil (Ultiva)

Drug class: A 4-anilidopiperidine derivative of fentanyl.

Route of administration: Intravenous.

Unlike other opioids, remifentanil is rapidly metabolized by hydrolysis of the propanoic acid-methyl ester linkage by nonspecific blood and tissue esterases. This metabolite has minimal activity. The pharmacokinetics of remifentanil is unaffected by the presence of renal or hepatic impairment [268].

The pharmacokinetics of remifentanil in children has been described [269, 270].

Contraindications: Due to the presence of glycine in the formulation, remifentanil is contraindicated for epidural or intrathecal administration. Remifentanil is also contraindicated in patients with known hypersensitivity to fentanyl analogs.

Clinical application: Remifentanil has been shown to be effective in providing analgesia-based sedation in pediatric ICU patients requiring mechanical ventilation, in newborns requiring mechanical ventilation, and in another group of children who were being mechanically ventilated postoperatively [271].

The use of remifentanil in children (in Europe) has recently been reviewed [272, 273].

Common adverse events include nausea, vomiting, and shivering in children. Other adverse events reported in children include onset of rhonchi, postoperative complication, stridor, and cough.

S-Ketamine (Ketanest, Ketaset, Ketalar)

Drug class: Phencyclidine derivative; S-ketamine is the active isomer of ketamine [274].

Route of administration: Primarily intravenous, although intranasal [275], caudal block [276–282] and rectal [14, 283, 284] administration in children have been reported.

Ketamine is rapidly absorbed following parenteral administration and rapidly distributed into body tissues [275].

The pharmacodynamics [285] and the pharmacokinetics [286, 287] of S-ketamine in children have been described.

Contraindications: S-ketamine is contraindicated in those in whom a significant elevation of blood pressure would constitute a serious hazard and in those who have shown hypersensitivity to the drug.

Clinical application: Clinically, the anesthetic potency of the S(+)-isomer is approximately three to four times that of the R(−)-isomer.

Ketamine is a rapid-acting general anesthetic that produces an anesthetic (dissociative anesthesia) state characterized by profound analgesia, normal pharyngeal–laryngeal reflexes, normal or slightly enhanced skeletal muscle tone, cardiovascular and respiratory stimulation, and occasionally a transient and minimal respiratory depression.

Like ketamine, S(+)-ketamine is used for premedication, sedation, and induction and maintenance of general anesthesia, which is then termed "dissociative anesthesia." Ketamine and its S(+)-isomer are ideal anesthetic agents for trauma victims, patients with hypovolemic and septic shock, and patients with pulmonary diseases. Even subanesthetic doses have analgesic effects, so ketamine is also recommended for postoperative analgesia and sedation. The combination of ketamine with midazolam or propofol can be extremely useful and safe for sedation and pain relief in intensive care patients, especially during sepsis and cardiovascular instability.

Common adverse events are similar to those reported for ketamine.

Sufentanil (Sufenta)

Drug class: Opioid.

Route of administration: Intravenous. Sufentanil has an immediate onset of action, with relatively limited accumulation. Rapid elimination from tissue storage sites allows for relatively more rapid recovery as compared with equipotent dosages of fentanyl. Within anesthetic dosages, recovery times are more rapid compared to equipotent fentanyl dosages. The liver and small intestine are the major sites of biotransformation. Approximately 80 % of the administered dose is excreted within 24 h and only 2 % of the dose is eliminated as unchanged drug [288].

The elimination half-life of sufentanil is shorter in infants and children, and longer in neonates compared to that of adolescents and adults. The pharmacokinetics of sufentanil in children has been described [289–292].

Contraindications: Sufentanil is contraindicated in patients with known hypersensitivity to the drug or known intolerance to other opioid agonists.

Clinical application: Sufentanil has been reported to be as much as 5–10 times as potent as fentanyl.

At intravenous doses of up to 8 mg/kg, sufentanil is an analgesic component of general anesthesia; at intravenous doses >8 mg/kg, sufentanil produces hypnosis and a deep level of anesthesia.

Common adverse events include respiratory depression, skeletal muscle rigidity (particularly of the truncal muscles), and hypotension. The return of normal bladder activity may be delayed.

Reversal Agents

Flumazenil (Flumazenil, Anexate, Lanexat, Mazicon, Romazicon, Anexate)

Drug class: Imidazobenzodiazepine.

Route of administration: Primarily intravenous [293], although intramuscular [294], intranasal [295, 296], oral [294], and rectal [290–300] administration in children have been reported.

Flumazenil is completely metabolized in the liver. Elimination is essentially complete within 72 h, with 90–95 % appearing in urine and 5–10 % in feces.

The pharmacokinetics of flumazenil in children has been described [300, 301].

Contraindications: Flumazenil is contraindicated in patients with a known hypersensitivity to flumazenil or benzodiazepines, patients who have been given a benzodiazepine for control of a potentially life-threatening condition (e.g., control of intracranial pressure or status epilepticus), and in patients who are showing signs of serious cyclic antidepressant overdose.

Clinical application: Flumazenil is a benzodiazepine receptor antagonist. Its primary use in sedation is to reverse sedation resulting from the administration of benzodiazepines such as diazepam, lorazepam, midazolam, and temazepam.

Common adverse events include convulsions in patients with severe hepatic impairment and in patients who were relying on benzodiazepine effects to control seizures, who were physically dependent on benzodiazepines, or who had ingested large doses of other drugs (mixed-drug overdose). Serious adverse reactions include deaths, the majority of which occurred in patients with serious underlying disease or in patients who had ingested large amounts of nonbenzodiazepine drugs (usually cyclic antidepressants), as part of an overdose [293].

Naloxone (Narcan, Nalone, Narcanti)

Drug class: Opioid, a synthetic congener of oxymorphone.

Route of administration: Primarily intravenous, although naloxone may be administered intramuscularly or subcutaneously.

Naloxone has also been administered orally for nonsedating purposes (e.g., constipation).

Naloxone is metabolized in the liver, primarily by glucuronide conjugation. The drug is excreted in the urine.

The pharmacokinetics of naloxone in newborns has been described [302–304].

Contraindications: Naloxone is contraindicated in patients known to be hypersensitive to naloxone hydrochloride or to any of the other ingredients.

Clinical application: Naloxone is an opioid antagonist. Its primary use in sedation is to reverse sedation resulting from the administration of opioids such as fentanyl and morphine.

It is indicated for the complete or partial reversal of opioid depression, including respiratory depression, induced by opioids such as propoxyphene, methadone, and certain mixed agonist–antagonist analgesics: nalbuphine, pentazocine, butorphanol, and cyclazocine.

The American Academy of Pediatrics, Committee on Drugs issued guidelines on the use of naloxone in children in 1990 [305].

Common adverse events (in postoperative patients) include hypotension, hypertension, ventricular tachycardia and fibrillation, dyspnea, pulmonary edema, and cardiac arrest. Death, coma, and encephalopathy have been reported as sequelae of these events. Excessive doses of naloxone in postoperative patients may result in significant reversal of analgesia and agitation. For patients in whom naloxone is administered for opioid depression, abrupt reversal of opioid depression may result in nausea, vomiting, sweating, tachycardia, hypertension, tremulousness, seizures, ventricular tachycardia and fibrillation, pulmonary edema, and cardiac arrest, which may result in death.

Local Anesthetics

Lidocaine (Lignocaine)

Drug class: Aminoethylamide.

Route of administration: Topical; also administered intravenously as an antiarrhythmic agent

Lidocaine is metabolized in the liver through CYP450 enzymes [306].

The pharmacokinetics of lidocaine administered topically in children has been described [307–312].

Contraindication: Lidocaine is contraindicated in patients with a known history of hypersensitivity to local anesthetics of the amide type.

Clinical application: Lidocaine has a wide range of clinical uses as a local anesthetic of intermediate duration. The combination of lidocaine (2.59 %) and prilocaine (2.5 %) in an occlusive dressing (EMLA anesthetic disk) is used as an anesthetic prior to venipuncture, skin graft harvesting, and infiltration of anesthetics into genitalia.

Common adverse events [313] are, in general, dose-related and may result from high plasma levels caused by excessive dosage, rapid absorption, or inadvertent intravascular injection or may result from a hypersensitivity, idiosyncrasy, or diminished tolerance on the part of the patient. Serious adverse experiences are generally systemic in nature.

Central nervous system manifestations are excitatory and/or depressant and may be characterized by light-headedness, nervousness, apprehension, euphoria, confusion, dizziness, drowsiness, tinnitus, blurred or double vision, vomiting, sensations of heat, cold or numbness, twitching, tremors, convulsions, unconsciousness, and respiratory depression and arrest. The excitatory manifestations may be very brief or may not occur at all, in which case the first manifestation of toxicity may be drowsiness merging into unconsciousness and respiratory arrest. Drowsiness following the administration of lidocaine is usually an early sign of a high blood level of the drug and may occur as a consequence of rapid absorption.

Cardiovascular manifestations are usually depressant and are characterized by bradycardia, hypotension, and cardiovascular collapse, which may lead to cardiac arrest.

Allergic reactions are characterized by cutaneous lesions, urticaria, edema, or anaphylactoid reactions. Allergic reactions as a result of sensitivity to lidocaine are extremely rare.

Lidocaine hydrochloride injection should be employed only by physicians who are well versed in diagnosis and management of dose-related toxicity and other acute emergencies that might arise and then only after ensuring the immediate availability of oxygen, other resuscitative drugs, cardiopulmonary equipment, and the personnel needed for the proper management of toxic reactions and related emergencies. Delay in proper management of dose-related toxicity, underventilation from any cause, and/or altered sensitivity may lead to the development of acidosis, cardiac arrest and, possibly, death.

The mechanisms and treatment of local anesthetic systemic toxicity has been reviewed [314].

Antiemetics

Ondansetron (Zofran)

Drug class: Selective serotonin 5-HT3 receptor antagonist.

Route of administration: Intravenous. Ondansetron is extensively metabolized, with approximately 5 % of a radiolabeled dose recovered as the parent compound from the urine. The primary metabolic pathway is hydroxylation on the indole ring followed by glucuronide or sulfate conjugation. In vitro metabolism studies have shown that ondansetron is a substrate for human hepatic cytochrome P-450 enzymes, including CYP3A4 (predominantly), CYP1A2, and CYP2D6 [315].

The pharmacokinetics of ondansetron in children has been described [316–318].

Contraindication: Ondansetron is contraindicated for patients known to have hypersensitivity to the drug.

Clinical application: Ondansetron is administered for the prevention of nausea and vomiting associated with initial and repeat courses of emetogenic cancer chemotherapy, and the prevention of postoperative nausea and/or vomiting.

Common adverse events in pediatric patients are wound problems, anxiety or agitation, headache, drowsiness/sedation, pyrexia, bronchospasm, postprocedural pain, and diarrhea.

Metoclopramide (Maxolon, Reglan, Degan, Maxeran, Primperan, Pylomid, Cerucal, Pramin)

Drug class: Dopaminergic blocking agent.

The antiemetic properties of metoclopramide appear to be a result of its antagonism of central and peripheral dopamine receptors. Dopamine produces nausea and vomiting by stimulation of the medullary chemoreceptor trigger zone (CTZ), and metoclopramide blocks stimulation of the CTZ by agents like L-dopa or apomorphine, which are known to increase dopamine levels or to possess dopamine-like effects. Metoclopramide also abolishes the slowing of gastric emptying caused by apomorphine.

Route of administration: Intravenous and oral.

Metoclopramide is rapidly and well absorbed. There is extensive distribution of drug to the tissues. Renal impairment affects the clearance of metoclopramide [319].

The pharmacokinetics of metoclopramide in children has been described [319–321].

Contraindications: Metoclopramide should not be used in the presence of gastrointestinal hemorrhage, mechanical obstruction, or perforation.

Metoclopramide is contraindicated in patients with pheochromocytoma because the drug may cause a hypertensive crisis.

Metoclopramide should not be used in patients with epilepsy or those receiving other drugs that are likely to cause extrapyramidal reactions, since the frequency and severity of seizures or extrapyramidal reactions may be increased.

Clinical application: Metoclopramide stimulates motility of the upper gastrointestinal tract, resulting in accelerated gastric emptying and intestinal transit.

Common adverse events include restlessness, drowsiness, fatigue, and lassitude. Insomnia, headache, confusion, dizziness, or mental depression with suicidal ideation occurs less frequently. There are isolated reports of convulsive seizures without clear-cut relationship to metoclopramide. Rarely, hallucinations have been reported.

Extrapyramidal reactions (EPS): Acute dystonic reactions, the most common type of EPS associated with metoclopramide, have been reported in a few patients treated daily with metoclopramide. Symptoms include involuntary movements of limbs, facial grimacing, torticollis, oculogyric crisis, rhythmic protrusion of tongue, bulbar type of speech, trismus, opisthotonus (tetanus-like reactions), and, rarely, stridor and dyspnea possibly due to laryngospasm; ordinarily these symptoms are readily reversed by diphenhydramine. Parkinsonian-like symptoms may include bradykinesia, tremor, cogwheel rigidity, and masklike facies. Tardive dyskinesia is often characterized by involuntary movements of the tongue, face, mouth, or jaw, and sometimes of the trunk and/or extremities; movements may be choreoathetotic in appearance. Motor restlessness (akathisia) may consist of feelings of anxiety, agitation, jitteriness, and insomnia, as well as inability to sit still, pacing, and foot tapping. These symptoms may disappear spontaneously or respond to a reduction in dosage.

Rare occurrences of neuroleptic malignant syndrome have been reported. This potentially fatal syndrome includes hyperthermia, altered consciousness, muscular rigidity, and autonomic dysfunction. In general, the incidence of adverse reactions correlates with the dose and duration of metoclopramide administration.

Scopolamine (Levo-duboisine, Hyoscine)

Drug class: Belladonna alkaloid.

Route of administration: Transdermal (at the postauricular area only).

The system is programmed to deliver in vivo approximately 1.0 mg of scopolamine at an approximately constant rate to the systemic circulation over 3 days.

Scopolamine is well absorbed percutaneously. Following application to the skin behind the ear, circulating plasma levels are detected within 4 h with peak levels being obtained, on average, within 24 h.

The pharmacokinetics of scopolamine administered transdermally in children has not been described.

Contraindications: Scopolamine is contraindicated in persons who are hypersensitive to the drug or to other belladonna alkaloids, to any ingredient or component in the formulation or delivery system, or in patients with angle-closure (narrow-angle) glaucoma.

Clinical application: Scopolamine is indicated for prevention of nausea and vomiting associated with motion sickness and recovery from anesthesia and surgery. The patch should be applied only to skin in the postauricular area.

The use of scopolamine in children is off-label [322].

Common adverse events include dry mouth and dizziness.

Other adverse events reported include acute angle-closure (narrow-angle) glaucoma, confusion, difficulty urinating, dry, itchy, or conjunctival injection of eyes, restlessness, hallucinations, memory disturbances, rashes and erythema, and transient changes in heart rate.

Drug withdrawal/postremoval symptoms: Symptoms such as dizziness, nausea, vomiting, headache, and disturbances of equilibrium have been reported following discontinuation. More serious symptoms include muscle weakness, bradycardia, and hypotension.

Diphenhydramine (Benadryl, DPH, DHM, Dimedrol, Daedalon)

Drug class: Ethanolamine H-receptor antagonist.

It is thought that the antiemetic properties of diphenhydramine are due to its ability to suppress motion-enhanced vestibular neuronal firing.

Route of administration: Intravenous, oral.

Diphenhydramine in the injectable form has a rapid onset of action. It is widely distributed throughout the body, including the CNS. A portion of the drug is excreted unchanged in the urine, while the rest is metabolized via the liver.

The pharmacokinetics of diphenhydramine in children has been described [323].

Contraindications: Diphenhydramine should not be used in neonates or premature infants. Because of the higher risk of antihistamines for infants generally, and for neonates and premature infants in particular, antihistamine therapy is contraindicated in nursing mothers. Because of the risk of local necrosis, this drug should not be used as a local anesthetic.

Clinical application: Diphenhydramine has significant anticholinergic and sedative effects that contribute to its efficacy as an antiemetic [324].

Common adverse events include diminished mental alertness or excitation in children. Overdosage may cause hallucinations, convulsions, or death [325].

Dexamethasone (Decadron)

Drug class: Steroid.

Route of administration: Intravenous and oral.

The pharmacokinetics of dexamethasone in children has been described [326–328].

Contraindications: Dexamethasone is contraindicated in patients with systemic fungal infections and in patients who are hypersensitive to any components of this product.

Clinical application: Dexamethasone is a well-established antiemetic in patients receiving highly emetogenic cancer chemotherapy. Its antiemetic mechanism of action is not well understood, however.

Common adverse events include hypertension, weight gain, increased intraocular pressure, infection, psychosocial disturbances, thromboembolism, peptic ulcers, cataracts, and osteoporosis [329].

Pediatric patients who are treated with corticosteroids by any route, including systemically administered corticosteroids, may experience a decrease in their growth velocity. The linear growth of pediatric patients treated with corticosteroids should be monitored, and the potential growth effects of prolonged treatment should be weighed against clinical benefits obtained and the availability of treatment alternatives. In order to minimize the potential growth effects of corticosteroids, pediatric patients should be titrated to the lowest effective dose.

The adverse reactions that have been reported with dexamethasone or other corticosteroids encompass almost every system in the body such as allergic reactions, cardiovascular, dermatologic, endocrine, fluid and electrolyte disturbances, gastrointestinal, metabolic, musculoskeletal, neurological/psychiatric, and ophthalmic.

References

1. American Academy of Pediatrics, American Academy of Pediatric Dentistry, Coté CJ, Wilson S, Work Group on Sedation. Guidelines for monitoring and management of pediatric patients during and after sedation for diagnostic and therapeutic procedures: an update. Pediatrics. 2006;118(6):2587–602.
2. American Society of Anesthesiologists Task Force on Sedation and Analgesia by Non-Anesthesiologists. Practice guidelines for sedation and analgesia by nonanesthesiologists. Anesthesia. 2002;96:1004–17.
3. Dial S, Silver P, Bock K, Sagy M. Pediatric sedation for procedures titrated to a desired degree of immobility results in unpredictable depth of sedation. Pediatr Emerg Care. 2001;17(6):414–20.
4. Maxwell LG, Yaster M. The myth of conscious sedation. Arch Pediatr Adolesc Med. 1996;150(7):665–7.
5. American Academy of Pediatrics, Committee on Drugs. Guidelines for monitoring and management of pediatric patients during and after sedation for diagnostic and therapeutic procedures. Pediatrics. 1992;89(6 Pt 1):1110–5.
6. Yaster M, Nichols DG, Deshpande JK, Wetzel RC. Midazolam-fentanyl intravenous sedation in children: case report of respiratory arrest. Pediatrics. 1990;86(3):463–7.
7. Dallimore D, Herd DW, Short T, Anderson BJ. Dosing ketamine for pediatric procedural sedation in the emergency department. Pediatr Emerg Care. 2008;24(8):529–33.
8. Coté CJ, Karl HW, Notterman DA, Weinberg JA, McCloskey C. Adverse sedation events in pediatrics: analysis of medications used for sedation. Pediatrics. 2000;106(4):633–44.
9. Lopez JM, Valeron M, Perez O, Consuegra E, Urquia L, Moron A, et al. Safety and effectiveness of the sedoanalgesia with fentanyl and propofol. Experience in a pediatric intensive medicine unit. Med Intensiva. 2007;31(8):417–22.
10. Oraishi SA, Girdharry TD, Xu SG, Orkin FK. Prolonged retrograde amnesia following sedation with propofol in a 12-year old boy. Paediatr Anaesth. 2007;17(4):375–9.
11. Veselis RA, Reinsel RA, Feshchenko VA, Wronski M. The comparative amnestic effects of midazolam, propofol, thiopental and fentanyl at equisedative concentrations. Anesthesiology. 1997;87(4):749–64.
12. Wagner BK, O'Hara DA, Hammond JS. Drugs for amnesia in the ICU. Am J Crit Care. 1997;6(3):192–201.
13. Koirala B, Pandev RK, Saksen AK, Kumar R, Sharma S. A comparative evaluation of newer sedatives in conscious sedation. J Clin Pediatr Dent. 2006;30(4):273–6.
14. Heinrich M, Wetzstein V, Muensterer OJ, Till H. Conscious sedation: off-label use of rectal S(+)-ketamine and midazolam for wound dressing changes in paediatric heat injuries. Eur J Pediatr Surg. 2004;14(4):235–9.
15. Buffett-Jerrott SE, Stewart SH, Finley GA, Loughlan HL. Effects of benzodiazepines on explicit memory in a paediatric surgery setting. Psychopharmacology (Berl). 2003;168(4):377–86.
16. Pringle B, Dahlquist LM, Eskenazi A. Memory in pediatric patients undergoing conscious sedation for aversive medical procedures. Health Psychol. 2003;22(3):263–9.
17. Henry DW, Burwinkle JW, Klutman NE. Determination of sedative and amnestic doses of lorazepam in children. Clin Pharm. 1991;10(8):625–9.
18. Kennedy RM, Porter FL, Miller JP, Jaffe DM. Comparison of fentanyl/midazolam with ketamine/midazolam for pediatric orthopedic emergencies. Pediatrics. 1998;102(4 Pt 1):956–63.
19. Smith MC, Williamson J, Yaster M, Boyd GJ, Heitmiller ES. Off-label use of medications in children undergoing sedation and anesthesia. Anesth Analg. 2012;115(5):1148–54.
20. Mathis LL, Yao LP. Pediatric sedatives and the food and drug administration: challenges, limitations, and drugs in development. In: Mason K, editor. Pediatric sedation outside of the operating room: a multispecialty collaboration. 2nd ed. New York: Springer; 2015, p. 539–548.
21. http://www.fda.gov/ScienceResearch/SpecialTopics/RunningClinicalTrials/GuidancesInformationSheets andNotices/ucm116355.htm. Accessed 10 Jan 2010.
22. American Academy of Pediatrics, Committee on Drugs. Alternative routes of drug administration—advantages and disadvantages (subject review). Pediatrics. 1997;100(1):143–52.
23. American Academy of Pediatrics Committee on Drugs. Policy statement: off-label use of drugs in children. Pediatrics. 2014;133(3):563–7.
24. Soriano SG, Vutskits L. Is there evidence for long-term neurocognitive effects of sedatives? In: Mason K, editor. Pediatric sedation outside of the operating room: a multispecialty collaboration. 2nd ed. New York: Springer; 2015, p. 549–552.

Alfentanil

25. Brenchley J, Ramlakhan S. Intranasal alfentanil for acute pain in children. Emerg Med J. 2006;23(6):488.
26. Schwagmeier R, Boerger N, Meissner W, Striebel HW. Pharmacokinetics of intranasal alfentanil. J Clin Anesth. 1995;7(2):109–13.
27. http://dailymed.nlm.nih.gov/dailymed/drugInfo.cfm?id=6884. Accessed 14 Dec 2013
28. Baririan N, Van Obbergh L, Desager JP, Verbeeck RK, Wallemacq P, Starkel P, et al. Alfentanil-induced miosis as a surrogate measure of alfentanil pharmacokinetics in patients with mild and moderate liver cirrhosis. Clin Pharmacokinet. 2007;46(3):261–70.
29. Fiset P, Mathers L, Engstrom R, Fitzgerald D, Brand SC, Hsu F, et al. Pharmacokinetics of computer-controlled alfentanil

administration in children undergoing cardiac surgery. Anesthesiology. 1995;83(5):944–55.
30. den Hollander JM, Hennis PJ, Burm AG, Vletter AA, Bovill JG. Pharmacokinetics of alfentanil before and after cardiopulmonary bypass in pediatric patients undergoing cardiac surgery: part I. J Cardiothorac Vasc Anesth. 1992;6(3):308–12.
31. Marlow N, Weindling AM, Van Peer A, Heykants J. Alfentanil pharmacokinetics in preterm infants. Arch Dis Child. 1990;65 (4 Spec No):349–51.
32. Davis PJ, Stiller RL, Cook DR, Brandom BW, Davis JE, Scierka AM. Effects of cholestatic hepatic disease and chronic renal failure on alfentanil pharmacokinetics in children. Anesth Analg. 1989;68(5):579–83.
33. Davis PJ, Killian A, Stiller RL, Cook DR, Guthrie RD, Scierka AM. Pharmacokinetics of alfentanil in newborn premature infants and older children. Dev Pharmacol Ther. 1989;13(1):21–7.
34. den Hollander JM, Hennis PJ, Burm AG, Bovill JG. Alfentanil in infants and children with congenital heart defects. J Cardiothorac Anesth. 1988;2(1):12–7.
35. Roure P, Jean N, Leclerc AC, Cabanel N, Levron JC, Duvaldestin P. Pharmacokinetics of alfentanil in children undergoing surgery. Br J Anaesth. 1987;59(11):1437–40.
36. Goresky GV, Koren G, Sabourin MA, Sale JP, Strunin L. The pharmacokinetics of alfentanil in children. Anesthesiology. 1987; 67(5):654–9.
37. Meistelman C, Saint-Maurice C, Lepaul M, Levron JC, Loose JP, Mac Gee K. A comparison of alfentanil pharmacokinetics in children and adults. Anesthesiology. 1987;66(1):13–6.
38. Van Peer A, Levron JC, Noorduin H, Heykants J. Overview of the clinical pharmacokinetics of alfentanil. Acta Anaesthesiol Belg. 1984;35(Suppl):261–3.
39. Gutstein HB, Akil H. Opioid analgesics. In: Brunton LL, Lzo JS, Parker KL, editors. Goodman and Gilman's the pharmacological basis of therapeutics. 11th ed. New York: McGraw-Hill; 2006. p. 547–90.

Chloral Hydrate

40. Lovinger DM, Zimmerman SA, Levitin M, et al. Trichloroethanol potentiates synaptic transmission mediated by g-aminobutyric acid receptors in hippocampal neurons. J Pharmacol Exp Ther. 1993;264:1097–103.
41. Treluyer JM, Andre C, Carp PF, Chalumeau M, Tonnelier S, Cuq C, et al. Sedation in children undergoing CT scan or MRI: effect of time-course and tolerance of rectal chloral hydrate. Fundam Clin Pharmacol. 2004;18(3):347–50.
42. Sakaguchi M, Inouye S. Anaphylaxis to gelatin-containing rectal suppositories. J Allergy Clin Immunol. 2001;108(6):1033–4.
43. Dacher JN, Neuenschwander S, Monroc M, Vanier A, Eurin D, Le Dosseur P. Sedation with oral hydroxyzine and rectal chloral hydrate in pediatric MRI and CT. J Radiol. 1996;77(12):1189–92; discussion 1193–4 (article in French).
44. Moody Jr EH, Mourino AP, Campbell RL. The therapeutic effectiveness of nitrous oxide and chloral hydrate administered orally, rectally, and combined with hydroxyzine for pediatric dentistry. ASDC J Dent Child. 1986;53(6):425–9.
45. Baselt RC. Disposition of toxic drugs and chemicals in man. 7th ed. Foster City: Biomedical; 2004.
46. Mayers DJ, Hindmarsh KW, Sankaran K, Gorecki DK, Kasian GF. Chloral hydrate disposition following single-dose administration to critically ill neonates and children. Dev Pharmacol Ther. 1991;16(2):71–7.
47. Reimche LD, Sankaran K, Hindmarsh KW, Kasian GF, Gorecki DK, Tan L. Chloral hydrate sedation in neonates and infants-clinical and pharmacologic considerations. Dev Pharmacol Ther. 1989;12(2):57–64.
48. Pershad J, Palmisano P, Nichols M. Chloral hydrate: the good and the bad. Pediatr Emerg Care. 1999;15(6):432–5.
49. American Academy of Pediatrics, Committee on Drugs and Committee on Environmental Health. Use of chloral hydrate for sedation in children. Pediatrics. 1993;92(3):471–3.

Codeine

50. http://www.fda.gov/Drugs/DrugSafety/ucm313631.htm. Accessed 14 Dec 2013.
51. http://www.fda.gov/Drugs/DrugSafety/ucm339112.htm. Accessed 14 Dec 2013.

Dexmedetomidine

52. http://www.precedex.com/wp-content/uploads/Precedex_PI.pdf. Accessed 14 Dec 2013.
53. Sakurai Y, Obata T, Odaka A, Terui K, Tamura M, Miyao H. Buccal administration of dexmedetomidine as a pre-anesthetic in children. J Anesth. 2010;24(1):49–53.
54. Karaaslan D, Peker TT, Alaca A, Ozmen S, Kirdemir P, Yorgancigil H, et al. Comparison of buccal and intramuscular dexmedetomidine premedication for arthroscopic knee surgery. J Clin Anesth. 2006;18(8):589–93.
55. Anttila M, Penttilä J, Helminen A, Vuorilehto L, Scheinin H. Bioavailability of dexmedetomidine after extravascular doses in healthy subjects. Br J Clin Pharmacol. 2003;56(6):691–3.
56. Penttilä J, Helminen A, Anttila M, Hinkka S, Scheinin H. Cardiovascular and parasympathetic effects of dexmedetomidine in healthy subjects. Can J Physiol Pharmacol. 2004;82(5): 359–62.
57. Talon MD, Woodson LC, Sherwood ER, Aarsland A, McRae L, Benham T. Intranasal dexmedetomidine premedication is comparable with midazolam in burn children undergoing reconstructive surgery. J Burn Care Res. 2009;30(4):599–605.
58. Yuen VM, Hui TW, Irwin MG, Yuen MK. A comparison of intranasal dexmedetomidine and oral midazolam for premedication in pediatric anesthesia: a double-blinded randomized controlled trial. Anesth Analg. 2008;106(6):1715–21.
59. Yuen VM, Irwin MG, Hui TW, Yuen MK, Lee LH. A double-blind, crossover assessment of the sedative and analgesic effects of intranasal dexmedetomidine. Anesth Analg. 2007;105(2): 374–80.
60. Mason KP, Lubisch NB, Robinson F, Roskos R. Intramuscular dexmedetomidine sedation for pediatric MRI and CT. AJR Am J Roentgenol. 2011;197(3):720–5.
61. Mason KP, Lubisch N, Robinson F, Roskos R, Epstein MA. Intramuscular dexmedetomidine: an effective route of sedation preserves background activity for pediatric electroencephalograms. J Pediatr. 2012;161(5):927–32.
62. Petroz GC, Sikich N, James M, van Dyk H, Shafer SL, Schily M, et al. A phase I, two-center study of the pharmacokinetics and pharmacodynamics of dexmedetomidine in children. Anesthesiology. 2006;105(6):1098–110.
63. Díaz SM, Rodarte A, Foley J, Capparelli EV. Pharmacokinetics of dexmedetomidine in postsurgical pediatric intensive care unit

patients: preliminary study. Pediatr Crit Care Med. 2007;8(5): 419–24.
64. Vilo S, Rautiainen P, Kaisti L, Aantaa R, Scheinin M, Manner T, et al. Pharmacokinetics of intravenous dexmedetomidine in children under 11 years of age. Br J Anaesth. 2008;100(5):697–700.
65. Potts AL, Warman GR, Anderson BJ. Dexmedetomidine disposition in children: a population analysis. Paediatr Anaesth. 2008;18(8):722–30.
66. Potts AL, Anderson BJ, Warman GR, Lerman J, Diaz SM, Vilo S. Dexmedetomidine pharmacokinetics in pediatric intensive care—a pooled analysis. Paediatr Anaesth. 2009;19(11): 1119–29.
67. Evers AS, Crowder CM, Balser JR. General anesthetics. In: Brunton LL, Laso JS, Parker KL, editors. Goodman and Gilman's the pharmacological basis of therapeutics. 11th ed. New York: McGraw-Hill; 2006. p. 341–68.

Diazepam

68. http://dailymed.nlm.nih.gov/dailymed/lookup.cfm?setid=09c6e0a1-85ad-4450-cb99-7a6b7b0d3aff. Accessed 14 Dec 2013.
69. Blumer JL. Clinical pharmacology of midazolam in infants and children. Clin Pharmacokinet. 1998;35(1):37–47.

Etomidate

70. http://dailymed.nlm.nih.gov/dailymed/lookup.cfm?setid=b7ed5bf8-ba75-44dc-8f81-96b4ad5766be. Accessed 14 Dec 2013.
71. Sfez M, Le Mapihan Y, Levron JC, Gaillard JL, Rosemblatt JM, Le Moing JP. Comparison of the pharmacokinetics of etomidate in children and in adults. Ann Fr Anesth Reanim. 1990;9(2):127–31.
72. Baxter AL, Mallory MD, Spandorfer PR, Sharma S, Freilich SH, Cravero J, et al. Etomidate versus pentobarbital for computed tomography sedations: report from the Pediatric Sedation Research Consortium. Pediatr Emerg Care. 2007;23(10):690–5.
73. Di Liddo L, D'Angelo A, Nguyen B, Bailey B, Amre D, Stanciu C. Etomidate versus midazolam for procedural sedation in pediatric outpatients: a randomized controlled trial. Ann Emerg Med. 2006;48(4):433–40, 440.e1.
74. Kienstra AJ, Ward MA, Sasan F, Hunter J, Morriss MC, Macias CG. Etomidate versus pentobarbital for sedation of children for head and neck CT imaging. Pediatr Emerg Care. 2004;20(8): 499–506.
75. Cotten JF, Husain SS, Forman SA, Miller KW, Kelly EW, Nguyen HH, et al. Methoxycarbonyl-etomidate: a novel rapidly metabolized and ultra-short-acting etomidate analogue that does not produce prolonged adrenocortical suppression. Anesthesiology. 2009;111:240–9.
76. Cotten JF, Forman SA, Laha JK, Cuny GD, Husain SS, Miller KW, et al. Carboetomidate: a pyrrole analog of etomidate designed not to suppress adrenocortical function. Anesthesiology. 2010;112:637–44.

Fentanyl

77. http://www.accessdata.fda.gov/drugsatfda_docs/label/2005/19813s039lbl.pdf. Accessed 14 Dec 2013.
78. Zernikow B, Michel E, Anderson B. Transdermal fentanyl in childhood and adolescence: a comprehensive literature review. J Pain. 2007;8(3):187–207.
79. Finkel JC, Finley A, Greco C, Weisman SJ, Zeltzer L. Transdermal fentanyl in the management of children with chronic severe pain: results from an international study. Cancer. 2005;104(12): 2847–57.
80. Noyes M, Irving H. The use of transdermal fentanyl in pediatric oncology palliative care. Am J Hosp Palliat Care. 2001;18(6): 411–6.
81. Hunt A, Goldman A, Devine T, Phillips M; FEN-GBR-14 Study Group. Transdermal fentanyl for pain relief in a paediatric palliative care population. Palliat Med. 2001;15(5):405–12.
82. Mannerkoski MK, Heiskala HJ, Santavuori PR, Pouttu JA. Transdermal fentanyl therapy for pains in children with infantile neuronal ceroid lipofuscinosis. Eur J Paediatr Neurol. 2001;5(Suppl A):175–7.
83. Collins JJ, Dunkel IJ, Gupta SK, Inturrisi CE, Lapin J, Palmer LN, et al. Transdermal fentanyl in children with cancer pain: feasibility, tolerability, and pharmacokinetic correlates. J Pediatr. 1999; 134(3):319–23.
84. Clotz MA, Nahata MC. Clinical uses of fentanyl, sufentanil, and alfentanil. Clin Pharm. 1991;10(8):581–93.
85. Chung S, Lim R, Goldman RD. Intranasal fentanyl versus placebo for pain in children during catheterization for voiding cystourethrography. Pediatr Radiol. 2010;40(7):1236–40.
86. Holdgate A, Cao A, Lo KM. The implementation of intranasal fentanyl for children in a mixed adult and pediatric emergency department reduces time to analgesic administration. Acad Emerg Med. 2010;17(2):214–7.
87. Cole J, Shepherd M, Young P. Intranasal fentanyl in 1-3-year-olds: a prospective study of the effectiveness of intranasal fentanyl as acute analgesia. Emerg Med Australas. 2009;21(5):395–400.
88. Herd D, Borland M. Intranasal fentanyl paediatric clinical practice guidelines. Emerg Med Australas. 2009;21(4):335.
89. Borland ML, Clark LJ, Esson A. Comparative review of the clinical use of intranasal fentanyl versus morphine in a paediatric emergency department. Emerg Med Australas. 2008;20(6):515–20. Erratum in: Emerg Med Australas. 2009;21(3):246. (Dosage error in article text).
90. Voronov P, Tobin MJ, Billings K, Coté CJ, Iyer A, Suresh S. Postoperative pain relief in infants undergoing myringotomy and tube placement: comparison of a novel regional anesthetic block to intranasal fentanyl–a pilot analysis. Paediatr Anaesth. 2008;18(12):1196–201.
91. Ali S, Klassen TP. Intranasal fentanyl and intravenous morphine did not differ for pain relief in children with closed long-bone fractures. Evid Based Med. 2007;12(6):176.
92. Wolfe T. Intranasal fentanyl for acute pain: techniques to enhance efficacy. Ann Emerg Med. 2007;49(5):721–2.
93. Borland M, Jacobs I, King B, O'Brien D. A randomized controlled trial comparing intranasal fentanyl to intravenous morphine for managing acute pain in children in the emergency department. Ann Emerg Med. 2007;49(3):335–40.
94. Borland ML, Bergesio R, Pascoe EM, Turner S, Woodger S. Intranasal fentanyl is an equivalent analgesic to oral morphine in paediatric burns patients for dressing changes: a randomised double blind cross-over study. Burns. 2005;31(7):831–7.
95. Borland ML, Jacobs I, Geelhoed G. Intranasal fentanyl reduces acute pain in children in the emergency department: a safety and efficacy study. Emerg Med (Fremantle). 2002;14(3):275–80.
96. Manjushree R, Lahiri A, Ghosh BR, Laha A, Handa K. Intranasal fentanyl provides adequate postoperative analgesia in pediatric patients. Can J Anaesth. 2002;49(2):190–3.
97. Finkel JC, Cohen IT, Hannallah RS, Patel KM, Kim MS, Hummer KA, et al. The effect of intranasal fentanyl on the emergence characteristics after sevoflurane anesthesia in children undergoing surgery for bilateral myringotomy tube placement. Anesth Analg. 2001;92(5):1164–8.

98. Galinkin JL, Fazi LM, Cuy RM, Chiavacci RM, Kurth CD, Shah UK, et al. Use of intranasal fentanyl in children undergoing myringotomy and tube placement during halothane and sevoflurane anesthesia. Anesthesiology. 2000;93(6):1378–83.
99. Mahar PJ, Rana JA, Kennedy CS, Christopher NC. A randomized clinical trial of oral transmucosal fentanyl citrate versus intravenous morphine sulfate for initial control of pain in children with extremity injuries. Pediatr Emerg Care. 2007;23(8):544–8.
100. Zernikow B, Michel E, Craig F, Anderson BJ. Pediatric palliative care: use of opioids for the management of pain. Paediatr Drugs. 2009;11(2):129–51.
101. Robert R, Brack A, Blakeney P, Villarreal C, Rosenberg L, Thomas C, et al. A double-blind study of the analgesic efficacy of oral transmucosal fentanyl citrate and oral morphine in pediatric patients undergoing burn dressing change and tubbing. J Burn Care Rehabil. 2003;24(6):351–5.
102. Howell TK, Smith S, Rushman SC, Walker RW, Radivan F. A comparison of oral transmucosal fentanyl and oral midazolam for premedication in children. Anaesthesia. 2002;57(8):798–805.
103. Klein EJ, Diekema DS, Paris CA, Quan L, Cohen M, Seidel KD. A randomized, clinical trial of oral midazolam plus placebo versus oral midazolam plus oral transmucosal fentanyl for sedation during laceration repair. Pediatrics. 2002;109(5):894–7.
104. Moore PA, Cuddy MA, Magera JA, Caputo AC, Chen AH, Wilkinson LA. Oral transmucosal fentanyl pre-treatment for outpatient general anesthesia. Anesth Prog. 2000;47(2):29–34.
105. Sharar SR, Carrougher GJ, Selzer K, O'Donnell F, Vavilala MS, Lee LA. A comparison of oral transmucosal fentanyl citrate and oral oxycodone for pediatric outpatient wound care. J Burn Care Rehabil. 2002;23(1):27–31.
106. Howell TK, Smith S, Rushman S, Walker RW. A comparison of oral transmucosal fentanyl and oral midazolam for premedication in children. Paediatr Anaesth. 2000;10(6):697.
107. Sharar SR, Bratton SL, Carrougher GJ, Edwards WT, Summer G, Levy FH, et al. A comparison of oral trans-mucosal fentanyl citrate and oral hydromorphone for inpatient pediatric burn wound care analgesia. J Burn Care Rehabil. 1998;19(6):516–21.
108. Ginsberg B, Dear RB, Margolis JO, Dear GD, Ross AK. Oral transmucosal fentanyl citrate as an anaesthetic premedication when dosed to an opioid effect vs total opioid consumption. Paediatr Anaesth. 1998;8(5):413–8.
109. Dsida RM, Wheeler M, Birmingham PK, Henthorn TK, Avram MJ, Enders-Klein C, et al. Premedication of pediatric tonsillectomy patients with oral trans-mucosal fentanyl citrate. Anesth Analg. 1998;86(1):66–70.
110. Weisman SJ, Bernstein B, Schechter NL. Consequences of inadequate analgesia during painful procedures in children. Arch Pediatr Adolesc Med. 1998;152(2):147–9.
111. Malviya S, Voepel-Lewis T, Huntington J, Siewert M, Green W. Effects of anesthetic technique on side effects associated with fentanyl Oralet premedication. J Clin Anesth. 1997;9(5):374–8.
112. Epstein RH, Mendel HG, Witkowski TA, Waters R, Guarniari KM, Marr AT, et al. The safety and efficacy of oral transmucosal fentanyl citrate for preoperative sedation in young children. Anesth Analg. 1996;83(6):1200–5.
113. Schutzman SA, Liebelt E, Wisk M, Burg J. Comparison of oral transmucosal fentanyl citrate and intramuscular meperidine, promethazine, and chlorpromazine for conscious sedation of children undergoing laceration repair. Ann Emerg Med. 1996;28(4):385–90.
114. Brenn BR. Side effects with use of oral transmucosal fentanyl. Pediatrics. 1995;96(3 Pt 1):544.
115. Schechter NL, Weisman SJ, Rosenblum M, Bernstein B, Conard PL. The use of oral transmucosal fentanyl citrate for painful procedures in children. Pediatrics. 1995;95(3):335–9.
116. Friesen RH, Carpenter E, Madigan CK, Lockhart CH. Oral transmucosal fentanyl citrate for preanaesthetic medication of paediatric cardiac surgery patients. Paediatr Anaesth. 1995;5(1):29–33.
117. Schutzman SA, Burg J, Liebelt E, Strafford M, Schechter N, Wisk M, et al. Oral transmucosal fentanyl citrate for premedication of children undergoing laceration repair. Ann Emerg Med. 1994;24(6):1059–64.
118. Friesen RH, Lockhart CH. Oral transmucosal fentanyl citrate for preanesthetic medication of pediatric day surgery patients with and without droperidol as a prophylactic anti-emetic. Anesthesiology. 1992;76(1):46–51.
119. Lind GH, Marcus MA, Mears SL, Ashburn MA, Peterson BJ, Bernhisel KT, et al. Oral transmucosal fentanyl citrate for analgesia and sedation in the emergency department. Ann Emerg Med. 1991;20(10):1117–20.
120. Goldstein-Dresner MC, Davis PJ, Kretchman E, Siewers RD, Certo N, Cook DR. Double-blind comparison of oral transmucosal fentanyl citrate with oral meperidine, diazepam, and atropine as preanesthetic medication in children with congenital heart disease. Anesthesiology. 1991;74(1):28–33.
121. Ashburn MA, Streisand JB, Tarver SD, Mears SL, Mulder SM, Floet Wilms AW, et al. Oral transmucosal fentanyl citrate for premedication in paediatric out-patients. Can J Anaesth. 1990;37(8):857–66.
122. Stanley TH, Leiman BC, Rawal N, Marcus MA, van den Nieuwenhuyzen M, Walford A, et al. The effects of oral transmucosal fentanyl citrate premedication on preoperative behavioral responses and gastric volume and acidity in children. Anesth Analg. 1989;69(3):328–35.
123. Feld LH, Champeau MW, van Steennis CA, Scott JC. Preanesthetic medication in children: a comparison of oral transmucosal fentanyl citrate versus placebo. Anesthesiology. 1989;71(3):374–7.
124. Streisand JB, Stanley TH, Hague B, van Vreeswijk H, Ho GH, Pace NL. Oral transmucosal fentanyl citrate premedication in children. Anesth Analg. 1989;69(1):28–34.
125. Nelson PS, Streisand JB, Mulder SM, Pace NL, Stanley TH. Comparison of oral transmucosal fentanyl citrate and an oral solution of meperidine, diazepam, and atropine for premedication in children. Anesthesiology. 1989;70(4):616–21.
126. Katz R, Kelly HW. Pharmacokinetics of continuous infusions of fentanyl in critically ill children. Crit Care Med. 1993;21(7):995–1000.
127. Paut O, Camboulives J, Viard L, Lemoing JP, Levron JC. Pharmacokinetics of transdermal fentanyl in the peri-operative period in young children. Anaesthesia. 2000;55(12):1202–7.
128. Wheeler M, Birmingham PK, Lugo RA, Heffner CL, Coté CJ. The pharmacokinetics of the intravenous formulation of fentanyl citrate administered orally in children undergoing general anesthesia. Anesth Analg. 2004;99(5):1347–51.
129. Sahyoun C, Krauss B. Clinical implications of pharmacokinetics and pharmacodynamics of procedural sedation agents in children. Curr Opin Pediatr. 2012;24(2):225–32.

Fospropofol

130. Moore GD, Walker AM, MacLaren R. Fospropofol: a new sedative-hypnotic agent for monitored anesthesia care. Ann Pharmacother. 2009;43(11):1802–8.
131. Garnock-Jones KP, Scott LJ. Fospropofol. Drugs. 2010;70(4): 469–77.
132. http://dailymed.nlm.nih.gov/dailymed/lookup.cfm?setid=8cc837aa-14f0-4809-9ca1-6cc7ff84646b. Accessed 14 Dec 2013.

Ketamine

133. http://dailymed.nlm.nih.gov/dailymed/lookup.cfm?setid=bb912318-2e22-4469-b0a2-774803ee1bb8. Accessed 14 Dec 2013.

134. Herd D, Anderson BJ. Ketamine disposition in children presenting for procedural sedation and analgesia in a children's emergency department. Paediatr Anaesth. 2007;17(7):622–9.
135. Maliknovsky JM, Servin F, Cozian A, Lepage JY, Pinaud M. Ketamine and norketamine plasma concentrations after i.v., nasal and rectal administration in children. Br J Anaesth. 1996; 77(2):203–7.
136. Pedraz JL, Calvo MB, Lanao JM, Muriel C, Santos Lamas J, Domínguez-Gil A. Pharmacokinetics of rectal ketamine in children. Br J Anaesth. 1989;63(6):671–4.
137. Grant IS, Nimmo WS, McNicol LR, Clements JA. Ketamine disposition in children and adults. Br J Anaesth. 1983;55(11): 1107–11.
138. Idvall J, Holassek J, Stenberg P. Rectal administration for induction of anesthesia in children. Anesthesia. 1983;38(1):60–4.
139. Sinner B, Graf BM. Ketamine. Handb Exp Pharmacol. 2008;182: 313–33.
140. Roelofse JA. The evolution of ketamine applications in children. Paediatr Anaesth. 2010;20(3):240–5.

Ketofol

141. Rapeport DA, Martyr JW, Wang LP. The use of "ketofol" (ketamine-propofol admixture) infusion in conjunction with regional anaesthesia. Anaesth Intensive Care. 2009;37:121–3.
142. Loh G, Dalen D. Low-dose ketamine in addition to propofol for procedural sedation and analgesia in the emergency department. Ann Pharmacother. 2007;41:485–92.
143. Andolfatto G, Abu-Laban RB, Zed PJ, Staniforth SM, Stackhouse S, Moadebi S, et al. Ketamine-propofol combination (ketofol) versus propofol alone for emergency department procedural sedation and analgesia: a randomized double-blind trial. Ann Emerg Med. 2012;59:504–12.e1-2.
144. Aouad MT, Moussa AR, Dagher CM, Muwakkit SA, Jabbour-Khoury SI, Zbeidy RA, et al. Addition of ketamine to propofol for initiation of procedural anesthesia in children reduces propofol consumption and preserves hemodynamic stability. Acta Anaesthesiol Scand. 2008;52:561–5.
145. Green SM, Andolfatto G, Krauss B. Ketofol for procedural sedation? Pro and con. Ann Emerg Med. 2011;57(5):444–8.

Lorazepam

146. http://dailymed.nlm.nih.gov/dailymed/lookup.cfm?setid=ad2a0633-50fe-4180-b743-c1e49fc110c6. Accessed 14 Dec 2013.
147. Muchohi SN, Obiero K, Newton CR, Ogutu BR, Edwards G, Kokwaro GO. Pharmacokinetics and clinical efficacy of lorazepam in children with severe malaria and convulsions. Br J Clin Pharmacol. 2008;65(1):12–21.
148. Relling MV, Mulhern RK, Dodge RK, Johnson D, Pieper JA, Rivera GK, et al. Lorazepam pharmacodynamics and pharmacokinetics in children. J Pediatr. 1989;114(4 Pt 1):641–6.

Meperidine

149. http://dailymed.nlm.nih.gov/dailymed/lookup.cfm?setid=987a91b8-dd9e-47ce-bd43-f8189a54838e Accessed Dec 14, 2013.
150. Hamunen K, Maunuksela EL, Seppälä T, Olkkola KT. Pharmacokinetics of i.v. and rectal pethidine in children undergoing ophthalmic surgery. Br J Anaesth. 1993;71(6):823–6.

Methohexital

151. http://dailymed.nlm.nih.gov/dailymed/lookup.cfm?setid=eccd8340-ead3-4363-8902-0c19d33aa2ac. Accessed 14 Dec 2013.
152. Forbes RB, Murray DJ, Dillman JB, Dull DL. Pharmacokinetics of two percent rectal methohexitone in children. Can J Anaesth. 1989;36(2):160–4.
153. Kestin IG, McIlvaine WB, Lockhart CH, Kestin KJ, Jones MA. Rectal methohexital for induction of anesthesia in children with and without rectal aspiration after sleep: a pharmacokinetic and pharmacodynamic study. Anesth Analg. 1988;67(11):1102–4.
154. Björkman S, Gabrielsson J, Quaynor H, Corbey M. Pharmacokinetics of i.v. and rectal methohexitone in children. Br J Anaesth. 1987;59(12):1541–7.
155. Quaynor H, Corbey M, Björkman S. Rectal induction of anaesthesia in children with methohexitone. Patient acceptability and clinical pharmacokinetics. Br J Anaesth. 1985;57(6):573–7.
156. Kraus G, Frank S, Knoll R, Prestele H. Pharmacokinetic studies following intravenous, intra- muscular and rectal administration of methohexital in children. Anaesthesist. 1984;33(6):266–71.
157. Stimmesse B, Barale F, Lassauge F, Truong Than T, Arbez-Gindre F, Adloff M, Succi C, Guichard C, Belon JP. Pharmacokinetics of methohexital administered rectally in pediatric anesthesia. Agressologie. 1987;28(10):1015–7 (French).
158. Michel-Guéroult P, Benoit I, Grellet J, Meynat Y, Merlet JP, Saux MC. Pharmacokinetic and clinical evaluation of rectal hydrophilic gel of methohexital in pediatric surgery. Therapie. 1993;48(1): 27–32 (French).
159. Liu LMP, Gaudreault P, Firedman PA. Methohexital plasma concentrations in children following rectal administration. Anesthesiology. 1985;62:567–70.

Midazolam

160. http://dailymed.nlm.nih.gov/dailymed/lookup.cfm?setid=0be63f63-6a93-4782-8f9c-d13ca5ae44bd. Accessed 14 Dec 2013.
161. Johnson TN, Rostami-Hodjegan A, Tucker GT. Prediction of the clearance of eleven drugs and associated variability in neonates, infants and children. Clin Pharmacokinet. 2006;45(9):931–56.
162. Minagawa K, Watanabe T. A pharmacokinetic study of midazolam for the treatment of status epilepticus in children: a preliminary report. No To Hattatsu. 2006;38(4):301–3.
163. Björkman S. Prediction of drug disposition in infants and children by means of physiologically based pharmacokinetic (PBPK) modelling: theophylline and midazolam as model drugs. Br J Clin Pharmacol. 2005;59(6):691–704.
164. de Wildt SN, de Hoog M, Vinks AA, van der Giesen E, van den Anker JN. Population pharmacokinetics and metabolism of midazolam in pediatric intensive care patients. Crit Care Med. 2003; 31(7):1952–8.
165. Johnson TN, Rostami-Hodjegan A, Goddard JM, Tanner MS, Tucker GT. Contribution of midazolam and its 1-hydroxy metabolite to preoperative seda- tion in children: a pharmacokinetic-pharmacodynamic analysis. Br J Anaesth. 2002;89(3):428–37.
166. Reed MD, Rodarte A, Blumer JL, Khoo KC, Akbari B, Pou S, et al. The single-dose pharmacokinetics of midazolam and its primary metabolite in pediatric patients after oral and intravenous administration. J Clin Pharmacol. 2001;41(12):1359–69.
167. Nahara MC, McMorrow J, Jones PR, Anglin D, Rosenberg R. Pharmacokinetics of midazolam in critically ill pediatric patients. Eur J Drug Metab Pharmacokinet. 2000;25(3–4): 219–21.
168. Scott RC, Besag FM, Boyd SG, Berry D, Neville BG. Buccal absorption of midazolam: pharmacokinetics and EEG pharmacodynamics. Epilepsia. 1998;39(3):290–4.

169. Jones RD, Visram AR, Kornberg JP, Irwin MG, Gunawardene WM. Premedication with oral midazolam in children—an assessment of psychomotor function, anxiolysis, sedation and pharmacokinetics. Anaesth Intensive Care. 1994;22(5):539–44.
170. Malinovsky JM, Lejus C, Servin F, Lepage JY, Le Normand Y, Testa S, et al. Plasma concentrations of midazolam after i.v., nasal or rectal administration in children. Br J Anaesth. 1993;70(6): 617–20.
171. Tolia V, Brennan S, Aravind MK, Kauffman RE. Pharmacokinetic and pharmacodynamic study of midazolam in children during esophagogastroduodenoscopy. J Pediatr. 1991;119(3):467–71.
172. Walbergh EJ, Wills RJ, Eckhert J. Plasma concentrations of midazolam in children following intranasal administration. Anesthesiology. 1991;74(2):233–5.
173. Rey E, Delaunay L, Pons G, Murat I, Richard MO, Saint-Maurice C, et al. Pharmacokinetics of midazolam in children: comparative study of intranasal and intravenous administration. Eur J Clin Pharmacol. 1991;41(4):355–7.
174. Kraus GB, Gruber RG, Knoll R, Danner U. Pharmacokinetic studies following intravenous and rectal administration of midazolam in children. Anaesthesist. 1989;38(12):658–63.
175. Payne K, Mattheyse FJ, Liebenberg D, Dawes T. The pharmacokinetics of midazolam in paediatric patients. Eur J Clin Pharmacol. 1989;37(3):267–72.
176. Mathews HM, Carson IW, Lyons SM, Orr IA, Collier PS, Howard PJ, et al. A pharmacokinetic study of midazolam in paediatric patients undergoing cardiac surgery. Br J Anaesth. 1988;61(3): 302–7.
177. Salonen M, Kanto J, Iisalo E, Himberg JJ. Midazolam as an induction agent in children: a pharmacokinetic and clinical study. Anesth Analg. 1987;66(7):625–8.
178. Saint-Maurice C, Meistelman C, Rey E, Esteve C, de Lauture D, Olive G. The pharmacokinetics of rectal midazolam for premedication in children. Anesthesiology. 1986;65(5):536–8.
179. Jochemsen R, Breimer DD. Pharmacokinetics of benzodiazepines: metabolic pathways and plasma level profiles. Curr Med Res Opin. 1984;8 Suppl 4:60–79.

Morphine

180. http://dailymed.nlm.nih.gov/dailymed/lookup.cfm?setid=22055b20-bc20-4e45-8574-4b218e0901e4. Accessed 14 Dec 2013.
181. Lugo RA, Kern SE. Clinical pharmacokinetics of morphine. J Pain Palliat Care Pharmacother. 2002;16(4):5–18.
182. Mashayekhi SO, Ghandforoush-Sattari M, Routledge PA, Hain RD. Pharmacokinetic and pharmacodynamic study of morphine and morphine 6-glucuronide after oral and intravenous administration of morphine in children with cancer. Biopharm Drug Dispos. 2009;30(3):99–106.
183. Peters JW, Anderson BJ, Simons SH, Uges DR, Tibboel D. Morphine pharmacokinetics during veno- arterial extracorporeal membrane oxygenation in neonates. Intensive Care Med. 2005;31(2):257–63.
184. Bouwmeester NJ, Anderson BJ, Tibboel D, Holford NH. Developmental pharmacokinetics of morphine and its metabolites in neonates, infants and young children. Br J Anaesth. 2004; 92(2):208–17.
185. Hunt A, Joel S, Dick G, Goldman A. Population pharmacokinetics of oral morphine and its glucuronides in children receiving morphine as immediate-release liquid or sustained-release tablets for cancer pain. J Pediatr. 1999;135(1):47–55.
186. Hain RD, Hardcastle A, Pinkerton CR, Aherne GW. Morphine and morphine-6-glucuronide in the plasma and cerebrospinal fluid of children. Br J Clin Pharmacol. 1999;48(1):37–42.
187. Kart T, Christrup LL, Rasmussen M. Recommended use of morphine in neonates, infants and children based on a literature review: part 1—pharmacokinetics. Paediatr Anaesth. 1997;7(1):5–11.
188. Lundeberg S, Beck O, Olsson GL, Boreus LO. Rectal administration of morphine in children. Pharmacokinetic evaluation after a single-dose. Acta Anaesthesiol Scand. 1996;40(4):445–51.
189. Olkkola KT, Hamunen K, Maunuksela EL. Clinical pharmacokinetics and pharmacodynamics of opioid analgesics in infants and children. Clin Pharmacokinet. 1995;28(5):385–404.
190. Dampier CD, Setty BN, Logan J, Ioli JG, Dean R. Intravenous morphine pharmacokinetics in pediatric patients with sickle cell disease. J Pediatr. 1995;126(3):461–7.
191. Nichols DG, Yaster M, Lynn AM, Helfaer MA, Deshpande JK, Manson PN, Carson BS, Bezman M, Maxwell LG, Tobias JD, et al. Disposition and respiratory effects of intrathecal morphine in children. Anesthesiology. 1993;79(4):733–8. discussion 25A.
192. Dagan O, Klein J, Bohn D, Barker G, Koren G. Morphine pharmacokinetics in children following cardiac surgery: effects of disease and inotropic support. J Cardiothorac Vasc Anesth. 1993;7(4):396–8.
193. Choonara I, Lawrence A, Michalkiewicz A, Bowhay A, Ratcliffe J. Morphine metabolism in neonates and infants. Br J Clin Pharmacol. 1992;34(5):434–7.
194. McRorie TI, Lynn AM, Nespeca MK, Opheim KE, Slattery JT. The maturation of morphine clearance and metabolism. Am J Dis Child. 1992;146(8):972–6. Erratum in: Am J Dis Child. 1992;146(11):1305.
195. Nahata MC. Plasma concentrations of morphine in children with chronic pain–comparison of controlled release and regular morphine sulphate tablets. J Clin Pharm Ther. 1991;16(3):193–5.
196. Choonara IA, McKay P, Hain R, Rane A. Morphine metabolism in children. Br J Clin Pharmacol. 1989;28(5):599–604.
197. Attia J, Ecoffey C, Sandouk P, Gross JB, Samii K. Epidural morphine in children: pharmacokinetics and CO2 sensitivity. Anesthesiology. 1986;65(6):590–4.
198. Shelly MP, Cory EP, Park GR. Pharmacokinetics of morphine in two children before and after liver transplantation. Br J Anaesth. 1986;58(11):1218–23.
199. Nahata MC, Miser AW, Miser JS, Reuning RH. Variation in morphine pharmacokinetics in children with cancer. Dev Pharmacol Ther. 1985;8(3):182–8.
200. Vandenberghe H, Mac Leod S, Chinyanga H, Endrenyi L, Soldin S. Pharmacokinetics of intravenous morphine in balanced anesthesia: studies in children. Drug Metab Rev. 1983;14(5):887–903.

Nitrous Oxide

201. Koren G, Sloan I. The pharmacokinetics of inhaled NO in children. Res Commun Chem Pathol Pharmacol. 1985;49(1):95–108.
202. O'Callaghan AC, Koren G, Sloan IA. Effects of age and cardiac shunts on the measured uptake of nitrous oxide in children. Res Commun Chem Pathol Pharmacol. 1991;74(3):299–315.
203. Mace SE, Brown LA, Francis L, Godwin SA, Hahn SA, Howard PK, Kennedy RM, Mooney DP, Sacchetti AD, Wears RL, Clark RM; EMSC Panel (Writing Committee) on Critical Issues in the Sedation of Pediatric Patients in the Emergency. Clinical policy: critical issues in the sedation of pediatric patients in the emergency department. Ann Emerg Med. 2008;51(4):378–99, 399.e1–57.
204. Babl FE, Oakley E, Seaman C, Barnett P, Sharwood LN. High-concentration nitrous oxide for procedural sedation in children: adverse events and depth of sedation. Pediatrics. 2008;121(3): e528–32.
205. Bar-Meir E, Zaslansky R, Regev E, Keidan I, Orenstein A, Winkler E. Nitrous oxide administered by the plastic surgeon for repair of

facial lacerations in children in the emergency room. Plast Reconstr Surg. 2006;117(5):1571–5.
206. Luhmann JD, Schootman M, Luhmann SJ, Kennedy RM. A randomized comparison of nitrous oxide plus hematoma block versus ketamine plus midazolam for emergency department forearm fracture reduction in children. Pediatrics. 2006;118(4):e1078–86.
207. Onody P, Gil P, Hennequin M. Safety of inhalation of a 50% nitrous oxide/oxygen premix: a prospective survey of 35,828 administrations. Drug Saf. 2006;29(7):633–40.
208. Ekbom K, Jakobsson J, Marcus C. Nitrous oxide inhalation is a safe and effective way to facilitate procedures in paediatric outpatient departments. Arch Dis Child. 2005;90(10):1073–6.
209. Burnweit C, Diana-Zerpa JA, Nahmad MH, Lankau CA, Weinberger M, Malvezzi L, et al. Nitrous oxide analgesia for minor pediatric surgical procedures: an effective alternative to conscious sedation? J Pediatr Surg. 2004;39(3):495–9. discussion 495–9.
210. Kanagasundaram SA, Lane LJ, Cavalletto BP, Keneally JP, Cooper MG. Efficacy and safety of nitrous oxide in alleviating pain and anxiety during painful procedures. Arch Dis Child. 2001;84(6):492–5.
211. Luhmann JD, Kennedy RM, Porter FL, Miller JP, Jaffe DM. A randomized clinical trial of continuous-flow nitrous oxide and midazolam for sedation of young children during laceration repair. Ann Emerg Med. 2001;37(1):20–7.
212. Burton JH, Auble TE, Fuchs SM. Effectiveness of 50% nitrous oxide/50% oxygen during laceration repair in children. Acad Emerg Med. 1998;5(2):112–7.
213. Gregory PR, Sullivan JA. Nitrous oxide compared with intravenous regional anesthesia in pediatric forearm fracture manipulation. J Pediatr Orthop. 1996;16(2):187–91.
214. Evans JK, Buckley SL, Alexander AH, Gilpin AT. Analgesia for the reduction of fractures in children: a comparison of nitrous oxide with intramuscular sedation. J Pediatr Orthop. 1995;15(1):73–7.
215. Hennrikus WL, Shin AY, Klingelberger CE. Self- administered nitrous oxide and a hematoma block for analgesia in the outpatient reduction of fractures in children. J Bone Joint Surg Am. 1995;77(3):335–9.
216. Hennrikus WL, Simpson RB, Klingelberger CE, Reis MT. Self-administered nitrous oxide analgesia for pediatric fracture reductions. J Pediatr Orthop. 1994;14(4):538–42.
217. Henderson JM, Spence DG, Komocar LM, Bonn GE, Stenstrom RJ. Administration of nitrous oxide to pediatric patients provides analgesia for venous cannulation. Anesthesiology. 1990;72(2):269–71.
218. Wattenmaker I, Kasser JR, McGravey A. Self- administered nitrous oxide for fracture reduction in children in an emergency room setting. J Orthop Trauma. 1990;4(1):35–8.
219. Gamis AS, Knapp JF, Glenski JA. Nitrous oxide analgesia in a pediatric emergency department. Ann Emerg Med. 1989;18(2):177–81.
220. Benedetti C, Chapman CR, Colpitts YH, Chen AC. Effect of nitrous oxide concentration on event-related potentials during painful tooth stimulation. Anesthesiology. 1982;56(5):360–4.
221. Ruben H. Nitrous oxide analgesia in dentistry. Its use during 15 years in Denmark. Br Dent J. 1972;132(5):195–6.
222. Parbrook GD. The levels of nitrous oxide analgesia. Br J Anaesth. 1967;39(12):974–82.
223. Tobias JD. Applications of nitrous oxide for procedural sedation in the pediatric population. Pediatr Emerg Care. 2013;29(2):245–65.
224. Zier JL, Tarrago R, Liu M. Level of sedation with nitrous oxide for pediatric medical procedures. Anesth Analg. 2010;110(5):1399–405.

Pentobarbital

225. Mason KP, Zurakowski D, Connor L, et al. Infant sedation for MR imaging and CT: oral versus intravenous pentobarbital. Radiology. 2004;233:723–8.
226. http://dailymed.nlm.nih.gov/dailymed/lookup.cfm?setid=f302ddf5-0213-43b3-b6c1-b3edf2bafbcd. Accessed 14 Dec 2013.
227. Schaible DH, Cupit GC, Swedlow DB, Rocci Jr ML. High-dose pentobarbital pharmacokinetics in hypothermic brain-injured children. J Pediatr. 1982;100(4):655–60.
228. Wermeling DP, Blouin RA, Porter WH, Rapp RP, Tibbs PA. Pentobarbital pharmacokinetics in patients with severe head injury. Drug Intell Clin Pharm. 1987;21(5):459–63.

Propofol

229. Nelson LE, Guo TZ, Lu J, Saper CB, Franks NP, Maze M. The sedative component of anesthesia is mediated by GABA(A) receptors in an endogenous sleep pathway. Nat Neurosci. 2002; 5:979–84.
230. http://dailymed.nlm.nih.gov/dailymed/lookup.cfm?setid=28d7ba00-f824-4e55-139a-03f509c099db. Accessed 14 Dec 2013.
231. Engelhardt T, McCheyne AJ, Morton N, Karsli C, Luginbuehl I, Adeli K, et al. Clinical adaptation of a pharmacokinetic model of propofol plasma concentrations in children. Paediatr Anaesth. 2008;18(3):235–9.
232. Allegaert K, Peeters MY, Verbesselt R, Tibboel D, Naulaers G, de Hoon JN, et al. Inter-individual variability in propofol pharmacokinetics in preterm and term neonates. Br J Anaesth. 2007; 99(6):864–70.
233. Mazoit JX. Pharmacokinetic/pharmacodynamic modeling of anesthetics in children: therapeutic implications. Paediatr Drugs. 2006;8(3):139–50.
234. Shangguan WN, Lian Q, Aarons L, Matthews I, Wang Z, Chen X, et al. Pharmacokinetics of a single bolus of propofol in Chinese children of different ages. Anesthesiology. 2006;104(1):27–32.
235. Zuppa AF, Helfaer MA, Adamson PC. Propofol pharmacokinetics. Pediatr Crit Care Med. 2003;4(1):124–5.
236. Rigby-Jones AE, Nolan JA, Priston MJ, Wright PM, Sneyd JR, Wolf AR. Pharmacokinetics of propofol infusions in critically ill neonates, infants, and children in an intensive care unit. Anesthesiology. 2002;97(6):1393–400.
237. Knibbe CA, Melenhorst-deJong G, Mestrom M, Rademaker CM, Reijnvaan AF, Zuideveld KP, et al. Pharmacokinetics and effects of propofol 6% for short-term sedation in paediatric patients following cardiac surgery. Br J Clin Pharmacol. 2002;54(4):415–22.
238. Sakai T, Mi WD, Ebina T, Kudo T, Kudo M, Matsuki A. Pharmacokinetics of propofol and ketamine during and after total intravenous anesthesia with propofol, fentanyl and ketamine for pediatric patients. Masui. 1998;47(3):277–80.
239. Reed MD, Yamashita TS, Marx CM, Myers CM, Blumer JL. A pharmacokinetically based propofol dosing strategy for sedation of the critically ill, mechanically ventilated pediatric patient. Crit Care Med. 1996;24(9):1473–81.
240. Murat I, Billard V, Vernois J, Zaouter M, Marsol P, Souron R, et al. Pharmacokinetics of propofol after a single dose in children aged 1–3 years with minor burns. Comparison of three data analysis approaches. Anesthesiology. 1996;84(3):526–32.
241. Raoof AA, van Obbergh LJ, Verbeeck RK. Propofol pharmacokinetics in children with biliary atresia. Br J Anaesth. 1995; 74(1):46–9.
242. Short TG, Aun CS, Tan P, Wong J, Tam YH, Oh TE. A prospective evaluation of pharmacokinetic model controlled infusion of propofol in paediatric patients. Br J Anaesth. 1994;72(3):302–6.
243. Fisher DM. Propofol in pediatrics. Lessons in pharmacokinetic modeling. Anesthesiology. 1994;80(1):2–5.
244. Kataria BK, Ved SA, Nicodemus HF, Hoy GR, Lea D, Dubois MY, et al. The pharmacokinetics of propofol in children using three different data analysis approaches. Anesthesiology. 1994; 80(1):104–22.
245. Shafer SL. Advances in propofol pharmacokinetics and pharmacodynamics. J Clin Anesth. 1993;5(6 Suppl 1):14S–21.

246. Jones RD, Chan K, Andrew LJ, Lawson AD, Wong P. Comparative pharmacokinetics of propofol in Chinese adults and children. Methods Find Exp Clin Pharmacol. 1992;14(1):41–7.
247. Jones RD, Chan K, Andrew LJ. Pharmacokinetics of propofol in children. Br J Anaesth. 1990;65(5):661–7.
248. Saint-Maurice C, Cockshott ID, Douglas EJ, Richard MO, Harmey JL. Pharmacokinetics of propofol in young children after a single dose. Br J Anaesth. 1989;63(6):667–70.
249. Vandermeersch E, Van Hemelrijck J, Byttebier G, Van Aken H. Pharmacokinetics of propofol during continuous infusion for pediatric anesthesia. Acta Anaesthesiol Belg. 1989;40(3):161–5.
250. http://www.hospira.com/Images/EN-2029_32-5641_1.pdf. Accessed 14 Dec 2013.
251. De Leon-Casasola OA, Weiss A, Lema MJ. Anaphylaxis due to propofol. Anesthesiology. 1992;77:384–6.
252. Laxenaire MC, Mata-Bermejo E, Moneret-Vautrin DA, Gueant JL. Life-threatening anaphylactoid reactions to propofol (Diprivan). Anesthesiology. 1992;77:275–80.
253. McHale SP, Konieczko K. Anaphylactoid reaction to propofol. Anaesthesia. 1992;47(10):864–5.
254. Hofer KN, McCarthy MW, Buck ML, Hendrick AE. Possible anaphylaxis after propofol in a child with food allergy. Ann Pharmacother. 2003;37:398–401.
255. Murphy A, Campbell DE, Baines D, Mehr S. Allergic reactions to propofol in egg-allergic children. Anesth Analg. 2011;113(1): 140–4.
256. Dewachter P, Mouton-Faivre C, Castells MC, Hepner DL. Anesthesia in the patient with multiple drug allergies: are all allergies the same? Curr Opin Anaesthesiol. 2011;24(3):320–5.
257. Gemma M, de Vitis A, Baldoli C, Calvi MR, Blasi V, Scola E, et al. Functional magnetic resonance imaging (fMRI) in children sedated with propofol or midazolam. J Neurosurg Anesthesiol. 2009;21(3):253–8.
258. Lightdale JR, Valim C, Newburg AR, Mahoney LB, Zgleszewski S, Fox VL. Efficiency of propofol versus midazolam and fentanyl sedation at a pediatric teaching hospital: a prospective study. Gastrointest Endosc. 2008;67(7):1067–75.
259. Mallory MD, Baxter AL, Kost SI, Pediatric Sedation Research Consortium. Propofol vs pentobarbital for sedation of children undergoing magnetic resonance imaging: results from the Pediatric Sedation Research Consortium. Paediatr Anaesth. 2009;19(6):601–11.
260. Pershad J, Wan J, Anghelescu DL. Comparison of propofol with pentobarbital/midazolam/fentanyl sedation for magnetic resonance imaging of the brain in children. Pediatrics. 2007;120(3):e629–36.
261. Rai K, Hegde AM, Goel K. Sedation in uncooperative children undergoing dental procedures: a comparative evaluation of midazolam, propofol and ketamine. J Clin Pediatr Dent. 2007;32(1): 1–4.
262. Gottschling S, Meyer S, Krenn T, Reinhard H, Lothschuetz D, Nunold H, et al. Propofol versus midazolam/ketamine for procedural sedation in pediatric oncology. J Pediatr Hematol Oncol. 2005;27(9):471–6.
263. Koroglu A, Teksan H, Sagir O, Yucel A, Toprak HI, Ersoy OM. A comparison of the sedative, hemodynamic, and respiratory effects of dexmedetomidine and propofol in children undergoing magnetic resonance imaging. Anesth Analg. 2006;103(1):63–7.
264. Mahmoud M, Gunter J, Donnelly LF, Wang Y, Nick TG, Sadhasivam S. A comparison of dexmedetomidine with propofol for magnetic resonance imaging sleep studies in children. Anesth Analg. 2009;109(3):745–53.
265. Prabhakar H, Bindra A, Singh GP, Kalaivani M. Propofol versus thiopental sodium for the treatment of refractory status epilepticus (Review). Evid Based Child Health. 2013;8(4):1488–508.
266. Cravero JP, Beach ML, Blike GT, Gallagher SM, Hertzog JH, Pediatric Sedation Research Consortium. The incidence and nature of adverse events during pediatric sedation/anesthesia with propofol for procedures outside the operating room: a report from the Pediatric Sedation Research Consortium. Anesth Analg. 2009;108(3):795–804.
267. Mayette M, Gonda J, Hsu JL, Mihm FG. Propofol infusion syndrome resuscitation with extracorporeal life support: a case report and review of the literature. Ann Intensive Care. 2013; 3(1):32.

Remifentanil

268. http://dailymed.nlm.nih.gov/dailymed/lookup.cfm?setid=dbc63b6e-f8c5-4fd0-8ec3-4f5e19125313. Accessed 14 Dec 2013.
269. Ross AK, Davis PJ, Dear Gd GL, Ginsberg B, McGowan FX, Stiller RD, et al. Pharmacokinetics of remifentanil in anesthetized pediatric patients undergoing elective surgery or diagnostic procedures. Anesth Analg. 2001;93(6):1393–401.
270. Davis PJ, Wilson AS, Siewers RD, Pigula FA, Landsman IS. The effects of cardiopulmonary bypass on remifentanil kinetics in children undergoing atrial septal defect repair. Anesth Analg. 1999;89(4):904–8.
271. Battershill AJ, Keating GM. Remifentanil: a review of its analgesic and sedative use in the intensive care unit. Drugs. 2006;66(3):365–85.
272. Sammartino M, Garra R, Sbaraglia F, De Riso M, Continolo N. Remifentanil in children. Paediatr Anaesth. 2010;20(3):246–55.
273. Marsh DF, Hodkinson B. Remifentanil in paediatric anaesthetic practice. Anaesthesia. 2009;64(3):301–8.

S-Ketamine

274. Kharasch ED, Labroo R. Metabolism of ketamine stereoisomers by human liver microsomes. Anesthesiology. 1992;77(6):1201–7.
275. Weber F, Wulf H, el Saeidi G. Premedication with nasal s-ketamine and midazolam provides good conditions for induction of anesthesia in preschool children. Can J Anaesth. 2003;50(5):470–5.
276. Almenrader N, Passariello M, D'Amico G, Haiberger R, Pietropaoli P. Caudal additives for postoperative pain management in children: S(+)-ketamine and neostigmine. Paediatr Anaesth. 2005;15(2):143–7.
277. Passariello M, Almenrader N, Canneti A, Rubeo L, Haiberger R, Pietropaoli P. Caudal analgesia in children: S(+)-ketamine vs S(+)-ketamine plus clonidine. Paediatr Anaesth. 2004;14(10):851–5.
278. Martindale SJ, Dix P, Stoddart PA. Double-blind randomized controlled trial of caudal versus intravenous S(+)-ketamine for supplementation of caudal analgesia in children. Br J Anaesth. 2004;92(3):344–7.
279. Weber F, Wulf H. Caudal bupivacaine and s(+)-ketamine for postoperative analgesia in children. Paediatr Anaesth. 2003; 13(3):244–8.
280. Hager H, Marhofer P, Sitzwohl C, Adler L, Kettner S, Semsroth M. Caudal clonidine prolongs analgesia from caudal S(+)-ketamine in children. Anesth Analg. 2002;94(5):1169–72.
281. De Negri P, Ivani G, Visconti C, De Vivo P. How to prolong postoperative analgesia after caudal anaesthesia with ropivacaine in children: S-ketamine versus clonidine. Paediatr Anaesth. 2001; 11(6):679–83.
282. Marhofer P, Krenn CG, Plöchl W, Wallner T, Glaser C, Koinig H, et al. S(+)-ketamine for caudal block in paediatric anaesthesia. Br J Anaesth. 2000;84(3):341–5.

283. Marhofer P, Freitag H, Höchtl A, Greher M, Erlacher W, Semsroth M. S(+)-ketamine for rectal premedication in children. Anesth Analg. 2001;92(1):62–5.
284. Tanaka M, Nishikawa T. Rectal S(+)-ketamine for pediatric premedication. Anesth Analg. 2001;93(5):1363–4.
285. Herd DW, Anderson BJ, Keene NA, Holford NH. Investigating the pharmacodynamics of ketamine in children. Paediatr Anaesth. 2008;18(1):36–42.
286. Weber F, Wulf H, Gruber M, Biallas R. S-ketamine and s-norketamine plasma concentrations after nasal and i.v. administration in anesthetized children. Paediatr Anaesth. 2004;14(12):983–8.
287. Koinig H, Marhofer P, Krenn CG, Klimscha W, Wildling E, Erlacher W, et al. Analgesic effects of caudal and intramuscular S(+)-ketamine in children. Anesthesiology. 2000;93(4):976–80.

Sufentanil

288. http://dailymed.nlm.nih.gov/dailymed/lookup.cfm?setid=53dbe21e-0b97-4271-a7af-2d18986adcd8. Accessed 14 Dec 2013.
289. Guay J, Gaudreault P, Tang A, Goulet B, Varin F. Pharmacokinetics of sufentanil in normal children. Can J Anaesth. 1992;39(1):14–20.
290. Davis PJ, Stiller RL, Cook DR, Brandom BW, Davin-Robinson KA. Pharmacokinetics of sufentanil in adolescent patients with chronic renal failure. Anesth Analg. 1988;67(3):268–71.
291. Greeley WJ, de Bruijn NP, Davis DP. Sufentanil pharmacokinetics in pediatric cardiovascular patients. Anesth Analg. 1987;66(11):1067–72.
292. Davis PJ, Cook DR, Stiller RL, Davin-Robinson KA. Pharmacodynamics and pharmacokinetics of high-dose sufentanil in infants and children undergoing cardiac surgery. Anesth Analg. 1987;66(3):203–8.

Flumazenil

293. http://dailymed.nlm.nih.gov/dailymed/lookup.cfm?setid=442ed32b-b508-40cc-9915-ff05674566da. Accessed 14 Dec 2013.
294. Weinbroum AA, Flaishon R, Sorkine P, Szold O, Rudick V. A risk-benefit assessment of flumazenil in the management of benzodiazepine overdose. Drug Saf. 1997;17(3):181–96.
295. Heard C, Creighton P, Lerman J. Intranasal flumazenil and naloxone to reverse over-sedation in a child undergoing dental restorations. Paediatr Anaesth. 2009;19(8):795–7. Discussion 798–9.
296. McGlone R, Fleet T, Durham S, Hollis S. A comparison of intramuscular ketamine with high dose intramuscular midazolam with and without intranasal flumazenil in children before suturing. Emerg Med J. 2001;18(1):34–8.
297. Haret D. Rectal Flumazenil can save the day. Paediatr Anaesth. 2008;18(4):352.
298. Carbajal R, Simon N, Blanc P, Paupe A, Lenclen R, Oliver-Martin M. Rectal flumazenil to reverse midazolam sedation in children. Anesth Analg. 1996;82(4):895.
299. Lopez-Herce J, Lopez de Sa E, Garcia de Frias E. Reversal of midazolam sedation with rectal flumazenil in children. Crit Care Med. 1994;22(7):1204.
300. Jones RD, Chan K, Roulson CJ, Brown AG, Smith ID, Mya GH. Pharmacokinetics of flumazenil and midazolam. Br J Anaesth. 1993;70(3):286–92.
301. Scheepers LD, Montgomery CJ, Kinahan AM, Dunn GS, Bourne RA, McCormack JP. Plasma concentration of flumazenil following intranasal administration in children. Can J Anaesth. 2000;47(2):120–4.

Naloxone

302. http://dailymed.nlm.nih.gov/dailymed/lookup.cfm?setid=8535cc84-ad4a-4d67-8480-fb5a2e3406f8. Accessed 14 Dec 2013.
303. Moreland TA, Brice JE, Walker CH, Parija AC. Naloxone pharmacokinetics in the newborn. Br J Clin Pharmacol. 1980;9(6):609–12.
304. Stile IL, Fort M, Wurzburger RJ, Rodvold KA, Spector S, Hiatt IM, et al. The pharmacokinetics of naloxone in the premature newborn. Dev Pharmacol Ther. 1987;10(6):454–9.
305. American Academy of Pediatrics Committee on Drugs. Naloxone dosage and route of administration for infants and children: addendum to emergency drug doses for infants and children. Pediatrics. 1990;86(3):484–5.

Lidocaine

306. Catterall WA, Mackie K. Local anesthetics. In: Brunton LL, Lzo JS, Parker KL, editors. Goodman and Gilman's the pharmacological basis of therapeutics. 11th ed. New York: McGraw-Hill; 2006. p. 377–9.
307. Burrows FA, Lerman J, LeDez KM, Strong HA. Pharmacokinetics of lidocaine in children with congenital heart disease. Can J Anaesth. 1991;38(2):196–200.
308. Amitai Y, Zylber-Katz E, Avital A, Zangen D, Noviski N. Serum lidocaine concentrations in children during bronchoscopy with topical anesthesia. Chest. 1990;98(6):1370–3.
309. Leopold A, Wilson S, Weaver JS, Moursi AM. Pharmacokinetics of lidocaine delivered from a transmucosal patch in children. Anesth Prog. 2002;49(3):82–7.
310. Mazoit JX, Dalens BJ. Pharmacokinetics of local anaesthetics in infants and children. Clin Pharmacokinet. 2004;43(1):17–32.
311. Kopecky EA, Jacobson S, Bch MB, Hubley P, Palozzi L, Clarke HM, et al. Safety and pharmacokinetics of EMLA in the treatment of postburn pruritus in pediatric patients: a pilot study. J Burn Care Rehabil. 2001;22(3):235–42.
312. Elad S, Cohen G, Zylber-Katz E, Findler M, Galili D, Garfunkel AA, et al. Systemic absorption of lidocaine after topical application for the treatment of oral mucositis in bone marrow transplantation patients. J Oral Pathol Med. 1999;28(4):170–2.
313. http://dailymed.nlm.nih.gov/dailymed/lookup.cfm?setid=95e8a1e3-04c7-433f-ae8c-afa1c0d61deb. Accessed 14 Dec 2013.
314. Wolfe JW, Butterworth JF. Local anesthetic systemic toxicity: update on mechanisms and treatment. Curr Opin Anaesthesiol. 2011;24(5):561–6.

Ondansetron

315. http://dailymed.nlm.nih.gov/dailymed/archives/fdaDrugInfo.cfm?archiveid=12293. Accessed 14 Dec 2013.
316. Mondick JT, Johnson BM, Haberer LJ, Sale ME, Adamson PC, Coté CJ, et al. Population pharmacokinetics of intravenous ondansetron in oncology and surgical patients aged 1–48 months. Eur J Clin Pharmacol. 2010;66(1):77–86.
317. Spahr-Schopfer IA, Lerman J, Sikich N, Palmer J, Jorch U. Pharmacokinetics of intravenous ondansetron in healthy children undergoing ear, nose, and throat surgery. Clin Pharmacol Ther. 1995;58(3):316–21.
318. de Alwis DP, Aarons L, Palmer JL. Population pharmacokinetics of ondansetron: a covariate analysis. Br J Clin Pharmacol. 1998;46(2):117–25.

Metoclopramide

319. http://dailymed.nlm.nih.gov/dailymed/lookup.cfm?setid=ffa52dfa-8adf-4f70-39a7-461757f226e9. Accessed 14 Dec 2013.
320. Vauzelle-Kervroedan F, Rey E, D'Athis P, Badoual J, Olive G, Pons G. Metoclopramide plasma concentration in neonates. Int J Clin Pharmacol Ther. 1997;35(11):519–21.
321. Bateman DN, Craft AW, Nicholson E, Pearson AD. Dystonic reactions and the pharmacokinetics of metoclopramide in children. Br J Clin Pharmacol. 1983;15(5):557–9.

Scopolamine

322. http://dailymed.nlm.nih.gov/dailymed/lookup.cfm?setid=4d705c57-fa98-46e0-97f3-38e1b0ada76b. Accessed 14 Dec 2013.

Diphenhydramine

323. Simons KJ, Watson WT, Martin TJ, Chen XY, Simons FE. Diphenhydramine: pharmacokinetics and pharmacodynamics in elderly adults, young adults, and children. J Clin Pharmacol. 1990;30(7):665–71.
324. Altman DF. Drugs used in gastrointestinal diseases. In: Katzung BG, editor. Basic and clinical pharmacology. 8th ed. New York: McGraw-Hill; 2001. p. 1064–76.
325. http://dailymed.nlm.nih.gov/dailymed/lookup.cfm?setid=ec691492-a295-4b48-a1a3-5824931efa97. Accessed 14 Dec 2013.

Dexamethasone

326. Naylor MW, Greden JF, Alessi NE. Plasma dexamethasone levels in children given the dexamethasone suppression test. Biol Psychiatry. 1990;27(6):592–600.
327. Young MC, Cook N, Read GF, Hughes IA. The pharmacokinetics of low-dose dexamethasone in congenital adrenal hyperplasia. Eur J Clin Pharmacol. 1989;37(1):75–7.
328. Richter O, Ern B, Reinhardt D, Becker B. Pharmacokinetics of dexamethasone in children. Pediatr Pharmacol (New York). 1983;3(3–4):329–37.
329. http://dailymed.nlm.nih.gov/dailymed/lookup.cfm?setid=537b424a-3e07-4c81-978c-1ad99014032a. Accessed 14 Dec 2013.

Sedatives: Effects on Memory and Amnesia

10

Robert A. Veselis

Abstract

This chapter will focus on the memory effects of diverse sedative agents. To best understand the relationship between memory and sedation, an understanding of the physiology underlying not only sedation, but also sleep and memory is needed. This knowledge will not only ground a discussion of drug mechanisms but also will prepare for future developments providing the ability to put research and marketing initiatives into an appropriate context. One might consider the brain as two interacting sets of systems: A deep-seated, lower-level system containing subcortical/brainstem nuclei working in networks to control sleep and/or sedation interacts with a higher level, cortically based system of networks that mediate memory function and consciousness. To provide a contextual framework for understanding sedation, memory processes, amnesia, and sleep, terminology will be tackled. First will be the attempt to distinguish between sedation and anesthesia, only to become apparent through this chapter that there is actually little distinction between the two. The blurry distinction between sedation and anesthesia underlies the difficulty in producing coherent and consistent guidelines to match providers with sedation services. The key difference between sedation and anesthesia principally reflects the dose of drugs administered, and to a lesser extent the drugs administered.

Keywords

Sedation • Anesthesia • Memory • Sleep • Amnesia • Sleep pathways • Gamma amino butyric acid (GABA) • Locus ceruleus • Ventrolateral preoptic nucleus (VLPO) • Persistent vegetative state (PVS) • Hippocampus • Retrograde amnesia • Unconscious • Propofol • Midazolam • Benzodiazepine • Dexmedetomidine • Ketamine • Etomidate • *N*-Methyl-D-aspartate

Introduction: Sedation, Sleep, Memory, and Amnesia

"I don't want to remember a thing!" is a common admonition of the anxious patient, be they pediatric or adult. To provide such a service the practitioner must be facile with the properties of each sedative agent, including their side effects. These can be used to advantage especially when combined with other agents. This chapter will focus on the memory effects of diverse sedative agents. To best understand the relationship between memory and sedation, some understanding of the physiology underlying not only sedation, but also sleep and memory is needed. This knowledge will not only ground a discussion of drug mechanisms but also prepare for future developments and provide the ability to put research, and marketing initiatives, into an appropriate context. One might consider the brain as two interacting sets of systems. A deep-seated, lower-level system containing subcortical/brainstem nuclei

R.A. Veselis, M.D. (✉)
Department of Anesthesiology/CCM, Memorial Sloan Kettering Cancer Center, 1275 York Avenue, New York, NY 10065-6007, USA
e-mail: veselisr@mskcc.org

K.P. Mason (ed.), *Pediatric Sedation Outside of the Operating Room: A Multispecialty International Collaboration*, DOI 10.1007/978-1-4939-1390-9_10, © Springer Science+Business Media New York 2015

working in networks to control sleep and/or sedation interacts with a higher level, cortically based system of networks that mediate memory function and consciousness [1, 2].

Sedation Versus Anesthesia

In addition to providing a contextual framework for understanding sedation, memory processes, amnesia, and sleep, the not insignificant problem of terminology will be tackled. First will be the distinction between sedation and anesthesia, and it will become apparent through this chapter that there is actually little distinction between these two. Despite the caveat that this publication does not deal with anesthesia, the state of sedation we wish to produce in children is really next door, if not in the yard of anesthesia. The blurry distinction between sedation and anesthesia underlies the difficulty in producing coherent and consistent guidelines for matching providers with services. Is it justifiable for non-anesthetists to administer propofol (this rhetorical question serves to highlight these issues)?

The key difference between sedation and anesthesia principally reflects the dose of drugs administered, and to a certain extent which drugs are used [3, 4]. Anesthesia can be induced using high doses of sedative drugs, the best example being propofol (but also etomidate and ketamine), and sedation can be induced with low doses of prototypical anesthetic drugs, examples being volatile agents used with inhalers, a fashion that has come and gone ever since the first inhalers were used hundreds of years earlier.

To Sleep, Perchance to Sedate

With better understanding of sleep physiology, much focus has been placed on natural sleep pathways mediating the anesthetic (read "sedative") actions of drugs on arousal, defined as those brain processes necessary to stay awake [5–7]. The absence of arousal when it should be present leads to narcolepsy, the pathologic inability to stay awake [8]. Morpheus, the god of dreams, lends his name to one of the first sedative agents, morphine. Anesthesia is not sleep, as one cannot be aroused from this state, but great effort has been expended to develop drugs that can mimic the idyllic state of natural sleep while providing ideal sedative conditions, namely non-movement during invasive procedures without respiratory compromise. The propensity to move during sedation relates to analgesia and sedatives with analgesic properties (e.g., ketamine and nitrous oxide) can be administered in relatively lower doses to provide good procedural conditions. On the other hand, when analgesics with potent respiratory depression (i.e., opioids) are used in conjunction with sedative agents, inevitably some respiratory catastrophes will occur if close attention is not paid to drug synergies and potentiation.

Physiologic mechanisms responsible for sleep are important for both sedation and anesthesia, explaining why sedation is in the front yard of anesthesia. It is helpful to consider sedation as being the opposite of arousal, and the terminology of "arousal pathways" is frequently used to describe how sedation is expressed in the brain. Sedation is closely intertwined with memory, and will be discussed in detail subsequently. The opposite of sedation, namely arousal—or, in other contexts, "attention"—is a powerful mediator of memory performance. A substantial literature examines the effects of attention on memory [9–12]. The bottom line is that if no attention is paid to an outside stimulus, then it is not remembered, at least consciously. If we divert attention from what is happening—a state that may be termed "divided attention"—then memory for what is happening is impaired [10]. We routinely do this in clinical practice, for example, by having an assistant engage the patient in conversation when we are starting IVs. Thus, it should not be forgotten that psychology is an important component of our sedation armamentarium in addition to drugs themselves.

To stay awake, one needs arousal, and this is mediated by the aforementioned deep-seated and brainstem nuclei projecting to each other and other parts of the brain including the cortex (Fig. 10.1) [13]. Their effects on arousal are mediated via certain neurotransmitters, two important ones being norepinephrine (the adjective form being noradrenergic) and histamine. Salient examples of these neurotransmitter systems are the noradrenergic projections from the locus ceruleus in the brainstem and histaminergic projections from the tuberomammillary nucleus in the hypothalamus (just next to the pituitary gland at the base of the brain) [7]. These brain regions mediate certain of the side effects of drugs via actions on their neurotransmitter systems. For example, drugs that inhibit histamine (e.g., diphenhydramine) will cause drowsiness, and it stands to reason that drugs inhibiting output from the locus ceruleus will do the same. In fact, this is how dexmedetomidine mediates sedation [14]. The fact that the locus ceruleus is a critical component of sleep pathways also explains why dexmedetomidine produces a sedative state described as more "sleeplike" and seems different from that produced by other sedatives (e.g., benzodiazepines) that affect other receptor systems [15, 16].

On the opposite side of arousal are sleep-promoting nuclei, the most important example being a nucleus in the hypothalamus called the ventrolateral preoptic nucleus (VLPO), a brain region also referred to as the "preoptic area" to indicate how close it is to the optic nerves. This nucleus is active during sleep, and actually inhibits other arousal nuclei [17]. The neurotransmitter mediating VLPO's effects is gamma amino butyric acid (GABA), which happens to be the target of many sedatives (benzodiazepines, etomidate, propofol).

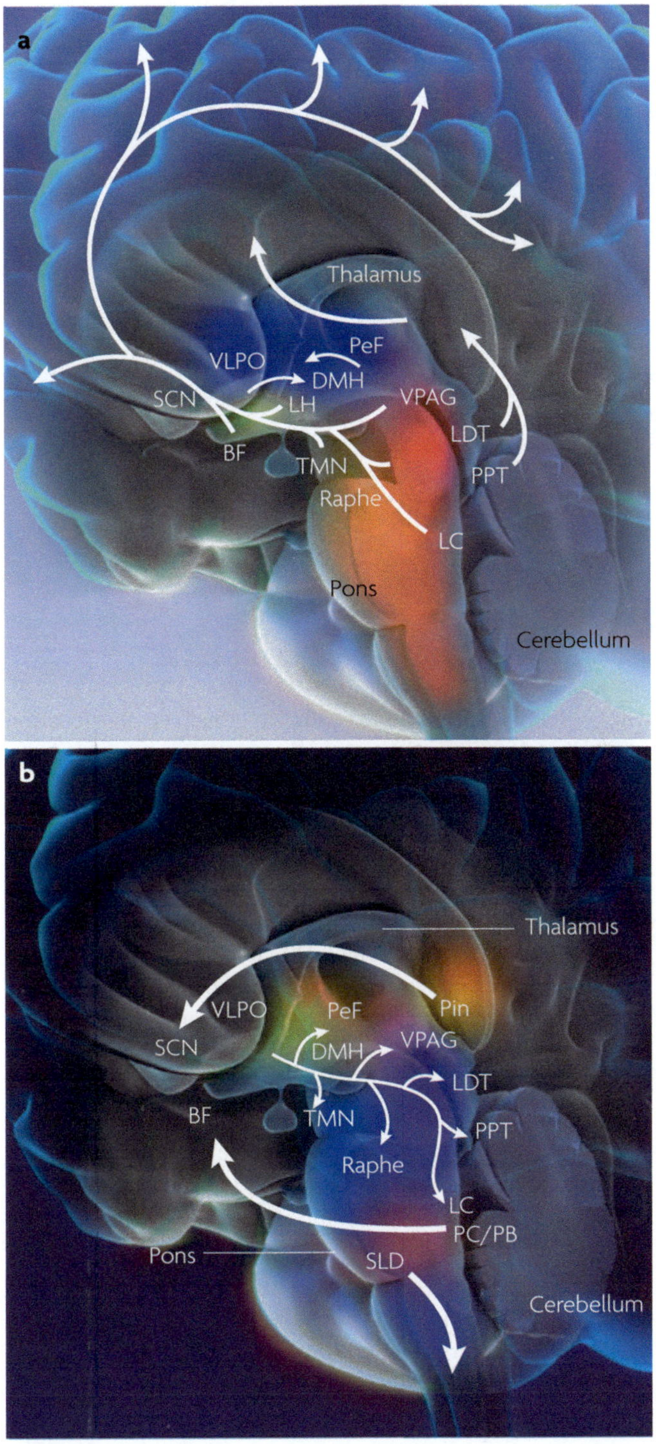

Fig. 10.1 Sleep and arousal centers in the human brain. (**a**) Artistic rendering of the human brain in the awake state illustrating important arousal and sleep centers and pathways of neurotransmission. Cholinergic input (*orange*) from the laterodorsal tegmental (LDT) and pedunculopontine (PPT) nuclei project through the thalamus and facilitate thalamocortical transmission of arousal signals. A second pathway projects through the hypothalamus to cortical centers and facilitates the processing of thalamocortical inputs arising from midbrain centers including the noradrenergic (*blue*) locus ceruleus (LC), the serotonergic (*purple*) dorsal raphe (Raphe), the histaminergic (*pink*) tuberomammillary nucleus (TMN), and the dopaminergic (*yellow*) ventral periaqueductal gray matter (VPAG). This pathway also receives input from the cholinergic (*orange*) basal forebrain (BF) and the peptidergic neurons of the lateral hypothalamus (LH) and perifornical neurons (PeF), which contain orexin or melanin-concentrating hormone (*light green*). The melatonergic (*red*) neural network affects arousal and sleep through the regulation of circadian rhythms. This internal biological clock originates in the suprachiasmatic nucleus (SCN) and projects through the dorsomedial hypothalamus (DMH) sending inhibitory signals to the GABAergic (*gray*) ventrolateral preoptic nucleus of the hypothalamus (VLPO). (**b**) Artistic rendering of the human brain in the sleeping state illustrating important sleep and arousal centers and pathways of neurotransmission. The VLPO of the hypothalamus sends descending GABAergic (*gray*) inhibitory signals to the midbrain arousal centers including the PeF, TMN, VPAG, Raphe, LDT and PPT, and LC. During the early hours of dark periods, the pineal gland (Pin) releases melatonin (*red*), which has inhibitory effects on the SCN and DMH of the melatonergic system. Nuclei that control neural activity during rapid eye movement (REM) sleep have been identified in the pontine midbrain. The pericoeruleus (PC) and parabranchial (PB) nuclei send glutaminergic (*green*) projections through the BF to affect cortical activity during REM sleep, and projections from the sublaterodorsal nucleus (SLD) send glutamatergic signals through the spinal cord to induce atonia that is characteristic of REM sleep (Reprinted with permission from Wafford KA, Ebert B. Emerging anti-insomnia drugs: tackling sleeplessness and the quality of wake time. Nat Rev Drug Discov. 2008 Jun;7(6):530–40)

However, GABA receptors are also widely distributed throughout the brain, being concentrated in certain brain regions such as the medial temporal lobe [18]. Thus GABAergic drugs act at many locations other than VLPO. GABA receptors are not only widely dispersed throughout the brain, but come in some 18 varieties, depending on which and how particular subunits making up the receptor are configured. Thus "GABAergic" drugs differ from each other depending on how they interact with receptor subspecies [19]. This will be further elaborated in the section on etomidate, which targets GABA receptors containing the alpha5 subunit [20]. GABA receptors are notably present in brain regions important in memory processing, namely medial temporal lobe structures comprising the hippocampus and amygdala [21]. These brain regions are located close by the brainstem and hypothalamus, and the collection of these structures may be considered as a functional unit upon which higher cortical centers depend. It is no surprise that one of these systems (e.g., sleep pathways) will influence function of other systems (e.g., memory). Thus, drugs acting at GABA receptors will have effects on memory as well as arousal (sedation).

The known physiology of sleep pathways is ever expanding, and increasingly complex interactions are teased out as new pathways, neurotransmitters, and nuclei are discovered. A recent example is the orexinergic pathway, so named because the transmitter in question is orexin [22]. This neurotransmitter may be familiar as a mediator of eating behaviors, and how this system relates to obesity is an active and exciting area of research [23]. Turning back to sedation and sleep, a lack of orexin leads to narcolepsy [8]. No doubt, in

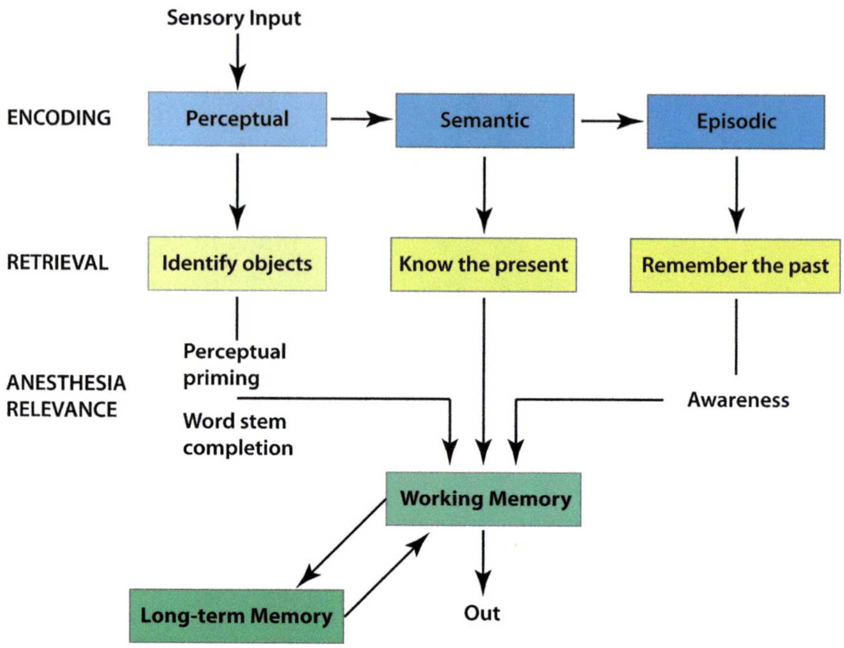

Fig. 10.2 Serial parallel independent memory (Adapted from Schacter DL, Tulving E. Memory systems 1994. Cambridge, Mass., MIT Press, 1994)

the future, sedative drugs targeting the orexinergic pathways will become part of our armamentarium, presumably after pharmacologic congeners have been marketed for treatment of obesity. It is fruitful to conceptualize arousal and sleep nuclei and their neurotransmitters dancing in a carefully choreographed harmony [24]. This careful seesaw balancing act allows transitions between states of sleep and arousal over short periods of time as one set of nuclei come on line and inhibit the others. The behavioral correlate of this activity is the seemingly rapid transitions between "nodding off" and startling back awake. These mechanisms may play a role in the quality of sedation experienced with dexmedetomidine as patients seem to pass through similar rapid transitions. It should be noted, however, that these transitions occur on top of a background of tonic inhibition. One is not fully awake and then suddenly asleep. Thus, nodding off occurs only when a certain level of background sedation (non-arousal) is present, such as occurs with sleep deprivation and the accumulation of melatonin in the brain. This also seems to be a characteristic when dexmedetomidine is given, and further detailed in the section on dexmedetomidine. Sleep (adequate sedation) is not possible until a given "tonic" state of sedation develops as the drug is being infused. Even then, arousal from dexmedetomidine sedation may occur quite easily compared with other sedative agents.

To Sedate, Perchance to Not Remember!

If a patient is sedated to the point that they do not respond to their surroundings, then they will also not remember what is happening in their surroundings. Implementation of "I don't want to remember anything!" relies on this fact, and sedation is usually administered at a dose that produces unresponsiveness. Clinically this is a much easier goal to target than producing "amnesia," where the patient is responsive, but will not subsequently remember (more on this later) [25, 26].

The heuristic of producing unresponsiveness to ablate memory formation naturally leads to the question of what is it to "experience" something? This is not a trivial question, and can certainly enter the realm of philosophy. For purposes of this chapter, conscious experience is defined in terms of brain processes [27]. Experience begins when information from the outside world registers in the brain, the initial portal being the sensory cortices via transmission through the thalamus. The thalamus is a deep-seated set of nuclei that one can consider as analogous to the key Internet hubs through which the world's information flows [28]. But sensory "experience" is by itself not sufficient for "Experience" with a capital E [29]. Information from different parts of the brain must be integrated into what is more formally termed a "percept." Integration occurs not only from sensory cortices, but also from memory areas that represent knowledge of the world, those being semantic memories. The integration of these memories allows the events just experienced to be deciphered as a conscious experience. After this percept forms, it has the chance to be (consciously) remembered [30, 31] (Fig. 10.2). As providers of sedation, we can interfere with any of these stages using our armamentarium of sedative potions. Our influence on these events may seem to be greater than it actually is. In fact, even when fully anesthetized, sensory experience still occurs, but as it happens that sensory input remains pretty much localized to the sensory cortices; how this happens will be explained later in this chapter [32–35]. The murky question is whether the arrival of sensory input during full anesthesia has any influence on anything afterwards—do we form unconscious memories of some sort [36, 37]? As sedation is really anesthesia using lower doses of drugs, this becomes even a more vexing issue assuming a dose–response relationship. To this point there is no literature to guide us. The state of affairs with auditory input during sedation may be analogous to the not-so-distant issue of whether neonates perceived pain, and whether this was important to prevent. When it became evident that neonates did, in fact, perceive pain, it was felt that it would be in the best interest of the patient to prevent this. Narcotics (or other methods of alleviating pain) became a requisite part of the anesthetic management of neonates during surgery. So, the philosophical question is whether children who are sedated, who no doubt receive auditory input that is registered in the sensory cortices of the brain, should also be afforded similar considerations. Fortunately for a significant percentage of pediatric patients, they have foam earplugs inserted for magnetic resonance (MR) scanning. But for others, should we not be aware of the nature of auditory input during sedation? This rhetorical question has no answer to date, but does set the groundwork for interesting research in the future. For example, at clinically relevant doses, pentobarbital is associated with auditory activation, whereas propofol does not seem to be [38].

The ability to influence information processing after sensory perception using sedative agents is much greater, as processes of information integration and subsequent memory formation are much more sensitive to drug action. Consciousness is the binding of information across different brain regions into a thought, if internally generated[1], or a percept generated from external sensory inputs. The percept incorporates sensory parameters (nature of the object/sound being experienced), previous knowledge (semantic memories; e.g., "This object is a red block"), and personal subjective memories of experiences (i.e., episodic memories; e.g., "I played with this block last time") [39]. Another way to think of sedation is that it is administered so as to prevent information integration; i.e., when the child is "asleep," they are not able to integrate information into a percept [2, 33, 40–45]. Sensory input may (and undoubtedly does) arrive in the brain, but it has nowhere to go. Processes connecting part A of the brain with part B are rendered largely nonfunctional by the sedative agent, so there is no chance for memory formation—at least of conscious memory (which is the form of memory we are most concerned with when we "don't remember a thing") [46, 47].

[1]Certain authorities consider dreaming as a form of consciousness as well.

Memory: What Is It, Really?

Memory is not a unitary process, but rather a complex set of interrelated physiologic processes, and as such is continually malleable over time. At its simplest level, there are two distinct forms of memory—conscious and unconscious—and this chapter will focus on the former [48]. Conscious memory requires the formation of a percept, which is the sine qua non of consciousness. In other words, one has to be conscious to form a conscious memory. Thus, when someone is unconscious, for the purposes of this chapter specifically as a result of sedation, conscious memories will not be formed. As an illustrative side point, questions of whether patients in persistent vegetative states (PVSs) are "conscious" revolve around the question of information integration, the ability to form a percept from external or internal experience [49]. As someone in a PVS cannot respond, electrophysiologic evidence of information integration is sought in these patients. Various approaches have been used to identify electrophysiologic signatures of information integration to use as a surrogate of "consciousness." However, even very sophisticated methods suffer from statistical artifacts, and one still cannot be sure whether consciousness is or is not present. On a much larger scale, this also is the case during sedation/anesthesia. To date, there is no reliable EEG-type monitor (or for that matter, any other type of monitor) that can tell us whether a patient is sufficiently sedated, sufficiently anesthetized, or sufficiently amnesic for a particular situation [50–53]. Thus, it is not surprising that even when we think a patient is well sedated, they can be "playing possum" and suddenly wake up; i.e., they have the ability to integrate information despite our best efforts. This fear of sudden arousal leads to even higher dosing of sedative agents, wandering dangerously close or actually into the state of anesthesia (by definition preventing arousal in 50 % of patients when a surgical incision is made). Thus, it would be desirable to utilize sedative agents that not only sedate but can also affect the last stage of memory formation, that of incorporation of the conscious percept into a lasting conscious memory. This last process is the most sensitive to drug effect, occurring at concentrations lower than those producing sedation, as long as the drug has specific amnesic properties [54–56]. These are much fewer in number than those producing sedation, but they are widely used, consisting of the benzodiazepines, propofol, and ketamine. These drugs have the ability to impair formation of long-lasting memories (defined as longer than 30–60 min) for conscious percepts formed during periods of arousal sufficient for information integration, a state often termed "awareness."

To be aware is to experience your surroundings and can be proven by responding appropriately to verbal commands (e.g., "Squeeze my hands twice." Parenthetically it is very difficult to prove or disprove awareness without any behavioral measures, and that is why it is difficult to know if patients in a PVS are conscious) [57, 58]. In fact, a significant proportion of patients who are "fully" anesthetized can be aware, but virtually none of them consciously remember this experience of awareness afterwards [59].

The Last Building Block of a Conscious Memory: Consolidation

This is the key section in which "amnesia" will be defined. To be clear, amnesia in this chapter is being used in the context of administration of sedative drugs [25, 60]. Amnesia generally refers to any pathologic state in which memory is affected (e.g., Alzheimer's dementia, transient ischemic amnesia, traumatic amnesia, etc.). These amnesias can be classified as either anterograde or retrograde, depending on which memories are affected. If the insult affects only memory after the insult, this is termed anterograde amnesia and is the type of amnesia produced by drugs (more on this later). A much more intriguing type of memory loss is retrograde amnesia, subject of many movies. This refers to loss of memories before the insult, usually some type of traumatic event (e.g., head injury, electroconvulsive therapy), where the time frame of loss of memory ranges from minutes (not remembering how the accident occurred, for instance) to months, possibly years. Retrograde memory loss has never been convincingly demonstrated for any drug to date. "Amnesia" as used in this chapter (and generally any investigation of acute drug administration) refers to the drug-induced inability to remember a conscious percept and in many studies is demonstrated by the lack of memory for pictures or words seen or heard while drug was being given [56]. The presence of conscious percepts allows one to be aware, in other words able to integrate information either from external or internal sources. We can only observe external awareness, as illustrated by the question of whether patients in a PVS are internally aware. Awareness is evidenced by appropriate behaviors to the environment (e.g., ability to follow commands in the presence of sedative drugs). Awareness occurs in the "here and now," but to remember being aware at some past point requires further processing of information into a memory. In order for this to occur, the conscious percept has to be consolidated into a lasting memory [55] (Fig. 10.3).

Consolidation is a fundamental area of neuroscience investigation, finding its roots in the works of Donald O. Hebb in the middle of the last century. Hebb was a psychologist keenly interested in the basis of memory and proposed that the brain was plastic; in other words, neurons changed their connections (synapses) with each other based on how they were activated [61]. In essence, a memory resides in the altered synaptic connections in the brain [62]. Thus, consolidation produces a brain different from what it was before and that difference is a memory. These specific changes, referred to as Hebbian learning, are the result of many dozens of physiologic and molecular processes, each having its own particular time frame [63, 64]. The sum total of these processes are termed consolidation and become active once a conscious percept is learned, defined as acquiring information from the outside world. Consolidative processes are present to varying degrees for the life of the memory. A corollary of the fact that consolidative processes are continuously active is that memories are continuously malleable [65–68]. The whole question of the reliability of eyewitness testimony revolves around this physiologic fact. Other times, malleable memories can get out of hand, resulting in "flashbacks" of increasing intensity producing post-traumatic distress syndrome where memories are closely linked to flight or fight fear responses [69–71]. But the most common fate of memories is that they decay over time [72].

Just as the thalamus is a key hub for sensory experience and integration that allows consciousness to exist, a seahorse-shaped structure in the medial temporal lobes (almost adjacent to the thalamus, as it turns out) called the hippocampus is a similarly important mediator of conscious memory [73–75]. The hippocampus connects incoming information with diverse locations in the brain, where previous memories reside, to allow new memories to be created (Fig. 10.4). Without the hippocampus, no conscious memories can be formed, and this was first appreciated in the famous neurologic case involving a patient with the pseudonym HM. HM had bilateral temporal lobectomies for the treatment of intractable epilepsy in 1956 [75]. This operation was a well-accepted form of treatment in the era where the brain was considered to operate under the principle of equivalency. This principle rests on the thought that if one part of the brain was damaged or removed, another part would take over that function, thus minimizing the impact of pathology or surgical intervention. Indeed, it was thought that surgical intervention could remove the diseased focus in the brain, thus ameliorating symptoms of the disease, in particular epilepsy [76]. To a large extent this was true for epileptic foci in many cortical regions. However, epileptic foci commonly reside in the temporal lobes, and it soon became apparent that significant removal of the medial temporal lobes bilaterally (which happened to contain the hippocampi) resulted in severe impairments of conscious memories. This was described most famously by Scolville and Milner [75]. For those interested, a quite accurate depiction of what life would be like without the ability to form conscious memories is made in the film *Memento* [77]. The hippocampus is also important in

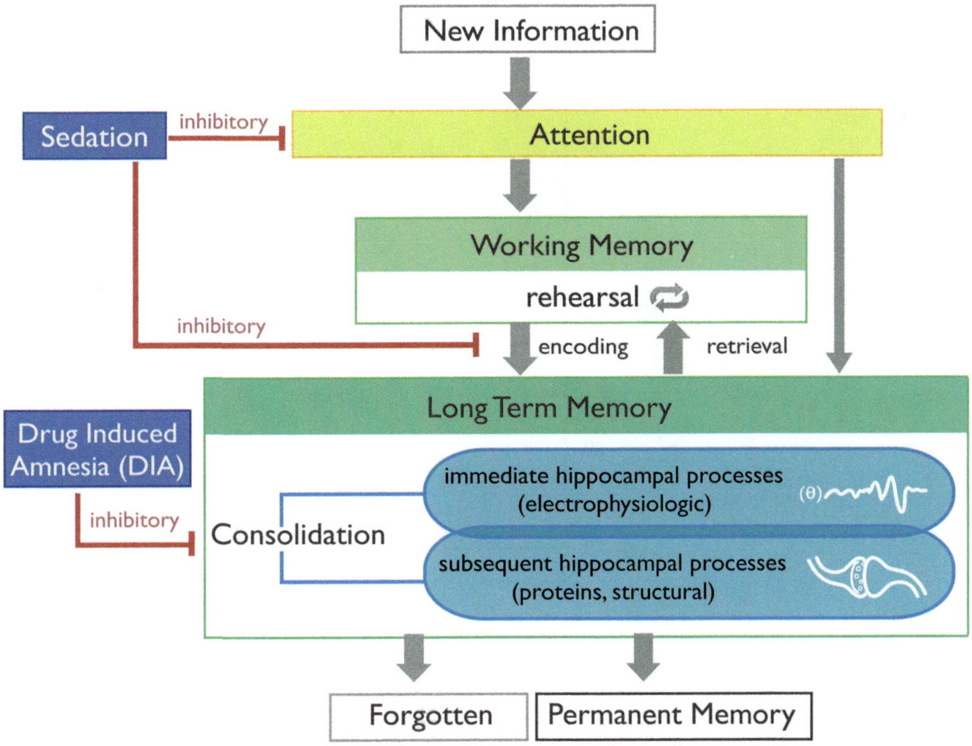

Fig. 10.3 Flow of sensory input comparing amnesia versus memory formation during sedation (Reprinted by permission © Memorial Sloan-Kettering Cancer Center)

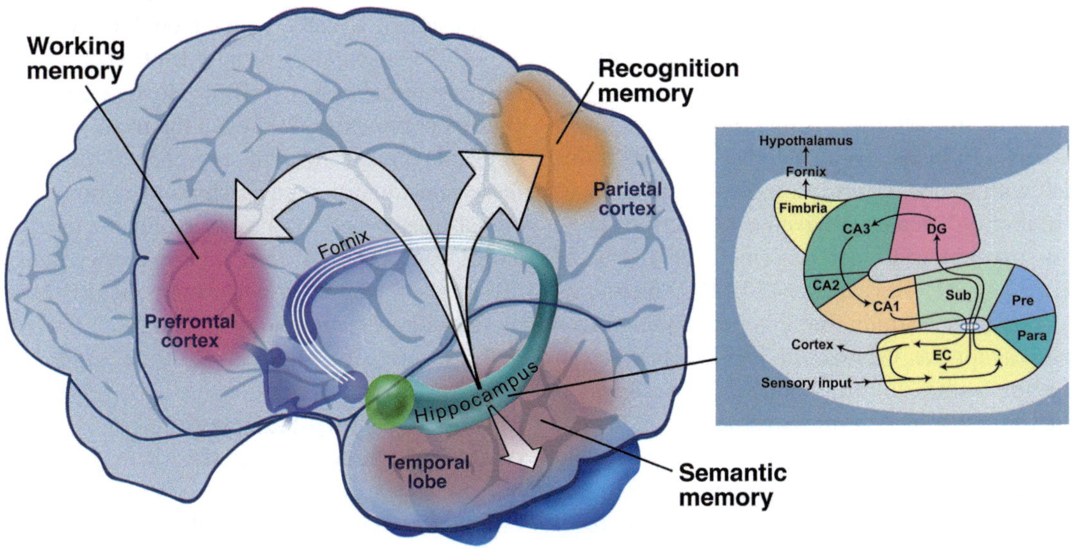

Fig. 10.4 Memory regions of the brain. *Inset* shows sensory pathway (Reprinted by permission © Memorial Sloan-Kettering Cancer Center)

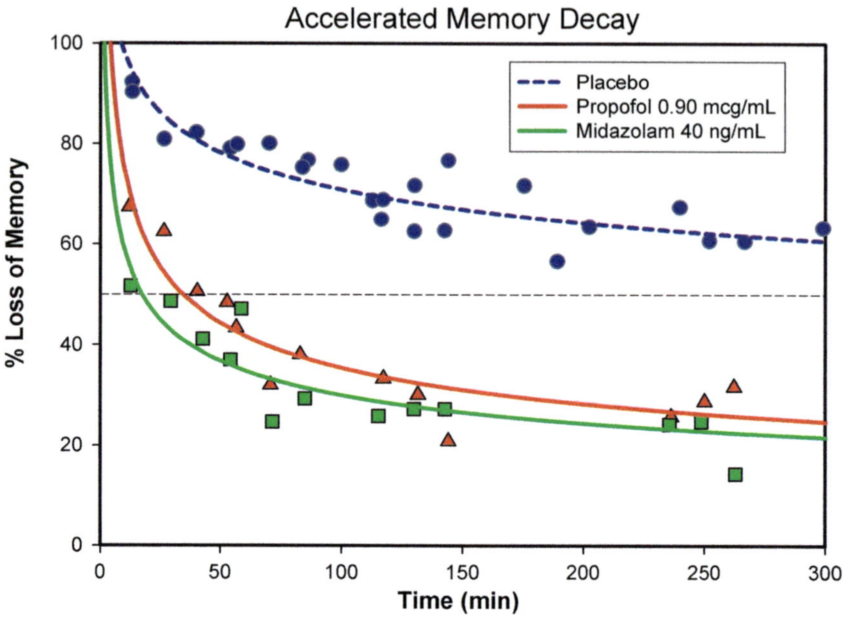

Fig. 10.5 Memory decay following propofol and midazolam compared to placebo (Reprinted by permission © Memorial Sloan-Kettering Cancer Center)

"readout" of newly formed memories, and in a sense this readout is "practiced" during certain stages of sleep [78–81]. Sleep will improve conscious memories, and the adage "get a good night's sleep" is not without merit [82]. Not surprisingly, detailed investigations of how hippocampal mechanisms interact with memory are ongoing topics of research.

The First Building Block of Amnesia: Forgetting

The fate of virtually all memories is that they are forgotten over time. This is a fortunate event, as otherwise our brains would be filled with useless information. Some rare cases of the inability to lose old memories have been described [83]. Ebbinghaus, a psychologist, first described the decay of memories over time over 150 years ago [84]. Most memories are forgotten soon after learning, but this process continues at a slower pace as long as we measure it [72]. They key to understanding the nature of drug-induced amnesia is to understand the forgetting of memories over time. For, in fact, memories can be and are formed in the presence of amnesic drugs [85]. The fact that at low concentrations of, for example, benzodiazepines, virtually all processes required to form a conscious memory are operational—namely, sensory perception, information integration, learning, and initial conscious memory formation—explains why behavior is visibly normal, other than possibly being affected by some sedation (e.g., being "drunk"). If we measure what happens to memories formed in the presence of an amnesic drug over time, we find that they disappear very rapidly [54]. In fact, in the case of midazolam or propofol, no discernible memory is present after 30–60 min (Fig. 10.5). Thus, drug-induced amnesia is typified by the inability of memories to be remembered over time. The mechanism(s) underlying this effect is (are) still unknown, but could be summarized as the inability of consolidation to function normally, so that the memory cannot be retained at its usual strength over time. These qualities set the stage for an event such as date rape, where a small amount of a substance active at GABAergic receptors is secretly administered, usually with alcohol to mask any sedative effect. No suspicion is aroused; observers note no particularly abnormal behavior [86]. However, the victim experiences a complete lack of even the most traumatic memories of events transpiring in the presence of the drug. Fortunately these same qualities are much more commonly used for beneficial uses, where propofol or midazolam (and likely ketamine) can produce amnesia for events transpiring in the presence of drug even when the patient is awake (or using more accurate terminology: aware).

Mechanistic Implications of Drug-Induced Amnesia

Long-term memory is the final stage of processing of information acquired from the outside world, a process termed "learning." Learned information has thus experienced sensory and cognitive manipulations located in diverse regions of the brain. Thus, a sine qua non of memory function is that different parts of the brain must be able to communicate amongst themselves. These processes of communication have become the mechanisms of most interest in terms of understanding anesthetic and sedative drug actions on cognition and consciousness [44–47, 87]. Using quite sophisticated measurement and analytic techniques, connectivity between different brain regions can be quantitated [88]. Measures of the complexity of information (information content) flowing between these regions can be obtained as well [89]. It is no surprise that such complex processes are inhibited at low doses of anesthetic sedatives. Memory impairment from sedation is based on these inhibitory mechanisms [90]. At higher drug doses, key brain regions participating in the maintenance of consciousness, namely, the thalamus, are disconnected from the rest of the brain (or, alternatively, the cortical brain becomes disconnected from itself (clustered) preventing information flow), and the person falls asleep, or more correctly is anesthetized [88, 91, 92].

Similar inhibitory mechanisms of information processing could be at play to produce amnesia when sedation is minimal. As explained previously, amnesia is best characterized as the inability to retain a memory over time, which means that a memory was formed in the first place—in other words, learning has occurred. Learning can only occur if all the processes important in the formation memory function well. Behaviorally, the person experiencing an amnesic concentration of drug will appear to be relatively normal, as most of their brain functions are working well. Specifically, information is transmitted through the thalamus to sensory cortices of the brain, and this information is forwarded to other brain regions for processing. The first way station after sensory perception is working memory, which can be considered a scratchpad containing information from different parts of the brain, which are then collated into a percept [93, 94]. These working memory processes are located in the front part of the brain (prefrontal cortex) and involve communications with the thalamus and hippocampus to process a memory [95]. Working memory processes are transient and are most sensitive to sedation [96, 97]. As sedation increases, these processes become increasingly impaired, and information cannot be then further processed and thus cannot be learned as a memory. We all experience this when we are too sleepy to remember some bit of information given to us (prototypically a telephone number, thus the popularity of napkins as external scratchpads in bars). Ergo, for the amnesic effect of a drug to be expressed, working memory must be intact. Newly acquired information must be transferred from working memory into long-term memory stores located in diffuse regions of the brain, with the hippocampus anchoring learning and retrieval of these memories [55]. The long-term memory that was just learned in the presence of amnesic drugs is then quickly forgotten. Both long-term and working memory processes can be indexed by electrophysiologic measurements. Indeed, amnesic drugs affect electrophysiologic measures of long term, but not working memory processes [85].

Memories We Don't Know We Have: The Unconscious Mind

This chapter will focus on conscious memory processes, as described so far. This is primarily related to the fact that it is much easier to study the effects of drugs on conscious memory, as behavioral changes (i.e., recognition of previously experienced stimuli, "Did you see this picture before?") are robustly measureable. Unconscious memories are hard to detect, as changes in behavior based on these memories can be quite subtle. It is especially difficult to determine if a change in a memory-related behavior is as a result of effects on conscious or unconscious processes. Thus, controversy usually surrounds the interpretation of these studies in terms of drug effects on unconscious versus conscious memories [37].

Clinical Practice

In clinical practice, it is unusual, particularly in pediatric patients, to produce a state where some quantity of drug is given, but at a dose where little sedation is apparent. Such a situation would amplify the differences between amnesic (e.g., propofol, midazolam, ketamine) and non-amnesic (pentobarbital, probably dexmedetomidine) drugs. Typically, in practice a deep state of sedation is produced, where little responsiveness is present. As detailed previously, if stimuli are not perceived, then they will not be remembered (at least as conscious memories). When propofol is administered in a similar fashion to dexmedetomidine, namely, giving a loading dose over a 10-min period, the effects on memory between these drugs are virtually indistinguishable, despite the fact that propofol has stronger and more specific amnesic properties. However, what is clinically relevant is if drug concentrations become low enough that patients wake up and become responsive while they still have some drug in their system. At these low concentrations, amnesic drugs such as propofol will prevent retention of any memories learned in this state, whereas dexmedetomidine will probably not.

Sedative Agents: Brief Considerations

The adjective "brief" is used to represent the fact that very few studies have been conducted to examine the interaction of drugs with sedation versus their amnesic effects. As discussed so far, both effects are closely related and are difficult to dissect out. The vast majority of studies examining the interaction of sedative drugs with memory have been conducted in healthy adult volunteers, in order to control the many factors that can affect memory other than the presence of drug. Remarkably fewer studies have been conducted in children, and to a large extent, as far as memory effects of drugs are concerned, children are considered as "small adults," which undoubtedly is not true. However, at this time, this is all we have to guide us.

Propofol

The story of how propofol's effects on memory were discovered mirrors the increased knowledge of potential mechanisms by which many anesthetics affect conscious memory processes. To a certain extent, this knowledge reflects the realization that anesthesia is not a unitary event affecting one neurobiologic target, but rather a blend of many effects [4]. Even for a given effect (e.g., memory impairment) probably, there are diverse targets of different anesthetics, but these likely lead to a final common pathway that is the critical effect causing amnesia. As conscious memory is dependent not only on certain neuroanatomical substrates but also distributed processes involved with information flow and communication, multiple potential targets are candidates for a critical common pathway designation. One example is the theta oscillations of brain activity associated with memory processes [98].

It is only recently that specific actions of anesthetics on memory have been generally appreciated. For many years, it was accepted that all sedative drugs were just that and any effect on memory was a "side effect" of sedation, such as one sees from alcohol and other commonly used sedative medications. As detailed above, sedation impairs memory when it is of a sufficient magnitude. A not-so-fortuitous conjunction of events initially branded propofol as a non-amnesic drug. The great advantage of propofol lies in its pharmacokinetics, such that the drug virtually disappears from the blood stream before one's eyes [99]. Propofol rapidly migrates from the blood (and thus the brain) into the vast pharmacologic reservoirs of the body, and so its effect is very transient after a single or even multiple boluses. Because of these properties, propofol could be used to induce deep sedation, with little or no accumulation of drug. Thus a rapid wake-up resulted even after substantial doses of drug were given with little, if any, hangover effect. Propofol quickly became the drug of choice in many situations, not only for sedation but anesthesia as well. But the very same pharmacokinetics could work against the provider. When propofol was administered by intermittent bolusing rather than continuous administration, a great likelihood existed of subtherapeutic drug concentrations being present between boluses because the drug disappeared so quickly from the blood. Subtherapeutic concentrations meant that there was very little chance of amnesia being present, as amnesia occurs only over a very small dose window. Inevitably, case reports describing this exact situation were published and supported the notion that propofol could not be used to reliably prevent memory formation [100–103]. However, it was not the drug that was the issue, but the way it was administered. When propofol is administered by continuous infusion and constant blood levels are maintained, propofol is as good as an amnesic drug as any other, most notably the benzodiazepines—the yardstick of amnesic agents [26, 55, 56, 85, 104]. Fortunately, drug infusion pumps are now much more commonly available and are routinely used to administer intravenous medications, which continue to evolve to be ever more short acting.

Propofol was an ideal agent to use in volunteer studies to dissect out how anesthetics might impact conscious memory because of the rapid onset and offset pharmacokinetics and, not insignificantly, its anti-nausea properties [105]. Initial studies focused on carefully measuring sedation, and when these were equated amongst different drugs, memory impairment for events occurring in the presence of drug differed substantially between amnesic and sedative drugs, namely, propofol and midazolam versus thiopental or fentanyl [56]. These observations indicated that two separable drug effects on memory were present and laid the groundwork to further delineate properties of drug-induced amnesia using propofol as a prototypical amnesic agent.

The next key observation was that propofol (and midazolam) did not prevent formation of memories, other than some mild impairment from associated sedation [54, 85, 106]. A most useful conceptualization of memory processing was that of memory being the end result of the flow of information from the outside world, through transient working memory processes into a final conscious memory (Fig. 10.3). Sedation affected initial working memory processes (just as divided attention does by diverting resources away from working memory) and indeed would prevent memory formation. However, the amnesic effect of propofol (and midazolam) occurred after the memory was formed, in other words during the consolidation process.

Further studies refined the nature of this amnesic effect. The loss of information over time could be modeled using a power decay curve, and the rapid loss of memories formed in the presence of amnesic drugs was reflected in the rapid decay constant of this curve. Initial strength of the memory was separable in another parameter and reflected the sedative effects of the drug in question (Fig. 10.6). These measures parameterized previous observations, namely, that sedation prevented memory formation (decreasing initial strength of the memory), whereas amnesic actions prevented the consolidation of any memories that were formed or, in other words, increased the rate of forgetting. In the case of propofol and midazolam, memory was lost within 30–60 min after being formed. A key question is: When exactly in the consolidation time frame do these drugs produce amnesia? In a sense the answer can be "back engineered" based on the following thought experiment.

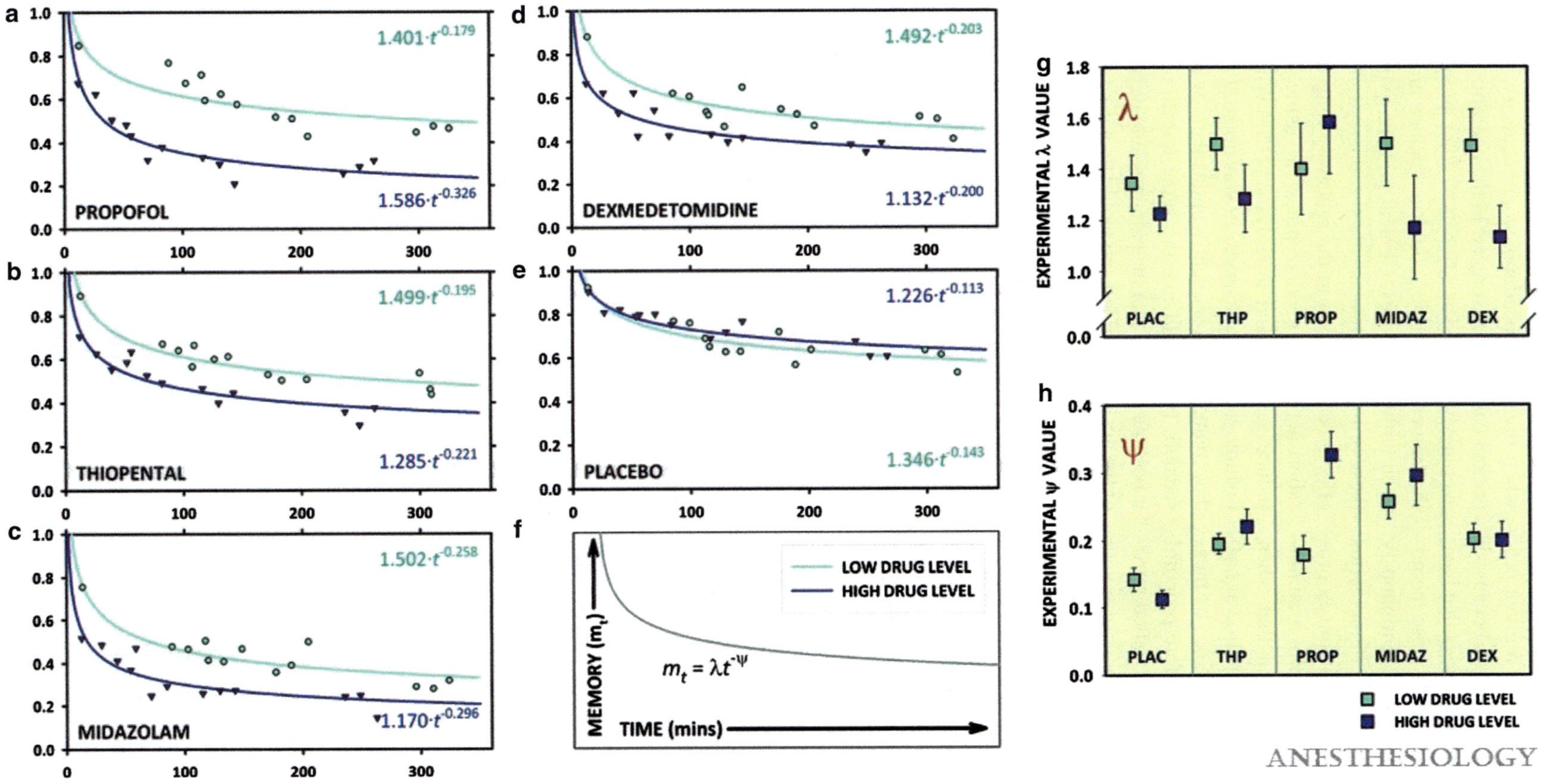

Fig. 10.6 Memory decay curves and estimates for λ (lambda) and ψ (psi) by drug and dose condition. (**a–f**) The power decay curves for each of the drug–dose combinations. The abscissa represents the duration from the final encoding exposure to the subsequent recognition exposure (the recognition interval). For each curve, recognition data were corrected for false positives, clustered into 13 time points, and then fit to the equation $mt=\lambda$ (lambda) $t-\psi$ (psi) using Marquardt–Levenberg nonlinear regression. The specific equations describing each curve are shown in the upper and lower *right* corners of panels **a–f**. (**g**, **h**) The values for λ (lambda) and ψ (psi) are shown, with *error bars* representing the SEM for the estimate derived from the nonlinear regression. However, statistical comparison of the decay functions was performed using a more robust nonlinear mixed effects model. For λ (lambda), independent effects were established for drug ($P<0.0001$) and level ($P<0.0001$) and significant fixed effects seen for the midazolam to level interaction ($P=0.014$), the dexmedetomidine to level interaction ($P=0.008$), and the propofol to level interaction ($P=0.008$). For ψ (psi), independent effects were established for drug ($P=0.027$) and drug–level interaction ($P<0.0001$), whereas fixed effects were established for midazolam ($P=0.008$) and propofol to level interaction ($P<0.0001$). *DEX* dexmedetomidine, *MIDAZ* midazolam, *PLAC* placebo, *PROP* propofol, *THP* thiopental (Reprinted with permission from Pryor KO, Reinsel RA, Mehta M, Li Y, Wixted JT, Veselis RA. Visual p2–n2 complex and arousal at the time of encoding predict the time domain characteristics of amnesia for multiple intravenous anesthetic drugs in humans. Anesthesiology. 2010 Aug;113(2):313-26)

As mentioned, consolidation represents dozens of physiologic processes, each coming online at a given time after learning. Let us say that this time is $T_{critical}$ for a given process, $P_{critical}$. If propofol exerts its amnesic effects because it impairs $P_{critical}$, then it will also block any memories that have not yet reached the $P_{critical}$ stage, in other words those memories "in the pipeline." Memories are being continuously formed, and at any given time, a certain number of memories are in the pipeline before $P_{critical}$. $P_{critical}$ is continuously processing memories, including the moment propofol is administered at time zero, $t=0$. It stands to reason that when propofol is given, then any memories in the pipeline at $t=0$ will be lost. In other words, we can determine $T_{critical}$ by measuring the time at which memories are lost before propofol was administered. This type of memory loss is called retrograde amnesia and is commonly observed in cases of severe head trauma (which might be considered in a sense as a "computer crash"). It is also observed in medically induced therapy that "reboots the computer," namely, electroconvulsive therapy [107, 108]. These major insults to memory processing can be thought of as stopping all consolidation processes at once, and the length of retrograde amnesia gives some indication of how long it takes for a new memory to become an old memory, resistant to various insults[2]. The key observation of drug-induced amnesia is that despite very careful observations, no significant retrograde amnesia has ever been measured [109]. Thus, the $P_{critical}$ affected by amnesic drugs must be a consolidation process that occurs within minutes after learning a new memory. A likely candidate process is one that is based on electrophysiologic processing of incoming information [98, 110, 111].

As discussed previously in the section "Clinical Practice", in reality propofol is rarely administered to produce amnesia; rather it is given at higher doses to produce sedation. Even then, no evidence of retrograde amnesia is present.

Benzodiazepines

The classic amnesic drug is the benzodiazepine originally marketed to manage anxiety, namely, diazepam. For many years, benzodiazepines were known to have side effects that included memory impairment. As these drugs were originally used to manage anxiety, this side effect was considered annoying, and great efforts were expended to eliminate this quality, which continue to this day [112, 113]. Initially, memory impairment was considered to be primarily related to the sedative effects of these drugs, and nonsedating benzodiazepines were sought [114]. Eventually these drugs were introduced into situations of extreme anxiety, such as when invasive procedures were necessary, treatment in the critical care unit, or surgery. In the operating room, benzodiazepines were used as adjuncts to other anesthetics as benzodiazepines themselves could not induce an anesthetic state even with large doses. Clinical practice evolved from using these drugs to induce anesthesia, where significant hangover effects occurred due to the relatively long half-life of even "short-acting" benzodiazepines, to using lower doses to induce sedation and anxiolysis [115]. When used in this fashion, a curious observation was noted. Patients receiving diazepam, and subsequently midazolam, would be calm and sedated, but would ask the same question over and over. It became evident that the patient would have no recollection of the answer provided and would then ask the same question repeatedly. This anecdotal observation started further detailed inquiry into the exact nature of the memory effects of sedative drugs used in the hospital setting. As has happened with so many drugs, an annoying side effect became the main therapeutic indication for that drug. These were ideal agents, more so in adults than pediatric patients, as when these drugs were given almost no recollection of events during sedation occurred. The distinction between sedation and actual amnesia was born rather dramatically. For example, after a few milligrams of midazolam, the patient could undergo a "rough" bronchoscopy with coughing, yet when they came back for their next procedure, they would comment how lovely their previous experience had been. Careful comparison of midazolam with propofol revealed essentially identical actions on memory processes [54, 56].

Midazolam is frequently used in clinical practice, and a key question is what to expect in terms of amnesia. How much drug to give and how "dense" will the amnesia be? Though the answer is deterministic, in practice response is much more variable. The degree of amnesia is related to the brain concentration of drug, and this can be determined fairly precisely using pharmacokinetic and pharmacodynamic relationships (as done in our volunteer studies). However, all these measures are after the fact. As noted elsewhere, the determination of amnesia is a retrospective measure. We do not know how much memory loss there was until after the fact when we have tested for recognition of events during drug effect. Thus, it is very difficult to determine before a drug is given exactly how much is needed to produce a satisfactory amnesic effect for a given stimulus/procedure in a particular patient. The best that can be done is to rely on previous experience, both personal and published literature. The most reliable effects will be obtained when a predictable blood concentration can be obtained. This is most likely when midazolam is administered intravenously or, a close second, intranasally. Oral administration is less reliable, and if dense amnesia is desired, then likely a relative overdose

[2]Memories of a certain age, autobiographical memories, are very resistant to any intervention (though they are malleable "sepia memories"). Thus HM who could form no new memories still had vivid recollections of memories of childhood.

will be needed that may produce substantial sedation and hangover effects. A few studies have been done in children where memory has been closely assessed in relation to dosing [116–119]. The dose of midazolam used in three of these studies was 0.2 mg/kg intranasally (buccally), and in the study by Kain et al., more than twice the dose, 0.5 mg/kg, was given orally. This study also assessed memory at multiple time points (5, 10, and 20 min). Memory impairment was quantitated as a percent of items recalled spontaneously or recognized (which is always more than recalled) versus a control (placebo or baseline) condition. With intranasal/buccal administration, approximately 25–30 % of items were recalled (recognition of about twice the number of stimuli occurred when tested), whereas 0 % were recalled (40 % recognized) for oral administration in the Kain et al. study. The peak effect for amnesia with oral administration was at 20 min (but further time points were not tested). Importantly, it should also be noted that items used in all these studies were non-salient (e.g., pictures). Thus, in summary, the published literature showed that with these doses and routes of administration for midazolam, amnesia was significant, but not necessarily "dense." It is likely that recall for emotive or painful stimuli would be greater. If dense amnesia is required with rapid recovery, propofol is a much easier drug to titrate, as the sedative effect can be used as a proxy for a likely amnesic effect in real time.

Dexmedetomidine

As described in the introduction, the ideal sedative agent would produce a state similar to natural sleep without any drug "hangover," be easily titratable, and be safe enough (i.e., minimal respiratory compromise), so that non-anesthesia personnel could administer it. Dexmedetomidine comes close to fulfilling these highly desirable goals [120] (however, see the study by Oto et al. [121] that demonstrated abnormal sleep patterns with dexmedetomidine sedation—but this was a study in ICU patients and may not be relevant to other patient populations). Of all the sedative agents available, dexmedetomidine comes closest to targeting natural sleep pathways, with primary actions upstream from modulation of GABAergic receptors in the sleep pathways [14]. However, as opposed to the GABAergic agents propofol and the benzodiazepines, there seems to be little effect on memory per se, other than that produced by sedation [54, 85, 122]. This is likely due to the fact that dexmedetomidine does not affect GABA receptors directly, thus having little effect on these receptors in the medial temporal lobe. The phrase "there seems" is used as very little investigation has been undertaken to determine if dexmedetomidine is an amnesic agent, as defined previously in this chapter. What little evidence there is supports dexmedetomidine as a sedative agent with little amnesic effect. If the "forgetting" characteristics of dexmedetomidine are compared side by side with midazolam, propofol, and thiopental (a short-acting barbiturate that has sedative actions on memory, no longer available for clinical use), it is found that these resemble thiopental more than the amnesic "forgetting" profile of midazolam or propofol [54]. Similarly, the electrophysiologic signature of the effect of dexmedetomidine on memory processes is again different than the amnesic drugs midazolam and propofol [85]. Thus, mechanistically, actions of dexmedetomidine on memory processes are different than typical amnesic drugs. Whether this translates into clinically appreciable differences is still an open question, but retrospective analysis of a large post-op Quality Assurance database revealed cases of recall of intraoperative events associated with dexmedetomidine, but not propofol (in this case, during cardiac surgery), providing indirect evidence of the lack of amnesic actions of dexmedetomidine [122].

Due to its upstream action at the locus ceruleus, in turn modulating GABA receptors in the VLPO, the quality of sedation is different than other GABAergic agents, notably midazolam and pentobarbital, which directly target GABA receptors [14, 17]. Similar to sleep, there can be rapid transitions from deep sedation to wakefulness, but these may not be entirely predictable. Also, during induction of sedation, which requires administration of a bolus of drug over about a 10-min period, the absence of stimulation is important in ensuring a smooth induction of sedation. As with its parent compound clonidine, which significantly potentiates but cannot act alone as an anesthetic drug, dexmedetomidine may find its most useful niche as a major component of a multidrug regimen. For example, the analgesic effect of ketamine may help prevent movement during procedures, and the side effect of tachycardia with ketamine may counteract the propensity for bradycardia from dexmedetomidine [123].

Ketamine

As with all drugs discussed in this chapter, what we know about ketamine's effects on cognition is derived from adults. Ketamine has a long history of use in pediatrics, with its use falling dramatically with the arrival of newer agents. The pendulum is swinging back with ketamine being used as an adjunct to other sedatives. Ketamine's side effects are often complementary with the side effects of other drugs. For instance, the amnesic properties of ketamine may be beneficial when used with dexmedetomidine, which seems to have poor amnesic effects beyond its sedative properties. Additionally, ketamine has potentially beneficial analgesic and antiinflammatory properties when given in low doses [124–126].

Ketamine has substantial effects on cognition, and these have been examined from the perspective of psychiatry and drug addiction fields. As a consequence, the cognitive effects of ketamine are much better understood than, for instance, dexmedetomidine or etomidate. Ketamine has been used to model the cognitive changes occurring in schizophrenia, such as hallucinations, delusions, idiosyncratic and illogical thinking, poverty of speech and thought, agitation, disturbances of emotion and affect, withdrawal, decreased motivation, and dissociation [127, 128]. It should be noted that many of these "disturbing" symptoms are uncommon in the clinical setting. These disturbing psychologic side effects are more likely to be seen when ketamine, which is one of the big three "club" drugs, is used in unmonitored settings (the "K-hole") [129–131].

There is good evidence that ketamine is a true amnesic drug as opposed to simply being a sedative agent. It produces substantial memory impairment, at doses 0.4–0.8 mg/kg that produce little sedation [132]. Some studies have administered ketamine as a continuous infusion that maintained fairly constant serum concentrations over the time period of memory encoding, similar to our studies measuring the memory effects of propofol [133, 134]. Results from these studies can be interpreted using the same schema for memory as used with propofol, as presented earlier. Doses of ketamine that produced serum concentrations of 129 ng/mL produced similar degrees of sedation as did propofol in our studies, as measured by increases in reaction times. In other words, these doses of ketamine were equi-sedative to the amnesic doses of propofol we have studied. In these studies, ketamine produced a similar characteristic of forgetting of memories encoded in the presence of drug over time as previously demonstrated for propofol.

Emphasis is made again that memory formation is the end result of information flow from the outside world, through sensory cortices, through working memory where information is collated with previous knowledge, to a final memory in long-term memory stores. The key characteristic of an amnesic drug appears to be that the amnesic effects occur after learning of long-term memory. A consequence of this schema of drug action is that the low drug concentrations that produce amnesia will not affect cognitive processes necessary to encode information into long-term memory. Measures of working memory should be relatively unaffected, and this is indeed the case for propofol (administered at approximately 5 mg/kg/h) and lower doses (0.4 mg/kg) of ketamine. Additional support is obtained from ketamine's effects on the electrophysiologic response of the brain to incoming information [111, 135]. These effects are similar to what we have measured for propofol and midazolam, namely, inhibition of signals related to long-term memory, but not working memory function [85]. Thus, the amnesic properties of ketamine are remarkably similar to actions of propofol and midazolam on memory, and it is likely that the mechanism of amnesic effect is also similar. All these drugs appear to affect some consolidation process necessary for the maintenance of a memory over time.

Etomidate

Etomidate is rarely used, but apparently has desirable properties when used at sedative doses in mice. This allows it to be an exemplar agent to investigate the molecular biology of sedation versus amnesia. Virtually no studies have been conducted on the memory effects of etomidate in humans. No doubt, part of the reason is the high incidence of myoclonus and the very unusual side effect of adrenal suppression even after one dose of drug [136]. Both of these qualities make it a difficult drug to use in human volunteer studies. At best, indirect evidence indicates a "favorable" memory profile in clinical practice [137, 138]. Thus, it is impossible to state whether etomidate is an amnesic or only a sedative drug in humans. However, animal data support the amnesic effects of etomidate, and how it has been used to dissect out a potential role of GABA receptors in producing amnesic versus sedative effects of a drug will now be outlined [20].

As mentioned before, GABA receptors come in many varieties, as the receptor is made of five subunits, each of which can be a different configuration, labeled alpha, beta, gamma, etc. [139, 140]. Thus GABA receptors are often referred to according to their subunit composition, for example, the most common GABA-A receptor can be referred to as alpha-1beta-2gamma-2. More commonly the receptor flavor is indicated by the subunit that is of particular interest, e.g., alpha5GABA-A, as the alpha subunit modulates memory function (alpha5GABA-A receptors are uncommon, 4 % in the brain, but are 25 % of the receptors in the hippocampus). GABA-A receptor subtypes are distributed differentially across the brain, as well as over individual neurons [18, 141]. Thus drugs that target certain receptor types would logically affect certain brain structures/functions simply based on the specific receptors interacting with the drug. Thus "GABAergic" agents could have very different effects on the basis of which particular GABA receptors they affect [3]. Thus, dissociable actions of a given drug on cognition can be mediated by differential effects of GABA receptor subpopulations. In particular, we are interested in explaining the dissociation of sedation from amnesia for amnesic drugs, and this has been convincingly demonstrated for etomidate in an animal model [20].

Before delving into the details, one more consideration is important. There are two modes of receptor activation by GABA. The "traditional" receptor interaction occurs at dendritic synapses, where receptors on axons are directly across from synaptic boutons releasing GABA from vesicles. This interaction is termed "phasic" as there is quick onset of

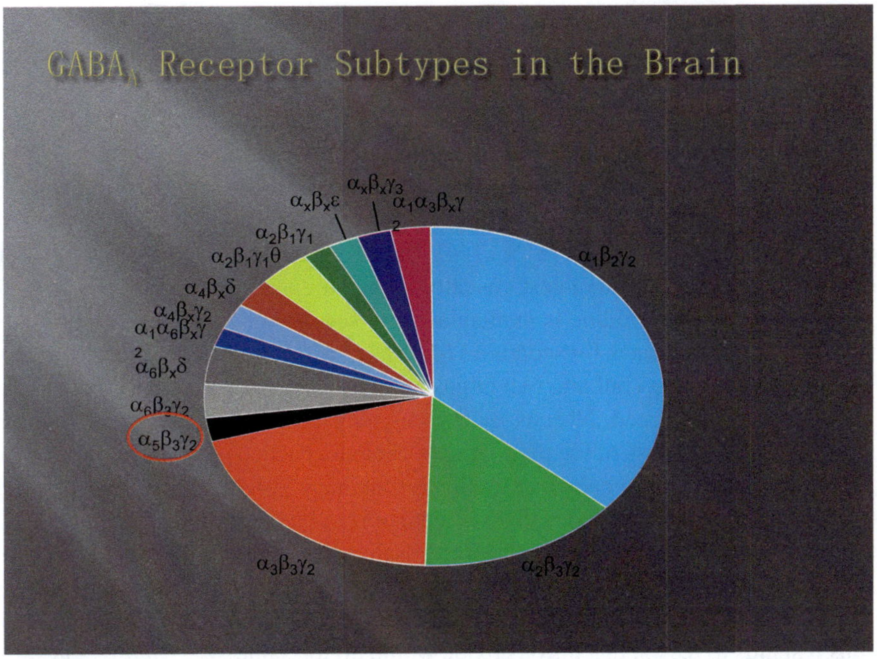

Fig. 10.7 The distribution is unequal with $\alpha\beta\gamma$ (alpha, beta, gamma) being the most ubiquitous. We are interested in the a5 receptors, which make up less than 5 % of the total population, but they are heavily expressed in the hippocampus. These are thus a plausible target if you wish to modify memory (Reprinted with permission from Whiting PJ. GABA-A receptor subtypes in the brain: a paradigm for CNS drug discovery? Drug Discovery Today. 2003;8(10):445-450)

action, and then the receptors quickly turn back on[3] after binding with GABA. This is the main inhibitory mechanism in the brain, and one can think of activation of phasic receptors as the graphite rods in a nuclear reactor, tamping down excitation produced by stimulating neurotransmitters, the most common one in the brain being glutamate. Overexcitation is manifested by, for example, seizures or, more commonly, ischemic injury of neurons. The latter can be thought of as burnout of neurons from overstimulation from masses of excitatory neurotransmitters released during ischemia, when cellular integrity breaks down.

More sophisticated cellular experiments revealed another type of receptor interaction. This mode of receptor activation is in the background and was more difficult to detect, as it involves sparse GABA receptors located away from synapses [141, 142]. Appropriately enough, this mode of activation is termed "tonic." It regulates the baseline resting state of the cell, upon which phasic actions occur. The key property of tonic receptors is that they need only small quantities of GABA to be affected [143]. In other words, low concentrations of drug that would have little if any effect on "classic" phasic GABA receptors would affect tonic receptors. And this is what seems to underlie the amnesic/sedation dissociation of etomidate. At low concentrations, tonic GABA receptors are affected, resetting cellular electrophysiology that ultimately results in some problem with consolidation of memories, quite possibly by affecting theta rhythms in the hippocampus (where these receptors are concentrated). The behavioral effect of these receptor interactions is expressed as "amnesia." At higher concentrations, traditional phasic inhibitory receptors are potentiated by etomidate, and likely other GABAergic drugs, and the end result is sedation (enhanced inhibition of the brain by potentiating the effect of the GABA "graphite rods"). Further proof of this very appealing hypothesis is the fact that tonic GABA receptors contain an alpha5 subunit, distinctive to this class of receptors (Fig. 10.7). Mice who lack this subunit do not experience the memory effects of etomidate, but will still experience sedation. Unfortunately, we do not know if a similar situation exists with propofol. These animal studies are complex, and repeating them with propofol would be a difficult undertaking. However, the behavioral evidence from humans would be entirely consistent with the same dichotomy of action of propofol on phasic and tonic GABA receptors.

Thus, etomidate provides a link from drug–receptor interactions to electrophysiology in the hippocampus, with other studies pointing to electrophysiologic impairments being important in the inability of long-term memories to be consolidated, thus leading to the state termed "amnesia." This attractive hypothesis needs much more study to determine if indeed such mechanisms underlie the amnesic effects of anesthetics.

Inhalational and Miscellaneous Agents

Barbiturates, popularized in film noir and spy movies as "truth serum" or "Mickey Finns," have been widely used in the years following the Second World War. Over time,

[3]GABA is an inhibitory neurotransmitter, so it turns the receptor "off."

chemical modifications to their structure have been made to make these drugs "short acting" by increasing the rate of their metabolism. Thus, we have a spectrum of drugs from barbital, originally synthesized in 1903 at Bayer, to phenobarbital, to thiopental, to methohexital. If results of studies using thiopental can be extrapolated to the other barbiturates, these drugs, which are active at GABA receptors, produce sedation but little amnesia [56, 144]. Increasingly these drugs are unavailable, the latest casualty being thiopental. Now that dexmedetomidine is available, there seems to be little use for barbiturates for sedation [145].

Inhalational agents fall into two large categories, as far as receptors are concerned. Nitrous oxide (laughing gas) and xenon act as a subclass of the predominant excitatory receptors in the brain, whose neurotransmitter is glutamate [146–148]. The subclass of receptors that are antagonized by these agents, *N*-methyl-D-aspartate (NMDA), are the same receptors antagonized by ketamine [149–151].[4] Ketamine has definite amnesic properties, as described previously, and thus it stands to reason that nitrous oxide would do the same. Nitrous oxide in low doses (10–30 %) does indeed impair memory [152, 153]. Whether the characteristics of the memory impairment produced by nitrous oxide are as those described previously for propofol and the benzodiazepines, producing rapid loss of newly formed memories, has not been thoroughly investigated.

All the other inhalational agents (e.g., isoflurane, sevoflurane) act predominantly at GABA receptors, though their actions have been described as "promiscuous," as these agents seem to affect many receptors [4, 154, 155]. When the memory effects of nitrous oxide are compared directly with these agents, all seem to produce similar forms of memory impairment, which occurs at about ¼ to ½ the dose required to produce unresponsiveness (to surgical incision in 50 % of patients) [152, 153, 156]. Whether memory impairment is the characteristic of amnesia or is a result purely from sedation is unknown at this time.

Self-administered inhalers using these agents have been used as long as there has been anesthesia [157, 158]. Nitrous oxide inhalers were available from after the 1870s, and through the years almost all inhalational agents have been administered in this fashion for various reasons, primarily for analgesia during short procedures, labor, and delivery [157]. The great advantage of nitrous oxide is that it is odorless, washes in and out very quickly, and has undisputed analgesic properties [153, 156, 159, 160].

[4]The hypothesis that nitrous oxide could be used as an alternative to ECT to treat major depression is intriguing [149], as ketamine (or its oral cogeners) is a drug of keen interest to rapidly treat major depression while drugs targeting other receptor systems are ramping up to their antidepressant effect [150, 151].

Case Studies

Case 1

A 4-year-old boy scheduled for magnetic resonance imaging (MRI) sedation received dexmedetomidine sedation after oral premedication of midazolam for anxiolysis. For the first 45 min of the MRI study, the patient remained motionless. The scan was more lengthy than expected and eventually required that the child be physically adjusted in order to accommodate further imaging studies. Upon moving the child, he woke up and started to cry out for his mother. The child immediately received a repeat loading dose of dexmedetomidine, following which he achieved successful (re)sedation within 10 min. The nurse, who was present for this entire scenario, asked whether the physician who administered the sedation should discuss this "wake-up" event with the family and, furthermore, what are the chances that this child will have recall of awakening in the MRI scanner.

Recommendation

A number of issues are raised by this clinical scenario. These include the predictability of amnesia and the management of potential "awareness." The question of whether amnesia is present is most relevant when a patient is awake and responsive. If unresponsive, particularly if the drug-producing unresponsiveness is an amnesic agent such as midazolam, propofol, or ketamine, then the patient will undoubtedly be amnesic. Amnesia occurs at lower drug concentrations than unresponsiveness. It is likely that dexmedetomidine is not an amnesic agent, and thus the question is whether the effect of midazolam is still present 45 min after administration. This is made more difficult by the fact that midazolam is administered orally, and absorption is less predictable than with intravenous or intranasal administration. In any case, even after intravenous administration, depending on the dose, the period of likely amnesia would be 30–45 min.

Thus, with these considerations in mind, there is a reasonable likelihood that the child could remember the instance of "wake-up." The child could potentially be traumatized by this event, and pretending it did not happen would just make any psychological sequelae worse. Whether awareness occurs following general anesthesia or during sedation seems to make little difference [161]. A good operational definition of "awareness" is when a patient recalls events during a period of time they were expecting to be asleep. Thus, awareness could occur during sedation for an imaging study if the expectation of the patient was that they would be

(continued)

"asleep for the whole procedure." This occurrence would be potentially more traumatic than someone undergoing surgery where they were expecting to be awake during a portion of the surgery (e.g., wake-up test to check neurologic function during spine or neurosurgery). In the latter situation, the patient had every expectation that they would be awake, and nothing unusual occurred from their expectations.

In the current situation, the possibility of recall of events during sedation should be explained. These may not be recalled directly, but could be evidenced in the form of unusual dreams, or in the play behavior of the child. A full explanation of what happened, why it happened, and how it can be prevented in the future should be done. Resources for psychological support should be offered to the child.

Case 2

A 12-year-old girl with a history of bipolar disease, schizophrenia, and anxiety presents to the emergency department with a deep head laceration in need of suture. She is anxious, screaming, and unable to be approached by healthcare providers. Her parents request that she receives an intramuscular injection of sedation, stating that she will not be amenable to nitrous oxide by face mask or the initiation of an intravenous catheter for administration of sedation. In reviewing the sedation agents available, you consider ketamine for its potent analgesic and sedative effects. Would you have any hesitations about administering this child ketamine, particularly with her history of schizophrenia? Furthermore, how would you discuss the risks of ketamine and possible side effects with the child and her parents, given her medical history?

Recommendation

Parents often know best, and it is wise to entertain their requests seriously. Intramuscular (IM) induction of sedation does seem to be the best option for this necessary procedure. IM ketamine for pediatric sedation has a long track record. It has additional advantages of minimal respiratory compromise along with its likely amnesic effects (in the fullest sense of the word). One might consider the addition of atropine with ketamine to avoid hypersalivation.

The critical issue in this particular patient is the psychiatric history, particularly schizophrenia. Ketamine has been used extensively to model the effects of schizophrenia on cognition [127, 162]. The question that is less studied is the cognitive effects of ketamine in patients who themselves have schizophrenia. Would we be adding fuel to the fire? Again, there is no literature in the pediatric population (though, schizophrenia tends to be diagnosed in patients of an older age). Conflicting results are reported in adult patients with schizophrenia who undergo ketamine challenge. Subanesthetic doses (0.3–0.5 mg/kg) have been variously reported to exacerbate psychotic symptoms, or to have no effect compared with placebo [163–165]. A meta-review of a number of studies where doses of 0.1–0.5 mg/kg were administered revealed an acceptable incidence of these effects [166]. In sum, volunteers might experience a worsening of their symptoms, but these were of a nature similar to episodes experienced during periods of exacerbation of their disease and were of limited duration.

Importantly, review of these studies from an ethical standpoint revealed informed consent was possible in this patient population, and conduct of these studies was justified [166]. Thus, in this clinical scenario, the parents should be informed that ketamine is a suitable, and probably necessary, intervention to best treat the patient. There is a strong possibility that symptoms of schizophrenia would be exacerbated, but that this effect in all likelihood would be of limited duration (similar to that experienced in the past with her disease exacerbation).

A new wrinkle is now present. There is substantial literature supporting the combined use of dexmedetomidine with ketamine. The side effects of these drugs in a sense balance each other out, and thus smaller doses of each drug can be used [123, 167–169]. A recent study demonstrated the efficacy of IM dexmedetomidine for sedation [170]. The aforementioned studies using a ketamine/dexmedetomidine combination administered medications IV. It is an interesting question of whether a combination of IM ketamine and IM dexmedetomidine would be better in this patient, but there is no literature directly addressing this mode of administration.

Case 3

A 9-year-old boy with autism and a brain tumor presents for his regular blood sampling by hematology for routine follow-up of his tumor. He is always apprehensive and recently has become so fearful that he screams upon entering the hospital lobby and has to be dragged into phlebotomy and held down during the blood sampling. His mother states that through this process, her son has become more anxious and fearful. She requests that sedation be administered to her son for the blood sampling and venipuncture. She would like to be sure that this child has no recall of these future events. You are considering the options available for sedation for this

(continued)

short procedure. She is requesting both anxiolysis and amnesia. You consider nitrous oxide and propofol. What are the chances of amnesia associated with each agent? Would one agent be better than another in terms of ensuring lack of memory of the subsequent venipuncture? Should you consider midazolam as an alternative or supplement? Is there a difference in recall dependant on the route of midazolam administration? For example, are the chances of memory recall of the event the same whether you administer midazolam by oral versus intravenous route? If you administer it orally, how long should you wait before performing the procedure, in order to maximize chances of anterograde amnesia?

Recommendation

This clinical scenario highlights the most vexing problem associated with amnesic drugs and that is we do not know when amnesia is occurring! As opposed to most other acute medications—for example, vasopressors—where we keep giving a drug and measuring a response, there is no response to measure for the amnesic state. Memory can only be assessed retrospectively. We can only determine amnesia *after* the fact. With better understanding of how memory processes are embodied in brain physiology (e.g., theta rhythms, information transfer between brain regions, etc.), there may come a time when some monitor will prospectively predict the occurrence of amnesia. But the likelihood is that the application of the monitor itself will be a cumbersome affair and even if available would be of little use in this situation.

Thus we are left with giving amnesic medications on the basis of known pharmacology and previous experience using our best clinical judgment. All the drugs mentioned in this scenario are amnesic agents when given at the appropriate concentration. We know from previous volunteer studies that the concentration of drug-producing amnesia is invariably lower than that producing sedation. Sedation is something we *can* measure in real time and can act as a good surrogate for the presence of amnesia (for amnesic agents). Thus, whatever drug we choose, we can be reasonably sure amnesia will occur for events occurring in the presence of drug when it is being given at doses that cause some drowsiness. As the patient has a brain tumor, one wants to avoid excessive sedation, with carbon dioxide retention with resultant potential for increased intracranial pressure.

The particular problem with an anxious pediatric patient is getting the drug to the brain. Intravenous administration is the most reliable but also the most difficult to achieve in this anxious child. Propofol in this situation is basically useless. Although an ideal amnesic agent with relatively rapid onset and clearance, it requires intravenous access. Thus, alternative routes will need to be considered. Blood vessels are close to the surface and will readily absorb drug into the circulation in the lung, the nose, and under the tongue (and the rectum, a route not often used anymore). Thus inhalational agents are terrific if the child will cooperate with breathing through a device, and nitrous oxide is a good choice in this situation. It also provides analgesia at subanesthetic concentrations and will be ideal for painful procedures such as venipuncture [153]. Both amnesic and analgesic concentrations can be achieved when nitrous oxide concentration is greater than 35 %, and substantially higher concentrations can be given while maintaining adequate oxygenation. Remember that nitrous oxide dissipates as quickly as it achieves its action. Thus, if nitrous oxide is used, it must be administered throughout the entire period during which amnesia is sought. Forcibly holding a mask over the child's face may induce as much psychic trauma as the venipuncture itself, and indeed when anesthesia is induced in this manner, posttraumatic stress disorder (PTSD) may be the result. Parents report children in this situation tying down their dolls onto the bed after such experiences. The cure may be worse than the disease.

Administering a drug in a bolus fashion so that is absorbed and will be around in the circulation at sufficient concentrations during the period in question has advantages. Intranasal or sublingual administration of drugs that have reasonably long half-lives (e.g., midazolam or ketamine) is a fairly predictable method of doing this [171]. Intranasal administration is more predictable than sublingual administration and has the advantage of a single intervention (though the dose has to be carefully considered ahead of time). The bitter taste of midazolam can be masked with sweet juice, but gastric absorption is the least predictable and also has the slowest time to onset. The peak amnesic effect of midazolam occurs approximately 5 min after intravenous administration, and onset will take at least this long using alternative routes. If the dose is high enough to cause drowsiness, this will be a good marker that amnesia is present. The disadvantage of midazolam is the "hangover effect": Once the 30 s venipuncture is done, the child is still under the influence of drug for a significant period of time following this.

A combination approach with intranasal midazolam and inhaled nitrous oxide may be most suitable. The midazolam will relieve some anxiety and may produce amnesia, subsequently facilitating cooperation and acceptance of inhaled nitrous oxide for the short venipuncture procedure. Nitrous oxide will have rapid onset/offset, provide amnesia for the venipuncture (which may be enhanced by the presence of midazolam), and, in combination with the smaller dose of midazolam, will have little lingering effect following the procedure.

References

1. Mashour GA (2011) Sleep, anesthesia, and consciousness. Sleep 34(3):247–248
2. Mashour GA, Alkire MT (2013) Consciousness, anesthesia, and the thalamocortical system. Anesthesiology 118(1):13–15. doi:10.1097/ALN.1090b1013e318277a318279c318276
3. Rudolph U, Antkowiak B (2004) Molecular and neuronal substrates for general anaesthetics. Nat Rev Neurosci 5(9):709–720
4. Campagna JA, Miller KW, Forman SA (2003) Mechanisms of actions of inhaled anesthetics. N Engl J Med 348(21):2110–2124 [Review]
5. Franks NP (2008) General anaesthesia: from molecular targets to neuronal pathways of sleep and arousal. Nat Rev Neurosci 9(5): 370–386
6. Brown EN, Lydic R, Schiff ND (2010) General anesthesia, sleep, and coma. N Engl J Med 363(27):2638–2650 [Research Support, N.I.H., Extramural Research Support, Non-U.S. Gov't Review]
7. Brown EN, Purdon PL, Van Dort CJ (2011) General anesthesia and altered states of arousal: a systems neuroscience analysis. Annu Rev Neurosci 34:601–628 [Research Support, N.I.H., Extramural Research Support, Non-U.S. Gov't Review]
8. Burgess CR, Scammell TE (2012) Narcolepsy: neural mechanisms of sleepiness and cataplexy. J Neurosci 32(36):12305–12311 [Research Support, N.I.H., Extramural Research Support, Non-U.S. Gov't Review]
9. Kim H (2011) Neural activity that predicts subsequent memory and forgetting: a meta-analysis of 74 FMRI studies. Neuroimage 54(3):2446–2461
10. Uncapher MR, Rugg MD (2008) Fractionation of the component processes underlying successful episodic encoding: a combined FMRI and divided attention study. J Cogn Neurosci 20(2):240–254
11. Hasselmo ME, Stern CE (2006) Mechanisms underlying working memory for novel information. Trends Cogn Sci 10(11):487–493
12. Wager TD, Jonides J, Reading S (2004) Neuroimaging studies of shifting attention: a meta-analysis. Neuroimage 22(4):1679–1693
13. Wafford KA, Ebert B (2008) Emerging anti-insomnia drugs: tackling sleeplessness and the quality of wake time. Nat Rev Drug Discov 7(6):530–540 [Review]
14. Nelson LE, Lu J, Guo T, Saper CB, Franks NP, Maze M (2003) The alpha2-adrenoceptor agonist dexmedetomidine converges on an endogenous sleep-promoting pathway to exert its sedative effects. Anesthesiology 98(2):428–436
15. Huupponen E, Kulkas A, Tenhunen M, Saastamoinen A, Hasan J, Himanen SL (2008) Diffuse sleep spindles show similar frequency in central and frontopolar positions. J Neurosci Methods 172(1):54–59
16. McCarley RW (2007) Neurobiology of REM and NREM sleep. Sleep Med 8(4):302–330 [Research Support, N.I.H., Extramural Research Support, U.S. Gov't, Non-P.H.S. Review]
17. Morairty S, Rainnie D, McCarley R, Greene R (2004) Disinhibition of ventrolateral preoptic area sleep-active neurons by adenosine: a new mechanism for sleep promotion. Neuroscience 123(2):451–457
18. Fritschy JM, Mohler H (1995) GABAA-receptor heterogeneity in the adult rat brain: differential regional and cellular distribution of seven major subunits. J Comp Neurol 359(1):154–194
19. Cunha C, Monfils MH, Ledoux JE (2010) GABA(C) receptors in the lateral amygdala: a possible novel target for the treatment of fear and anxiety disorders? Front Behav Neurosci 4:6
20. Cheng VY, Martin LJ, Elliott EM, Kim JH, Mount HTJ, Taverna FA et al (2006) {alpha}5GABAA receptors mediate the amnestic but not sedative-hypnotic effects of the general anesthetic etomidate. J Neurosci 26(14):3713–3720
21. Squire LR, Wixted JT (2011) The cognitive neuroscience of human memory since H.M. Annu Rev Neurosci 34:259–288
22. Kelz MB, Sun Y, Chen J, Cheng Meng Q, Moore JT, Veasey SC et al (2008) An essential role for orexins in emergence from general anesthesia. Proc Natl Acad Sci U S A 105(4):1309–1314 [Research Support, N.I.H., Extramural Research Support, Non-U.S. Gov't]
23. Kotz C, Nixon J, Butterick T, Perez-Leighton C, Teske J, Billington C (2012) Brain orexin promotes obesity resistance. Ann N Y Acad Sci 1264(1):72–86 [Review]
24. Mantz J, Hemmings HC Jr (2011) Sleep and anesthesia: the histamine connection. Anesthesiology 115(1):8–9
25. Ghoneim MM, Hinrichs JV (1997) Drugs, memory and sedation: specificity of effects. Anesthesiology 87(Oct):734–736
26. Veselis RA (2006) The remarkable memory effects of propofol. Br J Anaesth 96(3):289–291
27. Sanders RD, Tononi G, Laureys S, Sleigh JW (2012) Unresponsiveness not equal unconsciousness. Anesthesiology 116(4):946–959 [Research Support, N.I.H., Extramural Research Support, Non-U.S. Gov't Review]
28. Blum A (2012) Tubes: a journey to the center of the internet, 1st edn. Ecco, New York
29. Mashour GA (2006) Integrating the science of consciousness and anesthesia. Anesth Analg 103(4):975–982
30. Tulving E (1995) Organization of memory: quo vadis. Cogn Neurosci 839–847
31. Tulving E (2001) Episodic memory and common sense: how far apart? Philos Trans R Soc Lond B Biol Sci 356(1413):1505–1515
32. Liu X, Lauer KK, Ward BD, Rao SM, Li SJ, Hudetz AG (2012) Propofol disrupts functional interactions between sensory and high-order processing of auditory verbal memory. Hum Brain Mapp 33(10):2487–2498 [Research Support, N.I.H., Extramural Research Support, Non-U.S. Gov't]
33. Imas OA, Ropella KM, Wood JD, Hudetz AG (2006) Isoflurane disrupts anterio-posterior phase synchronization of flash-induced field potentials in the rat. Neurosci Lett 402(3):216–221
34. Veselis R, Reinsel R, Feshchenko V, Beattie B, Akhurst T (2004) Auditory rcbf covariation with word rate during drug-induced sedation and unresponsiveness: a h2015 pet study. Brain Cogn 54(2):142–144
35. Plourde G, Belin P, Chartrand D, Fiset P, Backman SB, Xie G et al (2006) Cortical processing of complex auditory stimuli during alterations of consciousness with the general anesthetic propofol. Anesthesiology 104(3):448–457
36. Ghoneim MM, Block RI (1997) Learning and memory during general anesthesia. Anesthesiology 87(2):387–410
37. Hadzidiakos D, Horn N, Degener R, Buchner A, Rehberg B (2009) Analysis of memory formation during general anesthesia (propofol/remifentanil) for elective surgery using the process-dissociation procedure. Anesthesiology 111(2):293–301
38. Di Francesco MW, Robertson SA, Karunanayaka P, Holland SK (2013) Bold fMRI in infants under sedation: comparing the impact of pentobarbital and propofol on auditory and language activation. J Magn Reson Imaging 38(5):1184–1195
39. Saksida LM (2009) Neuroscience. Remembering outside the box. Science 325(5936):40–41
40. Alkire MT, Hudetz AG, Tononi G (2008) Consciousness and anesthesia. Science 322(5903):876–880
41. Hudetz AG, Imas OA (2007) Burst activation of the cerebral cortex by flash stimuli during isoflurane anesthesia in rats. Anesthesiology 107(6):983–991
42. Hudetz AG, Pearce R (2010) Suppressing the mind: anesthetic modulation of memory and consciousness. Humana, Totowa
43. Hudetz AG, Vizuete JA, Imas OA (2009) Desflurane selectively suppresses long-latency cortical neuronal response to flash in the rat. Anesthesiology 111(2):231–239. doi:10.1097/ALN.0b013e3181ab671e
44. Lee U, Muller M, Noh GJ, Choi B, Mashour GA (2011) Dissociable network properties of anesthetic state transitions. Anesthesiology 114(4):872–881
45. Lee U, Oh G, Kim S, Noh G, Choi B, Mashour GA (2010) Brain networks maintain a scale-free organization across consciousness,

anesthesia, and recovery: evidence for adaptive reconfiguration. Anesthesiology 113(5):1081–1091
46. Lewis LD, Weiner VS, Mukamel EA, Donoghue JA, Eskandar EN, Madsen JR et al (2012) Rapid fragmentation of neuronal networks at the onset of propofol-induced unconsciousness. Proc Natl Acad Sci 109(49):E3377–E3386
47. Boveroux P, Vanhaudenhuyse A, Bruno M-A, Noirhomme Q, Lauwick S, Luxen A et al (2010) Breakdown of within- and between-network resting state functional magnetic resonance imaging connectivity during propofol-induced loss of consciousness. Anesthesiology 113(5):1038–1053. doi:10.1097/ALN.0b013e3181f697f5
48. Tulving E, Schacter DL (1990) Priming and human memory systems. Science 247(4940):301–306
49. Mashour GA, Avidan MS (2013) Capturing covert consciousness. Lancet 381(9863):271–272 [Comment]
50. Russell IF (2013) The ability of bispectral index to detect intra-operative wakefulness during total intravenous anaesthesia compared with the isolated forearm technique. Anaesthesia 68(5):502–511
51. Russell IF (2006) The narcotrend 'depth of anaesthesia' monitor cannot reliably detect consciousness during general anaesthesia: an investigation using the isolated forearm technique. Br J Anaesth 96(3):346–352
52. Schneider G, Hollweck R, Ningler M, Stockmanns G, Kochs EF (2005) Detection of consciousness by electroencephalogram and auditory evoked potentials. Anesthesiology 103(5):934–943
53. Schneider G, Kochs EF, Horn B, Kreuzer M, Ningler M (2004) Narcotrend does not adequately detect the transition between awareness and unconsciousness in surgical patients. Anesthesiology 101(5):1105–1111
54. Pryor KO, Reinsel RA, Mehta M, Li Y, Wixted JT, Veselis RA (2010) Visual p2-n2 complex and arousal at the time of encoding predict the time domain characteristics of amnesia for multiple intravenous anesthetic drugs in humans. Anesthesiology 113(2): 313–326
55. Veselis RA, Reinsel RA, Feshchenko VA, Johnson R Jr (2004) Information loss over time defines the memory defect of propofol: a comparative response with thiopental and dexmedetomidine. Anesthesiology 101(4):831–841
56. Veselis RA, Reinsel RA, Feshchenko VA, Wronski M (1997) The comparative amnestic effects of midazolam, propofol, thiopental, and fentanyl at equisedative concentrations. Anesthesiology 87(4):749–764
57. Russell IF (1995) Intraoperative awareness and the isolated forearm technique [letter] [see comments]. Br J Anaesth 75(6):819–821 [Letter] [See comments]
58. Russell IF (2013) Fourteen fallacies about the isolated forearm technique, and its place in modern anaesthesia. Anaesthesia 68(7):677–681
59. Nordstrom O, Sandin R (1996) Recall during intermittent propofol anaesthesia. Br J Anaesth 76(5):699–701
60. Ghoneim MM, Dembo JB, Block RI (1989) Time course of antagonism of sedative and amnesic effects of diazepam by flumazenil. Anesthesiology 70:899–904
61. Hebb DO (1949) The organization of behavior; a neuropsychological theory. Wiley, New York
62. Fernandez G, Effern A, Grunwald T, Pezer N, Lehnert K, Duempelmann M et al (1999) Real-time tracking of memory formation in the human rhinal cortex and hippocampus. Science 285:1582–1585
63. McGaugh JL (2000) Memory—a century of consolidation. Science 287(5451):248–251
64. Izquierdo I, Bevilaqua LR, Rossato JI, Bonini JS, Medina JH, Cammarota M (2006) Different molecular cascades in different sites of the brain control memory consolidation. Trends Neurosci 29(9):496–505
65. Johansson M, Aslan A, Bauml K-H, Gabel A, Mecklinger A (2006) When remembering causes forgetting: electrophysiological correlates of retrieval-induced forgetting. Cereb Cortex 17(6): 1335–1341
66. Miller G (2004) Forgetting and remembering. Learning to forget. Science 304(5667):34–36
67. Wagner AD, Davachi L (2001) Cognitive neuroscience: forgetting of things past. Curr Biol 11(23):964–967
68. Wixted JT (2005) A theory about why we forget what we once knew. Curr Dir Psychol Sci 14(1):6–9
69. Cahill L (1997) The neurobiology of emotionally influenced memory. Implications for understanding traumatic memory. Ann N Y Acad Sci 821:238–246
70. Leslie K, Chan MTV, Myles PS, Forbes A, McCulloch TJ (2010) Posttraumatic stress disorder in aware patients from the b-aware trial. Anesth Analg 110(3):823–828
71. Reist C, Duffy JG, Fujimoto K, Cahill L (2001) Beta-adrenergic blockade and emotional memory in PTSD. Int J Neuropsychopharmacol 4(4):377–383
72. Wixted JT, Carpenter SK (2007) The Wickelgren power law and the Ebbinghaus savings function. Psychol Sci 18(2):133–134
73. Zola-Morgan S, Squire LR (1993) Neuroanatomy of memory. Annu Rev Neurosci 16:547–563
74. Zola-Morgan S, Squire LR, Amaral DG (1986) Human amnesia and the medial temporal region: enduring memory impairment following a bilateral lesion limited to field ca1 of the hippocampus. J Neurosci 6(10):2950–2967
75. Scoville WB, Milner B (1957) Loss of recent memory after bilateral hippocampal lesions. J Neurol Neurosurg Psychiatry 20:11–21
76. Hebb DO, Penfield W (1940) Human behavior after extensive bilateral removal from the frontal lobes. Arch Neurol Psych 44(2):421–438
77. Anonymous. [June 1, 2013]; Available from: http://en.wikipedia.org/wiki/Memento_(film)
78. Marshall L, Born J (2007) The contribution of sleep to hippocampus-dependent memory consolidation. Trends Cogn Sci 11(10):442–450
79. Andrade KC, Spoormaker VI, Dresler M, Wehrle R, Holsboer F, Sämann PG et al (2011) Sleep spindles and hippocampal functional connectivity in human nrem sleep. J Neurosci 31(28):10331–10339
80. Gais S, Albouy G, Boly M, Dang-Vu TT, Darsaud A, Desseilles M et al (2007) Sleep transforms the cerebral trace of declarative memories. Proc Natl Acad Sci 104(47):18778–18783
81. Gais S, Born J (2004) Declarative memory consolidation: mechanisms acting during human sleep. Learn Mem 11(6):679–685
82. Rudoy JD, Voss JL, Westerberg CE, Paller KA (2009) Strengthening individual memories by reactivating them during sleep. Science 326(5956):1079
83. Parker ES, Cahill L, McGaugh JL (2006) A case of unusual autobiographical remembering. Neurocase 12(1):35–49
84. Ebbinghaus H. Memory: a contribution to experimental psychology. 1885 [June 1, 2013]; Available from: http://psychclassics.yorku.ca/Ebbinghaus/memory7.htm
85. Veselis RA, Pryor KO, Reinsel RA, Li Y, Mehta M, Johnson R Jr (2009) Propofol and midazolam inhibit conscious memory processes very soon after encoding: an event-related potential study of familiarity and recollection in volunteers. Anesthesiology 110(2):295–312
86. Schwartz RH, Milteer R, LeBeau MA (2000) Drug-facilitated sexual assault ('date rape'). South Med J 93(6):558–561
87. Lee U, Ku S, Noh G, Baek S, Choi B, Mashour GA (2013) Disruption of frontal-parietal communication by ketamine, propofol, and sevoflurane. Anesthesiology 118(6):1264–1275. doi:10.1097/aln.0b013e31829103f5
88. Monti MM, Lutkenhoff ES, Rubinov M, Boveroux P, Vanhaudenhuyse A, Gosseries O et al (2013) Dynamic change of global and local information processing in propofol-induced loss and recovery of consciousness. PLoS Comput Biol 9(10): e1003271

89. Tononi G (2012) Integrated information theory of consciousness: an updated account. Arch Ital Biol 150(2–3):56–90 [Research Support, Non-U.S. Gov't Review]
90. Ferrarelli F, Massimini M, Sarasso S, Casali A, Riedner BA, Angelini G et al (2010) Breakdown in cortical effective connectivity during midazolam-induced loss of consciousness. Proc Natl Acad Sci U S A 107(6):2681–2686
91. Hudetz AG, Vizuete JA, Pillay S (2011) Differential effects of isoflurane on high-frequency and low-frequency γ oscillations in the cerebral cortex and hippocampus in freely moving rats. Anesthesiology 114(3):588–595. doi:10.1097/ALN.0b013e31820ad3f9
92. Liu X, Lauer KK, Ward BD, Li S-J, Hudetz AG (2013) Differential effects of deep sedation with propofol on the specific and nonspecific thalamocortical systems: a functional magnetic resonance imaging study. Anesthesiology 118(1):59–69. doi:10.1097/ALN.1090b1013e318277a318801
93. Baddeley A (1996) The fractionation of working memory. Proc Natl Acad Sci U S A 93(24):13468–13472
94. Baddeley A (2000) The episodic buffer: a new component of working memory? Trends Cogn Sci 4(11):417–423
95. Schlosser RG, Wagner G, Sauer H (2006) Assessing the working memory network: studies with functional magnetic resonance imaging and structural equation modeling. Neuroscience 139(1): 91–103
96. Miller GA (1956) The magical number seven, plus or minus two: some limits on our capacity for processing information. Psychol Rev 63:81–97
97. Lisman JE, Idiart MA (1995) Storage of 7 +/- 2 short-term memories in oscillatory subcycles. Science 267(5203):1512–1515
98. Perouansky M, Rau V, Ford T, Oh SI, Perkins M, Eger EI 2nd et al (2010) Slowing of the hippocampal theta rhythm correlates with anesthetic-induced amnesia. Anesthesiology 113(6):1299–1309
99. Hughes MA, Glass PS, Jacobs JR (1992) Context-sensitive half-time in multicompartment pharmacokinetic models for intravenous anesthetic drugs. Anesthesiology 76(3):334–341
100. Rupreht J (1989) Awareness with amnesia during total intravenous anaesthesia with propofol. Anaesthesia 44(12):1005 [Letter]
101. Bennett S (1992) Propofol and awareness. Anesthesiology 77(6):1232–1233; discussion 1233-1234; [Letter; Comment]
102. Cox RG (1992) Propofol and awareness. Anesthesiology 77(6):1232; discussion 1233-1234; [Letter; Comment]
103. Tasch MD (1992) Propofol and awareness. Anesthesiology 77(6):1232; discussion 1233-1234; [Letter; Comment]
104. Veselis RA, Reinsel RA, Wronski M, Marino P, Tong WP, Bedford RF (1992) EEG and memory effects of low-dose infusions of propofol. Br J Anaesth 69(3):246–254
105. Gan TJ, Ginsberg B, Grant AP, Glass PS (1996) Double-blind, randomized comparison of ondansetron and intraoperative propofol to prevent postoperative nausea and vomiting. Anesthesiology 85(5):1036–1042
106. Veselis RA, Pryor KO, Reinsel RA, Mehta M, Pan H, Johnson R Jr (2008) Low-dose propofol-induced amnesia is not due to a failure of encoding: left inferior prefrontal cortex is still active. Anesthesiology 109(2):213–224
107. McDaniel WW, Sahota AK, Vyas BV, Laguerta N, Hategan L, Oswald J (2006) Ketamine appears associated with better word recall than etomidate after a course of 6 electroconvulsive therapies. J ECT 22(2):103–106
108. Gregory-Roberts EM, Naismith SL, Cullen KM, Hickie IB (2010) Electroconvulsive therapy-induced persistent retrograde amnesia: could it be minimised by ketamine or other pharmacological approaches? J Affect Disord 126(1–2):39–45 [Research Support, Non-U.S. Gov't Review]
109. Ghoneim MM, Block RI (2007) Immediate peri-operative memory. Acta Anaesthesiol Scand 51(8):1054–1061
110. Grunwald T, Beck H, Lehnertz K, Blumcke I, Pezer N, Kurthen M et al (1999) Evidence relating human verbal memory to hippocampal n-methyl-d-aspartate receptors. Proc Natl Acad Sci U S A 96(21):12085–12089
111. Grunwald T, Kurthen M (2006) Novelty detection and encoding for declarative memory within the human hippocampus. Clin EEG Neurosci 37(4):309–314
112. Low K, Crestani F, Keist R, Benke D, Brunig I, Benson JA et al (2000) Molecular and neuronal substrate for the selective attenuation of anxiety. Science 290(5489):131–134
113. Whiting PJ (2006) Gaba-a receptors: a viable target for novel anxiolytics? Curr Opin Pharmacol 6(1):24–29 [Review]
114. Curran HV (1986) Tranquillising memories: a review of the effects of benzodiazepines on human memory. Biol Psychol 23(2):179–213
115. Reves JG, Fragen RJ, Vinik HR, Greenblatt DJ (1985) Midazolam: pharmacology and uses. Anesthesiology 62:310–324
116. Twersky RS, Hartung J, Berger BJ, McClain J, Beaton C (1993) Midazolam enhances anterograde but not retrograde amnesia in pediatric patients. Anesthesiology 78(1):51–55
117. Kupietzky A, Holan G, Shapira J (1996) Intranasal midazolam better at effecting amnesia after sedation than oral hydroxyzine: a pilot study. Pediatr Dent 18(1):32–34
118. Kain ZN, Hofstadter MB, Mayes LC, Krivutza DM, Alexander G, Wang SM et al (2000) Midazolam: effects on amnesia and anxiety in children. Anesthesiology 93(3):676–684
119. Millar K, Asbury AJ, Bowman AW, Hosey MT, Martin K, Musiello T et al (2007) A randomised placebo-controlled trial of the effects of midazolam premedication on children's postoperative cognition. Anaesthesia 62(9):923–930
120. Huupponen E, Maksimow A, Lapinlampi P, Sarkela M, Saastamoinen A, Snapir A et al (2008) Electroencephalogram spindle activity during dexmedetomidine sedation and physiological sleep. Acta Anaesthesiol Scand 52(2):289–294
121. Oto J, Yamamoto K, Koike S, Onodera M, Imanaka H, Nishimura M (2012) Sleep quality of mechanically ventilated patients sedated with dexmedetomidine. Intensive Care Med 38(12):1982–1989
122. Pollard RJ, Coyle JP, Gilbert RL, Beck JE (2007) Intraoperative awareness in a regional medical system: a review of 3 years' data. Anesthesiology 106(2):269–274
123. Tobias JD (2012) Dexmedetomidine and ketamine: an effective alternative for procedural sedation? Pediatr Crit Care Med 13(4): 423–427 [Review]
124. Loix S, De Kock M, Henin P (2011) The anti-inflammatory effects of ketamine: state of the art. Acta Anaesthesiol Belg 62(1):47–58 [Review]
125. Anand KJ, Garg S, Rovnaghi CR, Narsinghani U, Bhutta AT, Hall RW (2007) Ketamine reduces the cell death following inflammatory pain in newborn rat brain. Pediatr Res 62(3):283–290
126. Hudetz JA, Iqbal Z, Gandhi SD, Patterson KM, Byrne AJ, Hudetz AG et al (2009) Ketamine attenuates post-operative cognitive dysfunction after cardiac surgery. Acta Anaesthesiol Scand 53(7):864–872 [Randomized Controlled Trial Research Support, N.I.H., Extramural]
127. Fletcher PC, Honey GD (2006) Schizophrenia, ketamine and cannabis: evidence of overlapping memory deficits. Trends Cogn Sci 10(4):167–174
128. Newcomer JW, Farber NB, Jevtovic-Todorovic V, Selke G, Melson AK, Hershey T et al (1999) Ketamine-induced NMDA receptor hypofunction as a model of memory impairment and psychosis. Neuropsychopharmacology 20(2):106–118
129. De La Torre R (2010) Commentary on Morgan et al. (2010): Ketamine abuse: first medical evidence of harms we should confront. Addiction 105(1):134–135 [Comment]
130. Muetzelfeldt L, Kamboj SK, Rees H, Taylor J, Morgan CJ, Curran HV (2008) Journey through the k-hole: phenomenological aspects of ketamine use. Drug Alcohol Depend 95(3):219–229
131. McKie D. Date rape drug busts put china at top of border agency's list. CBC News. 2013

132. Morgan CJ, Curran HV (2006) Acute and chronic effects of ketamine upon human memory: a review. Psychopharmacology (Berl) 188(4):408–424
133. Morgan CJ, Mofeez A, Brandner B, Bromley L, Curran HV (2004) Ketamine impairs response inhibition and is positively reinforcing in healthy volunteers: a dose-response study. Psychopharmacology (Berl) 172(3):298–308
134. Morgan CJ, Mofeez A, Brandner B, Bromley L, Curran HV (2004) Acute effects of ketamine on memory systems and psychotic symptoms in healthy volunteers. Neuropsychopharmacology 29(1):208–218
135. Grunwald M, Weiss T, Krause W, Beyer L, Rost R, Gutberlet I et al (1999) Power of theta waves in the EEG of human subjects increases during recall of haptic information. Neurosci Lett 260(3):189–192
136. Forman SA (2011) Clinical and molecular pharmacology of etomidate. Anesthesiology 114(3):695–707 [Research Support, N.I.H., Extramural Research Support, Non-U.S. Gov't Review]
137. Ghoneim MM, Yamada T (1977) Etomidate: a clinical and electroencephalographic comparison with thiopental. Anesth Analg 56(4):479–485
138. Gallagher CS Jr, Hann JR (1985) Clinical assessment of etomidate for outpatient general anesthesia: a preliminary evaluation. J Oral Maxillofac Surg 43(11):860–864
139. Jacob TC, Moss SJ, Jurd R (2008) Gaba(a) receptor trafficking and its role in the dynamic modulation of neuronal inhibition. Nat Rev Neurosci 9(5):331–343 [Research Support, N.I.H., Extramural Research Support, Non-U.S. Gov't Review]
140. Farrant M, Nusser Z (2005) Variations on an inhibitory theme: phasic and tonic activation of GABA(A) receptors. Nat Rev Neurosci 6(3):215–229 [Research Support, Non-U.S. Gov't Review]
141. Banks MI, Pearce RA (2000) Kinetic differences between synaptic and extrasynaptic GABA(A) receptors in ca1 pyramidal cells. J Neurosci 20(3):937–948
142. Caraiscos VB, Elliott EM, You-Ten KE, Cheng VY, Belelli D, Newell JG et al (2004) Tonic inhibition in mouse hippocampal ca1 pyramidal neurons is mediated by alpha5 subunit-containing gamma-aminobutyric acid type a receptors. Proc Natl Acad Sci U S A 101(10):3662–3667
143. Mortensen M, Patel B, Smart TG (2012) Gaba potency at GABAA receptors found in synaptic and extrasynaptic zones. Front Cell Neurosci 20:6 [Review]
144. Osborn AG, Bunker JP, Cooper LM, Frank GS, Hilgard ER (1967) Effects of thiopental sedation on learning and memory. Science 157(788):574–576
145. Mason KP, Prescilla R, Fontaine PJ, Zurakowski D (2011) Pediatric ct sedation: comparison of dexmedetomidine and pentobarbital. AJR Am J Roentgenol 196(2):W194–W198
146. de Sousa SL, Dickinson R, Lieb WR, Franks NP (2000) Contrasting synaptic actions of the inhalational general anesthetics isoflurane and xenon. Anesthesiology 92(4):1055–1066 [See comments]
147. Mennerick S, Jevtovic-Todorovic V, Todorovic SM, Shen W, Olney JW, Zorumski CF (1998) Effect of nitrous oxide on excitatory and inhibitory synaptic transmission in hippocampal cultures. J Neurosci 18(23):9716–9726
148. Jevtovic-Todorovic V, Todorovic SM, Mennerick S, Powell S, Dikranian K, Benshoff N et al (1998) Nitrous oxide (laughing gas) is an NMDA antagonist, neuroprotectant and neurotoxin. Nat Med 4(4):460–463 [See comments]
149. Milne B (2010) Nitrous oxide (laughing gas) inhalation as an alternative to electroconvulsive therapy. Med Hypotheses 74(5):780–781
150. Berman RMCA, Anand A, Oren DA, Heninger GR, Charney DS, Krystal JH (2000) Antidepressant effects of ketamine in depressed patients. Biol Psychiatry 47(4):351–354
151. Zarate CA SJ Jr, Carlson PJ, Brutsche NE, Ameli R, Luckenbaugh DA, Charney DS, Manji HK (2006) A randomized trial of an n-methyl-d-aspartate antagonist in treatment-resistant major depression. Arch Gen Psychiatry 63(8):856–864
152. Dwyer R, Bennett HL, Eger EI 2nd, Heilbron D (1992) Effects of isoflurane and nitrous oxide in subanesthetic concentrations on memory and responsiveness in volunteers. Anesthesiology 77(5):888–898 [Clinical Trial Randomized Controlled Trial Research Support, Non-U.S. Gov't]
153. Duarte R, McNeill A, Drummond G, Tiplady B (2008) Comparison of the sedative, cognitive, and analgesic effects of nitrous oxide, sevoflurane, and ethanol. Br J Anaesth 100(2):203–210 [Comparative Study Randomized Controlled Trial Research Support, Non-U.S. Gov't]
154. Hemmings HC Jr, Akabas MH, Goldstein PA, Trudell JR, Orser BA, Harrison NL (2005) Emerging molecular mechanisms of general anesthetic action. Trends Pharmacol Sci 26(10):503–510
155. Hemmings H (2010) Molecular anesthetic targets. In: Hudetz AG, Pearce R (eds) Suppressing the mind: anesthetic modulation of memory and consciousness. Humana, Totowa, pp 11–31, 252 pp
156. Galinkin JL, Janiszewski D, Young CJ, Klafta JM, Klock PA, Coalson DW et al (1997) Subjective, psychomotor, cognitive, and analgesic effects of subanesthetic concentrations of sevoflurane and nitrous oxide. Anesthesiology 87(5):1082–1088
157. Ball C (1993) Hewitt's nitrous oxide-oxygen inhaler. Anaesth Intensive Care 21(6):733 [Biography Historical Article]
158. Ball C (1993) Clover's nitrous oxide/ether inhaler 1876. Anaesth Intensive Care 21(3):273 [Biography Historical Article]
159. Janiszewski DJ, Galinkin JL, Klock PA, Coalson DW, Pardo H, Zacny JP (1999) The effects of subanesthetic concentrations of sevoflurane and nitrous oxide, alone and in combination, on analgesia, mood, and psychomotor performance in healthy volunteers. Anesth Analg 88(5):1149–1154
160. Pirec V, Patterson TH, Thapar P, Apfelbaum JL, Zacny JP (1995) Effects of subanesthetic concentrations of nitrous oxide on cold-pressor pain in humans. Pharmacol Biochem Behav 51(2–3): 323–329
161. Kent CD, Mashour GA, Metzger NA, Posner KL, Domino KB (2013) Psychological impact of unexpected explicit recall of events occurring during surgery performed under sedation, regional anaesthesia, and general anaesthesia: data from the anesthesia awareness registry. Br J Anaesth 110(3):381–387 [Comparative Study Research Support, Non-U.S. Gov't]
162. Neill E, Rossell SL, McDonald S, Joshua N, Jansen N, Morgan CJ (2011) Using ketamine to model semantic deficits in schizophrenia. J Clin Psychopharmacol 31(6):690–697 [Randomized Controlled Trial Research Support, Non-U.S. Gov't]
163. Lahti AC, Weiler MA, Tamara Michaelidis BA, Parwani A, Tamminga CA (2001) Effects of ketamine in normal and schizophrenic volunteers. Neuropsychopharmacology 25(4):455–467
164. LaPorte DJ, Lahti AC, Koffel B, Tamminga CA (1996) Absence of ketamine effects on memory and other cognitive functions in schizophrenia patients. J Psychiatr Res 30(5):321–330
165. Lahti AC, Koffel B, LaPorte D, Tamminga CA (1995) Subanesthetic doses of ketamine stimulate psychosis in schizophrenia. Neuropsychopharmacology 13(1):9–19
166. Carpenter WT Jr (1999) The schizophrenia ketamine challenge study debate. Biol Psychiatry 46(8):1081–1091
167. Ulgey A, Aksu R, Bicer C, Akin A, Altuntas R, Esmaoglu A et al (2012) Is the addition of dexmedetomidine to a ketamine-propofol combination in pediatric cardiac catheterization sedation useful? Pediatr Cardiol 33(5):770–774
168. Raman V, Yacob D, Tobias JD (2012) Dexmedetomidine-ketamine sedation during upper gastrointestinal endoscopy and biopsy in a patient with Duchenne muscular dystrophy and egg allergy. Int J Crit Illn Inj Sci 2(1):40–43
169. Mester R, Easley RB, Brady KM, Chilson K, Tobias JD (2008) Monitored anesthesia care with a combination of ketamine and dexmedetomidine during cardiac catheterization. Am J Ther 15(1):24–30
170. Mason KP, Lubisch N, Robinson F, Roskos R, Epstein MA (2012) Intramuscular dexmedetomidine: an effective route of sedation preserves background activity for pediatric electroencephalograms. J Pediatr 161(5):927–932
171. Ghali AM, Mahfouz AK, Al-Bahrani M (2011) Preanesthetic medication in children: a comparison of intranasal dexmedetomidine versus oral midazolam. Saudi J Anaesth 5(4):387–391

Pharmacokinetics and Pharmacodynamics in the Pediatric Population

11

Brian J. Anderson

Abstract

Regulations encouraging pediatric investigation of new drugs are advancing the therapeutic pharmacopoeia, but for many commonly used medicines the lack of well-conducted pharmacokinetic–pharmacodynamic (PKPD) studies is replaced by extrapolation from adult or nonhuman data. While neonates, infants, and children have different psychology, social structure, behavior, and disease spectrum from adults, they also share many similarities. Growth and developmental aspects account for major differences between neonates and infants and adults. However, once out of infancy, body size alone can account for many of the pharmacokinetic differences between children and adults. Pharmacodynamic factors that may influence response in early life remain poorly defined. Most PK and PD differences occur in the first few years of postnatal life with major changes occurring during the neonatal period that are mature by the end of infancy (i.e., 2 years of age). Knowledge of pediatric PKPD and changes seen during growth and maturation are essential for dosing sedatives in children.

Keywords

Pharmacokinetics • Pharmacodynamics • Allometry • Population modeling • Covariates • Maturation • Drug metabolism • Interactions • Pharmacogenomics • Bioavailability • Distribution • Blood–brain barrier (BBB) • Body surface area (BSA) • Remifentanil • Clearance • Hepatic elimination • Organ function (OF) • Pulmonary elimination • Single nuclear polymorphism (SNP) • Minimal alveolar concentration • Neuromuscular locking drug • Bispectral index (BIS) • Electroencephalogram (EEG) • Target-controlled infusion (TCI) • Volume of distribution

Introduction

Many pharmacological maturational changes involving pharmacokinetics, pharmacodynamics, and toxicity are complete within the first few years of postnatal life. The time course of drug concentration after administration is determined by three processes: input (absorption, bioavailability), distribution, and elimination (metabolism and excretion).

PK Differences in the First Year of Life

Absorption

Absorption characteristics will impact on amount of drug available, maximum concentration, speed of onset of effect, duration of effect, and time to offset of effect.

B.J. Anderson, PhD, FANZCA, FJFICM (✉)
Department of Anaesthesiology, University of Auckland School of Medicine, Auckland, New Zealand
e-mail: briana@adhb.govt.nz

K.P. Mason (ed.), *Pediatric Sedation Outside of the Operating Room: A Multispecialty International Collaboration*,
DOI 10.1007/978-1-4939-1390-9_11, © Springer Science+Business Media New York 2015

Enteral

The rate at which most drugs are absorbed when given by the oral route is slower in neonates than in older children because gastric emptying is delayed and normal adult rates may not be reached until 6–8 months [1–4]. Slow gastric emptying and reduced clearance may dictate both reduced doses and reduced frequency of administration. This has been demonstrated for both cisapride [5] and acetaminophen [6]. Chloral hydrate used as a sedative will have delayed onset in those less than 6 months of age. This slow absorption combined with reduced clearance causes a prolonged effect that contributes to respiratory depression and death in this age group [7]. Enteral administration through the rectum (e.g., thiopentone, methohexitone) takes approximately 8 min in children but is speedier for neonates undergoing cardiac catheter study or radiological sedation [8, 9]. Diazepam (0.3 mg/kg) is also rapidly absorbed rectally with peak concentrations at 16 min [10].

Intramuscular

The intramuscular route is commonly frowned upon in children. It retains high bioavailability but absorption is delayed compared to the intravenous route. Ketamine, however, remains popular and peak concentrations are reached within 10 min after 4 mg/kg [11]. Dexmedetomidine has a similar absorption profile [12, 13].

Nasal

Exploration of alternative delivery routes in young children has centered on the nasal passages [14]. Nasal diamorphine 0.1 mg/kg is used in the United Kingdom for forearm fracture pain in the emergency room [15–18]. It is rapidly absorbed as a nasal spray (0.1 mg/kg) in 0.2 mL sterile water, with peak morphine plasma concentrations (T_{peak}) occurring at 10 min [18]. Nasal S-ketamine 2 mg/kg results in peak plasma concentrations of 355 ng/ mL within 18 min. Nasal fentanyl (150 μg/mL) 1.5 μg/kg given to children (3–17 years) for fracture pain resulted in good analgesia. Peak concentrations were at 13 min [19, 20]. Similar results are reported for nebulized fentanyl (4 μg/kg) given through a standard nebulizer [21]. Flumazenil concentrations peak within a few minutes after nasal administration [22], while midazolam takes approximately 12 min [23]. Dexmedetomidine is somewhat slower and peak concentrations were not reached until 38 min [24]. Clonidine administered as nasal aerosol (3–8 μg/kg) was not found to achieve adequate preoperative sedation within 30 min of administration [25], attributable to slow absorption (T_{peak} 1.5–3 h) [26]. There remain concerns that intranasal drugs may pass through the posterior nasopharynx or irritate the vocal cords [27].

Advances in aerosol delivery devices have improved dosing accuracy. Administration of ketorolac15 mg (weight <50 kg) or 30 mg (weight >50 kg) by the intranasal route resulted in a rapid increase in plasma concentration (time to peak concentration was 52 min, standard deviation 6 min) and may be a useful therapeutic alternative to IV injection. A target concentration of 0.37 mg/L in the effect compartment was achieved within 30 min and remained above that target for 10 h [28]. The nasal passages change with age and so it would be unsurprising if absorption by that route did not also change with age.

Cutaneous

The larger relative skin surface area, increased cutaneous perfusion, and thinner stratum corneum in neonates [29] increase absorption and exposure of topically applied drugs (corticosteroids, local anesthetic creams, antiseptics). Neonates have a tendency to form methemoglobin because they have reduced levels of methemoglobin reductase and fetal hemoglobin is more readily oxidized compared to adult hemoglobin. This, combined with increased absorption through the neonatal epidermis, resulted in reluctance to use lidocaine–prilocaine cream for repeat use in this age group [30, 31].

Alveolar

Anesthetic delivery to the alveoli is determined largely by alveolar ventilation and functional residual capacity (FRC). Neonates have increased alveolar ventilation. They also have a smaller FRC compared to adults because of increased chest wall compliance; this causes an increase in the speed of delivery. Pulmonary absorption is generally more rapid in infants and children than in adults [32]. The greater cardiac output and greater fraction of the cardiac output distributed to the vessel-rich tissue group (i.e., a clearance factor) and the lower tissue/blood solubility (i.e., a volume factor) also affect the more rapid wash-in of inhalational anesthetics in the younger age group [33]. Solubility determines volume of distribution. An inhalational agent with a greater volume of distribution will take longer to reach a steady-state concentration when delivered at a constant rate. The solubility in blood of halothane, isoflurane, enflurane, and methoxyflurane is 18 % less in neonates than in adults [34], attributable to altered serum albumin, globulin, cholesterol, and triglyceride concentrations. The solubility of these same agents in the vessel-rich tissue group in neonates is approximately one-half of those in adults [34]. The latter may be due to the greater water content and decreased protein and lipid concentration in neonatal tissues. Infants, with their decreased solubility would be expected to have a shorter time to reach a predetermined F_E/F_I ratio because of a smaller volume of distribution. Age has little effect on the solubility of the less-soluble agents, nitrous oxide and sevoflurane [35]. These principles also apply to new sedative techniques using inhalational drugs delivered by disposable anesthetic conserving devices (e.g., AnaConDa®,

Sedana Medical, Uppsala, Sweden). The wash-in kinetics for sevoflurane delivered by the AnaConDa are similar to those delivered by vaporizer [36]. Such devices have been used for sedation in the intensive care ward [37, 38] and may soon be used out of this locale [39].

Induction of anesthesia may be slowed by right-to-left shunting of blood in neonates suffering cyanotic congenital cardiac disease or intrapulmonary conditions. This slowing is greatest with the least soluble anesthetics [40]. Left to right shunts usually have minimal impact on uptake because cardiac output is increased so that systemic tissue perfusion is maintained at normal levels. The flow of mixed venous blood returning to the right heart ready for anesthetic uptake is normal. If cardiac output is not increased, and peripheral perfusion is reduced, then there will be less anesthetic uptake in the lung. Although alveolar anesthetic partial pressure may be observed to rise rapidly, there is a slower rise in tissue partial pressure and anesthetic effect is delayed.

Bioavailability

The oral bioavailability may be affected by interactions with food when feeding is frequent in the neonate (e.g., phenytoin [41]), by use of adult formulations that are divided or altered for pediatric use (nizatidine [42]), and by lower cytochrome P450 enzyme activity in the intestine. The latter may cause an increased bioavailability of midazolam because CYP3A activity is reduced [43]. The use of adult vials for pediatric use may result in dose inaccuracy, causing a relative increase or decrease in assumed bioavailability [44].

Analgesic medications and delivery systems commonly used in adults may not be possible or practicable in children because they do not have behavioral maturity. Infants are unable to use patient-controlled analgesia devices. Dose accuracy is lost when buccal and sublingual administration is attempted because those routes require prolonged exposure to the mucosal surface. Infants find it difficult to hold drug in their mouth for the requisite retention time (particularly if taste is unfavorable), and this results in more swallowed drug or drug spat out than in adults [45]. If the drug has a high first-pass effect, then the lower relative bioavailability results in lower plasma concentrations. Although many analgesics are available in an oral liquid formulation, taste is a strong determinant of compliance and unpalatable preparations may be refused [46]. Taste changes with age.

First-pass effect impacts on bioavailability and contribution of active metabolites to effect. The oral bioavailability of clonidine is low ($F=0.55$) in children 3–10 years. Consequently, higher oral doses of clonidine (per kg) are required when this formulation is used to achieve concentrations similar to those reported in adults [47]. Oral absorption is slow (absorption half-time 0.45 h) and peak concentrations are not reached until 1 h. Similarly, oral ketamine needs to be given in doses of up to 10 mg/kg to achieve therapeutic effect in children 1–8 years suffering burns [48]. Not only was bioavailability reduced ($F=0.45$) but absorption was also slow; absorption half-time was 59 min and had high between-subject variability in this cohort [48]. Analgesic effect, however, may be contributed by the increased concentration of the active metabolite norketamine.

The frequent passage of stools in the neonate may render suppository use ineffective. Variable absorption and bioavailability has resulted in respiratory arrest when repeat opioids are administered by the rectal route to children [49].

Distribution

At its simplest, volume of distribution determines the initial dose of a drug. The bigger the volume of distribution, the bigger the dose required to achieve a target concentration. However, many drugs used in anesthesia distribute to more than one compartment and do not have one simple volume of distribution. Bigger doses may cause bigger adverse effects, e.g., hypotension with propofol. Distribution is influenced by body composition, protein binding, hemodynamics (e.g., regional blood flow), and membrane permeability.

Body Composition

Total body water and extracellular fluid (ECF) [50] are increased in neonates, and reduction tends to follow postnatal age (PNA). Polar drugs such as the non-depolarizing neuromuscular blocking drugs (NMBDs) and aminoglycosides distribute rapidly into the ECF, but enter cells more slowly. The initial dose of such drugs is consequently higher in the neonate compared to the infant, older child, or adult.

The percentage of body weight contributed by fat is 3 % in a 1.5 kg premature neonate and 12 % in a term neonate; this proportion doubles by 4–5 months of age. "Baby fat" is lost when infants start walking and protein mass increases (20 % in a term neonate, 50 % in an adult). These body component changes affect volumes of distribution of drugs. Volume of distribution influences initial dose estimates. Fentanyl has an increased volume of distribution in neonates. The volume of distribution at steady state is 5.9 (standard deviation 1.5) L/kg in a neonate under 1 month of age compared to 1.6 (standard deviation 0.3) L/kg in an adult [51]. This may contribute to the reduced degree of respiratory depression seen after single doses as high as 10 μg/kg in older term neonates. The dramatic increase in muscle bulk in children from 3 years until adolescence influences drug dose required for neuromuscular blockade. The ED_{95} of vecuronium, for example, is 47 μg/kg standard deviation

11 μg/kg in neonates and infants, 81 μg/kg standard deviation 12 μg/kg in children between 3 and 10 years of age, and 55 μg/kg standard deviation 12 μg/kg in patients aged 13 years or older [52]. Dose is greater than anticipated in neonates who have immaturity of the neuromuscular junction because the ECV is increased but the duration of neuromuscular blockade is greater in neonates because of immature clearance pathways. The plasma concentration required in neonates to achieve the same level of neuromuscular block as in children or adults is 20–50 % less [53].

Reduction of propofol concentrations after induction is attributable to redistribution rather than rapid clearance because its pharmacokinetics is described using more than one compartment. Neonates have low body fat and muscle content and so less propofol is apportioned to these tissues. Delayed awakening occurs because central nervous system (CNS) concentration remains higher than that observed in older children as a consequence of reduced redistribution.

Plasma Proteins

Albumen and alpha-1 acid glycoprotein (AAG) concentrations are reduced in neonates but are similar to those in adults by 6 months, although between patient variability is high (e.g., AAG 0.32–0.92 g/L) [54, 55]. Bupivacaine is bound to AAG. The recommended bolus epidural dose of bupivacaine in neonates is lower than in children (1.5–2 mg/kg versus 2.5 mg/kg) because a greater proportion will be unbound drug and it is unbound drug that exerts effect. AAG is an acute phase reactant that increases after surgical stress. This causes an increase in total plasma concentrations for low to intermediate extraction drugs such as bupivacaine [56]. The unbound concentration, however, will not change because clearance of the unbound drug is affected only by the intrinsic metabolizing capacity of the liver. Any increase in unbound concentrations observed during long-term epidural is attributable to reduced clearance rather than AAG concentration [57, 58].

Plasma albumin concentrations are lowest in premature infants, and other fetal proteins such as alpha-fetoprotein (synthesized by the embryonic yolk sac, fetal gastrointestinal tract, and liver that has 40 % homology with albumin) have reduced affinity for drugs. In addition, increased concentrations of free fatty acids and unconjugated bilirubin compete with acidic drugs for albumin binding sites. Neonates also have a tendency to manifest a metabolic acidosis that alters ionization and binding properties of plasma proteins. Serum albumin concentrations approximate adult values by 5 months of age and binding capacity approaches adult values by 1 year of age. The induction dose of thiopentone is lower in neonates than older children. It is possible that this is related to decreased binding of thiopentone to plasma albumin; 13 % of the drug is unbound in newborns compared to 7 % in adults [59].

Regional Blood Flows

The initial phase of distribution after intravenous administration reflects regional blood flow. Consequently, the brain, heart, and liver are the tissues first exposed to the drug. Drug is then redistributed to other relatively well-perfused tissues, such as the skeletal muscle. There is a much slower tertiary distribution to relatively underperfused tissues of the body that is noted with long-term drug infusions. These changes contribute to a shorter context-sensitive half-time in infants with quicker "awakening" after sedative drugs; these infants have less fat and muscle bulk that drug can redistribute to and later leach out from. Clearance, however, is typically reduced in neonates and contributes to the longer observed context-sensitive half-time.

Apart from the neonatal circulatory changes that occur at birth (e.g., secondary to functional closure of the ductus venosus and ductus arteriosus), there are differences in relative organ mass and regional blood flow change with growth and development during the first few months of life. Blood flow, relative to cardiac output, to the kidney and brain increases, while that to the liver decreases through the neonatal period [60]. Cerebral and hepatic mass as a proportion of body weight are much higher in the infant than in the adult [61].

Mean cerebral blood flow is highest in early childhood (70 mL/min/100 g) at about 3–8 years of age [62]. It is reduced before this age in neonates and later in adults, where flows are similar (50 mL/min/100 g) [63]. The highly lipophilic induction agents diffuse rapidly across the blood–brain barrier (BBB) to achieve concentration equilibrium with brain tissue. Reduced cardiac output in neonates and reduced cerebral perfusion means that onset time after intravenous induction is slower in neonates that in early childhood. Offset time is also delayed because redistribution to the well-perfused and deep, underperfused tissues is less.

Blood–Brain Barrier

The BBB is an elaborate network of complex tight junctions between specialized endothelial cells that restricts the paracellular diffusion of hydrophilic molecules from the blood to the brain substance. Confusion over the importance of this barrier in the neonate exists, partly because of early studies comparing respiratory depression caused by the opioids, morphine, and pethidine. Greater respiratory depression was evident in neonates after morphine given as an adult equipotent dose of pethidine [64]. This finding is consistent with pethidine, unlike morphine, being lipid soluble and therefore crossing the immature or mature BBB equally [64]. However, plasma opioid concentrations were not measured in that study, and the increased neonatal respiratory depression observed after morphine when given the same dose (mg/kg) as adults could be due to reduced volume of distribution of morphine in term neonates 1–4 days (1.3 L/kg) compared to those at 8–60 days (1.8 L/kg), 61–180 days (2.4 L/kg), and adults (2.8 L/kg) [65]. Consequently we might expect initial concentrations of morphine to be higher in neonates than in adults and consequent respiratory depression greater. Respiratory depression, as measured by carbon dioxide response curves or by arterial oxygen tension, is similar in children from 2 to 570 days of age at the same morphine concentration [66].

The BBB may have impact in other ways. There are specific transport systems selectively expressed in the barrier endothelial cell membranes that mediate the transport of nutrients into the CNS and of toxic metabolites out of the CNS. Small molecules access fetal and neonatal brains more readily than they do adult brains [67]. BBB function improves gradually throughout fetal brain development, possibly reaching maturity at term [67]. Kernicterus, for example, is more common in the premature neonate than the term neonate. Pathological conditions within the CNS can cause BBB breakdown or alterations in transport systems play an important role in the pathogenesis of many CNS diseases. Proinflammatory substances and specific disease-associated proteins often mediate BBB dysfunction [68].

Fentanyl is actively transported across the BBB by a saturable ATP-dependent process, while ATP-binding cassette proteins such as P-glycoprotein actively pump out opioids such as fentanyl and morphine [69]. P-glycoprotein modulation significantly influences opioid brain distribution and onset time, magnitude, and duration of analgesic response [70]. Modulation may occur during disease processes, increased temperature, or other substances (e.g., verapamil, magnesium) [69]. Genetic polymorphisms affecting P-glycoprotein-related genes may explain some individual differences in CNS-active drug sensitivity [71].

Drug Metabolism

The main routes by which drugs and their metabolites leave the body are the hepatobiliary system, the kidneys, and the lungs. Elimination rate is commonly described by clearance. Clearance is the important pharmacokinetic parameter that is used to determine maintenance dose or infusion rate at steady state. The liver is the primary organ for clearance of most drugs, although the lungs have a major role for anesthetic vapors. Nonpolar, lipid-soluble drugs are converted to more polar and water-soluble compounds. Water-soluble drugs and metabolites rendered water soluble by the liver are excreted by the kidneys. Both hepatic and renal systems are immature in the neonate and mature within the first year of life. The impact of birth as an accelerator or temporal switch in the maturation of these processes remains uncertain. Maturation of these processes is commonly measured against postmenstrual age (PMA), although PNA may also have impact [72, 73] on maturation. The impact of birth on enzyme maturation is probably minor [74].

Descriptors for Metabolism Maturation

Three descriptors (size, maturation, and organ function) have been used to describe changes in clearance with age [75, 76]. There is a nonlinear relationship between clearance and size. Clearance in children 1–2 years of age, expressed as L/h/kg, is commonly greater than that observed in older children and adolescents. Consequently, infusion rates of propofol or remifentanil are higher in young children than in adolescents.

Size is commonly standardized using body surface area (BSA), and although the calculation of BSA commonly involves height and weight, it can also be expressed using weight alone [77]:

$$\text{BSA} \propto \text{weight}^{2/3}$$

However, in all species studied, including humans, the log of basal metabolic rate (BMR) plotted against the log of body weight produces a straight line with a slope of ¾. This is different to the BSA, which is described using body weight with an exponent of 2/3 [77]. Fractal geometry is used to mathematically explain this phenomenon known as allometry [78]. A great many physiological, structural, and time-related variables scale predictably within and between species with weight (W) exponents (PWR) of 3/4, 1, and 1/4, respectively [76].

These exponents have applicability to pharmacokinetic parameters such as clearance (CL), volume (V), and half-time [76]. The factor for size (F_{size}) for total drug clearance may be expected to scale weight with an exponent of ¾:

$$F_{size}\left(W/70\right)^{3/4}$$

The use of these allometric models allows prediction of dose in children from that of adult dose; such prediction is not possible using the mg/kg scaling. Pediatric doses in children out of the neonatal age group are greater than adults.

Remifentanil clearance in children 1 month–9 years is similar to adult rates when scaled using an allometric exponent of ¾ [79]. Remifentanil is hydrolyzed by nonspecific tissue and plasma esterases that do not appear to be influenced by age after scaling for size. Plasma esterases responsible for clearance are mature at birth [80].

The effect of size on the dose of remifentanil tolerated during spontaneous ventilation under anesthesia has been investigated in children undergoing strabismus surgery ($n=45$, age 6 months–9 years). The propofol infusion was titrated using state entropy as a pharmacodynamic endpoint and remifentanil infused, using a modified up-and-down method, with respiratory rate depression as a pharmacodynamic endpoint. A respiratory rate of just greater than 10, stable for 10 min, determined the final remifentanil infusion rate [81]. This influence of age on the remifentanil infusion requirement is shown in Fig. 11.1 [81–83]. Superimposed on this figure are clearance estimates for age, determined by size using an allometric model with a standardized clearance

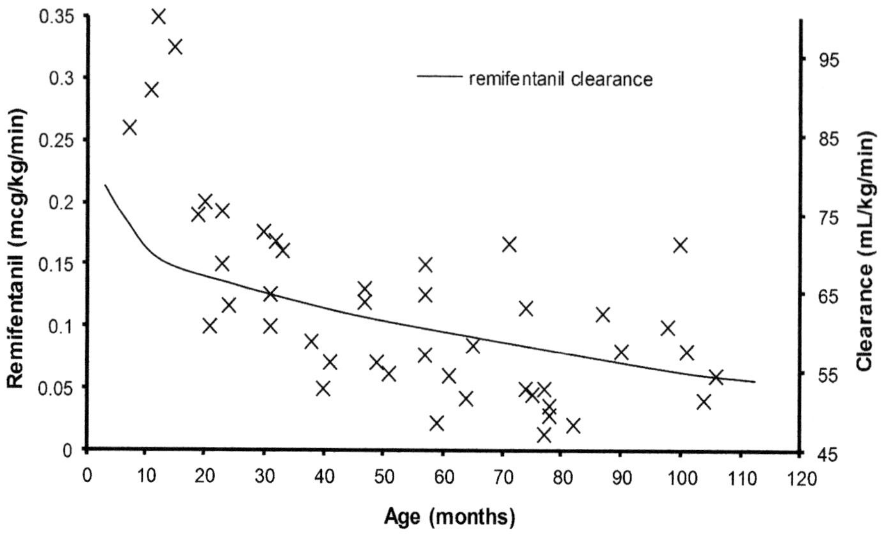

Fig. 11.1 The effect of age on the dose of remifentanil tolerated during spontaneous ventilation under anesthesia in children undergoing strabismus surgery [81]. Superimposed on this plot is estimated remifentanil clearance determined using an allometric model [82]. There is a mismatch between clearance and infusion rate for those individuals still in infancy (Reprinted with permission from Anderson BJ. Pediatric models for adult target-controlled infusion pumps. Paediatr Anaesth 2010 Mar;20(3):223-32)

of 2,790 mL/min for a 70 kg person. Clearance mirrors infusion rate in children over the age of 1 year. There is a divergence between clearance estimate and infusion rate in those children in infancy. The higher infusion rates recorded in those infants can be attributed to greater suppression of respiratory drive in this age group than the older children during the study; a respiratory rate of ten breaths per minute in an infant is disproportionately slow compared to the same rate in a 7-year-old child, suggesting excessive dose.

For most drugs, however, allometry alone is insufficient to predict clearance in neonates and infants from adult estimates. Most clearance systems are not mature at birth. The addition of a model describing clearance maturation with age is required. The sigmoid hyperbolic function (also known as the Hill equation) [84] (also used to describe the oxygen saturation curve) has also been found useful for describing this maturation process (MF).

$$\mathrm{MF} = \frac{\mathrm{PMA}^{\mathrm{Hill}}}{\mathrm{TM}_{50}^{\mathrm{Hill}} + \mathrm{PMA}^{\mathrm{Hill}}}$$

The TM_{50} describes the maturation half-time, while the Hill coefficient relates to the slope of this maturation profile. Maturation of a considerable number of drugs has now been described using this equation [85]. The maturation profile for dexmedetomidine expressed using allometric scaling, and this maturation model is shown in Fig. 11.2 [86].

Organ function (OF) remains the other major covariate influence on clearance. While renal pathology may be reflected by assessment such as creatinine clearance, distinguishing this from normal physiology in infants may be difficult unless ordinary renal maturation is understood [75]. Although specific organ dysfunction of the kidney or liver is well recognized as having effect on clearance, other processes (sepsis, malnutrition, disease severity scores) can also be used as markers of reduced clearance. Midazolam clearance was noted to be reduced in critically ill children. This was assumed to be due to reduced CYP3A activity, although reduced hepatic blood flow is more likely [87]. Pharmacokinetic parameters (P) can be described in an individual as the product of size (F_{size}), maturation (MF), and organ function (OF) influences where P_{std} is the value in a standard size adult without pathological changes in organ function:

$$P = P_{\mathrm{std}} \cdot F_{\mathrm{size}} \cdot \mathrm{MF} \cdot \mathrm{OF}$$

This methodology is increasingly used to describe clearance changes with age [85]. An understanding of these principles can be used to predict dose in children using target concentration methodology [88].

When maturation changes have not been described using real data, then an alternative method known as the physiological-based pharmacokinetic (PBPK) model can be used to predict changes with age. Organ maturation, body composition, and ontogeny of drug elimination pathways have marked effects on pharmacokinetic parameters in the first few years of life. PBPK models require detailed physiological data. Data on ontogeny of individual clearance pathways, derived from measurements of enzyme expression and activity in postmortem livers, and from in vivo data from drugs that are cleared by similar pathways are useful. Continued input of information concerning genetic, physiological, organ and tissue size and composition, protein binding, demographic and clinical data into the library, and algorithms for PBPK modeling programs has progressively improved their prediction ability. These models have been used to assist with first-time dosing in children [89–91]. The introduction of population variability in enzyme abundance and activity contributes to between-individual variability estimates [92]. This approach has been recently used to investigate fentanyl maturation changes with age in neonates [93].

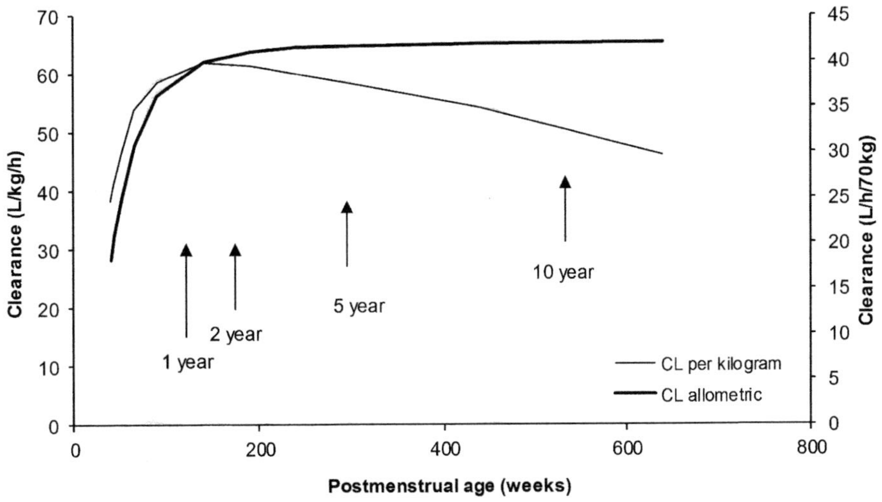

Fig. 11.2 Dexmedetomidine clearance changes with age, expressed both as per kilogram and using allometric scaling with a maturation model. The per kilogram model (L/h/kg) demonstrates an increased clearance in infants that explains the observed increased infusion (mg/min/kg) required for sedation in this age group. The use of the allometric model allows better understanding of the clearance maturation process (Data from Potts et al. [86])

Hepatic Elimination

Phase 1

The mixed function P450 (CYP, so named because these enzymes absorb light at wavelengths near 450 nm) oxidases are reduced [94, 95]. Enzyme maturation occurs at different rates. Individual hepatic drug-metabolizing enzymes have been categorized into one of three classes based on developmental trajectories [96]. Class 1 enzymes are expressed at their highest levels in the fetus during the first trimester (e.g., CYP3A7 that may have a role in retinoic metabolism); enzymes belonging to the second class are expressed at relatively constant levels throughout gestation and into adulthood (e.g., sulfotransferase, SULT1A1, responsible for most of paracetamol clearance in neonates). The vast majority of enzymes (Class 3, e.g., CYP3A4, UGT2B7; see below) are expressed at low levels at birth and mature with time.

The activity of the CYP2E1 enzyme surges after birth [97], CYP2D6 (e.g., codeine, tramadol) becomes detectable soon thereafter, and the CYP3A4 (e.g., midazolam) and CYP2C (e.g., diclofenac) family appear during the first week, whereas CYP1A2 (e.g., caffeine) is the last to appear [98]. Neonates are dependent on the immature CYP3A4 for levobupivacaine clearance and CYP1A2 for ropivacaine clearance, dictating reduced epidural infusion rates in this age group [99–101]. Some of these maturation rates have been described, e.g., midazolam [102] and levobupivacaine [103].

If a drug has a high extraction ratio, then intrinsic clearance may be very much greater than liver blood flow, and in these situations, hepatic clearance is primarily determined by liver blood flow characteristics. Fentanyl clearance (CYP3A4) is 70–80 % of adult values in term neonates and, standardized to a 70-kg person, reaches adult values within the first few weeks of life [57]. Omphalocele repair may be associated with raised intra-abdominal pressure (an organ function effect) resulting in reduced fentanyl clearance attributable to decreased hepatic blood flow.

Phase 2

Some phase II pathways are mature in term neonates at birth (sulfate conjugation), while others are not (acetylation, glycination, glucuronidation) [104]. Allometric body-size scaling complimented by maturation models [76, 105] has been used to unravel the developmental PK of drugs cleared by glucuronosyltransferase. Paracetamol and morphine are cleared by individual isoforms of glucuronosyltransferase (UGT1A6 and UGT2B7), as is bilirubin (UGT1A1). Clearance of both drugs [106–108] is immature in the premature 24-week PMA neonate and mature to reach adult rates by the first year of life. Dexmedetomidine is also cleared predominantly by the UGT system and has a similar maturation profile [109]. Glucuronidation is also the major metabolic pathway of propofol metabolism, although multiple cytochrome P450 isoenzymes, including CYP2B6, CYP2C9, or CYP2A6, contribute to its metabolism and cause a faster maturation profile (Fig. 11.3) [105, 109–113] than expected from glucuronide conjugation alone [73].

This maturation process can be difficult to discern because other factors such as illness impact on observed clearance. Morphine clearance is greater in infants undergoing noncardiac surgery than in those after cardiac surgery [114], or in those receiving extracorporeal membrane oxygenation [115] or positive pressure ventilation [110]. Similarly clearance of propofol was reduced after cardiac surgery in children admitted to a pediatric intensive care [116]. Dexmedetomidine clearance is reduced with low cardiac output, consistent with reduced hepatic blood flow [117]. A circadian night rhythm effect was noted in an investigation of infant propofol sedation after major craniofacial surgery [118].

Renal Elimination

Drugs and their metabolites are excreted by the kidneys by two processes—glomerular filtration and tubular secretion—that mature at different rates [119]. Glomerular filtration rate

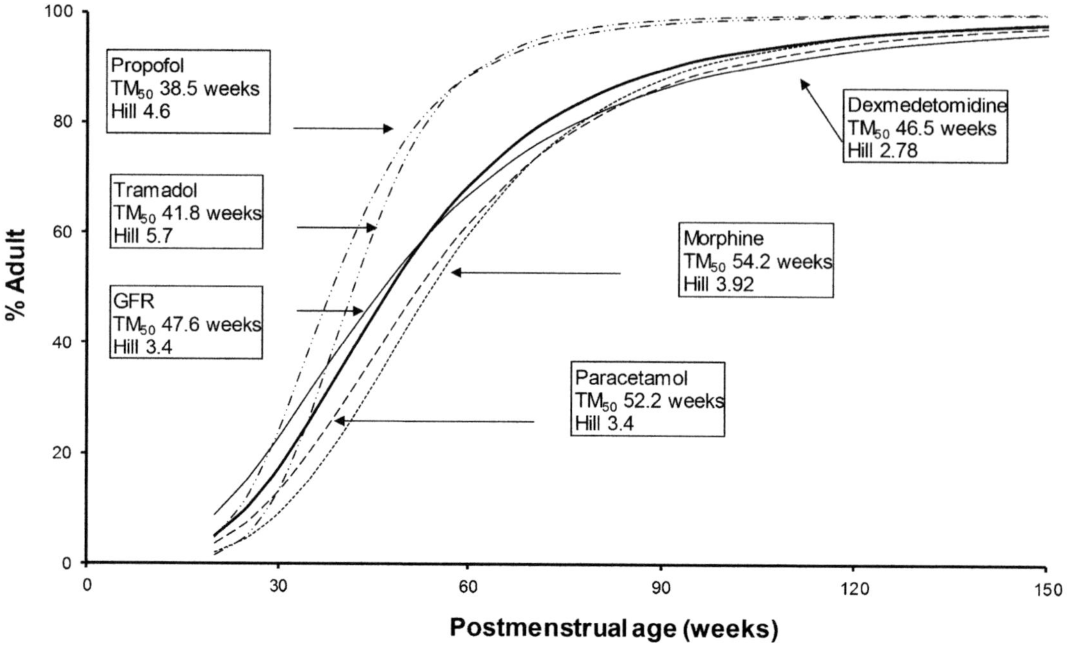

Fig. 11.3 Clearance maturation, expressed as a percentage of mature clearance, of drugs where glucuronide conjugation (paracetamol, morphine, dexmedetomidine) plays a major role. These profiles are closely aligned with glomerular filtration rate (GFR). In contrast, cytochrome P450 isoenzymes also contribute to propofol metabolism and cause a faster maturation profile than expected from glucuronide conjugation alone. Tramadol clearance maturation (phase I, CYP2D6, CYP3A) is also rapid. Maturation parameter estimates were taken from references [105, 109–113]

(GFR) is only 10 % that of mature value at 25 weeks, 35 % at term, and 90 % of the adult GFR at 1 year of age [111]. Tubular secretion maturation lags behind that of GFR [119]. Aminoglycosides are almost exclusively cleared by renal elimination, and maintenance dose is predicted by PMA because it predicts the time course of development of renal function [120]. The clearance of the old NMBD, D-tubocurarine, can be directly correlated with GFR [121].

Immaturity of clearance pathways can be used to our advantage when managing apnea after anesthesia in the premature nursery graduate. N_7-methylation of theophylline in the newborn to produce caffeine is well developed whereas oxidative demethylation (CYP1A2) responsible for caffeine metabolism is deficient and develops over the ensuing months. Theophylline is effective for the management of postoperative apnea in the premature neonate, partly because it is a prodrug of caffeine, which is effective controlling apnea. Caffeine can only be slowly cleared by the immature kidney and is mature by 60 weeks PMA [122].

Pulmonary Elimination

The factors determining anesthetic absorption (alveolar ventilation, FRC, cardiac output, tissue/blood solubility) also contribute to elimination. We might anticipate more rapid washout in neonates than adults for any given duration of anesthesia because there is less distribution to fat and muscle content. The greater decrease in cardiac output induced by halothane in neonates might be expected to speed elimination, but brain perfusion will also be reduced and this slows recovery. Halothane, in particular, and to a far lesser extent isoflurane and sevoflurane undergo hepatic metabolism, but contribution is small compared to pulmonary elimination [123].

Metabolites

Many drugs have active metabolites that contribute to effect. Examples include norketamine from ketamine [124], 4′-hydroxydiclofenac from diclofenac [125], *O*-demethyl tramadol from tramadol [112], hydroxymidazolam from midazolam [126], and morphine 6-glucuronide (M6G) from morphine [127].

Contributions to both the desired effect (analgesia) and the undesired effects (nausea, respiratory depression) of M6G remain uncertain [128]. The EC_{50} for both morphine and M6G appear similar [129, 130], but M6G takes greater time (4–8 h versus 16 min) to equilibrate with the effect site [129, 131]. The relative ratios of morphine to M6G vary in neonates and early infancy, depending on relative maturation of UGT2B7 (formation of M6G) and GFR (elimination of M6G). Term neonates less than 7 days old have a lower ratio of plasma morphine/M6G than those over 1 year despite similar doses [74, 132]. The impact of this is unclear.

Pharmacogenomics

Pharmacogenomics (PG) is the investigation of variations of DNA and RNA characteristics as related to drug response that incorporates both PK and PD. There is large between-individual PK variability that is contributed to by polymorphisms of the genes encoding for metabolic enzymes [133]. Genetic variability influencing plasma cholinesterase activity and its influence on succinylcholine is a well-known example. Another example is the CYP2D6 single nuclear polymorphism (SNP) that is inherited as an autosomal recessive trait. Homozygous individuals are deficient in the metabolism of a variety of important groups of drugs: β(beta)-adrenoceptor blocking agents, antidepressants, neuroleptic agents, and opioids. Poor metabolizers have reduced morphine production from codeine [134, 135]. Tramadol is also metabolized by O-demethylation in the liver (CYP2D6) to *O*-desmethyl tramadol (M1), and the M1 metabolite has a mu-opioid affinity approximately 200 times greater than tramadol.

An SNP is only important if it contributes greater than 50 % metabolism, has an active metabolite, a steep dose–response relationship, and a narrow therapeutic index. These polymorphisms may have little impact during the neonatal period when metabolism is developmentally limited [5, 112, 136–138]. SNPs will certainly have impact in infants and children. Impact will be dependent on the rate of maturation of the specific enzyme system. Certainly ultra-extensive metabolizers of codeine (CYP2D6) may suffer respiratory depression resulting from the rapid formation of morphine [139]. Reports of death due to respiratory compromise in children given codeine for pain relief after tonsillectomy may limit the future use of this drug [140].

Pharmacogenomic differences also have impact on PD. Candidate genes involved in pain perception, pain processing, and pain management like opioid receptors, transporters, and other targets of pharmacotherapy are under investigation [141]. Genetic differences (e.g., G118 allele) may explain why some patients need higher opioid doses and the adverse effects profile may be modified by these mutations [142]. Some genes (e.g., fetal hemoglobin) are expressed much more in early life than in adults, and gene switching may mean a drug is effective at one age and not another.

In adults, gene testing may prove valuable for reducing adverse drug effects [143, 144]. However, most drug responses involve a large number of proteins regulated by multiple genes. Genotype does not equate with phenotype; environment, concomitant therapy, and disease have impact, and allele prevalence varies among ethnic groups [145]. The situation in children is more complex. Allelic variants may remain unchanged throughout life, but transcriptomic, proteomic, and metabolomic data in children are continuously changing throughout the development.

Pharmacodynamic Differences in the First Year of Life

Children's responses to drugs have much in common with the responses in adults [146]. For example, acetaminophen analgesia appears similar in both neonates and children [147]. The perception that drug effects differ in children arises because the drugs have not been adequately studied in pediatric populations who have size- and maturation-related effects as well as different diseases. Neonates and infants, however, often do have altered pharmacodynamics.

The minimal alveolar concentration (MAC) for almost all anesthetic vapors is less in neonates than in infancy, which is in turn greater than that observed in children and adults [33]. MAC of isoflurane in preterm neonates less than 32 weeks gestation was 1.28 %, and MAC in neonates 32–37 weeks gestation was 1.41 % [148]. This value rose to 1.87 % by 6 months before decreasing again over childhood [148]. The cause of these differences is uncertain and may relate to maturation changes in cerebral blood flow, gamma-aminobutyric acid ($GABA_A$) receptor numbers, or developmental shifts in the regulation of chloride transporters. Delivery of halothane to neonates at a MAC suitable for adults contributed to bradycardia and increased mortality in neonates [149].

The dose of thiopentone varies with age, e.g., 3.4 mg/kg in neonates, 6.3 mg/kg in infants, and 4.5 mg/kg in children 4–7 years [150, 151]. It remains uncertain whether altered pharmacokinetics or pharmacodynamic responses explain the reduced dose requirements in neonates. The effect site concentration of thiopentone for induction of anesthesia in neonates may be less than that in infants because the neonate has relatively immature cerebral cortical function, rudimentary dendritic arborizations, and relatively few synapses, but there are no studies to support or refute this premise.

Neonates have an increased sensitivity to the effects of NMBDs [121]. The reason for this is unknown but it is consistent with the observation that there is a threefold reduction in the release of acetylcholine from the infant rat phrenic nerve [152, 153]. The increased volume of distribution, however, means that a single NMBD dose is the same as the older child; reduced clearance prolongs duration.

Cardiac calcium stores in the endoplasmic reticulum are reduced in the neonatal heart because of immaturity. Exogenous calcium has greater impact on contractility in this age group than in older children or adults. Conversely, calcium channel blocking drugs (e.g., verapamil) can cause life-threatening bradycardia and hypotension [154]. There are some data to suggest greater sensitivity to warfarin in children, but the mechanism is not determined [155]. Amide local anesthetic agents induce shorter block duration and require a larger weight-scaled dose to achieve similar dermatomal levels when given by subarachnoid block to infants.

This may be due, in part, to myelination, spacing of nodes of Ranvier, and length of nerve exposed as well as size factors and cerebrospinal fluid volume changes with age. There is an age-dependent expression of intestinal motilin receptors and the modulation of gastric antral contractions in neonates. Prokinetic agents may not be useful in very preterm infants, partially useful in older preterm infants, and useful in full-term infants. Similarly, bronchodilators in infants are ineffective because of the paucity of bronchial smooth muscle that can cause bronchospasm.

Measurement of PD Endpoints

Outcome measures are more difficult to assess in neonates and infants than in children or adults. Measurement techniques, disease and pathology differences, inhomogeneous groups, recruitment issues, ethical considerations, and endpoint definition for establishing efficacy and safety confuse data interpretation [156].

Common effects measured include anesthesia depth, pain, and sedation and neuromuscular blockade. A common effect measure used to assess depth of anesthesia is the electroencephalogram or a modification of detected EEG signals (spectral edge frequency, bispectral index [BIS], entropy). Physiological studies in adults and children indicate that EEG-derived anesthesia depth monitors can provide an imprecise and drug-dependent measure of arousal. Although the outputs from these monitors do not closely represent any true physiological entity, they can be used as guides for anesthesia and in so doing have improved outcomes in adults. In older children, the physiology, anatomy, and clinical observations indicate the performance of the monitors may be similar to that in adults. In infants their use cannot yet be supported in theory or in practice [157, 158]. During anesthesia, the EEG in infants is fundamentally different from the EEG in older children; there remains a need for specific neonate-derived algorithms if EEG-derived anesthesia depth monitors are to be used in neonates [159, 160].

New monitoring devices continue to be investigated. For example, a mid-latency auditory evoked potential-derived index of depth of hypnosis was recently investigated, but found inferior to BIS for differentiating different levels of sedation [161]. Alternative EEG signal-processing devices show promise and have been used to deliver closed-loop anesthesia [162].

The Children's Hospital of Wisconsin Sedation Scale [163] has been used to investigate ketamine in the emergency department [164]. However, despite the use of such scales in procedural pain or sedation studies, few behavioral scales have been adequately validated in this setting [165, 166]. Interobserver variability can be high [167]. The COMFORT sedation scale [168] is one scoring system that is finding increasing usefulness in the pediatric intensive care setting. It is well validated [169], appears useful in different cultures, and has even been extended to premature neonates [170] and children with Trisomy 21 [171]. Changing patterns of drug use and reconsideration of what constitutes important adverse events may result in new definitions of the sedation continuum [172, 173]. Unfortunately, most pain scores are validated for the acute, procedural setting and perform less for subacute or chronic pain or stress. Postoperative nausea is difficult to quantify in neonates and infants who cannot verbalize; this makes comparison with adult postoperative nausea and vomiting scales tenuous.

Population Modeling

Mathematical models describe complex systems in simple terms, enabling us to describe, predict, and explain observations. Pharmacokinetic (PK) and pharmacodynamic (PD) models are used to improve pediatric anesthetic and sedation management. They quantify the exposure–response relationship, often providing clarity and insight into complex systems as well as a mechanistic understanding of the drug effect. Dose selection can be rationalized. Models may enable extrapolation beyond observed data. Modeling is a knowledge management tool; it captures and integrates data from all studies. Models can also be used for hypothesis testing and can drive decision-making during drug development.

Population PK and PD modeling using nonlinear mixed effects models has had enormous impact in adult anesthetic pharmacology. This methodology has particular applicability in children where the blood volume available for sampling is limited. Sparse data from multiple subjects can be used. Sampling times are not crucial for population methods and can be fitted around clinical procedures or outpatient appointments. Sampling time bands rather than exact times are equally effective and allow flexibility in neonates. Sampling cannulae used for PK studies may block or tissue, parents may refuse repeat sampling, and repeat venipuncture is frowned upon. Missing data, however, can still be used in a pediatric population analysis. Data from different studies can be pooled [174, 175].

The Target Concentration Approach

The goal of treatment is the target effect. (Refer to Chap. 31.) A pharmacodynamic model is used to predict the target concentration given a target effect. Population estimates for the PD model parameters and covariate information are used to predict typical PD values in a specific patient. Population estimates of PK model parameter estimates and covariate information are then used to predict typical PK values in a typical patient. For example, a dexmedetomidine steady-state target concentration of 0.6 μg/L may be achieved with an infusion of 0.33 μg/kg/h in a neonate, 0.51 μg/kg/h in a 1-year-old, and 0.47 μg/kg/h in an 8-year-old [109]. This target concentration strategy is a powerful tool for determining clinical dose [176]. Monitoring of serum drug concentrations and Bayesian forecasting may be used to improve dosing in individual patients.

This target effect approach is intrinsic to pediatric anesthetists using target-controlled infusion systems. These devices target a specific plasma or effect site concentration in a typical individual, and this concentration is assumed to have a typical target effect. The target concentration is one that achieves target therapeutic effect (e.g., anesthesia or a sedation level) without excessive adverse effects (e.g., hypotension). Effect monitoring (e.g., BIS) can be used to refine the target effect.

Pharmacokinetic Models

Compartment models dominate the sedative and analgesic literature. Standard compartment models may be unable to accurately describe drug concentrations immediately after bolus administration of an anesthetic induction agent because mixing in the central compartment is not instantaneous, making it difficult to model the fast blood-to-brain concentration equilibrium [177], and pulmonary uptake may also occur [178]. Recirculatory models help explain these early phase PK [179]. Such models have proved valuable determining anesthetic induction doses [180] and NMBD pharmacodynamics [181]. Physiologically based pharmacokinetic (PBPK) modeling has been used to assist with first-time dosing in children. A general PBPK model for drug disposition in infants and children, covering the age range from birth to adulthood, has been successfully evaluated using theophylline and midazolam as model drugs [60].

A single compartment is often insufficient to characterize the time-concentration profile, and further compartments are required (mammillary models). Drug is administered into a central compartment (V1) and redistributes to peripheral compartments (V2, V3, etc.; Fig. 11.4a). In a two-compartment model, transfer of drug between the central and peripheral compartment is relatively fast compared with the rate of elimination. Such models can be applied to both intravenous and inhalational drugs. The anesthetic conserving device (AnaConDa) delivering sevoflurane has also been described using compartment models [182]. A plot of the natural log of concentration after bolus reveals two distinct slopes (rate constants, α[alpha] and β[beta], Fig. 11.4b). Consequently the time-concentration profile is commonly described using a polyexponential function:

$$C(t) = A \cdot e^{-\alpha \cdot t} + B \cdot e^{-\beta \cdot t}$$

These polyexponential parameters have little connection with underlying physiology, and an alternative parameterization is the use of a central volume and three rate constants (k_{10}, k_{12}, k_{21}) that describe drug distribution between compartments. Another common method is to use two volumes (V_1, V_2) and two clearances (CL, Q). Q is the intercompartment clearance.

Students are commonly taught to estimate compartment model PK parameters through interpretation of graphs representing time-concentration profiles. Conversion of concentration to a log scale allows estimation of elimination constants and compartment volumes (Fig. 11.4c). Integration of the function describing this profile yields an AUC (area under the curve), from which CL can be determined:

$$\mathrm{CL} = \mathrm{Dose} / \mathrm{AUC}$$

Computers have made the use of nonlinear regression to directly estimate parameters through iterative techniques using least squares curve fitting. Models with two or more compartments are now commonly solved using differential equations.

Parameter estimates (CL, Q, V_1, V_2) can be used to predict dose. A loading dose raises concentration in the plasma to target concentration promptly and may be desirable in anesthesia when rapid effect is required. In a one-compartment model, the volume of distribution is the proportionality factor that relates total amount of drug in the body to plasma concentration (TC = target concentration):

$$\text{Loading dose} = V.\mathrm{TC}$$

This calculation may not be applicable to many sedative drugs that are characterized using multi-compartment models. The use of V_1 results in a loading dose too high; too high a dose may cause transient toxicity.

An alternative technique is to use the target effect dose. The time to peak effect (T_{peak}) is dependent on clearance and effect site equilibration half-time ($T_{1/2keo}$). At a submaximal dose, T_{peak} is independent of dose. At supramaximal doses, maximal effect will occur earlier than T_{peak} and persist for longer duration. The T_{peak} concept has been used to calculate optimal initial bolus doses [183].

Clearance is the most important parameter when defining a rational steady-state dosage regimen. At steady state:

Dosing rate_{ss} = rate of elimination_{ss} = CL · TC

When a drug is given intermittently:

$$\text{Dosing rate} = \text{maintenance dose} \times \text{dosing interval}$$

When a drug is given by constant infusion:

$$\text{Infusion rate}_{ss} = \text{dosing rate}_{ss}$$

Once the target concentration of a drug is defined, the infusion rate is determined by CL at steady state. Many sedative drugs distribute to peripheral compartments and steady state may

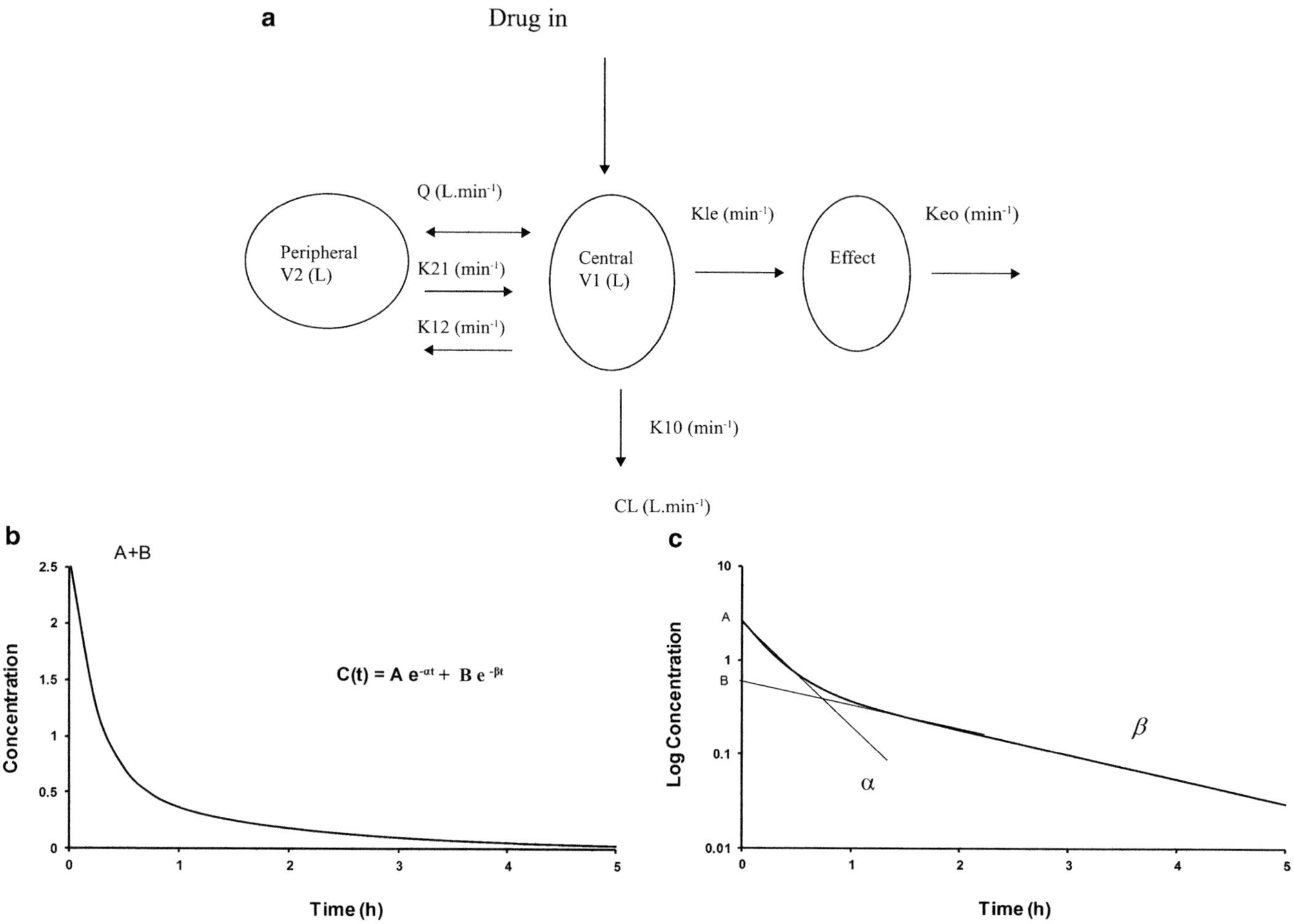

Fig. 11.4 (**a**) A mammillary two-compartment PK model with additional compartment for effect. (Reprinted with permission from Anderson BJ. Pediatric models for adult target-controlled infusion pumps. Paediatr Anaesth 2010 Mar;20(3):223-32.) (**b**) Time-concentration profile for a two-compartment model. (**c**) Conversion of concentration to a log scale allows estimation of elimination constants and compartment volumes

not be achieved during the time of infusion. Dose adjustment is required to achieve constant effect until steady-state conditions are reached.

Propofol PK are usually described using a three-compartment mammillary model. In order to achieve steady state, 3 μg/mL in children 3–11 years, dosing changes are required, e.g., a loading dose of 2.5 mg/kg followed by an infusion rate of 15 mg/kg/h for the first 15 min, 13 mg/kg/h from 15 to 30 min, 11 mg/kg/h from 30 to 60 min, 10 mg/kg/h from 1 to 2 h, and 9 mg/kg/h from 2 to 4 h. Target-controlled infusion (TCI) pumps are capable of fine-tuning by making adjustments at 10 s intervals [184].

The PK of drug disposition confined to a one-compartment model is often expressed in terms of half-life. Half-life ($T_{1/2}$) is the time required to change the amount of drug in a body compartment by one-half:

$$T_{1/2} = \text{In}(2) \cdot \frac{\text{V}}{\text{CL}}$$

This half-life is related to the elimination rate constant (k), a parameter representing the slope of the exponential decay curve:

$$k = \frac{\text{CL}}{\text{V}}$$

Elimination half-life is of no value in characterizing disposition of intravenous anesthetic drugs with multiple compartments during dosing periods relevant to anesthesia. A more useful concept is that of the context-sensitive half-time where "context" refers to infusion duration. This is the time required for the plasma drug concentration to decline by 50 % after terminating infusion [185]. The context-sensitive half-time is the same as the elimination half-life for a one-compartment model and does not change with infusion duration.

Context-sensitive half-time may be independent of infusion duration (e.g., remifentanil 2.5 min), moderately affected (propofol 12 min at 1 h, 38 min at 8 h), or display marked prolongation (e.g., fentanyl 1 h at 24 min, 8 h at 280 min). This is due to return of drug to plasma from peripheral compartments after ceasing infusion. Peripheral compartment size differs in children from adults, so that at termination of infusion, more drug may remain in the body for any given plasma concentration than in adults. The context-sensitive half-time for children given propofol, for example, is longer [184]. The context-sensitive half-time gives insight into PK of a hypnotic drug, but the parameter may not be clinically relevant because the percentage decrease in concentration required for recovery is not necessarily 50 %.

Pharmacodynamic Models

Pharmacokinetics is what the body does to the drug, while pharmacodynamics is what the drug does to the body. The precise boundary between these two processes is ill defined and often requires a link describing movement of drug from the plasma to the effect site and its target. Drugs may exert effect at nonspecific membrane sites, by interference with transport mechanisms, by enzyme inhibition or induction, or by activation or inhibition of receptors.

The Sigmoid E_{max} Model

The relation between drug concentration and effect may be described by the Hill equation (see maturation model above), well known to anesthesiologists through the oxygen dissociation curve [84], according to the equation:

$$\text{Effect} = E_0 = \frac{\left(E_{\max} \cdot C_e^{\,N}\right)}{\left(\text{EC}_{50}^{N} + C_e^{\,N}\right)}$$

where E_0 is the baseline response, E_{max} is the maximum effect change, C_e is the concentration in the effect compartment, EC_{50} is the concentration producing 50 % E_{max}, and N is the Hill coefficient defining the steepness of the concentration–response curve. Efficacy is the maximum response on a dose or concentration–response curve. EC_{50} can be considered a measure of potency relative to another drug, provided N and E_{max} for the two drugs are the same. A concentration–response relationship for acetaminophen has been described using this model. An EC_{50} of 9.8 mg/L, $N=1$, and an E_{max} of 5.3 pain units (VAS 0–10) was reported [186]. Midazolam PD in adults has been similarly defined using EEG response [187, 188]. Adverse effects can also be described using this model; the reduced cardiac output observed as dexmedetomidine concentration increases has been expressed using a sigmoid E_{max} model with a EC_{50} of 2.4 μg/L and N 3.15 [117]. Blood pressure changes in children given dexmedetomidine have also been described using Emax models [189].

Quantal Effect Model

The potency of anesthetic vapors may be expressed by MAC (minimum alveolar concentration), and this is the concentration at which 50 % of subjects move in response to a standard surgical stimulus. MAC appears at first sight to be similar to EC_{50}, but is an expression of quantal response rather than magnitude of effect. There are two methods of estimating MAC. Responses can be recorded over the clinical dose range in a large number of subjects and logistic regression applied to estimate the relationship between dose and quantal effect; the MAC can then be interpolated. Large numbers of subjects may not be available and so an alternative is often used. The "up-and-down" method described by Dixon [190, 191] estimates only the MAC rather than the entire sigmoid curve. It involves a study of only one concentration in each subject and, in a sequence of subjects, each receives a concentration depending upon the response of the previous subject; the concentration is either increased if the previous subject did not respond or decreased if they did. The MAC is usually calculated either as the mean concentration of equal numbers of responses and no-responses or is the mean concentration of pairs of "response-no response." This method has also been applied to drugs other than inhalation vapors, e.g., local anesthesia dose for spinal block [192, 193].

Logistic Regression Model

When the pharmacological effect is difficult to grade, then it may be useful to estimate the probability of achieving the effect as a function of plasma concentration. Effect measures such as movement/no movement or rousable/non-rousable are dichotomous. Logistic regression is commonly used to analyze such data, and the interpolated EC_{50} value refers to the probability of response. For example, an EC_{50} of 0.52 mg/L for arousal after ketamine sedation in children has been estimated using this technique [164].

Linking PK with PD

A simple situation in which drug effect is directly related to concentration does not mean that drug effects parallel the time course of concentration. This occurs only when the concentration is low in relation to EC_{50}. In this situation, the half-life of the drug may correlate closely with the half-life of drug effect. Observed effects may not be directly related to serum concentration. Many drugs have a short half-life but a long duration of effect. This may be attributable to induced physiological changes (e.g., aspirin and platelet function) or may be due to the shape of the E_{max} model. If the initial concentration is very high in relation to the EC_{50}, then drug concentrations 5 half-lives later, when we might expect minimal concentration, may still exert considerable effect [74]. There may be a delay due to transfer of the drug to effect site (NMBD), a lag time (diuretics), physiological response (antipyresis), active metabolite (propacetamol), or synthesis of physiological substances (warfarin).

A plasma concentration–effect plot can form a hysteresis loop because of this delay in effect. Hull [194] and Sheiner [195] introduced the effect compartment concept for muscle relaxants. The effect compartment concentration is not the same as the blood or serum concentration and is not a real measurable concentration. It has negligible volume and contains negligible blood. A single first order parameter ($T_{1/2keo}$) describes the equilibration half-time. This mathematical trick assumes concentration in the central compartment is the same as that in the effect compartment at equilibration, but that a time delay exists before drug reaches the effect compartment. The concentration in the effect compartment is used to describe the concentration–effect relationship [196].

Adult $T_{1/2keo}$ values are well described, e.g., morphine 16 min, fentanyl 5 min, alfentanil 1 min, and propofol 3 min. This $T_{1/2keo}$ parameter is commonly incorporated into TCI pumps in order to achieve a rapid effect site concentration. The adult midazolam $T_{1/2keo}$ of 5 min [197] may be prolonged in the elderly [198, 199], resulting in overdose if this is not recognized during dose titration.

Onset of drug effect is quicker with decreasing age. We might expect a shorter propofol $T_{1/2keo}$ with decreasing age based on size models [200], and this is exactly what has been described by Jeleazcov et al. [201]. Similar results have been demonstrated for sevoflurane and BIS [202]. If unrecognized, this will result in excessive dose in a young child if the effect site is targeted and peak effect (T_{peak}) is anticipated to be later than it actually is because it was determined in a teenager or adult. Unfortunately, integrated PKPD studies in children are lacking. Available pediatric propofol $T_{1/2keo}$ values have been determined by application of published PK data to PD observations only [203–205].

Adverse Effects

Neonates and young children may suffer permanent effects resulting from a stimulus applied at a sensitive point in development. For example, congenital hypothyroidism, if untreated, causes lifelong phenotypic changes. The incidence of vaginal carcinoma is high in children of mothers treated with stilboestrol during pregnancy [206]. There are concerns that neonatal exposure to some anesthetic agents (e.g., ketamine, midazolam) may cause widespread neuronal apoptosis and long-term memory deficits [207, 208].

Anesthesia, analgesia, or sedation generally involves examination of immediate adverse effects such as PONV, hypotension, or respiratory depression. A dose–response curve for intravenous morphine and vomiting was investigated in children having day-stay tonsillectomy. Doses above 0.1 mg/kg were associated with a greater than 50 % incidence of vomiting [209]. These data are similar to those in children undergoing inguinal herniorrhaphy [210], suggesting that lower doses of morphine are associated with a decreased incidence of emesis after day-stay surgery, and encourage the use of alternative analgesic drugs.

Therapeutic use of drugs balances beneficial effects against adverse effects. Adverse effects, however, may be simply consequent upon a poor understanding of pharmacokinetics. Propofol infusion dose in neonates, if based on adult dose (mg/kg/h), will overdose and cause hypotension; propofol infusion dose in 1–2-year-olds (where clearance is increased expressed as mg/kg/h) may underdose and result in awareness. Morphine dose in the very young was traditionally limited by fears of respiratory compromise; postoperative arterial oxygen desaturation continues to be reported with sedative drugs in neonates [211]. These are a result of poor pharmacokinetic understanding. However, there are also pharmacodynamic differences. Premature neonates are more prone to apnea. Sympathetic–parasympathetic tone is immature in neonates, and the use of propofol in neonates has recently been associated with profound hypotension [212], questioning our understanding of the dose–effect relationships of this common drug [213]. Such information allows informed dosing.

Drug Interactions

Drug interactions can increase or decrease response mediated through either PK or PD routes. Phenobarbitone induces a number of other pathways responsible for drug clearances, e.g., CYP1A2, CYP2C9, CYP2C19, CYP3A4, and UDP-glucuronosyltransferase (UGT) [214]. Ketamine in humans is metabolized mainly by CYP3A4. The steep concentration–response curve described for ketamine [164] means that small changes in the plasma concentration attributed to increased clearance can have dramatic impact on the degree of sedation [215].

An increase in the $T_{1/2keo}$ of D-tubocurarine with increasing inspired halothane concentrations has been demonstrated [216]. Halothane is a negative inotrope [217] and reduces skeletal muscle blood flow [218], so it seems reasonable to interpret changes in $T_{1/2keo}$ as due to changes in blood flow. Inhalation anesthetic agents can also prolong duration of block and this effect is agent specific. Sevoflurane potentiated vecuronium more than halothane; when compared to balanced anesthesia, the dose requirements of vecuronium were reduced by approximately 60 % and 40 %, respectively [219].

Anesthetic drug interactions traditionally have been characterized using isobolographic analysis or multiple logistic regression. Minto et al. [220] have proposed a model based on response surface methodology. Computer simulations based on interactions at the effect site predicted that the maximally synergistic three-drug combination (midazolam, propofol, and alfentanil) tripled the duration of effect compared with propofol alone. Response surfaces can describe anesthetic interactions, even those between agonists, partial agonists, competitive antagonists, and inverse agonists [220].

Synergism between propofol and alfentanil has been demonstrated using response surface methodology. Remifentanil alone had no appreciable effect on response to shaking and shouting or response to laryngoscopy while propofol could ablate both responses. Modest remifentanil concentrations dramatically reduced the concentrations of propofol required to ablate both responses [221]. When comparing the different combinations of midazolam, propofol, and alfentanil, the responses varied markedly at each endpoint assessed and could not be predicted from the responses of the individual agents [222]. Similar response surface methodology has been taken for investigation of the combined administration of sevoflurane and alfentanil [223] and remifentanil and propofol [224] on ventilation control. These combinations have a strikingly synergistic effect on respiration, resulting in severe respiratory depression in adults. These synergistic associations can be extended to pediatric sedation techniques. It is little wonder that the use of three or more sedating medications compared with one or two medications was strongly associated with adverse outcomes [7].

"Ketofol" is a mixture of ketamine and propofol (1:1) that is finding a niche for procedural sedation in the emergency room. Stable hemodynamics, analgesia, and good recovery are reported [225]. The additive interaction for anesthesia induction in adults has been reported [226], but not for continued sedation. It is probable that the "ideal mix" for sedation will depend on the duration of sedation required [227]. The context-sensitive half-time of ketamine increases with infusion duration, probably resulting in delayed recovery [228]. Ketamine, added to dexmedetomidine, mitigates sinus and atrioventricular nodal dysfunction [229]. (Refer to Chap. 9.)

Defining Target Concentration

An effect site target concentration has been estimated for many drugs used in anesthesia, analgesia, and sedation. For example, a propofol target concentration of 3 mg/L in a typical patient can be achieved using preprogrammed target-controlled infusion devices. A BIS monitor can then be used to manually adjust infusion rate to achieve a desired target effect in the specific individual. The luxury of such a feedback system is not available for most drugs. Sedation doses using scales such as that of Ramsey [230] are harder to quantify and are further modified by drug interactions. The ED_{50} of propofol hypnoses in adult females is reduced from 1.1 to 0.63 mg/kg in the presence of ketamine 0.21 mg/kg.

A target concentration of 10 μg/L is used for morphine analgesia. Observations in children after cardiac surgery suggested that steady-state serum concentrations greater than 20 mg/L resulted in hypercarbia ($PaCO_2 > 55$ mmHg) and depressed CO_2 response curve slopes. During washout, morphine concentrations more than 15 μg/L resulted in hypercarbia in 46 %, whereas concentrations less than 15 μg/L were associated with hypercarbia in 13 % of children. No age-related differences in respiratory effect were seen in these studies at the same serum morphine concentration [66]. Observation or self-reporting pain scales are used as part of the feedback loop for dose incremental changes.

The target concentration may vary, depending on the desired target effect. The target concentration for ketamine analgesia (0.25 mg/L) is quite different from that of anesthesia (2 mg/L) [231].

Conclusion

Children can be considered as small adults; size factors alone can explain many differences between children and adults. Neonates are developing children; maturation processes over the first few years of life have dramatic impact on both pharmacokinetics (PK) and pharmacodynamics (PD). Size, age, and organ function models can be used to characterize PK changes in the pediatric population. Although PD differences between neonates and children are recognized, there is little information describing maturation of these PD differences. Achievement of a target effect with minimal adverse effect is the key to anesthetic, analgesic, and sedation drug use. Pharmacodynamic models are useful tools to identify a target effect and concentration at which that occurs. Pharmacokinetic models, in turn, point to dosing that will achieve that target concentration. The population approach to modeling has proven beneficial to exploring PKPD differences in children. The impact of other drugs, active metabolites, stereoisomer interactions, and pharmacogenomics on the concentration–response relationship remains undefined for many drugs.

An understanding of PK and PD of drugs commonly used in children of all ages is vital for sensible sedation regimens. Simple infusion regimes for morphine, targeting a plasma concentration of 10 μg/L, that vary with age have been proposed [127]. Ketamine regimens that target an effect (e.g., arouses slowly to consciousness with sustained painful stimulus) are reported [232]. Target-controlled infusion pumps are dependent on an accurate knowledge of PK and PD parameters. Currently this technique is unavailable for even propofol and remifentanil in infants under 2 years of age because such information is lacking. Once this information is available, it will be possible to program these TCI pumps to deliver any adequately investigated drug to any specific target concentration in either plasma or effect site [83].

However, even with a good knowledge of PK and PD parameter estimates, there remains considerable between patient variability of both PK and PD parameters. This variability can result is some patients not achieving the desired sedation level because they are "too light" or "too deep." Concentration monitoring (e.g., propofol in expired breath) may reduce target concentration scatter attributable to PK parameter variability. Infusions can be increased or decreased to achieve the desired target. Unfortunately, the concentration–response curve is also associated with considerable variability, and target effect monitoring (e.g., modified EEG signaling) can be used to further modulate drug delivery for the individual. Modified EEG signaling and feedback loops that automatically regulate infusion rates to achieve desired effect are already available in adult practice and widely used for propofol. Children should not be denied similar levels of sophistication. This level of sophistication will only come once we have elucidated and understood pediatric PK and PD and the factors that contribute to their variability (e.g., age, size, pharmacogenomics).

References

1. Gupta M, Brans Y. Gastric retention in neonates. Pediatrics. 1978;62:26–9.
2. Grand RJ, Watkins JB, Torti FM. Development of the human intestinal tract: a review. Gastroenterology. 1976;70:790–810.
3. Liang J, Co E, Zhang M, Pineda J, Chen JD. Development of gastric slow waves in preterm infants measured by electrogastrography. Am J Physiol. 1998;274:G503–8.
4. Carlos MA, Babyn PS, Marcon MA, Moore AM. Changes in gastric emptying in early postnatal life. J Pediatr. 1997;130:931–7.
5. Kearns GL, Robinson PK, Wilson JT, et al. Cisapride disposition in neonates and infants: in vivo reflection of cytochrome P450 3A4 ontogeny. Clin Pharmacol Ther. 2003;74:312–25.
6. Anderson BJ, van Lingen RA, Hansen TG, Lin YC, Holford NH. Acetaminophen developmental pharmacokinetics in premature neonates and infants: a pooled population analysis. Anesthesiology. 2002;96:1336–45.
7. Cote CJ, Karl HW, Notterman DA, Weinberg JA, McCloskey C. Adverse sedation events in pediatrics: analysis of medications used for sedation. Pediatrics. 2000;106:633–44.
8. Pomeranz ES, Chudnofsky CR, Deegan TJ, Lozon MM, Mitchiner JC, Weber JE. Rectal methohexital sedation for computed tomography imaging of stable pediatric emergency department patients. Pediatrics. 2000;105:1110–4.
9. Burckart GJ, White 3rd TJ, Siegle RL, Jabbour JT, Ramey DR. Rectal thiopental versus an intramuscular cocktail for sedating children before computerized tomography. Am J Hosp Pharm. 1980;37:222–4.
10. Saint-Maurice C, Meistelman C, Rey E, Esteve C, de Lauture D, Olive G. The pharmacokinetics of rectal midazolam for premedication in children. Anesthesiology. 1986;65:536–8.
11. Herd D, Anderson B. Lack of pharmacokinetic information in children leads clinicians to use experience and trial-and-error to determine how best to administer ketamine. Ann Emerg Med. 2007;49:824, e1; author reply 5.
12. Mason KP, Lubisch N, Robinson F, Roskos R, Epstein MA. Intramuscular dexmedetomidine: an effective route of sedation preserves background activity for pediatric electroencephalograms. J Pediatr. 2012;161:927–32.
13. Mason KP, Lubisch NB, Robinson F, Roskos R. Intramuscular dexmedetomidine sedation for pediatric MRI and CT. AJR Am J Roentgenol. 2011;197:720–5.
14. Grassin-Delyle S, Buenestado A, Naline E, et al. Intranasal drug delivery: an efficient and non-invasive route for systemic administration: focus on opioids. Pharmacol Ther. 2012;134:366–79.
15. Hadley G, Maconochie I, Jackson A. A survey of intranasal medication use in the paediatric emergency setting in England and Wales. Emerg Med J. 2010;27:553–4.
16. Kendall JM, Latter VS. Intranasal diamorphine as an alternative to intramuscular morphine: pharmacokinetic and pharmacodynamic aspects. Clin Pharmacokinet. 2003;42:501–13.
17. Kendall JM, Reeves BC, Latter VS. Multicentre randomised controlled trial of nasal diamorphine for analgesia in children and teenagers with clinical fractures. BMJ. 2001;322:261–5.
18. Kidd S, Brennan S, Stephen R, Minns R, Beattie T. Comparison of morphine concentration-time profiles following intravenous and intranasal diamorphine in children. Arch Dis Child. 2009;94:974–8.
19. Borland M, Jacobs I, King B, O'Brien D. A randomized controlled trial comparing intranasal fentanyl to intravenous morphine for managing acute pain in children in the emergency department. Ann Emerg Med. 2007;49:335–40.
20. Borland M, Milsom S, Esson A. Equivalency of two concentrations of fentanyl administered by the intranasal route for acute analgesia in children in a paediatric emergency department: a randomized controlled trial. Emerg Med Australas. 2011;23:202–8.
21. Furyk JS, Grabowski WJ, Black LH. Nebulized fentanyl versus intravenous morphine in children with suspected limb fractures in the emergency department: a randomized controlled trial. Emerg Med Australas. 2009;21:203–9.
22. Scheepers LD, Montgomery CJ, Kinahan AM, Dunn GS, Bourne RA, McCormack JP. Plasma concentration of flumazenil following intranasal administration in children. Can J Anaesth. 2000;47:120–4.
23. Rey E, Delaunay L, Pons G, et al. Pharmacokinetics of midazolam in children: comparative study of intranasal and intravenous administration. Eur J Clin Pharmacol. 1991;41:355–7.
24. Iirola T, Vilo S, Manner T, et al. Bioavailability of dexmedetomidine after intranasal administration. Eur J Clin Pharmacol. 2011;67:825–31.
25. Larsson P, Eksborg S, Lonnqvist PA. Onset time for pharmacologic premedication with clonidine as a nasal aerosol: a double-blind, placebo-controlled, randomized trial. Paediatr Anaesth. 2012;22:877–83.
26. Almenrader N, Larsson P, Passariello M, et al. Absorption pharmacokinetics of clonidine nasal drops in children. Paediatr Anaesth. 2009;19:257–61.
27. Hippard HK, Govindan K, Friedman EM, et al. Postoperative analgesic and behavioral effects of intranasal fentanyl, intravenous morphine, and intramuscular morphine in pediatric patients undergoing bilateral myringotomy and placement of ventilating tubes. Anesth Analg. 2012;115:356–63.
28. Drover DR, Hammer GB, Anderson BJ. The pharmacokinetics of ketorolac after single postoperative intranasal administration in adolescent patients. Anesth Analg. 2012;114:1270–6.
29. Ginsberg G, Hattis D, Miller R, Sonawane B. Pediatric pharmacokinetic data: implications for environmental risk assessment for children. Pediatrics. 2004;113:973–83.
30. Taddio A, Shennan AT, Stevens B, Leeder JS, Koren G. Safety of lidocaine-prilocaine cream in the treatment of preterm neonates. J Pediatr. 1995;127:1002–5.
31. Taddio A, Stevens B, Craig K, et al. Efficacy and safety of lidocaine-prilocaine cream for pain during circumcision. N Engl J Med. 1997;336:1197–201.

32. Salanitre E, Rackow H. The pulmonary exchange of nitrous oxide and halothane in infants and children. Anesthesiology. 1969;30: 388–94.
33. Lerman J. Pharmacology of inhalational anaesthetics in infants and children. Paediatr Anaesth. 1992;2:191–203.
34. Lerman J, Schmitt Bantel BI, Gregory GA, Willis MM, Eger EI. Effect of age on the solubility of volatile anesthetics in human tissues. Anesthesiology. 1986;65:307–11.
35. Malviya S, Lerman J. The blood/gas solubilities of sevoflurane, isoflurane, halothane, and serum constituent concentrations in neonates and adults. Anesthesiology. 1990;72:793–6.
36. Sturesson LW, Johansson A, Bodelsson M, Malmkvist G. Wash-in kinetics for sevoflurane using a disposable delivery system (AnaConDa) in cardiac surgery patients. Br J Anaesth. 2009;102: 470–6.
37. Sackey PV, Martling CR, Granath F, Radell PJ. Prolonged isoflurane sedation of intensive care unit patients with the Anesthetic Conserving Device. Crit Care Med. 2004;32:2241–6.
38. Sackey PV, Martling CR, Radell PJ. Three cases of PICU sedation with isoflurane delivered by the 'AnaConDa'. Paediatr Anaesth. 2005;15:879–85.
39. Marcos-Vidal JM, Gonzalez R, Garcia C, Soria C. Out-of-operating room anesthesia: use of the AnaConDa vaporizer with anesthesia. J Clin Anesth. 2012;24:346–7.
40. Eger 2nd EI. Anesthetic uptake and action. Baltimore: Williams & Wilkins; 1974.
41. Albani M, Wernicke I. Oral phenytoin in infancy: dose requirement, absorption, and elimination. Pediatr Pharmacol (New York). 1983;3:229–36.
42. Abdel-Rahman SM, Johnson FK, Connor JD, et al. Developmental pharmacokinetics and pharmacodynamics of nizatidine. J Pediatr Gastroenterol Nutr. 2004;38:442–51.
43. de Wildt SN, Kearns GL, Hop WC, Murry DJ, Abdel-Rahman SM, van den Anker JN. Pharmacokinetics and metabolism of oral midazolam in preterm infants. Br J Clin Pharmacol. 2002;53: 390–2.
44. Allegaert K, Anderson BJ, Vrancken M, et al. Impact of a paediatric vial on the magnitude of systematic medication errors in preterm neonates: amikacin as an example. Paediatr Perinat Drug Ther. 2006;7.
45. Karl HW, Rosenberger JL, Larach MG, Ruffle JM. Transmucosal administration of midazolam for premedication of pediatric patients. Comparison of the nasal and sublingual routes. Anesthesiology. 1993;78:885–91.
46. Herd DW, Salehi B. Palatability of two forms of paracetamol (acetaminophen) suspension: a randomised trial. Paediatr Perinat Drug Ther. 2006;7:189–93.
47. Larsson P, Nordlinder A, Bergendahl HT, et al. Oral bioavailability of clonidine in children. Paediatr Anaesth. 2011;21:335–40.
48. Brunette KE, Anderson BJ, Thomas J, Wiesner L, Herd DW, Schulein S. Exploring the pharmacokinetics of oral ketamine in children undergoing burns procedures. Paediatr Anaesth. 2011;21: 653–62.
49. Gourlay GK, Boas RA. Fatal outcome with use of rectal morphine for postoperative pain control in an infant. BMJ. 1992;304: 766–7.
50. Friis-Hansen B. Body water compartments in children: changes during growth and related changes in body composition. Pediatrics. 1961;28:169–81.
51. Johnson KL, Erickson JP, Holley FO, et al. Fentanyl pharmacokinetics in the paediatric population. Anesthesiology. 1984;61:A441.
52. Meretoja OA, Wirtavuori K, Neuvonen PJ. Age-dependence of the dose-response curve of vecuronium in pediatric patients during balanced anesthesia. Anesth Analg. 1988;67:21–6.
53. Fisher DM, Canfell PC, Spellman MJ, Miller RD. Pharmacokinetics and pharmacodynamics of atracurium in infants and children. Anesthesiology. 1990;73:33–7.
54. Luz G, Innerhofer P, Bachmann B, Frischhut B, Menardi G, Benzer A. Bupivacaine plasma concentrations during continuous epidural anesthesia in infants and children. Anesth Analg. 1996;82:231–4.
55. Luz G, Wieser C, Innerhofer P, Frischhut B, Ulmer H, Benzer A. Free and total bupivacaine plasma concentrations after continuous epidural anaesthesia in infants and children. Paediatr Anaesth. 1998;8:473–8.
56. Erichsen CJ, Sjovall J, Kehlet H, Hedlund C, Arvidsson T. Pharmacokinetics and analgesic effect of ropivacaine during continuous epidural infusion for postoperative pain relief. Anesthesiology. 1996;84:834–42.
57. Anderson BJ, McKee AD, Holford NH. Size, myths and the clinical pharmacokinetics of analgesia in paediatric patients. Clin Pharmacokinet. 1997;33:313–27.
58. Calder A, Bell GT, Andersson M, Thomson AH, Watson DG, Morton NS. Pharmacokinetic profiles of epidural bupivacaine and ropivacaine following single-shot and continuous epidural use in young infants. Paediatr Anaesth. 2012;22:430–7.
59. Russo H, Bressolle F. Pharmacodynamics and pharmacokinetics of thiopental. Clin Pharmacokinet. 1998;35:95–134.
60. Bjorkman S. Prediction of drug disposition in infants and children by means of physiologically based pharmacokinetic (PBPK) modelling: theophylline and midazolam as model drugs. Br J Clin Pharmacol. 2005;59:691–704.
61. Johnson TN, Tucker GT, Tanner MS, Rostami-Hodjegan A. Changes in liver volume from birth to adulthood: a meta-analysis. Liver Transpl. 2005;11:1481–93.
62. Schoning M, Hartig B. Age dependence of total cerebral blood flow volume from childhood to adulthood. J Cereb Blood Flow Metab. 1996;16:827–33.
63. Chiron C, Raynaud C, Maziere B, et al. Changes in regional cerebral blood flow during brain maturation in children and adolescents. J Nucl Med. 1992;33:696–703.
64. Way WL, Costley EC, Way EL. Respiratory sensitivity of the newborn infant to meperidine and morphine. Clin Pharmacol Ther. 1965;6:454–61.
65. Pokela ML, Olkkola KT, Seppala T, Koivisto M. Age-related morphine kinetics in infants. Dev Pharmacol Ther. 1993;20:26–34.
66. Lynn AM, Nespeca MK, Opheim KE, Slattery JT. Respiratory effects of intravenous morphine infusions in neonates, infants, and children after cardiac surgery. Anesth Analg. 1993;77:695–701.
67. Engelhardt B. Development of the blood-brain barrier. Cell Tissue Res. 2003;314:119–29.
68. Persidsky Y, Ramirez SH, Haorah J, Kanmogne GD. Blood-brain barrier: structural components and function under physiologic and pathologic conditions. J Neuroimmune Pharmacol. 2006;1:223–36.
69. Henthorn TK, Liu Y, Mahapatro M, Ng KY. Active transport of fentanyl by the blood-brain barrier. J Pharmacol Exp Ther. 1999;289:1084–9.
70. Hamabe W, Maeda T, Kiguchi N, Yamamoto C, Tokuyama S, Kishioka S. Negative relationship between morphine analgesia and P-glycoprotein expression levels in the brain. J Pharmacol Sci. 2007;105:353–60.
71. Choudhuri S, Klaassen CD. Structure, function, expression, genomic organization, and single nucleotide polymorphisms of human ABCB1 (MDR1), ABCC (MRP), and ABCG2 (BCRP) efflux transporters. Int J Toxicol. 2006;25:231–59.
72. Allegaert K, Vanhole C, Vermeersch S, Rayyan M, Verbesselt R, de Hoon J. Both postnatal and postmenstrual age contribute to the interindividual variability in tramadol glucuronidation in neonates. Early Hum Dev. 2008;84:325–30.
73. Allegaert K, Peeters MY, Verbesselt R, et al. Inter-individual variability in propofol pharmacokinetics in preterm and term neonates. Br J Anaesth. 2007;99:864–70.
74. Anderson BJ, Holford NH. Tips and traps analyzing pediatric PK data. Paediatr Anaesth. 2011;21:222–37.

75. Tod M, Jullien V, Pons G. Facilitation of drug evaluation in children by population methods and modelling. Clin Pharmacokinet. 2008; 47:231–43.
76. Anderson BJ, Holford NH. Mechanism-based concepts of size and maturity in pharmacokinetics. Annu Rev Pharmacol Toxicol. 2008;48:303–32.
77. Dreyer G, Ray W. Further experiments upon the blood volume of mammals and its relation to the surface area of the body. Philos Trans R Soc Lond B Biol Sci. 1912;202:191–212.
78. West GB, Brown JH, Enquist BJ. A general model for the origin of allometric scaling laws in biology. Science. 1997;276:122–6.
79. Rigby-Jones AE, Priston MJ, Thorne GC, Tooley MA, Sneyd JR, Wolf AR. Population pharmacokinetics of remifentanil in critically ill post cardiac neonates, infants and children. Br J Anaesth. 2005;95:578P–9.
80. Welzing L, Ebenfeld S, Dlugay V, Wiesen MH, Roth B, Mueller C. Remifentanil degradation in umbilical cord blood of preterm infants. Anesthesiology. 2011;114:570–7.
81. Barker N, Lim J, Amari E, Malherbe S, Ansermino JM. Relationship between age and spontaneous ventilation during intravenous anesthesia in children. Paediatr Anaesth. 2007;17: 948–55.
82. Rigby-Jones AE, Priston MJ, Sneyd JR, et al. Remifentanil-midazolam sedation for paediatric patients receiving mechanical ventilation after cardiac surgery. Br J Anaesth. 2007;99:252–61.
83. Anderson BJ. Pediatric models for adult target-controlled infusion pumps. Paediatr Anaesth. 2010;20(3):223–32.
84. Hill AV. The possible effects of the aggregation of the molecules of haemoglobin on its dissociation curves. J Physiol. 1910;14: iv-vii.
85. Holford NHG, Heo Y-A, Anderson BJ. A pharmacokinetic standard for babies and adults. J Pharm Sci. 2013;102(9):2941–52.
86. Potts A, Warman G, Anderson BJ. Dexmedetomidine pharmacokinetics in pediatric intensive care—a pooled analysis. Paediatr Anaesth. 2009;19:1119–29.
87. Vet NJ, de Hoog M, Tibboel D, de Wildt SN. The effect of critical illness and inflammation on midazolam therapy in children. Pediatr Crit Care Med. 2012;13:e48–50.
88. Anderson BJ, Holford NH. Understanding dosing: children are small adults, neonates are immature children. Arch Dis Child. 2013;98:737–44.
89. Johnson TN. The problems in scaling adult drug doses to children. Arch Dis Child. 2008;93:207–11.
90. Johnson TN, Rostami-Hodjegan A, Tucker GT. Prediction of the clearance of eleven drugs and associated variability in neonates, infants and children. Clin Pharmacokinet. 2006;45:931–56.
91. Edginton AN, Schmitt W, Voith B, Willmann S. A mechanistic approach for the scaling of clearance in children. Clin Pharmacokinet. 2006;45:683–704.
92. Edginton AN, Theil FP, Schmitt W, Willmann S. Whole body physiologically-based pharmacokinetic models: their use in clinical drug development. Expert Opin Drug Metab Toxicol. 2008;4:1143–52.
93. Encinas E, Calvo R, Lukas JC, Vozmediano V, Rodriguez M, Suarez E. A predictive pharmacokinetic/pharmacodynamic model of fentanyl for analgesia/sedation in neonates based on a semi-physiologic approach. Paediatr Drugs. 2013;15:247–57.
94. Hines RN, McCarver DG. The ontogeny of human drug-metabolizing enzymes: phase I oxidative enzymes. J Pharmacol Exp Ther. 2002;300:355–60.
95. Koukouritaki SB, Manro JR, Marsh SA, et al. Developmental expression of human hepatic CYP2C9 and CYP2C19. J Pharmacol Exp Ther. 2004;308:965–74; Epub 2003 Nov 21.
96. Hines RN. Developmental expression of drug metabolizing enzymes: Impact on disposition in neonates and young children. Int J Pharm. 2013;452(1–2):3–7.
97. Johnsrud EK, Koukouritaki SB, Divakaran K, Brunengraber LL, Hines RN, McCarver DG. Human hepatic CYP2E1 expression during development. J Pharmacol Exp Ther. 2003;307:402–7.
98. Kearns GL, Abdel-Rahman SM, Alander SW, Blowey DL, Leeder JS, Kauffman RE. Developmental pharmacology—drug disposition, action, and therapy in infants and children. N Engl J Med. 2003;349:1157–67.
99. Berde C. Convulsions associated with pediatric regional anesthesia. Anesth Analg. 1992;75:164–6.
100. Anderson BJ, Hansen TG. Getting the best from pediatric pharmacokinetic data. Paediatr Anaesth. 2004;14:713–5.
101. Chalkiadis GA, Anderson BJ. Age and size are the major covariates for prediction of levobupivacaine clearance in children. Paediatr Anaesth. 2006;16:275–82.
102. Anderson BJ, Larsson P. A maturation model for midazolam clearance. Paediatr Anaesth. 2011;21:302–8.
103. Chalkiadis GA, Abdullah F, Bjorksten AR, et al. Absorption characteristics of epidural levobupivacaine with adrenaline and clonidine in children. Paediatr Anaesth. 2013;23:58–67.
104. McCarver DG, Hines RN. The ontogeny of human drug-metabolizing enzymes: phase II conjugation enzymes and regulatory mechanisms. J Pharmacol Exp Ther. 2002;300:361–6.
105. Anderson BJ, Holford NHG. Mechanistic basis of using body size and maturation to predict clearance in humans. Drug Metab Pharmacokinet. 2009;24:25–36.
106. Holford NH, Shu Chin M, Anderson BJ. Prediction of morphine dose in humans. Paediatr Anaesth. 2012;22.
107. Anderson BJ, Woollard GA, Holford NH. A model for size and age changes in the pharmacokinetics of paracetamol in neonates, infants and children. Br J Clin Pharmacol. 2000;50:125–34.
108. Anderson BJ, Pons G, Autret-Leca E, Allegaert K, Boccard E. Pediatric intravenous paracetamol (propacetamol) pharmacokinetics: a population analysis. Paediatr Anaesth. 2005;15:282–92.
109. Potts AL, Warman GR, Anderson BJ. Dexmedetomidine disposition in children: a population analysis. Paediatr Anaesth. 2008; 18:722–30.
110. Anand KJ, Anderson BJ, Holford NH, et al. Morphine pharmacokinetics and pharmacodynamics in preterm and term neonates: secondary results from the NEOPAIN trial. Br J Anaesth. 2008;101:680–9.
111. Rhodin MM, Anderson BJ, Peters AM, et al. Human renal function maturation: a quantitative description using weight and postmenstrual age. Pediatr Nephrol. 2009;24:67–76.
112. Allegaert K, Anderson BJ, Verbesselt R, et al. Tramadol disposition in the very young: an attempt to assess in vivo cytochrome P450 2D6 activity. Br J Anaesth. 2005;231–9.
113. Allegaert K, de Hoon J, Verbesselt R, Naulaers G, Murat I. Maturational pharmacokinetics of single intravenous bolus of propofol. Paediatr Anaesth. 2007;17:1028–34.
114. Lynn A, Nespeca MK, Bratton SL, Strauss SG, Shen DD. Clearance of morphine in postoperative infants during intravenous infusion: the influence of age and surgery. Anesth Analg. 1998;86:958–63.
115. Peters JW, Anderson BJ, Simons SH, Uges DR, Tibboel D. Morphine pharmacokinetics during venoarterial extracorporeal membrane oxygenation in neonates. Intensive Care Med. 2005;31:257–63.
116. Rigby-Jones AE, Nolan JA, Priston MJ, Wright PM, Sneyd JR, Wolf AR. Pharmacokinetics of propofol infusions in critically ill neonates, infants, and children in an intensive care unit. Anesthesiology. 2002;97:1393–400.
117. Iirola T, Ihmsen H, Laitio R, et al. Population pharmacokinetics of dexmedetomidine during long-term sedation in intensive care patients. Br J Anaesth. 2012;108:460–8.
118. Peeters MY, Prins SA, Knibbe CA, et al. Propofol pharmacokinetics and pharmacodynamics for depth of sedation in nonventilated infants after major craniofacial surgery. Anesthesiology. 2006;104:466–74.

119. DeWoskin RS, Thompson CM. Renal clearance parameters for PBPK model analysis of early lifestage differences in the disposition of environmental toxicants. Regul Toxicol Pharmacol. 2008;51:66–86.
120. Langhendries JP, Battisti O, Bertrand JM, et al. Adaptation in neonatology of the once-daily concept of aminoglycoside administration: evaluation of a dosing chart for amikacin in an intensive care unit. Biol Neonate. 1998;74:351–62.
121. Fisher DM, O'Keeffe C, Stanski DR, Cronnelly R, Miller RD, Gregory GA. Pharmacokinetics and pharmacodynamics of d-tubocurarine in infants, children, and adults. Anesthesiology. 1982;57:203–8.
122. De Carolis MP, Romagnoli C, Muzii U, et al. Pharmacokinetic aspects of caffeine in premature infants. Dev Pharmacol Ther. 1991;16:117–22.
123. Sawyer DC, Eger 2nd EI, Bahlman SH, Cullen BF, Impelman D. Concentration dependence of hepatic halothane metabolism. Anesthesiology. 1971;34:230–5.
124. Herd DW, Anderson BJ, Holford NH. Modeling the norketamine metabolite in children and the implications for analgesia. Paediatr Anaesth. 2007;17:831–40.
125. van der Marel CD, Anderson BJ, Romsing J, Jacqz-Aigrain E, Tibboel D. Diclofenac and metabolite pharmacokinetics in children. Paediatr Anaesth. 2004;14:443–51.
126. Crevoisier C, Ziegler WH, Eckert M, Heizmann P. Relationship between plasma concentration and effect of midazolam after oral and intravenous administration. Br J Clin Pharmacol. 1983;16 Suppl 1:51S–61.
127. Bouwmeester NJ, Anderson BJ, Tibboel D, Holford NH. Developmental pharmacokinetics of morphine and its metabolites in neonates, infants and young children. Br J Anaesth. 2004;92:208–17.
128. Wittwer E, Kern SE. Role of morphine's metabolites in analgesia: concepts and controversies. AAPS J. 2006;8:E348–52.
129. van Dorp EL, Romberg R, Sarton E, Bovill JG, Dahan A. Morphine-6-glucuronide: morphine's successor for postoperative pain relief? Anesth Analg. 2006;102:1789–97.
130. Romberg R, Sarton E, Teppema L, Matthes HW, Kieffer BL, Dahan A. Comparison of morphine-6-glucuronide and morphine on respiratory depressant and antinociceptive responses in wild type and mu-opioid receptor deficient mice. Br J Anaesth. 2003;91:862–70.
131. Hannam JA, Anderson BJ. Contribution of morphine and morphine-6-glucuronide to respiratory depression in a child. Anaesth Intensive Care. 2012;40:867–70.
132. Bouwmeester NJ, van den Anker JN, Hop WC, Anand KJ, Tibboel D. Age- and therapy-related effects on morphine requirements and plasma concentrations of morphine and its metabolites in postoperative infants. Br J Anaesth. 2003;90:642–52.
133. de Wildt SN, Kearns GL, Leeder JS, van den Anker JN. Cytochrome P450 3A: ontogeny and drug disposition. Clin Pharmacokinet. 1999;37:485–505.
134. Williams DG, Hatch DJ, Howard RF. Codeine phosphate in paediatric medicine. Br J Anaesth. 2001;86:413–21.
135. Fagerlund TH, Braaten O. No pain relief from codeine…? An introduction to pharmacogenomics. Acta Anaesthesiol Scand. 2001;45:140–9.
136. Pariente-Khayat A, Rey E, Gendrel D, et al. Isoniazid acetylation metabolic ratio during maturation in children. Clin Pharmacol Ther. 1997;62:377–83.
137. Carrier O, Pons G, Rey E, et al. Maturation of caffeine metabolic pathways in infancy. Clin Pharmacol Ther. 1988;44:145–51.
138. Allegaert K, van den Anker JN, de Hoon JN, et al. Covariates of tramadol disposition in the first months of life. Br J Anaesth. 2008;100:525–32.
139. Voronov P, Przybylo HJ, Jagannathan N. Apnea in a child after oral codeine: a genetic variant—an ultra-rapid metabolizer. Paediatr Anaesth. 2007;17:684–7.
140. Anderson BJ. Is it farewell to codeine? Arch Dis Child. 2013;98:986–8.
141. Sadhasivam S, Chidambaran V. Pharmacogenomics of opioids and perioperative pain management. Pharmacogenomics. 2012;13:1719–40.
142. Lotsch J, Skarke C, Liefhold J, Geisslinger G. Genetic predictors of the clinical response to opioid analgesics: clinical utility and future perspectives. Clin Pharmacokinet. 2004;43:983–1013.
143. Phillips KA, Veenstra DL, Oren E, Lee JK, Sadee W. Potential role of pharmacogenomics in reducing adverse drug reactions: a systematic review. JAMA. 2001;286:2270–9.
144. Ensom MH, Chang TK, Patel P. Pharmacogenetics: the therapeutic drug monitoring of the future? Clin Pharmacokinet. 2001;40:783–802.
145. Naguib M, Bie B, Ting AH. Fundamental concepts of epigenetics for consideration in anesthesiology. Curr Opin Anaesthesiol. 2012;25:434–43.
146. Stephenson T. How children's responses to drugs differ from adults. Br J Clin Pharmacol. 2005;59:670–3.
147. Allegaert K, Naulaers G, Vanhaesebrouck S, Anderson BJ. The paracetamol concentration-effect relation in neonates. Paediatr Anaesth. 2013;23:45–50.
148. LeDez KM, Lerman J. The minimum alveolar concentration (MAC) of isoflurane in preterm neonates. Anesthesiology. 1987;67:301–7.
149. Keenan RL, Shapiro JH, Kane FR, Simpson PM. Bradycardia during anesthesia in infants. An epidemiologic study. Anesthesiology. 1994;80:976–82.
150. Jonmarker C, Westrin P, Larsson S, Werner O. Thiopental requirements for induction of anesthesia in children. Anesthesiology. 1987;67:104–7.
151. Westrin P, Jonmarker C, Werner O. Thiopental requirements for induction of anesthesia in neonates and in infants one to six months of age. Anesthesiology. 1989;71:344–6.
152. Meakin G, Morton RH, Wareham AC. Age-dependent variation in response to tubocurarine in the isolated rat diaphragm. Br J Anaesth. 1992;68:161–3.
153. Wareham AC, Morton RH, Meakin GH. Low quantal content of the endplate potential reduces safety factor for neuromuscular transmission in the diaphragm of the newborn rat. Br J Anaesth. 1994;72:205–9.
154. Radford D. Side effects of verapamil in infants. Arch Dis Child. 1983;58:465–6.
155. Takahashi H, Ishikawa S, Nomoto S, et al. Developmental changes in pharmacokinetics and pharmacodynamics of warfarin enantiomers in Japanese children. Clin Pharmacol Ther. 2000;68:541–55.
156. Baber NS. Tripartite meeting. Paediatric regulatory guidelines: do they help in optimizing dose selection for children? Br J Clin Pharmacol. 2005;59:660–2.
157. Davidson AJ. Measuring anesthesia in children using the EEG. Paediatr Anaesth. 2006;16:374–87.
158. Davidson AJ, Huang GH, Rebmann CS, Ellery C. Performance of entropy and Bispectral Index as measures of anaesthesia effect in children of different ages. Br J Anaesth. 2005;95:674–9.
159. Davidson AJ, Sale SM, Wong C, et al. The electroencephalograph during anesthesia and emergence in infants and children. Paediatr Anaesth. 2008;18:60–70.
160. Jeleazcov C, Schmidt J, Schmitz B, Becke K, Albrecht S. EEG variables as measures of arousal during propofol anaesthesia for general surgery in children: rational selection and age dependence. Br J Anaesth. 2007;99:845–54.

161. Cheung YM, Scoones GP, Hoeks SE, Stolker RJ, Weber F. Evaluation of the aepEX monitor of hypnotic depth in pediatric patients receiving propofol-remifentanil anesthesia. Paediatr Anaesth. 2013;23:891–7.
162. West N, Dumont GA, van Heusden K, et al. Robust closed-loop control of induction and maintenance of propofol anesthesia in children. Paediatr Anaesth. 2013;23:712–9.
163. Hoffman GM, Nowakowski R, Troshynski TJ, Berens RJ, Weisman SJ. Risk reduction in pediatric procedural sedation by application of an American Academy of Pediatrics/American Society of Anesthesiologists process model. Pediatrics. 2002;109: 236–43.
164. Herd DW, Anderson BJ, Keene NA, Holford NH. Investigating the pharmacodynamics of ketamine in children. Paediatr Anaesth. 2008;18:36–42.
165. Crellin D, Sullivan TP, Babl FE, O'Sullivan R, Hutchinson A. Analysis of the validation of existing behavioral pain and distress scales for use in the procedural setting. In: Paediatr Anaesth; 2007. p. 720–33.
166. von Baeyer CL, Spagrud LJ. Systematic review of observational (behavioral) measures of pain for children and adolescents aged 3 to 18 years. Pain. 2007;127:140–50.
167. Schade JG, Joyce BA, Gerkensmeyer J, Keck JF. Comparison of three preverbal scales for postoperative pain assessment in a diverse pediatric sample. J Pain Symptom Manage. 1996;12: 348–59.
168. van Dijk M, Peters JW, van Deventer P, Tibboel D. The COMFORT Behavior Scale: a tool for assessing pain and sedation in infants. Am J Nurs. 2005;105:33–6.
169. Bai J, Hsu L, Tang Y, van Dijk M. Validation of the COMFORT Behavior scale and the FLACC scale for pain assessment in Chinese children after cardiac surgery. Pain Manag Nurs. 2012; 13:18–26.
170. van Dijk M, Roofthooft DW, Anand KJ, et al. Taking up the challenge of measuring prolonged pain in (premature) neonates: the COMFORTneo scale seems promising. Clin J Pain. 2009;25: 607–16.
171. Valkenburg AJ, Boerlage AA, Ista E, Duivenvoorden HJ, Tibboel D, van Dijk M. The COMFORT-behavior scale is useful to assess pain and distress in 0- to 3-year-old children with Down syndrome. Pain. 2011;152:2059–64.
172. Green SM, Mason KP. Stratification of sedation risk—a challenge to the sedation continuum. Paediatr Anaesth. 2011;21:924–31.
173. Mason KP, Green SM, Piacevoli Q. Adverse event reporting tool to standardize the reporting and tracking of adverse events during procedural sedation: a consensus document from the World SIVA International Sedation Task Force. Br J Anaesth. 2012;108: 13–20.
174. Anderson BJ, Allegaert K, Holford NH. Population clinical pharmacology of children: general principles. Eur J Pediatr. 2006;165: 741–6.
175. Anderson BJ, Allegaert K, Holford NH. Population clinical pharmacology of children: modelling covariate effects. Eur J Pediatr. 2006;165:819–29.
176. Holford NH. The target concentration approach to clinical drug development. Clin Pharmacokinet. 1995;29:287–91.
177. Hull CJ. How far can we go with compartmental models? Anesthesiology. 1990;72:399–402.
178. Boer F. Drug handling by the lungs. Br J Anaesth. 2003;91:50–60.
179. Reekers M, Boer F, Vuyk J. Basic concepts of recirculatory pharmacokinetic modelling. Adv Exp Med Biol. 2003;523:19–26.
180. Krejcie TC, Avram MJ. What determines anesthetic induction dose? It's the front-end kinetics, doctor! Anesth Analg. 1999;89: 541–4.
181. Kuipers JA, Boer F, Olofsen E, Bovill JG, Burm AG. Recirculatory pharmacokinetics and pharmacodynamics of rocuronium in patients: the influence of cardiac output. Anesthesiology. 2001;94: 47–55.
182. Enlund M, Kietzmann D, Bouillon T, Zuchner K, Meineke I. Population pharmacokinetics of sevoflurane in conjunction with the AnaConDa: toward target-controlled infusion of volatiles into the breathing system. Acta Anaesthesiol Scand. 2008;52:553–60.
183. Wada DR, Drover DR, Lemmens HJ. Determination of the distribution volume that can be used to calculate the intravenous loading dose. Clin Pharmacokinet. 1998;35:1–7.
184. McFarlan CS, Anderson BJ, Short TG. The use of propofol infusions in paediatric anaesthesia: a practical guide. Paediatr Anaesth. 1999;9:209–16.
185. Hughes MA, Glass PS, Jacobs JR. Context-sensitive half-time in multicompartment pharmacokinetic models for intravenous anesthetic drugs. Anesthesiology. 1992;76:334–41.
186. Anderson BJ, Woollard GA, Holford NH. Acetaminophen analgesia in children: placebo effect and pain resolution after tonsillectomy. Eur J Clin Pharmacol. 2001;57:559–69.
187. Mould DR, DeFeo TM, Reele S, et al. Simultaneous modeling of the pharmacokinetics and pharmacodynamics of midazolam and diazepam. Clin Pharmacol Ther. 1995;58:35–43.
188. BuhrerM,MaitrePO,HungO,StanskiDR.Electroencephalographic effects of benzodiazepines. I. Choosing an electroencephalographic parameter to measure the effect of midazolam on the central nervous system. Clin Pharmacol Ther. 1990;48:544–54.
189. Potts AL, Anderson BJ, Holford NH, Vu TC, Warman GR. Dexmedetomidine hemodynamics in children after cardiac surgery. Paediatr Anaesth. 2010;20:425–33.
190. Dixon WJ. Efficient analysis of experimental observations. Annu Rev Pharmacol Toxicol. 1980;20:441–62.
191. Dixon WJ. Staircase bioassay: the up-and-down method. Neurosci Biobehav Rev. 1991;15:47–50.
192. Frawley G, Skinner A, Thomas J, Smith S. Ropivacaine spinal anesthesia in neonates: a dose range finding study. Paediatr Anaesth. 2007;17:126–32.
193. Frawley GP, Farrell T, Smith S. Levobupivacaine spinal anesthesia in neonates: a dose range finding study. Paediatr Anaesth. 2004;14:838–44.
194. Hull CJ, Van Beem HB, McLeod K, Sibbald A, Watson MJ. A pharmacodynamic model for pancuronium. Br J Anaesth. 1978; 50:1113–23.
195. Sheiner LB, Stanski DR, Vozeh S, Miller RD, Ham J. Simultaneous modeling of pharmacokinetics and pharmacodynamics: application to D-tubocurarine. Clin Pharmacol Ther. 1979;25:358–71.
196. Holford NH, Sheiner LB. Understanding the dose-effect relationship: clinical application of pharmacokinetic-pharmacodynamic models. Clin Pharmacokinet. 1981;6:429–53.
197. Buhrer M, Maitre PO, Crevoisier C, Stanski DR. Electroencephalographic effects of benzodiazepines. II. Pharmacodynamic modeling of the electroencephalographic effects of midazolam and diazepam. Clin Pharmacol Ther. 1990;48:555–67.
198. Albrecht S, Ihmsen H, Hering W, et al. The effect of age on the pharmacokinetics and pharmacodynamics of midazolam. Clin Pharmacol Ther. 1999;65:630–9.
199. Platten HP, Schweizer E, Dilger K, Mikus G, Klotz U. Pharmacokinetics and the pharmacodynamic action of midazolam in young and elderly patients undergoing tooth extraction. Clin Pharmacol Ther. 1998;63:552–60.
200. Anderson BJ, Meakin GH. Scaling for size: some implications for paediatric anaesthesia dosing. Paediatr Anaesth. 2002;12: 205–19.
201. Jeleazcov C, Ihmsen H, Schmidt J, et al. Pharmacodynamic modelling of the bispectral index response to propofol-based anaesthesia during general surgery in children. Br J Anaesth. 2008;100: 509–16.

202. Cortinez LI, Troconiz IF, Fuentes R, et al. The influence of age on the dynamic relationship between end-tidal sevoflurane concentrations and bispectral index. Anesth Analg. 2008;107:1566–72.
203. Munoz HR, Cortinez LI, Ibacache ME, Altermatt FR. Estimation of the plasma effect site equilibration rate constant (ke0) of propofol in children using the time to peak effect: comparison with adults. Anesthesiology. 2004;101:1269–74.
204. Munoz HR, Leon PJ. Fuentes RS. Cortinez LI. Prospective evaluation of the time to peak effect of propofol to target the effect site in children. Acta Anaesthesiol Scand: Echevarria GC; 2009.
205. Absalom AR, Vereecke HE, Eleveld DJ. A hitch-hiker's guide to the intravenous PK/PD galaxy. Paediatr Anaesth. 2011;21:915–8.
206. Linden G, Henderson BE. Genital-tract cancers in adolescents and young adults. N Engl J Med. 1972;286:760–1.
207. Fredriksson A, Archer T, Alm H, Gordh T, Eriksson P. Neurofunctional deficits and potentiated apoptosis by neonatal NMDA antagonist administration. Behav Brain Res. 2004;153: 367–76.
208. Wang C, Sadovova N, Fu X, et al. The role of the N-methyl-D-aspartate receptor in ketamine-induced apoptosis in rat forebrain culture. Neuroscience. 2005;132:967–77.
209. Anderson BJ, Ralph CJ, Stewart AW, Barber C, Holford NH. The dose-effect relationship for morphine and vomiting after day-stay tonsillectomy in children. Anaesth Intensive Care. 2000;28:155–60.
210. Weinstein MS, Nicolson SC, Schreiner MS. A single dose of morphine sulfate increases the incidence of vomiting after outpatient inguinal surgery in children. Anesthesiology. 1994;81:572–7.
211. Ansermino M, Basu R, Vandebeek C, Montgomery C. Nonopioid additives to local anaesthetics for caudal blockade in children: a systematic review. Paediatr Anaesth. 2003;13:561–73.
212. Welzing L, Kribs A, Eifinger F, Huenseler C, Oberthuer A, Roth B. Propofol as an induction agent for endotracheal intubation can cause significant arterial hypotension in preterm neonates. Paediatr Anaesth. 2010;20:605–11.
213. Lerman J, Heard C, Steward DJ. Neonatal tracheal intubation: an imbroglio unresolved. Paediatr Anaesth. 2010;20:585–90.
214. Strolin Benedetti M, Ruty B, Baltes E. Induction of endogenous pathways by antiepileptics and clinical implications. Fundam Clin Pharmacol. 2005;19:511–29.
215. Eker HE, Yalcin Cok O, Aribogan A, Arslan G. Children on phenobarbital monotherapy requires more sedatives during MRI. Paediatr Anaesth. 2011;10:998–1002.
216. Stanski DR, Ham J, Miller RD, et al. Pharmacokinetics and pharmacodynamics of d-tubocurarine during nitrous oxide-narcotic and halothane anesthesia in man. Anesthesiology. 1979;51:235–41.
217. Prys-Roberts C, Lloyd JW, Fisher A, et al. Deliberate profound hypotension induced with halothane: studies of haemodynamics and pulmonary gas exchange. Br J Anaesth. 1974;46:105.
218. Pauca AL, Hopkins AM. Acute effects of halothane, nitrous oxide and thiopentone on upper limb blood flow. Br J Anaesth. 1972;43:326–33.
219. Taivainen T, Meretoja OA. The neuromuscular blocking effects of vecuronium during sevoflurane, halothane and balanced anaesthesia in children. Anaesthesia. 1995;50:1046–9.
220. Minto CF, Schnider TW, Short TG, Gregg KM, Gentilini A, Shafer SL. Response surface model for anesthetic drug interactions. Anesthesiology. 2000;92:1603–16.
221. Bouillon TW, Bruhn J, Radulescu L, et al. Pharmacodynamic interaction between propofol and remifentanil regarding hypnosis, tolerance of laryngoscopy, bispectral index, and electroencephalographic approximate entropy. Anesthesiology. 2004;100:1353–72.
222. Short TG, Plummer JL, Chui PT. Hypnotic and anaesthetic interactions between midazolam, propofol and alfentanil. Br J Anaesth. 1992;69:162–7.
223. Dahan A, Nieuwenhuijs D, Olofsen E, Sarton E, Romberg R, Teppema L. Response surface modeling of alfentanil-sevoflurane interaction on cardiorespiratory control and bispectral index. Anesthesiology. 2001;94:982–91.
224. Nieuwenhuijs DJ, Olofsen E, Romberg RR, et al. Response surface modeling of remifentanil-propofol interaction on cardiorespiratory control and bispectral index. Anesthesiology. 2003;98: 312–22.
225. Andolfatto G, Abu-Laban RB, Zed PJ, et al. Ketamine-propofol combination (ketofol) versus propofol alone for emergency department procedural sedation and analgesia: a randomized double-blind trial. Ann Emerg Med. 2012;59:504-12e1-2.
226. Hui TW, Short TG, Hong W, Suen T, Gin T, Plummer J. Additive interactions between propofol and ketamine when used for anesthesia induction in female patients. Anesthesiology. 1995;82: 641–8.
227. Dallimore D, Anderson BJ, Short TG, Herd DW. Ketamine anesthesia in children-exploring infusion regimens. Paediatr Anaesth. 2008;18:708–14.
228. Coulter FL, Hannam J, Anderson BJ. Ketofol simulations for dosing in pediatric anesthesia. Pediatr Anesth. 2014;24:806–12.
229. Char D, Drover DR, Motonaga KS, et al. The effects of ketamine on dexmedetomidine-induced electrophysiologic changes in children. Paediatr Anaesth. 2013;23:898–905.
230. Ramsay MAE. Intensive care: problems of over- and undersedation. Best Pract Res Clin Anaesthesiol. 2000;14:419–32.
231. Herd D, Anderson BJ. Ketamine disposition in children presenting for procedural sedation and analgesia in a children's emergency department. Paediatr Anaesth. 2007;17:622–9.
232. Dallimore D, Herd DW, Short T, Anderson BJ. Dosing ketamine for pediatric procedural sedation in the emergency department. Pediatr Emerg Care. 2008;24:529–33.

Billing and Reimbursement for Sedation Services in the United States

12

Devona J. Slater

Abstract

Sedation is intended to provide safe and effective administration of drugs to relieve anxiety and reduce pain. The aim of any sedation service is to maximize patient comfort, while monitoring the patient continuously, so that the procedure can be completed in a safe environment. The billing for sedation services has to be representative of the actual services that the physician delivers. When pediatric sedation services are hospital-based (the sedation providers are employed by the hospital), the activity of the hospital-employed nurses cannot be included in the professional charges: only the actual services that the physician alone performs can be utilized in billing for his/her professional service. Professional services should be billed by the entity that employs the physician. No matter whether the physician is in private practice or is employed by a large entity, the billing rules for professional services apply.

Keywords

Billing • Coding • Revised Hospital Anesthesia Services Interpretive Guidelines • CPT-4, Current Procedural Terminology (CPT®) • Monitored anesthesia care (MAC) • Minimal sedation • Moderate sedation • Deep sedation • General anesthesia • Regional anesthesia • Center for Medicare and Medicaid Services (CNS) • American Medical Association (AMA)

Introduction

Sedation is the safe and effective administration of drugs that relieve anxiety and reduce pain. The aim of any sedation service is to make the patient as comfortable as possible, while monitoring the patient continuously, so that the procedure can be accomplished in a completely safe environment. The billing for sedation services has to be representative of the actual services that the physician delivers. Most pediatric sedation services are hospital-based (meaning the nurses are employed by the hospital), so the activity of hospital-employed nurses cannot be included in the professional charges; only the actual services that the physician alone performs can be utilized in billing for his/her professional service. Professional services should be billed by the entity that employs the physician. No matter whether the physician is in private practice or is employed by a large entity, the billing rules for professional services apply.

The Centers for Medicare & Medicaid Services (CMS), previously known as the Health Care Financing Administration (HCFA), is a federal agency within the United States Department of Health and Human Services (DHHS) that administers the Medicare program and works in partnership with state governments to administer Medicaid, the State Children's Health Insurance Program (SCHIP), and health insurance portability standards. In addition to these programs, CMS has other responsibilities, including the administrative simplification standards from the Health Insurance Portability and Accountability Act of 1996 (HIPAA), quality standards in long-term care facilities (more commonly

D.J. Slater, C.H.A., C.H.C., C.M.C.P. (✉)
Auditing for Compliance and Education, Inc. (ACE),
10561 Barkley Street, Suite 610, Overland Park, KA 66212, USA
e-mail: devonas@aceauditors.com

K.P. Mason (ed.), *Pediatric Sedation Outside of the Operating Room: A Multispecialty International Collaboration*,
DOI 10.1007/978-1-4939-1390-9_12, © Springer Science+Business Media New York 2015

referred to as nursing homes) through its survey and certification process, and clinical laboratory quality standards under the Clinical Laboratory Improvement Amendments. CMS provides health coverage for more than 100 million people in the United States and is charged with overseeing the delivery of services, improving health care quality, and controlling health care costs in the United States.

Within the CMS Medicare benefit structure there are four different parts that cover specific services. Medicare Part A (Hospital Insurance) covers inpatient care in hospitals, skilled nursing facilities, hospice, and home health care. Medicare Part B (Medical Insurance) covers physician and other health care provider services, outpatient care, durable medical equipment, and some preventive services. It is Medicare Part B that we will be referencing throughout this chapter in regards to CMS reimbursement. Medicare Part C (Medicare Advantage) offers health plan options that are administered by Medicare-approved private insurance companies. Medicare Advantage Plans typically offer one plan that combines the coverage offered from Part A, Part B and Part D coverage. Finally, Medicare Part D (Prescription Drug Coverage) was set up to assist Medicare beneficiaries cover the cost of prescription medications.

In December of 2009, the Revised Hospital Anesthesia Services Interpretive Guidelines, which are issued by CMS for clarification regarding requirements for participation for payment of services, clearly outlined that all services involving anesthesia must be organized under a single anesthesia department [1]. The memorandum specifically states that all services along the continuum of anesthesia services must be organized under a single anesthesia service and implemented in every hospital department that provides any type of anesthesia service. These services, which must be directed by a qualified physician and consistently implemented in every hospital department, will require sedation departments to work closely with the hospital-based anesthesia department to credential providers and assess airway management skills.

The guidelines also specifically address qualified providers for deep sedation and the requirements for pre- and postoperative visits. One note of importance is the guidelines are specific in what is expected for pre-anesthesia and post-anesthesia evaluations to determine if the services are considered as general, regional, deep sedation, or monitored anesthesia care (MAC). Any of these services restrict the providers to only allow for a "qualified" anesthesia provider to perform the evaluation within a 48-h window. They clearly define qualified anesthesia providers as an anesthesiologist, a certified registered nurse anesthetist (CRNA), or an anesthesia assistant (AA) within scope of practice. Their interpretation extends the qualified providers to physicians who have been credentialed to deliver sedation services (anesthesia service privileges). These guidelines directly impact the way anesthesia departments will be judged when the CMS site visit occurs. During these site visits by the government agency, auditors look for elements in which to judge the hospital on whether they will be allowed to continue participation in the Medicare program. Hospitals will look to physicians to ensure that documentation meets the criteria sent out in the memo. While the interpretative guidelines are not physician payment rules, hospitals could not survive if they were not allowed to participate in government programs. Physicians do have a duty to ensure that the services they deliver meet the guidelines expected for hospital participation.

The Interpretative Guidelines are specific to expecting only anesthesiologists to provide the medical oversight of CRNAs and AAs in these cases that are considered to be under the jurisdiction of anesthesia. These recent CMS guidelines are especially important for those sedation services that use non-anesthesia providers to administer sedation services. Based on these guidelines, one might conclude from the Interpretive Guidelines that all general, regional, deep sedation, and MAC should only be delivered by qualified anesthesia professionals. Please reference the current CMS interpretive guidelines for anesthesia services before making decisions regarding qualified providers [2, 3].

The second item of importance in the Interpretive Guidelines is the definition of "immediately available." This phrase has often been the center of different interpretation and some consternation. The transmittal states that the CRNA/AA must be supervised by a physician who is physically located within the same area. Although this definition is a bit restrictive as it is still vague, the intention and expectations of the government are clear. The government is expecting an area to be defined as the same labor and delivery unit, the same operative suite or a procedural area, like radiology, gastroenterology (GI) or cardiac catheterization suite. In the strict definition, the guidelines would require a qualified anesthesiologist to be in each area. While no specific mention was singled out for sedation services, one could conclude that the physician overseeing the sedation services would need to remain present in the same area that the deep sedation services are delivered to fulfill the guideline.

While these guidelines specifically address the hospital's participation in Medicare and Medicaid services, they have not been applied to Part B reimbursement methodology—the physician component of payment for Medicare services. History tells us that once applied to the hospital side of reimbursement, it is only a matter of time before these regulations make their way to physician payment rules. Physicians should expect that these guidelines may be applied to Medicare Part B reimbursement language for professional services in the future.

The American Medical Association (AMA) allows any physician to use any code in the CPT-4 book. The CPT-4 reference book is the *Current Procedural Terminology*

(CPT®), Fourth Edition [4]. It is published annually by the AMA and is a set of codes, descriptions, and guidelines intended to describe procedures and services performed by physicians and other health care providers. Each procedure or service is identified with a five-digit code. The use of CPT codes is recognized industry-wide and simplifies the reporting of services. In addition to CPT codes, there are modifiers that are appended to the codes that simply describe certain aspects of the service. In anesthesia, these modifiers are required to explain the way the services are delivered (medical direction modifiers) and if services are for MAC.

As previously stated, any physician may use any code as long as the services that are delivered are reported accurately. Documentation is critical as to the reason for the service as well as what was actually performed by the physician. Many insurance companies have policies specifically addressing the use of anesthesia codes by non-anesthesiologists. Most will reimburse any non-anesthesia physician's billing for MAC services or those with greater depth of sedation when the physician bills the appropriate anesthesia code (00100-01999). Using these anesthesia codes, however, requires that the physician:

- Perform pre-evaluation and post-evaluation services
- Document the anesthesia time in minutes
- Normally reimburse these services regardless of place of service
- Meet the requirements for MAC

The service documentation for MAC or deep sedation services must mirror that of a general or regional anesthetic in order to be billed with the anesthesia codes. It is recommended that if billing anesthesia codes, physicians should document in the anesthesia record format. This would include constant monitoring and the notation of drugs delivered on a time-sensitive record.

With sedation services facing financial pressures, it is important to remember that while the AMA may allow the anesthesia codes to be billed by non-anesthesia providers, some states have regulations regarding the scope of practice and who may administer specific anesthesia drugs, such as propofol. Several manufacturers of the specific regulated drugs have product labeling advising that only persons trained in the administration of general anesthesia should be allowed to utilize these drugs. While it is recognized that many physicians are skilled in the management of critically ill patients and have specialty training in cardiovascular resuscitation and airway management, the non-anesthesia provider must work with the anesthesia department to develop policies and procedures that will best protect the patient during sedation services. As stated previously, it is NOT the biller's responsibility to determine the codes that accurately describe the services provided. Only the provider knows what services were provided during the procedure and therefore it is their responsibility to determine the correct code. The biller may assist by educating the provider on which codes are available, but ultimately the provider must ensure the selected code(s) support the services performed.

In order to understand how best to bill for sedation services, it is important to first evaluate the services that are being provided for the patient. The documentation as well as the actual services rendered will direct how the service can be coded and billed. Sedation services are coded differently, based on the depth of sedation given. This is a medical decision made by a provider and cannot (and should not) be determined by a medical coder. The provider must be specific in his/her documentation as to whether they are providing minimal, moderate, or deep sedation, or a general anesthetic.

Minimal Sedation

Minimal sedation is a drug-induced state during which patients respond normally to verbal commands. Although cognitive function and coordination may be impaired, ventilatory and cardiovascular functions are unaffected. If providing minimal sedation services, there is no additional payment allowed. There are no codes to represent the service of minimal sedation. Minimal sedation is normally done under the direction of the surgeon and is bundled into the payment for a procedure. No additional payment is allowed for this service.

Moderate Sedation

Moderate sedation is a drug-induced depression of consciousness during which patients respond purposefully to verbal commands, either alone or accompanied by light tactile stimulation. No interventions are required to maintain the patient's airway and spontaneous ventilation is adequate.

Moderate sedation codes were introduced by the AMA in 2006 to recognize services that are in between minimal sedations and that of deep sedation (MAC). The services include: (1) a patient assessment, (2) establishment of IV access, (3) administrations of agents, (4) sedation maintenance, (5) monitoring of oxygen saturation, heart rate, and blood pressure; and (6) recovery of the patient. The AMA chose to keep with the logic of anesthesia billing, allowing the coding to be billed by time. The codes require the documentation of "intra-service" time. As defined, intra-service time starts with the delivery of the sedation agent and ends when the procedure is finished. Time-based codes must also follow the general instructions related to time-based services. CPT instructions specifically address the required definition of face-to-face time with the patient and explain that a unit of service may not be billed until the midpoint of time is passed. What this means in coding moderate sedation services is that

Table 12.1 Billing moderate sedation

99143	Moderate sedation services, provided by the same physician performing the diagnostic or therapeutic service that the sedation supports, requiring the presence of an independent trained observer to assist in the monitoring of the patient's level of consciousness and physiological status; younger than 5 years of age, first 30 min intra-service time
99144	Moderate sedation services, provided by the same physician performing the diagnostic or therapeutic service that the sedation supports, requiring the presence of an independent trained observer to assist in the monitoring of the patient's level of consciousness and physiological status; age 5 years or older, first 30 min intra-service time
99145	Each additional 15 min intra-service time
99148	Moderate sedation services, provided by a physician other than the health care professional performing the diagnostic or therapeutic service that the sedation supports; younger than 5 years of age, first 30 min intra-service time
99149	Moderate sedation services, provided by a physician other than the health care professional performing the diagnostic or therapeutic service that the sedation supports; age 5 years or older, first 30 min intra-service time
99150	Each additional 15 min intra-service time

the appropriate CPT code cannot be assigned unless 50 % or more of the time requirement is met.

The coding of moderate sedation services is reported by CPT codes 99143–99150. The actual coding is specific to the practitioner delivering the service, the age of the patient, the facility, and the amount of intra-service time. Surgeon supervision is allowed in all types of locations and requires an independent trained third-party person dedicated to monitor the patient. In contrast, CPT codes 99148–99150 are services provided by a second physician and are only allowed in a facility setting such as a hospital. The codes are specific to patients under or over the age of 5 and require it to be physician administered and require the physician to stay with the patient the entire time. Table 12.1 outlines each of these codes.

Currently the Medicare system and many commercial carriers allow additional payment for moderate sedation as long as it is not for a code that includes sedation services in the descriptor (see CPT-4 Book, current year, Appendix G). At the time of this writing, the moderate sedation codes have been assigned a status indicator of "C" under the Medicare Physician Fee Schedule, designating that these services are carrier priced—meaning that each individual Medicare intermediary determines the amount of payment appropriate for the service. At this time, CMS has not established relative value units for these services and payments vary based on the carrier and the region of the country. For commercial payors, rates range from $40 to 200 per unit, depending on the geographical area of the country and the specific carrier.

The confusion in billing for sedation services occurs when a separate physician delivers only a part of the sedation services, such as the triage, evaluation, and sedation plan followed by his supervision of a sedation nurse. There is no coding reference for this type of activity. However, it is important for the physician to support the need for sedation service. For example, it is understood that in young children, sedation services are necessary to perform procedures. Careful documentation is critical in the event that at a later period (maybe even years later), the reviewer disagrees with the necessity of having a separate physician provide the sedation service. Carriers may take up to 7 years to contest or disagree with a charge, but providers also should understand that if government agents believe fraud was involved, they may go back indefinitely. Therefore, a well-documented record that explains your thought process of why sedation is needed is the best protection you can have in defending health care scrutiny.

Key Components of Evaluation and Management Services Documentation

All evaluation and management services have specific components. There are seven components that assist coders in translating the documented work into the appropriate code selected, of which only three are required (key) components that must be documented for all visits. These three key components are: (1) patient history, (2) physical examination, and (3) medical decision-making.

The first specific key component is the *patient history*. The history section contains several elements, including:

- The chief complaint/presenting problem
- The history of present illness
- A review of systems
- The past medical, family, and social history of the patient

This history section should include the justification and rationale for requiring a separate physician to provide the sedation services.

The second of the key components is the *physical examination*. The examination documentation must contain up-to-date information regarding the patient's condition at the time of the exam and should describe the results and findings of body areas or organ systems that are actually examined by the physician during the encounter. It is specifically noted that this type of physical examination should be based on the physician's clinical judgment and directed toward that which is medically indicated to support the medical decision.

The final of the three key components is the *medical decision*. The medical decision is commonly referred to as "the thought process of the physician." It should be a statement (or statements) that represent the complexity of the decision-making process involved in selecting a plan for the management and delivery of sedation services. This assessment should include the critical elements that were considered in deriving the sedation plan as well as the intended depth of sedation required. There is not a clearly defined level of risk involved in providing sedation. The CMS guidelines best define the degree of risk involved in making these medical decisions within the low to moderate decision-making category, depending on the nature of the presenting problem(s) of the patient and the procedure.

If the evaluation and management plan of the sedation is performed by a provider separate from that who will be delivering and monitoring the sedation, it would be appropriate to charge for the initial services under evaluation and management codes. These concurrent care services are payable when the physician plays an active role in the patient's treatment or the treatment plan. The medical diagnosis should reflect the need for medical evaluation and management as a necessity for the delivery of subsequent sedation services.

Deep Sedation (MAC)

Deep sedation is defined as a drug-induced depression of consciousness during which patients cannot be easily aroused following repeated or painful stimulation. The ability to independently maintain ventilatory function during this time may be impaired and assistance may be required to maintain the airway.

One cannot discuss deep sedation and MAC without understanding the differences. MAC is light, moderate, or deep sedation where the provider of MAC must be prepared and qualified to convert to general anesthesia. Many MAC services do not require the delivery of any agents; although it is unlikely, the patient's risk level requires them to be prepared to convert to a general anesthetic.

Insurance companies are interested in addressing the rules surrounding medical necessity for the separate anesthesia provider as this adds to the cost of the service. The American Society of Anesthesiologists' (ASA) position statement defines medically necessary services as those that alleviate emotional or psychological duress or pain while undergoing a surgical, obstetrical, or other therapeutic/diagnostic procedure. The ASA supports that the level of sedation should be based on the medical judgment of a physician who is trained in anesthesia, in conjunction with the physician performing the procedure. The targeted level of sedation must consider all aspects of the patient's health as well as the procedure to be performed. Many insurance companies do not recognize this broad definition and relate the medical necessity to the ASA status of the patient, requiring additional diagnosis (ICD-9 codes) to accompany the reason for the procedure to support the need for separate anesthesia providers. The ASA status is the assignment of a P code to assess the degree of a patient's "sickness" or "physical state" prior to selecting the anesthetic or prior to performing surgery. It helps determine the "risk" that a patient presents, describing patients' preoperative physical condition. Some insurance companies designate an ASA status of P3 or higher to justify the need of a separate anesthesia provider.

In billing an anesthesia code from the CPT-4 book, physician providers are held to the same requirements of documentation as that which is required from an anesthesia provider. This includes:

1. A preoperative assessment that would review abnormalities of the major organ systems
2. An airway assessment
3. A history of any previous experience with sedation or anesthetics
4. A review of drug allergies and current medications
5. A review of tobacco, alcohol, or substance abuse
6. The time and nature of last oral intake
7. Assignment of the ASA physical status

During the actual medical procedure, the appropriate monitoring must be performed and would include:

1. Heart rates
2. Oxygenation
3. Respiratory frequency and adequacy of pulmonary ventilation
4. Blood pressure and cardiac monitoring

Vital signs should be documented at 5-min intervals.

A post-anesthesia assessment recording physiological status, mental status, and a pain level should be recorded prior to transferring care to post-anesthesia care unit personnel. The medical record should document that the patient was discharged from the recovery area only after meeting clinical criteria approved by the department of anesthesia or an anesthesiologist.

General, Regional, and Monitored Anesthesia Care

Billing done for anesthesia services allows the assignment of base units added to time units, usually assigned in 15-min increments, and then adding modifying circumstances or physical status units. The ASA base units are assigned to every surgical CPT code and reflect the difficulty of the anesthesia services, including the usual preoperative and postoperative care. The CPT procedure code is cross-walked to the appropriate anesthesia code based on region of the body, technique, and the age of the patient. Unlike with other specialties, anesthesia can only bill for a single procedure, even when multiple procedures are performed at the same setting. In these circumstances, the anesthesia may be billed for the procedure with the highest unit value. After the selection of base units has been established, anesthesia time is calculated and added to the base units. Anesthesia time starts when the provider begins to prepare the patient for anesthesia care in the operating room or equivalent area and ends when the patient is safely placed in the care of the post-anesthesia care unit. The total number of minutes is then divided by a number that is customary in the local area, which in most areas of the country is 15 min. This will convert the minutes into units that are then added to the base unit value. Qualifying circumstances and physical status modifiers carry a base unit value in certain circumstances. Patients with severe systemic disease or cases that meet the definition of qualifying circumstances may be allowed to add extra units. It is best to consult the ASA Current Year Relative Value Guide to establish billing for units.

In some circumstances, the insurance carrier may require "modifiers" that are meant to define "who provided the service" and, with other special modifiers, occasions when the services were MAC. Modifiers are simply additional two-digit codes that tell the carriers specific things about the anesthesia service. The first modifiers appended to the anesthesia service are termed as medical direction modifiers. *Only anesthesiologists are allowed to direct qualified anesthesia personnel and provide multiple services at one time.* The AA modifier designates that the physician alone provided the service. The QK modifier would represent medical direction services of a CRNA, AA, anesthesia resident/trainee or SRNA, and, if appropriate, would have a matching claim from those providers with the QX modifier.

When providing MAC, the second set of modifiers appended on the claim form should identify the MAC service with one of the following informational modifiers:

- QS: designates MAC
- G8: designates the MAC services are necessary because the procedure is noted as deep, complex, complicated, or markedly invasive
- G9: designates the MAC services are necessary because the patient has a personal history of cardiopulmonary disease

The final modifiers that may be appended would be the physical status modifiers denoting the condition of the patient. These are outlined in the CPT-4 instructions and all start with P.

Fee for Services

Payment for anesthesia services is determined on a unit basis. Payment is not restricted to specialty designation as long as the services are equal in nature. Unit values vary from a low of a few dollars (usually those paid by state or government programs) to more than $100.00 per unit.

Contracting with commercial payors for anesthesia services is a key element for success in a sedation program. Meeting with payors to explain the nature of the service and the allowance of non-anesthesia personnel to be paid under anesthesia codes are large hurdles for any sedation program. "Major" insurance carriers should be identified and then addressed individually. To support reimbursement, providers need to keep in mind the qualifications of the provider, the medical necessity of the service, and the cost benefit to the insurance company. Negotiations will require that the non-anesthesiologists demonstrate that they can provide the same level of care as the local anesthesiologists and that the care is medically necessary for the safety of the patient. The important thing for providers to remember is that quality of care is always assumed by insurance executives.

Payment for moderate sedation codes as well as evaluation and management codes are based on a flat fee service. These reimbursement amounts vary greatly by payor. Most non-governmental carriers will base reimbursement as a percentage of the Medicare Resource Based Relative Value System (RBRVS) reimbursement system. RBRVS is a payment methodology that was developed for the government back in 1988. RBRVS assigns a relative value to each procedure, which is then adjusted by geographic region. That value is then multiplied by a conversion factor, which changes every year, to determine the amount of payment. Management personnel should carefully evaluate reimbursement and negotiate rates with payors in order to reflect a fair and appropriate payment for the intensity and time required for the sedation services rendered.

Physician Quality Measure Reporting

There are category II codes in the CPT-4 book that coincide with the quality initiatives that have been developed by the CMS. The goal in reporting these codes is to decrease the need for clinical chart abstraction and to ease the burden on health care professionals in reporting the quality of patient care. CMS started the program in July of 2007 with incentive payments of 1.5 % for successful participation. At the time of this writing, the use of these codes and the program are optional and only for Medicare patients, although the program is scheduled to penalize physicians for not reporting starting in 2015.

There are currently 259 measures; 138 individual quality measures and the remaining measures are broken down into 12 measure groups. The codes actually describe clinical components that may occur during evaluation and management services or clinical services. There are some codes that actually describe results from clinical laboratory, radiology, or other diagnostic procedures relating to patient safety processes or reflecting compliance with state or federal laws during the service. The primary resource for these measures is found on the CMS Website [5], but additional resources can be found on the AMA Website [6]. The AMA Website has tools that review the indicators for each measure, the required elements in documentation, and the exact reporting instructions. Participation in this program encompasses a physician's entire practice. It is recommended that providers carefully review all of the information before selecting measures to report.

Physicians reporting sedation services, as discussed within this chapter with evaluation and management codes, have many reporting possibilities due to the patient history and examination options aligned with the evaluation and management codes. Popular measures reported by providers include reconciliation of medications, smoking status/tobacco use, and body mass indexing. For physicians who personally perform the sedation services (CPT-4 codes 99144-99150), there are no reporting options for those services. And finally, for those physicians who choose to report MAC services, there are limited category II options. Currently the anesthesia codes trigger measures on the timely administration of antibiotics and perioperative temperature management. Again, it is important before reporting any of the measures that providers thoroughly understand which CPT codes trigger the measure, what documentation is required in the patient's medical record, and how they are to be correctly reported.

Legal Consequences of Incorrect Coding/Documentation

If one is to choose billing for these services as an anesthesiologist, it is important to be compliant with documentation of billing for anesthesia time and concurrency. As defined, anesthesia time is face-to-face contact time with the patient. This is a concept that the enforcement agencies have paid particular attention to and will continue to do so. Using circulating nursing records, surgeon's operative reports, and post-anesthesia care unit records, auditors are able to verify if time reported is accurate. Concurrency again can only be reported by an anesthesiologist and even then close attention must be paid to exactly what services were being delivered at any one time. The government does not allow you to medically direct and personally perform services at any one given time. Knowing and understanding that an anesthesiologist cannot medically direct and personally perform services at the same time is crucial to staying out of compliance trouble. Deep sedation services will have the same constraints, remembering that one physician can only attend to one patient at a time.

No matter what specialty, the government's activities to recoup monies that have been paid inappropriately will continue. The realization is that the government has a tremendous return on fraud and abuse investment dollars and will continue to scrutinize services. Physicians can be penalized monetarily or, in some cases where fraud is involved, jail time, a loss of medical licensure, or exclusion from the Medicare and Medicaid programs prevail. It is for this reason that it is critical to implement compliance programs.

The implementation of a compliance program can be a challenge, as many physicians are still unclear as to "What makes an effective compliance program?" The most effective programs will have integrated the compliance into the day-to-day operations of the group and will incorporate the seven federal sentencing guidelines into simple day-to-day procedures.

The first of the sentencing guidelines requires written policies and procedures. The policies and procedures that have been written for the program need to be understood by all members of the group. It is important that employees have guidance in understanding the basic concepts discussed in the plan. Plan policies could be tested and results kept in personnel files to ensure that everyone knows the commitment of the group to the compliance plan and the intention to only bill for services that are appropriately documented.

Second, the guidelines specifically ask that a compliance officer be designated for the group. The group must evaluate the performance of the compliance officer and while the compliance officer does not necessarily have to be a physician, it does have to be someone who has the absolute authority to hire and fire personnel. The Board should assess whether the compliance officer has sufficient knowledge and education to deal with the assigned responsibilities. It would be important for them to judge whether appropriate auditing and education are being carried out to fulfill the requirements of compliance. Compliance committee minutes and processes of handling any reported violations should be reviewed to ensure all issues have been dealt with and recorded as to corrective action.

Education and training of all levels of employees must be done according to the sentencing guidelines. Courses and educational materials should reflect the important aspects of the group's compliance program. Ongoing training and demonstration of evaluation of knowledge should be recorded. Keeping accurate records of content, frequency, and attendees is very important in order to demonstrate educational efforts.

The sentencing guidelines stress open communication and it is considered an essential element in a compliance program. In today's environment, a provider cannot possibly have an effective compliance program if it receives minimal or no feedback from employees. Simply recording that there have not been any violations reported is not enough. A record of questions regarding policies, and any guidance given or research done by the compliance officer or committee, should be documented to show open lines of communication.

One of the key components of the sentencing guidelines stresses ongoing monitoring and auditing. Auditing, both internal and external, is critical to a successful compliance program. Frequency and the extent of the audit function will vary depending on the size and issues identified by the group. Audits must not discriminate between providers and must address issues that are considered "hot spots" in the specialty. Audits should ensure that elements set forth in the compliance plan are being monitored and that auditing techniques are valid and conducted by objective reviewers. For example, we know sedation programs may be using Evaluation and Management coding to bill for services. A compliance professional would want to audit these services to see if they meet the criteria for billing. If deep sedation programs are billing with anesthesia codes, an audit regarding anesthesia time, modifiers, and documentation of the components of an anesthesia service should be reviewed.

The sixth requirement of the federal sentencing guidelines requires suspected violations to be thoroughly investigated. When a provider learns of an issue, it is important to contact legal counsel to properly handle and circumvent any exposure to the group. If evidence exists that misconduct has occurred, counsel will be needed to work through the process of self-disclosure.

Finally, disciplinary action makes up the last key ingredient to the federal sentencing guidelines. Disciplinary action must be taken on those employees who fail to adhere to the group's standards set forth in the compliance program. Discipline must be applied consistently between employees, regardless of the employee's level in the corporation, and documented. Senior management must demonstrate a serious commitment to foster a climate that will require adherence to all federal and state regulations.

In summary, compliance is an activity that must be incorporated into the day-to-day practices of the group. Government investigations will continue. All new healthcare legislation mentions the need for continued efforts to fight fraud and abuse. The best protection for a group is an active compliance program.

Conclusion

Remember, there is no single way to bill "sedation" services. Anesthesia/sedation services must begin with careful documentation to adequately reflect the role of the sedation care provider throughout the entire sedation process. Careful consideration should be used to determine the appropriate coding methodology. In many instances, the coding should be determined on a case-by-case basis after careful review of the documentation and nature of physician services. It is recommended to regularly have an independent review of documentation, coding, and billing in order to avoid inadvertent mistakes that may be audited by authorities. A coding professional can assist in helping ascertain accurate coding and also determine the best way to achieve best reimbursement for service.

Case Scenarios

The following are scenarios of how cases may need to be billed based on the personnel involved, the level of sedation delivered, and the intensity of the service. These are hypothetical examples and in no way reflect medical care:

A pediatric radiologist in the outpatient hospital setting would like to have sedation services for the patient's magnetic resonance imaging (MRI) study.

1. If the radiologist supervises a registered nurse (non-physician) giving the moderate sedation, you would review codes 99143–99145.
2. If the radiologist requests another physician, such as a pediatrician, to perform the moderate sedation, you would review codes 99148–99150.
3. If the radiologist uses the hospital sedation service, which is headed by the hospitalist who sees the patient, clears the patient for the moderate sedation services, and then supervises a specially trained registered nurse (non-physician) to administer the moderate sedation, the physician may only bill for an evaluation and management service based on the evaluation and management elements documented and the medical decision-making performed.
4. If the radiologist requests that deep sedation be given and someone who has the credentials to deliver deep sedation provides the service, you should review the ASA code 01922 and review the anesthesia record for the appropriate time billing.
5. If a non-anesthesiologist or anesthesiologist is able to provide MAC for the radiologists, you should review ASA code 01922 and append the QS modifier designating that it is MAC and review the anesthesia record for the appropriate time billing.

References

1. Centers for Medicare and Medicaid Services. CMS Manual System. Pub 100-07 State Operations Provider Certification. Appendix A. 42 CFR. Section 482.52. Revised hospital anesthesia services interpretive guidelines, 11 Dec 2009. http://www.cms.gov/SurveyCertificationGenInfo/downloads/SCLetter10_09.pdf. Last accessed Dec 19, 2013
2. Department of Health & Human Services. Centers for Medicare & Medicaid Services. CMS Manual System. Pub. 100-07 State Operations Provider Certification. Transmittal 59. Clarification of the interpretive guidelines for the anesthesia services condition of participation, 21 May 2010. https://www.cms.gov/transmittals/downloads/R59SOMA.pdf. Last accessed Dec 19, 2013.
3. Centers for Medicare and Medicaid Services. CMS Manual System. Pub 100-07 State Operations Provider Certification. Appendix A. 42 CFR. Section 482.52. Revised hospital anesthesia services interpretive guidelines, 14 Jan 2011. http://www.cms.gov/SurveyCertificationgeninfo/downloads/SCLetter11_10.pdf. Last accessed Dec 19, 2013.
4. Current Procedural Terminology: CPT 2013. Professional edition. Chicago: AMA Press; 2012.
5. Centers for Medicare and Medicaid Services. http://www.cms.gov/Medicare/Quality-Initiatives-Patient-Assessment-Instruments/PQRS/MeasuresCodes.html. Last accessed Dec 19, 2013.
6. American Medical Association. http://www.ama-assn.org/ama/pub/physician-resources/clinical-practice-improvement/clinical-quality/physician-quality-reporting-system-2013.page. Last accessed Dec 19, 2013.

Part II

Sedation Models Delivered by Different Specialties: A Global Voyage

The Pediatric Hospital Medicine Service: Models, Protocols, and Challenges

13

Douglas W. Carlson and Suzanne S. Mendez

Abstract

Care of hospitalized patients often requires diagnostic and therapeutic procedures. Often, these procedures are best done using sedation and analgesia. It is the responsibility of the pediatric hospitalist to either perform or arrange for these procedures. It is also the responsibility of the pediatric hospitalist to guarantee that any sedation or analgesia needed to perform these procedures is delivered in the safest and most effective way possible. Pediatric hospitalists can either arrange for appropriately trained staff to deliver sedation or obtain the necessary skills to perform the sedations themselves.

Keywords

Pediatric hospitalist • Moderate sedation • Deep sedation • Training • Operating room • Simulations • Credentialing • Pre-sedation exam • Triage • Ketamine • Dexmedetomidine • Pentobarbital • Fentanyl • Midazolam • Nitrous oxide • Propofol • Dexmedetomidine • Pediatric advanced life support (PALS) • Upper respiratory tract infection (URI) • American Society of Anesthesiologists (ASA) • Laryngospasm

Introduction

The field of pediatric hospital medicine has grown rapidly over the past two decades. The term "hospitalist" was initially defined in an article in the New England Journal of Medicine in 1996; that definition included spending half or more of one's work in the area of inpatient care. There are now pediatric hospitalists on the medical staffs of most children's hospitals in the United States as well as on the medical staffs of an ever-increasing number of community hospitals.

D.W. Carlson, M.D. (✉)
Division of Pediatric Hospitalist Medicine,
Department of Pediatrics, St. Louis Children's Hospital,
Washington University, St. Louis, MO, USA
e-mail: carlson@wustl.edu

S.S. Mendez, M.D.
Department of Pediatrics, Santa Clara Valley
Medical Center, San Jose, CA, USA

Since pediatric hospitalists spend a majority of their time caring for hospitalized patients, they are in a position to fully understand the clinical needs of those patients. Pediatric hospitalists identify the needs of patients and work within systems to provide appropriate care. They also work to provide care safely, effectively, and efficiently.

Care of hospitalized patients often requires diagnostic and therapeutic procedures. Often, these procedures are best done using sedation and analgesia. It is the responsibility of the pediatric hospitalist to either perform or arrange for these procedures. It is also the responsibility of the pediatric hospitalist to guarantee that any sedation or analgesia needed to perform these procedures is delivered in the safest and most effective way possible.

The ability to provide safe procedural sedation is a core skill for pediatric hospitalists, as noted in the published Pediatric Hospital Medicine Core Competencies in 2010 [1]. In a survey conducted by the Pediatric Research in Inpatient Settings (PRIS) Network [2], 54 % of pediatric hospitalists reported providing moderate and/or deep sedation. The survey revealed that the majority of sedation is narcotic and

K.P. Mason (ed.), *Pediatric Sedation Outside of the Operating Room: A Multispecialty International Collaboration*,
DOI 10.1007/978-1-4939-1390-9_13, © Springer Science+Business Media New York 2015

Table 13.1 Sedation drugs reported by those pediatric hospitalists providing sedation [2]

94 %	Opioid/benzodiazepine combination
70 %	Chloral hydrate
51 %	Ketamine
46 %	Pentobarbital
16 %	Propofol
6 %	Nitrous oxide

Table 13.2 Location of sedations [2]

86 %	Inpatient wards
24 %	Radiology departments
16 %	Sedation centers
8 %	Emergency departments
5 %	PICU
4 %	Other: endoscopy suites, EEG, ambulatory surgery, and infusion centers

Table 13.3 Sedation training [2]

79 %	On the job
71 %	Residency training
44 %	Training under direct supervision
42 %	Postresidency educational courses following the completion of medical training
19 %	Operating room sedation during

benzodiazepine based, delivered on a hospital floor/ward, presumably at a patient's bedside. Furthermore, there is not always a specific designated training in sedation for pediatric hospitalists [2] (Tables 13.1, 13.2, and 13.3).

Training Hospitalists to Provide Moderate and Deep Sedation

There are no national standards for the training of non-anesthesiologists in the practice of safe delivery of sedation. The training should be established locally, and once established should be adhered to. The training should include evaluation of patients, establishing safe systems of care, decision-making on the most appropriate drugs, and ability to rescue patients from deeper levels of sedation than intended. There are different types of training that hospitalists use to obtain these skills. It is up to the individual hospitalist providing sedation to feel comfortable in their abilities to provide sedation, and it is up to the institutions where these hospitalists work to define the level of training necessary to develop and maintain sedation skills.

On-the-Job Training

In the PRIS survey, most hospitalists who provide sedation reported that they received on-the-job training. The intensity of this training varies widely, from being involved in a few sedations prior to performing them independently, to very structured programs. It is important that hospitalists have defined training prior to performing sedations and are never placed in a position of performing sedations simply because no one else is willing to [3].

Residency Training

Exposure to and training for safe sedation practice is highly variable during pediatric residencies. Many pediatric residents have significant exposure, and many pediatric residents perform sedations under direct supervision of pediatric-trained attendings. However, since the training is so highly variable, it should not be assumed that most pediatricians have adequate training in residency to perform sedations independently without further training and experience.

Training Under Direct Supervision

This is really part of on-the-job training but implies a more detailed and comprehensive program of gaining experience in safe sedation practice. This training can be done with anesthesiology staff or pediatricians with significant experience and proficiency in sedation. The number of directly supervised sedations and number performed with each drug used should be determined by the local institution.

Operating Room Time

This can be an important adjunct to other types of training. In the operating room (OR) there will likely be opportunities for airway management that are difficult to obtain elsewhere. This is particularly important with the concept of rescue. Most patients in the operating room need advanced airway management. Skills that can be practiced in the OR include maintaining airways with positioning, positive pressure ventilation with a bag, laryngeal mask airway (LMA) placement, and intubation. OR time allows improvement of airway management skills in a controlled environment. This type of training is not essential for everyone that is providing sedation but is something that should be strongly considered.

Simulation Time

There are an increasing number of simulation labs available for use in sedation training, particularly in academic medical centers. Training in a simulation lab can be very helpful in training for sedation. Mannequins are becoming more and more sophisticated and are more closely simulating real-life experiences. Simulation labs can be particularly helpful with management of difficult situations that are hopefully avoided in safe sedation practice on actual patients. Simulation can also be useful in training for rare events such as laryngospasm.

Pediatric Advance Life Support Training

Pediatric advanced life support (PALS) training is an important adjunct to the provision of safe sedation. However, it should not be used as a proxy for adequate training for those that are providing sedation. PALS should be a part of a training program for safe sedation, but should never be used alone as adequate indication of sufficient training to provide moderate and deep sedation.

Ongoing Competency

Once a hospitalist has been trained and credentialed in the provision of safe sedation, it is important to maintain the skill and have a method for measuring those competencies. There are no set standards for the number of sedations to be completed on an annual basis in order to maintain competencies. Each institution should establish a minimum number and type of sedations performed on an annual basis or develop a program that includes other methods of maintaining skills, such as OR time or simulation lab time. Some drugs, such as propofol, should have very defined minimum numbers of annual sedations provided by each provider in order to maintain credentialing. At St. Louis Children's Hospital, non-anesthesiologist providers who are credentialed to use propofol are required to document 25 propofol sedations on an annual basis. This number is not meant to be a guide for others but an example of one institution's decision [4, 5].

Credentialing Hospitalists to Provide Moderate and Deep Sedation in the United States

In the United States, most pediatric hospitalists have completed 3 years of pediatric training in a categorical pediatric residency. Some pediatric hospitalists have finished a combined residency in Pediatrics and Internal Medicine, and a few have completed family medicine residencies. Many pediatric residents have some exposure to the provision of moderate and deep sedation during their pediatric residency, but the provision of moderate and deep sedation is not part of the core competencies in pediatric residency as recognized by the Accrediting Council on Graduate Medical Education (ACGME). The training during pediatric residencies in sedation is highly variable, from very little formal training to several dedicated weeks in the operating room and on a sedation service. Training and experience with moderate and deep sedation is part of the core ACGME fellowship competencies for pediatric emergency medicine and pediatric critical care medicine.

Each hospital should develop its own criteria for credentialing physicians for the provision of moderate and deep sedation. The Joint Commission suggests that all individuals who provide moderate and deep sedation have a minimum level of competency based on education, training, and experience [6]. The Joint Commission outlines the following abilities and competencies for performing moderate and deep sedation:

1. Ability to evaluate patients before performing moderate and deep sedation
2. Ability to perform a moderate and deep sedation, including resuscitation of patients who move into a deeper-than-desired level of sedation or analgesia
   (a) Individuals providing moderate sedation are qualified to rescue patients from deep sedation and have the ability to manage a compromised airway and to provide adequate oxygenation and ventilation.
   (b) Individuals providing deep sedation are qualified to rescue patients from general anesthesia and are able to manage an unstable cardiovascular system as well as compromised airway, and to provide adequate oxygenation and ventilation.

Joint Commission standards also require that "individuals administering moderate and deep sedation are qualified and have the appropriate credentials to manage patients at whatever level of sedation is achieved, either intentionally or unintentionally" [6].

It is up to individual institutions to develop credentialing standards for moderate and deep sedation. Credentialing standards for physicians are set through an organized medical staff structure in most hospitals. This is done through the medical staff by laws and rules and regulations of the hospital. Most hospitals depend on their department of anesthesiology to establish the credentialing rules for the provision of moderate and deep sedation by non-anesthesiologists. The amount of education, training, and experience to provide privileges for the provision of moderate and deep sedation is an institution-by-institution decision.

Table 13.4 outlines the education, training, and experience necessary for moderate and deep sedation privileges at St. Louis Children's Hospital in the United States. It also outlines the experience and training necessary for the non-anesthesiologists that provide scheduled sedations on the sedation service. It also outlines the requirements for hospitalists to be granted specific privileges for the use of propofol. This information is presented as an example of a credentialing process.

Table 13.4 St. Louis Children's Hospital (SLCH) and Washington University (WU) credentialing requirements for hospitalists providing moderate and deep sedation

Credentials required for all non-anesthesiologist medical staff	
Successful completion of a postgraduate residency training program, approved by either the Accrediting Graduate Medical Education (AGME), the American Osteopathic Association (AOA), or the American Association of Dental Schools (AADS) with exposure to anesthesia and IV moderate and deep sedation including training in indications, contraindications, pre-sedation assessment, intra-sedation care, procedure monitoring, post-sedation care, and the pharmacology of sedation medication with associated reversal and resuscitative drugs *—OR—* If postgraduate training did not include exposure to anesthesia and sedation as stated above, demonstration of completion of an approved training sequence including both didactic and practical components that meet SLCH requirements and have documented clinical experience for at least 20 cases over the past 12 months with document and quality outcomes that meet guidelines as established by the anesthesiologist-in-chief and St. Louis Children's Hospital medical staff *—OR—* Performed at least 40 documented sedations over the prior 12 months at St. Louis Children's Hospital with documented quality outcomes that meet guidelines as established by the anesthesiologist-in-chief and St. Louis Children's Hospital	
Credentials required for hospitalists on sedation service	**Credentials required for propofol-certified hospitalists on sedation service**
1. St. Louis Children's Hospital moderate and deep sedation privileges	1. St. Louis Children's Hospital moderate and deep sedation privileges
2. Minimum of 1 year experience in SLCH/WU hospitalist program	2. Minimum of 2 years experience in SLCH/WU hospitalist program
3. Track record of strong clinical and interpersonal skills	3. Minimum of 1 year on our sedation service
4. Five operating room training days, including bag valve mask ventilation, LMA placements, and intubation	4. Didactic course and simulation lab time as directed by the department of anesthesiology
5. Documented experience with each sedative agent that will be used in our experience, including but not limited to ketamine, fentanyl/midazolam, dexmedetomidine, nitrous oxide, pentobarbital, and chloride hydrate	5. Ten intubations, 15 LMA placements, and 15 bag valve mask ventilations
	6. Twenty-five directly supervised propofol sedations

Logistics of Setting Up a Hospitalist-Run Sedation Service

Staffing

The number of hospitalists needed to provide sedation services will vary depending on the need that they are meeting. While some pediatric hospitalists provide sedation services full time, most involved in sedation services do it as one of several clinical responsibilities. The number of hospitalists needed to provide a sedation service needs to account for this, as well as the need to maintain a minimum number of sedations performed on an annual basis for competency. In general, pediatric hospitalists should perform a minimum of 25–50 sedations per year to maintain skills. With less than 25 sedations per year there should be a rigorous plan for further operating room time, simulation time, and supervised time. Further operating room time and simulation time is also an important part of maintaining skills for pediatric hospitalists who are performing more than 25 sedations per year.

Staffing Example

Providing a pediatric hospitalist for sedations 5 days per week, 10 h per day requires about 1.5 full-time equivalents (FTE) to staff the service. Therefore, if each pediatric hospitalist provides 4–5 days per month on a sedation service, four pediatric hospitalists would be needed to staff the service. Four to five days per month of providing sedation generally establishes a good balance between maintaining sedations skills and the other skills important to the clinical responsibilities of a pediatric hospitalist.

Sufficient time needs to be planned for training prior to starting a sedation service. It is important to plan for operating room time, supervised sedation time, and any other activities involved in training. If you underestimate the amount of time that it will take to establish a program, the start date will be delayed and promised expectations may not be met. It is also important to plan for turnover of staff. It is a good idea to get commitment of pediatric hospitalists for a prolonged period after the training while recognizing that some turnover is inevitable. Training of new personnel takes time and other resources that need to be accounted for in the planning stages [3].

Triaging Patients to Sedation by Pediatric Hospitalists

In general, pediatric hospitalists who are trained and credentialed to provide sedation do so on patients with mild sedation risk. Sedations performed by most pediatric hospitalists do not include planned airway intervention. However, it is essential that pediatric hospitalist have the ability to rescue patients from a deeper-than-intended level of sedation. Most often this includes skills of effective positive pressure ventilation and direct airway management through the LMA placement or endotracheal tube (ETT) placement. Patients must be properly triaged so that those with increased risk from sedation have the proper personnel attending the sedation. At St. Louis Children's Hospital, the conditions listed in Table 13.5 are referred to anesthesiologists for consultation.

At Santa Clara Valley Medical Center (SCVMC), with a hospitalist- and intensivist-based sedation service, the comorbidities in Table 13.5 are taken in context of the procedure to be performed.

This list is not meant to be comprehensive or complete. All patients should be carefully evaluated for the risk of needed air intervention and the ability to intervene. If there are any concerns about higher-than-usual risks, consultation with an anesthesiologist is recommended. Pediatric hospitalists providing sedation should be comfortable and have experience with rescue from complications of sedation, but should refer patients that are high risk for complications.

How and When Medical Evaluations Are Performed for Triage

Pediatric hospitalists provide sedations independently, and may also be asked to supervise sedations performed by others, including nurses. The responsibility for evaluation of patients undergoing sedation belongs with the supervising hospitalist when one is performing the procedure personally and when supervising someone else. Rules and regulations vary by hospital, but in most cases the sedating or supervising physician needs to perform a pre-sedation evaluation. This is not meant to replace a requirement for a pre-sedation physical exam performed by the ordering physician. This exam is meant to be focused on the risks of performing a scheduled sedation. This exam needs to be scheduled with ample time prior to the scheduled sedation. It is important to have the space and equipment to properly perform this exam. This exam is essential to the final decision-making of how and whether to proceed with a sedation. This exam is also essential in determining whether the sedation should proceed under the guidance of a pediatric hospitalist or whether it is best done by an anesthesiologist. Complication rates can increase when there is not ample time to evaluate patients immediately prior to sedation.

For elective sedations that allow performance of a test or procedure that is needed but not urgent, safety standards (including nil per os [NPO] times) should be carefully followed. If issues are found at the time of a pre-sedation exam, the sedation should be rescheduled unless rescheduling could increase risk to the patient. The risks of proceeding must be carefully measured against the risk in delaying diagnosis or treatment. At St. Louis Children's Hospital, the following are minimum recommendations for rescheduling elective sedations:

- Asthma exacerbation without underlying infectious ideology—7 days
- Asthma exacerbation with infectious etiology—3 weeks
- URI with cough or congestion—3 weeks
- Fever—when back to normal and off antipyretics 24 h
- Vomiting—when ceased for 24 h and tolerating clear liquids and evidence of good hydration
- Croup—3 weeks
- Pneumonia—4 weeks

Table 13.5 Medical criteria/conditions that initiate an anesthesiologist consult or referral at St. Louis Children's Hospital

Post-gestational age of less than 50 weeks
Evidence of sleep apnea
Tracheostomy
Anatomical airway abnormality
Cardiac abnormalities leading to decreased cardiac output
Pulmonary hypertension
Implanted pacemakers
Persistent vomiting
G-tube present
Swallowing difficulties
Chronic kidney disease
Sickle cell disease with complications
Frequent seizures
Cerebral palsy with respiratory compromise or airway abnormalities
Combative behavior
Significant congenital syndromes
Other considerations: – A patient with a body mass index (BMI) over 31 is evaluated closely by the sedation attending on the day of the procedure and may need to be referred to anesthesia, depending on body habitus and airway issues – Any patient with a BMI of 35 or greater is referred to anesthesia – Sedation on an infant with a post-gestational age of less than 50 weeks is usually deferred to anesthesia or, if possible, delayed until the infant is older

- Influenza—3 weeks
- RSV—6 weeks

NPO Guidelines for SCVMC and St. Louis Children's Hospital's Pediatric Sedation Units:

- 2 h for clears (water, apple juice, etc.)
- 3 h for breast milk
- 4 h for other liquids (formula, milk, sodas)
- 6 h for solids for children <36 months
- 8 h for solids for children >36 months

These are meant as general guidelines and not as absolute rules. This is one hospital's guidelines and does not mean that other guidelines are not valid. If the urgency of sedation requires that the test or procedure be performed in the presence of one of the aforementioned conditions or without inadequate NPO time, consultation with an anesthesiologist is generally recommended.

Funding Pediatric Hospitalist Sedation Programs

Pediatric hospitalist sedation programs are generally funded from two sources: (1) physician professional fees and (2) financial support from hospitals. Depending upon the number of sedations done, the ability to bill anesthesia codes, and reimbursement percentage, the level of funding of pediatric hospital sedation programs varies from institution to institution. In the United States, the Centers for Medicare and Medicaid (CMS) determines most rules in regard to physician billing [7]. CMS rules require that sedation services are overseen by a hospital's anesthesiology division/department. This generally requires a close working relationship between a hospital's anesthesiology group and others providing moderate and deep sedation. Most sedations performed reach the level of "deep sedation" as defined by the American Society of Anesthesiologists (ASA) and the American Academy of Pediatrics [8, 9]. In most cases, anesthesia codes can be used. Anesthesia codes are used appropriately by non-anesthesiologists when the level of care provided meets the standard of those codes. Ability to use anesthesia codes varies across the United States, sometimes on a state-by-state or local basis. Anesthesia codes are most often successfully billed when there is agreement within an institution about the appropriate use of these codes by non-anesthesiologists. If there is disagreement among departments of a hospital, it is often difficult to get reimbursed for these codes. Separate codes for moderate sedation were developed in 2006. These do not have RVUs attached. Each institution is responsible for determining the charges for these codes. Success in reimbursement for moderate sedation codes varies from region to region.

If pediatric hospitalist sedation programs have scheduled sedations each day, it is likely that the cost of providing this service will be met through the billing and collection of physician professional fees. If a sedation program is responsible to meet urgent demand and thus not able to schedule a full day, there is likely to be a shortfall in meeting the cost of the program. The ability to provide timely, safe sedation is important to many hospital services. Radiology, surgery, inpatient services, and outpatient services all benefit. Hospital administration and some services independently will likely be willing to provide financial support of sedation services outside of professional billing. It is important to understand who benefits from efficient sedations and to use that in negotiating support for those services.

The Future of Hospitalist Sedation Services

Based on estimates from the Society of Hospital Medicine, American Academy of Pediatrics, and Academic Pediatric Association, the number of pediatric hospitalists is 3,000–4,000 in the United States. Pediatric hospitalists can be a resource to meet the increasing demand for sedation. Exposure to safe sedation practices and training in safe sedation is becoming more common in pediatric residencies. It is likely that the need for sedation services will grow and also that the number of pediatric hospitalists will grow. Thus it is likely that the number of pediatric hospitalists in sedation programs will grow.

Developing National Standards for Training and Credentialing Pediatric Hospitalists in Sedation

As training for hospitalists is standardized, sedation training will likely become part of that standard. However, there are currently no national standards for training and credentialing pediatric hospitalists.

Most pediatric hospitalists gain competence for providing sedation after residency. Fifty percent of hospitalists report depending on continuing medical education (CME) as part of gaining and maintaining sedation skills. There are national conferences dedicated to pediatric sedation outside the operating room with full-day sedation workshops utilizing simulation. Core Competencies in Pediatric Hospital Medicine have been developed and providing safe sedation is part of those recommended competencies [1].

It is likely that national courses in sedation will be developed, but it is unlikely that a standardized training and certification process will emerge within the next few years. Credentialing for sedation will likely remain a local process. It is important that pediatric hospitalists providing sedation receive additional training, maintain skills, appropriately select patients, have the ability to rescue from deeper-than-intended levels of sedation, and work within systems where backup is available.

Planning, Monitoring, and Recovering from a Sedation

It is important for sedation to be performed in the safest possible manner. This begins by identifying that all personnel, equipment, and facilities needed to manage emergencies are immediately available. The safest place to perform sedation is in an area of the hospital where sedations are performed on a regular basis. Personnel in those areas will be familiar with all the equipment needed for monitoring and potential rescue and will have some experience to assist if necessary. If sedation is performed in an area of the hospital where sedation is not common, it is essential that the sedation provider have all necessary materials and personnel available before a sedation proceeds.

Pre-sedation Evaluation

All children undergoing sedation should be carefully screened for the potential of adverse events during sedation and recovery. A focused pre-sedation history and physical should be performed by the sedation provider. This evaluation should focus on characteristics that would indicate increased risk of sedation for the patient or the potential for difficult airway management. The history should include previous problems with sedation or anesthesia, stridor, snoring and sleep apnea, and recent respiratory illness. Significant physical exam findings include significant obesity, short neck, small mandible, dysmorphic facial features, small mouth opening, and large tonsils.

If a patient has significant history and physical exam findings indicating increased risk of providing sedation, the risks of providing the sedation need to be weighed against the absolute need for the procedure or diagnostic study. A hospitalist performing sedation should always feel comfortable providing rescue from a stage of sedation deeper than that intended to perform the procedure. If airway problems are anticipated, or are not anticipated but would be difficult to manage because of a patient's anatomy, consultation of an anesthesiologist is recommended.

The patient physical exam status endorsed by the ASA can be useful in assessing sedation risk. ASA class I and II children are at low risk for adverse events during sedation when carefully monitored. ASA III patients are by definition at increased risk. In general, for urgent hospital-based sedations most hospitalists should provide sedation only to ASA class I and II patients. Before providing sedation to ASA class III patients, consultation with anesthesiology is advised. Hospitalists working on a sedation service or providing sedation regularly can provide sedation to ASA class III patients safely as long as those patients are carefully evaluated and a backup system of care has been planned and is in place.

There is no proven relationship between fasting time prior to sedation and the risk of aspiration in humans. The general opinion is that fasting will likely reduce the risk of aspiration. For elective procedures, individual hospital guidelines for fasting should be followed just as they would be for general anesthesia. For urgent procedures, patients should be fasted as soon as the possible need for sedation is identified. The risk of clinically significant aspiration is small for most patients, but needs to be weighed carefully against the need to perform a diagnostic or therapeutic procedure quickly. In addition, even with proper NPO guidelines, there is still a risk of vomiting and aspiration, so the sedation provider needs to be able to monitor and respond quickly.

Personnel

For moderate sedation, a provider with adequate sedation training and experience needs to be responsible for the sedation and analgesia. This person may also perform the procedure, if patient safety and the unit policy allows. A second person with knowledge in basic pediatric life support is also required. This person is responsible for monitoring the patient's cardiopulmonary status. This person is also generally responsible for recording the data in a sedation record and may assist in brief, interruptible tasks once the level of sedation is stabilized.

For deep sedation, a provider trained in advanced pediatric life support must be in the room. The provider of the deep sedation should provide direct monitoring of the patient and must not be primarily responsible for the procedure. Problems with ventilation and oxygenation during deep sedation are generally easily managed when rapidly recognized. Deeper-than-intended sedation may occur in any patient; it is generally recommended that the sedation provider be prepared to manage deep sedation even when moderate sedation is expected and general anesthesia when deep sedation is intended.

Monitoring

For moderate sedation, a minimum of pulse oximetry is strongly recommended. In addition, continuous monitoring of heart rate, respiratory rate, and intermittent noninvasive blood pressure (NIBP) measurements are recommended. If intravenous access is not otherwise established, it is not required, but should be carefully considered.

For deep sedation, continuous electrocardiogram (ECG) heart rate, respiratory rate, pulse oximetry, and noninvasive blood pressure monitoring are strongly recommended. End-tidal carbon dioxide (CO_2) capnography monitoring is recommended. Intravenous access for patients receiving deep sedation is also recommended. Monitoring is needed throughout the sedation and recovery. In addition to electrophysiological monitoring, the child's color, airway patency, and rate and depth of respiration should be monitored by direct patient observation.

Medications

Medications used to provide moderate and deep sedation should be carefully chosen by the sedation provider to meet the goals of sedation. There can be many reasonable approaches to safe sedation and analgesia of patients. The goal of sedation should be to use the lowest dose and number of drugs with the widest therapeutic index. It is best for hospitalists to become familiar with a minimal number of drugs to provide pain relief and motionless sedation. These drugs may vary from provider to provider based on experience and availability. It is better to be comfortable with a small number of drugs that fit most circumstances than to use a large number of drugs to try to fit every clinical situation. In general, ketamine for painful procedures or for short motionless procedures and dexmedetomidine for long motionless, painless procedures will meet most needs for sedations that a hospitalist provides. Pentobarbital is a reasonable alternative for dexmedetomidine. There may be instances when sedation is best provided with a drug for which the hospitalist is uncomfortable or unfamiliar. In those cases, referral of the patient to another sedation provider is probably more prudent than proceeding with a drug that one uses infrequently.

Final Checklist Prior to Sedation

Just prior to the sedation, the sedation provider should go through a final checklist. This checklist should include a timeout, with patient identification and recheck of the patient's weight. The SOAPME acronym can be a useful tool for this final checklist:

- *Suction*: Equipment on and tested with properly sized Yankauer catheter.
- *Oxygen*: Nasal cannula, self-inflating ambu bag able to deliver continuous positive airway pressure (CPAP) bag available and hooked up, functioning ball supply, and oxygen tank if transporting patient.
- *Airway*: Size-appropriate nasopharyngeal and oral pharyngeal airways, ETTs, LMAs, functioning laryngoscope blades.
- *Pharmacy*: Medications for sedation, emergency medications for intubation, reversal agents if using opiates or benzodiazepines.
- *Monitors*: Pulse oximetry, NIBP, end-tidal CO_2 capnography, ECG, available stethoscope.
- *Equipment*: Crash cart/airway cart available nearby and other special equipment anticipated.

Recovery

It is important that patients be monitored and fully recovered from sedation prior to discharge home or placement back in an inpatient bed. Monitoring of recovery should be done by trained and experienced personnel familiar with the recovery phase of sedation. Hospitalists may need to do this themselves if properly trained nursing resources are not available. Patient handoffs should occur only if there are protocols in place for discharge or transfer by nonphysicians.

Some medications used for sedation have extremely long half-lives. Chloral hydrate PO or PR and pentobarbital IM are two such examples. Patients may seem to be nearly recovered with these medications and then have episodes of significant re-sedation with potential airway compromise.

Discharge/Transfer Criteria

In general, all of the following criteria should be met prior to discharge or transfer from the post-sedation recovery area:

1. Vital signs at baseline.
2. No respiratory distress.
3. SPO_2 at baseline.
4. Function at baseline; sits or stands with minimal assistance.
5. Hydration normal with no emesis or significant nausea.
6. Aldrete recovery score ≥ 9 for discharge ≥ 8 for admission.
7. Pain score ≤ 4 for discharge or ≤ 6 for transfer to inpatient bed.
8. Patient is awake and attentive or very easily aroused.
9. A clearly identified scale for identifying discharge "readiness" should be implemented. (Refer to Chap. 5.) A common scale used for determining appropriateness for discharge from recovery is the Aldrete recovery score (Table 13.6 [10, 11]).

Commonly Administered Sedation Drugs

There is a wide range of sedatives and analgesics available to pediatric hospitalists. Often, particularly with respect to propofol administration, it is the institution that determines whether to condone propofol administration by non-anesthesia providers. The commonly administered sedatives and analgesics administered, with a range of dosing and indications, is presented in Table 13.7 and detailed as follows. (Refer to Chap. 9.)

Ketamine

Ketamine is a very useful drug for short painful procedures and for short periods of decreased motion, such as needed by

Table 13.6 Aldrete recovery score (in general a total score ≥8 is needed for discharge) [10, 11]

Activity
• Able to move 4 extremities voluntarily or on command = 2
• Able to move 2 extremities voluntarily or on command = 1
• Able to move 0 extremities voluntarily or on command = 0
Respirations
• Able to deep breathe and cough freely = 2
• Dyspnea or limited breathing = 1
• Apneic = 0
Circulation
• BP ± 20 % of pre-sedation level = 2
• BP ± 20–50 % of pre-sedation level = 1
• BP =/–50 % or more pre-sedation level = 0
Consciousness
• Fully awake = 2
• Arousable with verbal stimulation = 1
• Not responding = 0
Color
• Pink = 2
• Pale, dusky, blotchy, jaundiced = 1
• Cyanotic = 0

computerized tomography (CT), if the child cannot tolerate the procedure without sedation. Ketamine can be given intravenous (IV), intranasal, or intramuscular (IM). When given IV, onset is usually within 30–60 s. When given IM, onset is usually within a few minutes. With a single dose of 1–2 mg/kg IV, initial deep effects last 5–10 min. Repeat doses of 0.5–1 mg/kg can be given at intervals of 5–10 min, based on effect, for longer procedures.

Ketamine given in small doses allows for the preservation of spontaneous respirations, and airway reflexes, while still providing unresponsiveness and analgesia. The relative lack of respiratory depression and sparing of airway reflexes have made ketamine a popular choice for a wide range of painful procedures. By most common definitions, the level of sedation most often achieved is deep. Since ketamine is a dissociative anesthetic, the level of sedation achieved is controversial. With preservation of airway reflexes some consider ketamine sedation to be in its own class. However, monitoring and personnel decisions should be based on the patient's likelihood to reach a level of deep sedation.

Laryngospasm is a rare but potentially serious adverse reaction to ketamine. Ketamine is generally contraindicated in patients with increased intracranial pressure. Ketamine can cause hypertension, tachycardia, significant irritability during emergence, and nystagmus. Nausea and vomiting commonly occur after larger doses of ketamine. Glycopyrrolate 5 mcg/kg IV may decrease oral secretions.

Coadministration with midazolam is a common practice. It has not been found to decrease the incidence of dysphoria or other unpleasant recovery phenomenon. Midazolam, however, may still be useful as an anxiolytic prior to the administration of ketamine. Ondansetron may be helpful if larger doses of ketamine are needed (>5 mg/kg) to prevent emesis or after the sedation, nausea or vomiting occurs [12]. There is no reversal agent for ketamine.

Dosing

Ketamine IV: Dose 1–2 mg/kg. Repeat doses of 0.5–1 mg/kg every 5–10 min as needed. There is no absolute upper limit of ketamine, but other methods of sedation should be considered for procedures lasting more than 30–45 min.
Ketamine IM: Dose 2–4 mg/kg. Onset 3–10 min [13].

Fentanyl and Midazolam

These drugs are often used in combination to provide analgesia and sedation. Midazolam and fentanyl when combined will most often lead to moderate to deep sedation. Personnel and monitoring decisions should be based on the likelihood deep sedation will be reached. Fentanyl/midazolam can cause respiratory depression that is out of proportion to the level of sedation achieved. Patients must be closely monitored for obstruction and apnea when these drugs are used in combination. These drugs have the advantage of being able to be titrated to effect.

Fentanyl is a high-potency opioid that has minimal adverse hemodynamic effects. Onset of action is 30–60 s, and duration of action is 5–10 min. The major side effect is respiratory depression that is dose related but sometimes can occur with low doses. The risk of respiratory depression is higher with benzodiazepines and barbiturates. Reversal agents for oversedation with fentanyl and midazolam are naloxone and flumazenil, respectively. Hypertension, hypotension, and chest wall rigidity are rare adverse events but can be difficult to deal with. Chest wall rigidity requires the use of a paralytic and endotracheal intubation.

Dosing

Midazolam: 0.1 mg/kg IV with subsequent doses of 0.05 mg/kg every 2–5 min to reach desired effect.
Fentanyl: 1–2 mcg/kg IV with subsequent doses of 1 mcg/kg every 2–5 min to reach desired effect.

Midazolam is often administered first with the goal of achieving anxiolysis to moderate sedation. This generally requires 0.1–0.2 mg/kg. Fentanyl is then added for analgesic effect and to achieve moderate to deep sedation.

Nitrous Oxide

Nitrous oxide when inhaled as 30–70 % mixed with oxygen can produce dissociative euphoria, drowsiness,

Table 13.7 Sedation drugs

Drug	Usage/sedation level	Dose	Onset/duration	Coadministration	Precautions
Ketamine	Short painful procedures, short periods of decreased motion	IV: 1–2 mg/kg	IV: onset 30–60 s	Midazolam as anxiolytic prior to ketamine administration has not been found to decrease incidence of dysphoria or other unpleasant emergency phenomenon	Laryngospasm (rare), contraindicated in patients with increased intracranial pressure
	Deep sedation	IM: 2–4 mg/kg Repeat doses of 0.5–1 mg/kg at intervals of 5–10 min, based on effect	IM: onset 3–10 min Duration 5–10 min deep sedation		Can cause hypertension tachycardia, significant irritability during emergence, nystagmus in most patients; glycopyrrolate 5 mCg/kg IV may decrease oral secretions
Fentanyl and midazolam	Combination provides analgesia and sedation for short painful procedures	Midazolam 0.1 mg/kg IV with subsequent doses of 0.05 mg/kg every 2–5 min until desired effect; fentanyl 1–2 mCg/kg IV with subsequent doses of 1 mCg/kg every 2–5 min to desired effect	Fentanyl IV: onset 30–60 s; duration 5–10 min	Midazolam is generally given first and titrated to provide anxiolysis to moderate sedation. Fentanyl is then added for analgesic effect and moderate to deep sedation	Can cause respiratory depression disproportionate to sedation level; patients should be closely monitored for obstruction and apnea
	Moderate to deep sedation		Midazolam IV: onset within 1 min, peak in 2–6 min; duration 30–60 min Midazolam PO: onset 15–20 min; duration 60–90 min		
Nitrous oxide	Analgesic and amnestic effect. Moderate sedation when given alone. Moderate to deep sedation when combined with other agents	30–70 % nitrous oxide mix with oxygen by inhalation		May be combined with oxycodone 0.2–0.3 mg/kg to max of 20 mg. This combination can result in deep sedation	
Pentobarbital	Long-term motionless sedation when pain control is not an issue	IV: 2.5–7.5 mg/kg. Can be given as initial dose of 2.5 mg followed by increments of 1.25 mg/kg until desired effect		Midazolam (0.05 mg/kg to max of 5 mg) to augment sedation and decreased motion	Prolonged post-sedation recovery period due to long half-life. Prolonged irritability up to 24 h

Propofol	Deep sedation to general anesthesia; can be used for short procedures needing deep sedation or prolonged motionless sedations	1–2 mg/kg followed by 1 mg/kg as needed for movement every 5–10 min for short procedures; for prolonged painless sedation, 1–2 mg/kg bolus, then as infusion of 150–200 mCg/kg/min	Onset <1 min/duration for single dose 5–10 min	Opioid or other pain medication if pain is likely	Should only be administered by experienced providers with advanced airway skills and significant experience with propofol. Airway obstruction and/or decreased respiratory effect is common; attention to airway is essential
Choral hydrate	Best for motionless sedation of children <12 months of age. Deep sedation	25–100 mg/kg orally or rectally to max of 3 g	Onset 30–60 min; recovery 60–120 min		Respiration depression and hypotension; due to half-life of 4–9 h, special precautions should be taken regarding discharge
Dexmedetomidine	Deep sedation	Bolus: 1–3 mCg/kg infused over 10 min Infusion: 1–2 mCg/kg/h	Onset by end of bolus delivery	Midazolam 0.05 mg/kg up to two times or pentobarbital 2 mg/kg to increase success of scan completion and safety	Bolus dose: bradycardia, sinus arrest, transient hypertension; infusion dose: hypotension, bradycardia; precaution needed for hypovolemia patients, patients receiving vasodilators or negative chronotropic agents, patients with arrhythmias, renal or hepatic insufficiency, and chronic hypertension

anxiolysis, and moderate amnesia and analgesia. Onset of effect is usually 2–3 min and recovery is complete 3–5 min after stopping inhalation. Children receiving nitrous oxide at 30–70 % are usually moderately sedated; a combination of nitrous oxide with a benzodiazepine or an opioid may cause deep sedation or even general anesthesia. Some children seem not to respond to nitrous oxide, probably due to psychological resistance. Vomiting occurs in about 10 % of patients receiving nitrous oxide. Nitrous oxide causes gas-filled cavities to expand; its use should be avoided if possible bowel obstruction, pneumothorax, or otitis media are suspected.

When nitrous oxide is used as a sole agent, monitoring should be at the level required for moderate sedation. If used with an oral opioid such as oxycodone (0.2–0.3 mg/kg, maximum 15 mg), deep sedation can sometimes be achieved and monitoring should be at the level required for such.

Special equipment is required for delivery of nitrous oxide. There are commercially available models with a mask, but effective nitrous oxide delivery requires a good mask seal and a patient generating significant negative pressure. Young patients may not be able to generate enough negative pressure to overcome the fountain nitrous apparatus. Nitrous for dental use is commercially available, but delivery of nitrous through the nasal cone may limit its use in medical settings. Institutions that have reported significant success with nitrous oxide often have internal support from their biomedical department.

Dosing

30–70 % nitrous oxide mix with oxygen by inhalation may be combined with oxycodone 0.2–0.3 mg/kg, max 15 mg. This combination can result in deep sedation; sedation providers need to be prepared for such [13].

Pentobarbital

Pentobarbital is a moderate long-acting barbiturate with sedative-hypnotic effects but no analgesia. The onset of action occurs in less than 60 s when given intravenously and after 10–30 min when given IM or PR. Recovery is dependent on redistribution and occurs in 50–75 min, even though the half-life is 15–20 h. Respiratory depression has been associated with pentobarbital and is dose dependent. Pentobarbital must be given slowly IV, as there is a high risk of apnea if delivered too quickly. At SCVMC, the sedation attending must be at the patient's side for the first 15 min after pentobarbital is given. There is no reversal agent for pentobarbital.

Pentobarbital has been shown to be highly effective for long-term motionless sedation when pain control is not an issue. Pentobarbital generally results in deep sedation. Airway reflexes and breathing are generally not significantly diminished. Monitoring, however, should be for the anticipated level of deep sedation and personnel with advanced airway skills should be available.

Midazolam given intravenously (0.05 mg/kg, maximum 5 mg) can be given if there is sustained motion.

The post-sedation period can be prolonged. It is important to give the patient adequate time to recover. Sometimes patients can be stimulated to the level of a wakefulness that supports discharge. Caregivers need to realize that there can be re-sedation because of the long half-life of pentobarbital. Patients often have prolonged irritability, ataxia, and nausea, sometimes lasting up to 24 h.

Dosing

Pentobarbital IV: 2.5–7.5 mg/kg. This can be given as an initial dose of 2.5 mg/kg followed by increments of 1.25 mg/kg until sedation is achieved.

Midazolam IV: 0.05 mg/kg, maximum 5 mg. Can be used to augment sedation and decreased motion, but can increase the chance of respiratory depression when combined with other medications that suppress the respiratory drive.

Propofol

Propofol is a nonbarbiturate sedative-hypnotic agent. It has no analgesic effect. Propofol is administered intravenously, and has an onset of less than 1 min. The duration of action for a single dose is 5–10 min. It can be used in doses of 1–2 mg/kg to provide sedation for short procedures. If pain is likely, propofol needs to be given with an appropriate dose of an opioid or other pain medication. For prolonged painless sedation, as is needed for magnetic resonance imaging (MRI) scans, it can be given as a 1–2 mg/kg bolus, then as an infusion of 150–200 μ(mu)g/kg/min. The quick onset of action and short duration make propofol an attractive drug for brief procedures; however, it can be difficult to titrate and it is easy to overshoot the intended level of sedation, leading to apnea and hypotension. If combined with opiates or benzodiazepines, there is an increased risk of respiratory depression.

Propofol should only be administered by experienced providers with advanced airway skills. Propofol leads to deep sedation or even a general anesthesia. Significant numbers of patients will have airway obstruction and/or decreased respiratory effect when given a bolus of 1–2 mg/kg of propofol. Attention to airway is essential.

In general, propofol should only be considered by providers who have significant skills and experience with deep sedation, along with advanced airway skills, including placement of LMA's and intubation [3].

Dosing

Prolonged sedation: 1–2 mg/kg initial bolus followed by 120–200 μ(mu)g/kg/min.

Short procedures: 1–2 mg/kg followed by 1 mg/kg as needed for movement every 5–10 min.

Dexmedetomidine

Dexmedetomidine is a selective alpha-2 receptor agonist. It has anesthetic, sedative, analgesic, and anti-shivering properties. It most commonly causes a level of sedation consistent with definitions of deep sedation. Electroencephalogram (EEG) activity while being sedated with dexmedetomidine resembles a non-rapid eye movement (NREM) sleep [14]. An advantage of dexmedetomidine is that it preserves respiratory parameters and does not cause respiratory depression [15].

Dexmedetomidine given IV has an initial half-life distribution of 6 min with terminal half-life of 2 h. Dexmedetomidine elicits a dose-dependent biphasic effect on blood pressure. At low serum concentrations there may be a slight drop in blood pressure and at high serum concentrations, hypertension may be observed [16]. Precautions should be taken for hypovolemia patients, patients receiving digoxin, vasodilators, or negative chronotropic agents, patients with arrhythmias, and patients with renal or a hepatic insufficiency and with chronic hypertension. (Refer to Chap. 9.)

Patients receiving dexmedetomidine for prolonged motionless sedation sometimes are sensitive to loud noises such as occur during a MRI exam. Ear plugs may be helpful. Midazolam, pentobarbital, or ketamine has been used successfully to increase the success of dexmedetomidine sedation as measured by completion of the scan and safety.

Dosing

IV Bolus: 1–3 mcg/kg infused over 10 min. Patients generally become sleepy after a few minutes and are generally able to begin the procedure when a bolus is done.

Infusion: 1–2 mcg/kg/h. Please note that this infusion is per hour, not per minute.

Intranasal: 2–4 mcg/kg divided into two doses (one for each nare).

Midazolam given to supplement sedation: 0.05 mg/kg IV may be given up to two times, or oral midazolam may be given prior to sedation with dexmedetomidine. Alternatively, pentobarbital may be given to supplement sedation: 2 mg/kg IV or ketamine 1 mg/kg IV [17–25].

Case Scenarios

Case 1

A 26-month-old male is referred to the outpatient sedation unit for a brain MRI study due to a history of multiple afebrile seizures. He was initially scheduled for the MRI 3 weeks ago but this was rescheduled due to the presence of a fever, cough, and rhinorrhea for 2 days. He is now in good health with no recent fevers or respiratory symptoms. He has speech delay and a mild delay in fine motor skills. There is no history of snoring nor obstructive sleep apnea. He is not on any medications and has no known medication nor food allergies. There is no prior history of sedation and no family history of sedation issues. NPO status: no solid food since 7 PM the night prior and no liquids since midnight. Pre-sedation exam: weight is 12 kg, heart rate is 150, respiratory rate is 35, BP is 105/60, and oxygen saturation on room air is 98 %. The child is an alert, interactive toddler in no apparent distress, though he is anxious and crying with exam. Airway exam shows 2+ tonsils and full range of motion of neck without lymphadenopathy. Heart/lung exam is normal, though limited by child's crying. The remainder of exam is normal.

Considerations

Given the child's developmental delay and multiple afebrile seizures, the neurologist has recommended an MRI to evaluate for brain anomalies. This may be a non-emergent study if the child has a non-focal neurologic exam and is otherwise well.

A special consideration with MRI is the decreased ability to visualize and touch the patient. Given this, airway issues and increased respiratory secretions may play a larger role for MRI sedation than for other sedations. The pre-sedation assessment must include a screen for airway or respiratory issues, and this child's non-urgent MRI was rescheduled until after his respiratory symptoms resolved. If the study is urgently needed despite the presence of respiratory or airway issues (including morbid obesity), referral to anesthesia should be considered.

An MRI also requires a child to remain still during the whole study, other non-painful procedures or studies may allow for some movement, so the level of sedation may need to be deeper-than-moderate level. Other considerations include the length of the study, whether intravenous contrast is necessary, and the ability to monitor the child and intervene for any respiratory or cardiovascular compromise. MRI scans tend to be of longer duration than CTs, which may more often be done without sedation. Many neonates and older children may be able to tolerate a short MRI study (less than 30–45 min) without sedation or with minimal sedation or anxiolysis. There are also rapid MRIs (less than 5–10 min), which may not require sedation, but this also depends on the child's level of cooperativeness and anxiety. For lengthier studies (over 90–120 min), the child may need sedation by an anesthesiologist.

(continued)

Monitoring is an important issue with any planned sedation, and there must be a way to monitor pulse oximetry and heart rate at a minimum while the child is in the scanner. End-tidal CO_2 monitoring is becoming a standard for monitoring for deep sedation and is strongly recommended if moderate to deep sedation is planned. Personnel should include a sedation nurse or physician to closely monitor and record vital signs and to rescue the child from any adverse events such as apnea, hypoxia, or hypotension. An MRI technician should also be present. These personnel should remain present throughout the study. Depending on the medication used and the sedation policy of the hospital, a sedation attending may need to be present in the MRI area or be immediately available for any possible complications.

Additional considerations include when and where the sedation medications are given, whether in a nearby sedation area or in the MRI scanner itself, and where the patient is to be monitored for recovery after the study. If the patient needs to be transported between locations and is not at his/her baseline status, the patient should be monitored with at minimum a portable pulse oximeter and should have a nurse or physician at the bedside who is capable of managing any sedation complication.

Sedative Options and Considerations

It is important to know more about the study, by discussion with either the MRI technician or radiologist. For this MRI, the plan is for a 30-min scan without intravenous contrast unless an anomaly is seen that requires its use. As with most MRI scans, it should not be painful.

For this sedation, an agent that will provide moderate to deep sedation for at least 30 min is the best choice. Analgesia is not necessary. Some medication options include IV propofol, IV or IM pentobarbital, or IV or intranasal dexmedetomidine, with or without midazolam. Other options such as IV or IM ketamine and fentanyl/midazolam have been used but are not ideal. Sedation with ketamine often produces a dissociative anesthesia, which may include spontaneous movement, and provides analgesia, so it is not generally the best choice for sedation for an MRI. With the combination of fentanyl and midazolam, it may be difficult to obtain an adequate level of sedation for enough time to obtain an MRI without causing respiratory compromise. Although for an older cooperative child or teen with anxiety or claustrophobia, a benzodiazepine (midazolam, lorazepam, or diazepam) or diphenhydramine may be adequate for anxiolysis/minimal sedation.

If intravenous contrast is required for the MRI, an IV sedation medication is often considered. Depending on the anxiety level of the child, oral midazolam (0.5 mg/kg) may be given 15–20 min prior to IV start. This may have the added benefit of providing amnesia at the IV start. Some centers are able to utilize nitrous oxide for IV placement. If available, a topical anesthetic such as a vapocoolant spray or topical lidocaine can be helpful to relieve the pain of IV starts and may help to increase the success rate of IV placement [26]. After the IV is placed, the child is brought to the MRI scanner and placed on MRI-compatible monitors and a small bolus of propofol may be given (1 mg/kg) and repeated if needed to induce moderate sedation. Then a propofol drip is started at 120 μ(mu)g/kg/min and is titrated as needed up to 150–200 μ(mu)g/kg/min to maintain a sedated state. Once the child is calm and will tolerate it, ear plugs are placed in both ears, and end-tidal CO_2 monitoring is recommended via a special nasal cannula. Toward the end of the study, the propofol drip may be stopped so that the child can awaken shortly after the MRI is completed.

Other IV alternatives include IV pentobarbital (2.5 mg/kg), given at the beginning of the MRI scanner without the need for a drip to maintain sedation. However, the recovery from IV pentobarbital tends to be longer than that from IV propofol. Ataxia and nausea may be present during the recovery period and up to 24 h later. IV dexmedetomidine is also a possible choice, with a bolus of 1–2 μ(mu)g/kg, followed by an infusion of 1–2 mcg/kg/h to maintain a sedated state. Side effects commonly noted include bradycardia, though perfusion often remains adequate, and BP issues (hypertension with the bolus dose, and hypotension during the infusion). Children may awaken and start moving in the MRI scanner due to the loud noises during the study, so IV midazolam (0.05 mg/kg), pentobarbital (1–2 mg/kg), or ketamine (0.5–1 mg/kg) may be needed as an adjunct.

For this case, intravenous contrast is not required, so a sedation provider may consider avoiding IV placement for medication administration. In the past for younger children, chloral hydrate po was a useful sedative-hypnotic agent, but this medication is no longer in production. Other alternatives include IM pentobarbital, 2–4 mg/kg, oral or intranasal midazolam, and intranasal dexmedetomidine, 2–3 mcg/kg, up to 4 mcg/kg. As noted previously, dexmedetomidine alone may produce an "arousable" sedated state, so children who appear to be sedated initially may awaken due to the noise in the MRI scanner.

To help potentiate the sedation for MRI, oral midazolam (0.5 mg/kg, maximum 20 mg po) may be given

(continued)

in addition to the intranasal dexmedetomidine. It is possible to give intranasal midazolam, but there may be a burning sensation on delivery of this medication. Extra time is needed to allow the oral midazolam to take effect if given at the same time as the intranasal dexmedetomidine. The taste of oral midazolam is unpleasant but is generally well tolerated.

Intranasal dexmedetomidine may take up to 30 min to take effect and there is generally a prolonged recovery time.

With intranasal medication administration, an atomizer device is recommended and, for doses over 0.2 mL, it is recommended to divide the dose between each nare (e.g., for a 0.4 mL dose, give 0.2 mL in the left nare and 0.2 mL in the right nare) to increase mucosal exposure and absorption. There may be reduced effectiveness if the amount of intranasal medication exceeds 1 mL, as some of the medication may be swallowed instead of atomized.

If needed, an additional dose of intranasal dexmedetomidine may be given (1–2 mcg/kg), but since this may take an additional 30 min for effect, IV placement and IV medication are often considered at this point. Options include IV propofol, IV pentobarbital, or IV midazolam and often only 1 dose is needed rather than an infusion, as once the child is sedated by the additional IV medication, the dose of intranasal dexmedetomidine that has already been given may be sufficient to maintain the sedated state.

For this case, intranasal dexmedetomidine 40 μ(mu) g is given (20 mcg in each nare; 3.3 mcg/kg total dose), along with 6 mg (0.5 mg/kg) of oral midazolam. The child is placed in an MRI-compatible gown, is placed on a monitor, and falls asleep 15 min later. He is brought to the MRI scanner on a portable monitor by a sedation-credentialed RN and is accompanied by his mother. He is transferred onto the MRI gurney, placed on MRI-compatible monitors, including an end-tidal CO_2 monitor/nasal cannula, and ear plugs are placed. The child briefly arouses due to the stimulation but then falls back asleep once placed in the MRI scanner. He is monitored continuously by the sedation-credentialed RN from the MRI control room, with vital signs (heart rate, respiratory rate, O_2 saturation, end-tidal CO_2, and blood pressure) recorded every 5 min. No intravenous contrast is required.

At the end of the scan, the child is brought out of the scanner and transferred back onto his hospital gurney. He is placed back on portable monitoring and begins to awaken, with his mother at his bedside. Once he is fully awake, he is allowed to drink water and eat and is monitored until back to his baseline. Once he meets discharge criteria, the mother is given discharge instructions and contact phone numbers for the sedation unit and provider, and the child is discharged home.

Case 2

A 5-year-old autistic child is referred for an outpatient EEG with sedation, as he did not tolerate lead placement on a prior attempt to get an EEG. He has staring spells and behaviors that may be consistent with focal seizure activity. His only medication is Ritalin, which he took this morning. NPO status: no solids since 10 PM last night and had apple juice with his Ritalin 3 h ago. He has had no recent illnesses or fevers. There is no snoring with sleeping or history of sleep apnea. His mother kept him up last night until 1 AM, so he has had 4 h less sleep than usual. He is allergic to eggs but has no known drug allergies. He had an MRI done under sedation with chloral hydrate 2 years ago and has had no other sedations or surgeries. He did well with that sedation and during recovery. On pre-sedation exam, his weight is 20 kg, and he is agitated when you approach him. Heart rate 124, respiratory rate 28, BP 107/72 (crying), O_2 saturation 98 % on room air. With his mother's assistance, you are able to complete the exam and find 2+ tonsils on exam of his oropharynx. No rhinorrhea, no lymphadenopathy. Heart/lung exam normal. You discuss sedation options versus attempting again without sedation, and the mother feels he will not allow lead placement without sedation.

Considerations

Some non-painful imaging procedures or studies can be done without sedation, and a trial without sedation may be warranted, depending on the urgency of the study and the ability to repeat it if the trial fails.

As with any study, the sedation provider must balance out the risks of the sedation versus the need for the procedure. For this case, the neurologist was planning to start antiepileptic medication if the EEG was positive for epileptiform activity, so the EEG results will alter the child's treatment plan.

Sedative Options and Considerations

For EEGs, a special consideration is that the study's findings may be altered by certain classes of medications. For example, benzodiazepines such as midazolam may suppress epileptiform activity and result in a falsely negative EEG. Barbiturates will have a similar effect. Ketamine may suppress seizure-like EEG discharges on patients during seizures and is not

(continued)

commonly used for EEGs as these are non-painful studies. Chloral hydrate has been used for younger children receiving EEGs and will alter the EEG slightly but is no longer in production. Hydroxyzine is another oral medication that has been used for EEG sedation, either alone or in combination with chloral hydrate. Two common medications used for sedated EEGs are propofol and dexmedetomidine. Propofol also has antiepileptic properties but can be given as a single small dose (1–2 mg/kg) to allow for lead placement, and the effects should wear off quickly with minimal changes on the EEG. Dexmedetomidine sedation resembles NREM sleep and does not suppress epileptiform activity.

Another consideration with EEG sedation is whether an IV is already present or not. IV placement is not necessary for the EEG itself, so the sedation provider needs to determine whether IV sedation is needed or not. If the preferred agent is propofol, an IV will be needed, and the child can be sedated briefly for lead placement and then allowed to awaken. If the leads are secured well and inaccessible to the patient, many children will tolerate the remainder of the EEG study. Dexmedetomidine may be given IV, IM, or intranasally.

With sedation for EEGs or other studies such as auditory brainstem responses (ABRs), some movement by the patient is tolerated, in contrast to studies such as MRI. This means the level of sedation can be minimal to moderate, and often a single agent and single dose of medication is sufficient.

An additional consideration in this case is the child's egg allergy. Some propofol preparations contain egg lecithin/phosphatide and soy oil, which means there is a small chance of an allergic reaction or anaphylaxis in children who have had severe allergic reactions or anaphylaxis after eating egg or soy products. One propofol preparation also contains trace amounts of peanut oil, so obtaining a food allergy history is important. The small risk of using propofol in these cases must be weighed against the risks of using alternative medications.

For This Case

The patient is given 60 μ(mu)g intranasal dexmedetomidine (3 μ[mu]g/kg) and falls asleep in 20 min. Vital signs stable on room air, with no bradycardia or blood pressure issues noted. He tolerates lead placement well and remains sedated for the EEG study and for an additional 40 min afterwards. Once he awakens, he is able to eat and his mother is given discharge instructions for home.

Case 3

A 15-month-old term female presents with left labial abscess for 1 day. She had a right buttock abscess, which was incised and drained in the emergency department 2 days ago, and she has been taking clindamycin for 2 days. The child is quite anxious with examination and the left labial area is erythematous and tender to the touch. The right buttock abscess continues to drain pus and is indurated without erythema. The pediatric surgeon evaluates the child and agrees that incision and drainage of the left labial abscess is necessary. The child has been admitted to the pediatric unit and has an intravenous (IV) in place.

Considerations

The first consideration with any sedation is whether the procedure or imaging study is necessary. In this case, both the pediatrician and pediatric surgeon agree that drainage is needed and would be of benefit to the child.

The second consideration is whether the procedure or study is needed emergently, urgently, or whether it can be scheduled later as an elective sedation. In this case, the child does not need emergent drainage on admission, but it should be done urgently rather than on an elective basis. It is recommended to follow the NPO guidelines for the institution.

The third consideration is where the procedure and sedation should be performed. The sedation must be performed with appropriate personnel trained in monitoring and airway management and in an area where resuscitation equipment is immediately available. The personnel involved should be trained in monitoring children with a level of moderate to deep sedation and should be prepared for a deeper level of sedation than planned. There should be at least one person assigned to monitor the child who is NOT involved in the procedure itself. In this case, there is a treatment room on the inpatient pediatric unit with appropriate monitors, including EKG monitors (required), respiratory rate (required), pulse oximetry (required), blood pressure cuff (required), and end-tidal capnography (strongly recommended). There is also appropriate resuscitation equipment (self-inflating bag with appropriate-sized mask, oxygen, suction, and a cart with intubation equipment and resuscitation medications).

Another issue to consider in the choice of location is any findings on the pre-sedation assessment: does the child have any other medical problems, a history of snoring or obstructive sleep apnea, or any other findings that would place her in a higher-risk category for

(continued)

sedation? (See list under "Triaging Patients to Sedation by Pediatric Hospitalists.")

Pre-sedation assessment: Vitals: 12 kg, heart rate 168, respiratory rate 45, oxygen saturation 98 % on room air, blood pressure 98/60. Child is alert and cooperative with parents but very fearful and resists exam. Exam of the airway is normal, and heart/lung exam is normal. There is no history of drug or food allergies and no prior history of sedations or surgeries. Home medications include clindamycin and acetaminophen. She ate a light lunch (few bites of a peanut butter sandwich, a few fries, and a cup of milk) 4 h ago.

Following standard NPO guidelines, the child should wait until 6 h have passed since her lunch, so all feedings and liquids should be stopped now and the sedation arranged in 2 h.

Sedative Options and Considerations

In this case, the child is likely to experience pain and anxiety due to the procedure, so sedation medications should be chosen that will address both these issues. Possible choices include fentanyl and midazolam, ketamine, propofol with fentanyl or ketamine, and nitrous oxide with opioids.

Another consideration is the goal level of sedation. For abscess drainage, the child may be in a level of moderate sedation rather than deep sedation, as some movement can be tolerated. Also, the procedure itself is relatively short in duration, so the sedation effects are not needed for a prolonged period as with an MRI. Medications of quick onset and short duration would be ideal.

In regard to which medication to choose, the decision depends on which medication the physician is most familiar with and on what is available for use at the location. For example, for nitrous oxide administration, a scavenger system is needed. If the child does not have an intravenous (IV) and the physician feels comfortable sedating without one, the most common options are nitrous oxide with opioids or intramuscular (IM) ketamine. Fentanyl and midazolam may be given via intranasal routes, but the absorption may not be reliable. The dose of IM ketamine ranges from 2 to 6 mg/kg. Below 3 mg/kg, a second IM injection is sometimes needed, though the child should be at a minimal to moderate sedation level and not as bothered by it. Above 4–5 mg/kg, the incidence of post-procedure nausea and vomiting increases.

For IV sedation, fentanyl and midazolam are one option, though the physician must be careful to avoid respiratory depression from this combination.

Ketamine is a common choice for relatively brief (less than 15–30 min), painful procedures. It provides analgesia and dissociative anesthesia with preservation of airway reflexes. For this patient, one may consider giving midazolam first due to the high level of anxiety from her prior procedure. If the parents stay for the procedure, it is best to warn them that the child's eyes will stay open at least initially and she will develop odd eye movements (nystagmus). Often ketamine will cause increased tears and saliva as well, which can be disturbing to family members. If high doses of ketamine are needed, the child may experience nausea and vomiting upon reemergence. Other reemergence phenomena can be tempered by allowing the child to awaken in a quiet, darkened room.

Propofol has the benefit of rapid onset and short duration but does not provide analgesia, so it is often not the first choice unless given with fentanyl, which increases the risk of respiratory depression and hypotension, or with ketamine.

Nitrous oxide has the benefit of providing anxiolysis and has rapid onset and short duration once stopped. For a painful procedure, it can be combined with oral oxycodone for deeper sedation and analgesia. The oxycodone should be given 20–30 min before the nitrous oxide is started.

In this case, the child is given IV midazolam (0.05–1 mg/kg), then ketamine (1 mg/kg), and the level of sedation is titrated to an effective level with repeat doses of 0.5 mg/kg ketamine every 3–5 min. The child is monitored by a sedation-trained nurse with vital signs every 5 min and continuous heart rate, respiratory rate, and pulse oximetry. Once nystagmus is noted, the patient is prepared and positioned for the procedure. The procedure is performed quickly and without complications, with a total of 2 mg/kg ketamine given.

The child is allowed to awaken gently with both parents present. She is monitored as for a deep level of sedation with frequent vital signs until back to her baseline functioning status. Once back at baseline, she is allowed to drink fluids and is observed closely for any signs of nausea or vomiting.

Case 4

A 7-month-old with hydronephrosis is referred to the hospitalist-run sedation service for a renal scan. The patient has recurrent urinary tract infections and the scan is indicated to look for kidney injury. The child is otherwise healthy. Physical exam is unremarkable

(continued)

except for a small amount of clear nasal discharge, which is reported to be unchanged over a 2-week period. There is no snoring but a mild intermittent cough that is improving is noted.

Considerations

It is important for diagnostic and therapeutic reasons for the patient to receive a renal scan. Evaluation of the patient is unremarkable except for chronic clear rhinitis and an occasional cough by history. While the renal scan is important, the potential increased risk of deep sedation in the face of possible resolving upper respiratory infection should be considered carefully. With an active upper respiratory infection or cough, elective sedation should be delayed until the patient is recovered. When any condition exists that may increase risk of sedation, that risk needs to be balanced against the urgency of the procedure or test being performed. After discussion with anesthesiology the sedation is performed.

Sedative Options and Considerations

The hospitalist proceeds with a bolus of propofol (2 mg/kg). The patient remains active and is given an additional 1 mg/kg of propofol. Five minutes later there is still movement and another 1 mg/kg of propofol is given. As the patient is placed on the nuclear medicine scanner stridor is noted, a chin lift is performed and an oral airway placed. The patient becomes apneic. Positive pressure is begun and a call for backup help is made. Oxygen saturations decrease to less than 90 % for 1 min and then are maintained above 94 %. The hospitalist and backup anesthesiologist elect to place a LMA. The anesthesiologist takes over the case, the scan is completed, and the patient recovers and is discharged to home.

It is essential for patient safety that all sedation providers are well trained to rescue from a deeper level of sedation than intended. It is also essential that there is a system to provide escalating care in the case of unintended sedation complications. Patient safety is dependent on well-trained providers working in safe systems of care.

Case 5

A 13-month-old female is referred for an MRI. The patient was born at 40 weeks estimated gestational age. She has persistent developmental delay and has been described as having poor muscle tone. She is able to sit without support but is not crawling and not able pull herself up to stand. She is described as being a poor feeder during the first few months of life. She had occasional coughing and gagging spells while feeding. At 6 months of age she was hospitalized with pneumonia. She otherwise has done well. She has no recent upper respiratory infections or other recent illnesses. An MRI of her brain and spine have been ordered as part of her evaluation for poor muscle tone and delayed motor development.

Considerations

This 13-month-old child has no recent illness but does have history and physical exam findings compatible with hypotonia. The etiology of her developmental delay is not known. An MRI is needed to help with diagnosis and prognosis. The poor muscle tone may increase her risk of sedation complication. She has some increased risk of airway complication and aspiration during a sedation. The history of poor feeding with coughing and gagging plus a history of pneumonia at 6 months of age may also indicate some difficulty with swallowing and handling oral secretions. There needs to be recognition of this increased risk for sedation. The provider of the sedation needs to be able to easily provide airway support including placement of a LMA or ETT. A referral or consultation to the anesthesia service may be indicated. Every sedation system needs to work out in advance how to best handle children that have an increased risk of sedation adverse events. Hospitalists that work in sedation systems should be capable of handling sedation complications including intubation, but if the risk of airway management is higher than usual the referral to an anesthesiologist is expected.

Sedation Options and Considerations

During the pre-sedation evaluation the mild hypotonia was again noted. It was thought that the patient did have an increased risk for sedation complication. The MRI had been scheduled to be done with propofol administered by a pediatric hospitalist. The hospitalist consulted anesthesiology and it was agreed that the case could be done that day but it should be done with LMA placement and be performed by an anesthesiologist. The sedation was performed using general anesthesia. The patient had no complications, was monitored throughout recovery and was discharged home.

References

1. Stucky ER, Maniscalco J, Ottolini MC, et al. The pediatric hospital medicine core competencies supplement: a framework for curriculum development by the society of hospital medicine with acknowledgement to pediatric hospitalists from the American academy of pediatrics and the Academic Pediatric Association. J Hosp Med. 2010; 5(Suppl 2):i–xv, 1–114
2. Marseille DJ, Maniscalco J, et al. Characteristics of pediatric hospitalists providing moderate to deep sedation: a study from the pediatric research in inpatient settings (PRIS) network. Honolulu: Pediatric Academic Societies; 2008.
3. Turmelle M, Moscoso LM, Hamlin KP, Daud YN, Carlson DW. Development of a pediatric hospitalist sedation service: training and implementation. J Hosp Med. 2012;7(4):335–9.
4. Srinivasan M, Turmelle M, Depalma LM, Mao J, Carlson DW. Procedural sedation for diagnostic imaging in children by pediatric hospitalists using propofol: analysis of the nature, frequency, and predictors of adverse events and interventions. J Pediatr. 2012;160(5):801–6.
5. Srinivasan M, Carlson DW. A proposed mechanism to assess knowledge of pediatric hospitalists to identify and manage rare events during procedural sedation. Hosp Pediatr. 2013;3(4):381–5.
6. Organizations JCoAoH. Hospital Accreditation Standards 2013.
7. Revised Hospital Anesthesia Services Interpretive Guidelines—State Operations Manual (SOM) Appendix A. In: Services DOHHSCfMM, ed. Baltimore; 2010.
8. Practice guidelines for sedation and analgesia by non-anesthesiologists. Anesthesiology. 2002;96(4):1004–17.
9. Cote CJ, Wilson S. Guidelines for monitoring and management of pediatric patients during and after sedation for diagnostic and therapeutic procedures: an update. Pediatrics. 2006;118(6):2587–602.
10. Aldrete J, Kroulik D. A postanesthetic recovery score. Anesth Analg. 1970;49(6):924–34.
11. Aldrete JA. The post-anesthesia recovery score revisited. J Clin Anesth. 1995;7(1):89–91.
12. Green SM, Roback MG, Krauss B, Brown L, McGlone RG, Agrawal D, McKee M, Weiss M, Pitetti RD, Hostetler MA, Wathen JE, Treston G, Garcia Pena BM, Gerber AC, Losek JD. Predictors of emesis and recovery agitation with emergency department ketamine sedation: an individual-patient data meta-analysis of 8,282 children. Ann Emerg Med. 2009;54(2):171–80. e1-4.
13. Srinivasan M, Carlson DW. Procedural sedation by pediatric hospitalists: analysis of the nature and incidence of complications during ketamine and nitrous oxide sedation. Hosp Pediatr. 2013;3(4): 342–7.
14. Mason KP, O'Mahony E, Zurakowski D, Libenson MH. Effects of dexmedetomidine sedation on the EEG in children. Paediatr Anaesth. 2009;19(12):1175–83.
15. Petroz GC, Sikich N, James M, van Dyk H, Shafer SL, Schily M, Lerman J. A phase I, two-center study of the pharmacokinetics and pharmacodynamics of dexmedetomidine in children. Anesthesiology. 2006;105(6):1098–110.
16. Potts AL, Anderson BJ, Warman GR, Lerman J, Diaz SM, Vilo S. Dexmedetomidine pharmacokinetics in pediatric intensive care—a pooled analysis. Paediatr Anaesth. 2009;19(11):1119–29.
17. Heard C, Burrows F, Johnson K, Joshi P, Houck J, Lerman J. A comparison of dexmedetomidine-midazolam with propofol for maintenance of anesthesia in children undergoing magnetic resonance imaging. Anesth Analg. 2008;107(6):1832–9.
18. Mason KP, Zurakowski D, Zgleszewski SE, Robson CD, Carrier M, Hickey PR, Dinardo JA. High dose dexmedetomidine as the sole sedative for pediatric MRI. Paediatr Anaesth. 2008;18(5): 403–11.
19. Mason KP, Zurakowski D, Zgleszewski S, Prescilla R, Fontaine PJ, Dinardo JA. Incidence and predictors of hypertension during high-dose dexmedetomidine sedation for pediatric MRI. Paediatr Anaesth. 2010;20(6):516–23.
20. Mason KP, Zgleszewski SE, Prescilla R, Fontaine PJ, Zurakowski D. Hemodynamic effects of dexmedetomidine sedation for CT imaging studies. Paediatr Anaesth. 2008;18(5):393–402.
21. Mason KP, Zgleszewski SE, Dearden JL, Dumont RS, Pirich MA, Stark CD, D'Angelo P, Macpherson S, Fontaine PJ, Connor L, Zurakowski D. Dexmedetomidine for pediatric sedation for computed tomography imaging studies. Anesth Analg. 2006;103(1):57–62.
22. Mason KP, Zgleszewski S, Forman RE, Stark C, DiNardo JA. An exaggerated hypertensive response to glycopyrrolate therapy for bradycardia associated with high-dose dexmedetomidine. Anesth Analg. 2009;108(3):906–8.
23. Hammer GB, Sam WJ, Chen MI, Golianu B, Drover DR. Determination of the pharmacodynamic interaction of propofol and dexmedetomidine during esophagogastroduodenoscopy in children. Paediatr Anaesth. 2009;19(2):138–44.
24. Mester R, Easley RB, Brady KM, Chilson K, Tobias JD. Monitored anesthesia care with a combination of ketamine and dexmedetomidine during cardiac catheterization. Am J Ther. 2008;15(1): 24–30.
25. Mason KP, Prescilla R, Fontaine PJ, Zurakowski D. Pediatric CT sedation: comparison of dexmedetomidine and pentobarbital. AJR Am J Roentgenol. 2011;196(2):W194–8.
26. Splinter W, Splinter K, Farion K, Newhook K, Tan S, Anderson J, Gaboury I. Pain ease vapocoolant spray versus placebo in reducing pain associated with intravenous insertion in children: RCT. Can J Anaesth. 2007;54(1 Supplement):44381.

The Anesthesia-Directed Sedation Service: Models, Protocols, and Challenges

14

Joss Thomas

Abstract

Anesthesiologists have made significant contributions to the specialty of pediatric sedation. In 1985, the first sedation guidelines were published by the American Academy of Pediatrics (AAP), with an anesthesiologist as the leading author. Although anesthesiologists may have led the pediatric sedation movements for the first two decades following this AAP publication, over the most recent decade, non-anesthesiologists have begun to replace anesthesiologists in some of the leading roles. In fact, anesthesia-directed sedation models may be on the decline. In 2005, only half of the respondents of a North American survey indicated that they had a formal sedation service. Only 26 % of institution-based sedation services involved either pediatric or general anesthesiologists.

Keywords

Anesthesia-directed sedation service • Anesthesia-directed sedation models • Nurse-assisted propofol sedation (NAPS) • Anesthesia physician assistants • Anesthesiology assistants • Sedation and anesthesia providers (SAP) • Certified registered nurse anesthetist (CRNA) • Objective risk assessment tool for sedation (ORATS) • Computer-assisted personalized sedation (CAPS) • Body mass index (BMI) • American Academy of Pediatrics (AAP) • American Society of Anesthesiologists (ASA) • American College of Emergency Physicians (ACEP) • American College of Gastroenterologists • Monitored anesthesia care • Joint Commission • Texan Children's Hospital • Center for Medicare and Medicaid Services (CMS) • Ketamine • Pentobarbital • Dexmedetomidine • Propofol • Food and Drug Administration (FDA) • University of Iowa

Background: The United States and Beyond

Anesthesiologists have made significant contributions to the specialty of pediatric sedation. In 1985, the first sedation guidelines were published by the American Academy of Pediatrics (AAP), with an anesthesiologist as the leading author [1]. Although anesthesiologists may have led the pediatric sedation movements for the first two decades following this AAP publication, over the most recent decade, non-anesthesiologists have begun to replace anesthesiologists in some of the leading roles. In fact, anesthesia-directed sedation models may be on the decline. In 2005, only half of the respondents of a North American survey indicated that they had a formal sedation service [2]. Only 26 % of institution-based sedation services involved either pediatric or general anesthesiologists [2].

Comparatively, outside of the United States, anesthesia-directed sedation models seem to be more common. The Hadassah University Hospital in Jerusalem is an example of a large-volume, international sedation program that has been organized and directed by its Department of Anesthesia.

J. Thomas, M.D., M.P.H., F.C.C.P. (✉)
Pediatric Anesthesia, Critical Care Medicine, Department of Anesthesia, University of Iowa Children's Hospital, Iowa City, IA, USA
e-mail: joss-thomas@uiowa.edu

K.P. Mason (ed.), *Pediatric Sedation Outside of the Operating Room: A Multispecialty International Collaboration*, DOI 10.1007/978-1-4939-1390-9_14, © Springer Science+Business Media New York 2015

This program initiated an anesthesia-supervised sedation service that directs nursing-administered sedation [3]. Another anesthesia-directed nurse-lead sedation service was developed in 1995 in the United Kingdom for magnetic resonance imaging (MRI). A collaboration between the Departments of Anesthesia, Radiology, and trained intensive care unit (ICU) nurses led to the creation of sedation protocols. The oral route was most common and included chloral hydrate, temazepam, and droperidol. These sedation nurses were trained in the operating room by anesthesiologists on airway skills and the evaluation of physiological vital signs from physiological monitors. These skills were assessed every 3 months [4]. In another UK hospital, a nurse-led cardioversion service, not under the direct supervision of anesthesiologists, has been in effect since 2004 [5]. Another unique example of anesthesia collaboration is the training of nurse anesthetists in resource-limited developing countries such as Haiti. Médecins Sans Frontières, a volunteer organization, has trained nurses using expatriate anesthesiologists for more than 10 years to provide anesthesia and sedation services in some of their hospitals [6].

It appears that globally, there seems to be a dearth of anesthesia-trained providers, and various models are emerging to address the shortage. Some of these sedation models have created disharmony between specialties, particularly as some non-anesthesiologists have assumed responsibility for propofol delivery. Currently, nurse-administered propofol sedation (NAPS) is practiced in the United States, Switzerland, and Japan [7]. In countries such as Japan and South Korea, the national health insurance refuses to approve medical reimbursement for anesthesiology care during endoscopic procedures [8]. NAPS has emerged, in part, out of necessity in areas deprived of adequate anesthesia resources. In the United States, the Food and Drug Administration (FDA) denied a petition from the gastroenterologists who sought revision of the propofol package insert that necessitated training in the delivery of anesthesia and, similarly, the European Society of Anesthesia (21 national societies of anesthesiology) signed a consensus statement confirming the same restrictions on propofol use [9]. This consensus statement, however, did not limit propofol administration to anesthesiologists in all European areas. Rather, in Europe, some areas embraced NAPS. Collaborative programs were developed to coordinate the training of non-anesthesia sedation providers under the auspices of the department of anesthesiology. One such example is the NAPS program in endoscopic units in Denmark [10, 11]. In this study about 15 patients (13 %) developed hypoxia that lasted more than 60 s. Although there was no mortality and most of the patients were American Society of Anesthesiologists (ASA) class I and II, about 119 of 2,527 patients developed short-lasting hypoxia (4.7 %), 61 (2.4 %) needed suction, 22 (0.9 %) required bag-mask ventilation, and 8 (0.3 %) procedures had to be discontinued. Also noted was that in 11 patients (0.4 %), anesthetic assistance was called due to short-lasting desaturation. Overall the authors maintain that NAPS is safe, and standardized training programs for nurses that are approved by the gastroenterology societies as well as anesthesia societies are necessary.

Non-anesthesia Sedation Providers

The delivery of sedation by non-anesthesia sedation providers has created a political debate between different specialty societies (American College of Emergency Physicians, American Society of Anesthesiology, and American College of Gastroenterologists). One primary issue of debate involves the depths of sedation, and how far a non-anesthesia provider should be allowed to sedate along the sedation continuum. Propofol "sedation," for many anesthesiologists, is believed to create a state of general anesthesia rather than moderate or deep sedation. The political debate has been compounded by the relative subjectivity of the sedation continuum and the accompanying definitions of the various depths (minimum, moderate, deep sedation, and anesthesia) [12]. American Society of Anesthesiologists has attempted to address these issues with statements and policies regarding the delivery of sedation by non-anesthesiologists [13–18].

Sedation delivery by non-anesthesiologists, however, is continuing to emerge globally: in Europe, unlike in the United States, anesthesia can only be delivered under the responsibility of an anesthesiologist. The limited availability of anesthesia personnel has forced the reconsideration of sedation delivery by nonphysician anesthesia providers [19]. This reconsideration may be influenced by the data from the US models that show no statistical differences in complication rates among non-anesthesia providers [20, 21]. In Europe (in countries such as Austria, Belgium, Cyprus, Finland, Germany, Ireland, Portugal, Spain, and the United Kingdom), there exists an entity identified as "circulation nurses/anesthetic nurses." These circulation nurses provide care in the operating rooms and are responsible for aiding the anesthesiologist during induction, maintenance, and emergence of anesthesia [22]. Another group of personnel include "anesthesia physician assistants" (in Switzerland and the United Kingdom) who can deliver both monitored anesthesia care (MAC) and induce general anesthesia for ASA I and II patients with indirect supervision by an anesthesiologist. They follow specific protocols and agreements [22].

In the United States, although anesthesiology assistants (AA) exist, they are trained and credentialed differently than are nurse anesthetists. Both AAs and nurse anesthetists undergo the same average duration of training (26 months), but their scope of training, education, and practice differs [23]. AAs have the ability to deliver anesthesia but only under the supervision of an anesthesiologist. In contrast, in some areas of the United States such as Iowa, Nebraska, Idaho, Minnesota, New Hampshire, New Mexico, Kansas, North Dakota, Washington, Alaska, Oregon, Montana, South Dakota, Wisconsin, California, Colorado, and Kentucky, the nurse anesthetists are able to function and bill independently in delivery of anesthesia care. These states have exercised the option of exemption of physician supervision for anesthesia delivery or "opt out" (42CFR part 416, 482, and 485). The request to "opt out" is usually carried out in a letter to the Center for Medicaid and Medicare Services (CMS) by a governor of the state in consultation with the state's Board of Medicine and Nursing.

In the United States, the sedation-delivery model appears to be evolving such that in the majority of models, the role of the anesthesiologist is to oversee, provide consultation for, or supervise the training of non-anesthesia providers, rather than to provide direct care. However, it is clear that such practitioners or non-anesthesia providers would need to have a minimum skill set to manage an airway and rescue patients who drift into deeper level of sedation than intended [24]. Lessons learned from the US models indicate that anesthetics would specifically advise and directly help other specialties who are interested in initiating or expanding sedation services. The Department of Anesthesia could help in the development of appropriate training and credentialing processes, training in airway skills, simulation training, and quality assurance.

In St. Louis Children's Hospital and Washington University, anesthesiologists provide airway skills training in the operating room for their hospitalists. At the University of Iowa, deep sedation credentialing requires airway skills (bag-mask) to be done every 2 years, in addition to a simulation and written examination. Another example is the creation of a sedation service using anesthesia oversight for urodynamic studies in children [25]. The credentialing of sedation and anesthesia providers (SAP), which could be a physician, a physician's assistant, or a nurse practitioner, occurred under the auspices of the director of anesthesiology, the surgeon-in-chief, or physician-in-chief. The requirements for credentialing involved a working knowledge of sedation principles and the hospital's sedation and analgesia policy. The SAP had to review and complete the SAP education module provided by the Department of Anesthesia, complete a qualifying examination, document adequate bag-mask airway management, and/or complete an appropriate life support skills course. Drugs used were primarily nasal midazolam and oral midazolam, and for moderate sedation, intravenous fentanyl, ketamine, and midazolam. All sedation outcomes were reviewed by the Department of Anesthesia.

In the United States, the Joint Commission mandates that sedation practices throughout the hospital be "monitored and evaluated by the Department of Anesthesia" [26]. In addition, in 2011, the CMS compelled institutions to place all sedation practices under the direction of one physician, which is usually deferred to the Chairman of the Department of Anesthesia. Current anesthesia models include sedation services that are run by anesthesiologists and certified registered nurse anesthetists (CRNAs). In some "opt out" states (states that have sought exemption from the physician oversight or supervision requirement for anesthesia delivery)—such as Iowa, Nebraska, Idaho, Minnesota, New Hampshire, New Mexico, Kansas, North Dakota, Washington, Alaska, Oregon, Montana, South Dakota, Wisconsin, California, Colorado, and Kentucky—CRNAs can practice independently. A recent publication by Parekh et al. showed that in 99,818 consecutive cases (of which 36,483 procedures were performed by CRNAs alone), CRNAs safely administered sedation for endoscopies without supervision of anesthesiologists [27].

In 2010, Boston Children's program transitioned from an anesthesia-supervised nurse sedation (RN) model to a CRNA-run sedation model in response to the changes effected by CMS in 2010 [28–30]. In a few institutions, such as the University of Iowa and Oregon Health Sciences, the sedation model is different. These institutions have anesthesiologists who supervise registered nurses (RNs) trained in procedural sedation. Rainbow Children's Hospital in Cleveland, Ohio has an established sedation service provided by intensivists. In response to the limited number of anesthesia providers, a multispecialty service model has evolved at many hospitals in the United States over the past decade [24]. An example of such a multispecialty-tiered sedation program is at Texas Children's Hospital.

Texas Children's Hospital

In response to a sedation-related death in 2005, the Chief of Anesthesia, Dean B. Andropoulos, MD, organized and mentored a comprehensive hospital-system-wide sedation program at Texas Children's Hospital.

The anesthesia department trains physicians to become credentialed in the administration of deep sedation. This training requires 2–7 days in the operating room under direct observation of a pediatric anesthesiologist. The physician must demonstrate skills in airway management (includes bag-mask ventilation, relieving upper airway obstruction, placement of a laryngeal mask airway, and endotracheal intubation). The physician must also pass an online sedation course (90 % correct answers to pass). Following completion of this training, the physician is then granted a secondary staff appointment in the department of anesthesiology. Recredentialing is required every 2 years and involves a complete repetition of the training. Maintenance of privileges requires a minimum of 20 successful deep sedation procedures a year without complications; physicians from multispecialties are eligible to be credentialed in deep sedation, intensive care medicine, emergency medicine, and hospital medicine. The sedation service is multitiered and has a distinct organization.

Two full-time sedation hospitalists are employed by the Department of Anesthesia. A third hospitalist, from the hospital medicine service, also participates in providing deep sedation services in MRI and to other out-of-operating room locations. They are allowed to administer propofol, ketamine, dexmedetomidine, and/or nitrous oxide to healthy ASA I and II children for specific procedures, such as MRIs, minor interventional procedures such as incision and drainage, dressing changes, bone marrow aspiration, and some gastroenterology procedures. The hospitalist sedation service is available during normal business hours, Monday–Friday (i.e., 7:30 A.M. to 5:00 P.M.), and they have immediate access to a pediatric anesthesiologist for consultation or in an emergency (by mobile phone). The sedation location is always collocated with an anesthesiologist sedation location or in close proximity to a designated backup anesthesiologist. A backup anesthesia response team has been set up which includes a second anesthesiologist and an "Anesthesia Stat" to the Anesthesia Clinical Coordinator.

Sedation for radiological procedures at Texas Children's Hospital is the primary responsibility of the hospital medicine physicians. The prescreening is done by a trained group of radiology scheduling staff. The staff integrates the child's electronic medical record information with the parent's response to a telephone interview of standardized questions, in order to triage the ASA I and II child to receive sedation from an anesthesiologist versus non-anesthesiologist. There are many ASA I and II patients who are referred to anesthesia, resulting in extended days that often extend into the evening, as well as Saturday and Sunday elective schedules. Children of ASA III or greater are referred directly to management by an anesthesiologist. Unanticipated emergencies are evaluated and triaged by the supervising anesthesiologist of that particular day.

Texas Children's Hospital also has a nursing-administered (registered nurses/RN) sedation program for procedures that are appropriate for minimal or moderate sedation. The sedation nurses must take an online sedation course and successfully pass an online examination. The nurse must renew their Basic Life Support (BLS) or Pediatric Advanced Life Support (PALS) certification every 2 years.

To ensure the safety of the protocols and to evaluate sedation outcomes, an anesthesiologist "Chairs" the multispecialty, multidisciplinary Sedation Oversight Committee. This committee is tasked with designing policies and procedures, and assessing quality and outcomes. Quality outcome data is mandatory for each patient and serious complications undergo Root Cause Analysis of the patient, sedation provider, environment, the institution, ancillary staff, and emergency response system.

The multitier service at Texas Children's Hospital has succeeded in addressing the huge demand for sedation services in such a busy hospital. In a 1-year period from September 2012 to August 2013, hospital medicine completed 545 cases, the critical care medicine team completed 210 cases, and 7 cases were done by the Emergency Medicine team. The Anesthesia Department completed 11, 914 cases (which include both procedural sedation cases and out of OR cases). The Department of Anesthesia was able to resolve ramifications particularly related to the use of anesthesia billing codes by non-anesthesiologists (hospitalists) by allowing them to be employed by anesthesia and or a joint appointment with the Department of Anesthesia.

Objective Risk Assessment Tool for Sedation

Though the anesthesia-delivered sedation model seems to be on a decline, anesthesia's presence in sedation is still very significant: the Institute of Medicine recognizes the field of anesthesia as a model of patient safety. Anesthesia-associated mortality is currently considered to be as low as 1 per 200,000–300,000 anesthetics [31]. Innovative ideas on improving or evolving the current practice of sedation usually involve collaboration with anesthesia. For example, Drs. Green (emergency medicine) and Mason (anesthesia) together introduced a new concept of assessing sedation levels not based on a patient's subjective response, but instead on objective physiological (vital signs) monitoring [12]. They identified this objective metric as ORATS (See Table 14.1) [32]. This is an Objective Risk Assessment Tool for Sedation (ORATS). Green and Mason suggested that the reformulated sedation continuum would be based on an objective means of stratifying sedation risk. This tool (ORATS) would guide training. It would also guide credentialing and quality indicators, as well as sedation outcomes. This new method of assessment is controversial, primarily founded on the financial costs that will be needed to implement the necessary physiological monitors [33]. Technology, however, is changing significantly.

Computer-Assisted Personalized Sedation

An emerging technology called a computer-assisted personalized sedation (CAPS) system has the potential to impact the practice of GI endoscopy, which looks promising [34]. Recently, a CAPS system was introduced in the SEDASYS® System (Ethicon Endo-Surgery, Inc., Cincinnati, OH). (Refer to Chaps. 31 and 38.) With the assistance of anesthesia consultants, SEDASYS was developed, trialed, and subsequently approved by the FDA in 2013. It is expected to be marketed in the United States in the early 2014. It is a CAPS-based intravenous propofol delivery system designed for

Table 14.1 Objective risk assessment tool for sedation (ORATS) [32]

New levels (as yet unnamed)	Escalating risk of serious adverse event	Physiological monitoring parameters (singular or combination)[a]	Recommended sedationist skill set	Recommended resources[b]
1	≤1:10,000	Consistent with normal awake pattern and frequency	Ability to observe and interpret the agreed-upon physiological monitoring parameters	Appropriate for risk level
2	1:1,000	← Objective monitoring predicts this level of risk	Skills appropriate for maintaining sedation at this risk level and for rescuing from the subsequent level	Appropriate for risk level
3	1:100	← Objective monitoring predicts this level of risk	Skills appropriate for maintaining sedation at this risk level and for rescuing from the subsequent level	Appropriate for risk level
4	≥1:10	← Objective monitoring predicts this level of risk	Skills appropriate for maintaining a patient at this risk level	Appropriate for risk level

Preliminary sample schematic. The choice of four levels here is arbitrary and for illustration purposes only. The final tool would contain the minimum number of discrete levels with independent predictive value

[a]Focused research would be required to validate the specific variables, parameters, and thresholds that predict the progressive levels of serious adverse event risk. Evaluation of capnography, for example, could include but not be limited to evaluation of waveform, frequency, pattern, and/or numerical value on inspiration or expiration

[b]To be determined at each level by consensus panel and would include but not be limited to recommendations on adjuvant personnel, intravenous access, availability of rescue medications, and airway equipment

ASA I and II adult patients undergoing endoscopy. The SEDASYS incorporates computer software that monitors vital signs (pulse oximetry, respiratory rate, capnography) and a patient's response (appropriate response to verbal command) in order to regulate the delivery of propofol. This was a non-blinded multicenter randomized comparative study (four ambulatory surgery centers, three endoscopy centers, and one academic center in the United States). One thousand ASA I to III class adults were enrolled and underwent routine colonoscopy or endoscopy. Sedation with propofol using the SEDASYS system and sedation with each site's current standard of care were compared (benzodiazepine/opioid combination). The results showed that the "area under the curve" for oxygen desaturation was significantly lower for the SEDASYS group (23.6 %) versus (88.0 %) for the comparative group $p=0.28$. In addition, patients who received propofol were more satisfied, and the recovery was expectedly faster than the comparison group [35]. Currently, the SEDASYS is approved for adults only, and there has not been any clinical application, nor studies performed with it in the pediatric population.

ASA Guidelines, Statements, and Education Modules

In summary, the American Society of Anesthesiology has, over the years, provided guidelines, statements, and education modules (Sedation and Analgesia by Non-anesthesiologists) [36]. This module is available online or as a DVD and includes carbon dioxide basic monitoring and advanced life support information. It also provides basic information and knowledge of sedative and analgesic drugs for moderate sedation. It emphasizes patient safety with proper training in sedation. The educational contents, training, and credentialing of these providers, however, vary from institution to institution. The remainder of this chapter will discuss and review the sedation protocols that have been established and delivered under the auspices of anesthesiologists.

Development of Protocols

Pediatric anesthesiologists have, at their disposal, a wide armamentarium of drugs for sedation. Anesthesiologists administer sedatives and analgesics independently—most commonly without set protocols. Typically, non-anesthesiologists follow protocols, many of which have been developed by anesthesiologists, with respect to sedation administration, monitoring, and recovery [37, 38]. Ironically, albeit anesthesiologists have supported the sedation training and protocol development of non-anesthesiologists, many also oppose the practice whereby non-anesthesiologists can use anesthesia billing codes and deliver propofol [39–42]. This chapter will continue by exploring the variety of protocols that have been established for various commonly administered sedatives.

Table 14.2 Exclusion criteria for ketamine-induced sedation [43]

Exclusion criteria for ketamine-induced sedation
Contraindications to the use of ketamine
1. Active pulmonary infection or disease
2. Known or potential (i.e., risk of) airway compromise
3. Pulmonary hypertension
4. Age of 3 months or younger
5. History of apnea or obstructive sleep apnea
6. Craniofacial defect that would make mask ventilation difficult
7. Complex cardiac disease
8. Acute globe injury
9. Prior adverse reaction to ketamine
10. History of bipolar disease or schizophrenia
11. Head injury associated with loss of consciousness, altered mental status, or emesis
12. Intracranial hypertension (i.e., CNS mass lesions, hydrocephalus, head injuries associated with increased intracranial pressure); *if there is any doubt, please have radiologist consult ordering physician to determine whether there is increased intracranial pressure risk*
13. Any child in whom there is a question of increased intracranial pressure
14. Child with potential ventriculoperitoneal shunt malfunction
15. Increased intraocular pressure
16. Patient or parent refusal

Ketamine

Ketamine has been used as an adjunct analgesic and hypnotic for radiological procedures, hearing tests, endoscopies, fracture reductions, suture insertion and removal, and oncological procedures such as lumbar puncture. Ketamine is versatile because it confers sedation, analgesia, and amnesia. A sedation protocol at Boston Children's Hospital allows radiology registered nurses (RN) to administer intravenous or intramuscular ketamine (under the auspices of a staff anesthesiologist or radiologist) for interventional, painful radiological procedures such as angiographies, percutaneous gastrostomy tubes, percutaneous inserted central catheters (PIC lines), and organ biopsies. There are clearly defined contraindications to the administration of ketamine, which guide the triage (screening) process (Table 14.2) [29, 43]. The advantage of these protocols was that it provided for the intramuscular (IM) route of administration for children who were not amenable to an intravenous (IV) initiation. This was particularly valuable for children who required a peripherally inserted central catheter (PIC) line for failure to achieve intravenous access. The Boston Children's Hospital protocol specified IM ketamine (using the concentrated form of ketamine 100 mg/kg) at an initial dose of 4 mg/kg for children under 5 years of age and 1 mg/kg above 5 years of age. Concomitantly, glycopyrrolate at 0.005 mg/kg was added to reduce the increased secretions associated with ketamine. Midazolam was administered to children over 5 years at 0.1 mg/kg to reduce the incidence of nightmares and hallucinations (Fig. 14.1 [29]). An intravenous ketamine protocol was also developed for administration by registered nurses. Ketamine IV 1 mg/kg and IV glycopyrrolate 0.005 mg/kg were administered together for procedures less than 10 min duration. Midazolam IV at 0.1 mg/kg was administered to those who were older than 5 years in order to decrease the incidence of hallucinations. For longer procedures, IV ketamine was delivered as a bolus followed by a continuous infusion of 50–125 mc/kg/min to maintain adequate depth of sedation (see Fig. 14.2 [29]). In oncology patients requiring procedures such as lumbar puncture, IV ketamine at an initial dose of 1 mg/kg (maximum of 75 mg), followed by additional boluses of 0.5 mg/kg as necessary (maximum of 2 mg/kg) was found to be effective [44].

Ketamine has also been used as an adjunct with propofol. Some have identified this combination using the term "ketofol" [45]. This combination is intended to decrease the dosing of each sedative, maintain hemodynamics, and decrease the risk of respiratory depression. A comparison of propofol versus propofol-ketamine combination for sedation during spinal anesthesia showed the combination provided better quality sedation with fewer complications as compared to propofol alone [46]. A protocol for auditory testing (ABR) of children age 1–13 years, demonstrated that the combination of 0.5 mg/kg ketamine and 1.5 mg/kg of propofol, decreased the need for additional boluses of propofol when compared to propofol alone (1.5 mg/kg). The ketamine and propofol (ketofol) combination decreased the total amount of propofol used. In addition no patients in the ketofol group had any desaturation or apneic events, whereas four patients had desaturation events and six had apneic events. Additional

INTRAMUSCULAR KETAMINE FOR PROCEDURES (ONLY FOR PICC LINE PROCEDURE OR AFTER ≥ 3 FAILED IV ATTEMPTS(FILL IN BELOW)

☐ <5 YEARS OF AGE

Glycopyrrolate 0.005 mg/kg x______kg = ______ mg IM x1

Ketamine 4 mg/kg x ______kg= ______ mg (max 200 mg/dose)Mx1

Mix together in one syringe and give IM x 1 in deltoid. Use concentrated form of ketamine (100 mg/mL).

May repeat Ketamine 2 mg/kg x ______kg = ______mg (max 100 mg/dose) IM x 1 after 45 minutes.

☐ ≥5 YEARS OF AGE

Glycopyrrolate 0.005 mg/kg x______kg = ______ mg IM x1

Midazolam 0.1 mg/kg x ______kg = ______ mg (max 3 mg/dose) IM x 1

Ketamine 1 mg/kg x ______kg = ______ mg (max 200 mg/dose) IM x 1

Mix together in one syringe and give IM x 1 in deltoid. Use concentrated form of ketamine (100 mg/mL).

May repeat Ketamine 2 mg/kg x ______ kg = ______ mg (max 100 mg/dose) IM x 1 after 45 minutes.

Fig. 14.1 This protocol is primarily for ketamine use when intravenous access is difficult or not attainable. The age groups are divided into children less than 5 years and children greater than 5 years [29]

INTRAVENOUS KETAMINE FOR PROCEDURES <10 MINUTES (FILL IN BELOW)

☐ <5 YEARS OF AGE

Glycopyrrolate 0.005 mg/kg x ______ kg = ______mg IV x1

Ketamine 1 mg/kg x ______kg = ______ mg (max 70 mg/dose) IV x1.
May repeat x 1 dose if patient still responsive to nailbed pressure after 1 minute.

☐ ≥5 YEARS OF AGE

Glycopyrrolate 0.005 mg/kg x ______ kg = ______mg IV x1

Midazolam 0.1 mg/kg x ______kg = ______mg (max 07 mg/dose) IV x1.

Ketamine 1 mg/kg x ______kg = ______mg (max 07 mg/dose) IV x1.
May repeat x1 dose if patient still responsive to nailbed pressure after 1 minute.

INTRAVENOUS KETAMINE FOR PROCEDURES >10 MINUTES (FILL IN BELOW)

☐ <5 YEARS OF AGE

Glycopyrrolate 0.005 mg/kg x ______ kg = ______mg IV x1

Ketamine 1 mg/kg x ______kg = ______ mg (max 70 mg/dose) IV x1.
May repeat x 1 dose if patient still responsive to nailbed pressure after 1 minute.

Ketamine 100 mcg/kg/minx ______kg = ______mcg/min IV drip to be iniated immediately after ketamine bolus above. Dilute ketamine to 10 mg/mL for continuous infusion. Assess patient Q10min for response to nailbed pressure. Titrate ketamine drip as necessary between 50 -125 mcg/kg/min.

Notify anesthesia if ketamine continuous infusion exceeds 60 minutes.

☐ ≥5 YEARS OF AGE

Glycopyrrolate 0.005 mg/kg x ______ kg = ______mg IV x1

Midazolam 0.1 mg/kg x ______kg = ______mg (max 07 mg/dose) IV x1.
May repeat x 1 dose after 60 to 80 minutes if sedation still needed.

Ketamine 1 mg/kg x ______kg = ______ mg (max 70 mg/dose) IV x1.
May repeat x 1 dose if patient still responsive to nailbed pressure after 1 minute.

Ketamine 100 mcg/kg/minx ______kg = ______mcg/min IV drip to be iniated immediately after ketamine bolus above. Dilute ketamine to 10 mg/mL for continuous infusion. Assess patient Q10min for response to nailbed pressure. Titrate ketamine drip as necessary between 50 -125 mcg/kg/min.

Notify anesthesia if ketamine continuous infusion exceeds 60 minutes.

Fig. 14.2 Intravenous administration of ketamine for pediatric radiological procedures [29]

Table 14.3 Medical conditions that contraindicate dexmedetomidine and nursing-administered sedation [59]

Medical conditions that contraindicate dexmedetomidine and nursing-administered sedation
1. Active, uncontrolled gastroesophageal reflux—an aspiration risk
2. Active, uncontrolled vomiting—an aspiration risk
3. Current (or within past 3 months) history of apnea requiring an apnea monitor
4. Active, current respiratory issues that are different from the baseline status (pneumonia, exacerbation of asthma, bronchiolitis, respiratory syncytial virus)
5. Unstable cardiac status (life-threatening arrhythmias, abnormal cardiac anatomy, significant cardiac dysfunction)
6. Craniofacial anomaly, which could make it difficult to effectively establish a mask airway for positive pressure ventilation if needed
7. Current use of digoxin
8. Moyamoya disease
9. New-onset stroke

doses were needed in the propofol group (21) versus (8) in the propofol-ketamine (ketofol) group [47]. A retrospective analysis of an IM ketamine-midazolam-atropine (5 mg/kg, 0.1 mg/kg, 0.01 mg/kg, respectively) combination for ABR sedation showed this combination to be effective with minimal side effects [48]. Another study demonstrated that a combination of propofol and ketamine was very effective for pediatric burn dressing changes [49]. In endoscopic procedures, there seems to be better tolerance during insertion of the scope when a combination of propofol-ketamine is used as opposed to ketamine-fentanyl [49].

Agents such as ketamine and dexmedetomidine have been used in combination for cardiac catheterizations but were not found to be superior to the ketamine-propofol combination with respect to analgesia and sedation conditions. The dexmedetomidine group had increased recovery time and a higher ketamine requirement than did the propofol-ketamine combination [50].

A protocol developed using intranasal sufentanil and ketamine was developed in Europe. The bioavailability of sufentanil and ketamine was 24.6 % and 35.8 %, respectively. A low dose of 0.5 mcg/kg intranasal sufentanil and 0.5 mg/kg ketamine was effective in 78 % of children undergoing painful procedures [51].

Pentobarbital

Although the drug has been in clinical use for more than 150 years and has an established safety record for sedation, the limitation is its relatively long half-life ranging between 15 and 48 h [52]. Pentobarbital given by the oral route (up to 8 mg/kg) has been shown to have a lower incidence of adverse events as compared to oral chloral hydrate [30]. An advantage of pentobarbital is that it may be administered by the oral and intravenous route with similar efficacy and adverse event profiles for each route [30]. Boston Children's Hospital still continues to have a nursing-administered pentobarbital sedation service. With clearly defined protocols, pentobarbital by the intravenous or oral route has been shown to be efficacious, predictable, and relatively safe. Although it has no analgesic properties, in conjunction with judicious administration of a narcotic, it may be used successfully for painful procedures [30, 53–55].

Dexmedetomidine

Dexmedetomidine is a selective alpha-2 adrenergic agonist that was approved in the United States in 1999 for intubated adults, and then in 2010 for the sedation of adults in areas outside of the operating room and ICU. It is not approved for pediatric usage although it is being used widely for this population in clinical practice. It was recently approved in September 2001, in Europe, for sedation in the ICUs. Although it does not carry pediatric labeling anywhere in the world, it has demonstrated itself to be effective and respiratory sparing as a sedative for non-painful radiological imaging studies, as well as a useful perioperative adjunct to improve analgesia and decrease emergence delirium [12, 54, 56–61].

Between 2005 and 2010, dexmedetomidine was incorporated into the nursing-administered sedation program for MRI at Boston Children's Hospital. It still continues to be administered by nurses for computerized tomography (CT) sedation, under the auspices of a physician from the Department of Anesthesia [54, 57–59, 61]. Clearly defined protocols have been established to guide administration: a list of contraindications to dexmedetomidine guided the triage/screening process (Table 14.3 and Fig. 14.3) [59]. An initial loading dose of 2–3 mcg/kg IV dexmedetomidine is administered over a 10-min period. Using the Ramsay Sedation Scoring System, the child would receive an additional bolus of 1–2 mcg/kg IV over another 10 min if he/she failed to achieve a Ramsay Sedation Score (RSS) of 4 after the first bolus. Once the child achieves this intended level

Boston Children's Hospital Intravenous Dexmedetomidine Sedation Order Sets

	Component	Order Details
	For CT/MRI/Nuclear Medicine [1.5 mcg/kg/hr continuous infusion]	
	dexmedetomidine IV bolus	
☐	Clinical Instructions	Instructions: Administer 1 bolus dose. Once the patient reaches adequate sedation, follow with the continuous infusion.
☐	dexmedetomidine	IV Loading Dose 2 mcg/kg, 1time Infuse Over 10 minute, Dose form = Injection
☐	Clinical Instructions	Instructions: If patient does not reach adequate sedation (Ramsey score 4) after one bolus of dexmedetomidine, notify prescriber via Spectra link
	dexmedetomidine IV infusion	
	RATE: 1.5 mcg/kg/hr	
☐	NS 50 mL + dexmedetomidine 200 mcg [1.5 mcg/kg/hr]	IV for 4 hr
☐	Clinical Instructions	Instructions: Please mix 200 mcg of Dexmedetomidine with 48 ml NS.
	pentobarbital IV: For patients requiring additional sedation	
☐	PENTobarbital	< 40 kg: IV 0.5 mg/kg, Q1min PRN Sedation for 4 dose, Dose Form = Injection
☐	PENTobarbital	>/= 40 kg: IV 20 mg, Q1min PRN Sedation for 4 dose, Dose Form = Injection
	PRN orders for hypotension	
	Hypotension Definition: **If Mean Arterial Blood Pressure (MAP) prior to sedation is within normal age-adjusted range - hypotension is defined as MAP below 20% of age adjusted normal value **If MAP prior to sedation is below normal age-adjusted range-hypotension is defined as a MAP below 20% of the pre-sedation MAP	
	Give 10 mL/kg of NS as a bolus for MAP < 20% age adjusted norms based on definition above (see attached reference information).	
☐	Sodium Chloride 0.9% (NS bolus)	IV 10 mL/kg Injection Q20min PRN Hypotension for 2 dose Infuse Over 10 minute
	Orders for Hypertension	
	Hypertension Definition: **If Mean Arterial Blood Pressure (MAP) is > 20% above normal age-based range and verified with repeat (MAP) discontinue dexmedetomidine infusion and notify sedating MD/NP. Infusion or bolus may be reinstated when MAP returns to age-adjusted normal range.	
☐	Clinical Instructions	Instructions: If MAP > 20% of age-adjusted normal and verified with repeat MAP, discontinue dexmedetomidine infusion. Infusion or bolus may be reinitiated when MAP returns to age-adjusted normal range, 1time, PRN, Reason: Other - See Order Comments
	Recovery Room IV fluid orders	
	NS bolus - Upon arrival to recovery room	
☐	Sodium Chloride 0.9% (NS bolus)	IV 20 mL/kg Injection 1time

Fig. 14.3 Boston Children's Hospital intravenous dexmedetomidine sedation order sets

of sedation, the sedation is maintained with an infusion dose of 1–2 mcg/kg/h. The infusion is stopped once the procedure is completed. The patient is then transported to a recovery area until discharge criteria (based on a modified Aldrete score) are met [58, 60]. In approximately 10 % of the cases, there was a need for adjuvant sedation with up to 2 mg/kg IV pentobarbital for optimal imaging conditions [60]. At the University of Iowa and St. Louis Children's Hospital, the dexmedetomidine protocols from Boston Children's Hospital have been adapted to include IV midazolam 0.1 mg/kg, IV ketamine 0.5 mg/kg, and propofol as alternatives to pentobarbital.

Propofol

Propofol is not FDA-approved as a sedative, but rather is considered an anesthetic agent [62]. In general, its administration should be reserved to only those who are skilled in the administration, recognition, and rescue from general anesthesia. Both the American Association of Nurse Anesthetists and American Society of Anesthesia made a joint statement on the need for restricting the use of propofol [63]:

> Whenever propofol is used for sedation/anesthesia, it should be administered only by persons trained in the administration of general anesthesia, who are not simultaneously involved in these

surgical or diagnostic procedures. This restriction is concordant with specific language in the propofol package insert, and failure to follow these recommendations could put patients at increased risk of significant injury or death.

Though the controversy on the use of propofol by non-anesthesia providers remains—especially in the United States—there is an increasing group of providers using it for sedation for endoscopic procedures [64].

Propofol protocols for upper gastrointestinal (GI) endoscopies have been developed in conjunction with other medications such as tramadol (used instead of fentanyl), which confers better respiratory stability than does fentanyl. A baseline level of sedation was provided with 1 mg/kg, and then patients were randomly assigned to receive fentanyl at 2 mcg/kg or tramadol at 2 mg/kg. It was found that tramadol provided sedation as efficient as fentanyl with better hemodynamic and respiratory stability (using propofol in the background as a steady dose) [65]. A meta-analysis of nine randomized controlled trials compared propofol in combination with other sedatives (such as midazolam, remifentanil, alfentanil, meperidine, fentanyl, and etomidate) to propofol alone. Propofol in combination was shown to decrease the total dose of propofol without affecting any change in cardiopulmonary complications [66]. Though the controversy of propofol use continues, the popularity of its use continues to grow with non-anesthesia providers. The recent first CAPS device using propofol was approved by the FDA in 2013 for commercial distribution in 2014 [67]. It has only been approved for use in healthy adult ASA I and II patients age 18 years and older. Although intended to allow non-anesthesiologists, gastroenterologists in particular, to deliver propofol for adult endoscopies, the FDA specifies that it requires the immediate availability of anesthesia [68]. The definition of "immediate availability" is not defined and is left to the discretion of the providers, institution, or facility.

A Close Examination of Some Unique Sedation Programs Developed in Conjunction with Anesthesia in the United States

Nursing-Delivered Propofol: The University of Iowa

Nursing-delivered propofol has been controversial because its use needs to be restricted (according to governing bodies such as the American Society of Anesthesiology and the FDA) to professionals trained in performing general anesthesia [69, 70].

The University of Iowa has a unique propofol model: registered nurses deliver propofol under the supervision of an anesthesiologist. A sedation protocol for endoscopy of children <10 years of age specifies a 10:1 combination of propofol and ketamine. The ketamine was intended to provide some analgesic and propofol sparing effect. Ketamine is not used as an adjunct to propofol for procedures in children >10 years of age for fear of hallucinations, nausea, and vomiting. Initially, the dosing interval between boluses was at 1 min intervals and slowly reduced to 15 s after the nurses gained experience. There are order sets that detail the dosing (see Table 14.4).

Nursing-Administered Sedation Program: The University of Iowa

In 2007, a nursing-administered sedation program was developed under the auspices of Dr. Joss Thomas. Prior, moderate, and deep sedation was administered by the anesthesia physicians. The program began with the training of five registered nurses (RNs) on bag-mask ventilation on anesthetized pediatric and adult patients, placement of a laryngeal mask airway, identification and rescue of airway obstruction and evaluation, and application of capnography. The nurses underwent simulation sessions on sedation-related events such as laryngospasm, airway obstruction, and equipment malfunction. They attended didactic sessions with anesthesia faculty who taught them important aspects of sedation: the pharmacology, pharmacokinetics and pharmacodynamics of sedatives and adjuvant medications, the concept of rescue, identifying levels of sedation, and recognizing that sedation is a continuum. They attended and worked in the Anesthesia Pre-evaluation Clinic to get skills in prescreening, and evaluating the past, current, and significant medical history. After 1 year of delay with the Iowa Board of Nursing, the University of Iowa began an unprecedented program: propofol-administered pediatric sedation administered by registered nurses under the supervision (but not continual presence) of anesthesia.

The credentialing requirements for these sedation nurses include a rigorous educational and didactic component, with a final exam to obtain final credentialing. The nurses must return to the operating room annually to demonstrate competency in the ability to independently mask ventilate five adults and children. They must also complete a minimum of 3–4 simulations annually. A designated anesthesiologist is assigned daily to supervise the nurses on the sedation service. The anesthesiologist is not in continuous attendance of each sedation, but is immediately available. All sedation is administered by predefined protocols, which may not be

Table 14.4 Propofol protocol for RN sedation (Merete Ibsen, MD, Department of Anesthesia, Carver College of Medicine, University of Iowa)

Propofol (P) - Ketamine (K) Infusion for Procedural Sedation	
P:K= 10:1	
Propofol = 200 mg of 10 mg/ml = 20 ml →	
Ketamine = 20 mg of 10 mg/ml = 2 ml →	
P-K total volume = 20 ml + 2 ml = 22 ml → • P-conc. = 9.1 mg/ml • K-conc = 0.91 mg/ml	
Example: 1. 8 kg child: 8 kg x 1 mg/kg = 8 mg = 8mg/9.1mg = 0.87 ml 2. 34 kg child: 34 kg x 1mg/kg = 34 mg = 34mg/9.1mg = 3.74 ml 3. 3. 50 kg child: 50 mg = 50/9.1 = 5.5 ml	
Propofol-Ketamine Infusion for Procedural Sedation And Propofol Infusion for Procedural Sedation	
Children < 10 years of age:	**Propofol-Ketamine Infusion**
• Midazolam:	0.1 mg/kg IV - (max 3 mg)
• Glycopyrrolate:	0.005 mg/kg IV (max 0.2 mg)
• Lidocaine:	1 mg/kg IV
• Initial P/K bolus:	0.5-1.0 mg/kg/0.05-0.1 mg/kg IV - (may be repeated)
• Infusion P/K:	100-125 mcg/kg/min
• As needed:	Bolus Propofol 0.5-1.0 mg/kg IV PRN
Children > 10 years of age:	**Propofol Infusion ONLY**
• Midazolam:	1-2 mg IV
• Lidocaine:	1 mg/kg IV before Propofol bolus
• Initial Propofol bolus:	0.5-1.0 mg/kg IV – (may be repeated)
• Infusion Propofol:	150 mcg/kg/min
• As needed:	Bolus Propofol 0.5-1.0 mg/kg IV PRN
Example: 1. 8 kg child: 8 kg x 1 mg/kg = 8 mg = 8 mg/9.1 mg = 0.87 ml 2. 34 kg child: 34 kg x 1 mg/kg = 34 mg = 34 mg/9.1 mg = 3.74 ml 3. 3. 50 kg child: 50 mg = 50/9.1 = 5.5 ml	

modified without approval of an anesthesiologist. All current requirements of sedation conform to policies of the Joint Commission and CMS [28, 71].

From January 2007 to April 2013, the University of Iowa has administered more than 9,000 pediatric sedations (an additional 1,000 in adults), 60 % of which were for radiological imaging and gastroenterology endoscopic procedures. Most patients were healthy ASA I and II medical status. There is an overall 4 % incidence of adverse events, which include oxygen desaturation (defined as less than 90 % saturation or decrease in saturation greater than 5 % of baseline for greater than 60 s) (not applicable to patients with congenital heart disease) not amenable to usual interventions such as blow by oxygen, position change, jaw thrust, short duration (less than 5 min) of bag-mask delirium/irritability, nausea and vomiting, airway obstruction, and inadequate sedation. The rate of significant adverse events was very low and involved unexpected admissions (17/10,000), allergic reactions (10/10,000), oxygen saturations less than 90 % (6/10,000), and reversal agent required (1/10,000). Through careful quality assurance and data review, modifications to protocols have led to improvements in outcome. For example, the reduction in ketamine usage and implementation of propofol reduced the rate of nausea and vomiting to approximately 4 % (manuscript in preparation). The preferred sedation for radiological imaging is dexmedetomidine, adopting the protocols developed at Boston Children's Hospital [54, 57–60].

The University of Iowa also trains non-anesthesiologists to administer deep sedation in the hospital. Training requires demonstration of bag-mask ventilation skills on anesthetized patients in the operating room and a 1-h simulation scenario in the presence of an anesthesiologist. Didactic learning occurs through a website with all the sedation-related material, which culminates with a written multiple choice exam. They are required to be current on their ACLS and/or PALS. This credentialing process is repeated every 2 years. All physicians must comply, regardless of past experience.

Conclusion

Under the leadership of anesthesia, sedation services can be created that rival the outcomes of anesthesia-delivered care. These models are uncommon both in the United States and abroad, in part because of political limitations but also because they require the commitment (time, intellectual, emotional) of anesthesiologists who are often limited in availability [35]. Training, credentialing, maintenance and demonstration of sedation skills, and collection and review of quality assurance data are all critical components of these sedation programs. The commitment of a Department of Anesthesia to partner with non-anesthesiologists in order to develop a non-anesthesia-delivered sedation service provides the opportunity for innovation and creativity.

Case Studies

Case One: Pulmonary Function Testing in an Infant

What are the Challenges?

1. The need to sedate a child who has very little respiratory reserve since the child only has one lung.
2. Spirometry chamber does not allow any other monitoring modality other than pulse oximetry.
3. Access to patient once in the spirometry chamber is difficult or compromised.
4. Child needs the test to evaluate whether surgery is indicated so the sedation should not compromise the normal breathing pattern of the child as much as possible.

Case Description

A 5-month-old baby with congenital agenesis of one lung and tracheal rings requires a pulmonary function test to assess lung function to plan whether surgical intervention of the tracheal rings is necessary at this age. In order to assess lung function, the baby requires sedation but needs to be spontaneously breathing. The baby is placed in a sealed chamber and, therefore, cannot be attached to monitors that have physical wires since the seal has to be "tight." The challenge here is that there are certain periods that the child would virtually have no conventional monitors (except for a pulse oximeter that is an integral part of the chamber). Though the process is not associated with noxious stimuli, there are episodes whereby the baby's lungs are inflated through a mask placed and sealed on the baby's face, which may be quite stimulating. We decide that dexmedetomidine would be the ideal drug to use since the baby would remain spontaneously breathing, and during the phases where the baby's lung was artificially inflated, we would bolus with a dose of ketamine. We used a protocol of 2 mcg/kg bolus over 10 min and 1.5 mcg/kg/h for dexmedetomidine, and used boluses of 0.5 mg/kg ketamine prior to the inflation of the lung. The whole process took about 45 min, and with these medications, the baby remained sedated, and the pulmonologists were able to get the data they needed to assess lung function. The information provided by

(continued)

the pulmonologists was enough to help the ENT surgeons to consider that intervention was not required immediately and they would continue to watch the baby for any signs of respiratory impairment as a result of the tracheal rings.

Case Two: Sedation for the Child Who Has Suffered from Burn Injury

What are the Challenges?

1. Access to areas to place monitors can be difficult due to burnt areas of the body usually covered with dressing.
2. Increased sweating on the patient due to the higher ambient temperatures, makes electrocardiogram (EKG) pads fall off easily making monitoring more difficult.
3. Increased chance of dislodgement of oxygen cannula and other monitors since the child needs to be moved for debridement and dressing changes.
4. The procedure is painful, and the child probably is highly tolerant to opioids and already is on relatively significant doses of pain-relieving medications.

Case Description

A 2-year-old sustained scalding injury to the hands and feet and requires dressing changes. The patient is transitioning from an inpatient to an outpatient and is likely not to have intravenous access. As an inpatient, the intravenous access is likely, and the sedation plan would involve intravenous ketamine and propofol. Some of the challenges include the problem of monitors not being able to stick to the patient, and one has to be vigilant to make sure that the reason why the monitors are not picking up the oxygen saturations or EKG is because of artifacts or problems with contact. During the transition phase to an outpatient, these patients are unlikely to have an intravenous line. In such situations, one can be placed using local anesthesia (cutaneous administration) and child life services. However, IM injections of ketamine and versed may work just as well. A mixture of 0.1 mg/kg or midazolam and 1–4 mg/kg of ketamine is used to provide adequate sedation for dressing changes. Some of these dressing changes occur in the room or in the bath area. Appropriate monitoring including end-tidal CO_2 is necessary to assure safety in monitoring as the pulse oximeter can sometimes fall off despite adequate securement at the time due to sweating. The use of nitrous oxide for this type of procedure can also be explored.

Case Three: Sedation for Multiple Procedures

What are the Challenges?

1. Different locations for different procedures so patients may have to be transported sedated through hallways and on elevators.
2. Some procedures may be more noxious stimulating than others, so one medication that usually works for sedation may not be ideal for the subsequent procedure. For example, if dexmedetomidine is used for radiological imaging but subsequently the child has to be sedated for a bone marrow, dexmedetomidine may not work for the bone marrow aspiration.
3. Procedures that depend on multiple different providers need exceptional coordination so that as each procedure is completed, subsequent providers are already available to complete their procedures in order to reduce time that the child is unnecessarily sedated.
4. Scheduling of multiple procedures depends on availability of different providers, which can be a challenge.

Case Description

Occasionally we get requests for children who need multiple procedures, some of which are associated with some discomfort or pain. In some cases, this is compounded by poor or difficult intravenous access. Depending on the age and cooperation of the child, procedures requiring noxious stimuli may deal with purely nitrous oxide sedation. The intravenous access can be less stressful to a child by using nitrous oxide and child life distraction techniques. If a child needs an MRI after a procedure such as a lumbar puncture, the nitrous oxide apparatus may not be MRI compatible. In such situations, we need to change the sedation to an intravenous mode using dexmedetomidine or propofol. In some instances where intravenous access is difficult, using inhalational anesthetics to get the intravenous access may be the most humane way of getting access (especially if the child is upset, agitated, or noncooperative). In such cases, the inhalational anesthetic can be continued to complete the procedure (in which case it becomes a general anesthetic case) or converted to a propofol or dexmedetomidine sedation where the inhalational gas is discontinued. The use of different sedation modalities allows the flexibility to undergo different serial procedures and allows for multiple procedures to be done in one sedation encounter.

References

1. Anonymous. Guidelines for the elective use of conscious sedation, deep sedation, and general anesthesia in pediatric patients. Committee on drugs. Section on anesthesiology. Pediatrics. 1985;76(2):317–21.
2. Lalwani K, Michel M. Pediatric sedation in North American children's hospitals: a survey of anesthesia providers. Paediatr Anaesth. 2005;15(3):209–13.
3. Gozal D, Drenger B, Levin PD, Kadari A, Gozal Y. A pediatric sedation/anesthesia program with dedicated care by anesthesiologists and nurses for procedures outside the operating room. J Pediatr. 2004;145(1):47–52.
4. Sury MR, Hatch DJ, Deeley T, Dicks-Mireaux C, Chong WK. Development of a nurse-led sedation service for paediatric magnetic resonance imaging. Lancet. 1999;353(9165):1667–71.
5. Boodhoo L, Bordoli G, Mitchell AR, Lloyd G, Sulke N, Patel N. The safety and effectiveness of a nurse led cardioversion service under sedation. Heart. 2004;90(12):1443–6.
6. Rosseel P, Trelles M, Guilavogui S, Ford N, Chu K. Ten years of experience training non-physician anesthesia providers in Haiti. World J Surg. 2010;34(3):453–8.
7. Luginbuhl M, Vuilleumier P, Schumacher P, Stuber F. Anesthesia or sedation for gastroenterologic endoscopies. Curr Opin Anaesthesiol. 2009;22(4):524–31.
8. Lee SH. Non-anesthesiologist administered propofol with or without midazolam for moderate sedation-the problem is not "which regimen" but "who's regimen". Dig Dis Sci. 2012;57(9):2243–5.
9. Perel A. Non-anaesthesiologists should not be allowed to administer propofol for procedural sedation: a consensus statement of 21 European national societies of anaesthesia. Eur J Anaesthesiol. 2011;28(8):580–4.
10. Slagelse C, Vilmann P, Hornslet P, Hammering A, Mantoni T. Nurse-administered propofol sedation for gastrointestinal endoscopic procedures: first Nordic results from implementation of a structured training program. Scand J Gastroenterol. 2011;46(12): 1503–9.
11. Jensen JT, Vilmann P, Horsted T, Hornslet P, Bodtger U, Banning A, et al. Nurse-administered propofol sedation for endoscopy: a risk analysis during an implementation phase. Endoscopy. 2011;43(8):716–22.
12. Green SM, Mason KP. Reformulation of the sedation continuum. JAMA. 2010;303(9):876–7.
13. Anesthesiologists ASo. Statement on safe use of propofol. 2009.
14. Anesthesiologists ASo. Statement on granting privileges for administration of moderate sedation to practitioners who are not anesthesia professionals. 2011.
15. Anesthesiologists ASo. Advisory on granting privileges for deep sedation to non anesthesiologist sedation practitioners. 2010.
16. Anesthesiology ASo. Statement on respiratory monitoring during endoscopic procedures. 2009.
17. Delegates AHo. Continuum of depth of sedation: Definition of general anesthesia and levels of sedation/analgesia. 2009.
18. American Society of Anesthesiologists ASA House of Delegates. Statement of granting privileges by the ad hoc committee on credentialing. 2004–2010. https://www.asahq.org/For-Members/Standards-Guidelines-and-Statements.aspx. Accessed 6 Jan 2014.
19. Clergue F. Time to consider nonphysician anaesthesia providers in Europe? Eur J Anaesthesiol. 2010;27(9):761–2.
20. Couloures KG, Beach M, Cravero JP, Monroe KK, Hertzog JH. Impact of provider specialty on pediatric procedural sedation complication rates. Pediatrics. 2011;127(5):e1154–60.
21. Cravero JP, Beach ML, Blike GT, Gallagher SM, Hertzog JH. The incidence and nature of adverse events during pediatric sedation/anesthesia with propofol for procedures outside the operating room: a report from the pediatric sedation research consortium. Anesth Analg. 2009;108(3):795–804.
22. Meeusen V, van Zundert A, Hoekman J, Kumar C, Rawal N, Knape H. Composition of the anaesthesia team: a European survey. Eur J Anaesthesiol. 2010;27(9):773–9.
23. Egger Halbeis CB, Schubert A. Staffing the operating room suite: perspectives from Europe and North America on the role of different anesthesia personnel. Anesthesiol Clin. 2008;26(4):637–63. vi.
24. Krauss B, Green SM. Training and credentialing in procedural sedation and analgesia in children: lessons from the United States model. Paediatr Anaesth. 2008;18(1):30–5.
25. Sweeney H, Marai S, Kim C, Ferrer F. Creating a sedation service for pediatric urodynamics: our experience. Urol Nurs. 2008;28(4): 273–8.
26. Organizations TJ CoAoH. Procedure for intravenous conscious sedation. Comprehensive Accreditation Manual for Hospitals: The Official Handbook. 1999:TX-73-79.
27. Parekh M. Do crnas need on-site md anesthesia supervision for safe propofol sedation in an ambulatory endoscopy center (aec)? A comparison of two sedation models: crna alone and crna with md anesthesia supervision in 99,818 consecutive procedures. San Diego: American College of Gastroenterology; 2013. Abstract 1.
28. Department of Health and Human Services CfMaMS. Revised hospital anesthesia services interpretive guidelines. State Operations Manual (SOM). 2010: Appendix A Ref: S&C-10-09-Hospital.
29. Mason KP, Michna E, DiNardo JA, Zurakowski D, Karian VE, Connor L, et al. Evolution of a protocol for ketamine-induced sedation as an alternative to general anesthesia for interventional radiologic procedures in pediatric patients. Radiology. 2002;225(2): 457–65.
30. Mason KP, Sanborn P, Zurakowski D, Karian VE, Connor L, Fontaine PJ, et al. Superiority of pentobarbital versus chloral hydrate for sedation in infants during imaging. Radiology. 2004;230(2):537–42.
31. Kohn LT, Corrigan JM, Donaldson MS. To err is human: building a safer health system. Committee on Quality of Health Care in America. Washington: National Academy Press; 2000.
32. Green SM, Mason KP. Stratification of sedation risk—a challenge to the sedation continuum. Paediatr Anaesth. 2011;21(9):924–31.
33. Cote CJ, Cravero J. Brave new world: do we need it, do we want it, can we afford it? Paediatr Anaesth. 2011;21(9):919–23.
34. Committee AT, Banerjee S, Desilets D, Diehl DL, Farraye FA, Kaul V, et al. Computer-assisted personalized sedation. Gastrointest Endosc. 2011;73(3):423–7.
35. Pambianco DJ, Vargo JJ, Pruitt RE, Hardi R, Martin JF. Computer-assisted personalized sedation for upper endoscopy and colonoscopy: a comparative, multicenter randomized study. Gastrointest Endosc. 2011;73(4):765–72.
36. Anesthesiologists ASo. Sedation and analgesia by non anesthesiologists. 2012.
37. Hoffman GM, Nowakowski R, Troshynski TJ, Berens RJ, Weisman SJ. Risk reduction in pediatric procedural sedation by application of an American Academy of Pediatrics/American Society of Anesthesiologists process model. Pediatrics. 2002;109(2):236.
38. Eichhorn V, Henzler D, Murphy MF. Standardizing care and monitoring for anesthesia or procedural sedation delivered outside the operating room. Curr Opin Anaesthesiol. 2010;23(4):494–9. doi:10.1097/ACO.0b013e32833b9c9f.
39. Cote CJ. Round and round we go: sedation—what is it, who does it, and have we made things safer for children? Paediatr Anaesth. 2008;18(1):3–8.
40. Aisenberg J, Brill JV, Ladabaum U, Cohen LB. Sedation for gastrointestinal endoscopy: new practices, new economics. Am J Gastroenterol. 2005;100(5):996–1000.
41. Green SM, Krauss B. Barriers to propofol use in emergency medicine. Ann Emerg Med. 2008;52(4):392–8.

42. Vargo JJ, Cohen LB, Rex DK, Kwo PY. Position statement: non-anesthesiologist administration of propofol for GI endoscopy. Gastrointest Endosc. 2009;70(6):1053–9.
43. Mason KP, Padua H, Fontaine PJ, Zurakowski D. Radiologist-supervised ketamine sedation for solid organ biopsies in children and adolescents. Am J Roentgenol. 2009;192(5):1261–5.
44. Evans D, Turnham L, Barbour K, Kobe J, Wilson L, Vandebeek C, et al. Intravenous ketamine sedation for painful oncology procedures. Paediatr Anaesth. 2005;15(2):131–8.
45. Andolfatto G, Abu-Laban RB, Zed PJ, Staniforth SM, Stackhouse S, Moadebi S, et al. Ketamine-propofol combination (ketofol) versus propofol alone for emergency department procedural sedation and analgesia: a randomized double-blind trial. Ann Emerg Med. 2012;59(6):504–12. e501–2.
46. Singh Bajwa SJ, Bajwa SK, Kaur J. Comparison of two drug combinations in total intravenous anesthesia: Propofol-ketamine and propofol-fentanyl. Saudi J Anaesth. 2010;4(2):72–9.
47. Akin A, Esmaoglu A, Tosun Z, Gulcu N, Aydogan H, Boyaci A. Comparison of propofol with propofol-ketamine combination in pediatric patients undergoing auditory brainstem response testing. Int J Pediatr Otorhinolaryngol. 2005;69(11):1541–5.
48. Bocskai T, Nemeth A, Bogar L, Pytel J. Sedation of children for auditory brainstem response using ketamine-midazolam-atropine combination—a retrospective analysis. Springerplus. 2013;2(1):178.
49. Tosun Z, Esmaoglu A, Coruh A. Propofol-ketamine vs propofol-fentanyl combinations for deep sedation and analgesia in pediatric patients undergoing burn dressing changes. Paediatr Anaesth. 2008;18:43–7.
50. Tosun Z, Akin A, Guler G, Esmaoglu A, Boyaci A. Dexmedetomidine-ketamine and propofol-ketamine combinations for anesthesia in spontaneously breathing pediatric patients undergoing cardiac catheterization. J Cardiothorac Vasc Anesth. 2006; 20(4):515–9.
51. Nielsen BN, Friis SM, Romsing J, Schmiegelow K, Anderson BJ, Ferreiros N, et al. Intranasal sufentanil/ketamine analgesia in children. Paediatr Anaesth. 2014;24(2):170–80.
52. Gilman A, Goodman L. The pharmacological basis of therapeutics. 6th ed. Gilman A, Meyer SE, Melmon KL, editors. New York: Macmillan Publishing Company.
53. Gozal D, Mason KP. Pediatric sedation: a global challenge. Int J Pediatr. 2010;2010:701257.
54. Mason KP, Prescilla R, Fontaine PJ, Zurakowski D. Pediatric CT sedation: comparison of dexmedetomidine and pentobarbital. Am J Roentgenol. 2011;196(2):W194–8.
55. Mason KP, Zurakowski D, Connor L, Karian VE, Fontaine PJ, Sanborn PA, et al. Infant sedation for MR imaging and CT: oral versus intravenous pentobarbital. Radiology. 2004;233(3):723–8.
56. Mason KP, Lerman J. Review article: dexmedetomidine in children: current knowledge and future applications. Anesth Analg. 2011;113(5):1129–42.
57. Mason KP, Lubisch NB, Robinson F, Roskos R. Intramuscular dexmedetomidine sedation for pediatric MRI and CT. Am J Roentgenol. 2011;197(3):720–5.
58. Mason KP, Zgleszewski SE, Dearden JL, Dumont RS, Pirich MA, Stark CD, et al. Dexmedetomidine for pediatric sedation for computed tomography imaging studies. Anesth Analg. 2006;103(1): 57–62. table of contents.
59. Mason KP, Zgleszewski SE, Prescilla R, Fontaine PJ, Zurakowski D. Hemodynamic effects of dexmedetomidine sedation for CT imaging studies. Paediatr Anaesth. 2008;18(5):393–402.
60. Mason KP, Zurakowski D, Zgleszewski SE, Robson CD, Carrier M, Hickey PR, et al. High dose dexmedetomidine as the sole sedative for pediatric MRI. Paediatr Anaesth. 2008;18(5):403–11.
61. Carollo DS, Nossaman BD, Ramadhyani U. Dexmedetomidine: a review of clinical applications. Curr Opin Anaesthesiol. 2008;21(4): 457–61.
62. Anonymous. American Academy of Pediatrics. "Inactive" ingredients in pharmaceutical products. Committee on drugs. Pediatrics. 1985;76(4):635–43.
63. Administration A-AJSRP. AANA-ASA joint statement regarding propofol administration. 2004.
64. Heuss LT, Froehlich F, Beglinger C. Nonanesthesiologist-administered propofol sedation: from the exception to standard practice. Sedation and monitoring trends over 20 years. Endoscopy. 2012;44(5):504–11.
65. Bedirli N, Egritas O, Cosarcan K, Bozkirli F. A comparison of fentanyl with tramadol during propofol-based deep sedation for pediatric upper endoscopy. Paediatr Anaesth. 2012;22(2):150–5.
66. Wang D, Wang S, Chen J, Xu Y, Chen C, Long A, et al. Propofol combined with traditional sedative agents versus propofol- alone sedation for gastrointestinal endoscopy: a meta-analysis. Scand J Gastroenterol. 2013;48(1):101–10.
67. Services DoHH. Sedasys computer-assisted personalized sedation system. 2013.
68. Administration FaD. Sedasys computer assisted personalized sedation system. 2013.
69. AANA-ASA Joint Statement Regarding Propofol Administration. 2004. http://sos.ga.gov/admin/files/propofol_admin.pdf. Accessed 6 Jan 2014.
70. AAP Pharmaceuticals LLC. Diprivan®. Propofol Injectable Emulsion. 2008. http://www.accessdata.fda.gov/drugsatfda_docs/label/2008/019627s046lbl.pdf. Accessed 6 Jan 2014.
71. Commission J. Sedation and anesthesia care standards. Joint Commission. 2010.

Sedation in the Neonatal Intensive Care Unit: International Practice

15

Karel Allegaert and John van den Anker

Abstract

Inadequate pain management in neonatal life impairs neurodevelopmental outcome because it alters pain thresholds, pain- or stress-related behavior, and physiological responses later in life. However, there are recently also emerging animal experimental and human epidemiological data on the impact of analgo-sedatives on neuro-apoptosis and impaired neurodevelopmental outcome. As a consequence, the management of neonatal pain is in search of a new balance, and these conflicting observations are the main drivers to tailor our pain management in neonates. Adequate pain management is based on prevention, assessment, and treatment with subsequent reassessment. Issues related to prevention and assessment tools are covered. Non-pharmacological (e.g., complementary interventions like facilitated tucking, nonnutritive sucking) and pharmacological (e.g., acetaminophen, opioids, ketamine, propofol) treatment modalities were reviewed and reflect the increased knowledge on neonatal pain management. Each topic ends with some *take-home messages* that in part also reflect our opinion on the current status of this topic.

Keywords

Neonatal Intensive Care Unit (NICU) • Neonate • Pain • Pain assessment tools • Premature Infant Pain Profile (PIPP) • Douleur Aiguë du Nouveau-né (DAN/EDIN) score • COMFORT score • The Modified Behavioral Pain Scale (MBPS) • Visual Analogue Scale (VAS) • Numeric Rating Scales (NRS) • Heart rate • Oxygen saturation • Facial expression • Limb movement • Vocalization • Nonnutritive sucking • Swaddling • Containment • Multisensorial stimulation • Analgesia • Sedation • Analgo-sedation • Bispectal index (BIS) • Near-infrared spectroscopy (NIRS) • American Academy of Pediatrics (AAP) • Neonatal Facial Coding Score (NFCS) • Ketamine • Eutectic Mixture of Local Anesthetics (EMLA) • Postnatal age • Postmenstrual age • Propofol • Pharmacokinetics • Pharmacodynamics • Remifentanil • Chloral hydrate • Morphine fentanyl • Benzodiazepines • Midazolam • Dexmedetomidine • Acetaminophen (paracetamol) • Infant-Centered Care index (ICC) • Infant Pain Management index (IPM) • Intubation–surfactant–extubation (INSURE) • Continuous positive airway pressure (CPAP)

K. Allegaert, M.D., Ph.D. (✉)
Department of Growth and Regeneration, KU Leuven and Neonatal Intensive Care Unit, University Hospitals Leuven, NICU, Herestraat 49, Leuven 3000, Belgium
e-mail: karel.allegaert@uzleuven.be

J. van den Anker, M.D., Ph.D.
Department of Pediatrics, Pharmacology and Physiology, Children's National Medical Center, 111 Michigan Ave NW, Washington, DC 20010, USA

Intensive Care, Erasmus Medical Center-Sophia Children's Hospital, Rotterdam, The Netherlands

Department of Pediatric Pharmacology, University Children's Hospital Basel, Basel, Switzerland
e-mail: jvandena@cnmc.org

K.P. Mason (ed.), *Pediatric Sedation Outside of the Operating Room: A Multispecialty International Collaboration*,
DOI 10.1007/978-1-4939-1390-9_15, © Springer Science+Business Media New York 2015

Introduction

Why Do Neonates Need Procedural Analgo-Sedation?

About 30 years ago, the myth that nervous system immaturity precluded neonates from pain perception and its negative effects was rejected by Anand et al. when he documented that inadequate analgesia during and following surgery resulted in both increased mortality and morbidity [1]. It subsequently became apparent that the negative effects of inadequate analgesia were not limited to neonatal life, but were also observed in later infancy. The ontogeny of the nervous system is based on a complex pattern of cell proliferation, migration, differentiation, and selective cell survival and includes apoptosis. Functional development relates to a balance of excitatory and inhibitory signals. Due to maturational plasticity of the nociceptive systems throughout infancy, nociceptive input may cause population-specific lasting alterations in pain processing [1–4].

However, these findings need a balanced approach. Experimental data from animals also provide evidence that chronic morphine exposure in perinatal life results in a reduced brain volume, decreased neuronal packing density, and less dendritic growth and branching. This is associated with learning and motor disabilities. In contrast, opioid receptor blockade through naloxone results in increased brain size and more pronounced dendritic arborisation. Similar animal experimental data have been reported for other analgo-sedatives, including benzodiazepines, ketamine, inhalational anesthetics, propofol, barbiturates, or combinations of such analgo-sedatives. Alterations are in part drug and dose dependent, and there is an age-related window of vulnerability for apoptosis on the one hand or dendritic changes on the other hand [5–8].

The extrapolation of these observations in animals to the human (pre)term newborn is obviously hampered by several limitations. An *association* between major neonatal surgery (number of interventions, disease severity) and neurodevelopmental impairment has been observed. However, exposure to analgo-sedatives is only one of the factors associated with this negative outcome [9, 10]. Others have extended these long-term impact research concepts to include medical procedure-related pain and nociception in later life in preterm neonates [2, 11]. Using functional magnetic resonance imaging (fMRI) during a tonic heat stimulus, the cerebral pain response in three sets (Neonatal Intensive Care Unit [NICU] preterm, NICU full term, no NICU admission) of each nine children were compared [11]. Former preterm infants had significantly higher activations than controls in primary somatosensory cortex, anterior cingulate cortex, and insula. This exaggerated brain response was pain-specific since this was not observed during non-painful warmth stimulation [11]. Similar, and using a term matched-control design in 43 former extreme preterm neonates, Walker et al. documented that there were differences in somatosensory perception in childhood [12]. Interestingly, these differences were in part local (e.g., thermal and mechanical hyposensitivity around a thoracotomy scar) and in part more general (thermal hyposensitivity).

The currently available observations strongly suggest that early pain contributes to neurodevelopmental outcome, pain thresholds, pain- or stress-related behavior, or physiological responses in later life. Effective pain management therefore remains an important indicator of the quality of care provided to neonates, not only from an ethical, but also from an outcome perspective [12, 13].

Although there is an obvious difference between sedation and analgesia, the available assessment tools and practices cannot always fully discriminate between sedation and analgesia. The increased awareness that neonates feel pain, the ethical obligation to treat this pain with analgesics, the growing body of evidence demonstrating that untreated neonatal pain can lead to altered reactivity to pain that persists throughout infancy and childhood, as well as the need for a humane management of neonates resulted in the development of guidelines to promote the use of analgesics in neonates [3, 14]. The main objectives of sedation and analgesia are reduction of pain, stress and irritability, and promotion of physiological stability. In the long term, reduced stress, as well as improved physiological stability, is believed to minimize the risks of neurological injury and death. Alleviation of pain is a fundamental human right, regardless of age [15, 16].

Despite the ethical issues, the increasing awareness regarding pain management in neonates and the availability of published guidelines for the treatment of procedural pain, preterm neonates still experience pain resulting in short- and long-term detrimental effects. The discrepancy between the available knowledge (relevance of adequate analgo-sedation, validation of techniques) and the bedside handling has been recently re-illustrated by Carbajal et al. [17]. This research group reported epidemiological data on the incidence of painful and stressful procedures and its management in the first 14 days of admission that were prospectively collected within a 6-week period (2005–2006) in 430 neonates admitted to tertiary care NICUs in the Paris region of France. This epidemiological study resulted in a median of 115 procedures for each neonate during the study period and 16 procedures per day. Of these, each neonate experienced a median of 75 painful procedures during the study period and 10 painful procedures per day of hospitalization. Of the 42,413 painful procedures, 2.1 % were performed with pharmacological-only therapy, 18.2 % with non-pharmacological-only therapy, 20.8 % with pharmacological and non-pharmacological therapy, and 79.2 % without specific analgesia; 34.2 % were performed while the neonate was receiving concurrent analgesic or anesthetic infusions for other reasons [17]. Prematurity, category of procedure, parental presence, surgery, daytime, and day of procedure after the first day of admission were associated with greater use of specific pre-procedural analgesia, whereas mechanical ventilation, noninvasive ventilation, and administration of nonspecific concurrent analgesia were associated with lower use of specific procedural analgesia [17]. Consequently, the authors concluded that large numbers of painful and stressful procedures were performed of which the majority were not accompanied by analgesia. The conclusions and epidemiological findings are very similar to the data published by Simons et al. that were collected 5 years earlier. Based on a dataset in 151 preterm neonates, each neonate was subjected to 14 (SD 4) procedures per day [18]. Despite the fact that most of these procedures were estimated to be painful, preemptive analgesia was provided to fewer than 35 % of neonates per study day, while about 40 % of the neonates did not receive any analgesic therapy during their NICU stay [18].

Similar results were reported when practices were compared between two time intervals in a same region. Survey data for the years 2004 and 2010 on analgesia policy and practices for common invasive procedures at Italian NICUs were compared to ascertain the extent to which neonatal analgesia for invasive procedures has changed since the publication of Italian guidelines [14, 19]. Based on paired data on 75 NICUs, the practice of pain monitoring became more common. However, only 21 and 17 % of NICUs routinely assess pain during mechanical ventilation and after surgery, respectively. Similarly, the routine use of medication for major invasive procedures was still limited (35 % of lumbar punctures, 40 % of tracheal intubations, 46 % during mechanical ventilation), and postoperative pain treatment was also inadequate. Consequently, the authors concluded that despite the improvements in neonatal analgesia practices in Italy since national guidelines were published, pain is still largely undertreated and underscored [14, 19].

Take-Home Messages: Why a Focused Chapter on Neonatal Analgo-Sedation?

Neonates do feel pain. It has even been described that neonates are even more vulnerable to pain. These more vulnerable neonates are precisely those that are most exposed to painful interventions. The subjectivity inherent to pain assessment in neonates probably further contributed to the wide variety of practices. The specific characteristics of neonates warrant a focused approach because:

- The lack of verbalization is likely one of the most important obstacles for the proper diagnosis and treatment of pain and distress in newborns. Pain in the newborn is usually not easily recognized and remains commonly under- or untreated [15, 16]. In general, if a procedure is painful in adults, it should be considered painful in neonates.
- Proper analgo-sedation in newborns is associated with a reduction in morbidity and mortality [1]. Compared with older children and adults, neonates, especially preterm neonates likely have a higher sensitivity to pain. This is due to a maturational delay in suppressive descending corticospinal tracts compared to ascending sensory spinocortical tracts. Moreover, the impact of inadequate managed pain during neurodevelopment results in a higher susceptibility to long-term effects of nociceptive stimulation [4].
- By virtue of their nature, newborns completely depend on their caregivers (parents, health-care professionals) to recognize their needs. This includes aspects related to comfort, stress reduction, and absence of pain and should cover evaluation/assessment, prevention, and managing of pain and distress [12].
- The appropriate use of environmental, behavioral, and pharmacological interventions can prevent, reduce, or eliminate pain and may improve comfort. This means that such interventions need to be validated, compared, and integrated in routine nursing and clinical care. Promotion of clinical research, knowledge diffusion, and validation of the effectiveness of implementation strategies to improve analgo-sedation remains crucial [5, 12].
- Simultaneously with this emerging evidence on the appropriate use of analgo-sedatives, neonatal care itself also is an evolving discipline. There is a shift toward less invasive care, reflected by introduction of minimal enteral feeding to shorten duration of parenteral nutrition, while duration of endotracheal ventilation was shortened through early nasal continuous positive airway pressure (CPAP) or the "INSURE" (*in*tubation–*sur*factant–*e*xtubation) approach. In the term neonates, systemic hypothermia became a valid technique to improve outcome following perinatal asphyxia. These shifts in clinical care induced a shift in pharmacokinetic covariates and pharmacodynamic endpoints [13].
- Neonatal drug dosing of analgo-sedatives should be based on the characteristics of the newborn and on the pharmacokinetics (PK, concentration-time) and pharmacodynamics (PD, concentration-effect) of the compound [5, 12]. Besides age and size, comorbidity, coadministration of drugs or genetic variations in drug-metabolizing enzymes, transporters, and receptors further contribute to the extensive interindividual variability in pharmacokinetics or pharmacodynamics [20]. When we apply the concept of developmental pharmacology to analgo-sedatives in neonates, this means that this should be a balanced decision based on systematic assessment of effects and side effects (PD), followed by a titrated administration of the most appropriate analgesic(s) (PK) with subsequent reassessment

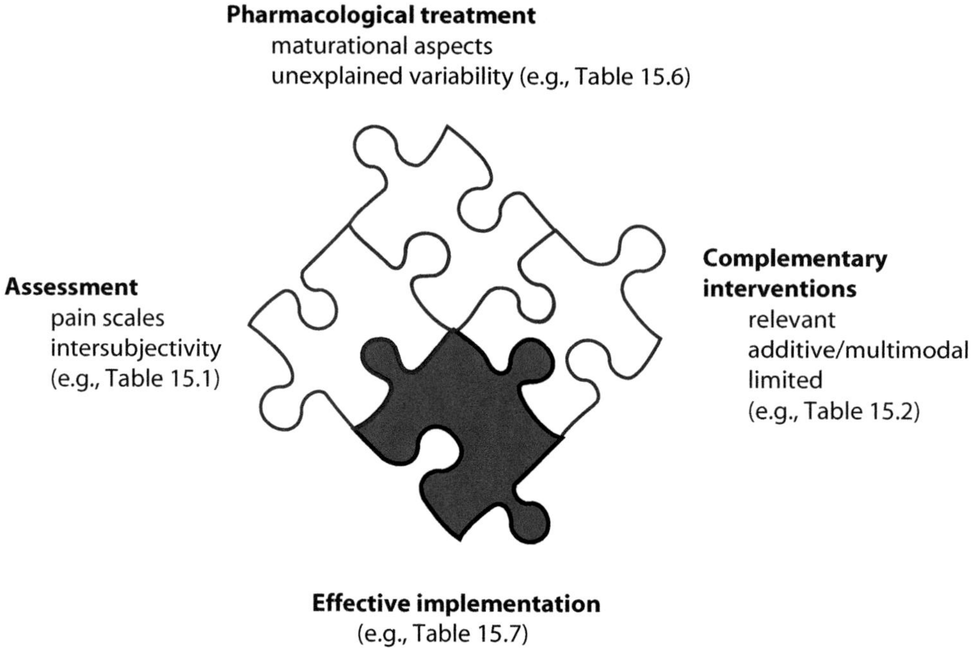

Fig. 15.1 Assessment, complementary interventions, pharmacological treatment, and effective implementation fit together like puzzle pieces for the effective management of pain in neonates

(PD) to adapt and further titrate exposure and effects [5, 12, 20].

- Inadequate management of pain in early human life contributes to impaired neurodevelopmental outcome and alters pain thresholds, pain- or stress-related behavior, and physiological responses. However, there are also emerging animal experimental data on the impact of exposure to analgo-sedatives on the incidence and extent of neuro-apoptosis [3, 9, 10]. Since this association has also been suggested in humans, the pharmacological treatment of neonatal pain is in search of a new equipoise since these "conflicting" observations are the main drivers to further reconsider our current treatment regimens.

Effective management of pain remains an important indicator of the quality of care provided to neonates. Effective treatment includes appropriate assessment, prevention when possible, and managing of pain and distress based on both non-pharmacological and pharmacological techniques with subsequent tailoring to the needs and characteristics of the individual newborn (Fig. 15.1). We will first discuss issues related to assessment, followed by illustrations on the potential relevance of preventive strategies. The main body of this chapter summarizes the available data on non-pharmacological (complementary) and pharmacological interventions in neonates. In the final part, there is a discussion about a research agenda on analgo-sedation in neonates, and this part finishes with a procedure-specific review (skin-breaking procedure, sedation for imaging). For each section, the available scientific information is provided, while the subsequent "key messages" in part also reflect our subjective opinion.

Assessment of Distress and Pain in Neonates

Limitations of Assessment of Distress and Pain in Neonates

Although this is still an area of active research, there are at present no easily applied, widely accepted, uniform techniques to assess either pain or distress in neonates. The gold standard of pain assessment (i.e., verbal report) cannot be used in preverbal patients: neonates can only display their distress or pain. It is up to the caregiver to read and recognize these signs [3, 21]. To structure this evaluation and to make this more objective, pain assessment tools have been constructed. However, assessing pain or distress in neonates remains one of the most challenging issues that caregivers, clinical researchers, and parents have to address. In the absence of a universally accepted, valid, reliable, and bedside-useful single biologic measure, we need to rely on pain assessment tools. Such assessment techniques are based on behavioral observations and/or physiological and hormonal measurements. In general, multidimensional assessment tools (i.e., both behavioral and physiological items) are used. Pain assessment tools that quantify pain-related behavior include but are not limited to muscle tone, facial expression, position of the eyebrows and mouth, crying, muscular activity, or consolability. Table 15.1 provides a list of commonly used multidimensional pain scales in neonates [22–30]. (Refer to Chaps. 5, 16, 17, and 20.)

Major limitations of pain scale are the impact of maturation and disease status on these indicators. In general, severe

Table 15.1 Characteristics of some frequently reported multidimensional pain assessment tools in (pre)term neonates and young infants [22–30]

PIPP [22]	PIPP=Premature Infant Pain Profile (Stevens et al. 1996). Procedural pain score. Indicators assessed are gestational age, behavioral state, heart rate, saturation, brow bulge, eye squeeze, and nasolabial furrow
DAN [23]	DAN=Douleur Aiguë du Nouveau Né (Carbajal et al. 2005). Procedural pain score. Indicators assessed are facial expression, limb movement, vocalizations, and attempts to vocalization
MBPS [24]	Modified Behavioral Pain Scale (Taddio et al. 1995). Procedural pain score. Indicators assessed are facial expression, cry, and body movements
COMFORT [25]	(van Dijk 2000). Prolonged pain, including postoperative pain. Alertness, calmness/agitation, respiratory response, crying (only in non-ventilated cases), physical movement, muscle tone, facial tension (initially behavioral and physiological measures)
COMFORT-neo [26]	(van Dijk 2009). Prolonged pain, adapted from the COMFORT score. Similar to the COMFORT score, seven behavioral items are scored, but muscular tone is scored based on observations (clenched toes/fists), while "no movement" was converted to "no or minor movement" to adapt for specific characteristics of neonates. One of the behavioral items is either crying (in non-ventilated cases) or respiratory response (in ventilated cases)
CRIES [27]	CRIES (Krechel et al. 1995)=Crying, requires increased oxygen, increased vital signs, expression, and sleeplessness. Prolonged pain, including postoperative pain
FLACC [28]	FLACC (Manworren et al. 2003)=Face, Legs, Activity, Cry, Consolability. Prolonged pain, including postoperative pain
N-PASS [29]	Neonatal Pain, Agitation, and Sedation Scale (Hummel et al. 2010). Procedural and prolonged pain, including ventilated or postoperative. Indicators assessed are crying/irritability, behavior state, facial expression, extremities (tone), and vital signs (heart rate, respiratory rate, blood pressure, oxygen saturation)
NIPS [30]	Neonatal Infant Pain Scale (Lawrence et al. 1993). Procedural pain. Indicators assessed are facial expression, cry, breathing patterns, arm movements, leg movements, and state of arousal

illness or immaturity will result in a less robust expression. In addition, these indicators have a limited specificity and even sensitivity for pain [31]. Distress or agitation (e.g., hunger, cold, wet diaper) will also result in similar behavioral responses, while Slater et al. nicely illustrated that there is a difference between nociception and pain expression (facial nonresponders) in neonates who underwent heel lancing. Pain assessment tools focus on aspects of pain expression, not necessary equal to or reflecting nociception [31, 32]. Finally, most of these assessment tools have been validated in a context of acute procedural pain, and may be less effective to unveil either acute persistent or chronic pain in neonates. Since most research focuses primarily on acute pain, in clinical practice, there remains the challenge of assessing prolonged and/or persisting pain [21].

Research can potentially provide more sophisticated measurement tools such as bispectral index (BIS) monitor, near-infrared spectroscopy (NIRS), or skin conductance to quantify sedation or pain in neonates [33]. BIS is a multifactorial tool derived from electroencephalographic findings and quantifies sedation, but has not been validated in infants in the first year of life. NIRS provides information on regional cerebral blood flow and oxygen extraction [33, 34]. However, this is only a surrogate marker for either sedation or pain. Skin conductance can be influenced by sweat glands and may hereby reflect autonomic activation, but in neonates also relates to differences in humidity of the incubator and maturational changes. Until such equipment becomes available following validation, we need to rely on clinical assessment tools [35, 36].

Despite the limitations discussed, there has been an extremely fast growth in the number of clinical assessment tools to quantify pain in neonates [21]. This proliferative growth likely reflects the dilemma related to the current absence of a universally accepted, valid, reliable, and bedside-useful single biologic measure. In the neonatal clinical setting, we suggest that the Premature Infant Pain Profile (PIPP) [22], the Douleur Aiguë du Nouveau-né (DAN/EDIN) score [23], and the COMFORT score [25, 26] are the most commonly used pain assessment tools. The Modified Behavioral Pain Scale (MBPS) has also been frequently used to assess pain expression in young infants [24]. Table 15.1 provides an overview of the variables included in these specific pain scores [22–30].

Despite the name, the PIPP score has been developed to measure procedural pain in both preterm and term neonates, but does consider gestational age (≥36, 32–35, 28–31, or <28 weeks, respectively) as one of the indicators to quantify the pain expression, hereby reflecting the fact that pain expression is less robust in more immature preterm infants. The PIPP score is based on seven indicators—three behavioral (all facial actions: brow bulge, eye squeeze, nasolabial furrow), two contextual (age, behavioral state), and two physiological (heart rate, oxygen saturation)—each with a four-point scale, resulting in a range of 0–28. The behavioral state is classified based on 15 s of observations, while (changes in) heart rate, oxygen saturation, brow bulge, eye squeeze, and nasolabial furrow are observed in a 30-s time interval [22]. The Douleur Aiguë du Nouveau-né (DAN/EDIN) score is a multidimensional *behavioral* pain assessment tool, initially developed to assess procedural pain in preterm and term neonates without a priori differentiation between both subpopulations [23]. It hereby combines issues related to facial expression (0–4 points), limb movements (0–3 points), and vocal expression (0–3 points) characteristics, resulting in a maximum total DAN score of 10. The scoring on vocal expression does contain specific instructions for intubated newborn infants.

The reliability and validity of the COMFORT scale as a postoperative pain instrument has been assessed in 158 neonates and toddlers following major abdominal or thoracic surgery [25]. Trained nurses rated the children's pain at 3, 6, and 9 h postoperatively in the Pediatric Surgical Intensive Care Unit using the COMFORT and a Visual Analogue Scale (VAS) for pain. Inter-rater reliability of the COMFORT items proved to be good for all items with the exception of the item "respiratory response," which was moderate (Kappa 0.54). Further analysis showed that the structure of the COMFORT data was best represented by three latent variables: COMFORT "behavior" with loadings from the behavioral items (alertness, calmness, respiratory response/crying, physical movement, muscle tone, and facial tension) and separate latent variables for "heart rate baseline" (HR) and "mean arterial blood pressure baseline" (MAP). Factor loadings of the items were invariant across time, indicating stability of the structure. The latent variables COMFORT "behavior" and VAS pain were highly interrelated, indicating congruent validity. Stability of COMFORT "behavior" and VAS pain was moderate [25]. Because prolonged pain in neonates remains a challenge, a modified version of the COMFORT-Behavior scale (COMFORT-neo) for its psychometric qualities in the NICU setting has more recently been assessed [26]. In a clinical observational study, nurses assessed patients with COMFORT-neo and Numeric Rating Scales (NRS) for pain and distress, respectively. Based on almost 3,600 triple ratings in 286 neonates, inter-rater reliability turned out to be good. Concurrent validity was demonstrated by adequate and good correlations, respectively, with NRS-pain and NRS-distress (r=0.52, 95 % confidence interval 0.44–0.59) and (r=0.70, 95 % confidence interval 0.64–0.75, respectively). COMFORT-neo cutoff scores of 14 or higher (score range is 6–30) had good sensitivity and specificity (0.81 and 0.90, respectively) using NRS-pain or NRS-distress scores of 4 or higher as criterion [26]. The Modified Behavioral Pain Scale (MBPS) quantifies facial expression, limb movements, and vocalizations or attempt at vocalizations and has mainly been developed and applied for procedural pain expression in young infants (2–6 months) (e.g., immunizations) [24].

Implementation of Assessment

Among others, the American Academy of Pediatrics states that ongoing assessment of pain is essential for adequate pain treatment. Despite this, there remains a gap between the available knowledge and the effective implementation of pain assessment in neonates [37]. The use of pain monitoring scales and the subsequent pain management undergo evaluation as part of the European project in neonates. To further illustrate the relevance of such epidemiological studies, we refer to three recently published observational studies from Italy, Australia, and the Netherlands [14, 19, 38, 39]. A recent report from Italian NICUs suggest that systematic assessment of pain is routinely applied in only 20 % of neonates on mechanical ventilation, in 12 % of neonates on nasal CPAP, and only 14 % of neonates in a postoperative setting [14, 19]. Similar observations were reported from Australia, based on data available from 196 hospitals. A clinical practice guideline informed the management of neonatal pain in 76 (39 %) of the hospitals. There was wide variation in their use between the states and a significantly higher use of such a guideline in higher-level care units. A pain assessment tool was only used in 21 (11 %) of the units with greater use in the higher-level care NICUs (50 %) and surgical NICUs (80 %). Awareness of breastfeeding for procedural pain was reported by 90 % of the 196 respondents, while 78 % reported that it was actually used. Awareness of sucrose for procedural pain was lower than breastfeeding at 79 %, with 53 % reporting that they used sucrose in their unit. Overall, 89 % of the respondents reported that either breastfeeding or sucrose was used for the management of procedural pain in their units [38]. Finally, Ceelie et al. assessed compliance to a pain management protocol in a cohort of 200 postoperative infants in the Rotterdam unit [39]. A mean of 11 assessments in the first 72 h postoperatively per patient had been recorded. A total of 2,103 pain assessments were retrieved, of which 1,675 (79.7 %) suggested comfort. Compliance to the protocol (reassessment and correct medication) was provided in 66 (15.4 %) of the 428 assessments suggesting pain or distress. Consequently, the authors concluded that the postoperative pain protocol applied in their ICU appeared to be effective, while full compliance to the protocol remained only marginal, possibly leading to undertreatment of pain.

Take-Home Messages on Pain Assessment

- Assessment of pain in neonates is an essential part of effective pain treatment [21].
- Multidimensional pain scales such as the PIPP, DAN, and COMFORT (neo) are the most commonly used pain assessment tools (Table 15.1) [22–30].
- Currently available assessment tools are suboptimal, since they are based on pain expression, not necessary reflecting nociception [31, 32].
- *Not the assessment, but the implementation of assessment is the problem*: strategies to optimize the implementation of systematic objective assessment of pain are urgently needed [37].

Preventive Strategies

Several complimentary interventions as well as adaptations of procedural techniques may be used to prevent pain and stress in newborn infants. In this way, such interventions may either reduce the need for pharmacological interventions or improve their effectiveness. Such strategies include light and noise reduction, nesting or swaddling, rationalizing and minimizing patient handling (e.g., preserving free periods for sleep, avoid consecutive blood sampling, clustered care), consider the use of central venous catheters instead of multiple peripheral perfusions, individualized monitoring techniques (vital signs registration, blood pressure measurement interval), tailoring nursing techniques (e.g., frequency endotracheal suctioning, skin and wound care, tape and wound dressing), and promoting skin-to-skin contact between the newborn and its parents. The growing body of evidence on specific non-pharmacological (complimentary) interventions is discussed later. We here would like to stress the relevance to consider methodological, procedural aspects as a potential powerful tool to reduce the need for analgosedation. This is illustrated by endotracheal suctioning and venous blood sampling.

Endotracheal suctioning is a painful and stressful procedure, commonly associated with pronounced fluctuations in vital signs in ventilated newborn infants. Cordero et al. compared two endotracheal suctioning frequencies in preterm neonates and concluded that there was no benefit of systematic, routine suctioning compared to suctioning as needed [40]. Based on these findings, an evidence-based protocol whereby ventilated newborn infants were suctioned only as needed based on clinical indicators was developed. This protocol was subsequently introduced as part of the collaborative quality improvement initiative earlier mentioned [41] and resulted in a significant decrease in the number of procedures performed. Four-handed care to facilitate containment during endotracheal suctioning was also associated with a decrease in stress and defense behavior and an increase in self-regulatory behavior [42]. Besides frequency of endotracheal suctioning or complimentary interventions, technical issues such as disconnection or deep versus shallow endotracheal suctioning have been evaluated in two recent Cochrane meta-analyses [43, 44]. Based on observations in 252 infants and using a crossover design in which suctioning with or without disconnection was compared, it was concluded that suctioning without disconnection resulted in a reduction in episodes of hypoxia (RR 0.48), and fewer infants experienced episodes where the transcutaneous partial pressure of oxygen ($TcPO_2$) decreased by >10 % (RR 0.39). Endotracheal suctioning without disconnection resulted in a more limited change in heart rate (weighted mean difference 6.77) and a reduction in the number of infants experiencing a decrease in heart rate by >10 % (RR 0.61). The number of infants having episodes of bradycardia was also reduced during closed suctioning (typical RR 0.38). There is evidence to suggest suctioning without disconnection from the ventilator improves the short-term outcomes when focusing on vital signs, likely reflecting reduced stress response [43]. In contrast, there is no evidence on the benefits or risks of deep versus shallow suctioning of endotracheal tubes in ventilated neonates [44].

Venous blood sampling is a commonly performed procedure in neonates. Besides complementary interventions such as nonnutritive sucking, sucrose, or containment, the technique used for blood sampling is also of relevance as illustrated in two studies in 120 and 100 healthy term neonates, respectively. In the study of Larsson et al. venipuncture was compared to a small or large lancet, respectively, in neonates who underwent testing for phenylketonuria. Successful sampling with only one skin puncture was successful in 86, 19, and 40 % of the cases, while median time to finalize collection was 191, 419, and 279 s, respectively. This also resulted in lower pain scores in the venipuncture group (Neonatal Facial Coding Score [NFCS]) (247) compared to both heel lancing techniques (333 and 460, respectively) [45]. Similar observations were reported by Ogawa et al. [46]. A population of 100 healthy term neonates were randomly allocated to 1 of 4 groups (venipuncture versus heel lancing, oral sucrose versus water). Using this design, the NFCS was significantly lower in the venipuncture group (230 versus 580). The lancing group with sucrose even still had higher scores compared to the venipuncture without sucrose (470 versus 230).

Take-Home Messages

- *Methods matter*: besides pharmacological and complimentary interventions, adaptations of techniques used can be a powerful tool to reduce pain and/or discomfort. This has been documented based on randomized controlled trials (RCTs) for both endotracheal suctioning and venous blood sampling [43–46].

Complementary Interventions

Increased awareness of a persistent high number of painful procedures routinely performed in neonates during their stay in the unit, combined with concerns regarding potential adverse effects of pharmacological agents, and the desire to actively involve parents in the care of their newborns resulted in a surge and evaluation of alternative, non-pharmacological interventions for acute, procedural pain in neonates [47, 48].

Non-pharmacological, such as environmental and behavioral, interventions have a wide applicability for neonatal pain management alone, or in combination with pharmacological treatments. These interventions are not necessarily substitutes or alternatives for pharmacological interventions but are complimentary. Non-pharmacological interventions can reduce neonatal pain indirectly by reducing the total amount of noxious stimuli to which infants are exposed and directly by blocking nociceptive transduction or transmission or activation of descending inhibitory pathways or by activating attention and arousal systems that modulate pain. In neonates, nonnutritive sucking, including sucrose, glucose ,or human milk, swaddling and containment procedures, sensory stimulation, and the kangaroo method can be considered as complementary interventions.

Nonnutritive Sucking, Sucrose, Glucose, and Human Milk

There is limited evidence to support the use of nonnutritive sucking in preterm and high-risk full-term infants as an intervention to promote behavioral outcomes and gastrointestinal function or feeding tolerance, but it has been linked to a reduced length of hospital stay and improved pain management. Nonnutritive sucking in preterm and high-risk full-term infants does not appear to have any short-term negative effects, but data on long-term outcome in high-risk full-term and preterm infants are not available. Based on the available results, it seems reasonable to utilize pacifiers for pain management in high-risk full-term and preterm infants [49, 50].

The most extensively evaluated non-pharmacological intervention for procedural pain relief in neonates is the oral administration of sucrose (12–24 %), glucose (30 %), or mother's milk, either or not combined with nonnutritive sucking (pacifier). It is believed that the effects of sucrose and nonnutritive sucking are mediated by both endogenous opioid and non-opioid systems. There is meta-analytical evidence in support of the use of oral administration of sucrose 24 %, glucose 30 %, or mother's milk in combination with a pacifier shortly before a painful procedure (e.g., blood sampling, nasogastric tube placement, immunization/vaccination) as an effective tool for procedural analgesia in neonates [51–56]. The observations on the use of sucrose during heel lancing hereby are much more common compared to other interventions or procedures.

Consequently, it became the most frequently applied intervention for procedural analgesia in neonates and, to a more limited extent, in infants. To make this more effective, this should be combined with the use of a pacifier, and the sweet solution should be administered on the tongue shortly (2 min) before the initiation of the procedure. This time interval is thought to coincide with the endogenous opioid release. When compared with local analgesia/EMLA or systemic acetaminophen (paracetamol) or morphine, glucose/sucrose results in the most prominent decrease in pain scores [51–56]. More moderate positive results were obtained during immunization in infancy (2–6 months), resulting in the guidelines to use sweet solution with a pacifier (or other facility to maintain suctioning) only up to the age of 4, max 6 months [57].

All these studies used neonatal pain scores to quantify pain expression, assuming that this also reflects differences in nociception. In the preverbal setting, the gold standard of pain assessment (i.e., verbal rapport of the individual patient) cannot be applied. The neonate is unable to say and can only show (express) his/her distress or pain. Consequently, it is up to the caregiver to recognize (read) these signs or to look for the absence of signs of comfort. To read these signs in a structured way, several sedation or pain scales have been developed and validated. In general, all currently clinical available tools focus on aspects of pain behavior or expression (e.g., motor activity, facial expression, motor tone, vital signs), not necessary reflecting pain perception or nociception [21–30]. This methodology-related conflict between different methods to assess pain in neonates has recently been illustrated in the paper of Slater et al. on sucrose during heel lancing in neonates [31, 32].

In a randomized controlled setting (sucrose versus water), the authors confirmed the significant decrease in PIPP scores when sucrose was applied. However, when more sophisticated assessment tools (spinal nociceptive reflex withdrawal activity or cortical evoked response, i.e., specific brain activity evoked by one time-locked heel lance with electroencephalography as identified by principal component analysis) were applied, no differences between both groups could be unveiled. We are aware that this study has been criticized on its sample size (insufficiently powered) and methods (electroencephalogram evaluated limited to 0.5 s before up to 1 s after the heel lance), but at least it re-illustrates that pain expression (as assessed by pain scores) is not equal to nociception [31, 32]. At least, the behavioral effect of sucrose can likely be explained by a pain modulation effect, and hereby provides evidence for the presence of pain modulating systems in neonates. In essence, caregivers responsible for neonates and infants are made aware of the fact that early pain experience is one of the covariates of interindividual variability in neurodevelopmental outcome (e.g., pain thresholds, pain- or stress-related behavior, and physiological responses in later life), while Slater et al. illustrated that sucrose or glucose are indeed not perfect as analgesics, and that they are likely in part effective through distraction and in part through endogenous opioid release [31, 32].

Swaddling and Containment Procedures

Van Sleuwen et al. performed a meta-analysis on the available knowledge on the impact of swaddling in excessively crying infants [58]. These authors concluded that swaddled

Table 15.2 Overview of studies to illustrate the effectiveness of facilitated tucking in preterm neonates, either or not combined with or compared to other complementary interventions (oral sucrose, nonnutritive sucking)

Reference	Study design and results
Liaw et al. [60]	Randomized, controlled crossover trial in 34 preterm (29–37 weeks) neonates to compare nonnutritive sucking to facilitated tucking with routine care on pain response (Premature Infant Pain Profile, PIPP score) after heel lancing. Both facilitated tucking and nonnutritive sucking resulted in a reduced pain response, but nonnutritive sucking was more effective as single intervention
Liaw et al. [61]	Randomized, controlled trial to assess the impact of nonnutritive sucking, sucrose, and facilitated tucking either alone or combined on infant's sleep–wake states before, during, and after heel-stick procedures in 110 infants (26.4–37 weeks gestational age). The combination of nonnutritive sucking, sucrose, and facilitated tucking resulted in the best preservation of the infant's sleep–wake states
Sundaram et al. [62]	Randomized controlled crossover pilot study in 20 preterm (28–36 weeks) neonates to compare the impact of facilitated tucking to no intervention on the PIPP score 30, 60, 90, and 120 s after the heel stick. Facilitated tucking resulted in significantly lower PIPP scores throughout time (8.8, 7.5, 7.2, 6.6, and 11.2, 10.7, 10.6, and 10.5)
Hill et al. [63]	Randomized, crossover study in 12 preterm (25–34 weeks) neonates to compare the impact of facilitated tucking to routine care on the stress response (PIPP) during routine nursing assessments. 9/12 infants received a lower PIPP score with facilitated tucking, reflecting the fact that the stress during routine nursing assessment can be reduced by facilitated tucking
Corff et al. [64]	Randomized, crossover study in 30 preterm (25–35 weeks) neonates to compare the impact of facilitated tucking with routine care on vital signs and sleep disruption following heel lancing. A lower heart rate, a shorter crying time and shorter sleep disruption times were documented during facilitated tucking
Cignacco et al. [65]	Randomized controlled trial in 71 (24–32 weeks) neonates to assess the effectiveness of sucrose, facilitated tucking, or both on the pain response following heel lancing, using the Bernese Pain Scale for Neonates. Facilitated tucking was less effective compared to sucrose, but combination of both interventions resulted in a further improvement in the recovery phase
Axelin et al. [66]	Prospective, randomized controlled trial in 20 preterm (24–33 weeks) neonates to assess the impact of facilitated tucking by parents on pain expression (Neonatal Infant Pain Scale, NIPS) and vital signs during endotracheal or pharyngeal suctioning. Facilitated tucking by parents resulted in a lower NIPS (median 3–5) score, and the infant calmed down more quickly (median: 5–17 s)
Ward-Larson et al. [67]	Prospective, randomized crossover trial in 40 (23–32 weeks) preterm neonates to assess the impact of facilitated tucking (second nurse) to routine nursing on procedural pain (PIPP) related to endotracheal suctioning. PIPP scores during facilitated tucking were significantly lower compared to routine nursing care
Fearon et al. [68]	The responses of preterm neonates to swaddling after a heel lance were quantified in 15 preterm neonates after blood sampling. Preterm infants aged 31 weeks or older showed protracted behavioral disturbances that were reduced by the use of swaddling. In younger infants, there was a return to behavioral patterns irrespective of the treatment conditions
Gabriel et al. [56]	NIPS scores in 136 healthy newborns. Skin-to-skin contact (SSC), combined with either sucrose (Sucr) of breastfeeding (BF) during heel prick. BF in addition to SSC provides superior analgesia to other kinds of non-pharmacological analgesia
Johnston et al. [69]	Therapeutic touch given immediately before and after heel lance in extreme preterm (<30 weeks) neonates in a randomized, blinded approach was ineffective (PIPP score) to reduce pain expression during and after heel lance

infants arouse less and sleep longer. Preterm infants have shown improved neuromuscular development, less physiological distress, better motor organization, and more self-regulatory ability when they are swaddled. When compared with massage, excessively crying infants cried less if swaddled, and swaddling can soothe pain in infants. It is supportive in cases of neonatal abstinence syndrome and infants with neonatal cerebral lesions. It can be helpful in regulating temperature but can also cause hyperthermia when misapplied. Another possible adverse effect is an increased risk of the development of hip dysplasia, which is related to swaddling with the legs in extension and adduction. In the neonatal intensive care setting, data are somewhat more contradictory. In a meta-analysis, it seems that swaddling has a pain-relieving effect, but it was maintained longer in term compared to preterm neonates [59].

In Table 15.2, we provide an illustrative overview of studies to illustrate the effectiveness of facilitated tucking in (pre)term neonates, either not combined with or compared to other complementary interventions, like oral sucrose, or non-nutritive sucking [56, 60–69]. Methodologically, the majority of these studies were not blinded and applied a crossover type of design, yet order effects are only rarely reported. However, the available evidence points to a modest reduction in pain scores and physiological fluctuations and a faster return to baseline [56, 60–69]. To test the comparative effectiveness of different non-pharmacological pain-relieving interventions, either applied alone or in combination to document potential synergism, effectiveness of oral sucrose, facilitated tucking, or both, a prospective study in 71 preterm (24–32 gestational age) neonates was performed in three NICUs in Switzerland [65]. Facilitated tucking alone was significantly less effective in relieving repeated procedural pain than sucrose 24 % (0.2 mL/kg). However, facilitated tucking in combination with sucrose had an added value in the recovery phase with lower pain scores compared to both single interventions.

Multisensorial Stimulation and Sensorial Saturation

Sensorial saturation is a multisensorial stimulation consisting of *simultaneous* delicate tactile, gustative, auditory, and visual stimuli. This procedure consists of simultaneously attracting the infant's attention by massaging the infant's face; speaking to the infant gently, but firmly; and instilling a sweet solution on the infant's tongue. Non-painful stimulation, by engaging a number of channels (i.e., auditory, tactile, visual, olfactory, vestibular, gustatory), is thought to compete with the painful sensory input. In a recent systematic review on this topic, ten studies were retrieved that evaluated at least partial sensorial saturation [47]. Based on the evidence collected, the use of an oral solution alone is less effective than sensorial saturation, while sensorial stimulation without oral sweet solution is ineffective. Consequently, it was concluded that sensorial saturation can be used for all newborns undergoing blood samples or other minor painful procedures. It is more effective than oral sugar alone and promotes interaction between the caregiver and infant [47, 56, 61, 65].

From Evidence to Practice: The Implementation Issue

Despite the available knowledge, deficits in the clinical management of pain remains. One reason is the gap between research evidence and translation of this knowledge into the clinical setting [70]. This is particularly true for non-pharmacological pain-relieving methods. Effective performance of some of these methods requires additional staffing and time. Although "facilitated tucking" is described as an efficient method for acute pain relief, the clinical facilitators required to successfully implement such a resource-consuming intervention remain unclear. In essence, the increased economic costs and organizational impact need to be balanced against possible (long-term) health gain benefits. Following the availability of studies on effectiveness of a given intervention, the subsequent implementation in the absence of allocation of appropriate means could provide caregivers with new knowledge and the burden not to be able to perform this good clinical practice. A report on the limited compliance with pain management guidelines for heel blood sampling in European NICUs confirms this gap between the available knowledge, the guidelines, and the bedside practices [71].

Another relevant question is how to integrate parents into these complementary interventions through either kangaroo care or facilitated tucking. Kangaroo care is defined as holding the newborn skin-to-skin against the mother's body with or without additional covering and in an upright 40–60° angle. Kangaroo care was documented to have some effect on pain expression (PIPP score) during heel lancing [72]. Similar, skin-to-skin contact, containment, and maternal voice resulted in a reduction in duration of crying or grimacing during and following heel lancing. However, the Johnston study had a 40 % refusal rate, indicating that not all parents are comfortable with these procedures and their contributions to the pain relief [72].

In two consecutive studies on parental-facilitated tucking, Axelin et al. first illustrated that facilitated tucking by parents is indeed effective (NIPS score: 3 [2–6] versus 5 [2–7]) and safe in preterm neonates that undergo endotracheal suctioning [66]. This was followed by an evaluation of the parental willingness to actively participate in their preterm infants' pain care through parental-facilitated tucking. The willingness to participate related to their internalized involvement, i.e., to what extent do the parents consider themselves skilled enough to take care of this responsibility [73].

Take-Home Messages

- Avoid procedural pain when possible or at least use the most appropriate technique [17, 18].
- Sucrose 24 %, glucose 30 %, or mother's milk, all, respectively, combined with a pacifier, are the most effective analgo-distractive techniques currently available for procedural pain relief in neonates. There is evidence in support of other non-pharmacological pain-relieving methods (e.g., swaddling, containment, multisensorial stimulation) [53–55, 61, 65].
- The sweet solution should be administered on the tongue shortly (2 min) before the initiation of the procedure. The illustration that this might not be as effective as anticipated should only enforce us to avoid procedural pain as much as possible [31, 32].
- Do not overestimate the analgesic effect of these compounds, and do not misuse these compounds to perform "minor" surgical interventions when more appropriate analgo-sedatives (local or systemic) are needed [15, 16].

Pharmacological Interventions

Pharmacological interventions focus either on analgesia, sedation, or both. We will first discuss agents commonly administered to attain analgesia with increasing potency (topical and local anesthesia, acetaminophen/paracetamol, morphine and fentanyl, remifentanil), followed by sedatives (benzodiazepines, chloral hydrate, propofol, dexmedetomidine), or both (ketamine, inhalational agents).

Topical and Local Anesthesia

Local anesthetics of the amide group (Ia) have effects on the central nervous system (depression or activation), peripheral nervous system (decreased conduction), and cardiovascular system (shortening action potential). Elimination is either through primary renal elimination or through hepatic metabolic clearance. Hepatic metabolism does result in intermediate metabolites, and these metabolites have also been linked to some of the observed toxic side effects [74]. However, the extent of the metabolic clearance compared to the primary renal elimination in neonates is unknown. Besides analgesia, there is also an increasing experience with lidocaine to treat neonatal seizures. However, this specific indication is beyond the scope of this chapter. In essence, there remains a delicate balance between effects and potential side effects in neonates with use of local anesthesia [74].

Topical local anesthetics are available in various forms such as a lidocaine ointment or gel, and amethocaine/tetracaine cream, but the Eutectic Mixture of Local Anesthetics (EMLA) as a cream, containing both 2.5 % of lidocaine and 2.5 % of prilocaine, is most commonly used and evaluated. We will first discuss efficacy data, followed by some observations on toxicity. In general, it provides good superficial (skin) anesthesia for 1–2 h when applied under an occlusive dressing. Application should be done about 1 h before the skin-breaking procedure. In neonates, this has been evaluated for heel lancing, venipuncture, lumbar puncture, and circumcision, but data for skin-breaking procedures are to a certain extent conflicting.

In a meta-analysis on *heel lancing*, there was no significant benefit of EMLA for any of the outcome measures used to assess pain (i.e., behavioral pain scores, infant crying, heart rate, blood pressure, respiratory rate, oxygenation) [75]. For *venipuncture*, infants treated with EMLA had significantly lower heart rates and crying duration compared with infants treated with a placebo. However, oral sucrose 24 % [76] or glucose 30 % [77] in combination with a pacifier seems to be more effective in reducing pain expression during venipuncture than EMLA application. However, the combination of sucrose and EMLA cream revealed a higher analgesic effect than sucrose 24 % alone during venipuncture in preterm infants [78]. Similar effects have been documented for pain relief during percutaneous venous catheter placement (heart rate, respiratory rate) and arterial puncture (behavioral pain score).

For *lumbar puncture*, we are aware of two studies with conflicting results. Kaur et al. provided evidence that supports the concept that EMLA is effective in reducing pain associated with needle insertion and withdrawal during lumbar puncture in newborn infants [79]. Unfortunately, compared with baseline observations, all newborn infants experienced pain as evidenced by increased heart rate, decreased oxygen saturation level, and total behavioral score [79]. In contrast, EMLA did not reduce physiological changes or behavioral pain scores in another RCT in neonates (>34 weeks GA) undergoing lumbar puncture [80]. Based on the available evidence, topical anesthetics may blunt the physiological markers of pain, but this does not result in a pain-free procedure [81].

Similar trends on limited to moderate effectiveness have been observed to treat pain during circumcision. EMLA cream (1–2 g) can be applied to the distal half of the penis with subsequent occlusive dressing 60–90 min before circumcision is performed. It is important to minimize systemic absorption by removing the cream just before the start of the surgical procedure. The first data on the efficacy and safety of this approach have been described by Taddio et al. [82]. Using an RCT approach, 38 neonates were treated with EMLA. Compared to 30 neonates in the placebo arm, the neonates in the lidocaine–prilocaine group had less facial activity, spent less time crying, and had smaller increases in heart rate than the neonates in the placebo group. Blood methemoglobin concentrations (expressed as a percentage of the hemoglobin concentration) were similar (1.3 %) in both groups. Lidocaine and prilocaine were detected in plasma in 61 and 55 % of the infants treated with lidocaine–prilocaine cream, respectively. However, when compared to other regional analgesic interventions (ring block, dorsal penile block), the ring block was equally effective through all stages of the circumcision, whereas dorsal penile nerve block and EMLA were less effective during foreskin separation and incision; methemoglobin levels were highest in the EMLA group, although not a single newborn required treatment [83].

Pretreatment with EMLA decreases infant pain related to routine vaccinations, but the application of these data is limited to healthy infants [84]. The combined use of EMLA and glucose 30 % was proven to be effective when compared to placebo, while combining sucrose, oral tactile stimulation, and parental holding was also associated with significantly reduced crying in infants receiving multiple immunization injections [85].

Besides EMLA cream, sprays (4 % lidocaine, max 0.1 mL/kg) or gel (2 %, max 0.3 mL/kg) for mucosal topical anesthesia (2) or local injection of lidocaine (up to 3 mg/kg max, equal to 0.3 of the 1 % formulation) are also commonly used. Data in infants documented that nebulized lidocaine is not effective to reduce the pain response to nasogastric tube placement [86]. In contrast, lingual 24 % sucrose is effective in reducing the behavioral and physiological pain response to nasogastric tube insertion in preterm infants [87]. We could not find data on the effects of mucosal spray to facilitate bronchoscopy or gastroscopy in neonates.

Table 15.3 Reported papers on the analgesic effects of tetracaine/amethocaine in neonates (type of procedure highlighted)

Reference	Study design and results
Shah et al. [88]	Randomized, double-blind, placebo-controlled trial, *intramuscular injection* (vitamin K) in 110 term neonates, topical amethocaine gel 4 %. There were no differences in crying duration, in pain score and only the latency to cry was somewhat longer in the treated group. Topical amethocaine gel 4 % was ineffective in reducing pain intramuscular injection of vitamin K in full-term neonates
Jain A et al. [89]	Randomized, double-blind, placebo-controlled trial in 40 (pre)term neonates during *venipuncture*. Topical amethocaine provided effective pain relief (crying, neonatal facial coding system) during venipuncture in the newborn when used as single technique for analgesia
Lemyre et al. [90]	Randomized, double-blind, placebo-controlled trial in 142 preterm (from 24 weeks onward) infants during *venipuncture*. Tetracaine did not significantly decrease procedural pain in infants undergoing a venipuncture, when used in combination with routine sucrose administration
Lemyre et al. [91]	Randomized, double-blind, placebo-controlled trial in 54 preterm neonates on the add-on effect of tetracaine gel in addition to sucrose to treat procedural pain related to *peripherally inserted central catheter (PICC) placement*. Tetracaine 4 % when applied for 30 min was not beneficial in decreasing procedural pain associated with a PICC in very small infants
Jain et al. [92]	Randomized, double-blind, placebo-controlled trial in 60 (pre)term neonates during *heel prick blood sampling*. Topical amethocaine gel does not have a clinically important effect on the pain of heel prick blood sampling. Its use for this purpose cannot therefore be recommended

Besides the overall limited benefit or add-on effect of lidocaine, there is a relevant concern about toxicity in neonates. Different case reports and case series on the association of EMLA application and seizures (lidocaine mediated) and/or methemoglobinemia (prilocaine mediated) have been described. Newborns are at higher risk to develop methemoglobinemia because of reduced NADH-dependent methemoglobin reductase. The same limited effect/potential side effect balance can be constructed for tetracaine. Some of the available reports on limited tetracaine effects in newborns were summarized in Table 15.3 [88–92]. However, contact dermatitis and cardiac arrhythmia has been described in neonates.

Take-Home Messages

- The overall evidence suggests a modest to moderate effect on procedural pain in neonates. This means that for most of the procedures, topical anesthesia should be considered as part of a multimodal analgesia [74].
- There remains a concern on absorption-related toxicity (seizures, methemoglobinemia). Maximal doses should be adhered to; absorption is more likely in the presence of disrupted skin. When applied for circumcision, EMLA should be removed just before the start of the surgical intervention [74].

Propofol

Propofol (2,6 di-isopropylphenol) is a highly lipophilic compound that exhibits rapid distribution from the blood to the subcutaneous fat and the central nervous system compartments with subsequent redistribution and metabolic clearance. It is considered to be a short-acting anesthetic (not an analgesic) that is both rapid in its onset and short in duration after cessation [93]. Because of these pharmacokinetic and dynamic characteristics, propofol became a frequently administered drug for induction and/or maintenance of anesthesia in children and, more recently, in neonates. However, continuous administration may result in serious, sometimes lethal metabolic complications (propofol infusion syndrome) in children and has more recently also been described in a preterm newborn following inadvertent dosing during surgery [94]. This is of relevance, since it took about 15 years of unlicensed, off-label administration before this serious side effect, and its risk factors in pediatric patients were unveiled.

Because propofol is a water-insoluble phenolic compound, propofol clearance is exclusively through metabolic clearance. In adults, metabolism is mainly through glucuronidation. Since glucuronidation capacity in neonates displays important ontogeny, pharmacokinetics in this specific population are of utmost relevance. Data on propofol pharmacokinetics in neonates are available [95]. Standardized propofol clearance at 38 weeks postmenstrual age (PMA) (CL_{std}) was 0.029 L/min. A fixed value in neonates with a postnatal age (PNA) of ≥10 days further improved the model and resulted in the equation:

$$\left[CL_{std}\cdot(PMA/38)11.5+0.03\right]1/\text{min for neonates} \geq 10\,\text{days}$$

When compared to adults (1.91 L/min^{-1}) following an IV bolus, the difference in clearance is impressive (65-fold) [95]. The complex interplay between size and maturation results in an overall low propofol clearance capacity at birth (estimated to be 0.029 L/min at 38 weeks PMA) with a subsequent PNA- and PMA-related increase. Consequently, both preterm and term neonates in the first week of postnatal life have an increased risk for accumulation following intermittent bolus or continuous administration of propofol due

Table 15.4 Summary of the reported studies on the use of propofol to facilitate endotracheal intubation in (pre)term neonates, reflecting the variability in clinical characteristics, outcome criteria, co-medication and doses (1–2.5 mg/kg) evaluated in the different studies

Reference	Study design and results
Welzing et al. [96]	Prospective, observational study on intubating conditions, vital signs, extubation times and outcome in 13 preterm neonates treated with propofol (1 mg/kg) for an INSURE (*in*tubation, *sur*factant, *e*xtubation) procedure. The study was stopped early because of significant cardiovascular side effects expressed as distinct drop in mean blood pressure (mean values = 38 mmHg to 24 mmHg 10 min after propofol exposure). Intubation conditions were reported to be good
Nauta et al. [97]	Retrospective analysis on trends in arterial blood pressure (invasive) in 21 preterm neonates (28.8, SD 3.5 weeks) exposed to propofol (2 mg/kg), 5/21 co-treated with atropine. The decline in mean arterial blood pressure before and after propofol administration (48–41 mmHg) was not significant, and the proportion of patients with hypotension was similar before and after propofol exposure
Ghanta et al. [98]	Randomized, open-label controlled trial comparing propofol (2.5 mg/kg) with morphine (100 μ[mu]g/kg)-atropine (10 μ[mu]g/kg)-suxamethonium (2 mg/kg) as induction agents for endotracheal intubation in 63 preterm neonates. There were no differences in vital signs, but trough oxygen saturation was significantly lower in the M-A-S group, and recovery time was shorter in the propofol group [recovery time = return of spontaneous muscle movement]
Papoff et al. [99]	Pilot study in 21 (pre)term neonates with severe respiratory distress syndrome. Fentanyl (1.5 μ[mu]g/kg) was coadministered with propofol (2 mg/kg over 20 s) and propofol was administered a second time if more than 1 attempt to intubate was needed. A subscore of ≤2 for all items of the Helbo-Hansen score system was qualified to reflect an easy intubation. Intubation was qualified as easy in all cases, intubation at first attempt in 18/21. Oxygen desaturation (all >60 %) was documented in 7/21 cases. These desaturation events were commonly associated with a transient decrease in systemic blood pressure (treated with crystalloids, 10 mL/kg)
Penido et al. [100]	Double-blinded, randomized controlled trial in 20 preterm (28–34 weeks) neonates, exposed to either propofol (2 mg/kg) or midazolam (0.2 mg/kg). Both (propofol/midazolam) were combined with remifentanil (1 μ[mu]g/kg). No differences in intubation conditions or number of attempts needed were observed

to the reduced clearing capacity. Secondly, there is still extensive unexplained variability in neonates after introducing PMA and PNA as covariates, making prediction in neonates more difficult [95].

Pharmacodynamics of propofol have been described, with specific emphasis on the (side) effects of propofol during endotracheal intubation (Table 15.4) [96–100]. Ghanta et al. reported on propofol (2.5 mg/kg) pharmacodynamics in 33 preterm neonates during semi-elective endotracheal intubation. Compared to a morphine/atropine/suxamethonium regimen, time until sleep, muscle relaxation, and time to achieve successful intubation were shorter [98]. These short-acting sedative effects were confirmed by others [96–100]. In contrast, however, a significant impact on blood pressure (decrease 20 %) and oxygenation have been reported in term neonates, in neonates with an associated cardiopathy, and in two cohorts of preterm neonates undergoing chest tube removal ($n=20$, 3 mg/kg^{-1}) or during INSURE ($n=13$, 1 mg/kg^{-1}). We hereby would like to remind the readers that there is an association between fluctuations in blood pressure and intracranial hemorrhage in the first days of postnatal life in preterm neonates [101].

Because spontaneous respiration can be maintained, propofol (intermittent bolus, 1 mg/kg, combined with topical anesthesia) has been used to facilitate diagnostic or therapeutic bronchoscopies. This approach is similar as in children, but reports in neonates are still limited to case reports. The use of a CPAP mask and maintaining spontaneous breathing significantly reduce the risk of relevant oxygen desaturation during the procedure.

Continuous administration of propofol has been used to facilitate procedural sedation during imaging procedures in neonates. Taking the aforementioned covariates (PNA and PMA) of propofol pharmacokinetics and the prolonged scanning times into account, we suggest to remain cautious with the use of prolonged propofol infusion in neonates. Although limited to one single case, Sammartino reported on the clinical and metabolic symptoms of "propofol infusion syndrome" in a preterm neonate [94].

In the absence of integrated PK-PD models in neonates, we can only speculate on the propofol concentration to aim for in neonates [102]. However, when we take the available pharmacokinetic estimates in early life into account, accumulation may occur even at "routine adult or pediatric" doses in early neonatal life. Although propofol seems to be a promising compound for versatile short-acting analgosedation, dose findings and safety studies are urgently needed. In a recent Cochrane review, Shah et al. concluded that no practice recommendation could be made based on the available evidence regarding the use of propofol in neonates [103]. Further research is therefore needed on the pharmacokinetics of propofol in neonates. Once a relatively safe dose range is identified, randomized controlled and comparative trials assessing the safety and efficacy of propofol are needed.

Take-Home Messages

- There is extensive variability in propofol clearance within the neonatal population, in part explained by both PNA and PMA [95, 102].
- There is conflicting information on the magnitude of hemodynamic (side) effects of propofol in (pre)term neonates [98, 101].
- There is experience with IV bolus propofol administration to facilitate endotracheal intubation, but there is important variability in clinical characteristics, outcome criteria, co-medication, and doses evaluated in the different studies [96–100].
- We do not recommend the use of propofol for sedation in ventilated neonates.

Ketamine

Ketamine is an anesthetic agent that provides amnesia, sedation, and analgesia. It can be administered by intravenous, intramuscular, nasal, rectal, or oral route with a systemic bioavailability of 93 %, 50 %, 25 %, and 17 %, respectively. It has an established role in pediatric anesthesia and is routinely used for induction and maintenance of anesthesia. This is in part due to the fast onset (30–60 s) and short duration of action, with limited hemodynamic and respiratory effects. The analgo-sedative effects are mediated through different mechanisms and contain both peripheral and central side effects. The contribution of *N*-methyl-D-aspartate (NMDA) receptor antagonism and interaction with cholinergic, adrenergic, serotonergic, opioid pathways, and local anesthetic effects remains to be fully elucidated. Hypersalivation is commonly observed during ketamine administration, resulting in the clinical practice to coadminister atropine or another antisialagogue. Ketamine is rarely used as a single anesthetic agent, is more commonly used as part of a multimodal anesthesia strategy, but can also be considered for procedural analgo-sedation [104, 105]. The cardiovascular stability observed with ketamine has made it a popular induction agent in infants with a congenital cardiopathy. In contrast, raised intracranial or intraocular pressure may be contraindications for ketamine analgo-sedation.

Pharmacokinetics

Ketamine is a highly lipid-soluble drug with rapid distribution from the systemic circulation to the brain. Due to these characteristics, systemic absorption of caudally or epidural-injected ketamine is also more likely [106]. It is a racemic (50/50) mixture of two enantiomers, and the S(+) enantiomer is four times more potent compared to the R(−) enantiomer. Ketamine undergoes *N*-demethylation to norketamine. This metabolite has limited analgo-sedative effects (30 % of the parent compound). Plasma protein binding is limited (47 %), and the metabolic clearance strongly relates to the hepatic blood flow with a high extraction ratio. Ketamine displays extensive first-pass drug metabolism, explaining the much higher doses suggested for oral as compared to intravenous administration, while rectal administration results in less predictable exposure. Consequently—when corrected for allometric differences—clearance in children and infants is similar to adults, but reduced (80–26 L/h/70 kg) in neonates [107]. In a randomized, crossover, trial in 16 preterm neonates plasma ketamine concentrations 15 min after intravenous administration (0.5, 1, or 2 mg/kg compared to placebo) were 103 (range 73–134), 189 (144–235), and 379 (320–437) ng/mL, respectively. Unfortunately, norketamine data were not collected, and sampling was limited to the 15 min time point [105]. The earlier discussed PK ketamine data explains that the dosing suggestions for analgo-sedation in neonates (0.5–1 mg/kg) are lower when compared to older children and much higher for oral as compared to intravenous administration (2–5 mg/kg oral).

Pharmacodynamics

The number of observations on effectiveness and safety of ketamine in neonates is limited. In the earlier-mentioned study of Saarenmaa et al., these authors evaluated the ketamine-related pain relief in an endotracheal suctioning model in 16 preterm (31, SD 3 weeks) neonates. The increase in heart rate, arterial blood pressure, and plasma catecholamines in response to endotracheal suctioning was not blunted when different (0.5, 1, and 2 mg/kg) doses of ketamine were compared to the response after placebo [105].

Another dataset relates to the use of ketamine sedation during the treatment of retinopathy of prematurity. In a NICU ward setting, ketamine sedation allowed laser therapy for retinopathy of prematurity in 11 preterm neonates (14 procedures). An empirical initial intravenous dose of 0.5 mg/kg was given, followed by further increments every 2 min if the child became distressed at insertion of the speculum. The median total dose was 2.4 mg/kg, the median duration of the intervention 1.6 h. Atropine was coadministered to minimize the salivation effect and to blunt reflex bradycardia [108]. We would also like to emphasize a single case report of a newborn with epidermolysis bullosa. Oral ketamine was used in this patient to facilitate dressing changes. Over 4 days, the dose was titrated from 0.125 to 0.75 mg/kg and resulted in sufficient sedation within 15 min after administration and dressing changes without crying or resisting for 45 min [108]. We hereby would like to mention that this oral dose is lower compared to the oral dosing suggested. In our opinion, differences in intestinal permeability support the need for dosing individualization [109].

Finally, there is growing concern about ketamine causing dose- and duration-related neuronal apoptosis in animal (mice, rat, rhesus monkey) experimental studies soon after

Table 15.5 Summary of the reported studies on remifentanil to facilitate endotracheal intubation in (pre)term neonates, reflecting the variability in clinical characteristics, outcome criteria, co-medication, and doses (1–4 μ[mu]g/kg, dose highlighted) evaluated

Reference	Study design and results
Norman et al. [110]	Randomized controlled trial in 34 preterm (<37 weeks) neonates for semi-urgent intubation. Atropine/morphine compared to RSI (rapid sequence intubation, based on glycopyrrolate, thiopental, suxamethonium, and remifentanil [1 μ(mu)g/kg]). Primary outcome: intubation score ≤10, secondary outcomes: procedural duration, physiological/biochemical variables, aEEG, and pain scores. Intubation score was superior in the RSI group [5 (IQR 5–6) compared to 12 (IQR 10–13.5)]. Plasma cortisol and pain scores were similar, but fluctuations in physiological variables were more pronounced and prolonged in the morphine group
Choong et al. [111]	Double blind, randomized controlled trial, 30 (pre)term neonates, semi-elective intubation. Remifentanil (3 μ[mu]g/kg) compared to fentanyl (2 μ[mu]g/kg) and succinylcholine (2 mg/kg). Primary outcome: time to successful intubation. Secondary outcomes: physiological variables, adverse events, survey on intubation conditions, and time until return of spontaneous respiration. There were no differences in time to successful intubation (156/247 s). Premedication with remifentanil attenuated physiological responses during intubation comparable to fentanyl and succinylcholine in neonates. Intubation condition were rated more favorably with fentanyl/succinylcholine. Muscular rigidity was observed in the remifentanil group ($n=2/15$)
Welzing et al. [112]	Prospective, descriptive pilot study in 21 preterm (29–31 weeks) neonates receiving remifentanil (2 μ[mu]g/kg, combined with atropine, 10 μ[mu]g/kg) as induction agent for the INSURE (intubation–surfactant–extubation) procedure. Outcome variables were intubation conditions, time until extubation, and complications. Intubation conditions were qualified as excellent or good. Average extubation time after surfactant administration was 16.9 (1–45 min), followed by a mean of 3.3 (1–8) days of respiratory support (CPAP)
Pereira e Silva et al. [113]	Double-blind randomized controlled trial in 20 preterm (28–34 weeks) neonates to evaluate intubation conditions following either morphine (150 μ[mu]g/kg) or remifentanil (1 μ[mu]g/kg), both combined with midazolam (0.2 mg/kg). Overall intubation conditions were better in the remifentanil group
Hume-Smith et al. [114]	Remifentanil dose-seeking study (sequential up-and-down design), including 20 neonates and young infants (0–<4 months, mean weight 5.9 kg). The ED_{50} was 3.1–3.7 μ(mu)g/kg when remifentanil was coadministered with glycopyrrolate (10 μ[mu]g/kg) and propofol (5 mg/kg)

birth. At present, it is unclear to what extent this also applies to human neonates and infants. Moreover, similar animal experimental observations have been reported for other analgo-sedatives (e.g., opioids, benzodiazepines, propofol, inhalational agents) [6–10].

Take-Home Messages

- Ketamine is rarely used as a single anesthetic agent, but is more commonly used as part of a multimodal anesthesia strategy.
- The clinical experience with ketamine in neonates is limited.
- There is growing concern about ketamine causing dose- and duration-related neuronal apoptosis in animal (mice, rat, rhesus monkey) experimental studies soon after birth [6–10].

Remifentanil

Besides morphine and fentanyl, there are also observations on shorter-acting opioids in neonates. Alfentanil, sufentanil, or more recently remifentanil have been used mainly for short procedures such as endotracheal intubation, retinal laser surgery, or percutaneous intravenous central catheter placement, while there is anecdotal experience during major surgery and to maintain analgo-sedation during mechanical ventilation [93]. Remifentanil hydrochloride is a short-acting, μ(mu)-receptor opioid agonist. It achieves its peak analgesic effect within a minute of administration, 3–4 times faster when compared to fentanyl and much faster when compared to morphine.

Table 15.5 provides a summary of the available studies on endotracheal intubation with remifentanil in neonates [110–114]. These studies do reflect the difference between the reported studies on remifentanil to facilitate endotracheal intubation in (pre)term neonates. There is variability in clinical characteristics (preterm or term, INSURE, or continuation of ventilator), outcome criteria (intubation score, duration of the procedure, physiological variables), co-medication, and doses (1–4 μ[mu]g/kg IV slow bolus) evaluated. The total number of neonates exposed to remifentanil in these studies suggests that further investigations on dose seeking and safety are clearly indicated.

Data on a dose–response for remifentanil to facilitate endotracheal intubation have only been published in two studies, with solely a focus on term neonates and young infants. Based on observations in 32 "term neonates," it was documented that the effective remifentanil dose in 50 % and 98 % ($ED_{50}=1.7$, SD 0.1 μ[mu]g/kg, and $ED_{98}=2.88$, SD 0.5 μ[mu]g/kg) were similar between "neonates" (mean weight 8 kg, SD 2.2) and children [115]. However, this remifentanil dose was part of a multimodal anesthesia in combination with propofol (4 mg/kg), and glycopyrrolate (10 μ[mu] g/kg) and the "neonates" were in fact infants (mean age 7 months, SD 3.3). In another dose–response study with sequential up-and-down design, 20 neonates and young infants (0–<4 months, mean weight 5.9 kg), the ED_{50} was significantly higher (3.1–3.7 μ[mu]g/kg) when remifentanil was coadministered with propofol (5 mg/kg) and glycopyrrolate (10 μ[mu]g/kg) [114].

To assess the analgesic and procedural efficacy of low-dose remifentanil infusion during percutaneous central catheter placement in preterm infants, 54 preterm neonates were randomly assigned to remifentanil infusion (0.03 μ[mu]g/kg/min) or placebo in addition to 0.3 mL of 12 % sucrose (oral) combined with nonnutritive sucking. Pain (PIPP = Premature Infant Pain Profile) scores were significantly lower in neonates exposed to remifentanil, suggesting better pain and distress control without significant difference in the time to complete the procedure and the number of attempts [116]. Sammartino et al. reported on their experience with remifentanil (0.75–1 μ[mu]g/kg/min at start, 3–5 μ[mu]g/kg/min during procedure) combined with intravenous midazolam (0.2 mg/kg) for retinal laser therapy in 6 preterm neonates [117]. The same group also reported on two cases of babies born at 26 weeks and 27 weeks gestation, weighing 580 g and 400 g, respectively, undergoing laparotomy for necrotizing enterocolitis [118]. Both received a midazolam bolus and continuous remifentanil infusion at high doses. Finally, this group also reported on their experience with remifentanil for analgo-sedation during mechanical ventilation. In their hands, remifentanil provided adequate analgesia, with a significant reduction of NIPS and COMFORT scores since 1 h after starting the infusion of remifentanil [119]. The drug was initially administered at a dose of 0.075 μ(mu)g/kg/min, but in 73 % of newborns, the latter had to be increased up to a dose of 0.094 (SD 0.03) μ(mu)g/kg/min. Using this dose, 97 % of the newborns were classified as having adequate analgesia and sedation. The time elapsed between the discontinuation of remifentanil infusion and extubation was 36 (SD 12) min, reflecting the short-acting character of this compound [119].

However, in the clinical setting, these short-acting and versatile characteristics need further considerations. A specific advantage of remifentanil is that this compound undergoes metabolic clearance by plasma esterases, resulting in fast and predictable clearance, irrespective of liver or renal function. The analgo-sedative effects disappear very soon after discontinuation of remifentanil since the drug is cleared very rapidly. This is perfect or optimal when used for procedural analgo-sedation without subsequent pain. However, the "short-acting" concept hereby refers to both its onset of action and end of action: remifentanil-related analgo-sedation disappears very soon after discontinuation. This warrants anticipation and its management may be dependent on the indication [120]. When used for major surgery, anticipation and replacement by another (longer) acting opioid or non-opioid analgesic is needed, or the remifentanil infusion should be prolonged. Further continuation will, however, more likely result in potential negative effects such as opioid-induced tolerance or hyperalgesia since these phenomena are much more common when opioids with a short elimination half-life are administered [120].

A recent trial in Europe, the RAPIP trial, examined whether remifentanil induced tolerance, withdrawal, or hyperalgesia in infants. An RCT of intubated infants between 36 and 60 weeks gestational age and PNA, respectively, compared the efficacy and safety of a remifentanil- to fentanyl-based sedation regimen. When administered for less than 96 h, remifentanil did not increase the risk of tolerance, withdrawal, or opioid-induced hyperalgesia [121].

Take-Home Messages

- Remifentanil is a very short-acting compound with still limited reported experience in neonates [93, 120].
- Its pharmacological profile seems suited for short procedural analgo-sedation, e.g., insure procedure (Table 15.5) [110–114].
- Good predictability, fast onset, and fast disappearance are suggested to be advantageous. Clinicians need to be aware of the potential fast-appearing tolerance, the phenomenon of hyperalgesia, and the potential risk of chest rigidity.
- Recent evidence suggests that when administered to ventilated infants for less than 96 h, remifentanil did not increase the risk of tolerance, withdrawal, or opioid-induced hyperalgesia [121].

Chloral Hydrate

Chloral hydrate is still widely used as (short) term sedative and hypnotic, but has no analgesic activity. In early infancy, indications commonly considered are procedural sedation for non-painful or noninvasive examinations (e.g., echocardiography, imaging techniques, hearing evaluation) or aspecific syndromes such as insomnia or non-opioid withdrawal syndrome. Chloral hydrate can be administered by either oral or rectal route. Following oral administration, absorption is rapid with subsequent hepatic metabolism to trichloroacetic acid or trichloroethanol (TCE). TCE subsequently undergoes conjugation and renal elimination. The TCE metabolite also has sedative effects, and because its elimination is delayed—most prominent in early life (elimination half-life is about 10 h in toddlers, but up to >50 h in preterm neonates)—accumulation and subsequent sedation may result from this metabolite [122, 123]. Preterm neonates and/or neonates with impaired renal or hepatic elimination are at an increased risk. Prolonged exposure may also result in gastritis, nausea and/or vomiting, overt overdosing or accumulation may also result in arrhythmia [124]. Finally, there is a concern that chloral hydrate may also have genotoxic effects. To illustrate this, sister chromatid exchange and micronucleus frequencies were determined in lymphocytes of infants before and after chloral hydrate exposure. After treatment, the frequencies of sister chromatid exchange and micronuclei were significantly increased, suggesting that chloral hydrate has moderate genotoxic potential in infants [125]. Because of all these side effects, prolonged repeated administration of chloral hydrate should be avoided. However, this does not mean that single-dose administration is without any risk.

The usual dose is 20–70 mg/kg by oral, nasogastric, or rectal route, with a tendency to go for relatively higher doses for rectal administration. Subsequent sedation can be anticipated within 30–45 min. Sedation may be prolonged, most common in preterm neonates because of the delayed TCE clearance. To further illustrate this, we refer to a study on the pharmacodynamics of chloral hydrate in 26 former preterm infants at term age. Sedation (COMFORT), feeding behavior, and cardiorespiratory events (bradycardic events, apneas) before and after administration of chloral hydrate (oral, 30 mg/kg) were prospectively evaluated in former preterm infants exposed to chloral hydrate to facilitate hearing screening [126]. We hereby were able to document a significant increase in sedation up to 12 h after administration, a minor but significant decrease in oral intake (161–156 mL/kg/day). Moreover, a significant increase in the number of bradycardic events and in the duration of the most severe bradycardic events was observed. Infants who displayed severe bradycardic (<60/min) events ($n=13$) after administration of chloral hydrate had a lower gestational age at birth. Based on the methodology applied, we were unable to discriminate between central or obstructive apnea [126].

Chloral hydrate-related sedation may result in central hypoventilation or apnea. Due to reduction in muscular tone and hypotonia of the upper airway maintaining muscles, obstructive apnea has also been described. In animal experimental setting, there was a significant decrease in electromyographic activity of the mouth floor muscles compared to the diaphragmatic muscle following chloral hydrate exposure [127, 128]. This may result in obstructive apnea, more common in infants or young children with obstructive apnea syndrome, or in neonates with malformations or microretrognathia. Obstructive apnea with secondary bradycardic episodes has been observed in young infants exposed to chloral hydrate to facilitate echocardiography [129]. Case reports on the association of chloral hydrate exposure and unanticipated "cod" death have been described. Since chloral hydrate—in part due to the TCE metabolite—is a long-acting compound, events may occur in the hours following the procedure. Once again, it seems that (pre)term neonates are more vulnerable to display relevant bradycardic events up to 24 h after exposure [126].

There are studies that reported on the efficacy and complications of chloral hydrate sedation, but these studies do not always report on the subgroup of (pre)term neonates in the first month(s) of life. Litman et al. reported on efficacy and complications following chloral hydrate (50–75 mg/kg) exposure to facilitate MRI examination in 1,394 infants [124]. Oxygen desaturation was more likely in hospitalized patients, in patients with a lower weight during drug administration, those who had a higher ASA status, and those who were younger (both related to postnatal as well as PMA). The incidence of desaturation (<90 %) or the need for supplemental oxygen was approximately 20 % in both preterm and term infants. There were 10 episodes of bradycardia in eight infants, six of whom involved preterm neonates. The predicted probability of post-procedural oxygen desaturation in early neonatal life is higher in preterm (0.1) compared to term neonates (0.05), with subsequent less decrease in predicted probability (at the PNA of 100 days = 0.035 as compared to 0.015) [124]. Heistein et al. reported on their experience with chloral hydrate (80 mg/kg, oral) to facilitate pediatric echocardiography, including 58 neonates and 398 young (1–6 months) infants. There was a moderate decrease in heart rate and blood pressure, while adverse events were observed in 10.8 %: apnea ($n=3$), airway obstruction ($n=15$), hypoxia ($n=65$), hypercarbia ($n=40$), hypotension with poor perfusion ($n=4$), vomiting ($n=4$), and prolonged sedation ($n=36$). Adverse events were more common in infants younger than 6 months [129].

The (side) effect profile of chloral hydrate has also been compared with other non-pharmacological and pharmacological techniques. The effect of fasting practice on sedation with chloral hydrate has been evaluated by Keidan et al. by comparing two different practices in two different hospitals for auditory brainstem response in neonates [130]. Fasting was associated with an increased failure rate of initial sedation. As a consequence, a higher total dose of chloral hydrate was required in the fasting group, also resulting in prolonged post-procedural sedation [130]. In contrast, compared to a "feed-and-scan" approach alone, chloral hydrate (50 mg/kg, oral or rectal) resulted in a shorter time until scanning and shorter scanning duration in 25 neonates, but no data on the post-scanning recovery were provided [131]. In essence, it is reasonable to conclude that a combined or stepwise approach (feeding and chloral hydrate or feeding followed by chloral hydrate when needed) seems to be the best approach [132]. Such a "feed-and-wrap" strategy has also been reported in 47 neonates with initial successful imaging in 42/47 cases, resulting in only 5 neonates exposed to chloral hydrate [133]. We hereby re-illustrate the add-on value of complementary interventions to reduce the exposure to analgo-sedatives or to improve the effectiveness of a pharmacological intervention.

Finally, there are some comparative studies. Oral pentobarbital (4 mg/kg) was compared to choral hydrate (50 mg/kg) for sedation in infants (<1 year) during neuroimaging. Based on observations collected in 1,316 infants, there was no difference in effectiveness, in time to sedation, and in time to discharge, but the overall adverse event rate was lower with pentobarbital (0.5 %) than with chloral hydrate (2.7 %) [134]. Unfortunately, data in the subgroup of neonates were not reported. In contrast, chloral hydrate (75 mg/kg) was more effective and had similar side effects when compared to midazolam (0.2 mg/kg intravenous) in a crossover study in seven term neonates [135].

Take-Home Messages

- Single-dose administration of chloral hydrate is a commonly used approach to facilitate non-painful procedural sedation, but focused studies in (pre)term neonates are limited.
- Initial sedation can be anticipated after 15–30 min. There is less certainty about the duration of this sedation, but sedative effects in neonates have been described up to 24 h afterward [122, 123, 126].
- It is reasonable to monitor (pre)term neonates to at least the equivalent of 46 weeks PMA after chloral hydrate exposure [126].
- A genotoxic risk has been linked to chloral hydrate exposure [125].

Morphine and Fentanyl

Morphine is probably the most extensive evaluated analgesic in neonates and can be administered either by oral (bioavailability is about 30 %) or by intravenous route. Morphine is a narcotic analgesic that stimulates opioid receptors, both within as well as outside the central nervous system. This explains effects (sedation, analgesia, miosis) and side effects (bladder retention, paralytic ileus, respiratory depression). It also necessitates appropriate monitoring (cardiorespiratory, sedation) during and following morphine exposure. It has been suggested that pain relief necessitates a morphine level of 120 ng/mL, while adverse effects appear at levels >300 ng/mL [136]. These levels are different in neonates, very likely due to both differences in opioid receptor expression/activity and maturational phenotypic glucuronidation activity. This is because morphine is converted to two glucuronide metabolites (morphine-3-glucuronide and morphine-6-glucuronide), and these metabolites subsequently are eliminated by renal route. While morphine-3-glucuronide is an antagonist to the effects of morphine, morphine-6-glucuronide also has analgesic and respiratory depressant effects. Morphine sulfation is only a very minor metabolic pathway [137].

Despite the fact that this compound has been used for at least three decades, important progress in the maturational pharmacokinetics of morphine in neonates has been made only more recently. The predictability of morphine disposition has been documented in a stepwise approach. Based on pooling of pharmacokinetic observations on morphine disposition, model-based simulations suggested that in preterm neonates, a loading dose (μ[mu]/kg) and a maintenance dose (μ[mu]$^{1.5}$/h), with an additional reduction (−50 %) of this maintenance dose in neonates younger than 10 days does result in a narrow range of morphine and morphine metabolites [138]. These simulations were subsequently validated on its pharmacokinetic predictability in other datasets of morphine observations in neonates [139]. These pharmacokinetic models can subsequently been applied to validate or reject the above suggested pharmacodynamic levels (120 and 300 ng/mL thresholds). Besides maturational weight (kg$^{1.5}$), specific disease characteristics such as systemic hypothermia or the type of surgery may further affect morphine pharmacokinetics [140, 141].

Fentanyl is the first of a sequence of synthetic, fat-soluble opioids (sufentanil, alfentanil). It penetrates faster into the central nervous system because of the fat solubility, resulting in a faster effect as compared to morphine. Fentanyl is a potent μ(mu)-opioid receptor agonist with a 70–125 times higher potency than that of morphine. Fentanyl is metabolized by *N*-dealkylation into non-active metabolites. It is considered to be "short" acting, but it has a prolonged elimination half-life in neonates when compared to older children and necessitates a similar level of monitoring in neonates. Tolerance is anticipated after about 3 days of exposure. Muscular (thoracic) rigidity has been reported occasionally. Short-term analgesia can be achieved with the administration of 5 μ(mu)/kg, but is associated with respiratory depression. Sustained use can be started with the same loading dose, followed by 1–5 μ(mu)/kg/h [93, 142].

Recommendations on the use of opioids in neonates mainly depend on the indications, i.e., postoperative pain relief, procedural pain, or analgo-sedation during mechanical ventilation. The treatment of opioid-related neonatal withdrawal/abstinence syndrome is outside the scope of this chapter.

In the setting of postoperative analgesia following "major" surgery, these compounds are recommended, either as monotherapy or as part of multimodal analgesia. There is even evidence from an RCT supporting the benefits of opioids on neonatal outcome [1]. Continuous infusions following a loading dose is most commonly applied for reasons of uniformity, safety, and simplicity, although similar outcome has been documented when continuous administration of morphine was compared to intermittent administration [143]. It has recently been documented that acetaminophen (paracetamol) does result in a clinically relevant reduction in morphine consumption when integrated in multimodal analgesia [144]. Because of its shorter elimination half-life, continuous administration after a loading dose is even more common practice for fentanyl. This practice—i.e., intermittent bolus versus continuous fentanyl in preterm neonates—has recently been evaluated on its effectiveness in mechanical-ventilated newborns [145].

In contrast, the evidence on the effective use of morphine for procedural analgesia is much more limited. Morphine administration does not blunt the pain scores related to endotracheal suctioning in ventilated newborns [146] and neither improves the pain response during venous blood sampling in neonates when compared to other interventions like oral sucrose [48].

This is at least in part due to the fact that morphine acts in the central nervous system. Consequently, there is a relevant lag time between the administration and the analgo-sedative effects. The same concept should be considered when morphine is administered to facilitate endotracheal intubation. In RCTs, morphine seems to perform worse if compared with remifentanil, fentanyl, or propofol [98, 110, 113]. Based on the clinical pharmacology of opioids, "fast-acting" opioids such as fentanyl or remifentanil (discussed previously) are more appropriate. The same limited evidence holds true for analgo-sedation during mechanical ventilation.

Routine use of morphine cannot be recommended for ventilated (pre)term neonates because no obvious beneficial short-term outcome effects have been documented in meta-analytic exercises [147]. Moreover, recent studies suggest that preemptive morphine in ventilated preterm infants is associated with suboptimal neurodevelopmental outcome variables at the age of 5 and 8 years, respectively, [148, 149]. The same advice can be provided for fentanyl. Based on a recently published study on the use of fentanyl in ventilated preterm neonates, there seems to be no place for the routine continuous fentanyl infusion in ventilated preterm newborns. This is because of the absence of continued pain score reduction and increased side effects of continuous infusion compared with the bolus administration of fentanyl. Moreover, the use of boluses of fentanyl before invasive procedures or on the basis of pain scores has demonstrated the same efficacy and an improved safety profile compared with the continuous infusion of fentanyl [150]. This conclusion can be made based on a recently published multicenter, double-blind, RCT where mechanically ventilated newborns ($\leq 32^{+6}$ weeks gestational age) were randomized to either fentanyl ($n = 64$, continuous infusion of fentanyl plus open-label boluses of fentanyl) or placebo ($n = 67$, continuous infusion of placebo plus open-label boluses of fentanyl). The primary endpoint was analgesic efficacy, as evaluated by the Echelle Douleur Inconfort Nouveau-Né (EDIN) and PIPP scales [145]. Interestingly, the need for open-label boluses of fentanyl was similar, and EDIN scores were comparable between both groups, while the median PIPP score was clinically and statistically higher in the placebo group compared with the fentanyl group on day 1 up to day 3 of treatment. When considering the side effects, mechanical ventilation at age 1 week was still required in 27 of 64 infants in the fentanyl group (42.2 %), compared with 17 of 67 infants in the placebo group (25.4 %) ($P = 0.042$). The first cycle of mechanical ventilation was longer, and the first meconium passage occurred later in the fentanyl group ($P = 0.019$ and 0.027, respectively). Based on the body of evidence collected, fentanyl does reduce acute pain, but does not reduce prolonged pain with an additional cost of an increase in duration of ventilation and paralytic ileus [145].

Take-Home Messages

- Data on the pharmacokinetics of morphine and fentanyl have been reported, resulting in dosing guidelines that result in predictable exposure [138, 139].
- There is strong evidence in support of the use of opioids in postoperative analgesia [1], but side effects include cardiorespiratory depression, bladder and intestinal paralysis, hypotension, and tolerance.
- For procedural pain relief during major interventions (e.g., endotracheal intubation), opioids are effective with a shorter effect time for fat-soluble synthetic opioids [98, 110, 113].
- In contrast, there is no evidence supporting the routine use of opioids in ventilated newborns. It seems that opioids should be solely used to reduce acute pain, but not to reduce prolonged pain because of an increased duration of ventilation and an increase in paralytic ileus. Moreover, follow-up data suggest a link between the extent of opioid exposure and impaired neurological outcome [145, 147].

Benzodiazepines

Benzodiazepines have their pharmacological interaction at the level of the gamma-aminobutyric acid (GABA) receptor in the central nervous system. This interaction results in sedation with associated hypnosis, anxiolysis, muscle relaxation, and anticonvulsant activity, but does not relieve pain. Importantly, it has been documented that the GABA receptor switches from an excitatory to an inhibitory mode during early development, equal to preterm age. This may explain age-related differences in pharmacodynamic side effects, such as agitation or muscular twitching. The most commonly used benzodiazepine is midazolam, with only very limited information on lorazepam or diazepam in neonates [151].

Midazolam's bioavailability is about 35 % when given as oral syrup and 50 % when absorbed directly through either buccal or nasal mucosa. Midazolam undergoes extensivemetabolicclearance,includinghydroxylationto1-OH-midazolam (cytochrome P450 3A), that also has some sedative effects and glucuronidation. Since these processes display maturation, clearance is reduced with an elimination half-life of 12 h in the neonate, compared to 2 h in the adult. Anderson and Larsson [152] recently described a maturational model of midazolam clearance and extrapolated that a steady-state infusion rate of 0.014 mg/kg/h is needed to attain a sedation target concentration similar to findings in adults. However, this dosing suggestion has not been validated while there are only a limited number of observations of midazolam in the neonate. Because major changes in phenotypic cytochrome P450 (CYP) 3A activity can be anticipated in the first few months of life, the maturation of in vivo CYP3A-mediated clearance of midazolam from preterm neonates of 26 weeks gestational age (GA) to adults has more recently been evaluated by Ince et al. [153]. This exercise was based on pooling of pharmacokinetic data after intravenous administration of midazolam from six previously reported studies, including premature neonates. Across the entire lifespan from premature neonates to adults, bodyweight was a significant covariate for midazolam clearance. The effect of bodyweight was best described by use of an allometric equation with an exponent changing with bodyweight in an exponential manner from 0.84 for preterm neonates (0.77 kg) to 0.44 for adults (89 kg). These findings confirm that indeed the most rapid maturation occurs during the youngest age range. Consequently, dosing should be lower in neonates and accumulation is more likely to occur in early life [153].

While midazolam is often used for premedication in children (oral, 0.5 mg/kg), a loading dose approach (intravenous, 0.05–0.1 mg/kg) in preterm neonates commonly results in hypoventilation, hypotension, and reduction in cerebral blood flow. Some units give 0.06 mg/kg/h for sedation in ventilated neonates, with a dose reduction after 24 h to avoid accumulation. However, this approach is now increasingly questioned because there is some anxiety to use benzodiazepines in preterm neonates following the NOPAIN study. The NOPAIN multicenter study aimed to assess the feasibility to test the effect of analgesia or sedation (morphine versus midazolam versus placebo) on mortality and neurological morbidity in a cohort of 67 preterm (24–32 weeks) neonates [154]. This pilot study suggested a statistically significant higher incidence of adverse neurological events with the use of midazolam (death, grade III or IV IVH, PVL). In addition, the most recent Cochrane meta-analysis of data from two studies showed a statistically significant longer duration of NICU stay in the midazolam group compared to the placebo group [154, 155].

Besides monotherapy for sedation during ventilation, there are also reports on the combined administration of midazolam with an opioid (morphine, fentanyl, or remifentanil) to achieve a more balanced analgo-sedation during ventilation. In a double-blind, RCT in mechanically ventilated newborns and young infants (<60 days), a low dose of midazolam (0.05 mg/kg/h) was combined with either remifentanil (3 μ[mu]/kg/h) or fentanyl (1 μ[mu]/kg/h). Both dosing schedules resulted in comparable efficacy, good hemodynamic stability, and comparably low incidence of adverse events. Interestingly, the median extubation time after interruption of the sedation was significantly shorter in the remifentanil when compared to fentanyl—median duration 80 (IQR 15–165) compared to 782 (250–1,875) minutes [156]. In conclusion and based on the currently available evidence, the *routine* use of midazolam to facilitate ventilation in (pre) term neonates cannot be recommended, while midazolam is often used as additional treatment when analgesia is considered insufficient or as a means to decrease exposure to analgesics. Similar to monotherapy, this strategy is associated with hypotension, hypoventilation, and hypoxemia [157].

Besides ventilation, there are also some reports on the use of benzodiazepines to facilitate endotracheal intubation. In a small ($n=20$) randomized study in preterm neonates, the number of attempts and overall intubation conditions was not significantly different when midazolam was compared to propofol [100]. Another randomized, double-blind trial in preterm neonates was stopped after 16 intubations because preterm neonates exposed to midazolam and atropine had more desaturations, and required more frequently cardiopulmonary resuscitation [158].

Midazolam causes hypotension in both preterm and term neonates, decreases cardiac output, and decreases cerebral blood flow velocity in preterm neonates. Consequently, it seems that midazolam use for endotracheal intubation in neonates seems to be limited. To further illustrate this, in a recent survey on the use of premedication for intubation in tertiary neonatal units in the United Kingdom, only a very limited number of units (6 %) used midazolam (median dose 0.1 mg/kg) to facilitate endotracheal intubation. Similarly, the American Academy of Pediatrics does not support the use of midazolam in preterm neonates, while it can be considered for use in term neonates and infants as part of the premedication sequence for elective intubation.

Finally, prolonged and cumulative doses of benzodiazepines have been associated with tolerance, physical dependency, and withdrawal syndrome also in neonates. Similar to approaches in children or adults, the feasibility of sedation and analgesia interruption following cannulation in neonates on extracorporeal membrane oxygenation (ECMO) has been described in a prospective observational study in 20 neonates on ECMO [159].

Take-Home Messages

- Midazolam clearance is much lower in neonates. Consequently, population-specific dosing is required, and accumulation is more likely in neonates [152, 153].
- The use of midazolam quite commonly results in side effects, including hypoventilation, hypotension, and cerebral hypoperfusion. Midazolam has been associated with poorer neurological outcome in former preterm neonates [154, 155, 158].
- Routine use of benzodiazepines for sedation is not indicated in neonates. Prescription needs to be individualized and is most commonly part of a multimodal analgo-sedative strategy [151, 155].

Dexmedetomidine

Ideal analgo-sedation should be rapid in its onset of action, be predictable in its duration and depth of action, not depending on active metabolites (effects or side effects), have rapid dissipation of effects on discontinuation of the agent, be non-addictive (physical dependence or withdrawal on discontinuation), without drug tolerance, nor have adverse effects on cardiopulmonary function [13]. Preferably, this should be combined with a wide therapeutic index, absence of drug interactions and incompatibilities with other drugs, and without influence of underlying comorbidities, like renal or hepatic disease. We are unaware of such an ideal compound for neonates, but dexmedetomidine may become a potential useful asset to attain these objectives in neonates [13].

Dexmedetomidine is a potent lipophilic α(alpha)2-adrenoreceptor agonist with a α(alpha)2/α(alpha)1 activity ratio of 1,620/1. Its mechanism of action is thought to result from activation of G proteins by central postsynaptic α(alpha)2-adrenoreceptors, increasing conductance through potassium ion channels, leading to inhibition of norepinephrine release. Through sympatholysis, dexmedetomidine exerts its sedative, analgesic, opioid-sparing, and anxiolytic properties, as well as its side effects such as hypotension or bradycardia. Of interest are also the cardioprotective properties through blunting stress-response effects after surgery, positive effects on facilitating extubation and (postoperative) delirium, and the claimed neuroprotective effects. Currently, dexmedetomidine is approved for short-term analgo-sedation (<24 h) in mechanically ventilated critical care adult patients and sedation of non-intubated adult patients prior to and/or during surgical and other procedures. Trials are underway to investigate its pharmacokinetics, clinical efficacy, and safety in long-term use, but there is already clinical experience with long-term administration of this drug in the adult ICU [160, 161].

In contrast, clinical experience with dexmedetomidine in the pediatric population is limited and anecdotal in neonates. Dexmedetomidine has many claimed theoretical advantages over standard sedative regimens with regard to adverse drug reactions. Dexmedetomidine does not affect respiratory drive. Neonates treated with dexmedetomidine have a shorter duration of mechanical ventilation compared to fentanyl-treated controls. Dexmedetomidine has minimal impact on gastric motility. Neonates treated with dexmedetomidine require a shorter time to reach full enteral feeds compared to neonates treated with fentanyl. Finally, in vitro and animal experimental studies suggest neuroprotective effects [13, 160, 161]. Unfortunately, dexmedetomidine has the potential for significant adverse drug reactions. The most concerning is hypotension, which is common with bolus doses of dexmedetomidine in both adult and pediatric patients. The incidence and degree of hypotension after bolus dosing appears to be similar to that typical of fentanyl and midazolam. Avoidance of bolus doses or rapid titration of dexmedetomidine attenuates this effect, at least in adults. Because of the pathophysiology of hypotension (related to central α[alpha]2-adrenoreceptor agonism), the subsequent treatment is more difficult and the duration prolonged.

Currently, the experience with dexmedetomidine in the pediatric population is limited and only anecdotal in neonates. The hemodynamics following dexmedetomidine (loading dose 1 μ[mu]g/kg within 10 min, followed by 0.5–0.8 μ[mu]g/kg/h) exposure during anesthesia for abdominal surgery in 16 neonates have recently been reported. As adjacent to sevoflurane anesthesia, hemodynamic stability (heart rate, diastolic and systolic blood pressure) was observed [161]. Shukry et al. reported on the use of dexmedetomidine to facilitate direct laryngoscopy and bronchoscopy in four infants, including one newborn (2 weeks to 11 months) [162]. The total dexmedetomidine dose used was 2–5 μ(mu) g/kg, and one patient (the newborn) needed one additional dose of propofol (3.7 mg/kg). Heart rate and mean arterial blood pressure remained stable throughout the procedure (7–38 min) [162]. Finally, there is a case report in a single newborn co-treated with dexmedetomidine (0.09–0.53 μ[mu] g/kg/h) in combination with midazolam (0.15 mg/kg/h) and fentanyl (0.8 μ[mu]g/kg/h) to facilitate analgo-sedation in a setting of airway compromise related to a congenital mediastinal neuroblastoma. Plasma dexmedetomidine concentrations were 0.25–0.65 ng/mL, and sedation (COMFORT score) was adequate [163].

Further studies to define the incidence and clinical impact of this effect in preterm neonates are necessary. Prospective studies of dexmedetomidine in preterm neonates must include continuous assessment of blood pressure and heart rate as well as utilize available technologies to assess perfusion. As a final warning, we refer to the case report on epileptic seizures related and likely induced by dexmedetomidine in one neonate [164]. This can be explained by the dexmedetomidine-related reduction in the anticonvulsant activity of the locus ceruleus.

Take-Home Messages

- Based on its pharmacokinetics and pharmacodynamics, dexmedetomidine holds the promise to become a useful tool for analgo-sedation in neonates [160–164].
- At present, data are not yet available to formulate any recommendation, except for the fact that this drug should only be used in clinical studies in order to get a valid impression on risk/benefit profile in neonates.

Inhalational Agents

The number of studies and the clinical application of inhalational agents for procedural analgo-sedation in neonates and young infants are—to the best of our knowledge—limited to equimolar nitrous oxide (N_2O)/oxygen mixture (retinopathy of prematurity screening, intramuscular palivizumab administration) and single unit experience with sevoflurane (central catheter placement, endotracheal intubation).

In concordance with the overall impression that equimolar nitrous oxide (N_2O) and oxygen display an age-dependent effectiveness with only limited analgo-sedation in the first year of life compared to children of 4 years or older [165], a recently reported RCT documented that this inhalational strategy does not produce any additional pain relief during eye screening examinations in preterm neonates [166]. The mean PIPP score at speculum insertion in the control group (8.4, 95 % CI 7.6–9.3) was comparable with the nitrous oxide-exposed group (8.5, 95 % CI 7.3–9.8). There were no significant differences in oxygen saturation or heart rate between both groups. Inhalation was tolerated without any measured side effects [166]. Using an at-random study design, infants receiving palivizumab administration received either nitrous oxide (50/50 mixture), EMLA application, or both. Pain assessment was based on the Modified Behavior Pain Scale (MBPS). Although there was a significant lower MBPS during nitrous oxide administration—most pronounced when combined with EMLA—the mean overall MBPS rating during immunization and recovery period were still 8 and 7, respectively [167]. These mean values are similar to those reported in another cohort of former preterm neonates during palivizumab immunization in which MBPS was assessed without any specific intervention [168].

The Montpellier unit reported the use of sevoflurane for procedural analgo-sedation in neonates [169–171]. Using a stepwise increase until loss of consciousness and motor response in 33 consecutive cases to facilitate central venous catheter placement, heart rate remained stable, but mean arterial blood pressure dropped, and none of the patients required intubation [169]. The ease of the procedure was scored as "average" 13 times and "excellent" 20 times [169]. This report followed an earlier reported RCT in 55 neonates, aimed at comparing efficacy and safety of sevoflurane with glucose and nonnutritive sucking (GNNS) analgo-sedation in reducing the duration of the procedure and in preventing pain-related effects during peripherally inserted central catheter (PICC) placement [170]. Sevoflurane exposure resulted in greater immobility, fewer episodes of hypertension, tachycardia, or bradycardia. Occurrences of hypotension were not different, while the glucose group showed more desaturation during the 4 h after the intervention. Finally, the same group reported on the use of sevoflurane for endotracheal intubation [171]. Thirty-three neonates were randomized to either sevoflurane (inspired concentrations 2–5 %) or no medication (preoxygenation with 100 % oxygen) before endotracheal intubation. No major differences in the incidence of adverse events were noted in the study group compared with the control group—hypotension (37.5–37.5 %), desaturations (37.5–44.5 %)—while hypertension (25–56.3 %) and bradycardic events (8.3–44.4 %) were more frequently observed in the control group. Moreover, intubation was easier in the sevoflurane group, with specific emphasis on the absence of movements (95.5–28 %), optimal glottis visualization (73–33 %), and failure rate (25–39 %). Because of the use of a "placebo-controlled" study design, it is not really possible to compare these outcome data with more commonly applied pharmacological strategies to facilitate endotracheal intubation.

Before we consider the use of inhalational agents for analgo-sedation in neonates, we should be aware of the maturational pharmacodynamic differences and of the logistics involved. To illustrate the age-dependent pharmacodynamics, we refer to the available data on halothane. Lerman et al. found that the minimum alveolar concentration (MAC) of halothane in neonates (0.87 %) was significantly lower than that in infants (1.20 %), while the MAC in infants were significantly higher when compared to older children [172]. With induction of anesthesia, the systolic blood pressure decreased 23 % in neonates and 34 % in infants. Similarly, the heart rate decreased 12 % in neonates and 22 % in infants, and hypotension was not significantly different (33–44 %). The authors concluded that the MAC of halothane for neonates is 25 % less as compared to infants and significantly less than was thought previously without any difference in the incidence of cardiovascular side effects. Secondly, the logistics needed mainly relate to the avoidance of air pollution, commonly in part achieved by the use of closed loop circuits. Consequently, this means that specific ventilation equipment is needed.

Take-Home Messages

- There are limited data on the use of inhalational agents in neonates.
- Because the logistics needed, its use will very likely remain limited.

Acetaminophen (Paracetamol)

Paracetamol, *N*-acetyl-*p*-aminophenol (acetaminophen), is a readily available antipyretic and analgesic agent. It is the most often prescribed drug for treatment of mild to moderate pain or fever in infants, including neonates, and can be administered by oral, rectal, but also by intravenous route [173]. Its peak concentration occurs approximately 60 min after oral dosing, while absorption after rectal administration is variable and prolonged. Acetaminophen is widely used in the management of pain, but has no antiinflammatory effects. In the therapeutic concentration range, acetaminophen is metabolized by the liver to acetaminophen glucuronide (47–62 %) and acetaminophen sulfate (25–36 %) as main metabolites, and subsequently eliminated by renal route. Only 1–4 % is excreted unchanged in urine, and about 8–10 % of acetaminophen is oxidized to 3-hydroxy-acetaminophen and the (hepatic) toxic metabolite *N*-acetyl-*p*-benzoquinone imine (NAPQI) [173]. Data on the clinical pharmacology of acetaminophen, including pharmacokinetics and tolerance (hepatic, hemodynamics) in neonates following either enteral or intravenous route, have been published. Clearance mainly relates to weight, age, and—to a limited extent—hyperbilirubinemia [174, 175]. Hepatic tolerance and hemodynamic tolerance have been documented during repeated administration [173]. Consequently, acetaminophen is perceived to have a good efficacy-to-safety ratio as analgesic in a wide range of patient populations. However, since acetaminophen is one of the most commonly used drugs to treat pain or fever, knowledge on the covariates of acetaminophen disposition remains crucial to avoid toxicity through unanticipated variability. In addition to oral and rectal formulations, several intravenous (IV) formulations became available more recently. Such a formulation enables the administration of acetaminophen when the enteral route cannot (yet) be used and should improve the predictability by the reduction in variability related to absorption [173–175].

Intermittent (p.r.n.) administration in response to perceived pain seldom provides optimal pain relief, while anticipatory use (preemptive) certainly helps to prevent postoperative pain. Visceral pain, however, commonly needs opioids. Compared to opioids, tolerance does not develop during repeated administration, but there is an analgesic ceiling effect. Based on these facts, the concept of multimodal analgesia has been introduced in the neonatal intensive care. However, it is only very recently that Ceelie et al. indeed documented a clinical significant (−66 %) morphine-sparing effect in neonates co-treated with IV acetaminophen compared to placebo following major, noncardiac surgery [144].

The data on acetaminophen analgesia during painful procedures are limited, but suggest an overall poor analgesic effect for procedural pain relief. Using a randomized, placebo-controlled study design in 75 term neonates, Shah et al. documented that acetaminophen administration (20 mg/kg, oral) was ineffective for pain relief related to heel prick [176]. Acetaminophen (15 mg/kg, oral) was neither found to ameliorate neither intraoperative nor the immediate postoperative pain of circumcision, although it seems that it may provide some benefit after the immediate postoperative period [177]. The effects of acetaminophen (20 mg/kg, rectal) on neonates following vacuum extraction has been documented by Van Lingen et al. [178]. Based on a randomized, placebo-controlled study design in 122 neonates delivered by vacuum extraction, one dose of acetaminophen significantly improved their clinical condition (e.g., drinking behavior), but did not result in a significant change in objective pain scores, and there were no positive effects following repeated administration. Very recently and using an preemptive approach and a placebo-controlled study design in 123 term neonates following assisted vaginal delivery, infants born by assisted vaginal delivery had low pain scores in the immediate period after birth, irrespective of acetaminophen exposure. However, acetaminophen (20–25 mg/kg, rectal) given to term newborns shortly after birth was associated with an aggravated subsequent stress response during heel lancing on day 2–3 of postnatal life [179].

The overall limited effects in neonates are somewhat in contrast to the documented analgesic effects of acetaminophen in infants and children, but may be attributed to inadequate serum concentrations due to, for example, low dose, delayed absorption, or variability in bioavailability. The fact that it has recently been described that the effect compartment concentration of 10 mg/L of acetaminophen, achieved following a loading dose administration (20 mg/kg, intravenous) in neonates, is effective for moderate pain relief further provides evidence that the absence of effects likely at least in part relates to insufficient dosing [180].

The hepatic tolerance during repeated administration has been mentioned earlier. However, there are case reports on hepatic failure following acetaminophen exposure in neonates. Unfortunately, most of these cases can be explained by the well-known tenfold overdosing error (intravenous formulation = 10 mg/mL). Other population-specific pharmacodynamic aspects that need to be mentioned are the recently described association between acetaminophen exposure and patent ductus closure and atopy in infancy, respectively. Reports of an association between acetaminophen exposure and patent ductus arteriosus closure in a limited number of extreme preterm neonates have been published. However, causality cannot yet be taken for granted because a link between the current knowledge of the clinical pharmacology of acetaminophen and (patho)physiology of ductal closure is not known. In contrast to nonselective cyclooxygenase inhibitors, acetaminophen has limited effects at peripheral sites, is a poor antithrombotic and antiinflammatory drug, and exerts its effects primarily within the central nervous system [181]. In early infancy, epidemiological data also suggest a link between acetaminophen exposure in early infancy and the risk to develop asthma similar to the link between maternal exposure and atopy in early infancy [182].

Take-Home Messages

- Data on acetaminophen pharmacokinetics/dynamics have been published and suggest that the same effect compartment concentration (10 mg/L) of acetaminophen should be aimed for in neonates [174, 175, 180].
- This means that a loading dose should be considered (intravenous or oral 20 mg/kg, rectal 30–40 mg/kg), followed by maintenance (intravenous or oral 10 mg/kg, rectal 1–18 mg/kg) doses—in term neonates q6h, in preterm (<32 weeks) neonates q8h [175].
- Data on safety suggest that acetaminophen has indeed a good safety profile in neonates when administered for a limited time (48–72 h).
- It has recently been published that—similar to children and adults—(IV) acetaminophen has indeed opioid-sparing (−66 %) effects in neonates after major noncardiac surgery [144].
- Acetaminophen is a very poor analgesic for procedural pain relief [176, 177].

Neonatal Analgo-Sedation: Balancing Between Scylla and Charybdis

Non-pharmacological as well as pharmacological treatment of pain became an indicator of quality of care in neonates following the pivotal publications by Anand et al. in the late 1980s, demonstrating the ability of newborn infants to feel pain [1]. It hereby was documented that ineffective treatment of pain in these vulnerable individuals was not only inhumane [15, 16], but likewise also resulted in negative health outcomes [2, 12]. In essence, these observations strongly suggest that early pain experience contributes to neurodevelopmental outcome, pain thresholds, pain- or stress-related behavior, and physiological responses in later life. Effective management of pain therefore remains an important indicator of the quality of care provided to neonates, not only from an ethical, but also from a short- and long-term outcome perspective [2, 12, 15, 16]. However, further adaptations and patient tailoring are needed because of both newly emerging data on neuroapoptosis associated with exposure to analgo-sedatives as well as simultaneous changes in neonatal care itself [7–10, 13].

The ontogeny of the nervous system is based on a complex pattern of cell proliferation, migration, differentiation, and selective cell survival and includes apoptosis. Functional development relates to a balance of excitatory and inhibitory signals. Due to maturational plasticity of the nociceptive systems throughout infancy, nociceptive input may cause population-specific lasting alterations in pain processing. Similarly, exposure of nociceptive and non-nociceptive nervous circuits to analgo-sedatives also modulates receptor signaling-related brain development. Experimental data from animals provide evidence that chronic morphine exposure in perinatal life results in reduced brain volume, decreased neuronal packing density, and less dendritic growth and branching. This is associated with learning and motor disabilities. In contrast, opioid receptor blockade through naloxone results in increased brain size and more pronounced dendritic arborisation. Similar animal experimental data have been reported for other analgo-sedatives, including benzodiazepines, ketamine, inhalational anesthetics, propofol, and barbiturates or combinations of such analgo-sedatives [7–10]. Alterations are in part drug- and dose-dependent, and there is an age-related window of vulnerability for apoptosis on the one hand or dendritic changes on the other hand. The extrapolation of these observations in animals to the human (pre)term newborn is obviously hampered by several limitations. Some authors report on an association between major neonatal surgery (number of interventions, disease severity) and neurodevelopmental impairment. However, exposure to analgo-sedatives is only one of the factors associated with this negative outcome [10].

The shifts in neonatal care refers toward less invasive care, as reflected by introduction of minimal enteral feeding to shorten duration of parenteral nutrition, while duration of endotracheal ventilation was shortened through early nasal CPAP or the "INSURE" approach [13].

First, adequate pain management is not an isolated activity. It should be an integrated part of developmental care. Behavior in former preterm infants was associated with the level of both developmental care ("Infant-Centered Care index" [ICC]—parents' involvement in the care of their infant and developmental-oriented care interventions) and pain management ("Infant Pain Management index" [IPM]—approach to and procedures used for reducing infant pain). A higher ICC was associated with higher scores for attention and regulation, less excitability, and low stress scores, while higher IPM scores were associated with higher attention, higher arousal, and lower lethargy. The association between both suggests that the combination of both practices (ICC and IPM) support better neurobehavioral stability [183]. In our opinion, non-pharmacological methods for analgesia in collaboration with different caregivers, including the parents, are the link between pharmacological analgesia and developmental-oriented care interventions.

Second, the introduction of analgo-sedatives and techniques also resulted in new clinical syndromes such as opioid-induced tolerance, neonatal drug withdrawal syndrome, and hyperalgesia or complications such as drug-related toxicities or toxicity due to locoregional techniques. Tenfold dosing errors with intravenous acetaminophen and propofol infusion syndrome were reported, and a case of hyperalgesia following opioid exposure in a newborn has

Table 15.6 Dosing suggestions for different analgo-sedatives as extracted from the Neofax

Topical/local anesthetics	*No dosing advice available*
Propofol	*No dosing advice available*
Ketamine	*No dosing advice available*
Remifentanil	*No dosing advice available*
Chloral hydrate	25–75 mg/kg per dose, orally or rectally
Morphine	*Intermittent*: 0.05–0.2 mg/kg per dose, IV/IM/SQ, q4h
	Continuous: loading 0.1–0.15 mg/kg over 1 h, followed by 0.01–0.02 mg/kg per hour
Fentanyl	*Intermittent*: 0.5–4 mcg/kg, iv slow push, as required (q2h–q4h)
	Continuous: 1–5 mcg/kg per hour
Midazolam	*Intermittent*: 0.05–0.15 mg/kg over at least 5 min, (q2h–q4h)
	Continuous: 0.01–0.06 mg/kg, per hour
Dexmedetomidine	*No dosing advice available*
Acetaminophen	*No dosing advice on intravenous administration available*
	Oral: loading dose 20–25 mg/kg, maintenance 12–15 mg/kg/dose
	Rectal: loading dose 30 mg/kg, maintenance 12–18 mg/kg/dose
	Maintenance intervals: q6h (term), q8h (32–36), q12h (<32 weeks)

This in part also reflects the overall limited information on dosing in neonates [183]

Table 15.7 A subjective opinion: how to improve pain management in neonates

Prevention

- Any effective pain relief program should be integrated in a more extensive program with focus on reduction of environmental stress and facilitation of neuromotor development. Parental involvement is hereby crucial
- Reduce the frequency of avoidable painful procedures
- Use the most appropriate technique to avoid stress or pain, as has been illustrated for blood sampling, endotracheal suctioning, or retinal surgery

Assessment

- Systematic evaluation of pain based on a validated pain scale is crucial. Delegate not only the responsibility to assess but also to act: delegate the treatment of pain and the titration of pharmacological treatment within predefined ranges to the bedside caregiver
- Systematic assessment of pain instead of ad hoc registration results in an increased awareness to treat and prevent pain

Treatment

- Introduce unit-specific recommendations for individual procedures, interventions, or clinical diagnoses based on validated non-pharmacological and pharmacological interventions. Such protocols should also consider weaning strategies, and assessment and treatment of withdrawal syndromes
- Titrated administration of analgesics in order to protect long-term neurological outcome should not only focus on a step-up, but also on a step-down strategy
- *You better know what you prescribe*: limit your pharmacological tools to some compounds and know their effects and side effects instead of introducing too many different compounds

been published. Caregivers should be aware of contemporary management of the aforementioned complications.

In the clinical setting, a structured approach is needed [37–39]. There is no doubt that all NICUs need to adapt a validated pain assessment tool and an algorithm outlining the responses of health-care providers if abnormal pain scores are detected. Reaching consensus within the NICU care team on the interpretation of an abnormal pain score and developing an algorithm of care for each pain scenario are crucially important. The same algorithm should also provide pathways for infants who do not respond to the treatment or develop adverse events. Although there is emerging information that there is a difference between pain expression and nociception, this structured approach should start with the routine use of a validated pain assessment score for a given age group and should be followed by a condition-specific pain management protocol with a limited number of compounds (tool box) of which caregivers are aware of (side) effects. Dosing guidelines as retrieved in the Neofax have been summarized in Table 15.6 [184]. This table hereby also reflects the relevant knowledge gaps on the clinical pharmacology in neonates, including the field on analgo-sedation.

These pain management protocols should also focus on the titration of analgesics, including a decision tree on when and how to increase and decrease exposure to analgesics. Until more advanced tools to assess pain become available, we can apply a validated pain assessment tool in clinical practice and train the NICU health-care providers in using these tools in a standardized way to guarantee an acceptable interobserver variation in assessing neonatal pain [37–39, 41].

A promising approach to facilitate more effective implementation of better practices to improve pain management of neonates has been described by Dunbar et al. [41]. Twelve NICUs in the Neonatal Intensive Care Quality Improvement Collaborative focused on improving neonatal pain management and sedation practices. Collaborative quality improvement techniques were used to facilitate local quality improvement in the management of pain in infants. In essence, these units developed and subsequently implemented evidence-based better practices for pain management and sedation in neonates. The group introduced changes through plan-do-study-act cycles and tracked performance measures throughout the process. Strategies for implementing potentially better practices varied between NICUs on the basis of local characteristics. Individual units identified their barriers to implementation, developed tools for improvement, and subsequently shared their experience with the collaborative. Using this approach of collaborative quality improvement techniques enhanced local quality improvement efforts and resulted in effective implementation of potentially better practices at participating NICUs [41]. Our intersubjective opinion on how to improve pain management in neonates has been summarized in Table 15.7.

Finally and obviously, further studies are needed. We suggest that this research agenda covers (1) the development and validation of more sophisticated pain assessment tools integrating neurobiological evaluation, (2) the collection of long-term outcome data after neonatal exposure to analgo-sedatives (pharmacovigilance), and (3) the use of an appropriate study design for neonatal pain studies. Besides more effective tools to assess pain, we encourage clinicians, but also ethical committees and other stakeholders involved, to design dose-finding studies needed to improve adequate (i.e., effective, neither overexposure nor underexposure) administration of analgo-sedatives in neonates. The experimental observations in animals concerning neuro-apoptosis force us to reconsider the modalities used, including both the drugs as well as the doses administered.

Case Studies

Case 1

The mother of a 2-month-old infant worries about immunization-related pain. She mentioned that the older sister of this infant is afraid of any medical intervention, while the mother herself has needle phobia, even resulting in avoidance of medical care when needed. In fact, the mother asks you to write a certificate that her infant does not tolerate any vaccination and consequently should not receive any vaccination. During the discussion, the mother wants to know if there is existing evidence for effective interventions to alleviate immunization-related pain in young infants.

Issues

Procedural analgesia: There is meta-analytical evidence on the effectiveness and tolerability of different pharmacological, physical, procedural technique-related, psychological interventions, and combination of these individual interventions to alleviate immunization-related pain. Pharmacological interventions relate to topical local anesthetics, sweet-tasting (sucrose 30 %, glucose 24 %) solutions, and combined analgesic interventions, including breastfeeding, were associated with reduced pain during childhood immunizations and should be recommended for use in clinical practice. Physical interventions: pain during immunization can be decreased by injecting the least painful formulation of a vaccine, having the child sit up or holding an infant, stroking the skin or applying pressure close to the injection site before and during injection. Other effective interventions relate to injecting the least painful vaccine first when two vaccines are being administered sequentially during a single office visit and performing a rapid intramuscular injection without aspiration. Psychological interventions related to parental breathing exercises, child-directed distraction, nurse-led distraction, and combined cognitive–behavioral interventions to reduce the pain and distress associated with routine childhood immunizations. Parents and health-care professionals should be advised to incorporate these psychological interventions to reduce the pain and distress experienced by children during immunization. Using a robust testing process, the HELPinKIDS program developed a parent-directed educational pamphlet and video about management of vaccination pain based on these aforementioned approaches. (Further reading: www.sickkids.ca/Learning/Stories/Knowledge-Translation/anna-taddio.html)

Relevance of postvaccination treatment of fever/pain: the administration of acetaminophen before immunization does not reduce the procedural-related pain. While prophylactic acetaminophen administration has been associated with a modest reduction in fuzziness or fever in the hours after immunization, this has also been linked with a reduction in the immunological response (antibodies). Consequently, systematic prophylactic administration of acetaminophen seems obsolete.

Case 2

Neonatal respiratory care has shifted from prolonged mechanical ventilation following endotracheal intubation toward nasal respiratory support through either nasal CPAP or high-flow nasal cannula. However, there is overwhelming evidence in support of early curative or even perhaps prophylactic endotracheal administration of surfactant in extreme low-birth-weight infants. This presents clinicians with a dilemma: endotracheal intubation warrants effective analgo-sedation in order to avoid mechanical trauma and pain, while prolonged analgo-sedation will result in failure to extubate shortly following surfactant administration. There is a growing body of evidence in support of such an "InSurE" (Intubate, Surfactant, Extubate) [184] approach. Still, clinicians struggle with the difficult balance between avoiding mechanical ventilation versus preventing pain or stress in preterm neonates.

Potential Options to Consider

Non-pharmacological interventions: Some groups consider to adapt the applied technique. Besides experimental research related to aerosol and inhalational disposition, this mainly translates into a less invasive technique by using a nasogastric tube to access the

(continued)

trachea instead of the commonly used endotracheal tubes. There is preliminary evidence (e.g., Kanmaz et al. [185]) showing the feasibility of early administration of surfactant via a thin catheter during spontaneous breathing (Take Care). This strategy further reduces the need for mechanical ventilation as compared to the InSurE [96] approach, but still needs prospective confirmatory studies.

Pharmacological interventions: Successful analgo-sedation for an InSurE approach not only relates to effective analgo-sedation during endotracheal intubation, but also relates to effective extubation shortly afterward. As a consequence, the usual combination strategies (e.g., morphine/atropine/suxamethonium) fail to a large extent because it does take time until morphine is sufficiently effective, and it does take time until morphine is sufficiently diffused out of the central nervous system. Alternative strategies based on remifentanil or propofol are much more suited to facilitate effective analgo-sedation for the InSurE approach. In the absence of randomized controlled evidence, we can only suggest the following doses to consider (remifentanil = 1–5 μ[mu]g/kg; propofol 1–3 mg/kg).

Case 3

Circumcision in the newborn is still in high demand in many countries across the globe including the United States. With the rapidly emerging information about the potential risks of exposure to inhalational or systemic anesthetic medications, especially the increased risk of neuro-apoptosis, there is more and more resistance in the medical community to perform circumcision under general anesthesia or even under conscious sedation with, for instance, the use of propofol. This clearly presents clinicians with a dilemma when parents want their (pre)term neonate to be circumcised. So, what are the potential options to consider if indeed parents want their newborn infant to be circumcised during their stay in the NICU?

Scenario: Parents of a clinically stable preterm neonate (gestational age, 24 weeks; PNA, 4 weeks; current weight 650 g) want their newborn infant to be circumcised and are very persistent in this request.

Potential Options to Consider

1. Try to convince the parents that circumcision in such a small male infant is not only technically challenging taking into consideration the size of the penis of an infant with a total weight of 650 g, but even more that adequate prevention of pain during and after the procedure might worsen the long-term outcome of their infant. Your advice is to postpone the circumcision to a later stage in infancy.
2. Perform the circumcision after explaining the parents all the aforementioned risks under local anesthesia. Use a penile block (technically very challenging in this size patient) or cream containing lidocaine–prilocaine. With the latter option, it is prudent to check methemoglobin concentrations in the infant because of the developmentally low expression of methemoglobin reductase. In a relatively small group of preterm infants with a gestational age of less than 32 weeks, no major issues have been detected. Therefore, based on the fact that this infant is already 4 weeks old, the risk is relatively low.
3. Perform the circumcision after explaining to the parents all the aforementioned risks under general anesthesia. In general, most institutions will require that the infant be a minimum of 60 weeks post-conceptual age (PCA) in order to undergo an anesthetic for this elective procedure [186].

References

1. Anand KJ, Hickey PR. Pain and its effects in the human neonate and fetus. N Engl J Med. 1987;317:1321–9.
2. Walker SM, Franck LS, Fitzgerald M, et al. Long-term impact of neonatal intensive care and surgery on somatosensory perception in children born extremely preterm. Pain. 2009;141:79–87.
3. Morton NS. The pain-free ward: myth or reality. Paediatr Anaesth. 2012;22:527–9.
4. Johnston CC, Fernandes AM, Campbell-Yeo M. Pain in neonates is different. Pain. 2011;152:S65–73.
5. Allegaert K, Tibboel D, van den Anker J. Pharmacological treatment of neonatal pain: in search of a new equipoise. Semin Fetal Neonatal Med. 2013;18:42–7.
6. Durrmeyer X, Vutskits L, Anand KJ, et al. Use of analgesic and sedative drugs in the NICU: integrating clinical trials and laboratory data. Pediatr Res. 2010;67:117–27.
7. Davidson AJ. Anesthesia and neurotoxicity to the developing brain: the clinical relevance. Paediatr Anaesth. 2011;21:716–21.
8. Davidson A, Flick RP. Neurodevelopmental implications of the use of sedation and analgesia in neonates. Clin Perinatol. 2013;40:559–73.
9. Nemergut ME, Aganga D, Flick RP. Anesthetic neurotoxicity: what to tell the parents? Paediatr Anaesth. 2014;24(1):120–6. doi:10.1111/pan.1235.
10. Marlow N. Anesthesia and long-term outcomes after neonatal intensive care unit. Paediatr Anaesth. 2014;24(1):60–7. doi:10.1111/pan.12304.
11. Hohmeister J, Kroll A, Wollgarten-Hadamek I, et al. Cerebral processing of pain in school-aged children with neonatal nociceptive input: an exploratory fMRI study. Pain. 2010;150:257–67.
12. Walker SM. Neonatal pain. Paediatr Anaesth. 2014;24(1):39–48. doi:10.1111/pan.12293.

13. Thewissen L, Allegaert K. Analgosedation in neonates: do we still need additional tools after 30 years of clinical research? Arch Dis Child Educ Pract Ed. 2011;96:112–8.
14. Lago P, Garetti E, Boccuzzo G, et al. Procedural pain in neonates: the state of the art in the implementation of national guidelines in Italy. Paediatr Anaesth. 2013;23:407–14.
15. Bellieni C, Buonocore G. Improve the struggle against babies' pain. Lancet. 2011;377:1315–6.
16. Guimaraes H, Sanchez-Luna M, Bellieni CV, et al. Ethical charter of Union of European Neonatal and Perinatal Societies. J Matern Fetal Neonatal Med. 2011;24:855–8.
17. Carbajal R, Rousset A, Danan C, et al. Epidemiology and treatment of painful procedures in neonates in intensive care units. JAMA. 2008;300:60–70.
18. Simons SH, van Dijk M, Anand KS, et al. Do we still hurt newborn babies? A prospective study of procedural pain and analgesia in neonates. Arch Pediatr Adolesc Med. 2003;157:1058–64.
19. Lago P, Boccuzzo G, Garetti E, et al. Pain management during invasive procedures at Italian NICUs: has anything changed in the last five years? J Matern Fetal Neonatal Med. 2013;26:303–5.
20. Allegaert K, Langhendries JP, van den Anker JN. Educational paper: do we need neonatal clinical pharmacologists? Eur J Pediatr. 2013;172:429–35.
21. Van Dijk M, Tibboel D. Update on pain assessment in sick neonates and infants. Pediatr Clin North Am. 2012;59:1167–81.
22. Stevens B, Johnston C, Taddio A, et al. The premature infant pain profile: evaluation 13 years after development. Clin J Pain. 2010;26:813–30.
23. Carbajal R, Paupe A, Hoenn E, et al. APN: evaluation behavioral scale of acute pain in newborn infants. Arch Pediatr. 1997;4:623–8.
24. Taddio A, Hogan ME, Moyer P, et al. Evaluation of the reliability, validity and practicality of 3 measures of acute pain in infants undergoing immunization injections. Vaccine. 2011;29:1390–4.
25. Van Dijk M, Peters JW, van Deventer P, et al. The COMFORT behavior scale: a tool for assessing pain and sedation in infants. Am J Nurs. 2005;105:33–6.
26. Van Dijk M, Roofthooft DW, Anand KJ, et al. Taking up the challenge of measuring prolonged pain in (premature) neonates: the COMFORT neo scale seems promising. Clin J Pain. 2009; 25:607–16.
27. Krechel SW, Bildner J. CRIES: a new neonatal postoperative pain measurement score. Initial testing of validity and reliability. Paediatr Anaesth. 1995;5:53–61.
28. Manworren RC, Hynan LS. Clinical validation of FLACC: preverbal patient pain scale. Pediatr Nurs. 2003;29:140–6.
29. Hummel P, Lawlor-Klean P, Weiss MG. Validity and reliability of the N-PASS assessment tool with acute pain. J Perinatol. 2010; 30:474–8.
30. Spasojevic S, Bregun-Doronjski A. A simultaneous comparison of four neonatal pain scales in clinical settings. J Matern Fetal Neonatal Med. 2011;24:590–4.
31. Slater R, Cantarella A, Franck L, et al. How well do clinical pain assessment tools reflect pain in infants? PLoS Med. 2008;24:e129.
32. Slater R, Cornelissen L, Fabrizi L, et al. Oral sucrose as an analgesic drug for procedural pain in newborn infants: a randomised controlled trial. Lancet. 2010;376:1225–32.
33. Hartley C, Slater R. Neurophysiological measures of nociceptive brain activity in the newborn infant—the next steps. Acta Paediatr. 2014;103(3):238–42. doi:10.1111/apa.12490.
34. Hyttel-Sorensen S, Austin T, van Bel F, et al. Clinical use of cerebral oximetry in extremely preterm infants is feasible. Dan Med J. 2013;60:A4533.
35. Munsters J, Wallström L, Agren J, et al. Skin conductance measurements as pain assessment in newborn infants born at 22–27 weeks gestational age at different postnatal age. Early Hum Dev. 2012;88:21–6.
36. Valkenburg AJ, Niehof SP, van Dijk M, et al. Skin conductance peaks could result from changes in vital parameters unrelated to pain. Pediatr Res. 2012;71:375–9.
37. Ista E, van Dijk M, van Achterberg T. Do implementation strategies increase adherence to pain assessment in hospitals? A systematic review. Int J Nurs Stud. 2013;50:552–68.
38. Foster J, Spence K, Henderson-Smart D, et al. Procedural pain in neonates in Australian hospitals: a survey update of practices. J Paediatr Child Health. 2013;49:E35–9.
39. Ceelie I, de Wildt SN, de Jong M, et al. Protocolized post-operative pain management in infants: do we stick to it? Eur J Pain. 2012;16:760–6.
40. Cordero L, Sananes M, Leona W. Mechanically ventilated VLBW infants: a comparison of two airway suctioning frequencies. Pediatr Res. 2001;49:273A.
41. Dunbar AE, Sharek PJ, Mickas NA, et al. Implementation and case-study results of potentially better practices to improve pain management of neonates. Pediatrics. 2006;118 Suppl 2: S87–94.
42. Cone S, Pickler RH, Grap MJ, McGrath J, Wiley PM. Endotracheal suctioning in preterm infants using four-handed versus routine care. J Obstet Gynecol Neonatal Nurs. 2013;42:92–104.
43. Taylor JE, Hawley G, Flenady V, Woodgate PG. Tracheal suctioning without disconnection in intubated ventilated neonates. Cochrane Database Syst Rev. 2011:CD003065.
44. Gillies D, Spence K. Deep versus shallow suction of endotracheal tubes in ventilated neonates and young infants. Cochrane Database Syst Rev. 2011:CD003309.
45. Larsson BA, Tannfeldt G, Lagercrantz H, Olsson GL. Venipuncture is more effective and less painful than heel lancing for blood tests in neonates. Pediatrics. 1998;101:882–6.
46. Ogawa S, Ogihara T, Fujiwara E, et al. Venepuncture is preferable to heel lance for blood sampling in term neonates. Arch Dis Child Fetal Neonatal Ed. 2005;90:F432–6.
47. Bellieni CV, Tei M, Coccina F, et al. Sensorial saturation for infants' pain. J Matern Fetal Neonatal Med. 2012;25 Suppl 1:79–81.
48. Cignacco E, Hamers JP, Stoffel L, et al. The efficacy of non-pharmacological interventions in the management of procedural pain in preterm and term neonates. A systematic literature review. Eur J Pain. 2007;11:139–52.
49. Karp H. The fourth trimester and the calming reflex: novel ideas for nurturing young infants. Midwifery Today Int Midwife. 2012; 102:25–6.
50. Pinelli J, Symington A, Ciliska D. Nonnutritive sucking in high-risk infants: benign intervention or legitimate therapy? J Obstet Gynecol Neonatal Nurs. 2002;31:582–91.
51. Harrison D, Bueno M, Yamada J, et al. Analgesic effects of sweet-tasting solutions for infants: current state of equipoise. Pediatrics. 2010;126:894–902.
52. Naughton KA. The combined use of sucrose and nonnutritive sucking for procedural pain in both term and preterm neonates: an integrative review of the literature. Adv Neonatal Care. 2013; 13:9–19.
53. Carbajal R, Chauvet X, Couderc S, et al. Randomised trial of analgesic effects of sucrose, glucose, and pacifiers in term neonates. BMJ. 1999;319:1393–7.
54. Bueno M, Yamada J, Harrison D, et al. A systematic review and meta-analyses of nonsucrose sweet solutions for pain relief in neonates. Pain Res Manag. 2013;18:153–61.
55. Stevens B, Yamada J, Lee GY, et al. Sucrose for analgesia in newborn infants undergoing painful procedures. Cochrane Database Syst Rev. 2013;1:CD001069.
56. Marin Gabriel MA, Del Rey Hurtado de Mendoza B, Jiménez Figueroa L, et al. Analgesia with breastfeeding in addition to skin-to-skin contact during heel prick. Arch Dis Child Fetal Neonatal Ed. 2013;98:F499–503.

57. Taddio A, Shah V, Leung E, et al. Knowledge translation of the HELPinKIDS clinical practice guideline for managing childhood vaccination pain: usability and knowledge uptake of educational materials directed to new parents. BMC Pediatr. 2013;13:23.
58. Van Sleuwen BE, Engelberts AC, Boere-Boonekamp MM, et al. Swaddling: a systematic review. Pediatrics. 2007;120:e1097–106.
59. Prasopkittikun T, Tilokskulchai F. Management of pain form heel stick in neonates: an analysis of research conducted in Thailand. J Perinat Neonatal Nurs. 2003;17:304–12.
60. Liaw JJ, Yang L, Katherine Wang KW, Chen CM, Chang YC, Yin T. Non-nutritive sucking and facilitated tucking relieve preterm infant pain during heel-stick procedures: a prospective, randomised controlled crossover trial. Int J Nurs Stud. 2012;49: 300–9.
61. Liaw JJ, Yang L, Lee CM, Fan HC, Chang YC, Cheng LP. Effects of combined use of non-nutritive sucking, oral sucrose, and facilitated tucking on infant behavioural states across heel-stick procedures: a prospective, randomised controlled trial. Int J Nurs Stud. 2013;50:883–94.
62. Sundaram B, Shrivatava S, Pandian JS, Singh VP. Facilitated tucking on pain in pre-term newborns during neonatal intensive care: a single blinded randomized controlled cross-over pilot trial. J Pediatr Rehabil Med. 2013;6:19–27.
63. Hill S, Engle S, Jorgensen J, Kralik A, Whitman K. Effects of facilitated tucking during routine care of infants born preterm. Pediatr Phys Ther. 2005;17:158–63.
64. Corff KE, Seideman R, Venkataraman PS, Lutes L, Yates B. Facilitated tucking: a nonpharmacologic comfort measure for pain in preterm neonates. J Obstet Gynecol Neonatal Nurs. 1995; 24:143–7.
65. Cignacco EL, Sellam G, Stoffel L, et al. Oral sucrose and 'facilitated tucking' for repeated pain relief in preterms: a randomized controlled trial. Pediatrics. 2012;129:299–308.
66. Axelin A, Salanterä S, Lehtonen L. 'Facilitated tucking by parents' in pain management of preterm infants-a randomized crossover trial. Early Hum Dev. 2006;82:241–7.
67. Ward-Larson C, Horn RA, Gosnell F. The efficacy of facilitated tucking for relieving procedural pain of endotracheal suctioning in very low birth weight infants. MCN Am J Matern Child Nurs. 2004;29:151–6.
68. Fearon I, Kisilevsky BS, Mains SM, Muir DW, Tranmer J. Swaddling after heel lance: age-specific effects on behavioral recovery in preterm infants. J Dev Behav Pediatr. 1997;18:222–32.
69. Johnston C, Campbell-Yeo M, Rich B, et al. Therapeutic touch is not therapeutic for procedural pain in very preterm neonates: a randomized trial. Clin J Pain. 2013;29:824–9.
70. Cignacco E, Axelin A, Stoffel L, et al. Facilitated tucking as a non-pharmacological intervention for neonatal pain relief: is it clinically feasible? Acta Paediatr. 2010;99:1763–5.
71. Losacco V, Cuttini M, Greisen G, et al. Heel blood sampling in European neonatal intensive care units: compliance with pain management guidelines. Arch Dis Child Fetal Neonatal Ed. 2011;96:F65–8.
72. Johnston CC, Stevens B, Pinelli J, et al. Kangaroo care is effective in diminishing pain response in preterm neonates. Arch Pediatr Adolesc Med. 2003;157:1084–8.
73. Axelin A, Lehtonen L, Pelander T, et al. Mothers' different styles of involvement in preterm infant pain care. J Obstet Gynecol Neonatal Nurs. 2010;39:415–24.
74. Lönnqvist PA. Regional anaesthesia and analgesia in the neonate. Best Pract Res Clin Anaesthesiol. 2010;24:309–21.
75. Taddio A, Ohlsson A, Einarson TR, et al. A systematic review of lidocaine-prilocaine cream (EMLA) in the treatment of acute pain in neonates. Pediatrics. 1998;101:E1.
76. Abad F, Diaz-Gomez NM, Domenech E, et al. Oral sucrose compares favourably with lidocaine-prilocaine cream for pain relief during venipuncture in neonates. Acta Paediatr. 2001; 90:160–5.
77. Gradin M, Eriksson M, Holmqvist G, et al. Pain reduction at venipuncture in newborns: oral glucose compared with local anesthetic cream. Pediatrics. 2002;110:1053–7.
78. Biran V, Gourrier E, Cimerman P, et al. Analgesic effects of EMLA cream and oral sucrose during venipuncture in preterm infants. Pediatrics. 2011;128:e63–70.
79. Kaur G, Gupta P, Kumar A. A randomized trial of eutectic mixture of local anesthetics during lumbar puncture in newborns. Arch Pediatr Adolesc Med. 2003;157:1065–70.
80. Enad D, Salvador A, Brodsky NL, Hurt H. Safety and efficacy of eutectic mixture of local anesthetics (EMLA) for lumbar puncture (LP) in newborns (NB). Pediatr Res. 1995;37:204A (Abstract 1212).
81. Madsen S. Towards evidence based emergency medicine: the BETs from the Manchester Royal Infirmary. BET1. Topical anaesthetic and pain associated with lumbar puncture in neonates. Emerg Med J. 2009;26:57–8.
82. Taddio A, Stevens B, Craig K, et al. Efficacy and safety of lidocaine-prilocaine cream for pain during circumcision. N Engl J Med. 1997;336:1197–201.
83. Brady-Fryer B, Weibe N, Lander JA. Pain relief for neonatal circumcision. Cochrane Database Syst Rev. 2004:CD004217.
84. Taddio A, Nulman I, Goldbach M, et al. Use of lidocaine-prilocaine cream for vaccination pain in infants. J Pediatr. 1994; 124:643–8.
85. Reis EC, Roth EK, Syphan JL, et al. Effective pain reduction for multiple immunization injections in young infants. Arch Pediatr Adolesc Med. 2003;157:1115–20.
86. Babl FE, Goldfinch C, Mandrawa C, et al. Does nebulized lidocaine reduce the pain and distress of nasogastric tube insertion in young children? A randomized, double-blind, placebo-controlled trial. Pediatrics. 2009;123:1548–55.
87. McCullough S, Halton T, Mowbray D, et al. Lingual sucrose reduces the pain response to nasogastric tube insertion: a randomised clinical trial. Arch Dis Child Fetal Neonatal Ed. 2008; 93:F100–3.
88. Shah VS, Taddio A, Hancock R, et al. Topical amethocaine gel 4 % for intramuscular injection in term neonates: a double-blind, placebo-controlled, randomized trial. Clin Ther. 2008;30:166–74.
89. Jain A, Rutter N. Does topical amethocaine gel reduce the pain of venipuncture in newborn infants? A randomised double blind controlled trial. Arch Dis Child Fetal Neonatal Ed. 2000;83: F207–10.
90. Lemyre B, Hogan DL, Gaboury I, et al. How effective is tetracaine 4 % gel, before a venipuncture, in reducing procedural pain in infants: a randomized double-blind placebo controlled trial. BMC Pediatr. 2007;7:7.
91. Lemyre B, Sherlock R, Hogan D, et al. How effective is tetracaine 4 % gel, before a peripherally inserted central catheter, in reducing procedural pain in infants: a randomized double-blind placebo controlled trial. BMC Med. 2006;4:11.
92. Jain A, Rutter N, Ratnayaka M. Topical amethocaine gel for pain relief of heel prick blood sampling: a randomised double blind controlled trial. Arch Dis Child Fetal Neonatal Ed. 2001; 84:F56–9.
93. Allegaert K. The clinical pharmacology of short acting analgo-sedatives in neonates. Curr Clin Pharmacol. 2011;6:222–6.
94. Sammartino M, Garra R, Sbaraglia F, et al. Propofol overdose in a preterm baby: may propofol infusion syndrome arise in two hours? Paediatr Anaesth. 2010;20:973–4.
95. Allegaert K, Peeters MY, Verbesselt R, et al. Inter-individual variability in propofol pharmacokinetics in preterm and term neonates. Br J Anaesth. 2007;99:864–70.
96. Welzing L, Kribs A, Eifinger F, et al. Propofol as an induction agent for endotracheal intubation can cause significant arterial

hypotension in preterm neonates. Paediatr Anaesth. 2010;20: 605–11.

97. Nauta M, Onland W, De Jaegere A. Propofol as an induction agent for endotracheal intubation can cause significant arterial hypotension in preterm neonates. Paediatr Anaesth. 2011;21:711–2.
98. Ghanta S, Abdel-Latif ME, Lui K, et al. Propofol compared with the morphine, atropine, and suxamethonium regimen as induction agents for neonatal endotracheal intubation: a randomized, controlled trial. Pediatrics. 2007;119:e1248–55.
99. Papoff P, Mancuso M, Caresta E, et al. Effectiveness and safety of propofol in newborn infants. Pediatrics. 2008;121:448.
100. Penido MG, de Oliveira Silva DF, Tavares EC, et al. Propofol versus midazolam for intubating preterm neonates: a randomized controlled trial. J Perinatol. 2011;31:356–60.
101. Vanderhaegen J, Naulaers G, Van Huffel S, et al. Cerebral and systemic hemodynamic effects of intravenous bolus administration of propofol in neonates. Neonatology. 2010;98:57–63.
102. Allegaert K, Peeters MY, Knibbe C. Propofol in (pre)term neonates: consider the extensive interindividual variability in clearance within the neonatal population. Paediatr Anaesth. 2011;21:174–5.
103. Shah PS, Shah VS. Propofol for procedural sedation/anaesthesia in neonates. Cochrane Database Syst Rev. 2011:CD007248.
104. Bhutta AT. Ketamine: a controversial drug for neonates. Semin Perinatol. 2007;31:303–8.
105. Saarenmaa E, Neuvonen PJH, Huttunen P, et al. Ketamine for procedural pain relief in newborn infants. Arch Dis Child Fetal Neonatal Ed. 2001;85:F53–6.
106. Lönnqvist PA, Walker SM. Ketamine as an adjunct to caudal block in neonates and infants: is it time to re-evaluate? Br J Anaesth. 2012;109:138–40.
107. Hartvig P, Larsson E, Joachimsson PO. Postoperative analgesia and sedation following pediatric cardiac surgery using a constant infusion of ketamine. J Cardiothorac Vasc Anesth. 1993;7:148–53.
108. Lyon F, Dabbs T, O'Meara M. Ketamine sedation during treatment of retinopathy of prematurity. Eye. 2008;22:684–6.
109. Anderson BJ, McKee AD, Holford NH. Size, myths and the clinical pharmacokinetics of analgesia in paediatric patients. Clin Pharmacokinet. 1997;33:313–27.
110. Norman E, Wilström S, Hellström-Wastas L, et al. Rapid sequence induction is superior to morphine for intubation of preterm infants: a randomized controlled trial. J Pediatr. 2011;159:893–9. e1.
111. Choong K, AlFaleh K, Doucette J, et al. Remifentanil for endotracheal intubation in neonates: a randomised controlled trial. Arch Dis Child Fetal Neonatal Ed. 2010;95:F80–4.
112. Welzing L, Kribs A, Huenseler C, et al. Remifentanil for INSURE in preterm infants: a pilot study for evaluation of efficacy and safety aspects. Acta Paediatr. 2009;98:1416–20.
113. Pereira e Silva Y, Gomez RS, Marcatto Ide O, et al. Morphine versus remifentanil for intubating preterm neonates. Arch Dis Child Fetal Neonatal Ed. 2007;92:F293–4.
114. Hume-Smith J, Cormack M, Montgomery C, et al. The effect of age on the dose of remifentanil for tracheal intubation in infants and children. Paediatr Anaesth. 2010;20:19–27.
115. Crawford MW, Hayes J, Jan JM. Dose-response of remifentanil for tracheal intubation in infants. Anesth Analg. 2005;100:1599–604.
116. Lago P, Tiozzo C, Boccuzzo G, et al. Remifentanil for percutaneous intravenous central catheter placement in preterm infant: a randomized controlled trial. Paediatr Anaesth. 2008;18:736–44.
117. Sammartino M, Bocci MG, Ferro G, Mercurio G, Papacci P, Conti G, et al. Efficacy and safety of continuous intravenous infusion of remifentanil in preterm infants undergoing laser therapy in retinopathy of prematurity: clinical experience. Paediatr Anaesth. 2003;13:596–602.
118. Sammartino M, Garra R, Sbaraglia F. Experience of remifentanil in extremely low-birth-weight babies undergoing laparotomy. Pediatr Neonatol. 2011;52:176–9.
119. Giannantonio C, Sammartino M, Valente E, et al. Remifentanil analgosedation in preterm newborns during mechanical ventilation. Acta Paediatr. 2009;98:1111–5.
120. Allegaert K, Thewissen L, van den Anker JN. Remifentanil in neonates: a promising compound in search of its indications? Pediatr Neonatol. 2012;53:387–8.
121. Welzing L, Link F, Junghaenel S, et al. Remifentanil-induced tolerance, withdrawal or hyperalgesia in infants: a randomized controlled trial. RAPIP trial: remifentanil-based analgesia and sedation of paediatric intensive care patients. Neonatology. 2013; 104(1):34–41.
122. American Academy of Pediatrics, Committee on Drugs, Committee on Environmental Health. Use of chloral hydrate for sedation in children. Pediatrics. 1993;92:471–3.
123. Reimche LD, Sankaran K, Hindmarsh KW, et al. Chloral hydrate sedation in neonates and infants—clinical and pharmacologic considerations. Dev Pharmacol Ther. 1989;12:57–64.
124. Litman RS, Soin K, Salam A. Chloral hydrate sedation in term and preterm infants: an analysis of efficacy and complications. Anesth Analg. 2010;110:739–46.
125. Ikbal M, Tastekin A, Dogan H, et al. The assessment of genotoxic effects in lymphocyte cultures of infants treated with chloral hydrate. Mutat Res. 2004;564:159–64.
126. Allegaert K, Daniels H, Naulaers G, et al. Pharmacodynamics of chloral hydrate in former preterm infants. Eur J Pediatr. 2005; 164:403–7.
127. Yu XQ, Suguihara C, Navarro H, et al. Effect of chloral hydrate on the cardiorespiratory response to hypoxia in newborn piglets. Biol Neonate. 1996;69:146–52.
128. Hershenson M, Brouillette RT, Olsen E, et al. The effect of chloral hydrate on genioglossus and diaphragmatic activity. Pediatr Res. 1984;18:516–9.
129. Heistein LC, Ramaciotti C, Scott WA, et al. Chloral hydrate sedation for pediatric echocardiography: physiologic responses, adverse events, and risk factors. Pediatrics. 2006;117:e434–41.
130. Keidan I, Gozal D, Minuskin T, et al. The effect of fasting practice on sedation with chloral hydrate. Pediatr Emerg Care. 2004; 20:805–7.
131. Beauve B, Dearlove O. Sedation of children under 4 weeks of age for MRI examination. Paediatr Anaesth. 2008;18:892–3.
132. Van Wezel-Meijler G, Leijser LM, de Bruine FT, et al. Magnetic resonance imaging of the brain in newborn infants: practical aspects. Early Hum Dev. 2009;85:85–92.
133. Bracken J, Heaslip I, Ryan S. Chloral hydrate sedation in radiology: retrospective audit of reduced dose. Pediatr Radiol. 2012; 42:349–54.
134. Mason KP, Sanborn P, Zurakowski D, et al. Superiority of pentobarbital versus chloral hydrate for sedation in infants during imaging. Radiology. 2004;230:537–42.
135. McCarver-May DG, Kang J, et al. Comparison of chloral hydrate and midazolam for sedation of neonates for neuroimaging studies. J Pediatr. 1996;128:573–6.
136. Olkkola KT, Hamunen K, Maunuksela EL. Clinical pharmacokinetics and pharmacodynamics of opioid analgesics in infants and children. Clin Pharmacokinet. 1995;28:385–404.
137. Taylor J, Liley A, Anderson BJ. The relationship between age an morphine infusion rate in children. Paediatr Anaesth. 2013; 23:40–4.
138. Knibbe CA, Krekels EH, van den Anker JN, et al. Morphine glucuronidation in preterm neonates, infants and children younger than 3 years. Clin Pharmacokinet. 2009;48:371–85.
139. Krekels EH, DeJongh J, van Lingen RA, et al. Predictive performance of a recently developed population pharmacokinetic model for morphine and its metabolites in new datasets of (preterm) neonates, infants and children. Clin Pharmacokinet. 2011;50:51–63.

140. Roka A, Melinda KT, Vasarhelyi B, et al. Elevated morphine concentrations in neonates treated with morphine and prolonged hypothermia for hypoxic ischemic encephalopathy. Pediatrics. 2008;121:e844–9.
141. Lynn A, Nespeca MK, Bratton SL, et al. Clearance of morphine in postoperative infants during intravenous infusion: the influence of age and surgery. Anesth Analg. 1998;86:958–63.
142. Walter-Nicolet E, Annequin D, Biran V, et al. Pain management in newborns: from prevention to treatment. Paediatr Drugs. 2010; 12:353–65.
143. Van Dijk M, Bouwmeester NJ, Duivenvoorden HJ, et al. Efficacy of continuous versus intermittent morphine administration after major surgery in 0–3 year old infants: a double-blind randomized controlled trial. Pain. 2002;98:305–13.
144. Ceelie I, de Wildt SN, van Dijk M, et al. Effect of intravenous paracetamol on postoperative morphine requirements in neonates and infants undergoing major noncardiac surgery: a randomized controlled trial. JAMA. 2013;309:149–54.
145. Ancora G, Lago P, Garetti E, et al. Efficacy and safety of continuous infusion of fentanyl for pain control in preterm newborns on mechanical ventilation. J Pediatr. 2013;163:645–51. e1.
146. Cignacco E, Hamers JP, van Lingen RA, et al. Pain relief in ventilated preterms during endotracheal suctioning: a randomized controlled trial. Swiss Med Wkly. 2008;138:635–45.
147. Bellu R, de Waal K, Zanini R. Opioids for neonates receiving mechanical ventilation: a systematic review and meta-analysis. Arch Dis Child Fetal Neonatal Ed. 2010;95:F241–51.
148. de Graaf J, van Lingen RA, Simons SH, et al. Long-term effects of routine morphine infusion in mechanically ventilated neonates on children's functioning: five-year follow-up of a randomized controlled trial. Pain. 2011;152:1391–7.
149. de Graaf J, van Lingen RA, Valkenburg AJ, et al. Does neonatal morphine use affect neuropsychological outcomes at 8 to 9 years of age? Pain. 2013;154:449–58.
150. van den Anker JN. Treating pain in newborn infants: navigating between Scylla and Charybdis. J Pediatr. 2013;163:618–9.
151. Hall RW. Anesthesia and analgesia in the NICU. Clin Perinatol. 2012;39:239–54.
152. Anderson BJ, Larsson P. A maturation model for midazolam clearance. Paediatr Anaesth. 2011;21:302–8.
153. Ince I, de Wildt SN, Wang C, et al. A novel maturation function for clearance of the cytochrome P450 3A substrate midazolam from preterm neonates to adults. Clin Pharmacokinet. 2013;52: 555–65.
154. Anand KJ, Barton BA, McIntosh N, et al. Analgesia and sedation in preterm neonates who require ventilatory support: results from the NOPAIN trial. Neonatal outcome and prolonged analgesia in neonates. Arch Pediatr Adolesc Med. 1999;153:331–8.
155. Ng E, Taddio A, Ohlsson A. Intravenous midazolam infusion for sedation of infants in the neonatal intensive care unit. Cochrane Database Syst Rev. 2012;6:CD002052.
156. Welzing L, Oberthuer A, Junghaenel S, et al. Remifentanil/midazolam versus fentanyl/midazolam for analgesia and sedation of mechanically ventilated neonates and young infants: a randomized controlled trial. Intensive Care Med. 2012;38:1017–24.
157. Burtin P, Daoud P, Jacqz-Aigrain E, et al. Hypotension with midazolam and fentanyl in the newborn. Lancet. 1991;337:1545–6.
158. Attardi DM, Paul DA, Tuttle DJ, et al. Premedication for intubation in neonates. Arch Dis Child Fetal Neonatal Ed. 2000;83:F161.
159. Wildschut ED, Hanekamp MN, Vet NJ, et al. Feasibility of sedation and analgesia interruption following cannulation in neonates on extracorporeal membrane oxygenation. Intensive Care Med. 2010;36:1587–91.
160. Chrysostomou C, Schulman SR, Herrera Castellanos M, et al. A phase II/III multicenter, safety, efficacy, and pharmacokinetic study of dexmedetomidine in preterm and term neonates. J Pediatr. 2014;164:276–82. doi:10.1016/jpeds.2013.10.002.
161. Dilek O, Yasemin G, Atci M. Preliminary experience with dexmedetomidine in neonatal anesthesia. J Anaesthesiol Clin Pharmacol. 2011;27:17–22.
162. Shukry M, Kennedy K. Dexmedetomidine as a total intravenous anesthetic in infants. Paediatr Anaesth. 2007;17:581–3.
163. Shiota M, Oda Y, Taniguchi M, et al. Dexmedetomidine infusion for sedation in the intensive care setting in an infant with airway compromise due to congenital mediastinal neuroblastoma. Paediatr Anaesth. 2012;22:603–5.
164. Kubota T, Fukasawa T, Kitamura E, et al. Epileptic seizures induced by dexmedetomidine in a neonate. Brain Dev. 2013; 35:360–2.
165. Reinoso-Barbero F, Pascual-Pascual SI, de Lucas R, et al. Equimolar nitrous oxide/oxygen versus placebo for procedural pain in children: a randomized trial. Pediatrics. 2011;127: e1464–70.
166. Mandel R, Ali N, Chen J, et al. Nitrous oxide analgesia during retinopathy screening: a randomised controlled trial. Arch Dis Child Fetal Neonatal Ed. 2012;97:F83–7.
167. Carbajal R, Biran V, Lenclen R, et al. EMLA cream and nitrous oxide to alleviate pain induced by palivizumab (Synagis) intramuscular injections in infants and young children. Pediatrics. 2008;121:e1591–8.
168. Allegaert K, Devlieger H, Bulckaert D, et al. Variability in pain expression characteristics in former preterm infants. J Perinat Med. 2005;33:442–8.
169. Vialet R, Michel F, Hassid S, et al. Sevoflurane for central venous catheterization in non-intubated neonates. Indian J Pediatr. 2009; 76:273–7.
170. Michel F, Vialet R, Hassid S, et al. Sevoflurane for central catheter placement in neonatal intensive care: a randomized trial. Paediatr Anaesth. 2010;20:712–9.
171. Hassid S, Nicaise C, Michel F, et al. Randomized controlled trial of sevoflurane for intubation in neonates. Paediatr Anaesth. 2007; 17:1053–8.
172. Lerman J, Robinson S, Willis MM, et al. Anesthetic requirements for halothane in young children 0–1 month and 1–6 months of age. Anesthesiology. 1983;59:421–4.
173. Cuzzolin L, Antonucci R, Fanos V. Paracetamol (acetaminophen) efficacy and safety in the newborn. Curr Drug Metab. 2013; 14:178–85.
174. Anderson BJ, Van Lingen RA, Hansen TG, et al. Acetaminophen developmental pharmacokinetics in premature neonates and infants: a pooled population analysis. Anesthesiology. 2002;96: 1336–45.
175. Allegaert K, Palmer GM, Anderson BJ. The pharmacokinetics of intravenous paracetamol in neonates: size matters most. Arch Dis Child. 2011;96:575–80.
176. Shah V, Taddio A, Ohlsson A. Randomised controlled trial of paracetamol for heel prick pain in neonates. Arch Dis Child Fetal Neonatal Ed. 1998;79:F209–11.
177. Howard CR, Howard FM, Weitzman ML. Acetaminophen analgesia in neonatal circumcision: the effect on pain. Pediatrics. 1994; 93:641–6.
178. Van Lingen RA, Quak CM, Deinum HT, et al. Effects of rectally administered paracetamol on infants delivered by vacuum extraction. Eur J Obstet Gynecol Reprod Biol. 2001;94:73–8.
179. Tinner EM, Hoesli I, Jost K, et al. Rectal paracetamol in newborn infants after assisted vaginal delivery may increase pain response. J Pediatr. 2013;162:62–6.
180. Allegaert K, Naulaers G, Vanhaesebrouck S, et al. The paracetamol concentration-effect relation in neonates. Paediatr Anaesth. 2013; 23:45–50.

181. Allegaert K, Anderson B, Simons S, et al. Paracetamol to induce ductus arteriosus closure: is it valid? Arch Dis Child. 2013;98: 462–6.
182. Wickens K, Beasley R, Town I, et al. The effects of early and late paracetamol exposure on asthma and atopy: a birth cohort. Clin Exp Allergy. 2011;41:399–406.
183. Montirosso R, Del Prete A, Bellu R, et al. Level of NICU quality of developmental care and neurobehavioral performance in very preterm infants. Pediatrics. 2012;129:e1129–37.
184. Thomson Reuters. Neofax®: a manual of drugs used in neonatal care. 24th ed. Montvale, NJ: Thomson Reuters; 2011.
185. Kanmaz HG, Erdeve O, Canpolat FE, Mutlu B, Dilmen U. Surfactant administration via thin catheter during spontaneous breathing: randomized controlled trial. Pediatrics. 2013;131(2): e502–9.
186. Smart Tots. Consensus statement on the use of anesthetics and sedatives in children. December 2012. http://www.smarttots.org/resources/consensus.html

16 Sedation in the Pediatric Intensive Care Unit: Challenges, Outcomes, and Future Strategies in the United States

Joseph D. Tobias

Abstract

Sedation and analgesia are required on a daily basis for infants and children in the pediatric intensive care unit (PICU). Regardless of the patient's age, cognitive level, underlying medical condition, or comorbid conditions, various factors may result in agitation, anxiety, and pain during the PICU process. One of the challenges of the PICU is the variability that is presented in patient type (age, weight, comorbid conditions, acute illness), procedure type and duration, and location (in the PICU versus off-site). The procedures may be brief (burn dressing changes, placement of central venous or arterial cannulae) or prolonged (mechanical ventilation) as well as non-painful requiring only sedation (imaging) or painful requiring both sedation and analgesia. When considering the patient who requires mechanical ventilation, the need for procedural sedation may last for days or even weeks as children may require prolonged sedation to overcome the pain and anxiety associated with the presence of an endotracheal tube and the requirement for ongoing mechanical ventilation. The pain and anxiety may be further magnified by psychological factors including periodic separation from parents, disruption of the day–night cycle and alterations of normal sleep patterns, unfamiliar people, the noise of imposing machines and monitoring devices, fear of death, and loss of self-control.

Keywords

Pediatric intensive care unit (PICU) • Sedation • American Society of Anesthesiologists (ASA) classification • Depth of sedation • Sedation scales • Bispectral index (BIS) • Agent • Route of delivery • Inhalational anesthetics • Benzodiazepines • Etomidate • Ketamine • Propofol • Propofol infusion syndrome • Barbiturates • Opioids • Phenothiazines • Butyrophenones • Alpha2-adrenergic agonists • Chloral hydrate • Tolerance • Dependency • Withdrawal • Delirium • Palliative care • End-of-life care • Observer's Assessment of Alertness/Sedation Scale (OAAS) • Modified Observer's Assessment of Altertness/Sedation Score (MOAASS) • COMFORT Scale • University of Michigan Sedation Scale (UMSS) • Modified Aldrete score • Bispectral index (BIS) • Aldrete score • Anesthetic Conserving Device (AnaConDa) • Gamma-aminobutyric acid (GABA) • Lorazepam • Midazolam • *N*-Methyl-D-aspartate (NMDA) • Electroencephalogram (EEG) • Intracranial pressure • Cerebral perfusion pressure • Remifentanil • Clonidine • Dexmedetomidine • Sophia Benzodiazepine and Opioid Withdrawal Checklist (SBOWC) • Neonatal abstinence syndrome (NAS) • Withdrawal and assessment tool (WAT) • Sedation withdrawal score (SWS) •

J.D. Tobias, M.D. (✉)
Department of Anesthesiology & Pain Medicine, Nationwide Children's Hospital, 700 Children's Drive, Columbus, OH 43205, USA
e-mail: Joseph.Tobias@Nationwidechildrens.org

K.P. Mason (ed.), *Pediatric Sedation Outside of the Operating Room: A Multispecialty International Collaboration*, DOI 10.1007/978-1-4939-1390-9_16, © Springer Science+Business Media New York 2015

Methadone • Intensive care delirium screening checklist (ICDSC) • Confusion assessment method for the ICU (CAM-ICU) • Opioid and benzodiazepine withdrawal scale (OBWS) • Sedation/agitation scale (SAS)

Introduction

Sedation and analgesia are required on a daily basis for infants and children in the pediatric intensive care unit (PICU). Regardless of the patient's age, cognitive level, underlying medical condition, or comorbid conditions, various factors may result in agitation, anxiety, and pain during the PICU process. One of the challenges of the PICU is the variability that is presented in patient type (age, weight, comorbid conditions, acute illness), procedure type and duration, and location (in the PICU versus off-site). The procedures may be brief (burn dressing changes, placement of central venous or arterial cannulae) or prolonged (mechanical ventilation) as well as non-painful requiring only sedation (imaging) or painful requiring both sedation and analgesia. When considering the patient who requires mechanical ventilation, the need for procedural sedation may last for days or even weeks as children may require prolonged sedation to overcome the pain and anxiety associated with the presence of an endotracheal tube and the requirement for ongoing mechanical ventilation. The pain and anxiety may be further magnified by psychological factors including periodic separation from parents, disruption of the day–night cycle and alterations of normal sleep patterns, unfamiliar people, the noise of imposing machines and monitoring devices, fear of death, and loss of self-control. In the adult population, a significant percentage of patients reported that they remembered mechanical ventilation with approximately 25 % noting that they would have chosen not to receive mechanical ventilation had it been any more painful [1].

Pre-procedure Preparation

Regardless of the setting, prior to the administration of pharmacologic agents for the control of procedure-related pain and anxiety, an evaluation of the patient and preparation of the environment is mandatory (Table 16.1). The latter is especially important for off-site procedures when the patient is transported out of the PICU to the radiology suite. Careful evaluation of the pediatric ICU patient is important in order to differentiate treatable and potentially life-threatening causes of agitation such as hypoxemia, hypercarbia, cerebral hypoperfusion, necrotic bowel, or a compartment syndrome from agitation that requires sedation. The injudicious use of sedative/analgesic agents without ongoing patient examination and monitoring may result in disaster. For example, a patient who has an abrupt increase in sedative/analgesic needs may need nothing more than a dose increase. A need for additional sedation should be carefully investigated and identified prior to delivering sedation, in order to establish that there is patient tolerance or the development of tachyphylaxis to the current sedation regimen. These concerns are less of an issue for a patient who is undergoing a brief invasive or noninvasive procedure, for which the pre-procedure evaluation is relatively the same as for patients outside of the PICU environment.

Table 16.1 Preparation for procedural sedation in the pediatric ICU

1. Rule out treatable causes of agitation
(a) Hypoxia and hypercarbia (b) Cerebral hypoperfusion (c) Bladder distention (d) Surgical lesion—necrotic bowel or compartment syndrome
2. Perform a presedation evaluation of the patient. This evaluation is similar to that performed prior to any surgical procedure performed in the operating room
3. Identify the etiology of the pain or agitation to guide the appropriate selection of the agent or agents as well as the need to provide sedation/anxiolysis/amnesia, analgesia, or both
4. Monitor patient according to the standards outlined by the American Academy of Pediatrics for procedural sedation and analgesia
5. Titrate the initial bolus dose of the medication and subsequent infusion rates based on the patient's clinical response with the use of formalized sedation/pain scales
6. Observe for adverse physiologic effects including the development of physical tolerance which necessitates increasing the dose of the agent used or switching to another agent that acts through a different receptor system

The basic components of the presedation assessment are outlined in Table 16.2. This assessment includes the performance of a focused history and physical examination. The history should focus on the child's current state of health as it relates to the reason for the procedure, the past medical history to identify significant comorbidities, as well as acute events that led to the PICU admission. Since the primary risks associated with sedation include adverse respiratory events (apnea, hypoxemia, hypercarbia, and upper airway obstruction) or cardiovascular events (hypotension, bradycardia, arrhythmias), the focus of the presedation evaluation and physical examination is placed on these systems or areas. The American Society of Anesthesiologists (ASA) emphasizes that the evaluation of the airway "should be conducted, whenever feasible, prior to the initiation of anesthetic care and airway management in all patients"[2]. The purpose of this examination is to detect physical characteristics that may indicate the presence of a difficult airway. (Refer to Chap. 7.) Although many patients may already have an endotracheal tube in place, the assessment of the upper airway should still be performed in the event that the endotracheal tube becomes dislodged at some time, such as during positioning for the procedure or patient transport. The upper airway assessment includes obtaining a history of signs and symptoms that indicate potential airway problems (noisy breathing, stridor, snoring, or obstructive sleep apnea). This is followed by an examination of the head and neck designed to identify the patient in whom airway management or endotracheal intubation may be difficult. An assessment is made of neck mobility (flexion and extension), mouth opening, the size of the oral cavity and tongue (presence of macroglossia), the presence of micrognathia, and the thyromental distance (distance from the thyroid cartilage to the tip of the mandible). In general, mouth opening should be greater than the width of two fingerbreadths, while the thyromental distance should be at least three. In both instances, the patient's own fingers can be used as the measuring instrument. In the adult population, an objective measure of the potential for difficult intubation is the Mallampati grading system (I through IV) (see Fig. 16.1) [3]. This system evaluates the ability to visualize the tonsillar pillars and the uvula when the patient opens their mouth. If the Mallampati grade is III or IV (tonsillar pillars and base of the uvula cannot be visualized with mouth opening and tongue protrusion), the trachea may be difficult to intubate and bag-mask ventilation may be problematic.

In the pediatric ICU patient, a thorough review of the patient's current medical regimen (both sedation/analgesic and others) is performed as well as a determination of the patient's current vascular access and which site will be used for the administration of the sedative/analgesic agents. Upon completion of the history and physical examination, an ASA (American Association of Anesthesiologist) classification may be assigned (Table 16.3) [4] to help guide the choice of sedation: Adverse events have been shown to have a greater incidence in patients with a higher ASA classification (III or IV versus I or II) [5]. During this evaluation, the child's previous experiences with procedural sedation are explored, identifying both their efficacy and the child's and parent's impressions of the experience. (Refer to Chap. 4.)

Table 16.2 The pre-procedure or presedation assessment

Patient's name, age, weight, and gender
Past medical history: Acute medical or surgical problems
Comorbid medical conditions: Previous sedation or anesthetic history including problems
Allergies
Current medications
Family history of anesthetic complications
Dietary history (*nil per os* status)
Pregnancy history
Physical examination: Baseline vital signs including room air oxygen saturation if feasible Airway examination with Mallampati grading system Focused cardiac and respiratory examination Current vascular access and infusion (to select site for medication administration)
Laboratory evaluation as appropriate
Summary: American Society of Anesthesiologists status (ASA I–V) Sedation and recovery plan Risks discussed and informed consent obtained from patients Perform formal, hospital-based time-out prior to the procedure

Table 16.3 ASA classification

ASA I	No associated comorbid disease
ASA II	Mild associated comorbid disease, mild asthma
ASA III	Severe associated comorbid disease, sickle cell anemia, obstructive sleep apnea, severe asthma
ASA IV	Comorbid disease that is a constant threat to life, dilated cardiomyopathy, septic shock
ASA V	Moribund patient that is not expected to survive 24 h
E	Modifier added for emergency procedure or surgery

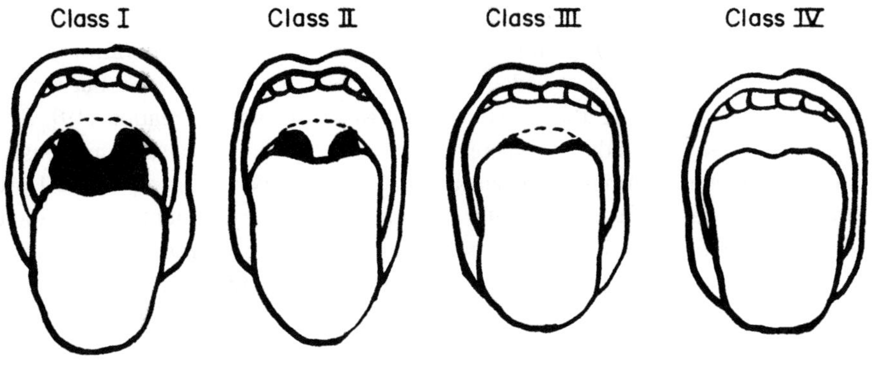

Fig. 16.1 Mallampati classification of pharyngeal structures. Reprinted with permission from Samsoon GL, Young JR. Difficult tracheal intubation: a retrospective study. *Anaesthesia*. May 1987;42(5):487–490

A final component of the presedation assessment is to minimize the risk of aspiration by adhering to the *nil per os* (NPO) status in order to limit gastric volume. In the PICU patient, factors other than NPO may affect gastric emptying and thereby both gastric volume and pH. The American Society of Anesthesiologists' recommendations for *per os* (NPO) are 2–3 h for clear liquids (including breast milk) and 4–8 h for infant formula [4]. The need to adhere to strict NPO guidelines for procedural sedation have been challenged, particularly by those working in acute care environments such as emergency rooms where procedures may need to be performed more urgently [6, 7]. While published reports from these environments have failed to show an effect of pre-procedure fasting on the incidence of adverse outcomes, these studies have been underpowered. If a patient is considered to be at significant risk of aspiration, consideration should be given to recruit anesthesia to perform a rapid sequence induction and endotracheal intubation. Following a careful assessment and prior to the start of the procedure, a formal "time out" should be performed and documented. This "time out" should include two patient identifiers (name and medical record number), validation that consents have been obtained and signed, a review of the procedure to be performed, and agreement on the site and laterality of the procedure.

Patients should be monitored in accordance with the guidelines set forth by the American Academy of Pediatrics (AAP) and/or the ASA both during and following the procedure [4, 8]. (Refer to Chap. 2.) As the PICU provides the optimal environment for the monitoring of a patient's physiologic functions, the monitoring should be continued when PICU patients are sedated outside of the PICU. Formal monitoring should include continuous pulse oximetry and heart rate (via the pulse oximeter or electrocardiography) as well as measurement of respiratory rate and blood pressure at 5 min intervals [4, 9, 10]. In 2011, the ASA amended the Standards for Basic Anesthesia Monitoring (first published in 1986) to specify that during moderate and deep sedation, ventilation should be followed by clinical observation and capnography [11]. Exceptions to capnography would be situations whereby patient, procedure, or equipment precludes or invalidates the monitoring. Adherence to these monitoring guidelines is mandatory as lack of appropriate monitoring has been shown to be a key failure in the analysis of adverse outcomes during procedural sedation [12]. Monitoring of ventilation via end-tidal carbon dioxide ($ETCO_2$) should also be considered under conditions where access to the patient is limited. $ETCO_2$ monitoring has been shown to detect hypercarbia in the absence of clinically apparent respiratory depression or desaturation if only pulse oximetry is used [13, 14]. $ETCO_2$ provides a tangible means to monitor and adjust ventilation in the intubated child. Ventilatory regulation in order to maintain a targeted $PaCO_2$ can be particularly important for patients with altered intracranial compliance, pulmonary hypertension, or those with compromised or cyanotic heart disease.

Assessing the Depth of Sedation

Some means for the ongoing evaluation of the depth of sedation should be incorporated into the procedural sedation routine. This monitoring allows for an increase or decrease in the doses used, based on the patient's depth of sedation rather than the hemodynamic parameters. Subjective scoring measures and assessments have been replaced by standardized pain and sedation scoring systems, which are monitored at regular intervals. (Refer to Chap. 5.) These scoring systems should be used both during prolonged sedation as well as brief periods of procedural sedation. The currently used PICU sedation scores evaluate physiologic variables, an objective assessment of the patient's depth of sedation, or a combination of the two. One commonly used scale, the COMFORT score, combines the scoring of a patient's response or movement in addition to various physiologic parameters (see Table 16.4) [15]. The COMFORT score assesses alertness, respiratory rate, blood pressure, muscle tone, agitation, movement, heart rate, and facial tension. It has been validated in the pediatric-aged patient and may have utility in the assessment of sedation during mechanical ventilation [15, 16]. Beware that scales based on physiologic parameters can be misleading in an ICU. Furthermore, patients with cardiovascular dysfunction requiring vasoactive medications may not manifest increases in heart rate and blood pressure normally seen with severe agitation or pain. Because of these concerns, Ista et al. have recently proposed the COMFORT-B score (see Table 16.5), a modification of the original COMFORT score, which eliminates physiologic variables and provides new cutoff points for the diagnosis of over- or undersedation [17].

Other scoring systems such as the sedation–agitation scale (SAS) (see Table 16.6) also eliminate the use of physiologic parameters by visually assessing the level of the patient's comfort and grades it from 1 (unarousable) to 7 (dangerous agitation such as pulling at the ETT) [18].

The Ramsay scale, a sedation scale used commonly in the adult ICU population, also assigns a value based on the observation of the patient, but also uses a tactile stimulus (a glabellar tap) to distinguish between the deeper levels of sedation [19]. Scoring for the Ramsey scale varies from 1 (awake, anxious, and agitated) to 6 (no response to a glabellar tap). The Hartwig score similarly uses a visual assessment of the patient, but as with the Ramsay scale includes a response to a noxious stimulus, in this case, tracheal suctioning thereby eliminating its use in non-intubated patients [20]. Scales such as the Ramsay and the Hartwig that assess the response to a tactile stimulus require disturbing the patient to differentiate between the deeper levels of sedation.

Table 16.4 The COMFORT Scale [15]

Characteristic	Evaluate	Points
Alertness	Deeply asleep	1
	Lightly asleep	2
	Drowsy	3
	Awake and alert	4
	Hyperalert	5
Agitation	Calm	1
	Slightly anxious	2
	Anxious	3
	Very anxious	4
	Panicky	5
Respiratory response	No coughing	1
	Spontaneous respiration with little response to ventilation	2
	Occasional coughing with little resistance to the ventilator	3
	Active breathing against the ventilator	4
	Actively fighting the ventilator and coughing	5
Physical movements	None	1
	Occasional, slight movements	2
	Frequent, slight movements	3
	Vigorous movements of extremities only	4
	Vigorous movements of extremities, torso, and head	5
Blood pressure (mean)	Below baseline	1
	Normal	2
	Infrequent elevations of 15 % or more	3
	Frequent elevations of 15 % or more	4
	Sustained elevation greater than or equal to 15 %	5
Heart rate	Below baseline	1
	Normal	2
	Infrequent elevations of 15 % or more	3
	Frequent elevations of 15 % or more	4
	Sustained elevation greater than or equal to 15 %	5
Muscle tone	Relaxed/none	1
	Reduced muscle tone	2
	Normal muscle tone	3
	Increased tone/flexion—fingers/toes	4
	Extreme rigidity/flexion—fingers/toes	5
Facial tension	Facial muscles relaxed	1
	Normal tone	2
	Some tension	3
	Full facial tension	4
	Facial grimacing	5
Total:		

Table 16.5 The COMFORT-B scale

Alertness	Ponits
Deeply asleep	1
Lightly asleep	2
Drowsy	3
Fully awake and alert	4
Hyperalert	5
Calmness/agitation	
Calm	1
Slightly anxious	2
Anxious	3
Very anxious	4
Panicky	5
Respiratory response (ventilated children)	
No coughing and no spontaneous respiration	1
Spontaneous respiration with little or no response to ventilation	2
Occasional cough or resistance to ventilator	3
Actively breathes against ventilator or coughs regularly	4
Fights ventilator, cough, or choking	5
Cry (non-ventilated children)	
Quiet breathing, no crying	1
Sobbing or gasping	2
Moaning	3
Crying	4
Screaming	5
Physical movement	
No movement	1
Occasional, slight movements	2
Frequent, slight movements	3
Vigorous movement limited to extremities	4
Vigorous movements including torso and head	5
Muscle tone	
Muscles totally relaxed, no muscle tone	1
Reduced muscle tone	2
Normal muscle tone	3
Increased muscle tone and flexion of fingers and toes	4
Extreme muscle rigidity and flexion of fingers and toes	5
Facial tension	
Facial muscle totally relaxed	1
Facial muscle tone normal; no facial muscle tension evident	2
Tension evident in some facial muscles	3
Tension evident throughout facial muscles	4
Facial muscles contorted and grimacing	5
Total:	

Additionally, scales that evaluate a patient's response to a stimulus or observe their behavior are not valid during the administration of neuromuscular blocking agents that prevent movement.

Various scales have also been developed for assessing the patient during procedural sedation. Given the potential morbidity associated with patients becoming too deeply sedated as well as concerns of inadequate sedation, tools that provide an accurate assessment of the response to sedative and analgesic agents during procedural sedation are also needed. During light sedation, this may be easily accomplished by assessment of the patient's ability to appropriately respond to questions. However, with deeper sedation, such assessments become of limited utility. The Observer's Assessment of Alertness/Sedation (OAAS) scale has been validated in children, but has been shown to have a limited ability to differentiate between the deeper levels of sedation [21].

Table 16.6 The sedation–agitation scale [17]

Scale	Agitation/sedation	Behavior
7	Dangerous agitation	Pulls at endotracheal tube, tries to remove catheters, climbs over bedrail, strikes at staff, thrashes side to side
6	Very agitated	Does not calm despite frequent verbal reminders of limits, requires physical restraint, bites endotracheal tube
5	Agitated	Anxious or mildly agitated, attempts to sit up, calms down to verbal instructions
4	Calm and cooperate	Calm, awakens easily, follows commands
3	Sedated	Difficult to arouse, awakens to verbal stimuli or gentle shaking but drifts off again, follows simple commands
2	Very sedated	Arouses to physical stimuli but does not communicate or follow commands, may move spontaneously
1	Unarousable	Minimal or no response to noxious stimuli, does not communicate or follow commands

Table 16.7 The University of Michigan Sedation Scale (UMSS)

Scale	Level of sedation
0	Awake and alert
1	Minimally sedated • Tired/sleepy • Appropriate response to verbal conversation and/or sounds
2	Moderately sedated • Somnolent/sleeping • Easily aroused with light tactile stimulation or simple verbal commands
3	Deeply sedated • Deep sleep • Arousable only with significant physical stimulation
4	Unarousable

The Vancouver Sedative Recovery Scale appears to be better able to differentiate deeper levels of sedation, although it is likely too cumbersome to be easily utilized during short procedures [22]. More recently, Malviya et al. developed and validated the University of Michigan Sedation Scale (UMSS) (see Table 16.7) [23]. This scale was developed to be a simple and efficient tool to assess depth of sedation over the entire sedation continuum and one that could easily be applied by various health-care providers. It utilizes a simple scale ranging from 0 (awake and alert) to 4 (unresponsive).

In addition to the classical sedation scales, there may be a role for monitoring technology to assess the depth of sedation through the analysis of the electroencephalogram (EEG). The bispectral index (BIS monitor, Covidien, Boulder, Colorado) uses an algorithm to interrogate the processed EEG pattern and provide a numeric value ranging from 0 (isoelectric) to 100 (awake with eyes open). Its predominant clinical use has been intraoperatively to monitor the effects of general anesthetic and sedative agents and provide a measure of the depth of anesthesia. (Refer to Chap. 6.) Although still somewhat controversial, it has been suggested that maintenance of a BIS value less than 60–70 correlates with a low probability of intraoperative awareness [24, 25]. The BIS monitor has also been used in settings outside of the operating room including the ICU where assessment of sedation is critical to interventions such as procedural sedation or mechanical ventilation [26–34]. Gill et al. compared BIS values with Ramsay sedation scores in 37 adults who received procedural sedation in the emergency room setting [26]. Although the BIS number correlated with the depth of sedation, there was a wide variability in BIS values at similar sedation scores. The BIS was most effective at differentiating moderate-to-deep sedation from general anesthesia. Brown-McDermott et al. compared BIS values with UMSS scores during procedural sedation administration in 86 children less than 12 years of age [27]. Although there was a good correlation between the BIS value and the sedation score even in patients less than 6 months of age, a wide variability in the range of BIS values for each level of sedation was again noted. Additionally, the BIS monitor was ineffective at determining the depth of sedation when specific agents were used, including ketamine or a combination of oral chloral hydrate, hydroxyzine, and meperidine. The latter is not surprising as the algorithm for the BIS monitor was developed during the use of general anesthetic agents such as propofol or the inhalational anesthetic agents that act through the GABA (gamma-aminobutyric acid) system.

Despite these shortcomings, the BIS monitor may be able to effectively identify patients who are becoming too deeply sedated and may therefore be at risk for adverse respiratory events. Motas et al. demonstrated that the depth of sedation as judged by the BIS monitor was predictive of adverse airway events during the administration of procedural sedation (either propofol, midazolam, or pentobarbital) by non-anesthesiologists [28]. The number of episodes of oxygen desaturation and airway events respectively increased from 1 and 0 of 20 patients when the BIS number was 71–90 to 2 and 3 of 17 patients when the BIS number was 61–70 and to 4 and 4 of 24 patients when the BIS number was less than 60.

BIS monitoring has also been evaluated as a means of evaluating the depth of sedation during prolonged mechanical ventilation. Although the results have been somewhat mixed, the majority of reports have demonstrated a clinically acceptable correlation between the BIS monitor and commonly used ICU sedation scores including the Ramsay or the COMFORT score [29–33]. As with its use during procedural, it has generally been shown that the BIS number correlates with the depth of sedation as assessed with the clinical sedation score, although there is significant variability in the BIS number at each level of sedation. Part of this variation may be related to interference from electromyographic (EMG) artifact from facial musculature, which may falsely elevate the BIS number [34, 35]. The more recent versions of the BIS probe incorporates a sensor that may be able to effectively eliminate EMG interference from the BIS algorithm and thereby address this issue. More importantly, the BIS algorithm was developed for use with propofol or the potent inhalational anesthetic agents that work through the GABA system. Therefore, the BIS monitor has not been shown to be an accurate means of judging the depth of anesthesia with the administration of etomidate or agents that act through the *N*-methyl-D-aspartate (NMDA) system including xenon or nitrous oxide [36–38].

Despite these issues, some form of depth of sedation monitoring may be clinically helpful in situations that preclude the use of conventional ICU scoring systems such as patients receiving neuromuscular blocking agents and/or medications that may alter heart rate and blood pressure responses and thereby negate the utility of clinical sedation scoring systems [39–42]. Additionally, technology such as the BIS monitor provides a continuous numeric readout using a simple 0–100 scale that is immediately available at the bedside as opposed to sedation scoring systems that provide only an intermittent assessment and require time to assess and add various parameters.

Basic Principles

Identification of the cause of the distress can be used to guide the selection of the most appropriate agent(s) for sedation and analgesia in the PICU. Tissue injury, an acute inflammatory process, or performance of a painful invasive procedure is generally best treated by an agent with analgesic properties, while emotional distress and anxiety may be more appropriately treated with agents that possess sedative, anxiolytic, and amnestic properties. Another variable is the duration of time during which sedation is required. Sedation may be required for less than 5 min for an invasive procedure, 1–2 h during an MRI scan, or days to weeks in a patient requiring prolonged mechanical ventilation or extracorporeal support. Short-acting drugs that provide rapid recovery may be chosen for brief procedures, while intermittent dosing of longer-acting agents or continuous infusions of short-acting agents can be used for prolonged procedures. There may be associated comorbid diseases that alter the end-organ effects of these agents, their adverse profile, and metabolism or elimination.

To date, there is limited evidence-based medicine from which to develop guidelines for the use of sedative and analgesic agents in the PICU setting. When compared with the adult population, there remains a paucity of data regarding the pharmacokinetics and pharmacodynamic properties of analgesic and sedative drugs in critically ill infants and children [43–45]. When available, these pharmacokinetic studies are generally performed in healthy adult volunteers with the attempted extrapolation of these results to critically ill infants and children. The comorbidities present in the PICU may affect the volume of distribution and elimination half-life, thereby further altering the pharmacokinetics of these agents. Additional variabilities in the PICU setting are likely to result from drug–drug interactions, end-organ (hepatic, renal) failure or dysfunction, malnutrition, low plasma proteins with altered drug binding, alterations in uptake of the medication if non-intravenous routes are used, and alterations in drug distribution.

Pharmacogenetic factors may also affect responses to medications including the response to acute illness and the metabolism and elimination of various medications [46, 47]. These genetic variations may also alter drug receptors and the patient's response to various sedative and analgesic agents [48, 49]. As there are currently limited means of identifying the impact of these many factors on the pharmacokinetics and pharmacodynamics of the medications that we use for sedation and analgesia in the PICU setting, it is imperative that the effects of these agents are continuously evaluated and the dose titrated based on the patient's response. An example of such variability, likely a multifactorial phenomenon in the PICU population, is demonstrated by an evaluation of fentanyl infusion requirements to provide sedation during mechanical ventilation in neonates and infants [50]. To achieve a similar level of sedation, the fentanyl infusion requirements varied from 0.47 up to 10.3 μ(mu)g/kg/h. Therefore, it is not feasible to approach the provision of sedation and analgesia in the PICU patient using a "cookbook" with specific guidelines concerning the medications to be used and their doses. Sedative and analgesic agents cannot be dosed on a per kilogram basis; rather, the infusion rate should be titrated up and down to achieve the desired level of sedation. The dosing recommendations provided in this chapter for the specific medications discussed are meant only as guidelines for starting doses. The actual dose should be titrated up or down to achieve the desired level of sedation or analgesia while attempting to avoid adverse effects [51].

More recently, the variability and the potential for adverse effects including prolonged sedation have led to the suggestion of using "drug holidays" on a daily basis. This process involves discontinuing the administration of sedative and analgesic agents until the patient awakens and then restarting the infusions at 50–75 % of the previous rate. In a prospective trial in 128 adults requiring mechanical ventilation, the median duration of mechanical ventilation was 4.9 days in the intervention group and 7.3 days in the control group ($p=0.004$) [52]. The median length of stay in the intensive care unit was 6.4 days as compared with 9.9 days, respectively ($p=0.02$). Six of the patients in the intervention group (9 %) underwent diagnostic testing to assess changes in mental status as compared with 16 or 27 % of the patients in the control group ($p=0.02$). Complications (including removal of the endotracheal tube by the patient) occurred in three of the patients in the intervention group and four of the patients in the control group ($p=$NS). The demonstration of improvements in outcome with such interventions has led to the widespread adoption of such practices in the adult population. Such therapy has been championed by the ICU physicians at Vanderbilt University with the development of the ABCDE bundle. This involves a group of ICU measures including spontaneous awakening and breathing coordination, attention to the choice of sedation, delirium monitoring, and early mobility and exercise. Additional work has demonstrated the potential impact of focusing on titration of ventilatory assistance to achieve synchrony with the patient rather than pushing sedation to eliminate spontaneous ventilation [53].

Despite the potential difficulties and risks of sedation and analgesia in the PICU patient, there may be significant benefits. Aside from humanitarian concerns, clinical trials have reported decreases in morbidity and mortality based on the analgesic regimen following cardiovascular surgery for congenital heart disease in neonates and infants [54, 55]. These effects are postulated to be the result of blunting of the endogenous physiologic stress response thereby decreasing release of endogenous catecholamines and adrenal cortical hormones. This physiologic stress response, when excessive, may have deleterious end-organ effects. Aside from its effects on the physiologic stress response, analgesia and sedation may provide benefits in other clinical scenarios in the PICU patient. Techniques for cardiac and respiratory support such as permissive hypercapnia, reverse I:E ratio ventilation, high-frequency ventilation, and extracorporeal support may be feasible only with effective control of the patient's agitation. Analgesia and sedation may also provide therapeutic benefits in the treatment of intracranial hypertension or to modulate pulmonary vascular resistance (PVR) in patients at risk for pulmonary hypertension. The effective use of sedation and analgesia may limit the need for neuromuscular blocking agents and their associated adverse effects [56].

Choice of Agent and Route of Delivery

The three primary decision points for sedation and analgesia in the PICU include the agent, its route of administration, and its mode of administration. The remainder of this chapter will focus on a brief discussion of each agent, its pharmacology, clinical applications, and adverse effect profile. Although the intravenous route is chosen in most clinical scenarios, alternative routes may be required in specific clinical scenarios or patient populations. Furthermore, there is expanding knowledge and interest regarding the use of alternative routes, especially inhalational anesthesia or subcutaneous administration in the PICU setting. These routes may be chosen as the primary route or used as an alternative when drug incompatibilities or limited venous access precludes intravenous administration. However, the availability of alternative routes is agent specific. Chloral hydrate must be administered by the oral or rectal route, isoflurane requires inhalation administration, while propofol is administered only via the intravenous route. Midazolam and ketamine provide the greatest options for route of administration with reports of intravenous, intramuscular, subcutaneous, oral, nasal, and sublingual administration. The third decision point is the mode of administration. Options include continuous administration, intermittent dosing, or patient-controlled techniques. When there is a prolonged need for sedation such as during mechanical ventilation, agents with long elimination half-times may be used by intermittent, bolus administration, while short-acting agents are generally best administered by a continuous infusion to maintain a steady-state serum concentration and thereby provide a stable level of sedation.

Inhalational Anesthetic Agents

Despite their introduction into clinical practice more than 150 years ago, the potent inhalational anesthetic agents remain one of the integral components for the provision of general anesthesia. They are used on a daily basis during the perioperative period to provide amnesia and analgesia during major and minor surgical procedures. Based on their chemical structure, these agents can be divided into alkanes such as halothane or substituted ethers. Although it was the mainstay of pediatric anesthesia for decades, halothane is no longer commonly used and will not be discussed in great detail. The agents in use include the methyl, ethyl ethers (isoflurane, desflurane) and the isopropyl ether, sevoflurane. The characteristics of these agents that may make them useful agents for ICU sedation include a rapid onset, rapid awakening upon discontinuation, and the ability to rapidly control the depth of sedation. As these agents are volatile substances, they are vaporized and administered by the inhalation route. The potent inhalational anesthetic agents also provide specific therapeutic end-organ effects including bronchodilation, myocardial preconditioning, and cerebral protection. Although experience with use of the potent inhalational anesthetic agents for ICU sedation in the United States is limited, certain centers in Europe and the United Kingdom have reported favorable experiences with these agents in adult ICU patients [57]. For a full review of the end-organ effects of these agents, their applications in the pediatric ICU, and techniques for their delivery, the reader is referred to the article by Tobias [58].

Although there are reports concerning the administration of all of the potent inhalational anesthetic agents as either therapeutic agents or for sedation in the ICU setting [59, 60], the majority of reports have used isoflurane. Despite the fact that these agents are all considered in the category of the potent inhalational anesthetic agents, their physiologic effects are distinctly different. Various adverse physiologic effects have been reported with halothane including a negative inotropic and chronotropic effect on myocardial function, the potential for a pro-arrhythmogenic effect especially in the setting of increased catecholamines or when used in conjunction with other medications (e.g., aminophylline), and the potential for the development of hepatitis related to an immunologic reaction directed against the oxidative metabolite, trifluoroacetic acid (TFA) [61, 62]. Hepatitis may occur with any of the inhalational anesthetic agents except for sevoflurane as its metabolic pathway does not result in the production of TFA. The incidence of hepatitis is extremely low with isoflurane compared to halothane due to its limited metabolism of 0.1–0.2 % compared with that of halothane (15–20 %). Given the potential for adverse effects on myocardial function and its association with perioperative cardiac arrests in infants and children, halothane is no longer in use in the United States [63, 64].

Metabolism of the inhalational anesthetic agents can also result in the release of inorganic fluoride and the potential for nephrotoxicity. This was primarily a concern with enflurane, which is no longer used in clinical practice. Although only 2 % of enflurane undergoes metabolic degradation, given its high fluoride content, serum fluoride concentrations increase with prolonged administration. Plasma fluoride concentrations in excess of 50 μ(mu)mol/L can have deleterious effects on renal function with a decreased glomerular filtration rate and renal tubular resistance to vasopressin with nephrogenic diabetes insipidus. Three to five percent of sevoflurane also undergoes metabolism, and like enflurane, sevoflurane is highly substituted with fluoride. Therefore, its prolonged administration can also result in elevated serum fluoride concentrations. Given limited experience with the prolonged administration of sevoflurane, there are no definite data on which to base decisions regarding the duration of administration.

Desflurane is the newest of the inhalational anesthetic agents. Its beneficial properties include low blood to gas and blood to fat solubility coefficients, thereby resulting in a rapid onset and rapid awakening upon its discontinuation. When compared with propofol for postoperative sedation of adults requiring mechanical ventilation, the emergence time was shorter and more predictable and there was a more rapid mental recovery with desflurane with no difference in the incidence of adverse effects [59]. Medication costs were lower with desflurane than with propofol (€95 Euros for desflurane versus €171 Euros for propofol per 24 h) with additional costs of soda lime (€5 Euros) being comparable to the costs of infusion tubing for propofol (€2.5 Euros). Adverse effects with desflurane include hypotension primarily from peripheral vasodilation, rebound tachycardia from stimulation of the sympathetic nervous system, direct irritant effects on the airway thereby making it less than optimal in patients with airway hyperreactivity, and rare reports of carbon monoxide formation due to desflurane's interaction with desiccated soda lime [65, 66].

Additional concerns with all of the inhalational anesthetic agents include their potential as a trigger agent for malignant hyperthermia, cost issues, effects on intracranial pressure (ICP), and alterations of the metabolism of other medications. As nonspecific vasodilators, all of the inhalational anesthetic agents cause cerebral vasodilation resulting in an increase in ICP in patients with compromised intracranial compliance. The effects on the cerebral vasculature and ICP can be blunted by modest hyperventilation [67, 68]. The inhalational anesthetic agents may alter hepatic blood flow and affect the metabolism of other medications including lidocaine and other local anesthetic agents, ß(beta)-adrenergic antagonists, and benzodiazepines [69].

There remains limited experience with the use of the potent inhalational anesthetic agents for sedation in the PICU setting. Arnold et al. reported their experience with isoflurane for sedation in ten pediatric patients, ranging in age from 3 weeks to 19 years, who required endotracheal intubation and mechanical ventilation for various reasons [70]. Sedation was initiated with isoflurane at an inspired concentration of 0.5 % and adjusted in 0.2 % increments as needed. The duration of administration varied from 29 to 769 h (245 ± 225 h). There was adequate sedation 75 % of the time, excessive sedation 4 % of the time, and inadequate sedation 21 % of the time. In the five patients who received isoflurane for at least 96 MAC (minimum alveolar concentration)-hours, there were no differences in blood urea nitrogen, serum creatinine, osmolality, bilirubin, and alanine aminotransferase between time 0 and 96 h. The duration of isoflurane administration correlated directly with the plasma fluoride concentration. The peak serum fluoride concentration averaged 11.0 ± 6.4 μ(mu)mol/L with a maximum value of 26.1 μ(mu)mol/L after 441 MAC-hours of isoflurane. One patient developed hemodynamic instability, which responded to fluid administration. When it was discontinued, five of the patients, who had received greater than 70 MAC-hours of isoflurane, manifested signs and symptoms of withdrawal including agitation and non-purposeful movements.

Despite the potential advantages of using these agents in the ICU setting, logistic problems regarding delivery continue to impede their widespread introduction into the ICU setting. The exhaled gas from the ventilator or anesthesia machine must be collected or scavenged and vented out of the ICU environment. Additional equipment required for the use of these agents in the ICU includes a vaporizer, which converts the liquid phase of the agent to a gas for delivery, and monitors to measure the end-tidal (exhaled) concentration of the drug. As a full discussion of these issues is beyond the scope of this chapter, the reader is referred to the article by Tobias [58] for a full discussion of delivery options and other considerations regarding the administration of the potent inhalational anesthetic agents in the ICU setting. Given these problems, novel means of delivering these agents are needed.

The Anesthetic Conserving Device or "AnaConDa®" (ACD, Hudson RCI, Upplands Väsby, Sweden) is a modified heat–moisture exchanger that may allow a simplified means of administering the inhalational anesthetic agents in the ICU setting. This device is not currently available in the United States. The device is placed between the Y-piece of the ventilator circuit and the endotracheal tube (ETT). There is also a port at the end of the device just proximal to its attachment to the ETT that allows gas sampling and monitoring of the agent concentration. The desired inspired concentration is titrated by adjusting the infusion rate on the syringe pump based on the manufacturer's recommendations. Exhaled isoflurane is adsorbed to the lipophilic carbon particle filter in the device and redelivered to the patient thereby limiting environmental pollution. Preliminary work has evaluated the ACD in the ICU setting in 40 adult patients requiring sedation for more than 12 h [71]. The patients were randomized to sedation with isoflurane administered with the ACD or a continuous infusion of midazolam. The inspired isoflurane concentration was started at 0.5 % (infusion rate on the syringe pump of 1–3.5 mL/h according to the manufacturer's recommendations) while midazolam was infused at 0.02–0.05 mg/kg/h. The infusion rates were adjusted as needed and opioids administered for analgesia. The percentage of time within the desired level of sedation was similar between the two groups (54 % with isoflurane and 59 % with midazolam) with no difference in opioid requirements or the need for bolus doses of sedative agents. The time to extubation (10 ± 5 versus 252 ± 271 min) and the time to follow verbal commands (10 ± 8 versus 110 ± 132 min) were shorter with isoflurane than with midazolam. Isoflurane-sedated patients had normal urine volumes and creatinine clearances. The inorganic fluoride concentration was greater than 50 μ(mu)mol/L in three patients with a maximum value of 64 μ(mu)mol/L during isoflurane sedation. Anecdotal experience with the device has also been reported in three pediatric patients who required sedation during mechanical ventilation or in the treatment of status epilepticus [72]. Effective sedation was achieved with isoflurane concentrations of 0.3–0.4 %, while 0.9 % was required to control status epilepticus. In 2 patients, who weighed 30 and 40 kg, respectively, the ACD was placed distal to the Y-piece as described in the adult population. In the third patient, who weighed 20 kg, when the ACD was placed in this position, the patient became tachypneic with an increase in his respiratory rate from 25 to 35 breaths per minute. Although several ventilatory changes were attempted to compensate for the dead space added by the ACD, effective ventilation could not be achieved. The ACD was removed and placed into the inspiratory limb of the ventilator circuit. This allowed effective ventilation and delivery of isoflurane; however, the authors commented that by using the ACD in this position, there would be a loss of the rebreathing function of the device and no conservation or scavenging of isoflurane. There was also an increase in the dead space of the system. The authors subsequently cautioned against the use of this device distal to the Y-piece in patients weighing less than 30 kg until a smaller model becomes available. They suggested that using the device in the inspiratory limb was a simpler technique than bringing a vaporizer into the PICU setting.

Benzodiazepines

The benzodiazepines remain the most commonly used agent for sedation during mechanical ventilation in the PICU patient. These agents produce amnesia, anxiolysis, and sedation through their effects on the inhibitory neurotransmitter, γ(gamma)-aminobutyric acid (GABA). Benzodiazepines bind to the α(alpha)-subunit of the GABA receptor thereby facilitating binding of the GABA molecule to the β(beta)-subunit resulting in increased chloride conduction across the neuronal membrane and hyperpolarization. Benzodiazepines in common clinical use for sedation in the PICU include midazolam and lorazepam.

Another benzodiazepine, although formerly a commonly used agent, is no longer used in the majority of pediatric ICUs across the country. Although its lipid solubility is greater than that of midazolam, thereby resulting in a more rapid penetration into the CNS and a more rapid onset, its low water solubility requires administration in a solution of propylene glycol. This diluent frequently results in pain and thrombophlebitis when administered through a peripheral vein. Alternatively, diazepam is available in a lipid-based formulation, which has been shown to alleviate the discomfort associated with the intravenous administration of the propylene glycol preparation [73, 74]. More importantly, diazepam is no longer used in the PICU because of its prolonged duration of action with repeated or continuous administration as well as its metabolism to active compounds including oxazepam and *N*-desmethyldiazepam. These active metabolites have elimination half-lives that far exceed the parent compound.

Midazolam is an imidazobenzodiazepine with a rapid onset of action and a short elimination half-life [75]. Given its rapid onset and water solubility with limited pain on injection, midazolam has found a role for both procedural sedation when administered by intermittent bolus dosing and sedation during mechanical ventilation when used as a continuous infusion except for brief procedures. Clinical experience and years of its use have demonstrated its efficacy for sedation in the PICU patient in doses ranging from 0.05 to 0.2 mg/kg/h [76, 77]. Although previously cost issues were significant, its availability in generic form makes it a cost-effective form of sedation. In a retrospective cohort of 55 pediatric patients requiring mechanical ventilation, sedation was provided by midazolam starting with a bolus dose of 0.25 mg/kg followed by a continuous infusion of 0.4–4 μ(mu)g/kg/min (0.02–0.2 mg/kg/h) [78]. Midazolam was effective in all patients without significant hemodynamic effects. Sedation was ineffective in one patient following the institution of extracorporeal membrane oxygenation (ECMO), which was postulated to be the result of midazolam binding to the membrane oxygenator. Similar efficacy has been reported by other investigators [79]. In the latter study, the investigators noted a significant variation of the plasma concentrations between the patients despite using the same infusion rate. Two infants with gestational ages less than 32 weeks had plasma concentrations greater than 1,000 ng/mL, thereby suggesting decreased clearance in preterm infants. This demonstrates the significant variability in the pharmacokinetics of medications that undergo hepatic metabolism given the immaturity of the hepatic microsomal P450 system.

Although intravenous administration is generally the route chosen in the PICU patient, midazolam remains unique among many of the other agents used for sedation in the ICU setting in that alternative, non-intravenous routes of delivery have been used clinically including oral, rectal, transmucosal (nasal, rectal, sublingual), and subcutaneous administration [80–83]. These non-intravenous routes (oral, rectal, and transmucosal) have generally been used in the arena of procedural sedation or as a premedicant prior to anesthetic induction, while subcutaneous administration has been used with a slow weaning protocol to prevent withdrawal following prolonged administration of benzodiazepines [84]. With all of these non-intravenous routes except for subcutaneous administration, increased doses are required due to decreased bioavailability. Bioavailability is approximately 60–70 % for nasal administration and as low as 30 % for oral administration.

In many centers in the United States, oral midazolam is currently the preferred agent for premedication in the operating room. Doses for oral administration have ranged from 0.25 up to 0.7 mg/kg. If the standard intravenous preparation is used for oral administration, the primary disadvantage is a bitter taste related to the preservative, benzyl alcohol. Although the taste can be masked by mixing the medication in some type of flavored solution, concern has been raised regarding the potential for the alteration of its absorption characteristics. Midazolam normally exists in an equilibrium of two chemical structures: an open and a closed ring form. The ratio of these two compounds in the solution is pH dependent so that with a lower pH, there is more of the open ring or the physiologically inactive configuration. A commercially available preparation of midazolam in a cherry-flavored solution for oral administration is available (Versed syrup, Roche Laboratories Inc, Nutley, NJ). Because of the control of pH during the manufacturing process, clinical data suggest that effective sedation can be achieved with doses as low as 0.25 mg/kg compared to the 0.5–1.0 mg/kg doses reported when using the IV preparation diluted in other solutions for oral administration [85].

Intranasal and sublingual administration has also been well described in the literature. With these routes, as the bioavailability is greater than with oral administration, the dose (0.2–0.4 mg/kg) is lower and the onset more rapid, occurring in as little as 5–10 min. This is avoided with sublingual administration, but issues of taste and patient cooperation may limit the usefulness of this route. With intranasal administration, the patient may object as the preservative, benzyl alcohol, irritates the nasal mucosa. Although the medication is frequently dripped into the nose from a tuberculin syringe, several devices (atomizers) are available that provide a fine mist to contact the mucosa. These may improve contact of the medication with the nasal mucosa, thereby increasing the absorption as well as decreasing the pain related to the diluent.

Midazolam is metabolized by isoforms of the hepatic $P_{450}3A$ enzyme system to the major hydroxylated metabolite, 1-OH midazolam. 1-OH midazolam is approximately equipotent with the parent compound. It undergoes further hepatic metabolism via the glucuronyl transferase system to 1-OH midazolam glucuronide, a water-soluble metabolite, which is renally excreted. In the presence of renal insufficiency, 1-OH midazolam glucuronide accumulates, thereby potentiating the effects of midazolam [86]. Several factors, including age and underlying illness, may also alter midazolam pharmacokinetics. With metabolism dependent on the hepatic P_{450} system, clearance changes from infancy to adult age and with alterations in hepatic function [87, 88]. Additional changes may occur related to critical illness. In a cohort of 21 PICU patients, midazolam clearance was significantly longer (5.5 ± 3.5 h) than that reported in healthy age-matched children (1.2 ± 0.3 h) [89, 90]. Another issue of clinical significance when continuous infusions are used is the context-sensitive half-time of the medication. Given the pharmacodynamics of many medications, although their half-lives are short and their clinical effects dissipate rapidly following a single bolus dose, the effects can be prolonged following a continuous infusion. This is especially true of drugs that follow a multi-compartmental model [91]. Given these concerns, there is a new benzodiazepine on the horizon, remimazolam, which, like remifentanil, undergoes ester metabolism with a plasma half-life of minutes [92]. Given this unique property, there may be limited context sensitivity in its pharmacokinetic parameters.

Lorazepam is a water-soluble benzodiazepine that is metabolized by glucuronyl transferase to pharmacologically inactive compounds. Medications known to alter the P_{450} system (anticonvulsants, rifampin, cimetidine) and genetic polymorphisms do not impact lorazepam's pharmacokinetics. In advanced liver disease, phase II reactions (glucuronyl transferase) are better preserved than phase I reactions (P_{450} system) so that the pharmacokinetics of lorazepam remain unchanged. Although the Society of Critical Care Medicine's initial guidelines for sedation of adult patients in the ICU setting recommended lorazepam as the preferred sedative, the most recent guidelines, which were published in 2013, have suggested that sedation with non-benzodiazepines (propofol or dexmedetomidine) may be preferred over lorazepam or midazolam [93, 94]. The guidelines relate this change in practice to the increasing literature suggesting that clinical outcomes are improved with non-benzodiazepine sedation including length of mechanical ventilation and the incidence of delirium.

In comparison to midazolam, there are a limited number of reports regarding the use of lorazepam for sedation in the PICU patient. When comparing lorazepam with midazolam in adult ICU patients, the mean infusion rates to achieve adequate sedation were 0.06 mg/kg/h for lorazepam and 0.15 mg/kg/h for midazolam [95, 96]. There were fewer infusion rate adjustments per day with lorazepam than with midazolam (1.9 for lorazepam versus 3.6 for midazolam). The mean time to return to baseline mental status was also shorter with lorazepam (261 min with lorazepam versus 1,815 min with midazolam). Three of six surviving patients in the midazolam group required more than 24 h to return to their baseline mental status, while all 7 patients in the lorazepam group returned to baseline in less than 12 h.

Prior to its availability as a generic medication, enteral lorazepam was suggested as a means to decrease intravenous midazolam dosing requirements and drug costs during mechanical ventilation in a cohort of 30 infants and children [97]. Midazolam was used for sedation until the requirements were stable for 24 h. Enteral lorazepam equivalence was calculated to be 1/6th of the total daily intravenous midazolam dose. Following the administration of enteral lorazepam, there was a significant reduction in midazolam requirements on day 1, and by day 3, the midazolam infusion was discontinued in 24 of 30 patients. When considering acquisition costs at the time of the study (late 1990s), the projected savings were more than $40,000 for the 30 patients. Enteral lorazepam has also been successfully used for the treatment or prevention of withdrawal following the prolonged administration of intravenous benzodiazepines for sedation during mechanical ventilation in the PICU population [98].

Each mL of the intravenous lorazepam solution (2 mg lorazepam per mL of solution) contains 0.8 mL or 800 mg of propylene glycol. With prolonged or high-dose intravenous administration, issues may arise related to the diluent used in the intravenous formulations, propylene glycol [99–101]. Signs and symptoms of propylene glycol toxicity include metabolic acidosis, renal failure/insufficiency, mental status changes, hemolysis, and an elevated osmolar gap (see later). Propylene glycol is metabolized in the liver to lactic acid and pyruvic acid, which, in part, accounts for lactic acidosis. Propylene glycol is also excreted unchanged in the urine, making toxicity more likely in patients with renal insufficiency. Attention to the propylene glycol infusion rate and periodic calculation of the osmolar gap (measured minus calculated serum osmolarity) may be indicated during high-dose or prolonged lorazepam infusions. An increasing osmolar gap has been shown to be predictive of increasing serum propylene glycol levels [101]. The osmolar gap is used to predict propylene glycol levels as actual plasma propylene glycol concentrations—although they can be measured by reference laboratories (concentrations greater than 18 mg/dL can be associated with toxicity)—are not routinely available in most hospitals. As neonates and especially preterm infants are unable to handle propylene glycol related to hepatic and renal immaturity, continuous infusions of lorazepam are not recommended in this population. In a cohort of 11 PICU patients, who received lorazepam infusions ranging from 0.1 to 0.33 mg/kg/h for 3–14 days, the propylene glycol concentration increased from 86 ± 93 μ(mu)g/mL at baseline to 763 ± 660 μ(mu)g/mL at the completion of the infusion [102]. The plasma propylene glycol concentration correlated with the cumulative dose of lorazepam. No end-organ effects, related to the increased propylene glycol concentrations such as acidosis or hyperosmolarity, were noted in these patients. The authors recommended periodic monitoring for lactic acidosis and hyperosmolarity during prolonged lorazepam infusions.

Etomidate

Etomidate (Amidate™, Abbott Pharmaceuticals) is an intravenous anesthetic agent, introduced into clinical practice in 1972. Its primary effects of sedation and amnesia are mediated through the GABA inhibitory neurotransmitter system. Unlike other sedative and hypnotic agents, only the R(+) enantiomer has clinical effects. Following intravenous administration, loss of consciousness is rapid (15–20 s), and as with propofol and the barbiturates, its duration of action following a single bolus dose is related to redistribution rather than metabolism and clearance. Etomidate undergoes hepatic metabolism with an elimination half-life that varies from 2.9 to 5.3 h [103]. Beneficial CNS effects include a decrease of the cerebral metabolic rate for oxygen ($CMRO_2$), cerebral blood flow (CBF), and ICP. Given its limited impact on myocardial function and blood pressure, cerebral perfusion pressure (CPP) is maintained even in patients with comorbid hemodynamic conditions. In an animal model, no hemodynamic changes were noted with etomidate (0.3 mg/kg), while propofol (2.5 mg/kg) decreased systolic blood pressure by 19.9 %, diastolic blood pressure by 25.3 %, cardiac output by 17.3 %, and systemic vascular resistance (SVR) by 11.6 % [104].

When compared with other sedative agents, there remains limited data regarding the use of etomidate in pediatric-aged patients with that observation that doses of 0.3 mg/kg are required for anesthetic induction [105, 106]. Other investigators found no clinically significant effects following anesthetic induction with etomidate (0.3 mg/kg) in a cohort of 30 pediatric patients with congenital heart disease (left-to-right and right-to-left shunts) [107]. Anecdotally, the successful use of etomidate has been reported in infants and children with depressed myocardial function [108, 109]. Despite the relatively limited clinical and outcome data, recent reviews continue to suggest its use as a single bolus dose for critically ill pediatric patients requiring endotracheal intubation [110, 111]. However, concerns remain regarding the universal use of etomidate for endotracheal intubation in the critically ill pediatric patient (see later).

Etomidate results in a dose-dependent depressant effect on respiratory function and can result in apnea depending on the dose used, concomitant use of other medications, and the patient's underlying status [112–115]. The effect on ventilator function has been shown to be similar to that which occurs with benzodiazepines and droperidol and less than that with the barbiturates. Etomidate results a shift of the CO_2 response curve to the right without a change in the slope. These effects have led some to suggest that etomidate can be used when maintenance of spontaneous ventilation is desirable. However, caution should be maintained; the effect is magnified by the concomitant administration of other sedative and analgesic agents including opioids of benzodiazepines.

Etomidate's place as an agent for procedural sedation (especially endotracheal intubation) results from its negligible effects on myocardial function, even in patients with significant alterations in myocardial function. This combined with its beneficial effects on the CNS (reduction of the $CMRO_2$ leading to cerebral vasoconstriction, decreased CBF, and decreased ICP) results in maintenance of CPP [116, 117]. Despite its ability to lower CBF and ICP, induction or sedative doses of etomidate can produce increased EEG activity and epileptic-like EEG potentials in patients with underlying seizure disorders [117–120]. Myoclonic movements are also a frequently observed effect following the rapid intravenous administration of etomidate [121]. Although these movements may simulate tonic–clonic seizure activity, no epileptiform discharges are noted. It has been suggested that the myoclonic movements are of spinal origin resulting from disinhibition of inhibitory neuronal pathways. Pretreatment with fentanyl, benzodiazepines, or a small dose of etomidate has been shown to be effective in decreasing the incidence of myoclonus. A trial of etomidate for sedation during computerized tomography was discontinued due to an unacceptably high incidence of involuntary motor movements preventing completion of the scan [122].

The most significant concern with etomidate and the factor that limits its long-term administration in the ICU and perioperative setting are its effects on the endogenous production of corticosteroids. This effect was initially identified when an increased risk of mortality was noted in adult ICU patients who were sedated with a continuous infusion of etomidate [123]. Etomidate inhibits the enzyme 11-β(beta)-hydroxylase which is necessary for a key step in the production of cortisol, aldosterone, and corticosterone. Although the implications of this effect are evident with prolonged infusions or repeated doses, there remains controversy regarding the clinical significance of adrenal suppression following a single dose. However, there are some authorities and investigators calling for the abandonment, or at least a reevaluation, of the use of etomidate [124–127]. The duration of adrenal suppression produced by a single induction dose of etomidate has varied from study to study. Duthie et al. demonstrated a decrease in plasma cortisol levels 1 h following an induction dose of etomidate; however, at 24 h no difference was noted between those patients receiving etomidate and those receiving other induction agents [128]. Other authors have suggested a more prolonged suppression of adrenocortical function. Following a single induction dose (0.3 mg/kg) in pediatric patients undergoing surgery for congenital heart disease, plasma cortisol levels were depressed during cardiopulmonary bypass (CPB), at the end of the operation, and at 24 h [129]. A similar effect with ongoing suppression of adrenal function at 24 h was reported in a cohort of critically ill adult patients [130]. The incidence of adrenal insufficiency (defined as a failure of the serum cortisol level to increase by 9 μ(mu)g/dL after a 250-μ(mu)g ACTH stimulation test) following a single dose of etomidate was 80 % at 12 h, 9 % at 48 h, and 7 % at 72 h [131]. Despite these findings, no difference in outcome was reported following etomidate administration even when there was accompanying effects on adrenal function, and, in fact, vasopressor therapy was required less frequently and in smaller doses when etomidate was used in a cohort of 159 adult patients with septic shock [132].

However, conflicting and more compelling data against the use of etomidate, at least in patients with possible sepsis, comes from the CORTICUS trial [133]. Although the trail was intended to evaluate the efficacy of corticosteroid therapy on outcome in adults with septic shock and adrenal insufficiency, post hoc analysis revealed that patients who had received etomidate had a significantly higher mortality rate. Additionally, this increased risk of mortality was not prevented by the administration of corticosteroids. These data suggest that etomidate should be avoided in patients with sepsis or septic shock; however, there are no definitive data to suggest its elimination from clinical use in other scenarios. Although the use of etomidate has decreased in many centers or has even been totally eliminated, given its beneficial effects on hemodynamic function and intracranial dynamics, until further data are available, it seems prudent to consider its use in critically ill patients outside of the sepsis arena. Perhaps the greater risk may be the potential for cardiovascular collapse when other agents that have significant cardiovascular effects are used in critically ill patients.

In addition to its effects on adrenal function, reports regarding continuous etomidate infusions with increased mortality suggested an association with infectious complications. Neutrophils incubated in vitro with etomidate demonstrate depressed chemiluminescence, an index of oxygen free radical generation, suggesting that etomidate may interfere with white blood cell bactericidal activity [134]. Even without effects on cortisol production, it has been suggested that the incidence of hospital-acquired pneumonia in adult trauma patients may be higher when etomidate is used. In a subset analysis of the HYPOLYTE study, a multicenter trial evaluating the use of hydrocortisone in trauma patients, 95 of the 149 patients enrolled in the trial received etomidate within 36 h of inclusion [135]. Forty-nine (51.6 %) patients who received etomidate developed hospital-acquired pneumonia compared to 16 patients (29.6 %) who did not receive etomidate ($p=0.009$). The hazard ratio for hospital-acquired pneumonia was 2.48 with etomidate, although there was no difference in the duration of mechanical ventilation.

Additional reported adverse effects with etomidate, related to the drug itself or the diluent, include anaphylactoid reactions, pain on injection, and an increased incidence of nausea and vomiting [136]. Issues related to the carrier vehicle (propylene glycol) include pain on injection, thrombophlebitis, and propylene glycol toxicity. The incidence of pain on injection has been reported to be as high as 50 %, is greater with injection into small veins on the dorsum of the head, and can be decreased by the preadministration of lidocaine (1.5 mg/kg) or fentanyl (2–3 μ(mu)g/kg). Olesen et al. evaluated the occurrence of pain on injection and the subsequent development of thrombophlebitis in 61 patients randomized to anesthetic induction with either etomidate or thiopentone [137]. Of the patients who received thiopentone, none complained of pain and 4 % developed thrombophlebitis. With etomidate, pain and the development of thrombophlebitis were noted in 24 %. A newer formulation, which contains etomidate dissolved in a fat emulsion of medium- and long-chain triglycerides, may limit the occurrence of injection pain and thrombophlebitis [138]. As with lorazepam, issues may arise with repeated dosing or continuous infusions of etomidate because of the diluent, propylene glycol (please note that given concerns regarding adrenal suppression, long-term etomidate infusions are no longer used in the ICU setting) [139–141].

Despite these issues, given its beneficial effects on CNS dynamics and myocardial function, etomidate has yet to be abandoned in critically ill patients and may still play a role as an effective agent to provide sedation and amnesia during endotracheal intubation [142]. Its lack of cardiovascular effects makes it particularly valuable in patients who may not tolerate a decrease in SVR or myocardial contractility. Given its effects on cerebral dynamics, it also should be considered for patients with increased ICP with or without associated myocardial dysfunction. Given the ongoing concerns regarding the potential for adrenal suppression, ongoing pharmacologic investigation has focused on the development of etomidate-like medications that lack the depressant effect on adrenal function. Carboetomidate was developed based on the hypothesis that the basic nitrogen in the imidazole ring of etomidate binds with high affinity to the heme site of the 11 β(beta)-hydroxylase enzyme [143]. This binding triggers a conformational transition in which the enzyme closes tightly around the bound ligand and becomes nonfunctional. Future clinical trials are needed to fully demonstrate the clinical applications and physiological properties of carbo-etomidate.

Ketamine

Ketamine was introduced into clinical practice during the 1960s [144]. The term *dissociative anesthesia* is used to describe the state of amnesia and analgesia that is achieved as patients may keep their eyes open and yet be unresponsive to painful stimuli. Ketamine's anesthetic (sedative, analgesic, and amnestic) properties are mediated through various postulated mechanisms including agonism at opioid receptors and antagonism of NMDA receptors. A unique attribute of ketamine, which separates it from the majority of other agents, is the provision of both amnesia and analgesia. Ketamine contains a chiral carbon in its structure, and the preparation currently used most commonly in clinical practice is a racemic mixture of the two optical isomers S(+) and R(−). However, in the United Kingdom and Europe, the enantiomer S(+) ketamine is available, with the suggestion from preliminary clinical trials that it may provide effective analgesia and sedation while limiting adverse effects including emergence phenomena (see later). Metabolism of ketamine occurs primarily by hepatic N-methylation to norketamine, which retains approximately one-third of the analgesic and sedative properties of the parent compound. Given its dependence on hepatic metabolism, doses should be adjusted in patients with hepatic dysfunction. Dose adjustments may also be required in patients with renal dysfunction since norketamine is dependent on renal elimination.

Beneficial properties of ketamine include preservation of cardiovascular function, limited effects on respiratory mechanics, and maintenance of central control of respiration. These properties make it an effective and popular agent in the arena of procedural sedation during painful, invasive procedures in the spontaneously breathing patient [145]. Incremental doses (0.5–1 mg/kg) can be administered every 1–2 min and titrated to achieve the desired level of sedation and analgesia while generally maintaining spontaneous ventilation. An anti-sialogogue such as glycopyrrolate to prevent salivation and a benzodiazepine to limit the occurrence of emergence phenomena are frequently used with ketamine.

Given its effects at the opioid and NMDA receptors, there is growing interest in the use of ketamine for the management of acute pain, especially during the postoperative period. When coadministered in low doses during morphine analgesia, ketamine has been shown to reduce postoperative opioid consumption and lower opioid-related adverse effects following major surgical procedures in the adult population [146–149]. As NMDA receptor stimulation may be one factor resulting in the development of tolerance to opioid-induced sedation and analgesia, there is interest in the potential benefits of using a low-dose ketamine infusion to delay tolerance during prolonged ICU infusions of morphine and other opioids. Despite the theoretical rationale behind this practice, to date there are no trials to demonstrate a clinically significant effect of this practice.

Ketamine's popularity in the arena of procedural sedation, especially painful invasive procedures, relates to its beneficial effects on cardiac and respiratory function. Ketamine generally increases heart rate and blood pressure as well as provides bronchodilation due to the release of endogenous catecholamines [150]. Although the indirect sympathomimetic effects from endogenous catecholamine release generally overshadow ketamine's direct negative inotropic properties, acting to maintain blood pressure and heart rate, hypotension and even cardiovascular collapse may occur in patients with diminished myocardial contractility as ketamine's direct negative inotropic properties may predominate when endogenous catecholamine stores have been depleted by stress or chronic illness [151–153].

An issue of potential concern and ongoing controversy regarding ketamine is its effects on PVR [154–157]. As these studies were generally performed without full mechanical ventilation support and control of the $PaCO_2$, it is not possible to determine whether the changes in PVR were directly related to ketamine or a consequence of increases in the $PaCO_2$. Most recently, Williams et al. evaluated the effects of ketamine on PVR during sevoflurane anesthesia (0.5 MAC) and spontaneous ventilation in 15 infants and children with pulmonary hypertension (mean PA pressure ≥25 mmHg, baseline PVR index of 11.3 Woods units) [158]. One-third of the patients had PA pressures that were suprasystemic. Ketamine was administered as a bolus of 2 mg/kg followed by an infusion at 10 μ(mu)g/kg/min. There were no significant changes in mean systemic arterial pressure, SVR index, mean pulmonary artery pressure, PVR index, cardiac index, and $PaCO_2$. The safety of ketamine in patients with congenital heart disease is further evidenced by experience with its use during spontaneous ventilation for sedation during cardiac catheterization [159, 160]. In a prospective evaluation of sedation during cardiac catheterization in infants and children, Lebovic et al. reported less hypotension with ketamine compared with propofol, although the recovery times were significantly longer with ketamine [160].

Ketamine has also been shown to have limited effects on several respiratory parameters including functional residual capacity, minute ventilation, and tidal volume [161, 162]. The release of endogenous catecholamines generally results in improved pulmonary compliance, decreased resistance, and prevention of bronchospasm [163]. These effects generally result in the clinical use of ketamine when endotracheal intubation is required in patients with status asthmaticus. Despite the fact that minute ventilation is maintained, hypercarbia with a rightward shift of the CO_2 response curve may occur [164]. However, like any sedative/analgesic/general anesthetic agent, ketamine can result in loss of protective airway reflexes, gastric aspiration, and apnea [165, 166]. These latter issues including the potential for respiratory depression are more likely to be clinically significant when ketamine is administered with opioids. An additional effect that may impact on airway patency and the potential for airway obstruction or laryngospasm is that ketamine may increase oral and airway secretions. These effects have resulted in the common clinical practice of administering an anticholinergic agent such as atropine (0.01 mg/kg) or glycopyrrolate (0.005 mg/kg) with ketamine. However, recent studies demonstrate that the actual risk of hypersalivation is low and that the use of these adjunct medications may be unnecessary, thereby resulting in an ongoing controversy regarding ketamine [167–169]. The incidence of airway problems such as laryngospasm with ketamine is higher when there is a history of an antecedent upper respiratory infection and perhaps in those patients chronically exposed to tobacco smoke. Despite the potential for increased airway secretions, reactivity, and even laryngospasm, ketamine has been used effectively for the sedation of infants during flexible fiberoptic bronchoscopy with the maintenance of spontaneous ventilation [170].

An additional area of controversy surrounding ketamine is its effect on ICP. These effects may be indirect, secondary to changes in $PaCO_2$, or the result of a direct effect on the cerebral vasculature. Clinical work from the 1970s reported that ketamine increased ICP, thereby suggesting that it was contraindicated in patients with altered intracranial compliance [171, 172]. These clinical studies were supported by animal investigations demonstrating that the alterations in ICP resulted from direct cerebral vasodilation, which was mediated through central cholinergic receptors [173, 174]. However, more recent data from both animal and human studies have shown no change or even a decrease in ICP following ketamine [175, 176]. Ketamine in doses of 1.5, 3, or 5 mg/kg decreased ICP when administered to adult head trauma patients who were sedated with propofol and mechanically ventilated to maintain a $PaCO_2$ of 35–38 mmHg [177]. The ICP decreased by 2 ± 0.5, 4 ± 1, and 5 ± 2 mmHg with doses of 1.5, 3, and 5 mg/kg respectively. There was no change in CPP, jugular bulb venous oxygen saturation, or middle cerebral artery blood flow velocity. Similar results were reported by Bourgoin et al. when comparing the effects of sedation with either a combination of ketamine and midazolam or sufentanil and midazolam in 25 adult patients with traumatic brain injury (TBI) [178]. The patients were receiving mechanical ventilation and modest hyperventilation. There were no differences in the number of ICP elevations during the study period. Patients receiving ketamine and midazolam had significantly higher heart rate values on days 3 and 4, decreased fluid requirements on day 1, as well as a trend toward decreased vasopressor use when compared with the sufentanil–midazolam group. Mayberg et al. reported that a 1 mg/kg bolus dose of ketamine (1 mg/kg) decreased ICP from 16 ± 1 to 14 ± 1 mmHg with no change in CPP in adult patients anesthetized with isoflurane and nitrous oxide [179]. An additional potentially beneficial effect of ketamine in patients with CNS trauma is an alteration of transmembrane calcium and magnesium currents through its effects on the NMDA receptor [180].

Another somewhat controversial issue related to the CNS effects of ketamine is its use in patients with an underlying seizure disorder. EEG recordings in children and laboratory animals during ketamine administration demonstrate increased frequency and amplitude with occasional paroxysmal seizure activity [181, 182]. However, no clinical evidence of seizure activity has been reported with ketamine administration. Studies in laboratory animals have demonstrated the anticonvulsant effects of ketamine, and there is at least one clinical report as well as animal data describing its use for the treatment of refractory status epilepticus [183–185].

With everyday clinical use, the adverse effect of ketamine that tends to attract the most attention is its potential to cause emergence phenomena or hallucinations. Because of these concerns, clinical practice generally includes the administration of a benzodiazepine (lorazepam or midazolam) along with or prior to the administration of ketamine. The ketamine solution that is in common clinical use is a racemic mixture of the two optically active enantiomers. The single enantiomer form, S(+) ketamine, has been released outside of the United States for clinical use [186–189]. The initial clinical trials have demonstrated that S(+) ketamine is twice as potent as the racemic formulation and offers the clinical advantages of fewer psychomimetic effects, less salivation, and a shorter recovery time [189].

To date, there are only anecdotal reports involving small case series regarding the use of a ketamine infusion for sedation of the PICU patient during mechanical ventilation [190–192]. The largest series included ten patients, ranging in age from 1 week to 30 months. A ketamine infusion, 1 mg/kg/h in five patients and 2 mg/kg/h in the other five patients, was used to provide sedation and analgesia following cardiac surgery in ten pediatric patients [191]. Supplemental doses of midazolam were administered as needed. The two groups had similar and acceptable levels of sedation. No adverse effects were noted. Ketamine has also been used as a therapeutic agent in pediatric patients with status asthmaticus requiring mechanical ventilation [193]. In a cohort of 17 pediatric patients, ketamine was administered as an intravenous bolus (2 mg/kg) followed by a continuous infusion of 20–60 μ(mu)g/kg/min to 17 pediatric patients without changing their preexisting bronchodilatory regimen. There was a significant increase in the PaO_2/FiO_2 ratio from 116 ± 55 to 174 ± 82, 269 ± 151, and 248 ± 124 at 1, 8, and 24 h, respectively, after the initiation of the ketamine infusion. There was also an improvement in the dynamic compliance as well as a decrease in the $PaCO_2$ and peak inspiratory pressure.

A final caveat with the use of ketamine either by bolus dosing or continuous infusion is that it is commercially available in three different concentrations (100, 50, and 10 mg/mL). Therefore, inadvertent overdosing or underdosing is possible without careful consideration of its concentration. Although it may never become a first-line agent for sedation in the PICU patient during mechanical ventilation, ketamine may be useful in patients who develop adverse cardiovascular effects with opioids or benzodiazepines, for the provision of sedation with the preservation of spontaneous ventilation when using noninvasive ventilation techniques, in patients with status asthmaticus in whom the release of endogenous catecholamines following ketamine administration may provide some therapeutic impact, in low doses by continuous infusion to delay or prevent the development of tolerance to opioids related to its effects at the NMDA receptor, and during the performance of brief, painful invasive procedures in the spontaneously breathing patient. Alternative, non-intravenous routes of delivery have been reported with ketamine including oral and transmucosal (nasal, rectal) administration [188, 194, 195]. These alternative routes of delivery have been used for one-time dosing of the agent for sedation during a procedure or as a premedicant to anesthetic induction. Additionally, ketamine is occasionally administered via the IM route in uncooperative patients without venous access.

Propofol

Propofol is an alkyl phenol compound (2,6-diisopropylphenol) with general anesthetic properties. Although its chemical structure is distinct from that of other intravenous anesthetic, its mechanism of action is similar as it acts through the GABA system [196]. Propofol facilitates the binding of GABA to membrane-bound receptors thereby increasing chloride conductance. Although propofol was initially introduced into anesthesia practice for the induction and maintenance of anesthesia, its rapid onset and recovery times led to its eventual use for sedation in the ICU setting [197, 198]. When compared with midazolam for sedation in adult patients, propofol has been shown to provide shorter recovery times, improved titration efficiency, reduced posthypnotic obtundation, and faster weaning from mechanical ventilation [199].

Propofol, in a manner similar to the barbiturates and etomidate, decreases cerebral metabolic rate of oxygen ($CMRO_2$) leading to reflex cerebral vasoconstriction and a lowering of ICP [200]. These beneficial effects on cerebral dynamics have been validated in animal studies [201, 202]. However, in some experimental studies, adverse hemodynamic effects of propofol required therapy with the direct-acting vasoconstrictor phenylephrine to maintain the mean arterial blood pressure (MAP). When used in clinical practice, the control of MAP has significant clinical impact on propofol's effect on the ICP. Although ICP is decreased in the majority of human trials, propofol's lowering of MAP may result in a decrease of the CPP. In patients with intact autoregulation of CBF, a decrease in CPP leads to reflex cerebral vasodilation to maintain CBF, which can secondarily increase ICP if intracranial compliance is altered. This effect negates the decrease in ICP related to the decrease in $CMRO_2$ induced by propofol. In an evaluation of the effects of propofol (2 mg/kg) on ICP and MAP in 6 adults with an ICP ≥25 mmHg, ICP decreased from a mean of 25 ± 3 mmHg to 11 ± 4 mmHg ($p<0.05$); however, the reduction of MAP resulted in a decrease of the CPP from 92 ± 8 mmHg to 50 ± 7 mmHg [203]. Similar results have been reported in adults with TBI or during cerebral aneurysm surgery [204–206]. However, if MAP is maintained at baseline with vasoactive agents, propofol may lower ICP and increase CPP. When propofol (2–4 mg/kg/h) was used for sedation during mechanical ventilation in 10 adult patients with TBI, ICP decreased by a mean of 2.1 mmHg at 2 h and the CPP increased by 9.8 mmHg at 24 h [207]. Additionally, beneficial effects of propofol in brain injury include animal data suggesting a protective effect of propofol in various types of hypoxic–ischemic injury models as well as the preservation of the CBF reactivity to carbon dioxide [208–210].

Although ketamine is generally considered the optimal agent for anesthetic induction in patients with active bronchospasm, both laboratory and clinical data support the beneficial effects of propofol on airway reactivity. When comparing the effects of anesthetic induction with propofol (2.5 mg/kg), etomidate (0.4 mg/kg), or thiopental (5 mg/kg) in 77 adults, respiratory resistance was lower after propofol (8.1 ± 3.4 cm H_2O/L/s) compared to thiopental (12.3 ± 7.9 cm H_2O/L/s) and etomidate (11.3 ± 5.3 cm H_2O/L/s) [211]. Pizov et al. randomized a cohort of asthmatic and non-asthmatic patients to anesthetic induction with thiopental/thiamylal (5 mg/kg), methohexital (1.5 mg/kg), or propofol (2.5 mg) [212]. Following endotracheal intubation, auscultation was performed to evaluate the presence of wheezing. In asthmatic patients, the incidence of wheezing was 45 % with thiopental/thiamylal, 26 % with methohexital, and 0 % with propofol. In non-asthmatic patients, the incidence of wheezing was 16 % with thiopental/thiamylal and 3 % with propofol. Propofol's beneficial effects on airway reactivity are further supported by animal studies showing attenuation of carbachol-induced airway constriction in canine tracheal smooth muscle and prevention of reflex bronchoconstriction to several provocative agents in isolated guinea pig trachea smooth muscle [213, 214]. However, the specific airway and respiratory effects may not be shared by all preparations of propofol. In both an animal model and a human study, these beneficial were present only with the propofol solution that has EDTA as the preservative and not the newer formulations containing sodium metabisulfite or benzyl alcohol [215, 216].

Propofol's cardiovascular effects resemble those of the barbiturates with the potential for hypotension from peripheral vasodilation and a negative inotropic effect. These effects are dose dependent and can be accentuated following rapid bolus administration and in patients with compromised cardiovascular function. Peripheral vasodilation may be detrimental in patients with a fixed stroke volume (aortic or mitral stenosis) or in the setting of pulmonary hypertension. The adverse hemodynamic profile of propofol administration can be prevented by the administration of calcium chloride [217]. Additional cardiovascular effects may be caused by augmentation of central vagal tone leading to bradycardia, conduction disturbances, and asystole [218–220]. These effects are more likely with the concomitant administration of other medications known to alter cardiac chronotropic function including fentanyl or succinylcholine.

Various neurological manifestations have been reported with the administration of propofol including opisthotonic posturing, myoclonic movements (especially in children), and movements that may resemble seizure-like activity [221–223]. Myoclonus, opisthotonic posturing, and other movements with propofol have been attributed to propofol's antagonism at glycine receptors in subcortical structures. To date, there is no formal evidence linking propofol with seizures, and its use in patients with seizures and other neurological disorders is acceptable. In a study evaluating the effects of propofol and thiopental on the surface electroencephalograms of 20 patients undergoing temporal lobe surgery, there was no difference between the two groups in the rate of discharge or extension of the irritative zone [224]. Propofol remains an effective agent for the termination of refractory status epilepticus and remains in various published algorithms regarding recommendations for its treatment [225, 226].

Despite its potential benefits in the ICU setting and its efficacy for providing sedation during mechanical ventilation, the routine use of propofol is not recommended and, in fact, is considered contraindicated by many authorities because of the potential for the development of what has been termed the "propofol infusion syndrome." First described in 1992, by Parke et al., the disorder includes metabolic acidosis, bradycardia, dysrhythmias, rhabdomyolysis, and fatal cardiac failure [227–229]. Eighteen children in the ICU setting with suspected propofol infusion syndrome were reviewed in a report by Bray [230]. The risk factors in the cohort for the development of the syndrome included propofol administration for ≥48 h or an infusion rate ≥4 mg/kg/h. However, not all patients meeting these risk factor criteria developed problems, suggesting that comorbid diseases or a genetic predisposition may be responsible for the development of the propofol infusion syndrome. Additionally, 13 of the 18 patients were ≤4 years of age while only 1 was ≥10 years of age. Subsequent to the initial reports and the review of Bray et al., the syndrome has been reported in older patients including a 17-year-old adolescent and adults [231–234]. In addition to metabolic acidosis and cardiovascular manifestations, additional clinical findings have included lipemic serum, hepatomegaly, rhabdomyolysis, and hyperkalemia. The suggested treatment includes the immediate discontinuation of the propofol combined with symptomatic treatment of cardiovascular dysfunction and acidosis.

Anecdotal evidence suggests that hemodialysis may be helpful as a therapeutic tool by removing a yet undiagnosed metabolite or toxin. Further study has provided insight into the mechanisms of the propofol infusion syndrome. In a guinea pig cardiomyocyte preparation, propofol has been shown to disrupt mitochondrial function [235]. Biochemical analysis of a 2-year-old boy who developed the propofol infusion syndrome revealed an increase in the concentration of C_5-acylcarnitine indicative of inhibition of mitochondrial function at complex II of the respiratory chain and an increased plasma concentration of malonylcarnitine [236]. This latter compound inhibits the transport protein necessary for the movement of long-chain fatty acids into the mitochondria. Hemofiltration was used in the treatment of this patient, which resulted in the reversal of the clinical manifestations and recovery of their patient. Similar findings with an elevated serum concentration of acylcarnitine were reported in a 5-month-old who developed propofol infusion syndrome [237]. Treatment was instituted with charcoal hemoperfusion, which resulted in the resolution of the signs and symptoms. These concerns led to the "Dear Healthcare Provider" letter issued in March 2001 by AstraZeneca (Wilmington, DE), the manufacturers of Diprivan®, one of the commercially available propofol preparations [238]. The letter summarized the results of a prospective clinical trial that compared propofol (a 1 or 2 % solution) to other agents used for PICU sedation. There were 12 (11 %) deaths in the 2 % propofol group, 9 deaths (8 %) in the 1 % propofol group, and 4 deaths (4 %) in the standard sedation group. Although subsequent review did not show a specific pattern to the deaths, there was enough concern that the company issued a letter stating: "propofol is currently not approved for sedation in PICU patients in the United States and should not be used for this purpose." In the majority of large pediatric centers, these concerns have eliminated the routine use of prolonged propofol infusions for sedation in the PICU.

Although propofol has been used safely and effectively for sedation in small cohorts of PICU patients [239–244], its routine use cannot be recommended. In specific clinical scenarios, propofol is still used as a therapeutic tool in the treatment of refractory status epilepticus or increased ICP. In such cases, intermittent analysis of acid–base status and creatinine phosphokinase is suggested. If a base deficit is noted with an increasing serum lactate, immediate discontinuation of the propofol is recommended. Additionally, the short-term administration of propofol (6–12 h) is still used in many centers to transition from other agents such as fentanyl and midazolam to allow for more rapid awakening for tracheal extubation. Short-term propofol infusions may also have a role in the arena of procedural sedation as a means of providing sedation during non-painful invasive procedures such as radiologic imaging. Given its lack of analgesic effects, additional agents (opioids or ketamine) may be required when invasive procedures are performed. Although rare, when such procedures are long, concern has also been expressed regarding the potential development of the propofol infusion syndrome. In a retrospective review of adult patients who received propofol infusion during radiofrequency ablation for atrial fibrillation or atrial flutter, 13 of 55 patients (24 %) had a base deficit of −2 or more compared to 22 of 267 (8.2 %, $p<0.01$) in a comparator group of patients undergoing carotid endarterectomy who did not receive propofol [245].

Additional concerns with propofol regarding its use for procedural sedation in spontaneously ventilating patients include a relatively high incidence of respiratory effects including hypoventilation, upper airway obstruction, and apnea, many of which required bag-mask ventilation or repositioning of the airway [246]. When used for procedural sedation, the depth of sedation, assessed using the bispectral index, may be similar to those achieved during general anesthesia. Reeves et al. demonstrated that the low BIS value achieved in children receiving propofol during the performance of a lumbar puncture or bone marrow aspiration was 29.7 ± 13.7 [247].

As propofol is delivered in a lipid emulsion, there may be allergic reactions, pain on injection, and elevated triglyceride levels or hypercapnia with prolonged infusions [248, 249]. It has been theoretically posted that cross-reactivity may occur in patients with allergies to egg, egg products, soybeans, or soy products. Soy allergy is rarely a systemic disease, more likely one limited to intolerance to the soy protein in the gastrointestinal tract. Additionally, although propofol is a soy-based emulsion, all protein components are removed during the manufacturing process. There is no concern in patients with peanut allergy other than the 5 % cross-reactivity with soy. The bigger question arises regarding the safety of propofol use in a patient with egg allergy. To date, there have been no immunologically validated anaphylactic reactions to propofol in this population. Propofol (Diprivan®) contains egg lecithin, which is derived from the egg yolk. The majority of true egg allergies are related to proteins in the egg white. Egg lecithin is a phospholipid compound, which has not been reported to be the provocative agent in allergic reactions. In fact, the literature confirms the safety of propofol use in patients that have been labeled with "egg allergies" and suggests that it is safe in the majority of egg-allergic patients who do not have a history of egg anaphylaxis [250, 251].

A propofol infusion of 2 mg/kg/h provides approximately 0.5 g/kg/day of fat. To limit the impact of the lipid component, a 2 % solution of propofol (twice the amount of propofol with the same amount of lipid per mL as the 1 % solution) has undergone clinical evaluations [252–256]. Although there were fewer problems with hypertriglyceridemia in patients receiving the 2 % solution, there may be an alteration in propofol's bioavailability as some of these studies have suggested an increased dose requirement and increased incidence of inadequate sedation when the 2 % solution is used compared with the 1 % solution. Given the concerns regarding the lipid component, its fat content should be considered into daily caloric requirements if prolonged infusions are used.

Pain with the injection of propofol remains a significant complaint especially when small veins on the dorsum of the hands or feet are used. Variable success in decreasing the incidence of pain has been reported with various maneuvers including the preadministration of lidocaine, mixing the lidocaine and propofol in a single solution, mixing the propofol with thiopental, diluting the concentration of the propofol, cooling it prior to bolus administration, or the administration of a small dose of ketamine (0.5 mg/kg) prior to the administration of propofol [257–261]. Since propofol has limited analgesic properties, ketamine and propofol can be administered together to take advantage of the analgesia provided by ketamine and the rapid recovery with propofol. There may also be some advantage to the use of a small dose of ketamine (0.5–1 mg/kg) along with a lower dose of propofol (1 versus 3 mg/kg) to initiate the sedation process as this may limit the respiratory and hemodynamic effects of propofol that frequently occur with the initial bolus dose. One final issue with the lipid component of propofol is its potential to serve as a viable growth media for bacteria with reports of bacteremia and postoperative wound infections linked to extrinsically contaminated propofol [262, 263]. Various preservatives are used in the currently available propofol solutions including disodium EDTA (ethylenediaminetetraacetic acid), sodium metabisulfite, and benzyl alcohol. The addition of these substances has dramatically reduced the incidence of bacterial contamination of the solution; however, strict attention to aseptic technique is mandatory. In clinical practice, there may be subtle yet clinically significant differences in these preparations including differential effects on airway reactivity, which have already been discussed in this chapter [215, 216]. The compatibility of various medications is also different with the various propofol preparations [264]. This is an important issue for pediatric patients in whom intravenous access may be limited when infusions may be administered via connectors attached to the same cannula.

Subtle differences in the anesthetic potency of the preparations have also been reported. Although a retrospective analysis of dose requirements during sedation for MRI demonstrated a decreased potency of the sodium metabisulfite propofol solution when compared to the EDTA solution [265], Fassoulaki et al. demonstrated no difference in the cardiovascular or hypnotic effects of the 2 solutions using BIS monitoring [266]. A theoretical disadvantage of the disodium EDTA preparation when used for prolonged infusions in the ICU setting is the chelation and depletion from the body of essential trace minerals such as zinc. Although there are no formal studies to demonstrate that this is a problem, concerns related to this issue are outlined in the manufacturer's package insert.

Barbiturates

The barbiturates were first synthesized in 1864 by von Baeyer. Thiopental, a short-acting barbiturate, was first administered for clinical use in 1934. This class of anesthetic agent can be classified according to their chemical structure or their duration of activity. The chemical structures of the barbiturates vary in that their ring structure can contain a sulfur atom (thiobarbiturates such as thiamylal and thiopental) or an oxygen atom (methohexital). The presence of a sulfur instead of an oxygen atom in the ring results in a more rapid onset and a shorter duration of action. Increasing the length of the carbon side chains at position 5 of the ring increases the potency of the compound. Short-acting agents such as methohexital, thiopental, and thiamylal have a clinical duration of action of 5–10 min and are used most commonly as a single bolus dose for the induction of anesthesia. When a more prolonged effect is needed, a continuous infusion may be used to maintain constant plasma levels. Long-acting agents with half-lives of 6–12 h include pentobarbital and phenobarbital. The clinical effects of the short-acting agents dissipate rapidly, related to their redistribution, although their hepatic metabolism may take hours. However, when this is done, the offset time will also be markedly prolonged and dependent on the duration of the infusion. In the PICU setting, the barbiturates are occasionally used by continuous infusion for sedation during mechanical ventilation (see later) although their more common use is based on their beneficial physiologic and therapeutic effects as anticonvulsants or to decrease ICP in patients with TBI [267–272].

Like propofol, the effects of the barbiturates on hemodynamic and respiratory function are dose dependent. In healthy patients, sedative doses have limited effects on cardiovascular function, respiratory drive, and airway protective reflexes, while larger doses, especially in patients with cardiorespiratory compromise, will result in respiratory depression, apnea, or hypotension. Hypotension results from peripheral vasodilation, a direct negative inotropic effect, and blunting of the sympathetic nervous system. On a cellular level, the barbiturates inhibit calcium fluxes across cell membranes and from the sarcoplasmic reticulum thereby depressing myocardial contractility. These effects are magnified in patients with comorbid cardiovascular diseases and in the presence of hypovolemia. These agents should be used cautiously, if at all, in patients with cardiovascular dysfunction. Additionally, the effects on cardiovascular and ventilatory function are additive with other agents such as opioids.

The ultrashort-acting barbiturates (thiopental and thiamylal) are used clinically in a 2.5 % solution with a pH of 10.5. The high pH results in a bacteriostatic solution limiting concerns of bacterial contamination as well as limiting the pain that may occur with intravenous injection. However, a pH of 10.5 leads to incompatibilities with other medications and parenteral alimentation solutions, thereby necessitating a separate infusion site if a continuous infusion is used. Of particular note is the potential for the barbiturates to form precipitates when administered with drugs such as rocuronium, mandating flushing the line during rapid administration of medications during maneuvers such as rapid sequence intubation to avoid loss of intravenous access during critical moments. Local erythema, thrombophlebitis, or skin sloughing may occur with subcutaneous infiltration. The barbiturates possess no analgesic properties and therefore should be used with an opioid in situations requiring analgesia.

The barbiturates' place in ICU sedation appears to be as an alternative or second-line agent when primary agents, either alone or in combination, fail to provide adequate sedation or result in untoward side effects [273]. There are a limited number of reports regarding the use of pentobarbital infusions for sedation in the PICU setting. A retrospective report described the use of pentobarbital for sedation during mechanical ventilation of 50 infants and children, ranging in age from 1 month to 14 years [274]. A pentobarbital infusion was started when a combination of a benzodiazepine (midazolam in doses of 0.4 mg/kg/h) and an opioid (either fentanyl in doses of 10 μ(mu)g/kg/h or morphine in doses of 100 μ(mu)g/kg/h) did not provide effective sedation. The midazolam infusion was discontinued when the pentobarbital infusion was started. In 12 patients, opioid infusion was continued for more than 48 h after starting the pentobarbital infusion to control pain related to a surgical procedure or an acute medical illness. In the other patients, the opioid infusion was discontinued. Pentobarbital was administered for a median duration of 4 days (range 2–37 days) at a median dose of 2 mg/kg/h (range 1–6 mg/kg/h). Once pentobarbital was started, neuromuscular blocking agents, which had been required in seven patients due to excessive movement and inadequate sedation, were discontinued. Additionally, there was no longer a need for direct-acting vasodilators (sodium nitroprusside or nicardipine) in the five patients who had previously required these agents. The cohort also included seven non-neonatal ECMO patients in whom pentobarbital provided effective sedation. Tolerance was noted with the administration of pentobarbital. In the 14 patients that received pentobarbital for ≥5 days, the dose requirements increased from 1.2 mg/kg/h on day #1 to 3.4 mg/kg/h on day #5. No significant adverse effects related to pentobarbital were noted. Six of the 36 patients who had received pentobarbital for more than 4 days manifested signs and symptoms of withdrawal. An opposing opinion is expressed by Yanay et al. who reported their retrospective experience with pentobarbital sedation for eight PICU patients [275]. Although pentobarbital provided effective sedation and allowed the discontinuation of neuromuscular blocking agents, they noted a relatively high incidence of adverse effects including blood pressure instability (25 %), oversedation (12.5 %), and neurologic sequelae (12.5 %) including withdrawal phenomena. These adverse effects led to the discontinuation of the drug in 25 % of their patients.

In addition to their role for therapeutic agents or perhaps for the provision of sedation during mechanical ventilation, there are several reports outlining the use of various barbiturates for procedural sedation. As they have no intrinsic analgesic properties, the barbiturates are used most commonly for sedation during non-painful procedures. The short-acting oxybarbiturate, methohexital, has been used extensively via both the oral and PR route as a sedative for CT or MR imaging with success rates of up to 80–85 % [276]. The standard dose per rectum is 20–30 mg/kg, which produces a rapid onset of sleep (6–10 min) with recovery to baseline status within 1.5–2 h. Adverse effects are uncommon with mild respiratory depression responsive to repositioning or the administration of supplemental oxygen occurring in up to 4 % of patients. The duration of action with intravenous use (0.75–1.0 mg/kg) is approximately 10 min, making the drug attractive for short procedures such as computerized tomography (CT imaging). However, the incidence of respiratory depression is greater with the intravenous route of administration, which may limit its usefulness. Unlike the other barbiturates, methohexital may activate the electroencephalogram (EEG) and has been reported to precipitate seizures in patients with underlying seizure disorders.

Although used most commonly by the intravenous route for the induction of anesthesia, thiopental has also been used as a rectal agent for sedation for radiologic procedures in doses of 25–50 mg/kg [277, 278]. When compared with methohexital, the depth of sedation achieved and reported success rates were somewhat higher (>90 %). The onset of action is slightly longer (15–30 min) with a similar duration of action (60–90 min) compared to methohexital. Pentobarbital has an intermediate duration of action and remains a popular choice for intravenous sedation during radiologic procedures such as MR imaging where sedation times may approach 60–90 min. Multiple delivery options are available including the IV, IM, and enteral routes, although IV administration remains the most commonly used route. Pentobarbital is administered in increments of 1–2 mg/kg every 3–5 min until sleep is induced (average total dose 4–5 mg/kg) [279, 280]. The average duration of sleep after a single intravenous dose is 60–90 min, which is adequate to perform most routine MRI evaluations. Respiratory depression and hypotension may occur, especially with rapid intravenous administration. Disadvantages with pentobarbital include prolonged recovery times (2–4 h) and emergence issues including agitation.

Opioids

Although generally used for analgesia, opioids also possess sedative properties, especially those with agonistic effects at the κ(kappa) opioid receptor [281]. Therefore, these agents may be effective for providing sedation during mechanical ventilation and remain second to the benzodiazepines as the most commonly used agents in the PICU setting. Although the opioids provide analgesia, even in settings such as anesthesia for cardiovascular surgery when high doses of specific agents (fentanyl 50–75 μ(mu)g/kg) are administered, amnesia is not provided. Therefore, additional agents are required in situations that demand amnesia such as a patient who is receiving a neuromuscular blocking agent. In patients with altered myocardial function or at risk for pulmonary hypertension, such as an infant with a large preoperative left-to-right shunt, particular benefit has been reported with the synthetic opioids as they provide cardiovascular stability, beneficial effects on PVR, and blunting of sympathetic stress response. Due to their prompt redistribution and resultant short plasma half-lives following bolus administration, the synthetic opioids are generally administered by a continuous infusion to maintain plasma concentrations adequate to provide sedation and analgesia.

The synthetic opioids that are currently in common clinical use include fentanyl, sufentanil, and remifentanil. Both fentanyl and sufentanil are dependent on hepatic metabolism, while remifentanil is depending on metabolism by nonspecific esterases (see later). Several clinical scenarios may alter hepatic metabolic function and thereby prolong the half-lives of these agents, including immaturity of the hepatic microsomal enzymes as is seen in term and especially preterm infants, decreased hepatic blood flow that occurs following intra-abdominal procedures, and primary hepatic diseases with hepatocellular dysfunction. Although these agents are short acting when administered as a single bolus dose, they also have a context-sensitive half-life so that the duration of their effect is prolonged when they are administered over an extended period of time. This effect is greater with fentanyl than sufentanil.

Remifentanil is metabolized by nonspecific esterases in the plasma. It has a clinical half-life of 5–10 min and a brief duration of effect even following 12–24 h of continuous infusion thereby not demonstrating changes related to a context-sensitive half-life [282]. These pharmacokinetic parameters hold true even in the neonatal population, making remifentanil the only opioid whose pharmacokinetics are not altered by gestational or chronologic age [283]. Given these properties, it is a potentially useful agent for providing a deep level of sedation and yet allowing for rapid awakening with discontinuation of the infusion even in the neonatal population. Although there is significant clinical experience with the use of remifentanil during surgical procedures in patients of all ages, to date there remains limited experience with its use in the ICU population. Cavaliere et al. evaluated the efficacy of a remifentanil infusion in doses starting at 0.02 μ(mu)g/kg/min and increasing up to 0.25 μ(mu)g/kg/min, in providing sedation during mechanical ventilation in a cohort of ten adult ICU patients [284]. Although sedation, assessed by clinical sedation scales, was adequate in the ten patients, the maximum infusion rate was achieved in only four of the ten patients due to the occurrence of adverse effects including hypotension and bradycardia at infusion rates ≥0.15 μ(mu)g/kg/min. Hypoventilation was noted at infusion rates as low as 0.1 μ(mu)g/kg/min. The authors concluded that low doses of remifentanil (0.05 μ(mu)g/kg/min) provided effective sedation in critically ill patients while the adverse effect profile limited the use of higher doses. In a prospective randomized trial, adults requiring mechanical ventilation received either a morphine infusion at 0.75 μ(mu)g/kg/min or a remifentanil infusion at 0.15 μ(mu)g/kg/min [285]. Although the percentage of optimal sedation hours was significantly greater with remifentanil with fewer dose adjustments, the duration of mechanical ventilation and extubation time was significantly longer with morphine. There was no difference in the incidence of adverse effects.

To date, there are limited data regarding the use of remifentanil for sedation during mechanical ventilation in the PICU population [286, 287]. Our preliminary clinical experience demonstrates that remifentanil may be useful in providing sedation during mechanical ventilation in patients with TBI who require frequent and intermittent neurological examination. In this population, the short half-life of remifentanil allows the successful neurological examination while providing a sedation plan of analgesia and sedation in the interim.

Although these anecdotal reports demonstrate that remifentanil may be an effective agent, providing a deep level of sedation with rapid awakening when the infusion is discontinued, an issue that needs further investigation prior to its widespread application in the ICU setting is the rapid development of tolerance. The development of tolerance has been demonstrated after even brief infusions of less than 60–90 min [288, 289]. This has translated into greater postoperative opioid requirements when remifentanil is used intraoperatively and the need to escalate doses rapidly when remifentanil is used for ICU sedation. Although tolerance may limit prolonged remifentanil infusions, there remains interest in the use of remifentanil in the arena of procedural sedation given that its effects dissipate rapidly when the infusion is discontinued [290–292]. Given its analgesic properties, remifentanil has been combined with midazolam or propofol as a means of providing analgesia during painful, invasive procedures. Despite its efficacy in this arena, reports demonstrate a significant incidence of respiratory depression and apnea, which may limit its applicability in this setting. However, given the ability of the opioids to blunt the cough reflex, remifentanil may have a role during bronchoscopy or when fiberoptic intubation of the trachea is necessary [291].

Two additional issues relevant to the synthetic opioids are potential effects on ICP and the risks of chest wall rigidity. Anecdotal reports suggested the potential for the synthetic opioids to increase ICP and decrease CPP in adults with altered intracranial compliance [293]. Rather than a direct effect, the mechanism responsible for the ICP increase has been shown to be a reflex cerebral vasodilation in response to the decrease in MAP or CPP [294]. A similar effect has been described with propofol (see earlier section). If the CPP or MAP is maintained with a direct-acting vasoconstrictor, no change in ICP is noted thereby making these agents safe and effective in patients with altered intracranial compliance. A second adverse effect specific to the synthetic opioids is chest wall and laryngeal rigidity [295, 296]. These effects are related to the dose and the rate of administration, are centrally mediated responses that can interfere with respiratory function, and their incidence can be decreased by premedication with the α(alpha)$_2$-adrenergic agonists, reversed with naloxone, and interrupted with neuromuscular blocking agents. Although rare, its occurrence should be considered if respiratory dysfunction is noted following the use of synthetic opioids. In severe cases, this effect may interfere with respiratory function resulting in rapid oxygen desaturation and hypoxemia [297].

Given the issues with the rapid development of tolerance following the use of the synthetic opioids, morphine has regained popularity for sedation and analgesia during mechanical ventilation in the PICU setting. As morphine has agonistic effects at both the mu and the kappa opioid receptor, it provides not only analgesia via the mu receptor but also sedation via the kappa receptor. Cardiovascular effects include dilation of the venous capacitance system with a decrease in preload, which may result in a modest decrease in blood pressure, especially in patients with decreased intravascular volume or comorbid cardiac diseases. When used by continuous infusion for sedation during mechanical ventilation in neonates, morphine has been shown to have no effect on intelligence, motor function, or behavior [298].

In infants, morphine infusions of 10–30 μ(mu)g/kg/h provided effective analgesia and sedation during mechanical ventilation after surgery for congenital heart disease without impairing the ability to wean mechanical ventilatory support [299]. Morphine infusions blunt the sympathetic response and reduce epinephrine levels in neonates requiring endotracheal intubation and mechanical ventilation for hyaline membrane disease [300]. In a cohort of infants requiring sedation and analgesia during ECMO (mean duration of ECMO 4–5 days), morphine and fentanyl provided equivalent levels of sedation while decreasing the need for supplemental bolus doses of opioid [301]. Infants receiving morphine had a lower incidence of withdrawal (13 of 27 with fentanyl versus 1 of 11 with morphine, $p<0.01$) and were hospitalized for fewer days after ECMO (31.1 ± 14 versus 21.5 ± 7.0 days, $p=0.01$).

Although administered most commonly via the intravenous route, rare circumstances, such as limited intravenous access or drug incompatibilities, may occur that preclude intravenous administration in the PICU setting. In such situations, the subcutaneous administration of opioids is feasible. Although used most commonly in the control of chronic cancer pain [302], there is experience with subcutaneous opioid infusions in the ICU setting. Bruera et al. successfully used subcutaneous opioids, administered by intermittent dosing or continuous infusions, in adult ICU patients [303]. The infusions were delivered through a 25 gauge butterfly needle inserted subcutaneously in the subclavicular area or the anterior abdominal wall. No infectious complications were noted and the insertion site was changed only three times due to local problems such as erythema. Although the authors expressed a theoretical concern over possible delays in the onset of activity or decreased absorption in patients with decreased peripheral perfusion, they noted no problems in their cohort.

There is also anecdotal experience with the use of subcutaneous opioids in the PICU population [304–306]. A retrospective evaluation regarding the subcutaneous administration of fentanyl in 24 PICU patients ranging in age from 2 weeks to 18 years demonstrated the efficacy of the technique in the control of postoperative pain, as a gradual weaning regimen following prolonged opioid use, or for the provision of comfort during the terminal stages of a disease [306]. The subcutaneous fentanyl infusions were administered when intravenous administration was not feasible due to lack of intravenous access or drug incompatibilities.

As with all of the previously described agents, opioids may have adverse effects on respiratory function with the potential for hypoventilation or apnea. However, an effect that appears to be relatively specific to the opioids is their potential impact on immune function. Opioid receptors have been found on immune cells that participate in the inflammatory response and various host defenses. Binding of opioids to these receptors decreases inflammation and may play some role in the control of acute pain by opioids. However, in specific circumstances, this effect may be deleterious. Increased viral loads have been noted in patients with HIV infections who are receiving methadone [307]. Opioids modulate cytokine production and in an animal model morphine has been shown to reduce reticuloendothelial cell function, phagocytic count, phagocytic index, killing properties, and superoxide anion production [308, 309]. Although there are no studies directly linking these effects to adverse clinical outcomes, additional studies are needed to define these effects, their mechanisms, and most importantly their impact on the PICU patient.

Phenothiazines and Butyrophenones

The phenothiazines and butyrophenones are classified as the "major tranquilizers." The majority of their clinical use is in the treatment of psychiatric disturbances or as antiemetics in various clinical scenarios. Of the several agents available, haloperidol is the agent that has been used most frequently for the sedation of adults in the ICU setting. Haloperidol acts through central dopamine receptors. With intravenous administration, its onset of action is within 10–20 min with a duration of action of 12–24 h given its long elimination half-life of 18–26 h [310]. Although not formally approved by the FDA for intravenous administration, there is significant and adequate clinical experience with its use by this route in the adult population [311]. Riker et al. reported their experience with the continuous infusion of haloperidol in doses ranging from 3 to 25 mg/h for sedation in eight adult ICU patients [312]. They proposed various benefits of haloperidol including a rapid onset, minimal respiratory depression, and lack of active metabolites. A retrospective report regarding haloperidol use in a cohort of 989 adult patients, who required mechanical ventilation for more than 48 h, reported not only efficacy in controlling agitation and delirium, but also a lower overall mortality in patients who received haloperidol [313]. Patients who received haloperidol within 48 h of the initiation of mechanical ventilation had a lower inhospital mortality (20.5 % versus 36.1 %, $p=0.004$) when compared with those who did not receive haloperidol. These differences persisted even when adjusted for age, comorbid features, severity of illness, degree of organ dysfunction, and admitting diagnosis. Because of the retrospective nature of the study and the potential risks associated with haloperidol (see below), the authors suggested that prospective randomized trials were needed before applying this therapy routinely to the ICU population.

Experience with haloperidol in the PICU population remains anecdotal. Harrison et al. reported their experience with haloperidol, administered by intermittent bolus dosing, in five critically ill children [314]. The patients ranged in age from 9 months to 16 years and had become difficult to sedate despite escalating doses of benzodiazepines and opioids. Haloperidol dosing included a loading dose of 0.025–0.1 mg/kg, repeated every 10 min until the patient was sedated. The total loading dose required ranged from 0.09 to 0.25 mg/kg. This was followed by intermittent doses of 0.015–0.15 mg/kg (daily maintenance dose of 0.06–0.45 mg/kg/day) administered every 8 h. Haloperidol's efficacy was demonstrated by a reduction of opioid and benzodiazepine requirements, decreased need for supplemental doses of sedative agents, decreased use of neuromuscular blocking agents, and improved clinical sedation. One patient developed a dystonic reaction, which resolved in 36 h without therapy as the haloperidol had already been discontinued.

Potential adverse effects associated with the butyrophenones and phenothiazines include hypotension related to peripheral α(alpha)-adrenergic blockade, dystonic and extrapyramidal effects, lowering of the seizure threshold, the neuroleptic malignant syndrome, and cardiac arrhythmias including *torsades de pointes* due to effects on cardiac repolarization. In the study of Riker et al., one of the eight adult patients developed atrial dysrhythmias, prolongation of the QT interval, and ventricular tachycardia [312]. The potential for cardiac dysrhythmias due to alterations in repolarization may be exacerbated in critically ill patients with altered sympathetic function related to fever, pain, or the stresses of an acute illness. Similar issues may occur with other drugs of this class including droperidol [315]. Through a black box warning issued by the US Food and Drug Administration, concern has been expressed regarding the potential association of droperidol and postoperative cardiac events including *torsades de pointes* in adult patients [316]. Prolonged postoperative electrocardiogram (ECG) monitoring is suggested in patients treated with droperidol during the perioperative period.

Alpha$_2$-Adrenergic Agonists

Although used initially for clinical effects such as the control of blood pressure, the α(alpha)$_2$-adrenergic agonists including clonidine and dexmedetomidine may also have a role in the PICU patient for the provision of sedation during mechanical ventilation, reduction of opioid requirements, control of pain of various etiologies, and provision of sedation during noninvasive procedures. The physiologic effects of these agents are mediated via stimulation of postsynaptic α(alpha)$_2$-adrenergic receptors that activate a pertussis toxin-sensitive guanine nucleotide regulatory protein (G protein), resulting in decreased activity of adenylyl cyclase [317, 318]. The subsequent reduction in intracellular cyclic adenosine monophosphate (cAMP) and cAMP-dependent protein kinase activity modifies membrane ion conductance resulting in decreased neuronal activation providing sedation and anxiolysis [319, 320].

Activation of receptors in the medullary vasomotor center reduces norepinephrine turnover and decreases central sympathetic outflow, resulting in alterations in sympathetic function with decreased heart rate and blood pressure. Additional effects result from the central stimulation of parasympathetic outflow and inhibition of sympathetic outflow from the locus ceruleus in the brainstem. The latter effect plays a prominent role in sedation and anxiolysis produced by these agents as decreased noradrenergic output from the locus ceruleus allows for increased firing of inhibitory neurons including the GABA system resulting in sedation and anxiolysis [321]. This effect has been shown to be similar to that which occurs during non-REM sleep [322, 323]. The lack of non-REM sleep with the use of other sedative agents including propofol, benzodiazepines, and barbiturates is one of the factors that may result in delirium in adult ICU patients. This mechanism of action has led to the increased use of this agent in adult ICUs where concerns regarding the impact of delirium on outcome have been emphasized in the recent literature. The α(alpha)$_2$-adrenergic agonists also potentiate the analgesic effects of opioids by regulating substance P release within the central nervous system [324].

Clonidine has been used as a premedicant in the operating room, for caudal and epidural analgesia, as an adjunct to opioid-induced analgesia during the postoperative period, and even for ICU sedation [325–328]. Although initially available only as a tablet, clonidine is now available as a transdermal patch and as a preparation for neuraxial administration. The latter has been administered intravenously in various clinical scenarios. In an open label evaluation in children in the PICU setting, a continuous clonidine infusion starting at 1 μ(mu)g/kg/min was added to a continuous midazolam infusion of 1 μ(mu)g/kg/min [328]. No significant change in heart rate, blood pressure, or cardiac index was noted. In 2 of the 20 patients, the clonidine infusion was increased to 2 μ(mu)g/kg/h. The clonidine infusion provided adequate sedation for 602 of the 672 study hours with no sedation failures. Arenas-Lopez et al. reported their experience with the addition of enteral clonidine (3–5 μ(mu)/kg every 8 h) as an adjunct to intermittent doses of morphine and lorazepam for sedation during mechanical ventilation in 14 children [329]. Adequate sedation was achieved during 82 % of the study period with an overall decrease in the requirements for both lorazepam and morphine. No adverse effects were noted. With the increased use of and accumulating clinical experience with dexmedetomidine, the use of clonidine has diminished in most pediatric ICUs [330].

Like clonidine, dexmedetomidine is a centrally acting, α(alpha)$_2$-adrenergic agonist and exhibits the same physiologic effects. However, it possesses an affinity eight times that of clonidine for the α(alpha)$_2$-adrenergic receptor, a differential α(alpha)$_1$ to α(alpha)$_2$ agonism of 1:1,600, and a half-life of 2–3 h thereby allowing its titration by intravenous administration. In healthy adult volunteers, the pharmacokinetic profile of dexmedetomidine includes a rapid distribution phase with a distribution half-life of approximately 6 min, an elimination half-life of 2 h, and a steady-state volume of distribution of approximately 118 L. Dexmedetomidine exhibits linear kinetics, is 94 % protein bound, and undergoes hepatic metabolism with minimal unchanged drug excreted in the urine and feces. Given its dependence on hepatic metabolism, dose adjustments are necessary in patients with altered hepatic function.

The pharmacokinetic profile of dexmedetomidine has been well studied in the pediatric population and in various clinical scenarios [331–336]. Diaz et al. studied the pharmacokinetics of dexmedetomidine in a cohort of 10 children ranging in age from 0.3 to 7.9 years following cardiac ($n=9$) or craniofacial procedures ($n=1$) [332]. Dexmedetomidine was administered as a bolus dose of 1 μ(mu)g/kg followed by an infusion of 0.2–0.7 μ(mu)g/kg/h for 8–24 h (median duration of administration of 19.6 h). In this cohort, the authors noted pharmacokinetics similar to those reported in the adult population and pediatric patients without CHD. Using a two-compartment model, the volume of distribution was

1.53 ± 0.37 L/kg, the clearance was 0.57 ± 0.14 L/kg/h (approximately 9.5 mL/kg/min), and the terminal elimination half-life was 2.65 ± 0.88 h. They also noted a low interpatient variability (coefficient of variation of 25 %) in their cohort of ten pediatric patients. Based on the clearance data from their study, it was determined that an infusion rate of 0.35 μ(mu)g/kg/h (range: 0.25–0.47 μ(mu)g/kg/h) should achieve a therapeutic plasma concentration of 600 pg/mL. Based on experience with several other pharmacologic agents, they cautioned that the pharmacokinetics of dexmedetomidine is likely to be significantly different in patients less than 4 months of age.

Potts et al. and Su et al. provide additional data regarding dexmedetomidine pharmacokinetics in the pediatric cardiac surgical population [334, 335]. The first of these studies administered a single bolus of dexmedetomidine over 10 min in a dose varying from 1 to 4 μ(mu)g/kg to a cohort of 45 pediatric patients, ranging in age from 4 days to 14 years [334]. As with previous investigations, the authors found that the pharmacokinetics best fits a two-compartment model. Clearance at birth was 15.55 L/h per 70 kg and matured with a half-time of 46.5 weeks to reach 87 % of adult values by 1 year of age. In distinction to other studies, no age-related changes in the volume of distribution were noted. Simulation of a bolus of 1 μ(mu)g/kg followed by an infusion of 0.7 μ(mu)g/kg/h suggested that children arouse from sedation at a plasma concentration of 0.304 μ(mu)g/mL (the suggested therapeutic level for sedation in adults is 0.600 μ(mu)g/mL). No comment was made regarding differences based on the type of congenital heart disease (single versus two ventricle, cyanotic versus non-cyanotic). Su et al. provide more specific information regarding the impact of CPB and the type of CHD on the pharmacokinetics of dexmedetomidine [335]. Sequential cohorts of 12 infants each who required mechanical ventilation following surgery for CHD were enrolled to receive one of three dosing regimens. The three regimens (loading dose and continuous infusion) included 0.35–0.25, 0.7–0.5, and 1–0.75 μ(mu)g/kg and μ(mu)g/kg/h respectively. The authors noted that dexmedetomidine clearance increased with weight, age, and single-ventricle physiology, while total CPB time was associated with a trend toward decreased clearance. Potts et al. performed a pooled analysis of four of the studies from the pediatric population in an attempt to provide a summary of the pharmacokinetics of dexmedetomidine in the pediatric-aged patient [336].

The effects of dexmedetomidine on sedation, hemodynamic and respiratory function were evaluated in a cohort of healthy adults [337]. The volunteers received either a bolus of saline followed by a saline infusion or 0.6 μ(mu)g/kg of dexmedetomidine infused over 10 min followed by a dexmedetomidine infusion at either 0.2 or 0.6 μ(mu)g/kg for 1 h. The level of sedation was graded by the patient (VAS level of sedation from 0 = asleep to 100 = wide awake), an observer, and by using the BIS monitor. The two dexmedetomidine infusions resulted in similar and significant degrees of sedation with limited changes in hemodynamic and respiratory function. In addition to its sedative properties, dexmedetomidine has been shown to decrease opioid requirements following surgical procedures. When compared with placebo in 119 adult patients who required mechanical ventilation following cardiac and general surgical procedures, patients receiving dexmedetomidine required 80 % less midazolam and 50 % less morphine [338]. Dexmedetomidine dosing included an initial bolus dose of 1 μ(mu)g/kg followed by an infusion of 0.2–0.7 μ(mu)g/kg/h. Eighteen of the 66 patients who received dexmedetomidine experienced hypotension (MAP less than 60 mmHg or a greater than 30 % decrease from baseline) or bradycardia (heart rate less than 50 beats per minute). The cardiovascular changes were noted during the bolus dose in 11 of the 18 patients.

To date, there remains only one prospective trial evaluating dexmedetomidine for sedation during mechanical ventilation in pediatric-aged patients [339]. Efficacy was evaluated using the Ramsay scale and by comparing the requirements for supplemental morphine. Dexmedetomidine at 0.25 μ(mu)g/kg/h provided sedation that was equivalent to midazolam at 0.22 mg/kg/h. Dexmedetomidine at 0.5 μ(mu)g/kg/h was more effective than midazolam, as demonstrated by a decreased need for supplemental morphine and a decrease in the number of Ramsay scores of 1 exhibited by the patients. Dexmedetomidine was somewhat less effective for patients ≤12 months of age as five of the six patients that exhibited a Ramsay score of 1 during dexmedetomidine were less than 12 months of age. The only adverse effect was bradycardia in one patient receiving dexmedetomidine who was also receiving digoxin [340].

In addition to its use for sedation during mechanical ventilation, other applications of dexmedetomidine have included procedural sedation, prevention of shivering, and treatment of iatrogenic opioid and benzodiazepine withdrawal following prolonged use in the ICU setting [336]. Koroglu et al. randomized 80 children (1–7 years of age) to dexmedetomidine or midazolam during MR imaging [341]. Dexmedetomidine was administered as a loading dose of 1 μ(mu)g/kg over 10 min followed by an infusion of 0.5 μ(mu)g/kg/h, while midazolam was administered as a loading dose of 0.2 mg/kg followed by an infusion of 6 μ(mu)g/kg/h. The quality of sedation was better and the need for rescue sedation was less (8 of 40 versus 32 of 40) with dexmedetomidine compared to midazolam. Similar efficacy was reported in an open label trial of dexmedetomidine for sedation during magnetic resonance (MR) imaging in 48 pediatric patients ranging in age from 5 months to 16 years, 15 of whom had failed sedation with another agent [342]. A second study by Koroglu et al. randomized 60 children to dexmedetomidine or propofol during MR imaging [343].

Although both of the agents were equally effective in providing sedation, propofol provided shorter induction times, recovery times, and discharge times. However, adverse effects including hypotension and oxygen desaturation were more common with propofol. Oxygen desaturation requiring intervention including a chin lift, discontinuation of the infusion, or supplemental oxygen occurred in 4 of 30 children receiving propofol versus 0 of 30 receiving dexmedetomidine.

In a retrospective review of data from their QA database, Mason et al. used escalating does of dexmedetomidine for sedation in 62 children during radiologic imaging [344]. Dexmedetomidine was administered as a loading dose of 2 μ(mu)g/kg over 10 min and repeated to achieve effective sedation after which an infusion was started at 1 μ(mu)g/kg/h. The mean loading dose was 2.2 μ(mu)g/kg with 52 patients requiring only the initial dose of 2 μ(mu)g/kg. The time to achieve sedation ranged from 6 to 20 min. Sinus arrhythmias were noted in ten patients (16 %). Heart rate and blood pressure decreased in all patients; however, no treatment was necessary and no hemodynamic value was less than the fifth percentile for age. No changes were observed in the $ETCO_2$ and no patient developed oxygen desaturation while breathing room air. Two patients developed agitation during the administration of the dexmedetomidine loading dose and were switched to other sedative agents (propofol or pentobarbital). More recently, preliminary data has suggested that dexmedetomidine may be administered via the intramuscular route when intravenous access is lacking. In two trials, intramuscular (IM) dexmedetomidine was shown to be effective for sedation during radiologic imaging and EEG analysis [345, 346].

Given its limited analgesic effects, dexmedetomidine may not to be the ideal agent when used alone for painful procedures. However, anecdotal experience suggests that a combination of dexmedetomidine with ketamine may be effective in such scenarios [347–349]. The reader is referred to Tobias [350] for a full review of the literature regarding the combination of these agents for procedural sedation. Although the data are limited, the combination of dexmedetomidine with ketamine makes pharmacologic sense as the two medications have the potential to balance the hemodynamic and adverse effects of one another. Dexmedetomidine may prevent the tachycardia, hypertension, salivation, and emergence phenomena from ketamine, while ketamine may prevent the bradycardia and hypotension that have been reported with dexmedetomidine [351]. When ketamine is included as part of the sedation induction regimen, it may speed the onset of sedation and eliminate the slow-onset times when dexmedetomidine is used as the sole agent.

Regardless of the agent or agents responsible for tolerance and withdrawal, the potential role of dexmedetomidine in treating such problems is supported by animal studies [352–355], case reports in adults and children [356–360], and one retrospective case series in infants [361]. The latter study retrospectively reviewed the clinical course of seven infants, ranging in age from 3 to 24 months, who had received sedation during mechanical ventilation with a continuous infusion of fentanyl supplemented with intermittent doses of midazolam. With the discontinuation of fentanyl and midazolam, withdrawal occurred as documented by a Finnegan score $\geq$12. Dexmedetomidine was administered as a loading dose of 0.5 μ(mu)g/kg/h followed by an infusion of 0.5 μ(mu)g/kg/h. The loading dose was repeated and the infusion increased to 0.7 μ(mu)g/kg/h in the two patients who had received the highest doses of fentanyl (8.5 ± 0.7 versus 4.6 ± 0.5 μ(mu)g/kg/h, $p < 0.0005$). Withdrawal was controlled and subsequent Finnegan scores were $\leq$7.

As with all of the medications discussed in this chapter, dexmedetomidine can have deleterious effects on ventilatory and cardiovascular function. The literature regarding dexmedetomidine's effects on respiratory function are somewhat divergent depending on the dose administered and the method of assessing ventilatory function. Belleville et al. reported a depression of the slope of the CO_2 response curve, a decrease in minute ventilation at an $ETCO_2$ of 55 mmHg, as well as irregular breathing patterns and short periods of apnea in some of the patients following a bolus dose of 2 μ(mu)g/kg [362]. When administered to a cohort of postoperative patients, 18 of 66 patients experienced adverse hemodynamic effects, which included hypotension ($MAP \leq 60$ mmHg or a greater than 30 % decrease from baseline) or bradycardia (heart rate $\leq$50 beats per minute) [338]. The adverse hemodynamic effects occurred during the bolus dose in 11 of the 18 patients. Talke et al. evaluated the efficacy of dexmedetomidine infusion in a cohort of 41 adults during vascular surgery [363]. There was a lower heart rate, a decreased incidence of tachycardia, and decreased norepinephrine levels during emergence from anesthesia in patients receiving dexmedetomidine. Adverse effects related to dexmedetomidine included one episode of postoperative hypotension and one patient that had a 5–10 s sinus pause after anesthetic induction with thiopental and fentanyl followed by endotracheal intubation. Electrophysiologic effects were also reported in an intraoperative study by Peden et al. [364]. Two patients who received dexmedetomidine experienced brief episodes of sinus arrest following laryngoscopy and propofol administration.

The previously discussed findings suggest that specific procedures (laryngoscopy), techniques (hypothermia to control ICP or for neuroprotection), and medications (propofol, fentanyl, digoxin) may potentiate the vagotonic effects of dexmedetomidine. Given these effects on cardiac conduction, it has been suggested that dexmedetomidine may not be a desirable agent for sedation in the cardiac catheterization suite when electrophysiological studies are planned [365]. The potential for these effects may be mitigated by the coadministration of ketamine [366]. Other authors have demonstrated that these negative chronotropic properties may be used as a therapeutic tool in infants and children who develop tachyarrhythmias following surgery for congenital heart disease [367]. A more in-depth review of this topic and the potential role of dexmedetomidine in the prevention or treatment of arrhythmias is presented by Tobias and Chrysostomou [368].

Data in animal and human studies demonstrate beneficial effects on cerebral dynamics including a decrease in CBF, cerebral metabolic rate for oxygen, and ICP [369–371]. However, given the potential effects on MAP, a decrease in CPP may occur [372]. Like the barbiturates, propofol, and the inhalational anesthetic agents, animal data suggest that dexmedetomidine may provide some degree of cerebral protection during periods of global or regional cerebral ischemia [373–375]. The data in animals regarding its effects on the seizure threshold are mixed depending on the provocative agent and the type of animal studied, with two studies suggesting a lowering of the seizure threshold and two suggesting an anticonvulsant effect [376–379]. Despite this, there is no reason for clinical concern regarding these effects.

Chloral Hydrate

Chloral hydrate, first synthesized in 1832, remains a commonly used agent for procedural sedation [380]. Its popularity results from several factors including its ease of administration by either the oral or rectal route, health-care providers' familiarity with it, and misconceptions regarding its margin of safety. It is not uncommon for health-care providers to believe that monitoring is not required when chloral hydrate is used. Unfortunately, these misconceptions regarding this agent have resulted in fatalities. The potential for respiratory effects is magnified when chloral hydrate is coadministered with other sedative agents. Following oral or rectal administration, chloral hydrate is rapidly and completely absorbed. It undergoes hepatic metabolism to its active metabolite: trichloroethanol (TCE). Although generally effective as a one-time agent for non-painful radiologic procedures, repeated dosing in the PICU setting leads to excessive and prolonged CNS depression due to a variable half-life ranging from 9 to 40 h as well as the accumulation of active metabolites [381]. These issues have resulted in recommendations against such practices from the AAP [382].

Respiratory and cardiovascular depression may occur with chloral hydrate. Despite the misconception that this agent is devoid of such adverse effects, apnea can occur with chloral hydrate and appropriate monitoring should always be used. Chloral hydrate is relatively contraindicated in neonates given its competition with bilirubin for protein binding sites. Additionally, the active metabolite, trichloroethanol, is related to the halogenated hydrocarbons and may cause ventricular arrhythmias especially in patients at risk for such problems (tricyclic antidepressant ingestions or underlying arrhythmia) [383, 384]. Given these issues, chloral hydrate has a limited role in sedation in the PICU setting; however, it may still have a place for sedation during non-painful radiologic imaging. When used for this purpose, doses of 75–100 mg/kg (maximum 2 g) can be administered by mouth or per rectum. Our clinical experience has suggested that chloral hydrate is less effective in patients older than 5 years of age and those with underlying CNS disorders such as autism. In a double-blind, randomized comparison with oral midazolam (0.5 mg/kg), chloral hydrate (75 mg/kg), the ability to complete the scan was higher with chloral hydrate (11 of 11 versus 11 of 22 with midazolam), and there was a decreased need for supplemental dosing (1 of 11 versus 12 of 22 with midazolam) [385]. Over the next few years, it is likely that there will be a continued decrease in the use of chloral hydrate. The liquid solution for oral administration is no longer available. Therefore, those centers that continue to use this agent have turned to their pharmacies as oral solutions must be prepared from powder preparations.

Tolerance, Physical Dependency, and Withdrawal

Over the past several years, data demonstrating the potential deleterious physiologic effects of untreated pain combined with ongoing humanitarian concerns have led to the increased use of sedative and analgesic agents. These initiatives have led to new consequences including physical dependency, tolerance, and withdrawal that require definition and effective treatment strategies. An appropriate place to begin the development of an effective approach to the patient with tolerance and physical dependency is a consensus on the definitions of these terms [386]. Tolerance is a decrease in a drug's effect over time or the need to increase the dose to achieve the same effect. Tolerance is related to changes at or distal to the receptor, generally at the cellular level. Some authorities have divided tolerance into various subcategories including innate tolerance referring to a genetically predetermined lack of sensitivity to a drug, pharmacokinetic or dispositional tolerance referring to changes in a drug's effect because of alterations in distribution or metabolism, learned tolerance or a reduction in a drug's effect as a result of learned or compensatory mechanisms (learning to walk a straight line while intoxicated by repeated practice at the task), and pharmacodynamic tolerance [386]. With pharmacodynamic tolerance, although the plasma concentration of the drug remains constant, there is a decreased effect. For the purpose of this discussion, the latter phenomenon will be referred to as tolerance as the other issues are not as relevant when considering the PICU patient.

Withdrawal includes the physical signs and symptoms that manifest when the administration of a sedative or analgesic agent is abruptly discontinued in a patient who is physically tolerant. The symptomatology of withdrawal varies from patient to patient and may be affected by several factors including the agent involved, the patient's age, cognitive state, and associated medical conditions. Physiologic (physical) dependence is the need to continue a sedative or analgesic agent to prevent withdrawal. Psychological dependence is the need for a substance because of its euphoric effects. Addiction is a complex pattern of behaviors characterized by the repetitive, compulsive use of a substance, antisocial or criminal behavior to obtain the drug, and a high incidence of relapse after treatment. Psychological dependency and addiction are extremely rare after the appropriate use of sedative or analgesic agents to treat pain or to relieve anxiety in the PICU setting.

The problems of opioid dependency and withdrawal in neonates and infants were first encountered in the 1970s and 1980s in infants of drug-addicted mothers [387, 388]. Despite the difference in the origin of the problem, these studies provided valuable information for dealing with today's PICU population. The studies from the 1970s and 1980s have provided various pharmacologic treatment regimens as well as scoring systems that may be used to grade the severity of withdrawal and to evaluate the efficacy of the treatment regimens. Arnold and colleagues were among the first to recognize the problems of dependency and withdrawal after prolonged opioid administration in the PICU population [389]. In a retrospective review of 37 neonates who required ECMO for respiratory failure and who had received intravenous fentanyl for sedation, they sought to identify the signs and symptoms of the neonatal abstinence syndrome (NAS) and risk factors for its occurrence. Fentanyl infusion requirements to achieve the desired level of sedation increased from 11.6±6.9 μ(mu)g/kg/h on day 1 to 52.5±19.4 μ(mu)g/kg/h on day 8. By measuring plasma fentanyl levels, they were able to demonstrate that there was an increase in the plasma fentanyl concentration required to achieve the same level of sedation, thereby demonstrating that the tolerance was pharmacodynamic and not pharmacokinetic (related to increased metabolism of the opioid). NAS was related to the total fentanyl dose and the duration of the infusion. A cumulative fentanyl dose ≥1.6 mg/kg and an ECMO duration ≥5 days were risk factors for the development of NAS (odds ratio of 7 and 13.9, respectively). The same investigators prospectively evaluated fentanyl dosing requirements and plasma fentanyl concentrations in a cohort of eight infants placed on ECMO [390]. Fentanyl infusion requirements increased from 9.2±1.9 μ(mu)g/kg/h on day 1 to 21.9±4.5 μ(mu)g/kg/h on day 6. As in their previous study, they noted an increase in the plasma fentanyl concentration from 3.1±1.1 ng/mL on day 1 to 13.9±3.2 ng/mL on day 6. In 1990, the potential for using oral methadone to treat or prevent opioid withdrawal after prolonged administration of fentanyl in the PICU patient was first suggested [391].

Subsequent reports demonstrated withdrawal from other agents used for prolonged sedation in the PICU patient including benzodiazepines, barbiturates, propofol, and even the inhalational anesthetic agents [392, 393]. Additional information concerning benzodiazepine withdrawal is provided by a retrospective review of Fonsmark et al. who evaluated 40 children who received sedation during mechanical ventilation. Sedation was provided by midazolam, pentobarbital, or a combination of the two [394]. Withdrawal symptoms occurred in 14 of 40 patients (35 %). Of the patients with withdrawal symptoms, eight had received both midazolam and pentobarbital, three received only midazolam, and three received only pentobarbital. A cumulative midazolam dose ≥60 mg/kg or a cumulative pentobarbital dose ≥25 mg/kg was associated with withdrawal whereas the duration of the infusion was not. Sedation was gradually tapered in only 1 of 14 patients who experienced withdrawal. Other anecdotal reports have noted withdrawal following the use of pentobarbital for sedation in the PICU population [273]. The potential for the development of tolerance to barbiturates is further supported by animal studies demonstrating the rapid development of tolerance after repeated administration and an increased susceptibility to pentylenetetrazol-induced seizures as a manifestation of barbiturate withdrawal [395, 396]. Anecdotal and retrospective reports have demonstrated similar withdrawal phenomenon following the prolonged administration of propofol and volatile anesthetic agents [397–400].

Clinical Signs and Symptoms of Withdrawal

The development of strategies to provide effective treatment of physical dependency and related problems requires the accurate identification and recognition of withdrawal symptoms. Ongoing or associated conditions that can manifest similar clinical signs and symptoms as withdrawal must be investigated and ruled out before concluding that the patient's symptoms are the result of withdrawal. In the PICU patient, these associated conditions may include central nervous system insults or infections, ICU psychosis, delirium, metabolic abnormalities, hypoxia, hypercarbia, and cerebral hypoperfusion from alterations in cardiac output or cerebral vascular disease.

Although many of the signs and symptoms of withdrawal are the same regardless of the agent, there may be subtle differences depending on the specific agent. The time to the onset of withdrawal symptoms varies depending on the half-life of the agent and the half-life of the active metabolites, which may be several times longer than the parent compound.

In general, the signs and symptoms of withdrawal from sedative and analgesic agents include signs and symptoms related to the CNS, the gastrointestinal tract, and the sympathetic nervous system. CNS manifestations are generally those of increased irritability including decreased sleep, tremulousness, hyperactive deep tendon reflexes, clonus, inability to concentrate, frequent yawning, sneezing, delirium, and hypertonicity. In neonates and infants, additional signs of central nervous system stimulation include a high-pitched cry and an exaggerated Moro reflex. Seizures have been reported with withdrawal from opioids, benzodiazepines, barbiturates, propofol, and inhalational anesthetic agents, while visual and auditory hallucinations have been described with opioid, benzodiazepine, barbiturate, and inhalational anesthetic withdrawal. GI manifestations include emesis, diarrhea, and feeding intolerance, which may be especially prominent in neonates and infants. When such problems occur in the absence of other signs and symptoms of withdrawal, they may be attributed to other problems and not withdrawal. Activation of the sympathetic nervous system with tachycardia, hypertension, dilated pupils, and tachypnea are prominent findings with withdrawal from any of the aforementioned sedative/analgesic agents. Additional signs and symptoms of sympathetic hyperactivity include nasal stuffiness, sweating, and fever.

Treatment of Withdrawal and Clinical Scoring Systems

As with most problems that arise in clinical medicine, effective treatment starts with prevention. Given that the incidence of withdrawal is related to the total amount of medication administered, careful titration of the sedative or analgesic agents using clinical sedation scales (discussed earlier) is suggested. In doing this, the minimal amount of medication required can be used. Although an increasing practice in the adult population, there are currently no data to support or refute the efficacy of the so-called drug holidays during the use of sedative and analgesic agents in the PICU setting. This practice involves turning off sedative and analgesic agents until the patient responds and then restarting the infusions at half of the previously used infusion rate. This practice effectively provides the same rationale as using clinical sedation scores in that excessive infusion rates are avoided. However, many physicians and certainly bedside nurses are hesitant to discontinue effective sedation and analgesia at times when painful processes may be present in the critically ill patient. Additionally, concerns have been raised that this practice may result in periods of excessive agitation in critically ill patients. Before such practices are universally embraced, prospective trials in the pediatric population are needed to demonstrate not only their efficacy, but also their safety.

Prospective studies are needed to better address the efficacy of rotating sedation regimens, intermittent versus continuous infusions of sedative/analgesic agents, and the role of other pharmacologic agents such as NMDA receptor antagonists and magnesium in preventing tolerance and dependency. Until further investigations provide additional insight into the factors controlling opioid dependency and ways of preventing or delaying it, PICU physicians will be faced with a group of patients who require specific actions to prevent the development of withdrawal symptoms. Treatment strategies and protocols are necessary so that the problems associated with tolerance, physical dependency, and withdrawals do not limit the administration of these agents in the PICU population.

In order to provide effective therapy for patients with withdrawal, it may be helpful to identify those patients who are most likely to manifest symptoms of withdrawal and also to have scoring systems to identify and quantitate the signs and symptoms of withdrawal. As noted previously in this chapter, risk factors that have been identified include not only the total dose of the sedative or analgesic agent that has been administered, but also the duration of the infusion. In a prospective trial of 23 infants and children who had received fentanyl infusions for sedation during mechanical ventilation, Katz et al. determined the factors that could be used to identify the group who was at risk of withdrawal [401]. Once sedation was no longer required, the fentanyl infusion was decreased by 50 % every 24 h times two and then discontinued. Withdrawal behavior was observed in 13 of 23 patients (57 %). The total fentanyl dose and the duration of the infusion correlated with the risk of withdrawal, whereas the maximum fentanyl infusion rate did not. A total fentanyl dose ≥1.5 mg/kg or an infusion duration ≥5 days was associated with a 50 % incidence of withdrawal, whereas a total fentanyl dose ≥2.5 mg/kg or an infusion duration ≥9 days was associated with a 100 % incidence of withdrawal.

Scoring systems may be helpful in the management of patients presenting with signs and symptoms of withdrawal, not only in identifying the behaviors of withdrawal, but also in grading its severity and judging the response to therapy. Unfortunately, the majority of scoring systems were developed to deal with neonates born to drug-addicted mothers and therefore may not be applicable to the PICU population [402]. To address such issues, Ista et al. reviewed the literature regarding withdrawal scoring systems and found that of the six available in the literature, only two were directed toward the PICU population [403]. The first of these included the sedation withdrawal score (SWS), which assigns 0–2 points to 12 withdrawal behaviors, thereby providing a maximum score of 24 (see Table 16.8). The signs and symptoms are grouped into the CNS (tremor, irritability, hypertonicity, high-pitched cry, convulsions, and hyperactivity), the GI system (vomiting and diarrhea), and the autonomic nervous system

Table 16.8 The sedation withdrawal score

Symptom	Score
Tremor	
Irritability	
Hypertonicity	
Hyperactivity	
Vomiting	
High-pitched cry	
Sneezing	
Respiratory distress	
Fever	
Diarrhea	
Sweating	
Convulsions	

For each symptom, score 0, absent; 1, mild; 2, severe. Maximum possible score, 24

(fever, sweating, sneezing, and respiratory rate) [404]. The decision regarding weaning of the current sedative and analgesic regimen is based on the score (0–6 wean, 6–12 no change, 12–18 revert to previous regimen, more than 18 reevaluate plan).

Ista et al. expressed concerns that this scale has not been validated in children and that, in particular, there are no data regarding its sensitivity, specificity, validity, and reliability. The other scale is the opioid and benzodiazepine withdrawal scale (OBWS) [405]. The OBWS is a 21-item checklist that evaluates 16 specific withdrawal behaviors. Franck et al. evaluated their scale by performing 693 assessments in 15 children who varied in age from 6 weeks to 28 months. Using 8 as a cutoff score for the presence of withdrawal, the sensitivity of the OBWS was only 50 % with a specificity of 87 %. The predictive value in terms of positive and negative ratios was 4.0 and 0.57 (considered moderate for a diagnostic tool), while the inter-rater reliability was acceptable at 0.8 (see Table 16.9) [405].

Because of these issues, Ista et al. concluded that a more appropriate scale was necessary in the PICU population and went on to use the data from their review to develop their own withdrawal scale [406]. Their withdrawal scale included all of the behaviors that had been reported in the literature as manifestations of withdrawal in the pediatric-aged patient. From this, they developed the Sophia Benzodiazepine and Opioid Withdrawal Checklist (SBOWC), which included 24 withdrawal symptoms. Over a 6-month period, they collected 2,188 observations in 79 children within 24 h of tapering off and discontinuing sedative and/or analgesic medication. They noted that specific symptoms including agitation, anxiety, muscle tension, sleeping for less than 1 h, diarrhea, fever, sweating, and tachypnea were observed most frequently and that longer duration of opioid or benzodiazepine use and high doses were risk factors for withdrawal. Twenty-three observations were scored simultaneously and

Table 16.9 Frequency of withdrawal symptoms measured with the OBWS [405]

	Nurse's assessment of withdrawal	
Sign or symptom	Present (%)	Absent (%)
Crying/agitated >75 % of interval	11.9	0.2
Crying/agitated 26–75 % of interval	33.8	11.8
Sleeping <25 % of the interval	51.7	10.7
Hyperactive Moro reflex	1.3	1.5
Pupils >4 mm	36.4	17.3
Tremors	35.7	17.4
Movement disorder	15.9	0.9
Hallucinations	0.7	0.4
Temperature >37.2 °C	81.5	67.9
Respiratory rate high for age	7.9	1.3
Frequent suction required	26.5	25.6
Sweating	10.6	1.8
Yawning	5.3	1.7
Sneezing	2.4	0.7
Nasal stuffiness	7.9	3.7
Vomiting	3.9	0.4
Diarrhea	42.4	20.3

resulted in an interobserver correlation coefficient of 0.85 with a range of 0.59–1.0 for the individual items.

Subsequent work by Franck et al. has resulted in the development of the WAT-1 (withdrawal and assessment tool) [407–409] (see Fig. 16.2). The components of this score, which is being used more frequently in pediatric ICUs around the country, are outlined by Franck et al. [409]. The score assigns a value of 0 for no or 1 for yes to the following questions: loose or watery stools; vomiting, retching, or gagging; and temperature ≥37.8 °C. The patient is then observed for 2 min to assess their state (asleep, awake, or calm versus distressed), the presence of a tremor, sweating, uncoordinated or repetitive motion, and yawning or sneezing. Again, these are scored as 0 for no and 1 for yes. The patient is then observed following a stimulus and during recovery for startle to touch and muscle as well as time to regain a calm state. These components result in a score from 0 to 12.

By maintaining a high index of suspicion and the use of withdrawal scores developed for the PICU patient, we may get closer to our goal of identifying patients who are manifesting withdrawal symptoms. As mentioned previously, the mainstay of preventing withdrawal must be the identification of high-risk patients and the slow weaning of sedative and analgesic agents. Withdrawal scales should still be applied to these patients in the event that withdrawal occurs despite our attempts to prevent it. Based on limited evidence-based medicine, it has been suggested that in patients who have received sedative and analgesic infusions for more than 5–7 days, weaning can be accomplished at a rate of 10–20 % per day [410, 411]. However, these studies have reported a significant

WITHDRAWAL ASSESSMENT TOOL VERSION 1 (WAT – 1)

© 2007 L.S. Franck and M.A.Q. Curley. All Rights reserved. Reproduced only by permission of Authors.

Patient Identifier														
	Date:													
	Time:													
Information from patient record, previous 12 hours														
Any loose /watery stools	No = 0 Yes = 1													
Any vomiting/wretching/gagging	No = 0 Yes = 1													
Temperature > 37.8°C	No = 0 Yes = 1													
2 minute pre-stimulus observation														
State	SBS[1] ≤ 0 or asleep/awake/calm = 0 SBS[1] ≥ +1 or awake/distressed = 1													
Tremor	None/mild = 0 Moderate/severe = 1													
Any sweating	No = 0 Yes = 1													
Uncoordinated/repetitive movement	None/mild = 0 Moderate/severe = 1													
Yawning or sneezing	None or 1 = 0 ≥2 = 1													
1 minute stimulus observation														
Startle to touch	None/mild = 0 Moderate/severe = 1													
Muscle tone	Normal = 0 Increased = 1													
Post-stimulus recovery														
Time to gain calm state (SBS[1] ≤ 0)	< 2min = 0 2 - 5min = 1 > 5 min = 2													
Total Score (0-12)														

WITHDRAWAL ASSESSMENT TOOL (WAT – 1) INSTRUCTIONS

- Start WAT-1 scoring from the **first day of weaning** in patients who have received opioids +/or benzodiazepines by infusion or regular dosing for prolonged periods (e.g., > 5 days). Continue twice daily scoring until 72 hours after the last dose.
- The Withdrawal Assessment Tool (WAT-1) should be completed along with the SBS[1] at least once per 12 hour shift (e.g., at 08:00 and 20:00 ± 2 hours). The progressive stimulus used in the SBS[1] assessment provides a standard stimulus for observing signs of withdrawal.

Obtain information from patient record (this can be done before or after the stimulus):

- ✓ **Loose/watery stools**: Score 1 if any loose or watery stools were documented in the past 12 hours; score 0 if none were noted.
- ✓ **Vomiting/wretching/gagging**: Score 1 if any vomiting or spontaneous wretching or gagging were documented in the past 12 hours; score 0 if none were noted
- ✓ **Temperature > 37.8°C**: Score 1 if the modal (most frequently occurring) temperature documented was greater than 37.8 °C in the past 12 hours; score 0 if this was not the case.

2 minute pre-stimulus observation:

- ✓ **State**: Score 1 if awake and distress (SBS[1]: ≥ +1) observed during the 2 minutes prior to the stimulus; score 0 if asleep or awake and calm/cooperative (SBS[1] ≤ 0).
- ✓ **Tremor**: Score 1 if moderate to severe tremor observed during the 2 minutes prior to the stimulus; score 0 if no tremor (or only minor, intermittent tremor).
- ✓ **Sweating**: Score 1 if any sweating during the 2 minutes prior to the stimulus; score 0 if no sweating noted.
- ✓ **Uncoordinated/repetitive movements**: Score 1 if moderate to severe uncoordinated or repetitive movements such as head turning, leg or arm flailing or torso arching observed during the 2 minutes prior to the stimulus; score 0 if no (or only mild) uncoordinated or repetitive movements.
- ✓ **Yawning or sneezing** > 1: Score 1 if more than 1 yawn or sneeze observed during the 2 minutes prior to the stimulus; score 0 if 0 to 1 yawn or sneeze.

1 minute stimulus observation:

- ✓ **Startle to touch**: Score 1 if moderate to severe startle occurs when touched during the stimulus; score 0 if none (or mild).
- ✓ **Muscle tone**: Score 1 if tone increased during the stimulus; score 0 if normal.

Post-stimulus recovery:

- ✓ **Time to gain calm state** (SBS[1] ≤ 0): Score 2 if it takes greater than 5 minutes following stimulus; score 1 if achieved within 2 to 5 minutes; score 0 if achieved in less than 2 minutes.

Sum the 11 numbers in the column for the total WAT-1 score (0-12).

[1]Curley et al. State behavioral scale: A sedation assessment instrument for infants and young children supported on mechanical ventilation. Pediatr Crit Care Med 2006;7(2):107-114.

Fig. 16.2 Withdrawal Assessment Tool Version 1 (WAT-1). Reprinted with permission from Franck LS, Harris S, Soetenga D, Amling J, Curley M. The withdrawal assessment tool (WAT-1): Measuring iatrogenic withdrawal symptoms in pediatric critical care. Pediatr Crit Care Med 2008;9(6):573–580

incidence of withdrawal using these protocols, thereby suggesting that a more reasonable approach may be a 5–10 % decrease per day as has been suggested for adult patients and supported by some in the PICU population [412, 413]. A more rapid wean can be accomplished when the patients have received these agents for less than 3–5 days.

After prolonged administration, the weaning process may require weeks to prevent withdrawal symptoms. Although the weaning process can be accomplished by slowly decreasing the intravenous infusion rate, this mandates the maintenance of intravenous access, ongoing hospitalization, and at times, continued monitoring in the PICU because, depending on hospital policies, certain medications such as fentanyl or midazolam cannot be administered by continuous infusion in settings other than the PICU. In these circumstances, options to consider include either switching to subcutaneous or oral administration.

If it is decided that tapering the infusion can be accomplished within a reasonable period of time that will not delay hospital discharge and that switching to oral medications will not expedite discharge home, the patient may be considered a candidate for subcutaneous administration (see previous) [84]. These patients are generally receiving moderate doses of fentanyl (5–10 μ(mu)g/kg/h) and/or midazolam (0.1–0.3 mg/kg/h). The switch to the subcutaneous route allows the removal of central venous access, eliminates the need to maintain peripheral intravenous access, and depending on individual hospital policies may eliminate the need for ongoing care in the ICU setting. Both fentanyl and midazolam can be effectively administered via the subcutaneous route and the infusions slowly tapered to prevent symptoms of withdrawal. Concentrated solutions of fentanyl (25–50 μ(mu)g/mL) and midazolam (2.5–5 mg/mL) are used so that the maximum subcutaneous infusion rate does not exceed 3 mL/h. Subcutaneous infusions are started at the same dose that is currently being used for intravenous administration. A topical dermal anesthetic cream can be placed over the site of anticipated subcutaneous cannulation. Several areas are suitable for subcutaneous administration, including the subclavicular region, abdomen, deltoid, or anterior aspect of the thigh. The site is cleaned and prepped with a sterile antiseptic solution, and then either a standard 22 gauge intravenous cannula or a 23 gauge butterfly needle is inserted into the subcutaneous tissue. Before placement, the tubing and needle are flushed with the opioid/benzodiazepine solution. The insertion site is then covered with a transparent, bio-occlusive dressing. The site should be changed every 7 days or sooner if erythema develops. The same infusion pumps that are used for intravenous administration can be used for subcutaneous administration. The pressure limit may need to be adjusted to allow for subcutaneous administration. Alternatively, a syringe pump can be used. If symptoms of withdrawal develop, additional boluses can be administered subcutaneously if necessary.

Several different opioids can be administered subcutaneously including the synthetic opioids, morphine, hydromorphone, and meperidine. Longer-acting agents such as methadone and levorphanol are not recommended because dose titration may be difficult given the long half-lives of these agents. Tissue reaction and erythema has been noted with methadone. Although there is limited experience with the use of subcutaneous infusions of opioids/benzodiazepines as a means of weaning patients and preventing withdrawal, the subcutaneous route has been used to treat chronic cancer-related pain as well as postoperative pain.

When prolonged administration of opioids or other sedative agents will be necessary, switching to the oral administration of long-acting agents such as methadone may allow for earlier hospital discharge. This is especially true in patients who have received weeks of therapy and are on large doses of opioids and/or benzodiazepines. Advantages of methadone include its longer half-life allowing for dosing 2–3 times per day, an oral bioavailability of 75–90 %, and availability as a liquid. Although the first report regarding the use of methadone suggested a starting dose of 0.1 mg/kg every 12 h, the three patients in the series were receiving relatively low opioid doses and, therefore, higher doses of methadone were not needed. The subsequent clinical experience has indicated that higher doses of methadone may be needed, depending on the dose of fentanyl.

When considering the appropriate dose transition from intravenous fentanyl to oral methadone, consideration should be given to the differences in the potency and half-life of the two medications as well as crossover tolerance [414]. Similar considerations are necessary when switching from intravenous midazolam to oral lorazepam. Lugo et al., in a study evaluating enteral lorazepam to decrease midazolam requirements during mechanical ventilation, suggested starting at a lorazepam dose that was 1/6th that of the total daily dose of intravenous midazolam [97]. Once the appropriate enteral/oral dose is determined and started, intravenous administration is tapered off quickly.

After the initial reports regarding the use of methadone, other authors have suggested variations in conversion ratios from fentanyl to methadone as well as dosing intervals and most importantly weaning schedules [410, 411, 415–417]. Some investigators have used intravenous methadone prior to oral methadone during the initial conversion process. Regardless of the protocol used, close observation during the conversion period is necessary to avoid adverse effects from oversedation or to recognize the early symptoms of withdrawal. There remain some stigmata concerning the use of methadone. Therefore, a thorough discussion with the parents is necessary to discuss why methadone is being used and to outline the differences between addiction and physical dependency. Because of these issues as well as familiarity with long-acting morphine preparations, which are used in the treatment of children with chronic cancer-related pain, some physicians prefer to use the latter agent. However, these agents are available only in tablets that cannot be crushed so that administration and subsequent weaning protocols may be more difficult in younger patients. Methadone on the other hand is available in a liquid formulation.

More recently, concern has been expressed in the adult population, who are on maintenance methadone for drug addiction regarding the potential for death and the potential for QT prolongation and arrhythmias [418]. To date, there are no reports from the pediatric population; however, these concerns have led to the consideration of obtaining periodic ECGs prior to and after instituting therapy with methadone. A final issue with methadone is its metabolism by the P_{450} isoenzyme system of the liver, making alterations in metabolism possible based on genetic factors and the coadministration of other medications. These factors should be considered when methadone is started or other medications are added to the patient's regimen.

In addition to opioids, non-opioid agents have been used to treat opioid withdrawal. In the author's opinion, this is less than optimal because it seems to make physiologic sense when dealing with the problems of tolerance and dependence to replace the missing agent rather than to treat the resulting symptoms. Given these concerns, our current clinical practice is to generally use a medication in the same class as the one resulting in withdrawal. In specific clinical scenarios, the centrally acting, α(alpha)$_2$-adrenergic agonists, clonidine and dexmedetomidine, have been used to treat and prevent opioid withdrawal [419–422].

Delirium

In addition to the myriad of issues surrounding the provision of sedation and analgesia to critically ill patients, recent attention in clinical practice and in the literature, especially in the adult ICU population, has been focused on the issue of delirium following critical illnesses. In the ICU setting, delirium has been described as an acute and fluctuating disturbance of consciousness and cognition. In more general terms, the American Psychiatric Association's (APA) Diagnostic and Statistical Manual of Mental Disorders (DSM-IV) has defined delirium as a disturbance of consciousness and cognition that develops over a short period of time and fluctuates over time. Over the years, several different terms and labels have been used to describe this syndrome in the ICU setting including ICU psychosis, ICU syndrome, acute confusional state, encephalopathy, and acute brain failure. However, with a greater appreciation of the importance of this syndrome on the outcomes of critically ill patients and the need to appropriately identify it, the critical care community has recently conformed to the recommendations of the APA that the term "delirium" be used uniformly to describe this syndrome of brain dysfunction.

Delirium may occur in up to 80 % of critically ill adults. Its short- and long-term consequences include prolonged hospitalization as well as other morbidities. It may also be either a marker for or a direct cause of both short-term and long-term mortality risk of ICU patients [423–425]. In a prospective evaluation meant to determine the immediate- and long-term consequences of delirium in a cohort of 224 adult ICU patients, 183 (81.7 %) developed delirium at some point during their ICU stay [426]. Demographics including age, comorbidity scores, dementia scores, activity of daily living scores, severity of illness, and admitting diagnoses were similar between those patients who developed delirium and those who did not. Patients who developed delirium had a higher 6-month mortality rate (34 % versus 15 %, $p=0.03$) and spent 10 days longer in the hospital than those patients who did not develop delirium ($p<0.001$). Additional morbidities related to delirium included prolonged ICU stay, prolonged duration of requirements for mechanical ventilation, and increased costs of care following hospital discharge.

Classification of Delirium

Given the difficulties with identification, even in the adult population, delirium may often go unrecognized or be attributed to other disease processes or comorbid conditions such as dementia and depression or be considered a natural, acceptable complication of a critical illness. Delirium can generally be divided into hypoactive and hyperactive subtypes, which outside of the ICU population have been shown to have some prognostic values. Hypoactive delirium, which tends to account for the majority of cases in the ICU setting, is characterized by decreased responsiveness, withdrawal behaviors, apathy, and depression. Hyperactive delirium, as the name implies, is characterized by agitation, restlessness, and emotional lability [427]. In a prospective evaluation of delirium in a cohort of adult medical ICU patients, Peterson et al. reported that purely hyperactive delirium was uncommon, occurring in 1.6 % of the patients, hypoactive delirium occurred in 43.5 % of the patients, while 54.1 % had mixed delirium [428]. Ouimet et al. proposed an alternative scheme for the categorization of delirium in the ICU setting, which is based on the number of symptoms of delirium that are present [429]. Six hundred ICU patients were observed for symptoms of delirium and then categorized according to the number of symptoms present. No delirium was present if there were no symptoms, patients with four or more symptoms were classified as having "clinical delirium," while an intermediate state, which the authors termed "subsyndromal delirium," was thought to be present in patients who manifested 1–3 symptoms.

Table 16.10 The intensive care delirium screening checklist (ICDSC)

Patient evaluation	Day 1	Day 2	Day 3	Day 4	Day 5
Altered level of consciousness (A–E)[a]					
If A or B, do not complete patient evaluation for the period					
Inattention					
Disorientation					
Hallucination–delusion–psychosis					
Psychomotor agitation or retardation					
Inappropriate speech or mood					
Sleep–wake cycle disturbance					
Symptom fluctuation					
Total score (0–8)					

[a]Level of consciousness:
A: No response, score: none
B: Response to intense and repeated stimulation (loud voice and pain), score: none
C: Response to mild or moderate stimulation, score: 1
D: Normal wakefulness, score: 0
E: Exaggerated response to normal stimulation, score: 1

Diagnosis of Delirium

Given its impact on short- and long-term outcome in the ICU patient, the accurate diagnosis of delirium is mandatory to identify its occurrence following critical illness and to facilitate trials to determine ways to limit its occurrence. As noted previously, the underdiagnosis and recognition of delirium remain a significant problem [430]. Such issues have led to the suggestion by the Society for Critical Care Medicine that some type of delirium screening tool should be used in all critically ill patients. As with the depth of sedation and withdrawal, there are instruments that have been validated for the assessment of delirium in ICU patients. To date, these instruments have only been studied in the adult population. Two such tools are (1) the intensive care delirium screening checklist (ICDSC) (see Table 16.10) and the confusion assessment method for the ICU (CAM-ICU) (see Table 16.11) [431, 432].

The scoring systems allow the assessment of and diagnosis of delirium in ICU patients by nonpsychiatric trained physicians and health-care workers in the ICU. These tools can be used even in patients who are unable to speak because of the presence of an ETT. Both scoring tools begin with an assessment of the patient's responsiveness, and no further evaluation is undertaken if the patient is obtunded or deeply sedated.

The ICDSC rates the level of consciousness from A to E, with A denoting no response and E denoting exaggerated response to normal stimulation. If an A (no response) or B (response to intense or repeated stimulation) is obtained, no further assessment is undertaken. For patients who manifest a C, D, or E level, a further evaluation for the presence of delirium is undertaken. This includes assessing inattentiveness, disorientation, hallucination–delusion–psychosis, psychomotor agitation or retardation, inappropriate speech or mood, sleep–wake cycle disturbances, and symptom fluctuation. These seven checklist items are added to altered level of consciousness to give eight possible items, which are scored as present or absent, to give a total delirium score of 0–8—with four or more considered diagnostic of delirium. More recently, this work has been extended into the pediatric population with the development of scoring systems for this population (see Fig. 16.3) [433, 434].

Risk Factors for the Development of Delirium

As with many outcomes in the ICU, the risk factors for the development of delirium include factors that may be present prior to the onset of the acute illness and those that relate directly to the acute illness or medications administered during it. Patient comorbidities that may increase the likelihood of delirium include advanced age, hypertension, the severity of illness, history of tobacco use, and baseline cognitive impairment. Other potential risk factors include metabolic disturbances (plasma levels of sodium, calcium, and blood urea nitrogen), acute infection, respiratory disease, acidosis, anemia, and hypotension. Additionally, there may be some genetic predisposition to the development of delirium. Ely et al. evaluated the possible association of the apolipoprotein E genotype and delirium among 53 mechanically ventilated medical ICU patients [435]. Patients with the apolipoprotein-4 polymorphism (a risk factor for Alzheimer's disease) manifested delirium twice as long as those without this polymorphism. The duration of delirium (median and interquartile range) was 4 days (3–4.5 days) versus 2 days (1–4 days, $p = 0.05$).

Also of significant concern in the ICU patient is the potential role that the use of sedative and analgesic agents may play in the development of delirium. Several studies have suggested an association between delirium and medications used for sedation or analgesia. To date, the most compelling evidence suggests that medications that act through the GABA system increase the likelihood of delirium. Most notable of the GABA-agonists in the role of delirium are the benzodiazepines, including both midazolam and lorazepam [436]. In distinction, there are little or no data to demonstrate any relationship between the use of opioids such as morphine or fentanyl and the risk of developing delirium. In fact, the appropriate use of opioids for analgesia may decrease its incidence, as Ouimet et al. reported that the mean daily dose of opioid was higher among patients without delirium than among those with delirium [437]. Similarly, in a cohort of

Table 16.11 The confusion assessment method for the ICU (CAM-ICU)

Features and descriptions	Absent	Present
I. Acute onset or fluctuating course[a] A. Is there evidence of an acute change in mental status from the baseline? Or B. Did the (abnormal) behavior fluctuate during the past 24 h? Come and go or increase and decrease in severity, as evidenced by fluctuations on the Richmond Agitation Sedation Scale (RASS) or the Glasgow Coma Scale?		
II. Inattention[b] Did the patient have difficulty focusing attention, as evidenced by a score of less than eight correct answers on either the visual or auditory components of the Attention Screening Examination (ASE)?		
III. Disorganized thinking Is there evidence of disorganized or incoherent thinking as evidenced by incorrect answers to three or more of the following four questions and inability to follow the commands? Questions 1. Will a stone float on water? 2. Are there fish in the sea? 3. Does 1 lb weigh more than 2 lb? 4. Can you use a hammer to pound a nail? Commands 1. Are you having unclear thinking? 2. Hold up this many fingers (examiner holds two fingers in front of the patient) 3. Now do the same thing with the other hand (without holding the two fingers in front of the patient) (If the patient is already extubated from the ventilator, determine whether the patient's thinking is disorganized or incoherent, i.e., rambling or irrelevant conversation, unclear or illogical flow of ideas, or unpredictable switching from subject to subject)		
IV. Altered level of consciousness Is the patient's level of consciousness anything other than alert? • *Alert*: spontaneously fully aware of the environment and interacts appropriately • *Vigilant*: hyperalert • *Lethargic*: drowsy but easily aroused, unaware of some elements in the environment or not spontaneously interacting with the interviewer; becomes fully aware and appropriately interactive when prodded minimally • *Stupor*: difficult to arouse, unaware of some or all elements in the environment or not spontaneously interacting with the interviewer; becomes incompletely aware when prodded strongly; can be aroused only by vigorous and repeated stimuli; as soon as the stimulus ceases, patient lapses into an unresponsive state • *Coma*: unarousable, unaware of all elements in the environment with no spontaneous interaction or awareness of the interviewer so that the interview is impossible even with maximal prodding		
Overall CAM-ICU Assessment (Features 1 and 2 or either Feature 3 or 4): Yes__ No__		

[a]The scores included in the 10-point RASS range from a high of 4 (combative) to a low of –5 (deeply comatose and unresponsive). Under the RASS system, patients who are spontaneously alert, calm, and not agitated were scored 0 (neutral). Anxious or agitated patients receive a range of scores depending upon their level of anxiety: 1, anxious; 2, agitated (fighting ventilator); 3, very agitated (pulling on or removing catheters); 4, combative (violent, a danger to staff). Scores of –1 to –5 are assigned to patients with varying degrees of sedation based on their ability to maintain eye contact: –1, more than 10 s; –2, less than 10 s; –3, eye opening but no eye contact. If physical stimulation is required, patients are scored as –4, eye opening or movement with physical or painful stimulation, and –5, no response to physical or painful stimulation

[b]In completing the visual ASE, patients are shown five simple pictures at 3-s intervals and asked to remember them. They are then immediately shown ten subsequent pictures and asked to nod "yes" or "no" to indicate whether they had or had not just seen each of the pictures. Because five pictures have been shown already and five pictures are new, a perfect score would be five "yes" and five "no" responses. For auditory ASE, patients are asked to squeeze the rater's hand whenever they heard the letter "A" during a recitation of ten letters, which are read in a normal tone at a rate of one letter per second: S A H E V A A R A T. A scoring method similar to the visual ASE is used for the auditory test

541 adult patients who were hospitalized for a hip fracture, those who received more than 10 mg/day of parenteral morphine or morphine equivalents were less likely to develop delirium than patients who received less analgesia [438]. Treatment with meperidine was an exception as meperidine has been shown to increase the risk of delirium when compared with other opioids.

Pathophysiology of Delirium

The exact cellular or physiologic mechanisms of delirium remain poorly defined. Additionally, it is likely that it may result from a multifactorial process, resulting from a combination of underlying patient factors, the critical illness, and medications used in the ICU setting. One theory that has

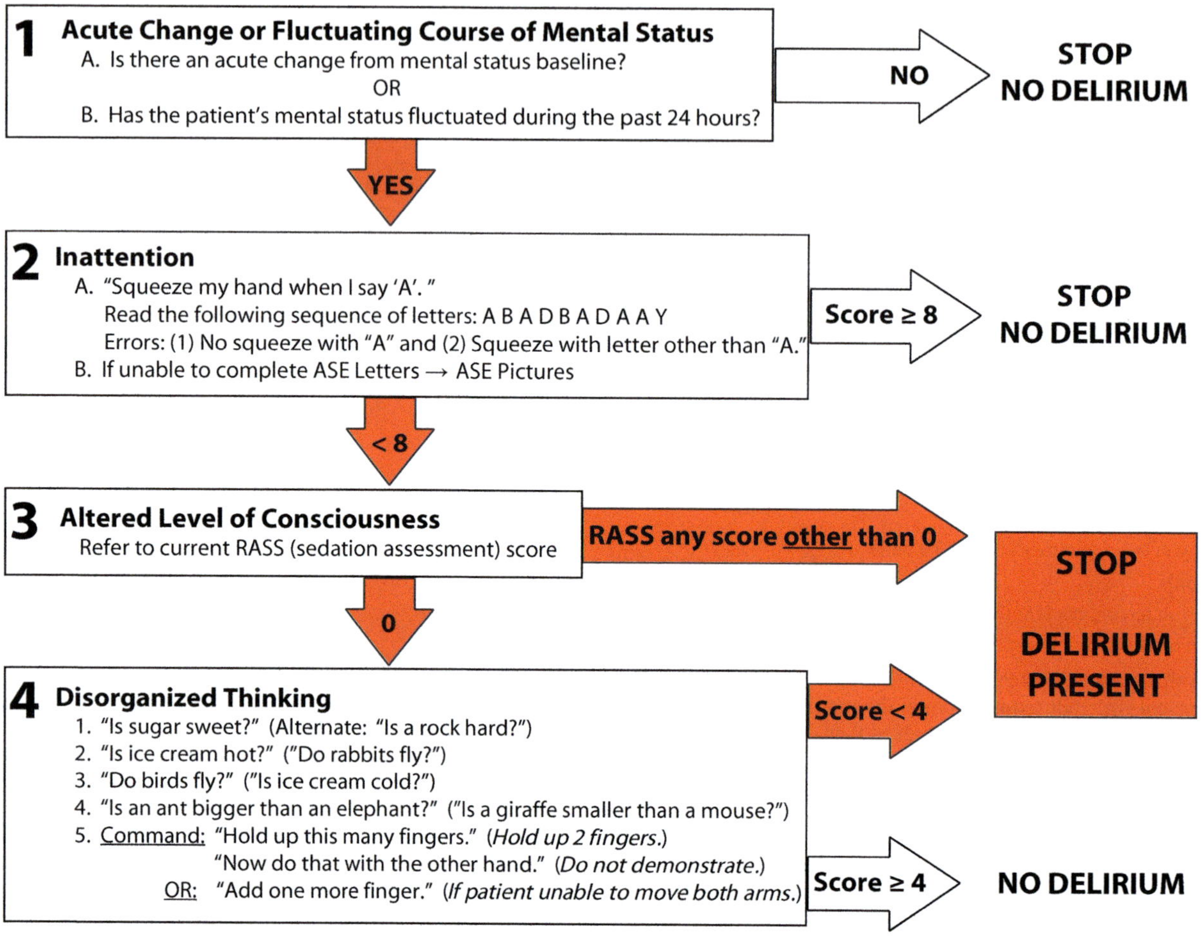

Fig. 16.3 Pediatric confusion assessment method for the intensive care unit: a practical time-saving approach to bedside implementation. Modified with permission from Smith HAB, Boyd J, Fuchs DC, et al. Diagnosing delirium in critically ill children: Validity and reliability of the Pediatric Confusion Assessment Method for the Intensive Care Unit. Crit Care 2011;39:150–157 [433]

been supported by clinical research is that delirium results from a neurotransmitter imbalance. Derangements of several different central neurotransmitters has been theorized to result in delirium, although the greatest focus has been on alterations in the central concentrations of dopamine and acetylcholine [439, 440]. Specifically, an excess of dopamine or relative deficiencies in acetylcholine may result in delirium. Other potential central neurotransmitters that may play a role in the pathogenesis of delirium include GABA, serotonin, endorphins, and glutamate. It has also been theorized that these alterations in neurotransmitter levels may be secondary to changes in plasma concentrations of amino acids such as tryptophan, tyrosine, leucine, or phenylalanine, which may occur during critical illnesses [441, 442]. Other evidence has pointed toward inflammation as a potential etiologic factor in the development of delirium.

As end-organ dysfunction in the ICU setting is known to result from a systemic inflammatory process resulting in multisystem organ failure, a generalized inflammatory process induced by endotoxins and cytokines may also result in CNS dysfunction and delirium. Animal studies have demonstrated that this inflammatory cascade may result in alterations in the blood–brain barrier, changes in vascular permeability within the CNS, and EEG changes consistent with those seen in ICU patients who develop delirium [443]. The end result of this inflammatory process may provoke delirium through alterations in CBF, by interfering with normal neurotransmitter function, or altering neurotransmitter concentrations within the CNS.

Prevention and Treatment of Delirium

Given the prevalence and adverse effects of delirium in the ICU setting, appropriate interventions include not only treatment once delirium has occurred, but potentially strategies to limit its incidence. Although performed in a non-ICU population, Inouye et al. nonrandomly assigned 852 hospitalized elderly patients to usual care or management with a multiple-component strategy aimed at decreasing the incidence of delirium [444]. Interventions included repeated reorientation of the patient, the provision of cognitively stimulating activities, a non-pharmacologic protocol to improve sleep, ambulation and mobilization activities, range of motion exercises, timely removal of catheters and physical restraints, and improvement in sensory input through the use of eyeglasses, magnifying lenses, and hearing aids. These interventions significantly reduced the incidence of delirium (15.0 % in the standard care group versus 9.9 % in the intervention group). Given the outcome of this and other similar trials, such protocols have been recommended for use in the ICU population as a means of potentially decreasing the incidence of delirium. Additionally, despite the recognition of the need for appropriate sedation and analgesic in the ICU setting, it must also be recognized that the use of sedative medications may increase the incidence of delirium. As such, the appropriate use of the lowest feasible dose of such medications has been suggested by titrating the level of sedation using sedation scores or more recently, in the adult ICU population, by the daily interruption of sedation [445].

Although there are no placebo-controlled trial, haloperidol has been recommended as the drug of choice for the treatment of ICU delirium by both the Society of Critical Care Medicine and the APA. Classified as a typical antipsychotic, haloperidol blocks dopamine$_2$ receptors thereby decreasing agitation, hallucinations, and delusions. Given the lack of prospective, clinical trials, the optimal dose regimen has not been defined. Recommendations from the Society of Critical Care Medicine for adults include an initial dose of 2 mg intravenously, followed by repeated doses (doubling the previous dose) every 15–20 min until the agitation is controlled. Once the agitation subsides, scheduled doses (every 4–6 h) are recommended for 2–3 days followed by a tapering of the dose once the problem has resolved. In addition to its use as treatment for acute delirium, haloperidol has been shown to be effective when used as a prophylactic agent to prevent delirium in a cohort of elderly patients, hospitalized for the treatment of hip fractures [446].

The atypical antipsychotics (risperidone, ziprasidone, quetiapine, and olanzapine) may also be helpful in the treatment of delirium, but only preliminary data exist supporting their use in the ICU [447]. These medications target dopamine receptors as well as receptors for other neurotransmitters within the CNS including serotonin, acetylcholine, and norepinephrine. Patients treated with haloperidol or other antipsychotics should be monitored for adverse effects including cardiac arrhythmias due to effects on repolarization (these effects are less common with the atypical antipsychotic agents), hypotension, dystonic reactions, extrapyramidal effects, malignant neuroleptic syndrome, and lowering of the seizure threshold. Given the potential for the development of lethal cardiac arrhythmias including torsades de pointes, these agents are contraindicated in patients with a prolonged QT interval. Anticholinergic effects such as dry mouth, constipation, and urinary retention may also occur.

Given the potential impact that delirium may have on outcome, there is significant interest in identifying its etiology, preventing its occurrence, or treating it once it has manifested. Given its impact on adult patients, there is increased interest in investigating it in the pediatric population during prolonged ICU stays. The reader is referred to Schieveld et al. [448] and Smith et al. [449] for recent information regarding delirium and the pediatric ICU patient.

Sedation During Palliative Care and End of Life

The majority of this chapter has focused on pain and sedation issues during the care of children in the pediatric ICU setting. The focus on such care is generally on providing humanitarian care during acute disease processes with the intent of returning these patients to their premorbid state of health. (Refer to Chap. 37.) However, given the complexities of ICU care, survival cannot always be ensured and at times the focus shifts to providing pain relief and comfort during the terminal stages of an illness. Palliative care includes the control of pain, relief of agitation, and treatment of other symptoms while addressing the psychological, social, or spiritual problems of children (and their families) living with life-threatening or terminal conditions [450, 451].

Given the ICU physicians' familiarity with potent and effective medications for analgesia and sedation, they may be involved in the care of pediatric patients in the palliative setting.

Despite the advances in pain management techniques, the palliative care or ICU physician is frequently confronted with a patient whose symptoms have been refractory to conventional therapies. In the early phases of terminal illness, opioids remain the mainstay of therapy given their efficacy in controlling pain. Furthermore, these agents remain the primary medication for the relief of dyspnea in this scenario [452]. Given the development of tolerance, dose escalations are frequently required over time or as disease progression occurs. As the use of opioids for this setting has been described in great detail elsewhere, this section will focus on medications that may be used when primary opioid therapy fails [453–455]. Escalation to other medications may be needed to treat adverse effects associated with high-dose opioid infusions, as adjunctive agents to control pain, to control agitation related to disease progression, or for terminal sedation/comfort care when opioids fail.

Although beyond the scope of this chapter, there are significant ethical issues to be considered and which likely need further refinement when considering the use of sedation in the terminally ill patient. (Refer to Chap. 37.) Decreasing the level of consciousness and the patient's ability to respond will decrease family interactions and limit their ability to participate in decisions regarding their care including limitations or escalations of care. Most importantly, rapid escalations of such medications may cross the line between symptom control and euthanasia. Such ethical issues must always be considered and discussed with the family in the context of state and societal legal implications [456, 457]. When considering the non-opioid choices for sedation, benzodiazepines, ketamine, dexmedetomidine, and propofol have been anecdotally reported to offer some benefit in this scenario. As their use is somewhat different from that already described in this chapter, a brief discussion will be provided of the latter three agents as they relate to palliative care.

Ketamine

Ketamine is generally classified as a general anesthetic agent; however, it can be administered at sub-anesthetic doses to provide analgesia or supplement opioid-based analgesic regimens in cancer-associated pain, neuropathic pain, ischemic pain, and regional pain syndromes [458, 459]. It is considered an integral medication for the management of refractory pain by the World Health Organization. Its analgesic effects are postulated to result primarily antagonism at the *N*-methyl-*D*-aspartate (NMDA) receptor. This effect may result in some reversal of opioid tolerance. Given its limited effects on hemodynamic and respiratory function, it has become a commonly used agent in refractory pain syndromes and palliative care [460]. It has been demonstrated that the psychomimetic effects may be blunted by gradual dose titration [461].

Although there will be alterations in its bioavailability, it can be effectively administered via intravenous, subcutaneous, and non-parenteral routes including oral. When oral administration is not be feasible due to the advanced stages of diseases, ketamine can be administered and effectively titrated by the subcutaneous route [462]. The techniques involved in the use of subcutaneous infusions are outlined by Tobias [463].

Propofol

Although also classified as an intravenous anesthetic agent, dose titration is feasible with propofol so that sedation can be achieved with lower doses. However, unlike ketamine, adverse effects on respiratory and hemodynamic function may be more common with propofol especially in patients with advanced terminal illnesses. These are significantly more common with bolus dosing, which is not recommended when propofol is used in the palliative care setting. Given its short half-life, rapid achievement of a steady-state serum concentration is achieved following its initiation or dose changes. As such, even for the initiation of sedation in this setting, bolus dosing is not needed. Propofol must be administered via the intravenous route, and depending on state regulations, it may need to be administered in the hospital setting. To date, the majority of experience remains anecdotal consisting of isolated case reports or small case series [464–466]. Despite the anecdotal nature of these reports, they uniformly demonstrate the efficacy of propofol in this scenario in providing sedation and symptom relief. There was a reduction in opioid needs or an avoidance of the need to escalate doses. In addition to reviewing their experience with propofol for palliative sedation in three children, Anghelescu et al. provide a useful algorithm for this scenario (see Fig. 16.4) [467].

Dexmedetomidine

Given that it was the last of these agents to be introduced into the clinical market, there remains a paucity of data regarding the use of dexmedetomidine in palliative care. However, given its relative lack of effects on end hemodynamic and respiratory, beneficial sedative properties, and the potential to act as an adjunct to opioid analgesia, dexmedetomidine may be a useful agent in this scenario [468–470]. Most importantly, as it is not classified as an intravenous anesthetic agent, its use outside of the hospital setting may be more feasible. Furthermore, evidence from the ICU setting has demonstrated its efficacy in both preventing and treating delirium. As with propofol, the literature regarding the use of dexmedetomidine in the palliative care setting remains anecdotal, with no reports regarding pediatric-aged patients [471, 472]. Although generally administered by the intravenous route in the ICU setting, there is increasing interest in the use of non-parenteral routes in the perioperative and procedural sedation arena including oral, intranasal, and buccal administration. Furthermore, anecdotal experience demonstrates its efficacy when administered by the subcutaneous route.

Conclusion

A cookbook approach to sedation and analgesia in the PICU is not feasible due to the wide variation in patients, ages, comorbid diseases, and clinical scenarios faced in this population. As no single agent will be effective in all patients

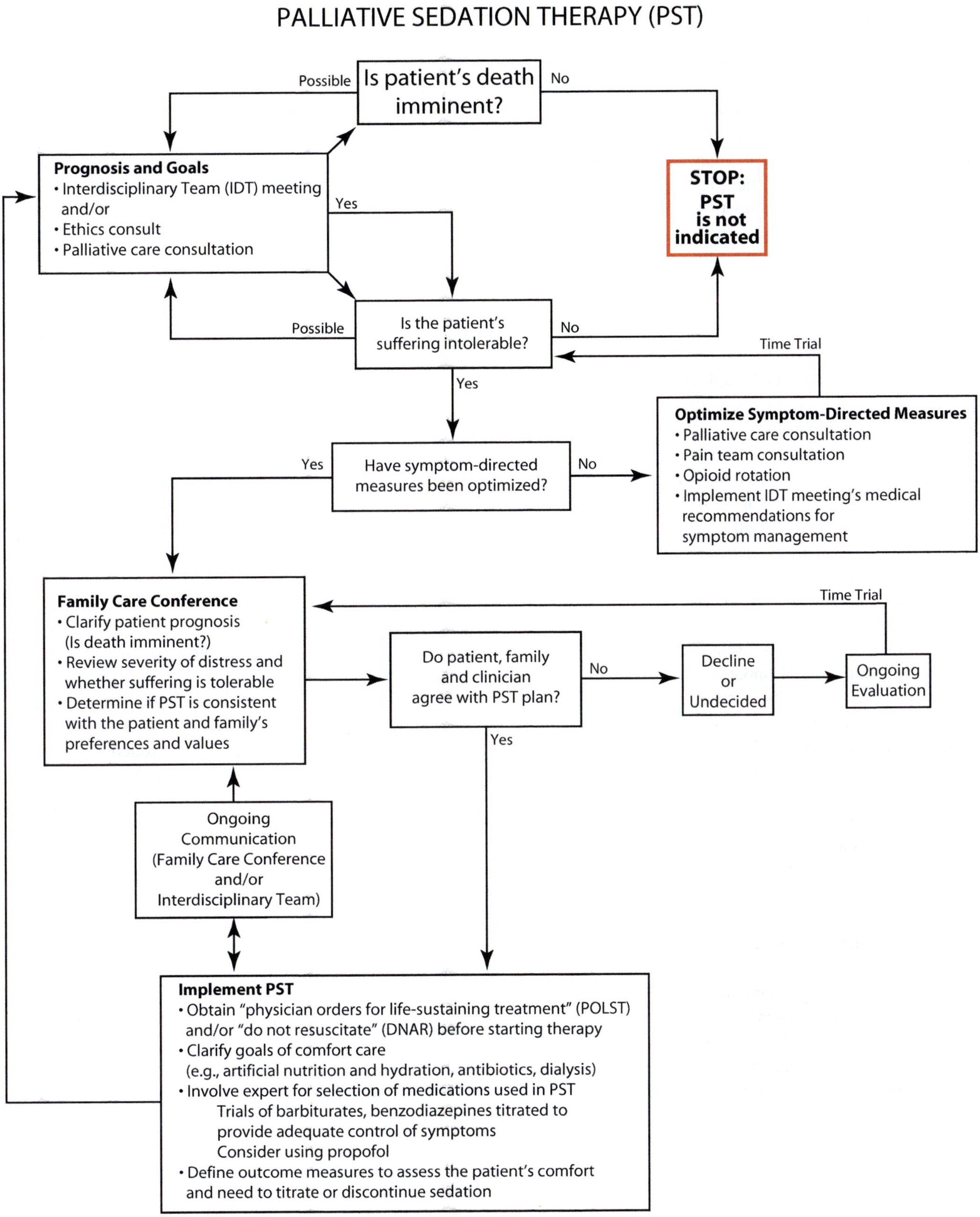

Fig. 16.4 Algorithm for initiation of palliative sedation therapy (PST), including selection of propofol [467]

and all scenarios, health-care providers must be facile with the use of a wide array of sedative and analgesic agents. The three primary choices that must be made when choosing a sedative/analgesic agent are the agent, its route or delivery, and the mode of delivery. In most scenarios, sedation during mechanical ventilation is initiated with either a benzodiazepine or an opioid. There is an abundance of clinical experience with midazolam in the PICU population, although lorazepam may provide an effective alternative with a longer half-life and more predictable pharmacokinetics without the concern of active metabolites. However, there are limited reports regarding its use in the PICU population and there may be concerns regarding accumulation of the diluent, propylene glycol.

Although fentanyl is frequently chosen because of its hemodynamic stability and beneficial effects on PVR, morphine is an effective alternative with data to suggest that the development of tolerance may be slower and that there may be fewer issues with withdrawal when compared to fentanyl. Long-term follow-up studies have demonstrated no adverse CNS developmental effects from morphine use in neonates and infants. In the critically ill infant at risk for pulmonary hypertension, the literature continues to support the use of the synthetic opioids given their ability to modulate PVR and prevent pulmonary hypertensive crisis. When these agents fail or lead to adverse effects, alternatives include ketamine, pentobarbital, or dexmedetomidine. Ketamine may be useful for the patient with hemodynamic instability or with increased airway reactivity as a component of their disease process. To date, there are limited reports regarding the use of pentobarbital in the PICU, with recent concerns being raised regarding a high incidence of adverse effects associated with its use. Propofol has gained great favor in the adult population as a means of providing deep sedation while allowing for rapid awakening. Similar beneficial properties are achieved in the pediatric-aged patient; however, concerns of the propofol infusion syndrome have significantly limited its use in the PICU population.

As the pediatric experience increases, it appears that there will be a role for newer agents such as dexmedetomidine. The use of dexmedetomidine may continue to increase as the incidence of delirium has been shown to be less with its use when compared to commonly used benzodiazepines [473]. Suggested starting guidelines for sedative and analgesic agents are outlined in Table 16.12. The second decision regarding PICU sedation includes the mode of administration. Effective sedation and analgesia is generally most easily achieved with the use of a continuous infusion of a benzodiazepine or opioid supplemented with as needed bolus doses to provide additional analgesia or sedation. These bolus doses are given during periods of breakthrough agitation or prior to noxious stimulation such as tracheal suctioning or other nursing interventions. Patients requiring frequent bolus doses should have the baseline infusion rate increased. As the infusion rate is increased, the bolus doses should be increased to equal the hourly rate. The titration of the infusion and use of supplemental bolus doses should be adjusted using clinical sedation scales. There may also be a role for newer devices that monitor awareness such as the bispectral index or BIS monitor. The third decision regarding sedative and analgesic agents is the route of administration. In the PICU setting, the intravenous route is used in the vast majority of patients. However, specific circumstances may exist that necessitate the use of a non-intravenous route. Although medications such as midazolam have been administered via many non-parenteral routes, including oral and transmucosal administration, these routes will have a limited role in the PICU population although they are viable options for procedural sedation. The subcutaneous route may be used in specific circumstances while future clinical trials with inhalational anesthetic agents may provide us with more information regarding these agents in infants and children.

When sedative and analgesic agents are administered, adverse effects on physiologic function may follow. Monitoring of the patient's physiologic function is mandatory whenever these agents are in use. There is also an increased understanding and recognition of withdrawal syndromes, which may occur following the prolonged administration of sedative and analgesic agents. Strategies are needed to identify those patients at risk for withdrawal followed by appropriate interventions to prevent or treat it. These may include a gradual tapering of the infusion rate or switching to oral or subcutaneous administration. As this is an increasing problem in the PICU setting, newer strategies to prevent its occurrence, such as the use of NMDA antagonists or rotating sedation regimens, warrant further investigations. With these caveats in mind, the goal of providing effective and safe sedation and analgesia for all of our patients is within reach.

Table 16.12 Suggested guidelines for dosing of sedative and analgesic agents

Agent	Dose	Comments
Fentanyl	2–3 μ(mu)g/kg/h	Modulates the postsurgical and sympathetic stress response thereby blunting increases in pulmonary vascular resistance. May have utility in neonates and infants at risk for pulmonary hypertension following surgery for congenital heart disease. Has limited effects on cardiac output and mean arterial pressure. May result in mild to moderate negative chronotropic effects
Morphine	10–30 μ(mu)g/kg/min	Cost-effective agent for sedation. Hemodynamic effects are generally related to vasodilation of capacitance vessels and a decrease in preload. These effects are exaggerated in the setting of hypovolemia. Delayed development of tolerance and less withdrawal issues when compared to fentanyl
Remifentanil	0.1–0.3 μ(mu)g/kg/min	Short (4–8 min) and consistent half-life across all age groups including neonates and infants due to esterase metabolism. Use for prolonged (more than 24 h) sedation limited by the rapid development of tolerance and cost
Midazolam	0.05–0.15 mg/kg/h	Abundant clinical experience as an agent for PICU sedation. Metabolism by the P_{450} may result in prolonged half-life in patients with hepatic dysfunction. Presence of an active metabolite may result in prolonged sedation with long-term administration. Generic form limits cost when compared with other agents
Lorazepam	0.025–0.05 mg/kg/h; 0.05–0.1 mg/kg every 3–4 h	Limited clinical experience as an agent for sedation in the PICU population. Generic preparations limit cost. A major consideration is the accumulation of its diluent, propylene glycol. Metabolism by glucuronyl transferase limits changes in pharmacokinetics even with hepatic dysfunction
Ketamine	1–2 mg/kg/h	Endogenous catecholamine release results in bronchodilation and cardiovascular stability. However, may cause cardiovascular collapse in patients whose endogenous catecholamines are depleted as its primary direct effect is a decrease in myocardial function. Controversial effects on intracranial pressure and pulmonary vascular resistance although the recent literature demonstrates no deleterious effects
Pentobarbital	1–2 mg/kg/h	Second-line agent after benzodiazepines and opioids. Alkaline pH leads to compatibility issues with other medications and may result in tissue irritation or sloughing of skin with extravasation. Hypotension may occur from vasodilation and negative inotropic effects
Propofol	1–3 mg/kg/h	Rapid awakening upon discontinuation of the infusion. Solution has a high lipid content. Prolonged use (≥12 h) for sedation contraindicated in the PICU population due to risk of propofol infusion syndrome. Increasing data suggests that this may also occur in the adult population. May still be used in rare circumstances as a therapeutic agent for the treatment of increased intracranial pressure or status epilepticus; however, intermittent monitoring of acid–base status is suggested to monitor for toxicity
Haloperidol	0.06–0.45 mg/kg/day	Limited clinical experience in the pediatric population. Anecdotal data in the adult population suggest benefits of a decreased incidence of withdrawal and delirium with its use. May have a role for the treatment of agitation and delirium in the PICU population. Hypotension may result from α-adrenergic blockade. Additional adverse effects include lowering of the seizure threshold and the potential for cardiac arrhythmias due to prolongation of the QT interval
Dexmedetomidine	0.25–1 μ(mu)g/kg/h	FDA approved for short-term (24 h) sedation in adults. Increasing experience in the pediatric population. Mechanism of action may limit delirium in the adult ICU setting. Adverse effects on hemodynamic function include bradycardia and hypotension

The listed infusion rates are suggestions for starting doses. The actual infusion rate should be titrated up or down based on the patient's actual requirements and the response to the agent

Case Scenarios

Case 1

A 12-year-old, 54 kg boy is brought to the emergency room following a seizure. His past medical history is significant for aortic stenosis with a gradient of 60 mmHg. He is scheduled for operative repair next month. His injuries included a closed head injury and a right femur fracture. His vital signs are stable and his Glasgow Coma Scale is 11. He ate lunch approximately 1 h before the seizure. He is sleepy but has intermittent periods of combative behavior. Sedation is requested for MR imaging.

Considerations

This patient's altered mental status and potential for a full-stomach make sedation without control of the airway potentially problematic in that loss of airway reflexes may result in upper airway obstruction, the need for bag-valve-mask ventilation with the risks of aspiration. Given these concerns, the decision is made not to provide sedation, but rather to protect the airway with endotracheal intubation and induce general anesthesia. Given the associated aortic stenosis, an agent with limited effects on hemodynamic function that will maintain contractility and SVR is indicated. Any decrease in SVR is likely to significantly decrease the MAP as the patient's aortic stenosis will cause a fixed stroke volume.

(continued)

Drugs

Etomidate is an intravenous anesthetic agent, introduced into clinical practice in 1972, whose primary effects of sedation and amnesia are mediated through the GABA inhibitory neurotransmitter system. Following intravenous administration, loss of consciousness is rapid (15–20 s), and as with propofol and the barbiturates, its duration of action following a single bolus dose is related to redistribution rather than metabolism and clearance. Beneficial CNS effects include a decrease of the cerebral metabolic rate for oxygen ($CMRO_2$), CBF, and ICP. CPP is maintained because of minimal effects on myocardial function and SVR. Although the barbiturates and propofol have similar effects on CNS dynamics, the latter agents are likely to decrease systemic vascular and MAP. The most significant concern with etomidate and the factor that limits its long-term administration in the ICU setting are its effects on the endogenous production of corticosteroids. This effect was identified when an increased risk of mortality was noted in adult ICU patients who were sedated with a continuous infusion of etomidate. Etomidate inhibits the enzyme, 11-β(beta) hydroxylase, which is necessary for the production of cortisol, aldosterone, and corticosterone. To date, significant controversy surrounds the clinical significance of adrenal suppression following a single induction dose of etomidate, with some authors calling for the abandonment or at least a reevaluation of the use of etomidate. The duration of adrenal suppression produced by a single induction dose of etomidate has varied from study to study, but may exceed 12 h. However, no study has demonstrated changes in clinical outcome based on adrenal suppression following a single dose of etomidate. Therefore, no definite decision can be reached regarding whether the use of etomidate should be eliminated from clinical practice, and even in the scenario presented, its use may be considered somewhat controversial. A modified, rapid sequence intubation is performed following the administration of etomidate and succinylcholine. This is followed by a propofol infusion starting at 25 μ(mu)g/kg/min and titrated up based on the hemodynamic response to allow for completion of the MRI. Following this, the patient is admitted to the pediatric ICU and his trachea is extubated once his mental status has returned to baseline.

Case 2

A 14-month-old infant is recovering from surgery for congenital heart disease. Following the surgical procedure, the infant is sedated with a morphine infusion with intermittent doses of midazolam for 7 days during mechanical ventilation. In anticipation of extubation, the fentanyl, which was infusing at 20 μ(mu)g/kg/min, and the intermittent doses of midazolam are discontinued. The patient's trachea is extubated and 3 h later, the infant is tachycardic, hypertensive, has dilated pupils, and a temperature of 38.6 °C.

Considerations

This infant is likely manifesting signs and symptoms of withdrawal; however, other possibilities must be excluded as the diagnosis of withdrawal is a diagnosis of exclusion. The work-up would include a thorough physical examination and perhaps laboratory evaluation including a complete blood count and blood gas analysis to rule out hypercarbia, hypoxemia, decreased cardiac output, and infection. Given the duration of sedation and analgesia (7 days), this patient is likely to manifest withdrawal if the sedative and analgesic agents are abruptly discontinued or decreased. The OBWS is a 21-item checklist that evaluates 16 specific withdrawal behaviors (see Table 16.9). The patient scores 12, indicative of withdrawal.

Drugs

Given that this patient is extubated and breathing spontaneously, it is decided to use dexmedetomidine, which may have less effect on ventilatory function than opioids or benzodiazepines. Dexmedetomidine is the pharmacologically active dextro-isomer of medetomidine. Like clonidine, it exerts its physiologic effects via α(alpha)$_2$-adrenergic receptors. Dexmedetomidine and clonidine are members of the imidazole subclass, which exhibits a high ratio of specificity for the α(alpha)$_2$ versus the α(alpha)$_1$ receptor. However, while clonidine exhibits an α(alpha)$_2$:α(alpha)$_1$ specificity ratio of 200:1, that of dexmedetomidine is 1,600:1, thereby making it a complete agonist at the α(alpha)$_2$-adrenergic receptor. Dexmedetomidine has a short half-life (2–3 h versus 12–24 h for clonidine) and is commercially available for intravenous administration. Adverse effects are generally limited with dexmedetomidine, although hemodynamic effects (bradycardia or hypotension) may occasionally be seen. As with clonidine, there is increasing experience and interest regarding the use of dexmedetomidine in the prevention and treatment of withdrawal following the prolonged administration of opioids and benzodiazepines in the PICU setting. Regardless of the agent or agents responsible for withdrawal, the role of dexmedetomidine in treating such problems is supported by animal studies, case reports in adults and children, and one retrospective case series in infants. A loading dose of dexmedetomidine

(continued)

(0.5 μ(mu)g/kg) was administered over 10 min followed by an infusion of 0.5 μ(mu)g/kg/h. Ongoing OBWS values decreased to 1–3 over the ensuring 3–4 h. Dexmedetomidine was decreased in increments of 0.1 μ(mu)g/kg/h with constant observation of the OBWS. Alternatively, dexmedetomidine can also be administered subcutaneously if there is a need to remove central lines and eliminate the need for vascular access. Given that gradual weaning may be required, a decision is made to calculate an equivalent dose of methadone based on the morphine infusion rate and to transition to enteral methadone, which can then be weaned following discharge from the pediatric ICU.

Case 3

A 15-month-old infant is admitted to the PICU following direct laryngoscopy and airway laser in the operating room. Direct laryngoscopy revealed a subglottic hemangioma, which was effectively treated with the laser, and the patient remains intubated with a 4.0 endotracheal tube given concerns of edema and airway swelling. The otolaryngologist requests overnight sedation (16–18 h) to ensure that the airway edema has resolved and that the trachea can be successfully extubated. On arrival in the PICU, the infant is initially comfortable with a Ramsay sedation score of 4. Sedation is initiated with morphine at 30 μ(mu)g/kg/h and midazolam at 0.5 mg/kg/h. The patient gradually becomes more awake and then agitated with Ramsay score of 1. Four bolus doses of midazolam (0.1 mg/kg) and two of morphine (0.05 mg/kg) are given, and the morphine infusion is increased to 50 and then ten 100 μ(mu)g/kg/h, while the midazolam infusion is increased to 0.25 mg/kg/h. Four hours later, the patient's Ramsay scores are 1–2 again.

Considerations

The goals of sedation in this patient are to maintain a deep level of sedation and then rapid awakening to ensure full respiratory function and upper airway control prior to endotracheal intubation. In a small subset of patients, the usual combination of an opioid (morphine or fentanyl) and midazolam fails to provide the needed depth of sedation. An additional concern with this combination is that these agents demonstrated a context-sensitive half-life whereby prolonged awakening may occur following a brief duration infusion of more than 12–24 h.

Drugs

Easily titratable agents whose effects dissipate rapidly would include propofol or remifentanil. Another option would be the short-term infusion of propofol. Propofol is an alkyl phenol compound (2,6-diisopropylphenol) with general anesthetic properties. Despite its potential benefits in the ICU setting and its efficacy for providing sedation during mechanical ventilation, the routine use of propofol is not recommended and in fact, is considered contraindicated by many authorities because of the potential for the development of what has been termed the "propofol infusion syndrome." In specific clinical scenarios, propofol may still be used short term (6–12 h) to transition from other agents such as fentanyl and midazolam to allow for more rapid awakening and tracheal extubation with limited residual effect.

The preferable option may be remifentanil. Remifentanil is a synthetic opioid that is metabolized by nonspecific esterases in the plasma. It has a clinical half-life of 5–10 min and a brief duration of effect even following 12–24 h of continuous infusion. These pharmacokinetic parameters hold true even in the neonatal population, making remifentanil the only opioid whose pharmacokinetics are not altered by gestational or chronologic age. Given these properties, it is a potentially useful agent for providing a deep level of sedation and yet allowing for rapid awakening with discontinuation of the infusion even in the neonatal population. However, the major limitation is that there is very limited experience with this agent in the pediatric ICU despite considerable experience in the operating room. The anecdotal reports regarding remifentanil in the ICU demonstrate rapid control of the depth of anesthesia and rapid awakening when the infusion is discontinued. Unlike other opioids, remifentanil does not demonstrate a context-sensitive half-life, and its duration of action remains constant even with a prolonged issue. Issues include the rapid development of tolerance, limiting its efficacy for more than 24 h, as well as cost.

Remifentanil is chosen to provide sedation. An infusion is started at 0.2 μ(mu)g/kg/min and the morphine infusion is discontinued after 15 min. Remifentanil is increased to 0.3 μ(mu)g/kg/min and the midazolam infusion is incrementally decreased and discontinued after 2 h. Over the next 12 h, the Ramsay scores are 4–5 and the infusion is increased to 0.4 μ(mu)g/kg/min. The next morning, an air leak is present around the ETT, and upper airway examination in the PICU reveals no concerns of airway edema. The remifentanil infusion is discontinued, and 15 min later, the patient's trachea is extubated without difficulty.

References

1. Mendelsohn AB, Belle SH, Fischhoff B, et al. How patients feel about prolonged mechanical ventilation 1 yr later. Crit Care Med. 2002;30:1439–45.
2. Practice guidelines for management of the difficult airway. An updated report by the American Society of Anesthesiologists task force on management of the difficult airway. Anesthesiology. 2013;118:251–70.
3. Mallampati SR, Gatt SP, Gugino LD, et al. A clinical sign to predict difficult tracheal intubation: a prospective study. Can Anaesth Soc J. 1985;32(4):429–34.
4. Practice guidelines for sedation and analgesia by non-anesthesiologists: a report by the American Society of Anesthesiologists Task Force on Sedation and Analgesia by Non-Anesthesiologists. Anesthesiology. 1996;84:459–71.
5. Malviya S, Voepel-Lewis T, Tait AR. Adverse events and risk factors associated with the sedation of children by non-anesthesiologists. Anesth Analg. 1997;85:1207–13.
6. Keidan I, Gozal D, Minuskin T, et al. The effect of fasting practice on sedation with chloral hydrate. Pediatr Emerg Care. 2004; 20:805–7.
7. Treston G. Prolonged pre-procedure fasting time is unnecessary when using titrated intravenous ketamine for paediatric procedural sedation. Emerg Med Australas. 2004;16:145–50.
8. Mace SE, Brown LA, Francis L, et al. Clinical policy : Critical issues in the sedation of pediatric patients in the emergency department. Ann Emerg Med. 2008;51:378–99.
9. Gottumukkala R, Street M, Fitzpatrick M, Tatineny P, Duncan JR. Improving team performance during the preprocedure time-out in pediatric interventional radiology. Jt Comm J Qual Patient Saf. 2012;38:387–494.
10. American Academy of Pediatrics and the American Academy of Pediatric Dentistry Work Group on Sedation. Guidelines for monitoring and management of pediatric patients during and after sedation for diagnostic and therapeutic procedures. *Pediatrics* 2006;118:2587–602.
11. American Society of Anesthesiologists. Standards for basic anesthetic monitoring. 2010. http://www.asahq.org/For-Members/~/media/For Members/documents/Standards Guidelines Stmts/Basic Anesthetic Monitoring 2011.ashx.
12. Cote CJ, Notterman DA, Karl HW, et al. Adverse sedation events in pediatrics: a critical incident analysis of contributing factors. Pediatrics. 2000;105:805–14.
13. Hart LS, Berns SD, Houck CS, et al. The value of end-tidal CO_2 monitoring when comparing three methods of conscious sedation for children undergoing painful procedures in the emergency department. Pediatr Emerg Care. 1997;13:189–93.
14. Tobias JD. End-tidal carbon dioxide monitoring during sedation with a combination of midazolam and ketamine for children undergoing painful, invasive procedures. Pediatr Emerg Care. 1999;15:173–5.
15. Ambuel B, Hamlett KW, Marx CM, Blumer JL. Assessing distress in pediatric intensive care environments: the COMFORT scale. J Pediatr Psychol. 1992;17:95–109.
16. Crain N, Slonim A, Pollack MM. Assessing sedation in the pediatric intensive care by using BIS and COMFORT scale. Pediatr Crit Care Med. 2002;3:11–4.
17. Ista E, van Dijk M, Tibboel D, de Hoog M. Assessment of sedation levels in pediatric intensive care unit patients can be improved by using the COMFORT "behavior" scale. Pediatr Crit Care Med. 2005;6:58–63.
18. Simmons LE, Riker RR, Prato BS, Fraser GL. Assessing sedation during intensive care unit mechanical ventilation with the Bispectral Index and Sedation-Agitation Scale. Crit Care Med. 1999;27:1499–504.
19. Ramsay M, Savage TM, Simpson ER, et al. Controlled sedation with aphalaxone-alphadone. BMJ. 1974;2:656–9.
20. Hartwig S, Roth B, Theisohn M. Clinical experience with continuous intravenous sedation using midazolam and fentanyl in the paediatric intensive care unit. Eur J Pediatr. 1991;150:784–8.
21. Chernik DA, Gillings D, Laine H, et al. Validity and reliability of the Observer's Assessment of Alertness/Sedation Scale: study with intravenous midazolam. J Clin Psychopharmacol. 1992; 12:43–8.
22. Macnab AJ, Levine M, Glick N, et al. A research tool for measurement of recovery from sedation: the Vancouver Sedative Recovery Scale. J Pediatr Surg. 1991;26:1263–7.
23. Malviya S, Voepel-Lewis T, Tait AR, et al. Depth of sedation in children undergoing computed tomography: validity and reliability of the University of Michigan Sedation Scale (UMSS). Br J Anaesth. 2002;88:241–5.
24. Flaishon RI, Windsor A, Sigl J, Sebel PS. Recovery of consciousness after thiopental or propofol. Bispectral index and isolated forearm technique. Anesthesiology. 1997;86:613–9.
25. Sebel PS, Lang E, Rampil IJ, White PF, Cork R, Jopling M, Smith NT, Glass PS, Manberg P. A multicenter study of bispectral electroencephalogram analysis for monitoring anesthetic effect. Anesth Analg. 1997;84:891–9.
26. Gill M, Green SM, Krauss B. A study of the Bispectral index monitor during procedural sedation and analgesia in the Emergency Department. Ann Emerg Med. 2003;41:234–41.
27. Brown McDermott N, VanSickle T, Motas D, Friesen RH. Validation of the Bispectral Index monitor during conscious and deep sedation in children. Anesth Analg. 2003;97:39–43.
28. Motas D, Brown McDermott N, VanSickle T, Friesen RH. Depth of consciousness and deep sedation attained in children as administered by nonanesthesiologists in a children's hospital. Pediatr Anaesth. 2004;14:256–9.
29. Berkenbosch JW, Fichter CR, Tobias JD. The correlation of the bispectral index monitor with clinical sedation scores during mechanical ventilation in the pediatric intensive care unit. Anesth Analg. 2002;94:506–11.
30. De Deyne C, Struys M, Decruyenaere J, Creupelandt J, Hoste E, Colardyn F. Use of continuous bispectral EEG monitoring to assess depth of sedation in ICU patients. Intensive Care Med. 1998;24:1294–8.
31. Aneja R, Heard AMB, Fletcher JE, Heard CMB. Sedation monitoring of children by the Bispectral Index in the pediatric intensive care unit. Pediatr Crit Care Med. 2003;4:60–4.
32. Arbour RB. Using the bispectral index to assess arousal response in a patient with neuromuscular blockade. Am J Crit Care. 2000;9:383–7.
33. Courtman SP, Wardugh A, Petros AJ. Comparison of the bispectral index monitor with the COMFORT score in assessing level of sedation of critically ill children. Intensive Care Med. 2003;29:2239–46.
34. Vivien B, Di Maria S, Ouattara A, Langeron O, Coirat P, Riou B. Overestimation of bispectral index in sedative intensive care unit patients revealed by administration of muscle relaxant. Anesthesiology. 2003;99:9–17.
35. Messner M, Beese U, Romstock J, Dinkel M, Tschaikowsky K. The Bispectral index declines during neuromuscular blockade in fully awake persons. Anesth Analg. 2003;97:488–91.
36. Goto T, Nakata Y, Saito H, et al. Bispectral analysis of the electroencephalogram does not predict responsiveness to verbal command in patients emerging from xenon anesthesia. Br J Anaesth. 2000;85:359–63.
37. Barr G, Jakobsson G, Owall A, Anderson RE. Nitrous oxide does not alter bispectral index: study with nitrous oxide as sole agent and as an adjunct to IV anaesthesia. Br J Anaesth. 1999;82:827–30.
38. Lallemand MA, Lentschener C, Mazoit JX, Bonnichon P, Manceau I, Ozier Y. Bispectral index changes following etomidate

induction of general anaesthesia and orotracheal intubation. Br J Anaesth. 2003;91:341–6.
39. Tobias JD, Grindstaff R. Bispectral index monitoring during the administration of neuromuscular blocking agents in the Pediatric ICU patient. J Intensive Care Med. 2005;20:233–7.
40. Grindstaff R, Tobias JD. Applications of bispectral index monitoring in the pediatric intensive care unit. J Intensive Care Med. 2004;19:111–6.
41. Tobias JD. Monitoring the depth of sedation in the pediatric ICU patient: where are we, or more importantly, where are our patients. Pediatr Crit Care Med. 2005;6:715–8.
42. Tobias JD, Berkenbosch JW. Tolerance during sedation in a Pediatric ICU patient: effects on the BIS monitor. J Clin Anesth. 2001;13:122–4.
43. Volles DF, McGory R. Pharmacokinetic considerations. Crit Care Clin. 1999;15:55–7.
44. Buck ML, Blumer JL. Opioids and other analgesics: adverse effects in the intensive care unit. Crit Care Clin. 1991;7:615–37.
45. Reed MD, Blumer JL. Therapeutic drug monitoring in the pediatric intensive care unit. Pediatr Clin North Am. 1994;41:1227–43.
46. de Wildt SN, de Hoog M, Vinks AA, van der Giesen E, van den Anker JN. Population pharmacokinetics and metabolism of midazolam in pediatric intensive care patients. Crit Care Med. 2003;31:1952–8.
47. Chua MV, Tsueda K, Doufas AG. Midazolam causes less sedation in volunteers with red hair. Can J Anaesth. 2004;51:25–30.
48. Katz R, Kelly HW. Pharmacokinetics of continuous infusions of fentanyl in critically ill children. Crit Care Med. 1993;21:995–1000.
49. Cohen M, Sadhasivam S, Vinks AA. Pharmacogenetics in perioperative medicine. Curr Opin Anaesthesiol. 2012;25:419–27.
50. Hajj A, Khabbaz L, Laplanche JL, Peoc'h K. Pharmacogenetics of opiates in clinical practice: the visible tip of the iceberg. Pharmacogenomics. 2013;14:575–85.
51. De Jonghe B, Bastuji-Garin S, Fangio P, et al. Sedation algorithm in critically ill patients without acute brain injury. Crit Care Med. 2005;33:120–7.
52. Kress JP, Pohlman AS, O'Connor MF, Hall JB. Daily interruption of sedative infusions in critically ill patients undergoing mechanical ventilation. N Engl J Med. 2000;342:1471–7.
53. Chanques G, Kress JP, Pohlman A, Patel S, Poston J, Jaber S, Hall JB. Impact of ventilator adjustment and sedation-analgesia practices on severe asynchrony in patients ventilated in assist-control mode. Crit Care Med. 2013;41:2177–87.
54. Anand KJS, Hansen DD, Hickey PR. Hormonal-metabolic stress responses in neonates undergoing cardiac surgery. Anesthesiology. 1990;73:661–70.
55. Anand KJS, Hickey PR. Halothane-morphine compared with high-dose sufentanil for anesthesia and postoperative analgesia in neonatal cardiac surgery. N Engl J Med. 1992;326: 1–9.
56. Hansen-Flaschen JH, Brazinsky S, Basile C, Lanken PN. Use of sedating drugs and neuromuscular blocking agents in patients requiring mechanical ventilation for respiratory failure. JAMA. 1991;266:2870–5.
57. Kong KL, Willatts SM, Prys-Roberts C. Isoflurane compared with midazolam for sedation in the intensive care unit. Br Med J. 1989;298:1277–80.
58. Tobias JD. Therapeutic applications and uses of inhalational anesthesia in the pediatric intensive care unit. Pediatr Crit Care Med. 2008;9:169–79.
59. Meiser A, Sirtl C, Bellgardt M, et al. Desflurane compared with propofol for postoperative sedation in the intensive care unit. Br J Anaesth. 2003;90:273–80.
60. Bedi A, Murray JM, Dingley J, Stevenson MA, Fee JPH. Use of xenon as a sedative for patients receiving critical care. Crit Care Med. 2003;31:2470–7.
61. Satoh H, Gillette JR, Takemura T, et al. Investigation of the immunological basis of halothane-induced hepatotoxicity. AdvExp Med Biol. 1986;197:657–773.
62. Kenna JG, Neuberger J, Williams R. Evidence for expression in human liver of halothane-induced neoantigens recognized by antibodies in sera from patients with halothane hepatitis. Hepatology. 1988;8:1635–41.
63. Morray JP, Geiduschek J, Ramamoorthy C, et al. Anesthesia-related cardiac arrest in children: initial findings of the POCA registry. Anesthesiology. 2000;93:6–14.
64. Bhanaker SM, Ramamoorthy C, Geiduschek JM, et al. Anesthesia-related cardiac arrest in children: update from the Pediatric Perioperative Cardiac Arrest Registry. Anesth Analg. 2007;105: 344–50.
65. Fan SZ, Lin YW, Chang WS, Tang CS. An evaluation of the contributions by fresh gas flow rate, carbon dioxide concentration and desflurane partial pressure to carbon monoxide concentration during low fresh gas flows to a circle anaesthetic breathing system. Eur J Anaesthesiol. 2008;25:620–6.
66. Ebert TJ, Muzi M. Sympathetic hyperactivity during desflurane anesthesia in healthy volunteers. A comparison with isoflurane. Anesthesiology. 1993;79:444–53.
67. Adams RW, Cucchiara RF, Gronert GA, Messick JM, Michenfelder JD. Isoflurane and cerebrospinal fluid pressure in neurosurgical patients. Anesthesiology. 1981;54:97–9.
68. Drummond JC, Todd MM, Scheller MS, Shapiro HM. A comparison of the direct cerebral vasodilating potencies of halothane and isoflurane in the New Zealand White Rabbit. Anesthesiology. 1986;65:462–7.
69. Reilly CS, Wood AJJ, Koshakji RP, Wood M. The effect of halothane on drug disposition: Contribution of changes in intrinsic drug metabolizing capacity and hepatic blood flow. Anesthesiology. 1985;63:70–6.
70. Arnold JH, Truog RD, Rice SA. Prolonged administration of isoflurane to pediatric patients during mechanical ventilation. Anesth Analg. 1993;76:520–6.
71. Sackey P, Martling CR, Granath F, Radell PJ. Prolonged isoflurane sedation of intensive care unit patients with the Anesthetic Conserving Device. Crit Care Med. 2004;32:2241–6.
72. Sackey PV, Martling CR, Radell PJ. Three cases of PICU sedation with isoflurane delivered the "AnaConDa®". Pediatr Anaesth. 2005;15:879–85.
73. Selander D, Curelaru I, Stefansson T. Local discomfort and thrombophlebitis following intravenous injection of diazepam. A comparison between a glycerol-water solution and a lipid emulsion. Acta Anaesthesiol Scand. 1981;25:516–8.
74. Forrest P, Galletly DC. A double-blind comparative study of three formulations of diazepam in volunteers. Anaesth Intensive Care. 1988;16:158–63.
75. Reves JG, Fragan RJ, Vinik R, et al. Midazolam: pharmacology and uses. Anesthesiology. 1985;62:310–7.
76. Lloyd-Thomas AR, Booker PD. Infusion of midazolam in paediatric patients after cardiac surgery. Br J Anaesth. 1986;58:1109–15.
77. Silvasi DL, Rosen DA, Rosen KR. Continuous intravenous midazolam infusion for sedation in the pediatric intensive care unit. Anesth Analg. 1988;67:286–8.
78. Rosen DA, Rosen KR. Midazolam for sedation in the paediatric intensive care unit. Intensive Care Med. 1991;17:S15–9.
79. Jacqz-Algrain E, Daoud P, Burtin P, Desplanques L, Beaufils F. Placebo-controlled trial of midazolam sedation in mechanically ventilated newborn babies. Lancet. 1994;344:646–50.
80. Beebe DS, Belani KG, Chang P, et al. Effectiveness of preoperative sedation with rectal midazolam, ketamine, or their combination in young children. Anesth Analg. 1992;75:880–4.
81. McMillian CO, Spahr-Schopfer IA, Sikich N, et al. Premedication of children with oral midazolam. Can J Anaesth. 1992;39:545–50.

82. Karl HW, Rosenberger JL, Larach MG, Ruffle JM. Transmucosal administration of midazolam for premedication of pediatric patients: comparison of the nasal and sublingual routes. Anesthesiology. 1993;78:885–91.
83. Theroux MC, West DW, Cordry DH, et al. Efficacy of midazolam in facilitating suturing of lacerations in preschool children in the emergency department. Pediatrics. 1993;91:624–7.
84. Tobias JD. Subcutaneous administration of fentanyl and midazolam to prevent withdrawal following prolonged sedation in children. Crit Care Med. 1999;27:2262–5.
85. Cote CJ, Cohen IT, Suresh S, et al. A comparison of three doses of a commercially prepared oral midazolam syrup in children. Anesth Analg. 2002;94:37–43.
86. Bauer TM, Ritz R, Haberthur C, et al. Prolonged sedation due to accumulation of conjugated metabolites of midazolam. Lancet. 1995;346:145–7.
87. Trouvin JH, Farinotti R, Haberer JP, et al. Pharmacokinetics of midazolam in anesthetized cirrhotic patients. Br J Anaesth. 1988;60:762–7.
88. Vinik HR, Reves JG, Greenblatt DJ, et al. The pharmacokinetics of midazolam in chronic renal failure patients. Anesthesiology. 1983;59:390–4.
89. de Wildt SN, de Hoog M, Vinks AA, et al. Population pharmacokinetics and metabolism of midazolam in pediatric intensive care unit patients. Crit Care Med. 2003;31:1952–8.
90. Payne K, Mattheyse FJ, Liebenberg D, et al. The pharmacokinetics of midazolam in paediatric patients. Eur J Clin Pharmacol. 1989;37:267–72.
91. Hughes MA, Glass PS, Jacobs JR. Context-sensitive half-time in multicompartment pharmacokinetic models for intravenous anesthetic drugs. Anesthesiology. 1992;76:334–41.
92. Rogers WK, McDowell TS. Remimazolam, a short-acting GABA(A) receptor agonist for intravenous sedation and/or anesthesia in day-case surgical and non-surgical procedures. Drugs. 2010;13:929–37.
93. Shapiro BA, Warren J, Egol AB, et al. Practice parameters for intravenous analgesia and sedation for adult patients in the intensive care unit: an executive summary. Crit Care Med. 1995;23:1596–600.
94. Barr J, Fraser GL, Puntillo K, et al. Clinical practice guidelines for the management of pain, agitation, and delirium in adult patients in the intensive care unit. Crit Care Med. 2013;41:263–306.
95. Pohlman AS, Simpson KP, Hall JCB. Continuous intravenous infusions of lorazepam versus midazolam for sedation during mechanical ventilatory support: a prospective, randomized study. Crit Care Med. 1994;22:1241–7.
96. Dundee JW, Johnston HM, Gray RC. Lorazepam as a sedative-amnestic in an intensive care unit. Curr Med Res Opin. 1976; 4:290–5.
97. Lugo RA, Chester EA, Cash J, et al. A cost analysis of enterally administered lorazepam in the pediatric intensive care unit. Crit Care Med. 1999;27:417–21.
98. Tobias JD, Deshpande JK, Gregory DF. Outpatient therapy of iatrogenic drug dependency following prolonged sedation in the Pediatric Intensive Care Unit. Intensive Care Med. 1994;20: 504–7.
99. Arbour R, Esparis B. Osmolar gap acidosis in a 60 year old man treated for hypoxemic respiratory failure. Chest. 2000;118:545–6.
100. Reynolds HN, Teiken P, Regan ME, et al. Hyperlactatemia, increased osmolar gap, renal dysfunction during continuous lorazepam infusion. Crit Care Med. 2000;28:1631–4.
101. Arroliga AC, Shehab N, McCarthy K, Gonzales JP. Relationship of continuous infusion lorazepam to serum propylene glycol concentration in critically ill adults. Crit Care Med. 2004;32:1709–14.
102. Chicella M, Jansen P, Parthiban A, et al. Propylene glycol accumulation associated with continuous infusion of lorazepam in pediatric intensive care patients. Crit Care Med. 2002;30:2752–6.
103. Sfez M, Le Mapihan Y, Levron JC, Gaillard JL, Rosemblatt JM, Le Moing JP. Comparison of the pharmacokinetics of etomidate in children and adults. Ann Fr Anesth Reanim. 1990;9:127–31.
104. Brussel T, Theissen JL, Vigfusson G, et al. Hemodynamic and cardiodynamic effects of propofol and etomidate: negative inotropic properties of propofol. Anesth Analg. 1989;69:35–40.
105. Kay B. A clinical assessment of the use of etomidate in children. Br J Anaesth. 1976;48:207–10.
106. Kay B. Total intravenous anesthesia with etomidate: evaluation of a practical technique for children. Acta Anaesthesiol Belg. 1977;28:115–21.
107. Dhawan N, Chauhan S, Kothari SS, Kiran U, Das S, Makhija N. Hemodynamic responses to etomidate in pediatric patients with congenital cardiac shunt lesions. J Cardiothorac Vasc Anesth. 2010;24:802–7.
108. Schechter WS, Kim C, Martinez M, Gleason BF, Lund DP, Burrows FA. Anaesthetic induction in a child with end-stage cardiomyopathy. Can J Anaesth. 1995;42:404–8.
109. Tobias JD. Etomidate: applications in pediatric anesthesia and critical care. J Intensive Care Med. 1997;12:324–6.
110. Ching KY, Baum CR. Newer agents for rapid sequence intubation: etomidate and rocuronium. Pediatr Emerg Care. 2009;25:200–7.
111. Martinon C, Duracher C, Bianot S, et al. Emergency tracheal intubation of severely head-injured children: changing daily practice after implementation of national guidelines. Pediatr Crit Care Med. 2011;12:65–70.
112. Lehman KA, Mainka F. Ventilatory CO_2-response after alfentanil and sedative premedication (etomidate, diazepam, and droperidol): a comparative study with human volunteers. Acta Anaesthesiol Belg. 1986;37:3–13.
113. Choi SD, Spaulding BC, Gross JB, Apfelbaum JL. Comparison of the ventilatory effects of etomidate and methohexital. Anesthesiology. 1985;62:442–7.
114. Giese JL, Stockham RJ, Stanley TH, et al. Etomidate versus thiopental for induction of anesthesia. Anesth Analg. 1985;64:871–6.
115. Morgan M, Lumley J, Whitwam JG. Respiratory effects of etomidate. Br J Anaesth. 1977;49:233–6.
116. Renou AM, Vernhiet J, Macrez P, et al. Cerebral blood flow and metabolism during etomidate anaesthesia in man. Br J Anaesth. 1978;50:1047–51.
117. Modica PA, Tempellhoff R. Intracranial pressure during induction of anesthesia and tracheal intubation with etomidate-induced EEG burst suppression. Can J Anaesth. 1992;39:236–41.
118. Gancher S, Laxer KD, Krieger W. Activation of epileptogenic activity by etomidate. Anesthesiology. 1984;61:616–8.
119. Ebrahim ZY, DeBoer GE, Luders H, Hahn JF, Lesser RP. Effect of etomidate on the electroencephalogram of patients with epilepsy. Anesth Analg. 1986;65:1004–6.
120. Ghoneim MM, Yamada T. Etomidate: a clinical and electroencephalographic comparison with thiopental. Anesth Analg. 1977;56:479–85.
121. Doenicke AW, Roizen MF, Kugler J, Kroll H, Foss J, Ostwald P. Reducing myoclonus after etomidate. Anesthesiology. 1999; 90:113–9.
122. Patel A, Dallas SH. A trial of etomidate infusion anaesthesia for computerized axial tomography (letter). Anaesthesia. 1981;36:63.
123. Wagner RL, White PF, Kan PB, et al. Inhibition of adrenal steroidogenesis by the anesthetic etomidate. N Engl J Med. 1984;310:1415–8.
124. Annane D. ICU physicians should abandon the use of etomidate. Intensive Care Med. 2005;31:325–6.
125. Cotton BA, Guillamondegui OD, Fleming SB, et al. Increased risk of adrenal insufficiency following etomidate exposure in critically injured patients. Arch Surg. 2008;143:62–7.
126. Markowitz BP. The drug that would not die (though patients receiving it do)(editorial). Pediatr Crit Care Med. 2009;10: 418–9.

127. Scherzer D, Leder M, Tobias JD. Pro-con debate: etomidate or ketamine for rapid sequence intubation in pediatric patients. J Pediatr Pharmacol Ther. 2012;17:142–9.
128. Duthie DJR, Fraser R, Nimmo WS. Effect of induction of anaesthesia with etomidate on corticosteroid synthesis in man. Br J Anaesth. 1985;57:156–9.
129. Donmez A, Kaya H, Haberal A, Kutsal A, Arslan G. The effect of etomidate induction on plasma cortisol levels in children undergoing cardiac surgery. J Cardiothorac Vasc Anesth. 1998;12:182–5.
130. Absalom A, Pledger D, Kong A. Adrenocortical function in critically ill patients 24 hour after a single dose of etomidate. Anaesthesia. 1999;54:861–7.
131. Vinclair M, Broux C, Faure P, et al. Duration of adrenal inhibition following a single dose of etomidate in critically ill patients. Intensive Care Med. 2008;34:714–9.
132. Ray DC, McKeown DW. Effect of induction agent on vasopressor and steroid use, and outcome in patients with septic shock. Crit Care. 2007;11:145–7.
133. Sprung CL, Annane D, Keh D, et al. CORTICUS study group: hydrocortisone therapy for patients with septic shock. JAMA. 2002;288:862–71.
134. Gelb AW, Lok P. Etomidate reversibly depresses human neutrophil chemiluminescence. Anesthesiology. 1987;66:60–3.
135. Asehnoune K, Mahe PJ, Sequin P, et al. Etomidate increases susceptibility to pneumonia in trauma patients. Intensive Care Med. 2012;38:1673–82.
136. Fazackerley EJ, Martin AJ, Tolhurst-Cleaver CL, Watkins J. Anaphylactoid reaction following the use of etomidate. Anaesthesia. 1988;43:953–4.
137. Olesen AS, Huttel MS, Hole P. Venous sequelae following the injection of etomidate or thiopentone IV. Br J Anaesth. 1984;56:171–3.
138. Nyman Y, Von Hofsten K, Palm C, et al. Etomidate-Lipuro® is associated with considerably less injection pain in children compared with propofol with added lidocaine. Br J Anaesth. 2006;97:536–9.
139. Bedicheck E, Kirschbaum B. A case of propylene glycol toxic reaction associated with etomidate infusion. Arch Intern Med. 1991;151:2297–8.
140. Levy ML, Aranda M, Selman V, Giannotta SL. Propylene glycol toxicity following continuous etomidate infusion for control of refractory cerebral edema. Neurosurgery. 1995;37:363–71.
141. Doenicke A, Roizen MF, Hoernecke R, Mayer M, Ostwald P, Foss J. Haemolysis after etomidate: comparison of propylene glycol and lipid formulations. Br J Anaesth. 1997;79:386–8.
142. Tobias JD. Airway management in the pediatric trauma patient. J Intensive Care Med. 1998;13:1–14.
143. Cotten JF, Forman SA, Laha JK, et al. Carboetomidate: a pyrrole analog of etomidate designed not to suppress adrenocortical function. Anesthesiology. 2010;112:637–44.
144. Domino EF, Chodoff P, Corssen G. Pharmacologic effects of CI-581, a new dissociative anesthetic in man. Clin Pharmacol Ther. 1965;6:279–91.
145. Tobias JD. End-tidal carbon dioxide monitoring during sedation with a combination of midazolam and ketamine for children undergoing painful, invasive procedures. Pediatr Emerg Care. 1999;15:173–5.
146. Adriaenssens G, Vermeyen KM, Hoffmann VLH, Mertens E, Adriaensen HF. Postoperative analgesia with iv patient-controlled morphine: effect of adding ketamine. Br J Anaesth. 1999;83:393–6.
147. Jahangir SM, Islam F, Aziz L. Ketamine infusion for postoperative analgesia in asthmatics: comparison with intermittent meperidine. Anesth Analg. 1993;76:45–9.
148. Himmelseher S, Durieux ME. Ketamine for perioperative pain management. Anesthesiology. 2005;102:211–20.
149. Lahtinen P, Kokki H, Hakala T, et al. S(+) ketamine as an analgesic adjunct reduces opioid consumption after cardiac surgery. Anesth Analg. 2004;99:1295–301.
150. Chernow B, Laker R, Creuss D, et al. Plasma, urine, and cerebrospinal fluid catecholamine concentrations during and after ketamine sedation. Crit Care Med. 1982;10:600–3.
151. Wayman K, Shoemaker WC, Lippmann M. Cardiovascular effects of anesthetic induction with ketamine. Anesth Analg. 1980;59:355–8.
152. Spotoft H, Korshin JD, Sorensen MB, et al. The cardiovascular effects of ketamine used for induction of anesthesia in patients with valvular heart disease. Can Anaesth Soc J. 1979;26:463–7.
153. Dewhirst E, Frazier WJ, Leder M, Fraser DD, Tobias JD. Cardiac arrest following ketamine administration for rapid sequence intubation. J Intensive Care Med. 2013;28:375–9.
154. Gooding JM, Dimick AR, Travakoli M, et al. A physiologic analysis of cardiopulmonary responses to ketamine anesthesia in non-cardiac patients. Anesth Analg. 1977;56:813–6.
155. Morray JP, Lynn AM, Stamm SJ, et al. Hemodynamic effects of ketamine in children with congenital heart disease. Anesth Analg. 1984;63:895–9.
156. Hickey PR, Hansen DD, Cramolini GM, et al. *Pulmonary* and systemic hemodynamic responses to ketamine in infants with normal and elevated pulmonary vascular resistance. Anesthesiology. 1985;62:287–93.
157. Wolfe RR, Loehr JP, Schaffer MS, Wiffins Jr JW. Hemodynamic effects of ketamine, hypoxia, and hyperoxia in children with surgically treated congenital heart disease residing ≥1,200 meters above sea level. Am J Cardiol. 1991;67:84–7.
158. Williams GD, Philip BM, Chu LF, et al. Ketamine does not increase pulmonary vascular resistance in children with pulmonary hypertension undergoing sevoflurane anesthesia and spontaneous ventilation. Anesth Analg. 2007;105:1578–84.
159. Singh A, Girotra S, Mehta Y, Radhakrishnan S, Shrivastava S. Total intravenous anesthesia with ketamine for pediatric interventional cardiac procedures. J Cardiothorac Vasc Anesth. 2000;14:36–9.
160. Lebovic S, Reich DL, Steinberg G, Vela FP, Silvay G. Comparison of propofol versus ketamine for anesthesia in pediatric patients undergoing cardiac catheterization. Anesth Analg. 1992;74:490–4.
161. Mankikian B, Cantineau JP, Sartene R, et al. Ventilatory and chest wall mechanics during ketamine anesthesia in humans. Anesthesiology. 1986;65:492–9.
162. Von Ungern-Sternberg BS, Regli A, Frei FJ, et al. A deeper level of ketamine anesthesia does not affect functional residual capacity and ventilation distribution in healthy preschool children. Pediatr Anaesth. 2007;17:1150–5.
163. Hirshman CA, Downes H, Farbood A, Bergman NA. Ketamine block of bronchospasm in experimental canine asthma. Br J Anaesth. 1979;51:713–8.
164. Bourke DL, Malit LA, Smith TC. Respiratory interactions of ketamine and morphine. Anesthesiology. 1987;66:153–6.
165. Lanning CF, Harmel MH. Ketamine anesthesia. Annu Rev Med. 1975;26:137–41.
166. Taylor PA, Towey RM. Depression of laryngeal reflexes during ketamine administration. Br Med J. 1971;2:688–9.
167. Brown L, Christian-Kopp S, Sherwin TS, Khan A, Barcega B, Denmark TK, Moynihan JA, Kim GJ, Stewart G, Green SM. Adjunctive atropine is unnecessary during ketamine sedation in children. Acad Emerg Med. 2008;15:314–8.
168. Kye YC, Rhee JE, Kim K, Kim T, Jo YH, Jeong JH, Lee JH. Clinical effects of adjunctive atropine during ketamine sedation in pediatric emergency patients. Am J Emerg Med. 2012;30:1981–5.
169. Chong JH, Chew SP, Ang AS. Is prophylactic atropine necessary during ketamine sedation in children? J Paediatr Child Health. 2013;49:309–12.
170. Berkenbosch JW, Graff GR, Stark JM. Safety and efficacy of ketamine sedation for infant flexible fiberoptic bronchoscopy. Chest. 2004;125:1132–7.

171. Shapiro HM, Wyte SR, Harris AB. Ketamine anesthesia in patients with intracranial pathology. Br J Anaesth. 1972;44:1200–4.
172. Gardner AE, Dannemiller FJ, Dean D. Intracranial cerebrospinal fluid pressure in man during ketamine anesthesia. Anesth Analg. 1972;51:741–5.
173. Reicher D, Bhalla P, Rubinstein EH. Cholinergic cerebral vasodilator effects of ketamine in rabbits. Stroke. 1987;18:445–9.
174. Oren RE, Rasool NA, Rubinstein EH. Effect of ketamine on cerebral cortical blood flow and metabolism in rabbits. Stroke. 1987;18:441–4.
175. Pfenninger E, Dick W, Ahnefeld FW. The influence of ketamine on both the normal and raised intracranial pressure of artificially ventilated animals. Eur J Anaesthesiol. 1985;2:297–307.
176. Pfenninger E, Grunert A, Bowdler I, Kilian J. The effect of ketamine on intracranial pressure during haemorrhagic shock under the conditions of both spontaneous breathing and controlled ventilation. Acta Neurochir. 1985;78:113–8.
177. Albanese J, Arnaud S, Rey M, et al. Ketamine decreases intracranial pressure and electroencephalographic activity in traumatic brain injury patients during propofol sedation. Anesthesiology. 1997;87:1328–34.
178. Bourgoin A, Albanese J, Wereszczynski N, Charbit M, Vialet R, Martin C. Safety of sedation with ketamine in severe head injury patients: comparison with sufentanil. Crit Care Med. 2003;31:711–7.
179. Mayberg TS, Lam AM, Matta BF, Domino KB, Winn R. Ketamine does not increase cerebral blood flow velocity of intracranial pressure during isoflurane/nitrous oxide anesthesia in patients undergoing craniotomy. Anesth Analg. 1995;81:84–9.
180. Shapira Y, Lam AM, Artru AA, Eng C, Soltow L. Ketamine alters calcium and magnesium in brain tissue following experimental head trauma in rats. J Cereb Blood Flow Metab. 1993; 13:962–9.
181. Rosen I, Hagerdal M. Electroencephalographic study of children during ketamine anesthesia. Acta Anaesthesiol Scand. 1976;20:32–9.
182. Manohar S, Maxwell D, Winters WD. Development of EEG seizure activity during and after chronic ketamine administration in the rat. Neuropharmacology. 1972;11:819–26.
183. Bourn WM, Yang DJ, Davisson JN. Effect of ketamine enantiomers on sound-induced convulsions in epilepsy prone rats. Pharmacol Res Commun. 1983;15:815–24.
184. Veliskova J, Velisek L, Mares P, Rokyta R. Ketamine suppresses both bicuculline and picrotoxin induced generalized tonic clonic seizures during ontogenesis. Pharmacol Biochem Behav. 1990; 37:667–74.
185. Sheth RD, Gidal BE. Refractory status epilepticus: response to ketamine. Neurology. 1998;51:1765–6.
186. Haeseler G, Zuzan O, Kohn G, et al. Anaesthesia with midazolam and S-(+) ketamine in spontaneously breathing paediatric patients during magnetic resonance imaging. Paediatr Anaesth. 2000;10: 513–9.
187. Pees C, Haas NA, Ewert P, et al. Comparison of analgesia and sedative effect of racemic ketamine and S(+) ketamine during cardiac catheterization in newborns and children. Pediatr Cardiol. 2003;24:424–9.
188. Marhofer P, Freitag H, Hochtl A, et al. S(+) ketamine for rectal premedication in children. Anesth Analg. 2001;92:62–5.
189. Koinig H, Marhoger P. S(+) ketamine in paediatric anaesthesia. Paediatr Anaesth. 2003;13:185–7.
190. Tobias JD, Martin LD, Wetzel RC. Ketamine by continuous infusion for sedation in the pediatric intensive care unit. Crit Care Med. 1990;18:819–21.
191. Hartvig P, Larsson E, Joachimsson PO. Postoperative analgesia and sedation following pediatric cardiac surgery using a constant infusion of ketamine. J Cardiothorac Vasc Anesth. 1993;7: 148–53.
192. Edrich T, Friedrich AD, Eltzschig HK, Felbinger TW. Ketamine for long-term sedation and analgesia of a burn patient. Anesth Analg. 2004;99:893–5.
193. Youssef-Ahmed MZ, Silver P, Nimkoff L, Sagy M. Continuous infusion of ketamine in mechanically ventilated children with refractory bronchospasm. Intensive Care Med. 1996;22:972–6.
194. Weksler N, Ovadia L, Muati G, et al. Nasal ketamine for paediatric premedication. Can J Anaesth. 1993;40:119–21.
195. Weber F, Wulf H, el Saeidi G. Premedication with nasal s-ketamine and midazolam provides good conditions for induction of anaesthesia in preschool children. Can J Anaesth. 2003;50:470–5.
196. Sebel PS, Lowdon JD. Propofol: a new intravenous anesthetic. Anesthesiology. 1989;71:260–77.
197. Harris CE, Grounds RM, Murray AM, et al. Propofol for long-term sedation in the intensive care unit. A comparison with papaveretum and midazolam. Anaesthesia. 1990;45:366–72.
198. Beller JP, Pottecher T, Lugnier A, et al. Prolonged sedation with propofol in ICU patients: recovery and blood concentration changes during periodic interruption in infusion. Br J Anaesth. 1988;61:583–8.
199. Ronan KP, Gallagher TJ, George B, Hamby B. Comparison of propofol and midazolam for sedation in intensive care unit patients. Crit Care Med. 1995;23:286–93.
200. Hemelrijck JV, Fitch W, Mattheussen M, Van Aken H, Plets C, Lauwers T. Effect of propofol on cerebral circulation and autoregulation in the baboon. Anesth Analg. 1990;71:49–54.
201. Nimkoff L, Quinn C, Silver P, Sagy M. The effects of intravenous anesthetic agents on intracranial pressure and cerebral perfusion pressure in two feline models of brain edema. J Crit Care. 1997;12:132–6.
202. Watts ADJ, Eliasziw M, Gelb AW. Propofol and hyperventilation for the treatment of increased intracranial pressure in rabbits. Anesth Analg. 1998;87:564–8.
203. Herregods L, Verbeke J, Rolly G, Colardyn F. Effect of propofol on elevated intracranial pressure. Preliminary results. Anaesthesia. 1988;43(Suppl):107–9.
204. Pinaud M, Lelausque J, Chetanneau A, Fauchoux N, Menegalli D, Souron R. Effects of propofol on cerebral hemodynamics and metabolism in patients with brain trauma. Anesthesiology. 1990;73:404–9.
205. Mangez JF, Menguy E, Roux P. Sedation par propofol a debit constant chez le traumatise cranien. Resultas preliminaires. Ann Fr Anesth Reanim. 1987;6:336–7.
206. Ravussin P, Guinard JP, Ralley F, Thorin D. Effect of propofol on cerebrospinal fluid pressure and cerebral perfusion pressure in patients undergoing craniotomy. Anaesthesia. 1988;43(suppl): 107–9.
207. Farling PA, Johnston JR, Coppel DL. Propofol infusion for sedation of patients with head injury in intensive care. Anaesthesia. 1989;44:222–6.
208. Yamaguchi S, Midorikawa Y, Okuda Y, et al. Propofol prevents delayed neuronal death following transient forebrain ischemia in gerbils. Can J Anaesth. 1999;46:593–8.
209. Young Y, Menon DK, Tisavipat N, et al. Propofol neuroprotection in a rat model of ischaemia reperfusion injury. Eur J Anaesthesiol. 1997;14:320–6.
210. Fox J, Gelb AW, Enns J, et al. The responsiveness of cerebral blood flow to changes in arterial carbon dioxide is maintained during propofol-nitrous oxide anesthesia in humans. Anesthesiology. 1992;77:453–6.
211. Eames WO, Rooke GA, Sai-Chuen R, Bishop MJ. Comparison of the effects of etomidate, propofol, and thiopental on respiratory resistance after tracheal intubation. Anesthesiology. 1996;84: 1307–11.
212. Pizov R, Brown RH, Weiss YS, et al. Wheezing during induction of general anesthesia in patients with and without asthma. A randomized, blinded trial. Anesthesiology. 1995;82:1111–6.

213. Chih-Chung L, Ming-Hwang S, Tan PPC, et al. Mechanisms underlying the inhibitory effect of propofol on the contraction of canine airway smooth muscle. Anesthesiology. 1999;91:750–9.
214. Pedersen CM, Thirstrup S, Nielsen-Kudsk JE. Smooth muscle relaxant effects of propofol and ketamine in isolated guinea-pig tracheas. Eur J Pharmacol. 1993;238:75–80.
215. Brown RH, Greenberg RS, Wagner EM. Efficacy of propofol to prevent bronchoconstriction. Anesthesiology. 2001;94:851–5.
216. Rieschke P, LeFleur BJ, Janicki PK. Effects of EDTA and sulfite-containing formulations of propofol on respiratory system resistance after tracheal intubation in smokers. Anesthesiology. 2003;98:323–8.
217. Tritapepe L, Voci P, Marino P, et al. Calcium chloride minimizes the hemodynamic effects of propofol in patients undergoing coronary artery bypass grafting. J Cardiothorac Vasc Anesth. 1999; 13:150–3.
218. Sochala C, Van Deenen D, De Ville A, Govaerts MJM. Heart block following propofol in a child. Paediatr Anaesth. 1999; 9:349–51.
219. Egan TD, Brock-Utne JG. Asystole and anesthesia induction with a fentanyl, propofol, and succinylcholine sequence. Anesth Analg. 1991;73:818–20.
220. Kannan S, Sherwood N. Termination of supraventricular tachycardia by propofol. Br J Anaesth. 2002;88:874–5.
221. Trotter C, Serpell MG. Neurological sequelae in children after prolonged propofol infusions. Anaesthesia. 1992;47:340–2.
222. Saunders PRI, Harris MNE. Opisthotonic posturing and other unusual neurological sequelae after outpatient anesthesia. Anaesthesia. 1992;47:552–7.
223. Finley GA, MacManus B, Sampson SE, Fernandez CV, Retallick I. Delayed seizures following sedation with propofol. Can J Anaesth. 1993;40:863–5.
224. Hewitt PB, Chu DLK, Polkey CE, Binnie CD. Effect of propofol on the electrocorticogram in epileptic patients undergoing cortical resection. Br J Anaesth. 1999;82:199–202.
225. McBurney JW, Teiken PJ, Moon MR. Propofol for treating status epilepticus. J Epilepsy. 1994;7:21–2.
226. Lowenstein DH, Alldredge BK. Status epilepticus. N Engl J Med. 1998;338:970–6.
227. Parke TJ, Stevens JE, Rice ASC, et al. Metabolic acidosis and fatal myocardial failure after propofol infusion in children: five case reports. Br Med J. 1992;305:613–6.
228. Strickland RA, Murray MJ. Fatal metabolic acidosis in a pediatric patient receiving an infusion of propofol in the intensive care unit: Is there a relationship? Crit Care Med. 1995;23:405–9.
229. Hanna JP, Ramundo ML. Rhabdomyolysis and hypoxia associated with prolonged propofol infusion. Neurology. 1998;50:301–3.
230. Bray RJ. Propofol infusion syndrome in children. Paediatr Anaesth. 1998;8:491–9.
231. Spitzfadden AC, Jimenez DF, Tobias JD. Propofol for sedation and control of intracranial pressure in children. Pediatr Neurosurg. 1999;31:194–200.
232. Cremer OL, Bouman EAC, Kruijswijk JE, et al. Long-term propofol infusion and cardiac failure in adult head-injured patients. Lancet. 2000;357:117–8.
233. Perrier ND, Baerga-Varela Y, Murray M. Death related to propofol use in an adult. Crit Care Med. 2000;28:3071–4.
234. Diedrich DA, Brown DR. Analytic reviews: propofol infusion syndromes in the ICU. J Intensive Care Med. 2011;26:59–72.
235. Schenkman KA, Yan S. Propofol impairment of mitochondrial respiration in isolated perfused guinea pig hearts determined by reflectance spectroscopy. Crit Care Med. 2000;28:172–7.
236. Wolf A, Weir P, Segar P, et al. Impaired fatty acid oxidation in propofol infusion syndrome. Lancet. 2001;357:606–7.
237. Withington DE, Decell MK, Al AT. A case of propofol toxicity: further evidence for a causal mechanism. Pediatr Anaesth. 2004;14:505–8.
238. Committee on Safety of Medicines, Medicines Control Agency. Propofol (Diprivan) infusion: sedation in children aged 16 years or younger. Curr Problems Pharmacovigilance. 2001;27:10.
239. Rigby-Jones AE, Nolan JA, Priston MJ, et al. Pharmacokinetics of propofol infusions in critically ill neonates, infants, and children in an intensive care unit. Anesthesiology. 2002;97:1393–400.
240. Reed MD, Yamashita TS, Marz CM, et al. A pharmacokinetically based propofol dosing strategy for sedation of the critically ill, mechanically ventilated pediatric patient. Crit Care Med. 1996;24:1473–81.
241. Norreslet J, Wahlgreen C. Propofol infusion for sedation of children. Crit Care Med. 1990;18:890–2.
242. Playfor SD, Venkatesh K. Current patterns of propofol use in the United Kingdom and North America. Paediatr Anaesth. 2004;14: 501–4.
243. Cornfield DN, Tegtmeyer K, Nelson MD, et al. Continuous propofol infusion in 142 critically ill children. Pediatrics. 2002;110: 1177–81.
244. Cray SH, Holtby HM, Kartha VM, Cox PN, Roy WL. Early tracheal extubation after paediatric cardiac surgery: the use of propofol to supplement low-dose opioid anesthesia. Paediatr Anaesth. 2001;11(4):465–71.
245. Cravens GT, Pcker DL, Johnson ME. Incidence of propofol infusion syndrome during noninvasive radiofrequency ablation for atrial flutter or fibrillation. Anesthesiology. 2007;106:1134–8.
246. Hertzog JH, Campbell JK, Dalton HJ, Hauser GJ. Propofol anesthesia for invasive procedures in ambulatory and hospitalized children: experience in the Pediatric Intensive Care Unit. Pediatrics. 1999;103:e30.
247. Reeves ST, Havidick JE, Tobin P. Conscious sedation of children with propofol is anything but conscious. Pediatrics. 2004;114:e74.
248. Laxenaire MC, Mata-Bermejo E, Moneret-Vautrin DA, Gueant JL. Life-threatening anaphylactoid reactions to propofol. Anesthesiology. 1992;77:275–80.
249. Gottardis M, Khunl-Brady KS, Koller W, et al. Effect of prolonged sedation with propofol on serum triglyceride and cholesterol concentrations. Br J Anaesth. 1989;62:393–6.
250. Baombe JP, Parvez K. Towards evidence-based emergency medicine: best BETs from the Manchester Royal Infirmary. BET 1: is propofol safe in patients with egg anaphylaxis? Emerg Med J. 2013;30:79–80.
251. Murphy A, Campbell DE, Baines D, Mehr S. Allergic reactions to propofol in egg-allergic children. Anesth Analg. 2011;113: 140–4.
252. Valente JF, Anderson GL, Branson RD, et al. Disadvantages of prolonged propofol sedation in the critical care unit. Crit Care Med. 1994;22:710–2.
253. Camps AS, Sanchez-Izquierdo Riera JA, Vazquez DT, et al. Midazolam and 2 % propofol in long-term sedation of traumatized, critically ill patients: efficacy and safety comparison. Crit Care Med. 2000;28:3612–9.
254. Barrientos-Vega R, Sanchez-Soria M, Morales-Garcia C, et al. Pharmacoeconomic assessment of propofol 2 % used for prolonged sedation. Crit Care Med. 2001;29:317–22.
255. Song D, Hamza MA, White PF, et al. Comparison of a lower-lipid propofol emulsion with the standard emulsion for sedation during monitored anesthesia care. Anesthesiology. 2004;100:1072–5.
256. Campos AS, Sanchez-Izquierdo R, Vazquez DT, et al. Midazolam and 2 % propofol in long-term sedation of traumatized, critically ill patients: efficacy and safety comparison. Crit Care Med. 2000;28:3612–9.
257. Griffin J, Ray T, Gray B, et al. Pain on injection of propofol: a thiopental/propofol mixture versus a lidocaine/propofol mixture. Am J Pain Manag. 2002;12:45–9.
258. Tobias JD. Prevention of pain associated with the administration of propofol in children: lidocaine versus ketamine. Am J Anesthesiol. 1996;23:231–2.

259. Picard P, Tramer MR. Prevention of pain on injection with propofol: a quantitative systematic review. Anesth Analg. 2000;90:963–9.
260. Mangar D, Holak EJ. Tourniquet at 50 mmHg followed by intravenous lidocaine diminishes hand pain associated with propofol injection. Anesth Analg. 1992;74:250–2.
261. Haugen RD, Vaghadia H, Waters T, Merick PM. Thiopentone pretreatment for propofol injection pain in ambulatory patients. Can J Anaesth. 1993;42:1108–12.
262. Sosis MB, Braverman B. Growth of Staphylococcus aureus in four intravenous anesthetics. Anesth Analg. 1993;77:766–8.
263. Postsurgical infections associated with extrinsically contaminated intravenous anesthetic agent—California, Illinois, Maine, and Michigan, 1990. MMWR. 1990;39:426–27, 433.
264. Trissel LA, Gilbert DL, Martinez JF. Drug compatibility differences with propofol injectable emulsion products with selected drugs during simulated Y-site administration. Am J Health Syst Pharm. 1997;54:1287–92.
265. Lewis TC, Janicki PK, Higgins MS, et al. Anesthetic potency of propofol with disodium edetate versus sulfite-containing propofol in patients undergoing magnetic resonance imaging: a retrospective analysis. Am J Anesthesiol. 2000;27:30–2.
266. Fassoulaki A, Paraskeva A, Papilas K, Patris K. Hypnotic and cardiovascular effects of proprietary and generic propofol formulations do not differ. Can J Anaesth. 2001;48:459–61.
267. Astrup J, Sorensen PM, Sorensen HR. Inhibition of cerebral oxygen and glucose consumption in the dog by hypothermia, pentobarbital and lidocaine. Anesthesiology. 1981;55:263–8.
268. Cormio M, Gopinath SP, Valadka A, et al. Cerebral hemodynamic effects of pentobarbital coma in head-injured patients. J Neurotrauma. 1999;16:927–36.
269. Krishnamurthy KB, Drislane FW. Depth of EEG suppression and outcome in barbiturate anesthetic treatment for refractory status epilepticus. Epilepsia. 1999;40:759–62.
270. Holmes GL, Riviello Jr JJ. Midazolam and pentobarbital for refractory status epilepticus. Pediatr Neurol. 1999;20:259–64.
271. Ishimaru H, Takahashi A, Ikarashi Y, et al. Effects of MK-801 and pentobarbital on cholinergic terminal damage and delayed neuronal death in the ischemic gerbil hippocampus. Brain Res Bull. 1997;43:81–5.
272. Morimoto Y, Morimoto Y, Nishihira J, et al. Pentobarbital inhibits apoptosis in neuronal cells. Crit Care Med. 2000;28:1899–904.
273. Tobias JD, Deshpande JK, Pietsch JB, Wheeler TJ, Gregory DG. Pentobarbital sedation in the Pediatric Intensive Care Unit patient. South Med J. 1995;88:290–4.
274. Tobias JD. Pentobarbital for sedation during mechanical ventilation in the Pediatric ICU patient. J Intensive Care Med. 2000;15: 115–20.
275. Yanay O, Brogan TV, Martin LD. Continuous pentobarbital infusion in children is associated with high rates of complications. J Crit Care. 2004;19:174–8.
276. Audenaert SM, Montgomery CL, Thompson DE, et al. A prospective study of rectal methohexital: efficacy and side effects in 648 cases. Anesth Analg. 1995;81:957–61.
277. Nguyen MT, Greenburg SB, Fitzhugh KR, et al. Pediatric imaging: sedation with an injection formulation modified for rectal administration. Radiology. 2001;221:760–2.
278. Alp H, Orbak Z, Guler I, et al. Efficacy and safety of rectal thiopental, intramuscular cocktail and rectal midazolam for sedation in children undergoing neuroimaging. Pediatr Int. 2002;44: 628–34.
279. Strain JD, Campbell JB, Harvey LA, et al. IV Nembutal: safe sedation for children undergoing CT. Am J Roentgenol. 1988;151:975–9.
280. Malviya S, Voepel-Lewis T, Tait AR, et al. Pentobarbital versus chloral hydrate for sedation of children undergoing MRI: efficacy and recovery characteristics. Paediatr Anaesth. 2004;14:589–95.
281. Dershwitz M, Rosow CE, DiBiase PM, Zaslavsky A. Comparison of the sedative effects of butorphanol and midazolam. Anesthesiology. 1991;74:717–24.
282. Burkle H, Dunbar S, Van Aken H. Remifentanil: a novel, short acting, mu opioid. Anesth Analg. 1996;83:646–51.
283. Kinder Ross A, Davis PJ, deL Dear G, et al. Pharmacokinetics of remifentanil in anesthetized pediatric patients undergoing elective surgery or diagnostic procedures. Anesth Analg. 2001;93:1393–401.
284. Cavaliere F, Antonelli M, Arcangeli A, et al. A low-dose remifentanil infusion is well tolerated for sedation in mechanically ventilated, critically ill patients. Can J Anaesth. 2002;49:1088–94.
285. Dahaba AA, Rabner T, Rehak PH, List WF, Metzler H. Remifentanil versus morphine analgesia and sedation for mechanically ventilated critically ill patients. Anesthesiology. 2004;101: 640–6.
286. Tobias JD. Remifentanil: Applications in the Pediatric ICU population. American Journal of Pain Management. 1998;8:114–7.
287. Akinci SB, Kanbak M, Guler A, Aypar U. Remifentanil versus fentanyl for short-term analgesia-based sedation in mechanically ventilated postoperative children. Paediatr Anaesth. 2005;15: 870–88.
288. Vinik HR, Kissin I. Rapid development of tolerance to analgesia during remifentanil infusion in humans. Anesth Analg. 1998; 86:1307–11.
289. Guignard B, Bossard AE, Coste C, et al. Acute opioid tolerance: intraoperative remifentanil increases postoperative pain and morphine requirement. Anesthesiology. 2000;93:409–17.
290. Keidan I, Berkenstadt H, Sidi A, et al. Propofol-remifentanil versus propofol alone for bone marrow aspiration in paediatric haemato-oncological patients. Paediatr Anaesth. 2001;11: 297–301.
291. Reyle-Hahn M, Niggemann B, Max M, et al. Remifentanil and propofol for sedation in children and young adolescents undergoing diagnostic flexible bronchoscopy. Paediatr Anaesth. 2000; 10:59–63.
292. Litman RS. Conscious sedation with remifentanil and midazolam during brief painful procedures in children. Arch Paediatr Adolesc Med. 1999;153:1085–8.
293. Sperry RJ, Bailey PL, Reuchman MV, et al. Fentanyl and sufentanil increase intracranial pressure in head trauma patients. Anesthesiology. 1992;77:416–20.
294. Milde LN, Milde JH, Gallagher WJ. Effects of sufentanil on cerebral circulation and metabolism in dogs. Anesth Analg. 1990;70:138–46.
295. Pokela ML, Ryhanen PT, Koivisto ME, et al. Alfentanil-induced rigidity in newborn infants. Anesth Analg. 1992;75:252–7.
296. Glick C, Evans OB, Parks BR. Muscle rigidity due to fentanyl infusion in the pediatric patient. South Med J. 1996;89:1119–20.
297. Dewhirst E, Naguib A, Tobias JD. Chest wall rigidity in two infants after low-dose fentanyl administration. Pediatr Emerg Care. 2012;28:465–8.
298. MacGregor R, Evans D, Sugden D, et al. Outcome at 5–6 years of prematurely born children who received morphine as neonates. Arch Dis Child Fetal Neonatal Ed. 1998;79:F40–3.
299. Lynn AM, Opheim KE, Tyler DC. Morphine infusion after pediatric cardiac surgery. Crit Care Med. 1984;12:863–6.
300. Quinn MW, Wild J, Dean HG, et al. Randomised double-blind controlled trial of effect of morphine on catecholamine concentrations in ventilated pre-term babies. Lancet. 1993;342:324–7.
301. Franck LS, Vilardi J, Durand D, et al. Opioid withdrawal in neonates after continuous infusions of morphine or fentanyl during extracorporeal membrane oxygenation. Am J Crit Care. 1998;7:364–9.
302. Bruera E, Brenneis C, Michaud M, et al. Use of the subcutaneous route for the administration of narcotics in patients with cancer pain. Cancer. 1988;62:407–11.

303. Bruera E, Gibney N, Stollery D, Marcushamer S. Use of the subcutaneous route of administration of morphine in the Intensive Care Unit. J Pain Symptom Manage. 1991;6:263–5.
304. Tobias JD, O'Connor TA. Subcutaneous administration of fentanyl for sedation during mechanical ventilation in an infant. Am J Pain Manage. 1996;6:115–7.
305. Dietrich CC, Tobias JD. Subcutaneous fentanyl infusions in the pediatric population. Am J Pain Manage. 2003;13:146–50.
306. Tobias JD. Subcutaneous administration of fentanyl and midazolam to prevent withdrawal after prolonged sedation in children. Crit Care Med. 1999;27:2262–5.
307. Suzuki S, Carlos MP, Chuang LF, et al. Methadone induces CCR5 and promotes AIDS virus infection. FEBS Lett. 2002; 519:173–7.
308. Carr DJ, Rogers TJ, Weber RJ. The relevance of opioids and opioid receptors on immunocompetence and immune homeostasis. Proc Soc Exp Biol Med. 1996;213:248–57.
309. Tubaro E, Borelli G, Croce C, Cavallo G, Santiangeli C. Effect of morphine on resistance to infection. J Infect Dis. 1983;148: 656–66.
310. Froemming JS, Lam YWF, Jann MW, Davis CM. Pharmacokinetics of haloperidol. Clin Pharmacokinet. 1989;17:396–423.
311. Harvey MA. Managing agitation in critically ill adults. Am J Crit Care. 1996;5:7–16.
312. Riker RR, Fraser GL, Cox PM. Continuous infusions of haloperidol controls agitation in critically ill patients. Crit Care Med. 1994;22:433–40.
313. Milbrandt EB, Alexander K, Kong L, et al. Haloperidol is associated with lower hospital mortality in mechanically ventilated patients. Crit Care Med. 2005;33:226–9.
314. Harrison AM, Lugo RA, Lee WE, et al. The use of haloperidol in agitated critically ill children. Clin Pediatr. 2002;41:51–4.
315. Schuderi PE. Droperidol: many questions, few answers. Anesthesiology. 2003;98:289–90.
316. US Food and Drug Administration MedWatch. http://www.fda/gov/medwatch/SAFETY/2001/inapsine.htm.
317. Correa-Sales C, Reid K, Maze M. Pertussis toxin mediated ribosylation of G proteins blocks the hypnotic response to an alpha$_2$ agonist in the locus coeruleus of the rat. Pharmacol Biochem Behav. 1992;43:723–7.
318. Correa-Sales C, Nacif-Coelho C, Reid K, Maze M. Inhibition of adenylate cyclase in the locus coeruleus mediates the hypnotic response to an alpha$_2$ agonist in the rat. J Pharmacol Exp Ther. 1992;263:1046–50.
319. Nacif-Coelho C, Correa-Sales C, Chang LL, Maze M. Perturbation of ion channel conductance alters the hypnotic response to the alpha$_2$ adrenergic agonist dexmedetomidine in the locus coeruleus of the rat. Anesthesiology. 1994;81:1527–34.
320. Sculptoreanu A, Scheuer T, Catterall WA. Voltage-dependent potentiation of L-type Ca^{2+} channels due to phosphorylation by cAMP-dependent protein kinase. Nature. 1993;364:240–3.
321. Correa-Sales C, Rabin BC, Maze M. A hypnotic response to dexmedetomidine, an alpha$_2$ agonist is mediated in the locus coeruleus in rats. Anesthesiology. 1992;76:948–52.
322. Doze VA, Chen BX, Maze M. Dexmedetomidine produces a hypnotic-anesthetic action in rats via activation of central alpha-2 adrenoceptors. Anesthesiology. 1989;71:75–9.
323. Nelson LE, Lu J, Guo T, Saper CB, Franks NP, Maze M. The alpha$_2$-adrenoceptor agonist dexmedetomidine converges on an endogenous sleep-promoting pathway to exert its sedative effects. Anesthesiology. 2003;98:428–36.
324. Maze MM, Tranquilli W. Alpha-2 agonists: defining the role in clinical anesthesia. Anesthesiology. 1991;74:581–91.
325. Mikawa K, Maekawa N, Nishina K, et al. Efficacy of oral clonidine premedication in children. Anesthesiology. 1993;79: 926–31.
326. De Kock MF, Pichon G, Scholtes JL. Intraoperative clonidine enhances postoperative morphine patient-controlled analgesia. Can J Anaesth. 1992;39:537–44.
327. Bohrer H, Bach A, Layer M, Werning P. Clonidine as a sedative adjunct in intensive care. Intensive Care Med. 1990;16:265–6.
328. Ambrose C, Sale S, Howells R, et al. Intravenous clonidine infusion in critically ill children: dose-dependent sedative effects and cardiovascular stability. Br J Anaesth. 2000;84:794–6.
329. Arenas-Lopez S, Riphagen S, Tibby SM, et al. Use of oral clonidine for sedation in ventilated pediatric intensive care patients. Intensive Care Med. 2004;30:1625–9.
330. Tobias JD. Dexmedetomidine: applications in pediatric critical care and pediatric anesthesiology. Pediatr Crit Care Med. 2007;8: 115–31.
331. Petroz GC, Sikich N, James M, van Dyk H, Shafer SL, Schily M, Lerman J. A phase 1, two center study of the pharmacokinetics and pharmacodynamics of dexmedetomidine in children. Anesthesiology. 2006;105:1098–110.
332. Diaz SM, Rodarte A, Foley J, Capparelli EV. Pharmacokinetics of dexmedetomidine in post-surgical pediatric intensive care unit patients: a preliminary study. Pediatr Crit Care Med. 2007;8: 419–24.
333. Vilo S, Rautiainen P, Kaisti K, Aantaa R, Scheinin M, Manner T, Olkkola KT. Pharmacokinetics of intravenous dexmedetomidine in children under 11 yr of age. Br J Anaesth. 2008;100:697–700.
334. Potts AL, Warman GR, Anderson BJ. Dexmedetomidine disposition in children: a population analysis. Paediatr Anaesth. 2008;18: 722–30.
335. Su F, Nicolson SC, Gastonguay MR, Barrett JS, Adamson PC, Kang DS, Godinez RI, Zuppa AF. Population pharmacokinetics of dexmedetomidine in infants following open heart surgery. Anesth Analg. 2010;110:1383–92.
336. Potts AL, Anderson BJ, Warman GR, Lerman J, Diaz SM, Vilo S. Dexmedetomidine pharmacokinetics in pediatric intensive care—a pooled analysis. Peadiatr Anaesth. 2009;19:1119–29.
337. Hall JE, Uhrich TD, Barney JA, et al. Sedative, amnestic, and analgesic properties of small-dose dexmedetomidine infusions. Anesth Analg. 2000;90:699–705.
338. Venn RM, Karol MD, Grounds RM. Pharmacokinetics of dexmedetomidine infusions for sedation of postoperative patients requiring intensive care. Br J Anaesth. 2002;88:669–75.
339. Tobias JD, Berkenbosch JW. Sedation during mechanical ventilation in infants and children: dexmedetomidine versus midazolam. South Med J. 2005;97:451–5.
340. Berkenbosch JW, Tobias JD. Development of bradycardia during sedation with dexmedetomidine in an infant concurrently receiving digoxin. Pediatr Crit Care Med. 2003;4:203–5.
341. Koroglu A, Demirbilek S, Teksan H, et al. Sedative, hemodynamic and respiratory effects of dexmedetomidine in children undergoing magnetic resonance imaging examination: preliminary results. Br J Anaesth. 2005;94:821–4.
342. Berkenbosch JW, Wankum P, Tobias JD. Prospective evaluation of dexmedetomidine for noninvasive procedural sedation in children. Pediatr Crit Care Med. 2005;6:435–9.
343. Koroglu A, Teksan H, Sagir O, et al. A comparison of the sedative, hemodynamic and respiratory effects of dexmedetomidine and propofol in children undergoing magnetic resonance imaging. Anesth Analg. 2006;103:63–7.
344. Mason KP, Zgleszewski SE, Dearden JL, et al. Dexmedetomidine for pediatric sedation for computed tomography imaging studies. Anesth Analg. 2006;103:57–62.
345. Mason KP, Lubisch NB, Robinson F, Roskos R. Intramuscular dexmedetomidine sedation for pediatric MRI and CT. AJR Am J Roentgenol. 2011;197:720–5.
346. Mason KP, Lubisch N, Robinson F, Roskos R, Epstein MA. Intramuscular dexmedetomidine: an effective route of seda-

tion preserves background activity for pediatric electroencephalograms. J Pediatr. 2012;161:927–32.
347. Scher CS, Gitlin MC. Dexmedetomidine and low-dose ketamine provide adequate sedation for awake fibreoptic intubation. Can J Anaesth. 2003;50:607–10.
348. Tosun Z, Akin A, Guler G, et al. Dexmedetomidine-ketamine and propofol-ketamine combinations for anesthesia in spontaneously breathing pediatric patients undergoing cardiac catheterization. J Cardiothorac Vasc Anesth. 2006;20:515–9.
349. Mester R, Easley RB, Brady KM, et al. Monitored anesthesia care with a combination of dexmedetomidine and ketamine during cardiac catheterization. Am J Ther. 2008;15:24–30.
350. Tobias JD. Dexmedetomidine and ketamine: an effective alternative for procedural sedation? Pediatr Crit Care Med. 2012;13: 423–7.
351. Levanen J, Makela ML, Scheinin H. Dexmedetomidine premedication attenuates ketamine-induced cardiostimulatory effects and postanesthetic delirium. Anesthesiology. 1995;82:1117–25.
352. Riihioja P, Jaatinen P, Oksanen H, et al. Dexmedetomidine, diazepam, and propranolol in the treatment of alcohol withdrawal symptoms in the rat. Alcohol Clin Exp Res. 1997;21:804–8.
353. Riihioja P, Jaatinen P, Haapalinna A, et al. Effects of dexmedetomidine on rat loceus coeruleus and ethanol withdrawal symptoms during intermittent ethanol exposure. Alcohol Clin Exp Res. 1999;23:432–8.
354. Riihioja P, Jaatinen P, Oksanen H, et al. Dexmedetomidine alleviates ethanol withdrawal symptoms in the rat. Alcohol. 1997;14:537–44.
355. Riihioja P, Jaatinen P, Haapalinna A, et al. Prevention of ethanol-induced sympathetic overactivity and degeneration by dexmedetomidine. Alcohol. 1995;12:439–46.
356. Maccioli GA. Dexmedetomidine to facilitate drug withdrawal. Anesthesiology. 2003;98:575–7.
357. Multz AS. Prolonged dexmedetomidine infusion as an adjunct in treating sedation-induced withdrawal. Anesth Analg. 2003;96: 1054–5.
358. Finkel JC, Elrefai A. The use of dexmedetomidine to facilitate opioid and benzodiazepine detoxification in an infant. Anesth Analg. 2004;98:1658–9.
359. Baddigam K, Russo P, Russo J, et al. Dexmedetomidine in the treatment of withdrawal syndromes in cardiothoracic surgery patients. J Intensive Care Med. 2005;20:118–23.
360. Finkel JC, Johnson YJ, Quezado YMN. The use of dexmedetomidine to facilitate acute discontinuation of opioids alter cardiac transplantation in children. Crit Care Med. 2005;33:2110–2.
361. Tobias JD. Dexmedetomidine to treat opioid withdrawal in infants and children following prolonged sedation in the Pediatric ICU. J Opioid Manag. 2006;2:201–6.
362. Belleville JP, Ward DS, Bloor BC, Maze M. Effects of intravenous dexmedetomidine in humans. Anesthesiology. 1992;77:1125–33.
363. Talke P, Chen R, Thomas B, et al. The hemodynamic and adrenergic effects of perioperative dexmedetomidine infusion after vascular surgery. Anesth Analg. 2000;90:834–83.
364. Peden CJ, Cloote AH, Stratford N, Prys-Roberts C. The effect of intravenous dexmedetomidine premedication on the dose requirement of propofol to induce loss of consciousness in patients receiving alfentanil. Anaesthesia. 2001;56:408–13.
365. Hammer GB, Drover DR, Cao H, et al. The effects of dexmedetomidine on cardiac electrophysiology in children. Anesth Analg. 2008;106:79–83.
366. Char D, Drover DR, Motonaga KS, et al. The effects of ketamine on dexmedetomidine-induced electrophysiologic changes. Paediatr Anesth. 2013;23:891–7.
367. Chrysostomou C, Beerman L, Shiderly D, et al. Dexmedetomidine: a novel drug for the treatment of atrial and junctional tachyarrhythmias during the perioperative period for congenital cardiac surgery: a preliminary study. Anesth Analg. 2008;107:1514–22.
368. Tobias JD, Chrysostomou C. Dexmedetomidine: antiarrhythmic effects in the pediatric cardiac patient. Pediatr Cardiol. 2013;34: 779–85.
369. Prielipp RC, Wall MH, Tobin JR, et al. Dexmedetomidine-induced sedation in volunteers decreases regional and global cerebral blood flow. Anesth Analg. 2002;95:1052–9.
370. Drummond JC, Dao AV, Roth DM, Cheng CR, Atwater BI, Minokadeh A, Pasco LC, Patel PM. Effect of dexmedetomidine on cerebral blood flow velocity, cerebral metabolic rate, and carbon dioxide response in normal humans. Anesthesiology. 2008; 108:225–32.
371. Zornow MH, Scheller MS, Sheehan PB, Strenat MA, Matsumoto M. Intracranial pressure effects of dexmedetomidine in rabbits. Anesth Analg. 1992;75:232–7.
372. Talke P, Tong C, Lee HW, et al. Effect of dexmedetomidine on lumbar cerebrospinal fluid pressure in humans. Anesth Analg. 1997;85:358–64.
373. Kuhmonen J, Haapalinna A, Sivenius J. Effects of dexmedetomidine after transient and permanent occlusion of the middle cerebral artery in the rat. J Neural Transm. 2001;108:261–71.
374. Hoffman WE, Kochs E, Werner C, Thomas C, Albrecht RF. Dexmedetomidine improves neurologic outcome from incomplete ischemia in the rat. Reversal by the alpha-2 adrenergic antagonist atipamezole. Anesthesiology. 1991;75:328–32.
375. Kuhmonen J, Pokorny J, Miettinen R, et al. Neuroprotective effects of dexmedetomidine in the gerbil hippocampus after transient global ischemia. Anesthesiology. 1997;87:371–7.
376. Miyazaki Y, Adachi T, Kurata J, Utsumi J, et al. Dexmedetomidine reduces seizure threshold during enflurane anaesthesia in cats. Br J Anaesth. 1999;82:935–7.
377. Whittington RA, Virag L, Vulliemoz Y, et al. Dexmedetomidine increases the cocaine seizure threshold in rats. Anesthesiology. 2002;97:693–700.
378. Tanaka K, Oda Y, Funao T, et al. Dexmedetomidine decreases the convulsive potency of bupivacaine and levobupivacaine in rats: Involvement of α_2-adrenoceptor for controlling convulsions. Anesth Analg. 2005;100:687–96.
379. Mirski MA, Rossell LA, McPherson RW, Traystman RJ. Dexmedetomidine decreases seizure threshold in a rat model of experimental generalized epilepsy. Anesthesiology. 1994;81: 1422–8.
380. Keeter S, Benator RM, Weinberg SM, Hartenberg MA. Sedation in pediatric CT. Radiology. 1990;175:745–52.
381. Reimche LD, Sankaran K, Hindmarsh KW, et al. Chloral hydrate sedation in neonates and infants—clinical and pharmacologic considerations. Dev Pharmacol Ther. 1989;12:57–64.
382. American Academy of Pediatrics Committee on Drugs and Committee on Environmental Health. Use of chloral hydrate for sedation in children. Pediatrics. 1993;92:471–3.
383. Rokicki W. Cardiac arrhythmia in a child after the usual dose of chloral hydrate. Pediatr Cardiol. 1996;17:419–20.
384. Seger D, Schwartz G. Chloral hydrate: a dangerous sedative for overdose patients? Pediatr Emerg Care. 1994;10:349–50.
385. D'Agostino J, Terndrup TE. Chloral hydrate versus midazolam for sedation of children for neuroimaging: a randomized clinical trial. Pediatr Emerg Care. 2000;16:1–4.
386. Collett BJ. Opioid tolerance: the clinical perspective. Br J Anaesth. 1998;81:58–68.
387. Finnegan LP. Effects of maternal opiate abuse on the newborn. Fed Proc. 1985;44:2314–7.
388. Finnegan LP, Connaughton Jr JF, Kron RE, et al. Neonatal abstinence syndrome: assessment and management. Addict Dis. 1975;2:141–58.
389. Arnold JH, Truog RD, Orav EJ, et al. Tolerance and dependence in neonates sedated with fentanyl during extracorporeal membrane oxygenation. Anesthesiology. 1990;73:1136–40.

390. Arnold JH, Truog RD, Scavone JM, et al. Changes in the pharmacodynamic response to fentanyl in neonates during continuous infusion. J Pediatr. 1991;119:639–43.
391. Tobias JD, Schleien CL, Haun SE. Methadone as treatment for iatrogenic opioid dependency in pediatric intensive care unit patients. Crit Care Med. 1990;18:1292–3.
392. Sury MRJ, Billingham I, Russell GN, et al. Acute benzodiazepine withdrawal syndrome after midazolam infusions in children. Crit Care Med. 1989;17:301–2.
393. van Engelen BGM, Gimbrere JS, Booy LH. Benzodiazepine withdrawal reaction in two children following discontinuation of sedation with midazolam. Ann Pharmacother. 1993;27:579–81.
394. Fonsmark L, Rasmussen YH, Carl P. Occurrence of withdrawal in critically ill sedated children. Crit Care Med. 1999;27:196–9.
395. Ho IK, Yamamoto I, Loh HH. A model for the rapid development of dispositional and functional tolerance to barbiturates. Eur J Pharmacol. 1975;30:164–71.
396. Jaffe JH, Sharpless SK. The rapid development of physical dependence on barbiturates. J Pharmacol Exp Ther. 1965;150: 140–6.
397. Cammarano WB, Pittet JF, Weitz S, et al. Acute withdrawal syndrome related to the administration of analgesic and sedative medications in adult intensive care unit patients. Crit Care Med. 1998;26:676–84.
398. Imray JM, Hay A. Withdrawal syndrome after propofol. Anaesthesia. 1991;46:704–5.
399. Arnold JH, Truog RD, Molengraft JA. Tolerance to isoflurane during prolonged administration. Anesthesiology. 1993;78:985–8.
400. Hughes J, Leach HJ, Choonara I. Hallucinations on withdrawal of isoflurane used as sedation. Acta Paediatr. 1993;82:885–6.
401. Katz R, Kelly W, Hsi A. Prospective study on the occurrence of withdrawal in critically ill children who receive fentanyl by continuous infusion. Crit Care Med. 1994;22:763–7.
402. Anand KJS, Arnold JH. Opioid tolerance and dependence in infants and children. Crit Care Med. 1994;22:334–42.
403. Ista E, van Dijk M, Gamet C, et al. Withdrawal symptoms in children after long-term administration of sedative and/or analgesics: a literature review. "Assessment remains troublesome". Intensive Care Med. 2007;33:1396–406.
404. Cunliffe M, McArthur L, Dooley F. Managing sedation withdrawal in children who undergo prolonged PICU admission after discharge to the ward. Paediatr Anaesth. 2004;14:293–8.
405. Franck LS, Naughton I, Winter I. Opioid and benzodiazepine withdrawal symptoms in paediatric intensive care patients. Intensive Crit Care Nurs. 2004;20:344–51.
406. Ista E, van Dijk M, Gamel C, et al. Withdrawal symptoms in critically ill children after long-term administration of sedatives and/or analgesics: a first evaluation. Crit Care Med. 2008;36:2427–32.
407. Fisher D, Grap MJ, Younger JB, Ameringer S, Elswick RK. Opioid withdrawal signs and symptoms in children: frequency and determinants. Heart Lung. 2013;42:407–13.
408. Franck LS, Scoppettuolo LA, Wypij D, Curley MA. Validity and generalizability of the Withdrawal Assessment Tool-1 (WAT-1) for monitoring iatrogenic withdrawal syndrome in pediatric patients. Pain. 2012;153:142–8.
409. Franck LS, Harris SK, Soetenga DJ, Amling JK, Curley MA. The Withdrawal Assessment Tool-1 (WAT-1): an assessment instrument for monitoring opioid and benzodiazepine withdrawal symptoms in pediatric patients. Pediatr Crit Care Med. 2008;9: 573–80.
410. Robertson RC, Darsey E, Fortenberry JD, et al. Evaluation of an opiate-weaning protocol using methadone in pediatric intensive care unit patients. Pediatr Crit Care Med. 2000;1:119–23.
411. Lugo RA, MacLaren R, Cash J, et al. Enteral methadone to expedite fentanyl discontinuation and prevent opioid abstinence syndrome in the PICU. Pharmacotherapy. 2001;21:1566–73.
412. Jacobi J, Fraser GL, Coursin DB, et al. Clinical practice guidelines for the sustained use of sedative and analgesics in the critically ill adult. Crit Care Med. 2002;30:119–41.
413. Playfor S, Jenkins I, Boyles C, et al. A consensus guidelines on sedation and analgesia in critically ill children. Intensive Care Med. 2006;32:1125–36.
414. Tobias JD. Outpatient therapy of iatrogenic drug dependency following prolonged sedation in the pediatric intensive care unit. Intensive Care Med. 1996;11:284–7.
415. Meyer MT, Berens RJ. Efficacy of an enteral 10-day methadone wean to prevent opioid withdrawal in fentanyl-tolerant pediatric intensive care unit patients. Pediatr Crit Care Med. 2001;2: 329–33.
416. Siddappa R, Fletcher JE, Heard AMB, et al. Methadone dosage for prevention of opioid withdrawal in children. Paediatr Anaesth. 2003;13:805–10.
417. Berens RJ, Meyer MT, Mikhailov TA, et al. A prospective evaluation of opioid weaning in opioid-dependent pediatric critical care patients. Anesth Analg. 2006;102:1045–50.
418. Atkinson D, Dunne A, Parker M. Torsades de pointes and self-terminating ventricular fibrillation in a prescription methadone user. Anaesthesia. 2007;62:952–5.
419. Gold MS, Redmond Jr DER, Kleber HD. Clonidine blocks acute opiate-withdrawal symptoms. Lancet. 1978;222:599–602.
420. Hoder EL, Leckman JF, Ehrenkranz R, et al. Clonidine in neonatal narcotic-abstinence syndrome. N Engl J Med. 1981;305:1284–5.
421. Deutsche ES, Nadkarni VM. Clonidine prophylaxis for narcotic and sedative withdrawal syndrome following laryngotracheal reconstruction. Arch Otolaryngol Head Neck Surg. 1996;122:1234–8.
422. Tobias JD. Subcutaneous dexmedetomidine infusions to treat or prevent drug withdrawal in infants and children. J Pain Symptom Manage. 2008;4:187–91.
423. Ely EW, Gautam S, Margolin R, Francis J, et al. The impact of delirium in the intensive care unit on hospital length of stay. Intensive Care Med. 2001;27:1892–900.
424. Jackson JC, Gordon SM, Hart RP, et al. The association between delirium and cognitive decline: a review of the empirical literature. Neuropsychol Rev. 2004;14:87–98.
425. Ely EW, Shintani A, Truman B, et al. Delirium as a predictor of mortality in mechanically ventilated patients in the intensive care unit. JAMA. 2009;291:1753–62.
426. Ely EW, Stephens RK, Jackson JC, et al. Current opinions regarding the importance, diagnosis, and management of delirium in the intensive care unit: a survey of 912 healthcare professionals. Crit Care Med. 2004;32:106–12.
427. Meagher DJ, Trzepacz PT. Motoric subtypes of delirium. Semin Clin Neuropsychiatry. 2000;5:75–85.
428. Peterson JF, Pun BT, Dittus RS, Thomason JW, Jackson JC, Shintani AK, Ely EW. Delirium and its motoric subtypes: a study of 614 critically ill patients. J Am Geriatr Soc. 2006;54:479–84.
429. Ouimet S, Riker R, Bergeon N, et al. Subsyndromal delirium in the ICU: evidence for a disease spectrum. Intensive Care Med. 2007;33:1007–13.
430. Spronk PE, Rickerk B, Hofhuis J, et al. Occurrence of delirium is severely underestimated in the ICU during daily care. Intensive Care Med. 2009;35:1276–80.
431. Bergeron N, Dubois MJ, Dumont M, et al. Intensive Care Delirium Screening Checklist: evaluation of a new screening tool. Intensive Care Med. 2001;27:859–64.
432. Ely EW, Inouye SK, Bernard GR, et al. Delirium in mechanically ventilated patients: validity and reliability of the confusion assessment method for the intensive care unit (CAM-ICU). JAMA. 2001;286:2703–10.
433. Smith HAB, Boyd J, Fuchs DC, et al. Diagnosing delirium in critically ill children: validity and reliability of the Pediatric Confusion

Assessment Method for the Intensive Care Unit. Crit Care. 2011;39:150–7.
434. Janssen NJ, Tan EYL, Staal M, Janssen EP, Leroy PL, Lousberg R, et al. On the utility of diagnostic instruments for pediatric delirium in critical illness: an evaluation of the Pediatric Anesthesia Emergence Delirium Scale, the Delirium Rating Scale 88, and the Delirium Rating Scale-Revised R-98. Intensive Care Med. 2011;37:1331–7.
435. Ely EW, Girard TD, Shintani AK, et al. Apolipoprotein E4 polymorphism as a genetic predisposition to delirium in critically ill patients. Crit Care Med. 2007;35:112–7.
436. Marcantonio ER, Juarez G, Goldman L, et al. The relationship of postoperative delirium with psychoactive medications. JAMA. 1994;272:1518–22.
437. Ouimet S, Kavanagh BP, Gottfried SB, et al. Incidence, risk factors and consequences of ICU delirium. Intensive Care Med. 2007;33:66–73.
438. Morrison RS, Magaziner J, Gilbert M, et al. Relationship between pain and opioid analgesics on the development of delirium following hip fracture. J Gerontol A Biol Sci Med Sci. 2003;58:76–81.
439. Tzepacz PT. Update on the neuropathogenesis of delirium. Dement Geriatr Cogn Disord. 1999;10:330–4.
440. Tzepacz PT. Delirium. Advances in diagnosis, pathophysiology, and treatment. Psychiatr Clin North Am. 1996;19:429–48.
441. Van Der Mast RC. Pathophysiology of delirium. J Geriatr Psychiatry Neurol. 1998;11:138–45.
442. Wurtman RJ, Hefti F, Melamed E. Precursor control of neurotransmitter synthesis. Pharmacol Rev. 1980;32:315–35.
443. Krueger JM, Walter J, Dinarello CA, et al. Sleep-promoting effects of endogenous pyrogen (interleukin-1). Am J Physiol. 1984;246:R994–9.
444. Inouye SK, Bogardus Jr ST, Charpentier PA, et al. A multicomponent intervention to prevent delirium in hospitalized older patients. N Engl J Med. 1999;340:669–76.
445. Kress JP, Pohlman AS, O'Connor MF, et al. Daily interruption of sedative infusions in critically ill patients undergoing mechanical ventilation. N Engl J Med. 2000;342:1471–7.
446. Kalisvaart KJ, de Jonghe JF, Bogaards MJ, et al. Haloperidol prophylaxis for elderly hip-surgery patients at risk for delirium: a randomized placebo-controlled study. J Am Geriatr Soc. 2005; 53:1658–66.
447. Skrobik YK, Bergeron N, Dumont M, et al. Olanzapine vs haloperidol: treating delirium in a critical care setting. Intensive Care Med. 2004;30:444–9.
448. Schieveld JNM, van der Valk JA, Smeets I, et al. Diagnostic considerations regarding pediatric delirium: a review and a proposal for an algorithm for pediatric intensive care units. Intensive Care Med. 2009;35:1843–9.
449. Smith HAB, Fuchs DC, Pandharipande PP, et al. Delirium: an emerging frontier in management of critically ill children. Crit Care Clin. 2009;25:593–614.
450. Frager G. Pediatric palliative care: building the model, bridging the gaps. J Palliat Care. 1996;12:9–12.
451. American Academy of Pediatrics, Committee on Bioethics. Ethics and the care of critically ill infants and children. Pediatrics. 1996; 98:149–52.
452. Lowey SE, Powers BA, Xue Y. Short of breath and dying: state of the science on opioid agents for the palliation of refractory dyspnea in older adults. J Gerontol Nurs. 2013;39:43–52.
453. Fielding F, Sanford TM, Davis MP. Achieving effective control in cancer pain: a review of current guidelines. Int J Palliat Nurs. 2013;19:584–91.
454. American Academy of Pediatrics, Committee on Bioethics and Committee on Hospital Care. Palliative care for children. Pediatrics. 2000;106:351–7.
455. Puntillo K, Nelson JE, Weissman D, et al. Palliative care in the ICU: relief of pain, dyspnea, and thirst-A report from the IPAL-ICU Advisory Board. Intensive Care Med. 2014;40(2):235–48.
456. Anquinet L, Rietjens JAC, Seale C, et al. The practice of continuous deep sedation until death in Belgium, the Netherlands, and the UK: a comparative study. J Pain Symptom Manage. 2012;44: 33–43.
457. Ten Have H, Welie JV. Palliative sedation versus euthanasia: an ethical assessment. J Pain Symptom Manage. 2014;47:123–36.
458. Salas S, Frasca M, Planchet-Barraud B, et al. Ketamine analgesic effect by continuous intravenous infusion in refractory cancer pain: considerations about the clinical research in palliative care. J Palliat Med. 2012;15:287–93.
459. Bell RF, Eccleston C, Kalso EA. Ketamin as an adjuvant to opioids for cancer pain. Cochrane Database Syst Rev. 2012;11, CD003351.
460. Prommer EE. Ketamine for pain: an update of uses in palliative care. J Palliat Med. 2012;15:474–83.
461. Okamoto Y, Tsuneto S, Tanimukai H, Matsuda Y, Ohno Y, Tsugane M, Uejima E. Can gradual dose titration of ketamine for management of neuropathic pain prevent psychotomimetic effects in patients with advanced cancer? Am J Hosp Palliat Care. 2013;30:450–4.
462. Benítez-Rosario MA, Salinas-Martín A, González-Guillermo T, Feria M. A strategy for conversion from subcutaneous to oral ketamine in cancer pain patients: effect of a 1:1 ratio. J Pain Symptom Manage. 2011;41:1098–105.
463. Tobias JD. Subcutaneous administration of fentanyl and midazolam to prevent withdrawal after prolonged sedation in children. Crit Care Med. 1999;27:2262–5.
464. Hooke MC, Grund E, Quammen H, Miller B, McCormick P, Bostrom B. Propofol use in pediatric patients with severe cancer pain at the end of life. J Pediatr Oncol Nurs. 2007;24:29–34.
465. Tobias JD. Propofol sedation for terminal care in a pediatric patient. Clin Pediatr. 1997;36:291–3.
466. Glover ML, Kodish E, Reed MD. Continuous propofol infusion for the relief of treatment-resistant discomfort in a terminally ill pediatric patient with cancer. J Pediatr Hematol Oncol. 1996;18:377–80.
467. Anghelescu DL, Hamilton H, Faughnan LG, Johnson LM, Baker JN. Pediatric palliative sedation therapy with propofol: recommendations based on experience in children with terminal cancer. J Palliat Med. 2012;15:1082–90.
468. Prommer E. Dexmedetomidine: does it have potential in palliative medicine? Am J Hosp Palliat Care. 2011;28:276–83.
469. Coyne PJ, Wozencraft CP, Roberts SB, Bobb B, Smith TJ. Dexmedetomidine: exploring its potential role and dosing guideline for its use in intractable pain in the palliative care setting. J Pain Palliat Care Pharmacother. 2010;24:384–6.
470. Jackson 3rd KC, Wohlt P, Fine PG. Dexmedetomidine: a novel analgesic with palliative medicine potential. J Pain Palliat Care Pharmacother. 2006;20:23–7.
471. Kent CD, Kaufman BS, Lowy J. Dexmedetomidine facilitates the withdrawal of ventilatory support in palliative care. Anesthesiology. 2005;103(2):439–41.
472. Soares LG, Naylor C, Martins MA, Peixoto G. Dexmedetomidine: a new option for intractable distress in the dying. J Pain Symptom Manage. 2002;24:6–8.
473. Riker RR, Shehabi Y, Bokesch PM, et al. Dexmedetomidine versus midazolam for sedation of critically ill patients: a randomized trial. JAMA. 2009;301:489–99.

Sedation in the Pediatric Intensive Care Unit: Current Practice in Europe

17

Ian A. Jenkins

Abstract

Of all the treatments that intensive care entails, the ones most commonly utilized are sedation and analgesia; yet many other treatments applied in intensive care are generally subject to far more scrutiny and debate. Sedation and analgesia are often seen as simply the means by which all other treatment can be facilitated; if only that were true and that sedation could be turned on and off at will—with no side effects, no tolerance, withdrawal, toxicity, and with no danger of producing neurologic and psychiatric effects well after the episode of intensive care has passed. So it is fortunate that there are enthusiastic workers in the specialty of pediatric intensive care who highlight the fact that this aspect of intensive care is far more complex than it first seems; and that advancing our understanding and critically revisiting entrenched habits in this field are also required for the conduct of responsible intensive care practice.

Keywords

Pediatric intensive care unit (PICU) • Europe • Sedation • Analgesia • Opioids • Benzodiazepines • Ketamine • Inhalation • Alpha-2 receptor agonists • Propofol • Neuropathology • Sedation scales • Delirium • Tolerance • Withdrawal • Withdrawal Assessment Tool (WAT) • State Behavioral Scale • Postmenstrual age • Morphine • Midazolam • Inhalational sedation • Anesthetic conserving device (AnaConDa) • Isoflurane • Sevoflurane • Xenon • Clonidine • Dexmedetomidine • University of Michigan Sedation Scale (UMSS) • Propofol infusion syndrome • Myopathy • COMFORT Scale • Hartwig scale • State sedation scale • Bispectral index (BIS) • Richmond Agitation-Sedation Scale (RASS) • Confusion assessment method (CAM) • Acute Physiology and Chronic Health Evaluation Scale (APACHE) • Addiction • Neonatal Abstinence Score • Sophia Observation Score (SOS)

Introduction

> Once you know a habit exists, you have the responsibility to change it…And once you understand that habits can change, you have the freedom and the responsibility to remake them.—Charles Duhigg [1]

I.A. Jenkins, M.B.B.S., F.R.C.A., F.R.C.P.E., F.F.I.C.M. (✉)
Department of Pediatric Intensive Care and Anesthesiology, Bristol Royal Hospital for Children,
Upper Maudlin Street, Bristol BS2 8BJ, UK
e-mail: ianajenkins@mac.com

Of all the treatments that intensive care entails, the ones most commonly utilized are sedation and analgesia; yet many other treatments applied in intensive care are generally subject to far more scrutiny and debate. Sedation and analgesia are often seen as simply the means by which all other treatment can be facilitated; if only that were true and that sedation could be turned on and off at will—with no side effects, no tolerance, withdrawal, toxicity, and with no danger of producing neurologic and psychiatric effects well after the episode of intensive care has passed. So it is fortunate that there are enthusiastic workers in the specialty of pediatric intensive care who highlight the fact that this aspect

K.P. Mason (ed.), *Pediatric Sedation Outside of the Operating Room: A Multispecialty International Collaboration*,
DOI 10.1007/978-1-4939-1390-9_17, © Springer Science+Business Media New York 2015

of intensive care is far more complex than it first seems; and that advancing our understanding and critically revisiting entrenched habits in this field are also required for the conduct of responsible intensive care practice [2].

Children who require intensive care will usually require both sedation and analgesia to combat pain and other noxious sensations from either surgery or trauma preceding their admission; distress and pain from other conditions; and the insertion and continuing presence of indwelling devices such as intravascular catheters, thoracic or abdominal drains, and particularly the presence of endotracheal tubes. However, greater doses will be required for endotracheal suction, chest, or other physiotherapy and procedures such as insertion of catheters or drains, wound inspection, debridement, and dressing changes.

The balance between sedation and analgesia will be dictated by the circumstances affecting the patient at the time. While it may be perfectly possible to conduct intensive care in adults with minimal or even no sedation, including ventilation via endotracheal intubation, this is only possible where sufficient maturity, orientation, and lack of painful stimuli may permit it [2]. In children, however, circumstances rarely permit intensive care to be carried out without obtunding the unpleasant combination of emotional, physical, and psychological noxious challenges [3].

If all the sedation and analgesia that were deemed to be necessary could be administered with no side effects, then not only would the intensive care staff be utterly free to concentrate purely on the underlying causes for their patients' admission to intensive care and treat the underlying pathophysiology, but there would be no necessity for the writing of this chapter. Unfortunately, both sedation and analgesia have great capacity to cause iatrogenic harm, in various guises, and the purpose of this chapter is to describe how this occurs and how strategies are being formulated to avoid, or minimize, these harmful effects and to concentrate on those areas that are receiving the most attention at the present time.

For the purposes of brevity and clarity in this chapter, references to sedation will refer to the combination of sedation and analgesia as "sedation" rather than the rather more cumbersome terms "sedo-analgesia" or "analgo-sedation" that are sometimes used elsewhere. Where there are agents that have distinct properties of either analgesia or sedation and need specific reference, then that distinction will be made when necessary.

Pharmacologic Aspects

General Aspects

Overall, relatively few studies specifically examine the effects of sedation, per se, on outcomes of pediatric ICU patients. The RESTORE group has recently delineated a set of criteria to facilitate a prospective study of sedation-related adverse events [4]. The variables they have identified include inadequate sedation defined by agitation measured on the "State Behavioral Scale" [5], pain (on published age-appropriate pain scales), withdrawal using the WAT-1 scale [6], and other surrogate markers such as unplanned extubation, post-extubation stridor, unplanned removal of any other device or catheter, ventilator-associated pneumonia, catheter-associated bloodstream infections, pressure ulcers, and new tracheostomies. It is hoped to use these criteria to construct a prospective, multicenter study [4].

It is recognized that sedation dampens normal physiological responses, such as the integrity of autonomic nervous system activity in response to the stressors of critical illness [7], although the importance, if any, of this is not clear yet.

Although it has been appreciated for many years that morphine and other opioids reduce gastrointestinal motility, the NEOPAIN group has shown that, in preterm infants, morphine delays the initiation and attainment of full enteral feeding. There did not, however, appear to be any effect on the incidence of acquired intestinal pathologies [8].

In adults, it has been shown that greater depth of sedation early in the admission to the ICU is associated time to extubation, time to delirium, and overall hospital and 180-day mortality, where sedation was analyzed by controlling for severity of illness and use of vasopressors [9]. When this was studied prospectively, the same association between early deeper sedation and longer duration of ventilation, increased ICU, in-hospital, and 180-day mortality was seen. This time there was also an association with greater use of vasopressors [10]. Whether or not the greater use of vasopressors in the more heavily sedated patients is a marker of greater illness or simply a side effect of these sedative agents remains a moot point.

The suggestion is that efforts should be made to use less sedation in the critically ill, but the practicalities of attempting this in the pediatric age group would need to be addressed.

There are many pharmacokinetic and pharmacodynamic factors that need to be considered in the context of prolonged infusions in intensive care. The advent of continuous infusions, as opposed to intermittent bolus sedation dosing, has enabled intensive care staff to busy themselves with other more pressing matters but has led to other unintended consequences, as will be explored in this chapter.

Pharmacokinetic factors that lead to long-term oversedation of patients include, firstly, a degree of hepatic and renal dysfunction decreasing the elimination of drugs and, secondly, the phenomenon of "context-sensitive half-life" which is, perhaps, an underappreciated factor in ICU patients' delayed recovery (Fig. 17.1). Fentanyl, when used in anesthetic practice, exhibits suitable properties for short-term infusions. However, when used on a long-term basis in the ICU, its fat solubility leads to loading of lipid-containing compartments to the extent that its context-sensitive half-life

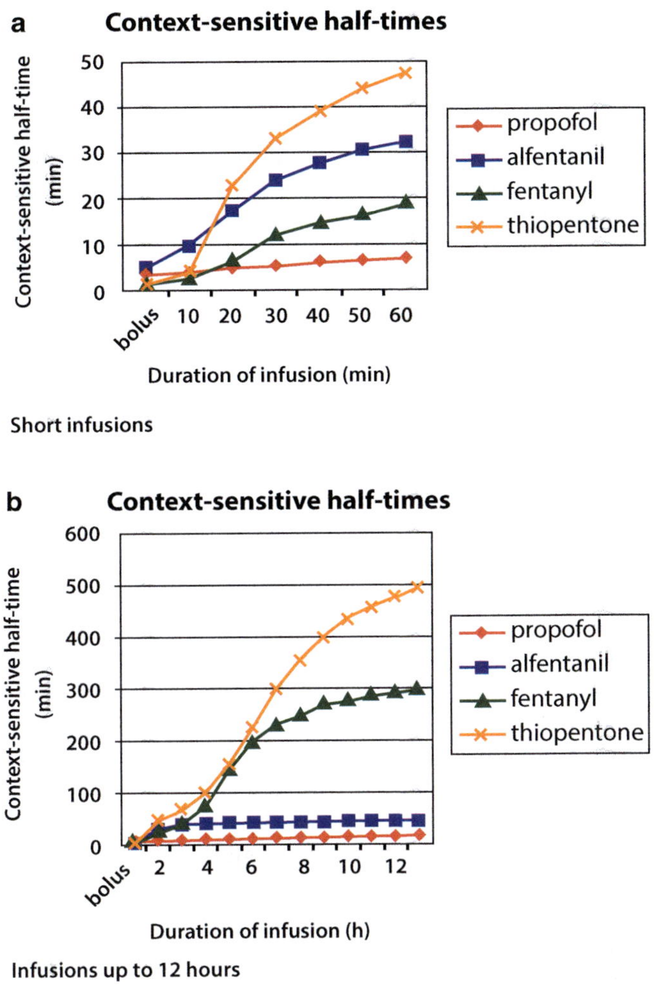

Fig. 17.1 Context-sensitive half-times [11] with permission of Oxford University Press

can be increased sixfold and therefore, arguably, is a poor drug for long-term infusions [11]. Alfentanil, by contrast, is more hydrophilic and thus is not associated with prolongation of its context-sensitive half-life.

Drugs commonly used in intensive care [12], such as morphine, midazolam, and vecuronium, all produce active metabolites that are dependent on adequate renal elimination. Morphine is converted in the liver to morphine-6-glucuronide, which is very active at opioid receptors, and morphine-3-glucuronide, which is active at NMDA receptors and is excitant and may be pro-convulsant [13, 14]. Midazolam is metabolized to alpha1-hydroxymidazolam, which, although less potent than the parent compound, has sedative activity and both compounds may accumulate [15]. Vecuronium has several active metabolites 3- and 17- hydroxyl- and 3,17-hydroxyl-vecuronium. All such compounds require renal elimination and thus often accumulate in the ICU patient. Consequently, there is a real danger of residual paralysis after cessation of muscle relaxants. Although this can be assessed using train-of-four nerve stimulation, caution must also be exercised in attempting to reverse this with sugammadex. Although sugammadex will clear the "accessible" ECF, it will not bind with drug that has crossed into other tissues. This enlarged volume of distribution is thought to be a function of disturbed capillary function in critical illness and length of time receiving the drug [16].

Another complicating factor is the post-conceptual age (or "postmenstrual" age [PMA]) of infants. The size of the child is only one consideration where other variables are important such as PMA and neurological maturation affecting pharmacodynamics and the pharmacokinetics affected by continuously developing organ maturation, although these factors are far from being fully understood [17, 18]. In infants with no renal compromise, glomerular filtration rates (GFR) have been studied. They appear to be at about 30 % of adult values at term and rise to approximately 90 % by 1 year of age, but the GFR of preterm infants may only be approximately 10 % [19].

A workaround for this complex situation may be to electively cease sedative infusions at a set time each day, which allows the patient to clear drugs, reduce accumulation in a variety of pharmacokinetic compartments, and emerge from sedation. This permits a practical recalibration of the level of sedation with the drugs being administered and prevents relentless loading of the patients' pharmacokinetic compartments. The clinical application of this in an adult ICU population was demonstrated by Kress where such interruptions were associated with decreased durations of ventilation and length of stay in the ICU [20]. More recently this has been reproduced in a pediatric population and, importantly, without any increase in adverse events, such as respiratory complications or accidental extubations [21].

Recent studies also suggest that the benefits of daily interruption of sedation can also be seen with nurse-led sedation protocols. It is possible that a combination of both strategies may lead to most benefit [22]. Generally, the greater the analgesia and sedation used, especially if this is combined with a degree of delirium, then the greater the length of time on the ventilator and in the ICU. This can be ameliorated if structure is given to sedation and analgesia administration [23]. Even where protocolization of sedation and analgesia resulted in greater doses of drugs being administered to neonates, it did not lead to increased durations of ventilation, length of ICU stay, or adverse outcomes [24]. This may be because there was greater structure for timeliness of increasing doses but also for decreasing them in conjunction with non-pharmacological measures.

Another strategy studied is the effect of automation on effective sedation ICU patients. Le Guen found that, when targeting a range of 40–60 bispectral index (BIS) using remifentanil and propofol, an automated system using a closed-loop controller linked directly to the BIS outperformed the staff-controlled system attempting to track the BIS manually [25]. This may indicate another avenue worthy of future study in the pediatric population.

Specific Aspects

Opioids

In the general population as a whole, there is an increasing appreciation that widespread complex genetic variation affects opioid absorption, distribution, metabolism, excretion, and toxicity [26]. This means that assumptions about drug effects and their elimination should be treated with caution.

The maturation of renal clearance of morphine in infants born preterm does not normalize at postmenstrual age of 40 weeks (i.e., term) but occupies a separate trajectory from those infants born at term [18]; thus, the administration of morphine to infants born preterm should reflect this difference in pharmacokinetics.

It has long been recognized that opioids induce tolerance and the need to increase doses to produce the same desired effect [27]. This is either "tolerance" where the μ-opioid receptor complex becomes desensitized, or "tachyphylaxis" where compensatory physiology—for example, activation of antagonist signaling systems such as the *N*-methyl-D-aspartate (NMDA) pathway—then runs unopposed when the opioid is removed. Whatever the underlying mechanism is, the acute removal of the opioid will thereby lead to withdrawal symptoms [28].

This effect of acute tolerance may well be more pronounced when the opioid has greater affinity for the opioid receptor, and this has been documented with the use of remifentanil [29, 30]. Theoretically, inhibition of the NMDA pathway with an agent such as ketamine may be expected to decrease the induced "compensatory" antagonism caused by that pathway against opioid effects at μ-receptors, but data from a study in children undergoing scoliosis surgery failed to demonstrate any benefit from co-administration of low-dose ketamine [31].

Benzodiazepines

Overall there is increasing evidence that benzodiazepine-based sedation is associated with longer length of stay and duration of ventilation, compared to non-benzodiazepine sedation regimens [32] and the introduction of propofol to adult ICU practice has been associated with shorter times on ventilation and decreased length of stay [33]. However, the use of propofol in pediatric practice remains low due to the concerns about outcomes associated with its use [34–38].

Midazolam remains one of the most commonly used benzodiazepines in ICU practice in both adults [39] and children [12], but there is a growing recognition that it is associated with significant morbidity. It is possible to measure plasma levels of midazolam and its metabolite alpha-1-hydroxymidazolam, but the concentration of these substances at which satisfactory clinical sedation is achieved varies sufficiently to preclude this form of monitoring from being practically useful [15].

Additional to general concerns about slowing the progress of patients off ventilators and discharge from the intensive care unit, there are specific concerns regarding side effects such as delirium [40, 41] and withdrawal phenomena [12, 42]. Both these subjects will be addressed more fully below.

Ketamine

Ketamine preparations may exist as one of two enantiomers, S(+)ketamine and R(−)ketamine. The S+ version is more potent and may have less side effects, and may be available singly, but the most prevalent preparation is still the mixed racemic R−/S+ form [43].

Ketamine, like other sedative agents, has been implicated in neurone apoptosis when used in infants. One study confirmed this, but by using large doses of ketamine in immature rates (20 mg kg^{-1}) [44]. Interestingly, this effect could be blocked either by the administration of vitamin D_3 or by "preconditioning" with ketamine at 5 mg kg^{-1}, a dose closer to that used in clinical practice.

However, there is also a possibility that ketamine may be neuroprotective in situations where neurological insults may be expected, as in cardiopulmonary bypass or frank hypoxic–ischemic damage, where resulting glutamate toxicity that would be mediated through NMDA receptors may be blocked by ketamine [45]. Antagonism of NMDA receptors also decreases the amounts of opioid necessary to attain satisfactory analgesia postoperatively [46] and decreases the rebound hyperalgesia ascribed to opioid tolerance induced by fentanyl and morphine [47].

There have been concerns that the use of ketamine in encephalopathies or traumatic brain injury might increase intracranial blood pressure (ICP) and thus compromise the injured brain [48]. However, these fears may not be well founded [49]. In 1997, Albanese and colleagues showed that incremental doses of ketamine, given to patients with intracranial monitoring, actually decreased the ICP [50]. Subsequent studies have similarly failed to show any detriment attributable to ketamine even if direct benefit has not been demonstrated [51].

The use of ketamine in asthma has also been evaluated. There is anecdotal evidence that ketamine may avert the need for intubation and ventilation at higher doses [52]. In a recent Cochrane review, only one study in children was eligible for inclusion, highlighting the paucity of good data in this area [53]. This study was conducted in unintubated children with relatively low doses of ketamine; a bolus of 0.2 mg kg^{-1} followed by an infusion at 0.5 mg kg^{-1} h^{-1} and showed no benefit in terms of hospital admission rate or need for mechanical ventilation [54].

It has been shown that ketamine does not raise pulmonary vascular resistance in children with cardiovascular disease and in those with preexisting pulmonary hypertension [55].

After an early case report of possible effectiveness of ketamine in resistant status epilepticus using quite low doses (a bolus of 2 μg kg^{-1} followed by 7.5 μg kg^{-1} h^{-1}) [56], a more recent study of children and adults with resistant status epilepticus has identified a possible role for ketamine in treating this disorder. The rationale for its potential effects is based on the fact that prolonged seizures are accompanied by a decline in effects from gamma-aminobutyric acid agonists (benzodiazepines) but not to NMDA antagonists [57]. There appeared to be some benefit, but only with doses superior to 0.9 mg kg^{-1} h^{-1}.

Inhalational Sedation

Isoflurane has been trialed over the last 20 years as an ICU sedative agent, particularly with interest in its possible beneficial effects in the management of asthma [58], but has proved itself to be free from neither logistic difficulties in delivery by ventilators adapted to deliver the agent with necessary scavenging [59, 60], nor in freedom from withdrawal phenomena [61].

The "Anaconda®" system (Sedana, Uppsala, Sweden) has been utilized to administer either isoflurane or sevoflurane and conserve the agents by "reflective" rebreathing. Unfortunately this adds 100 ml to the dead space, precluding its use in smaller children unless the device is moved to lie wholly within the inspiratory limb of the ventilator circuit [60, 62, 63]. However, this negates the rebreathing element of the device and raises consumption. End-tidal monitoring of the agent must be monitored and this is titrated against flow rates of liquid agent infused directly into the device using nomograms available as a guide. For isoflurane, end-tidal concentrations of isoflurane varying from 0.6 % to 1.2 % have been utilized [60, 62].

Both sevoflurane and isoflurane are metabolized within the body and cause fluoride ions to be excreted in the urine with the potential for renal tubular toxicity, particularly with more prolonged administration in the ICU. However, there has been little evidence of renal toxicity in studies of isoflurane in the ICU [64].

Xenon is proving to be an interesting element in regard to its use as an inhalational anesthetic and sedative agent. However, its anesthetic properties have been known since 1951 [65], including a very low blood-gas partition coefficient (leading to faster induction of effect and emergence), and with both hypnotic and analgesic effects. There are interesting and debatable aspects additional to these obvious advantages, when compared to the hydrofluorocarbon anesthetics; potential for greater cardiovascular stability [65], neuroprotection, and lack of greenhouse and ozone effects to be balanced against the increased costs in its production and utilization [66].

When isoflurane anesthesia was compared to xenon anesthesia in a multicenter trial, it was noted that xenon was safe, effective, and provided quicker recovery [67].

In a direct comparison to an intravenous propofol-alfentanil regimen, inhaled xenon at a mean inspired fraction of 28 % (range 9–62 %) provided satisfactory sedation with more cardiovascular stability and faster recovery times [68]. When xenon was compared to total intravenous anesthesia for adult vascular surgery, xenon was associated with dampening of autonomic responses [69].

Xenon has been shown to have neuroprotective effects by limiting the measurable effects of hypoxic–ischemic encephalopathy [70] and this has been borne out by histopathologic findings [71]. It is thought that xenon may produce its neuroprotective effect by competitive binding at the glycine site of the NMDA receptor [72].

In a prospective study on adult survivors of out-of-hospital cardiac arrests, it was found that xenon administered in hypothermic management reduced both markers of cardiac damage and cardiovascular instability [73].

While all the properties alluded to above may make xenon appear an attractive future anesthetic for cardiopulmonary bypass cases, it is equally capable of dissolving into any nitrogen bubbles in the circuit, in much the same way that has long been recognized for nitrous oxide. Thus, notwithstanding its demonstrated neuroprotective effects, this event would exacerbate "air" embolism [74] and, at least experimentally, this has been borne out with histopathology study [75].

It may have been hoped that the use of inhalational agents may have circumvented mechanisms causing withdrawal that was so evident from the intravenous agents. However, it became clear, that whatever the agent, compensatory mechanisms arise in the body to develop both tolerance and a degree of dependence, including isoflurane [61].

Alpha-2 Receptor Agonists

These agents work at several disparate sites where alpha-2 receptors exist [76]: presynaptically at sympathetic nerve endings (sympatholysis) [77], within the substantia gelatinosa [78] and affecting substance P release [79] (analgesia) and more centrally on the locus coeruleus (sedation and analgesia) [80] and potentially the nucleus ambiguus and dorsal motor nucleus of the vagus nerve (parasympathetic stimulation) [81]. The side effects that were anticipated as potential problems consequent to use in intensive care were primarily hypotension and bradycardia.

There is increasing information about the use of alpha-2 receptor agonists as sedatives in the ICU. The ones mostly studied in the ICU and PICU have been clonidine and dexmedetomidine, with the latter attracting the greater attention.

It has eight times the affinity of clonidine for the alpha-2 receptor [82] while having a half-life of 2–3 h compared to 12–24 h, respectively. The metabolic breakdown product of dexmedetomidine, "the H-3 metabolite," is thought to have only 0.5 % of the pharmacodynamic activity of the parent compound, which adds to the safety profile [83].

However, the effects of distribution on context-sensitive half-lives for both drugs have to be borne in mind, as indeed for many other sedatives in common use. When dexmedetomidine levels were measured in a cohort of critically ill patients, increasing the infusion rate to 2.5 μg kg^{-1} h^{-1} failed to show any accumulation and indeed circulating levels showed linearity with respect to the infusion rate [83]. However, the investigators point out that patients with known hepatic dysfunction were not included in this cohort so there remains a caveat in this regard.

When studied as an infused sedative of greater than 48 h duration, with loading of 3–6 μg kg^{-1}, followed by a modest rate of 0.1–0.25 μg kg^{-1} h^{-1}, its clearance was reduced in patients with decreased cardiac output and increasing age, and its volume of distribution was increased with hypoalbuminemia. Modeling suggested that context-sensitive half-times would be increased under these circumstances [84].

However, licensing processes, which vary internationally, have affected the distribution of use of dexmedetomidine in children. When the pharmacokinetics of clonidine in children were studied, it was found that clearance is dependent on renal function, with about 50 % being renally excreted unchanged and 50 % undergoing hepatic transformation. The clearance will therefore be dictated by renal function and, for small infants, on renal maturity [85]. In addition it was also found that the context-sensitive half-life may double with prolonged infusions, this being a function of its high lipid solubility and thus sequestration in peripheral tissues [85].

In an early study of the dose–response for clonidine in the PICU, it was found that doses of up to 2 μg kg^{-1} h^{-1} of clonidine when combined with midazolam at 50 μg kg^{-1} h^{-1} produced acceptable sedation and analgesia without adverse effects on cardiovascular performance, even after cardiac surgery [86]. Subsequently, also in a heterogeneous population of ventilated PICU patients, enterally administered clonidine 3–5 μg kg^{-1} 8 hourly was found to give adequate sedation, but this too was given with a background of both a benzodiazepine (in this study lorazepam) and morphine intravenously. However, there seemed to be increased sparing of both agents with time when combined with clonidine in this manner [87]. A multicenter, randomized, blinded trial comparing midazolam and clonidine has been carried out in the UK and results are awaited [88].

One emerging area is the possible benefits of alpha-2 agonist sedation in reducing delirium and other cognitive disorders associated with intensive care. When compared to lorazepam in adults, dexmedetomidine was shown to be associated with significantly less delirium and deep unconsciousness [89]. Additionally, the dexmedetomidine group appeared to have better preserved cognition in post-ICU neuropsychological testing.

When dexmedetomidine was compared to midazolam, there were similar findings; incidence of delirium and times to extubation were more favorable in the dexmedetomidine group. While bradycardia was more frequent in the dexmedetomidine group, the extent to which this needed treating was not significant statistically and the incidence of tachycardia and hypertension needing treatment was lower with dexmedetomidine [90].

When compared to propofol, dexmedetomidine is better at preserving cognition and "cooperative sedation" and thus may prevent the emergence of delirium [91].

When the dosing was increased to over 0.7 μg kg^{-1} h^{-1} in trauma patients, then hypotension was more frequent and hypertension was occasionally seen with loading [92]. This is thought to be due to the action of the different responses to stimulation of the two subtypes of alpha-2 receptors (alpha-2a and alpha-2b) producing hypotension and hypertension, respectively, and where alpha-2b-mediated activity is seen at the higher doses [93]. A dosing protocol in adults, titrating the infusion rate versus the Ramsay Sedation Score only every 30 min and not exceeding 0.7 μg kg^{-1} h^{-1} reduced the incidence of hypotension fourfold [93].

While it has been known for some time that clonidine does slow gastrointestinal transit [94], dexmedetomidine at 0.2 μg kg^{-1} h^{-1} appeared to be free from this side effect [95]. However, when given at the higher range, 0.7 μg kg^{-1} h^{-1}, there was quite a marked effect on slowing transit compared to morphine [96]. Thus, one potential advantage of this agent compared to opioids may be negated.

A large international multicenter study of dexmedetomidine use in adults has been carried out: one arm comparing it with midazolam, the other arm with propofol [97]. It was observed that dexmedetomidine provided equivalent quality of sedation compared to the other two agents and shorter duration of mechanical ventilation in the comparison with midazolam. Durations of ventilation were not significantly different in the comparison with propofol, but in both groups the time to extubation was shorter with dexmedetomidine. The ability of patients to interact with ICU staff appeared to be better with the use of dexmedetomidine than with either of the other two agents. Hypotension incidence was higher with dexmedetomidine compared with midazolam but not with propofol, the dexmedetomidine dose range in this study being permitted up to 1.4 μg kg^{-1} h^{-1}.

In a dose finding study of dexmedetomidine in ventilated PICU patients, Tobias found that a dose range of 0.25–0.5 μg kg^{-1} h^{-1} seemed to provide satisfactory conditions compared to midazolam and with the higher dose of 0.5 μg kg^{-1} h^{-1} perhaps providing more optimal conditions [98].

Doses up to 0.7 μg kg^{-1} h^{-1} were used in a subsequent observational study with little effect on blood pressure and heart rate, even when 76 % of the population studied had undergone cardiac surgery [99]. This contrasts with the findings of Hosokawa in an uncontrolled, sequential observational study in children after cardiac surgery; a mixed sedation regimen of chlorpromazine, fentanyl, and midazolam was compared with a subsequent sedative regimen based on dexmedetomidine but other agents such as midazolam, chlorpromazine, and fentanyl were added in as deemed necessary. The dexmedetomidine rate never exceeded 0.6 μg kg^{-1} h^{-1}. There were statistically significantly more episodes of hypotension but also faster times to extubation and less need for noninvasive respiratory support [100].

More recently an open-label, dose escalation pharmacokinetic and pharmacodynamic study in children after open heart surgery has been reported [101]. Three loading doses over ten minutes of either 0.35, 0.7, or 1 μg kg^{-1} were followed by respective continuous infusions of either 0.25, 0.5, or 0.75 μg kg^{-1} h^{-1} for 24 h. The frequency with which these different cohorts received supplemental sedation or analgesia with midazolam, morphine, fentanyl, or acetaminophen did not differ between the groups with any statistical significance. The level of sedation was monitored by the University of Michigan Sedation Scale [102] and this appeared to have moderate correlation with plasma levels of dexmedetomidine. The three cohorts showed no significant differences in cardiovascular or respiratory effects except a dose-dependent reduction in heart rate, although this was not felt to represent any clinical problem. Additionally, tracheal extubation was achieved within the 24-h infusion period amongst the three groups without any significant difference. When the pharmacokinetics of these dose ranges in children after open heart surgery were examined in detail, there did not appear to be any accumulation [103].

It may be that due to its effective partial sympatholysis, perhaps mediated through parasympathetic stimulation effects, dexmedetomidine may reduce the propensity to tachydysrhythmias. There are a few reports of possible beneficial effects in children in dealing with dysrhythmias such as junctional ectopic, supraventricular, and ventricular tachycardias [81].

It is not yet clear whether dexmedetomidine is associated with withdrawal symptoms that are seen with all other sedative and analgesic agents after prolonged administration. Darnell reported a sequence of events in an infant that would seem to indicate that withdrawal to dexmedetomidine can occur [104]. When dexmedetomidine was stopped in a cohort of children after at least 3 days of receiving cardiac intensive care, tachycardia, transient hypertension, and agitation were observed [105]. Earlier reports of the use of dexmedetomidine in children and adults suggested that it may not be associated with withdrawal [106–108]. There is some question therefore as to whether dexmedetomidine can be associated with withdrawal with these reports divided at the moment [109].

Dexmedetomidine has been reported as a "rescue" treatment for sedation withdrawal symptoms in children and it can be given subcutaneously, appropriately diluted, allowing removal of intravenous devices when they would not be otherwise indicated [110].

Propofol

This drug has many good attributes for a drug for sedation in intensive care. It has a good pharmacokinetic profile with minimal elevation of context-sensitive half-life with prolonged infusions. It is associated with fairly rapid reversal of sedation after cessation of the infusion. It reduces cerebral metabolism, reduces intracranial pressure, and—provided the blood pressure is supported, as is usual in ICU—has no deleterious effects on cerebral perfusion pressure [111], and has anti-inflammatory, antioxidant, and anticonvulsant properties [112].

It was not associated with any major problems until a small series of fatal myocardial failure in children was reported. This described metabolic acidosis and fatal myocardial failure in five children across three intensive care units in the UK [36]. The clinical picture in these children was remarkably similar, the salient features being an increasing metabolic acidosis, bradyarrhythmia, and progressive myocardial failure. The average infusion rate of propofol in these children was between 7.4 and 10 mg kg^{-1} h^{-1}.

At the same time, there were concerns that propofol administered as a sole agent, and thus at higher doses (6–18 mg kg^{-1} h^{-1}), could result in neurologic signs following cessation of the infusions. These consisted of abnormal myoclonic and choreiform activity although there were no long-term sequelae [37]. By 1998, with the emergence of additional similar case reports, the concept of a "propofol infusion syndrome" (PRIS) was taking root [113]. Nonetheless, there was another school of thought that was skeptical regarding the existence of PRIS and claiming that at the moderate doses many employed, backed up by pharmacokinetic data, there had been no occurrence of this syndrome [114, 115].

Subsequently, studies were conducted to explore whether propofol could be given safely under controlled conditions. It was suggested that infusion rates of ≤4 mg kg^{-1} h^{-1} for less than 48 h—while assiduously monitoring acid–base, lactate, and triglyceride levels—may be safe but acknowledging that further research was needed [35]; this was the position adopted by many in pediatric intensive care [34] and backed up by prospective studies [35, 116].

Clues to the etiology started to come from metabolic studies of children affected by what was termed PRIS. Wolf and colleagues studied a 2-year-old child who sustained head trauma, was given propofol up to 5.4 mg kg^{-1} h^{-1} and then developed renal failure and nodal bradycardia. After stopping the propofol and commencing transvenous pacing, the metabolic acidosis continued to worsen. Before starting hemofiltration, blood analysis showed raised malonylcarnitine, C5-acylcarnitine, creatine kinase, troponin-T, and myoglobinemia. The acidosis and cardiac function resolved after hemofiltration.

At a 9-month follow-up, all markers of fatty acid metabolism were normal. It was postulated that propofol had interfered with entry of long-chain acylcarnitine esters into mitochondria and caused failure of the mitochondrial respiratory chain at "complex II" and that this may have been exacerbated by low carbohydrate intake (39.8 kcal kg^{-1} day^{-1}) [38]. This was echoed by a subsequent case in Canada of a 5-month-old child sedated after a cleft lip repair. The carbohydrate intake had been restricted to 1.53–2.7 mg kg^{-1} min^{-1} and the propofol infusion rate had been increased sequentially to 15 mg kg^{-1} h^{-1} over 2 days. The child then developed wide complex tachydysrhythmias, metabolic acidosis, renal failure, hyperkalemia, hepatic dysfunction, and hypertriglyceridemia. Within 2 h of charcoal hemoperfusion the cardiac abnormalities showed marked improvement. Blood analysis prior to hemoperfusion also showed markedly abnormal acylcarnitine chemistry [117]. Further work also reinforced the notion that doses of propofol beyond 4 mg kg^{-1} h^{-1} seemed to be associated with the appearance of abnormal acylcarnitine biochemistry [118].

More recently, fatal PRIS occurred in an adult who had an underlying deficiency in skeletal muscle oxidative pathway, thus reinforcing the theory that the etiology of PRIS is likely to be due to abnormalities in mitochondrial functioning, whether this is congenital or acquired or a combination of these is still conjectural [119].

Despite guidance from various government drug agencies contraindicating its use in children following an unpublished study trialing 1 and 2 % propofol formulations versus conventional therapy [120, 121], propofol continues to be used in children but mostly with the aforementioned constraints and with a degree of caution [12]; but there is still no established consensus about what constitutes the safest dosage and under what circumstances [122].

After emergence of sporadic but serious outcomes in children, there followed similar reports in adults [123–125] even with relatively short infusions [126]. In a case report series, Cremer and colleagues identified adults who had head injuries but died with otherwise inexplicable cardiac arrests. This was attributed to the use of propofol with many of the associations of "propofol infusion syndrome" (metabolic acidosis, cardiac dysrhythmias, rhabdomyolysis, lipemia, and hyperkalemia) and it appeared to be associated with doses exceeding 5 mg kg^{-1} h^{-1} [127].

Further analysis of the electrocardiograms (ECGs) of these patients showed that they had developed ST segment elevation in leads V1 to V3 preceding the tachydysrhythmias that led to their deaths. The appearance of the ECG was similar to that found in Brugada syndrome and thus they speculated that PRIS could lead to an acquired version of this [128]. These ECG changes had also been noted elsewhere in young adults [129]. Despite recommendations regarding maximum propofol dosage rates [130], monitoring of the ECG, metabolic and biochemical markers, case reports of deaths in young adults still appear that describe a very similar picture [131].

In regard to the titratability of propofol to sedative effect, when formally studied in a randomized trial in children after cardiac surgery, there seemed to be some correlation between plasma levels and a derived EEG measure but not with clinical assessment of sedation status as measured by the COMFORT score. It was also noted that there was unpredictable variation in plasma levels with steady-state infusion rates [132].

Immunity

It has long been known that opioids affect the integrity of the immune system, but, arguably, the exact mechanism how this occurs is not yet fully elucidated. Possible mechanisms postulated are direct receptor-mediated effects on immune cells, via the hypothalamic–pituitary–adrenal axis or a combination of these [133].

Benzodiazepines have also been implicated in immunomodulatory effects. This can be mediated through inhibition of mast cells and reduction of pro-inflammatory mediator release and this appears also to be accounted for by direct binding sites on the walls of these cells [134].

Lymphocyte proliferation is diminished by morphine [135], thiopental, and midazolam, but appears to be well preserved by diazepam [136].

Propofol and midazolam were compared in terms of their effects on cytokine production in surgical ICU patients. Propofol was associated with higher levels of IL-1β(beta), IFN-γ(gamma), IL-6, and TNF-α(alpha), while midazolam was associated with decreases in these. IL-8 decreased in the presence of both agents, more with propofol. IL-2 also decreased with propofol. Some of these mediators are required for intact immune response rather than simply being an expression of inflammation, notably IFN-γ(gamma) and IL-2. Overall, it was felt that midazolam had less effect on the pro-inflammatory cytokines [137]. In an equine model, midazolam decreased phagocytosis and oxidative burst of neutrophils and macrophages [138].

Propofol inhibits human neutrophil chemotaxis, phagocytosis, and oxidative burst at clinically relevant blood concentrations. It is thought that this may be due to the inhibition of calcium influx into the cell [139]. These three aspects of neutrophil function were also depressed with clinically relevant concentrations of thiopental and midazolam while ketamine only affected phagocytosis [140].

Of relevance to the wider clinical usage of the alpha-2 agonists dexmedetomidine and clonidine, these two agents, by contrast, do not seem to affect neutrophil chemotaxis, phagocytosis, or superoxide production at clinically relevant concentrations [141].

Findings such as these have obvious potential implications for the use of such agents in the treatment of sepsis and systemic inflammation in the ICU.

Neuropathologic Effects

Considerable attention is currently being given to the role sedative, analgesic, and anesthetic agents may have on the developing brain. There is concern that apoptotic neurodegeneration may occur when exposed to certain agents. Volatile agents, midazolam and ketamine, have all been associated with apoptosis in immature rodents. However, doses studied in these experiments are often far in excess of those used in clinical human practice and in models of questionable analogy to pediatric anesthesia and intensive care [142]. A large prospective clinical study of preterm human infants ("EPIPAGE") failed to show any deleterious effects associated with the prolonged use of sedative and analgesia in the intensive care of preterm infants [143]. Indeed under certain circumstances, some agents are thought to have neuroprotective properties (e.g., xenon, sevoflurane, ketamine, clonidine, and dexmedetomidine) particularly where some other insult such as hypoxic injury may preexist or be imminent [142]. Untreated pain seems to lead to apoptosis too, and this can be offset by the use of ketamine [144]. There is also data that suggest that undertreatment of noxious stimuli, at least in the preterm infant, is associated with a range of persisting symptoms in the older child such as lowered pain thresholds and behavioral and emotional problems [17].

The overall situation, therefore, is rather unclear at present.

Another area of concern is the effect that sedation may play in the neuromyopathy seen in intensive care patients. Two phenotypes are currently identified: polyneuropathy and myopathy [145]. Electrophysiology is helpful in distinguishing between the two, but both may occur simultaneously in the same patient. In some cases, therefore, measurement of serum creatine kinase and even muscle biopsies may help with diagnosis where atrophy or pan-fascicular necrosis may be observed [146, 147].

As regards polyneuropathy, no single causative process has been identified. Putatively it has been suggested that such neuropathies are subject to degradation of the "blood–brain barrier"—or in this setting the blood–nerve barrier, much as other capillary beds lose integrity in inflammatory pathologies commonly seen in the ICU. Sepsis *per se* is associated with such polyneuropathic weakness. However, whereas axonal degeneration is seen, this is not associated with local histological evidence of inflammation, as is seen in Guillain–Barré Syndrome [148].

Myopathy is also seen where nerve conduction studies are otherwise normal. This seems to be associated with loss of myosin more than actin as "thick filament loss" [146]. Factors that lend themselves to producing muscle wasting include immobility (essentially diminution of neural stimulation and loss of antigravity activity), malnutrition, and hormonal factors, particularly the administration of glucocorticoids [148]; but emerging data suggests that inflammation, as in sepsis or systemic inflammation due to hypoxic and/or ischemic origins, disturbs muscle mitochondrial function [145]. There is no evidence that humoral factors are at play—at least those that might be expected to be blocked by the administration of immunoglobulins (if the model of Guillain–Barré were to be mirrored) [148].

The use of muscle relaxants reinforces the deafferentation of skeletal muscle thus exacerbating the tendency to lose the trophic stimulus of neural activity [146, 148]. Other agents that potentiate the action of muscle relaxants, such as aminoglycoside antibiotics, will also contribute and there is evidence of synergy between glucocorticoids and muscle relaxants in this regard [146].

Overall, sedation contributes to the problem by the relative immobilization of the patient and reduction of skeletal activity. It is no accident that the time-honored exhortation to mobilize patients as soon as possible holds very true, but of course this has to be balanced against the sheer practicalities of achieving this in very sick patients.

There is no specific therapy to avoid such neuropathies and myopathies once they have occurred, but diagnosis of these conditions is helpful in appreciating what the patient is up against in terms of weaning from the ventilator and also mobilization. Recovery may take up to several months [145].

Measuring Sedation

There are several clinical scoring scales reported in the literature, but until relatively recently few that have been rigorously assessed for suitability in the pediatric ICU population. (Refer to Chaps. 5, 16, 17, and 20.) The adult ICU community is now facing a rationalization of the various sedation scales available in the literature. A recent review has identified 11 such scales and then subjected these to psychometric analysis [149]. Two emerged with the most favorable profiles: the Richmond Agitation-Sedation Scale [150] and the Sedation-Agitation Scale [151, 152].

The COMFORT score has been widely applied in pediatric sedation research literature. Developed in 1992, it consists of an eight-domain scale based on observations of: spontaneous movement, calmness, facial tension, alertness, respiratory activity, muscle tone, heart rate, and blood pressure [153]. Each domain could be scored from 1 to 5; a score of 17–26 was associated with satisfactory sedation, neither too deep nor light [154]. However, subsequent studies showed that the "physiological" variables, heart rate and blood pressure did not play a significant part [155, 156]. As a result, the abbreviated version—the "behavioral" COMFORT-B using the 6 remaining domains—has been widely adopted and validated [157].

The Hartwig scale was developed in a study examining sedation in neonates and infants and consists of five domains, each scored 1–5 for motor activity, grimacing, eye opening, and respiratory activity, but the last domain is dependent on tracheal suctioning [158]. It has been validated in the neonate and under-1-year-old infant age group [159].

The State Behavioral Scale (SBS) uses a different method of incremental stimulation, commencing with observation, then voice, then noxious stimuli—either planned tracheal suctioning or <5 s of nail bed pressure [5]. Essentially five parameters are examined: movement, calmness, alertness, response to stimulus, cough (spontaneous or to stimulation), respiratory drive/coordination with ventilator. Scores are then given as +2 to −3, in line with the respective broader group headings: agitated, restless/inconsolable, awake/calmable, response to voice or touch, response to noxious stimuli, unresponsive.

The University of Michigan Sedation Scale was developed expressly for assessing sedation in children undergoing procedures such as computed tomography scans [102]. It consists of a five-point scale from 0 (awake and alert) to 4 (unarousable), with the intervening stages being judged against voice, touch, or "significant" physical stimulation. An advantage is simplicity but it must be remembered that it only assesses conscious level without any other corroborative information and was only designed for short procedures without intubation and ventilation. It appears to correlate poorly with bispectral index scoring (BIS) for such outpatient procedures [160].

The Richmond Agitation-Sedation Scale (RASS) was developed in adult ICU [150] but also appears in PICU delirium-related literature [41]. It consists of a ten-point scale from "combative" at +4, then down in stages through 0 for "alert and calm," and then further down to −5 for increasing sedation to "unrousable." It also uses incremental stimulation, starting at observation, voice, and then shaking shoulder, then sternal rub.

It has been hoped that a more objective method of assessing the sedation level of patients might be forthcoming on the ICU, rather than relying on "just" clinical observer assessment and scoring.

Bispectral index (BIS) was originally developed as a "measure" of anesthesia and has an empirical, derived output of 0–100 from mainly low-frequency EEG signals, where a measure of <40 is associated with deep sedation and >80 may be associated with recall [161]. It has been observed that BIS scoring differs between age groups due to the different spread of electrophysiologic frequencies. When BIS is measured at uniform sedative doses, the output varies with age when infants and older children are compared and that arousability to a uniform stimulus at a given BIS level also differs similarly [162].

BIS has been studied repeatedly in the PICU but, on balance, has yet to prove itself reliable with all patients, with all drugs, and in all circumstances [163]. Triltsch found that there was correlation between COMFORT scores and BIS, but that occurred at deeper levels of sedation but not so much in the "target" area of COMFORT scores of 17–26. Additionally a BIS score of 83 seemed to delineate between light and deeper sedation [163]. It may have a role in detecting deep sedation and assessing sedation under muscle relaxation [161, 165, 166].

Courtman found that BIS had moderate correlation to the COMFORT score but that it was only able to discriminate between light and deep sedation, but recognized its potential in children under muscle relaxation [167]. Others also found both the Ramsay Score and COMFORT behavioral scale correlated reasonably with BIS in the unparalyzed child [161, 165].

In older BIS models there may have been cross talk between electromyographic (EMG) signals and those from the EEG as changes in the BIS signal were noted with the administration of muscle relaxants [168]; however, more recent versions of BIS ("BIS-XP") have EMG compensation, although it is not clear to what extent this may alter how BIS readings correlate with levels of sedation [169].

Interestingly but importantly, when Froom and colleagues used twin BIS monitors in children on each side of the forehead, they found a discrepancy during stimulation. When they compared BIS to COMFORT scores, there was good correlation between COMFORT, mean BIS, and right and left BIS during light and moderate sedation; but during stimulation, the right BIS and COMFORT score did not correlate [170].

SNAP II Index is a more recent addition. This uses both low- and high-frequency electro-encephalogical (EEG) signals and is also expressed as an empiric scale 0–100. Previous experience has suggested that 50–65 was recommended for anesthesia. When this was studied in a PICU and compared to the COMFORT scores, a good correlation with COMFORT scoring was observed, particularly toward the deeper levels of sedation [171], though it is probably too early to draw any conclusions about an optimum SNAP II Index range. Previous work measuring a derived summed ratio (SR) of the EEG and comparing this with the COMFORT score during a staged emergence from propofol on the PICU showed that, with this agent at least, there was correlation with the SR, plasma levels of propofol, and the infusion rate, but the COMFORT score was a poor predictor of emergence—the children appearing to transition from deep sleep to very light sedation quite suddenly [132].

Delirium

There is an increasing appreciation of the role delirium plays in the management of the critically ill patient and the roles that primary pathologies and sedative practices play in this. Delirium is a disturbance of consciousness and cognition affecting the abilities to receive and process, store, and recall information. It is characterized by fluctuant symptoms, disorientation, hallucinations, and dysphoric elements such as fear, anger, or apathy and has been characterized as being either hyperactive (agitated) or hypoactive (lethargic). It is variously reported that the incidence of delirium in critically ill patients may be as high as 80 % in the more elderly populations in adult ICUs, at least at some point during an individual's ICU admission [172]. When reviewing research findings in the literature, it is clear that differences occur between languages and some attempt has been made to clarify terminology to facilitate sharing of research [173]. In a recent prospective study in adults, the incidence of delirium was an independent risk factor associated with higher hospital mortality and 6-month follow-up mortality and less favorable level of functioning after hospital discharge [174].

What is the cause of this delirium? Almost certainly this is multifactorial, consequent to the varied challenges, pharmacological and pathophysiological, to normal brain physiology.

In a study of adult critically ill patients on mechanical ventilation and receiving intravenous sedation, polysomnography with respect to rapid eye movement (REM) sleep was studied in concert with circadian rhythmicity as evidenced by hourly urine excretion of melatonin metabolites (6-sulphatoxymelatonin or "aMT6s"). Severe disorganization of sleep–wake regulation and circadian activity was observed [175]. Recently, it has been found that, in a series of patients undergoing noncardiac surgery followed by a period of mechanical ventilation in the ICU, delirium was observed in those patients whose melatonin levels dropped in the first hour following their surgery—but was not related to subsequent melatonin levels [176].

Hypothetically at least, there is the possibility that some aspects of delirium may be caused by disruption of normal signaling between a circuit made up of the posterior parietal cortex, the medial temporal lobe, and the prefrontal cortex. The integrity of this "circuit" is important for normal cognition. It is activated and maintained by the ascending reticular activating system. Disturbances in this may have knock-on effects at higher cognitive levels resulting in the disturbances in orientation and affect seen in delirium [177]. Additionally, fluctuant levels of sedation, as measured by the Richmond Agitation-Sedation Scale, were associated with a greater risk of developing delirium [178].

Clearly, it is helpful to have a structured and validated assessment tool and this was achieved over 10 years ago in adult practice with the Confusion Assessment Method for the ICU ("CAM-ICU") [172, 179]. In a recent survey of UK adult units, only 25 % screened for delirium. Of these, 55 % used a validated screening tool and of these, the majority (80 %) used the CAM-ICU [180].

S100B is a protein released into the blood in association with neurological injury. Routsi and colleagues showed that in adult patients without a primary neurological insult, over two-thirds of patients in their ICU had an elevated S100B level [181]. This was associated with elevated lactate levels, hemoglobin below 7 mg dL^{-1}, and decreased pH and mean arterial blood pressure. As delirium occurs with a similar incidence, the question arises if both phenomena—one laboratory, the other clinical—may reflect the same underlying pathologies [182].

When examining the potential role of the neurotransmitters serotonin, dopamine, norepinephrine, and acetylcholine and their precursors (phenylalanine, tryptophan, and tyrosine), it was found that high and low ratios of both tryptophan and tyrosine with respect to other large neutral amino acids were related to the transitioning into delirium. This transitioning, in the same study, was also found to be related to higher severity of illness scores (Acute Physiology and Chronic Health Evaluation II [APACHE II]) and exposure to fentanyl [183].

How may delirium be prevented and treated? In the recent UK survey of adult ICUs, the most common "rescue" treatment was haloperidol and the most common second-line treatment was benzodiazepines, particularly with hyperactive delirium; but, in hypoactive delirium, the most common approach was not to add in any further drugs, though some haloperidol was used [180].

It is worth questioning whether benzodiazepines are helpful or in fact may be part of the problem. In a prospective, randomized, double-blind study comparing midazolam against dexmedetomidine, equivalent levels of sedation were achieved, but with reduced incidence of delirium (and reduced ventilation times) in the dexmedetomidine group [90]. It has also been shown that lorazepam can be an independent risk factor for the development of delirium [40]. In a comparison of dexmedetomidine and lorazepam in adult ICU patients with or without sepsis, it was found that the septic group randomized to dexmedetomidine fared better with respect to less days ventilated, less days exhibiting brain dysfunction, and decreased mortality [184].

Such analyses of the situation affecting children are, at present, less well advanced, though delirium on emergence from anesthesia has been recognized for some years and a validated scoring system was developed by Sikich and Lerman in 2004, the "PAED Scale" [185]. More recently, some pioneering work is now forthcoming in addressing the evaluation of delirium in pediatric ICU patients [41, 186]. While the undercurrent etiologies may be quite similar, diagnostic methodology will differ in relation to age-related differences in brain and intellectual functions [41], although the broad principles remain the same [186]. In 2007, Schieveld described a 6-year series of PICU patients with an overall incidence of delirium of 5 %, where this was categorized into 25 % hypoactive, 35 % hyperactive, but with the largest group "emerging" or "veiled" in 40 % [187]. This latter category was characterized by anxiety, moaning, and/or restlessness. In all groups, treatment was mostly with haloperidol, but about 25 % with risperidone. In contrast to adult practice, pediatric delirium has a higher incidence of the more agitated version and this has been borne out in other work [186]. Since then scoring of pediatric delirium has been refined with the use of the Delirium Rating Scale [188] and, particularly regarding the PICU setting, the introduction of a validated pediatric version of the CAM-ICU, the "pCAM-ICU" [41].

There is a recent publication of guidelines by the American College of Critical Care Medicine for the management of pain, agitation, and delirium in adult ICU patients [189], but these are related to adult practice and further elucidation of delirium in the pediatric population will hopefully lead to similar guidelines. However, it is noteworthy that when previously the use of haloperidol had been suggested as an agent that might reduce the duration of delirium, this has now been dropped from the most recent version of these guidelines [189] and a recent study in adults seems to confirm lack of benefit of haloperidol in reducing delirium incidence or duration [190]. There is some interest, therefore, in finding other strategies or agents that may prevent or at least deal with delirium in ICU patients. In adult delirium patients, where rivastigmine had been shown to have some benefit in treating non-ICU patients, when this was examined in ICU patients, there was no apparent benefit and possibly some harm [191]. Presumably therefore, and perhaps unsurprisingly, there must be other confounding factors at play in what intensive care entails that complicates the etiology of delirium.

Tolerance and Withdrawal

There are a number of terms in this area of practice, some of which have overlapping and interrelated elements: tolerance, tachyphylaxis, addiction, dependence, and withdrawal.

Anand has attempted to delineate these [28]: addiction is characterized by psychological dependence and is a chronic and often relapsing disorder, rarely a facet of PICU practice. Tolerance and tachyphylaxis are, arguably, separated by their time course. Tachyphylaxis is seen with rapid loss of drug effects, e.g., with exhaustion of transmitters or activation of antagonistic systems such as the NMDA receptors. Tolerance is associated with more prolonged exposure and may reflect desensitization of receptors or up-regulation of compensatory intracellular processes (e.g., the cAMP pathway with opioid use [27]). Dependence is the physiological and biochemical adaptation of neurons where removal of a drug precipitates withdrawal or "abstinence" symptoms and signs. Withdrawal is a clinical syndrome of varied clinical symptoms that occurs after stopping a drug after prolonged exposure and where a form of dependence has been caused by adaptive physiology as outlined above.

Whereas tolerance and the reverse side of the coin, withdrawal, have long been associated with the use of opioids [28, 192], it has taken longer to appreciate that other agents used in the field of sedation and analgesia are capable of inducing tolerance and withdrawal [61, 192–194], including propofol [37, 195], midazolam [12, 42, 196, 197], isoflurane [61], clonidine [198], and dexmedetomidine [104, 105, 109].

Opioid tolerance appears to occur earlier in younger patients, perhaps exacerbated by background neurological insult [199], and with the shorter acting forms with high affinity for opioid receptors [28, 30, 200, 201] and this can occur quite rapidly, even during the course of anesthesia [29].

Benzodiazepine withdrawal seems to be associated with higher total doses, particularly regarding midazolam [12, 42]. However, these larger doses may reflect the underlying degree or nature of the illness affecting the child itself [12]. Additionally, these series were reported without cognizance of any underlying delirium—another emerging complication that needs to be considered and that, arguably, may have been present at the time [202].

Until recently, the assessment of withdrawal in children has been hampered by the lack of a tool constructed expressly for the pediatric ICU population. Historically, the literature in this area frequently utilized the Neonatal Abstinence Score. However, this was only devised to assess symptoms in neonates born to mothers suffering from addictions [203]. An adaptation of this, aimed at assessing children outside the infant group, the Sedation Withdrawal Score was described by Cunliffe. It compromised 12 clinical features, each scored from 0 to 2 (absent, mild, severe), giving a possible range of 0–24 [196].

Ista and colleagues described an array of 24 symptoms that were possibly associated with withdrawal in a pediatric ICU population, signposting the direction of future efforts at finding a suitable validated and reproducible tool [204].

Two validated scoring tools are now available: the Withdrawal Assessment Tool-1 (WAT-1) [6] and the Sophia Observation Score (SOS) [205]. Arguably the WAT-1 is more adept at picking up withdrawal from opioids than benzodiazepines [6, 205]. The WAT-1 consists of 11 domains: presence of loose stools, vomiting/gagging, pyrexia >37.8 °C, observation of "State" using the State Observation Scale [5], tremor, sweating, abnormal movements, yawning/

sneezing, startle to touch, muscle tone, and time to regain calm after stimulus. The test needs about 7 min for completion and gives a possible score range of 0–12, with high scores indicative of the extent of withdrawal with a score of >3 reflective of length of stay, necessity to wean of sedation, duration of mechanical ventilation, and ICU stay. These findings were confirmed by a recent validation exercise [206].

The SOS was constructed from a multidimensional analysis of co-occurrences between children who were divided into two groups by an experienced group of nurses and doctors depending on whether they were considered to have problems of withdrawal or not on weaning sedation. Out of an array of 21 potentially eligible symptoms, 15 were analyzed to be discriminatory. The score was then just present or absent ("1 or 0") for these symptoms without gradation, giving a potential range of 0–15 [205]. This has since received psychometric evaluation. A score of ≥4 was thought to reflect high probability of manifest withdrawal and other aspects of care were identified as statistically significant risk factors: "preweaning" duration and duration of weaning of both midazolam and morphine and the number of additional sedatives or opioids utilized [207]. The SOS at a level of ≥4 appears to be very reliable in predicting those children that will not develop overt withdrawal (specificity) but, like other scales, less sensitive in predicting those that will develop withdrawal. It is recognized that other factors such as pain, distress, and delirium may be confounding factors [207].

The time course for dealing with withdrawal symptoms covers a large reported range, up to 8 weeks in older children [196], but up to greater than 24 weeks in neonates after treatment with extracorporeal membrane oxygenation [197]. Given these prolonged time courses, some clinicians had managed these patients remotely at home with telephone and clinic support [194, 197]. Management may include stepwise reduction in the sedative agents ("tapering") [196] and this may include the use of subcutaneous infusions where necessary, which has the advantage of facilitating the removal of intravenous catheters and their attendant risk of infection [110, 194]; substitution of an intravenous agent with an oral agent of the same class—e.g., methadone or oral morphine replacing intravenous morphine or fentanyl [194], e.g., replacing intravenous midazolam with oral lorazepam; substitution of an agent that the child has become tolerant to another agent that sits on alternative receptors—e.g., replacing benzodiazepines or opioids with chlorpromazine [208], clonidine [196], or dexmedetomidine [110]. There is an argument for preemptive substitution rather than prolonged weaning [193], but this still has to be done in a closely monitored environment to ensure that the substitution agent is titrated appropriately. Now that we have validated scoring systems [206, 207] for assessing the presence and extent of sedation, tailoring of withdrawal treatment can occur with a greater degree of assurance.

Staff

It is not just patients who are vulnerable to the effects of the sedative and analgesic drugs used in the ICU.

A recent survey in the USA showed that of the academic anesthesiology departments contacted, 18 % had recorded one or more incidents of propofol abuse or "diversion" [209]. Of the individuals who had been identified, 28 % had died as a result of the propofol abuse. Propofol causes tolerance [195] and has psychotropic properties that lend themselves to abuse [210], and this has been corroborated in human volunteers [211]. Clearly, anesthesiology staff have greater access to such drugs than other health workers, and this results in greater drug abuse in this group [212], but next in line must surely come intensive care staff. What may be less well appreciated is that in a study utilizing mass spectrometry in operating room environments, aerosolized fentanyl has been detected in the air of an operating room, in patients' expiratory circuits, and in the headspace above sharps boxes, and aerosolized propofol was also detected in the expirations of a patient undergoing transurethral prostatectomy [213]. Given the potential of these drugs to exert effects at minute nanomolar concentrations [214], it may be that occupational exposure is not only a real hazard for addiction developing in operating room staff but also everywhere these drugs are commonly utilized, such as intensive care units and emergency departments. There needs to be institutional recognition of several aspects to this. Tracking of drugs with known addictive potential should be rigorous, and such drugs should have safe and irreversible disposal. This should now probably include propofol; and other drugs will undoubtedly emerge that have addictive properties. Lastly, the inherent vulnerability of health care staff to developing addiction is not solely due to their obvious access to these drugs but may also be due to subliminal as well as overt occupational environmental exposure.

Conclusion

> For every complex problem, there is a solution that is simple, neat and wrong.—H. L. Mencken [215]

The same could be said about our approach to sedation in the ICU. It looks like it should be simple, leaving us to concentrate on "more important" aspects of clinical care, but in fact there is abundant complexity, with ramifications that affect many aspects of intensive care for these children and their families. There is surely abundant scope for further exploration, but insofar as we are getting some understanding of where we are heading, we need to understand where we are. Concerning what we should do in the future with sedative and analgesic drugs, the horizon toward which we steer still recedes before us.

> By prevailing over all obstacles and distractions, we will unfailingly arrive at our chosen goal or destination.—Christopher Columbus

Clinical Case Samples

Case 1

A 15-year-old boy was treated for septic arthritis but worsened with apparent septic shock, necessitating volume resuscitation, inotropes, ventilation for 4 days, and hemofiltration for 5 days. A polyarthropathy appeared after 2 days, possibly a severe form of systemic juvenile connective tissue disease, and so he was treated with high-dose prednisolone. He had been difficult to sedate, needing a mixture of fentanyl; midazolam, with occasional clonidine; and chlorpromazine as required.

After extubation, he began vomiting, had frequent loose bowel actions, a new low-grade pyrexia appeared, and he had dilated pupils and some jitteriness. He was started on a clonidine infusion at 2 μg kg^{-1} h^{-1}, having been loaded with 2.5 μg kg^{-1}, but these symptoms did not settle until the fentanyl infusion was recommenced at 5 μg kg^{-1} h^{-1} shortly afterwards.

After this, all the aforementioned symptoms attributed to withdrawal resolved, although he was noted to be "jittery" when mobilized for a few more days. A day later, he was able to eat and drink, and his bowels had settled. Two days later, oral morphine was commenced and the fentanyl infusion halved and later that day it was stopped.

The next day the IV clonidine was converted to the enteral route with a plan to wean both this and morphine over 10 days, which was accomplished successfully. Subsequent investigations regarding juvenile arthritis proved negative, but neither was there any evidence of infection demonstrated on culture or polymerase chain reaction.

Consideration

Withdrawal

This was the principal problem here. A duration of ventilation of 4 days might not be expected to lead to withdrawal phenomena, but data from several papers indicates that this may be expected even after such short duration, particularly where larger doses of sedatives have been used and where this comprises midazolam. He had been "difficult to sedate" adequately and on cessation of sedative agents he demonstrated good evidence of withdrawal. If the SOS is applied, then the score was 7, well above the threshold of 4 that has been shown to be reliably associated with withdrawal.

One strategy is to cover the decreasing patient drug levels of midazolam and opioids with other agents, principally α(alpha)$_2$ receptor agonists such as clonidine and dexmedetomidine. However, it is important to realize that both drugs—with half-lives of 12–24 h and 2–3 h, respectively—will need loading before any expectation that steady-state infusion rates will exert any effect. Notwithstanding the loading of clonidine before running the infusion, it became necessary to reintroduce fentanyl. The effect of this was dramatic with immediate reversal of agitation and gastrointestinal symptoms, although some residual jitteriness remained.

It is possible that the jitteriness might have been best addressed by more specific cover of the withdrawal of the midazolam with, for example, enteral lorazepam.

Having overcome the immediate problem, the next objective, if possible, is to convert to drugs that can be given enterally to facilitate removal of intravenous catheters, although some clinicians have used the subcutaneous route. For this enteral strategy to succeed, three preconditions need to be satisfied: the enteral route needs to be fully and reliably working, the bioavailability of the new drug must be satisfactory, and, thirdly, the pharmacodynamic efficacy of the new drug must be matched to that of the intravenous drug it replaces.

In this case administration of enteral morphine at 0.5 mg kg^{-1} 4 hourly was sufficient to replace the effects of the fentanyl, and the clonidine infusion was replaced with a similar 4 hourly regimen of enteral clonidine at 2.5 μg kg^{-1} per dose. Both these drugs need to be weaned progressively where the rate of this takes account of the duration of the sedation the child initially received.

Case 2

A 4-year-old boy was admitted with pseudomonas pneumonia, empyema, septicemia, and neutropenia, having received chemotherapy induction for leukemia 2 weeks previously. He became difficult to ventilate and quickly progressing to high-frequency oscillation ventilation with inhaled nitric oxide.

After 10 days, high-dose methylprednisolone was given to treat ARDS and then reduced over 21 days. He later developed cystic pneumatoceles and air leaks.

(continued)

Muscle relaxation with rocuronium was used for 2 weeks while sedated with midazolam and fentanyl.

His condition only slowly improved and a tracheostomy was performed after a month in order to facilitate weaning of ventilation and sedation. Due to concerns about underlying delirium associated with unexplained episodes of hypertension and tachycardia requiring frequent changes in substantial sedative drug dosing, he had already been started on haloperidol. This permitted decreasing sedation and a gradual wean of ventilation. On emergence from sedation, a hemiparesis was noted and CT showed a small cerebral infarct. Peripheral neurophysiology was consistent with myopathy but no defect in nerve conduction. He was transferred from intravenous agents to oral clonidine and morphine, and these, with the haloperidol, were weaned over a month with melatonin administered at night.

Considerations

Delirium

There was a clinical concern that there was a degree of delirium underlying his sedation, these suspicions being prompted by episodic hypertension and tachycardia unrelated to direct stimulation and resultant fluctuant dosing of substantial sedation. Added to this is the known risk factor of severe critical illness, particularly sepsis.

Delirium is characterized by disorganized brain functioning, essentially manifest in conscious patients as "confusion." Unfortunately, there is at present no method of clinically assessing such brain dysfunction while the patient is sedated, and although work has been done on clinical assessment scores in adults and children over 5 years of age, there is, as yet, no method for assessing children under the age of 5. The efficacy of haloperidol in delirium, as well as other agents such as rivastigmine and more particularly risperidone in pediatric patients, is by no means established and in need of further evaluation.

The later diagnosis of a cerebral infarct and thus organic brain pathology may go some way to explaining the earlier symptoms of brain dysfunction that had been suspected earlier.

Sleep Cycle

A concern in this boy's later care was the evident disturbance in normal diurnal sleep patterns. This is an extremely common phenomenon in intensive care and not least in a child who had been ventilated for a month. It is very important to try to recreate a more physiological environment for such a patient to try and maintain the external factors involved in the pineal axis governing the sleep–wake cycle. Such physical measures would include darkening the ICU and reduction of noise and other physical interference at night. Other more subtle measures such as attempting to give the bulk of feeds during the day may contribute to normal cycling. An additional measure is to administer melatonin at night to replicate normal secretion patterns, but although there are some favorable reports, the definitive research is yet to be done.

Neuromyopathy

Two phenotypes are recognized: polyneuropathy and myopathy. Electrophysiology can often delineate which pathology predominates, although they may often occur together. Polyneuropathy is predominantly associated with sepsis. Myopathy is also seen consequent to factors that produce muscle wasting, disuse atrophy, malnutrition, and administration of glucocorticoids. All these would apply in this case, but the use of muscle relaxants of 2 weeks duration seen here would be expected to de-afferent the muscles even further and thus contribute to muscle wasting. In this case, although no specific therapy is currently available, neurophysiologic studies were helpful to characterize the extent of the problem, alert physiotherapy staff to his future mobilization challenges, and to direct rehabilitation.

Case 3

A 4-day-old neonate underwent a Norwood surgical operation for hypoplastic left heart. After the operation, the chest was left open till the second postoperative day to allow recovery of the heart and some clearance of generalized tissue edema with diuresis and peritoneal dialysis. During this time, she received fentanyl and rocuronium (a neuromuscular blocker) infusions. After chest closure, the muscle relaxant and fentanyl infusions were stopped to maximize clearance. The following day, there appeared to be little spontaneous respiratory activity, and it was noted there was a degree of renal impairment. A train-of-four test showed that there was considerable residual neuromuscular blockade.

Sugammadex, a neuromuscular blocker reversal agent, was administered in 2 mg kg^{-1} increments, and observations for spontaneous movements and response to train-of-four were commenced. There was no response to the first two boluses. It was not until a total of 6 mg kg^{-1} was given that spontaneous movement and respiratory drive evident by triggering of the ventilator became apparent. The patient was then observed

(continued)

closely for any evidence of recurarization in the next few hours after the reduction in ventilation. The child then progressed without further incident but emerged from residual sedation slowly over a few days.

Consideration

Context-Sensitive Half-Life

This pharmacokinetic property is often overlooked. In this case, fentanyl, once administered for more than 24 h, exhibits a steady and quite steep rise in its context-sensitive half-life due to its lipid solubility, becoming increasingly sequestered in vessel-poor, lipid-rich tissues. Even when the infusion is stopped, the drug can leak out from other compartments thus maintaining plasma levels. These effects are exacerbated in cases with capillary leakage, increased interstitial fluid formation, and reduced hepatorenal elimination. Consideration should therefore be given to the use of drugs with more favorable pharmacokinetic profiles such as alfentanil. The best profile probably belongs to remifentanil; however, this drug is particularly associated with the induction of acute tolerance.

Although rocuronium is not associated with production of active metabolites, it is still vulnerable to decreased hepatic and renal elimination. Additionally, all muscle relaxants, although predominantly hydrophilic and usually constrained to the intravascular space, may accumulate in the tissues in conditions associated with capillary leakage. Whereas sugammadex has been shown to be very effective in the binding of muscle relaxants, this will not be so effective where the drug may be sequestered in other compartments. The use of sugammadex in the context of patients with potential sequestering must therefore be done with careful titration and observation for potential recurarization.

References

1. Duhigg C. The power of habit—why we do what we do in life and business. New York: Random House; 2012.
2. Peitz GJ, Balas MC, Olsen KM, Pun BT, Ely EW. Top 10 myths regarding sedation and delirium in the ICU. Crit Care Med. 2013;41(9 Suppl 1):S46–56.
3. Wolf AR, Jackman L. Analgesia and sedation after pediatric cardiac surgery. Paediatr Anaesth. 2011;21(5):567–76 [Review].
4. Grant MJ, Balas MC, Curley MA. Defining sedation-related adverse events in the pediatric intensive care unit. Heart Lung. 2013;42(3):171–6.
5. Curley MA, Harris SK, Fraser KA, Johnson RA, Arnold JH. State behavioral scale: a sedation assessment instrument for infants and young children supported on mechanical ventilation. Pediatr Crit Care Med. 2006;7(2):107–14.
6. Franck LS, Harris SK, Soetenga DJ, Amling JK, Curley MA. The Withdrawal Assessment Tool-1 (WAT-1): an assessment instrument for monitoring opioid and benzodiazepine withdrawal symptoms in pediatric patients. Pediatr Crit Care Med. 2008;9(6):573–80.
7. Bradley BD, Green G, Ramsay T, Seely AJ. Impact of sedation and organ failure on continuous heart and respiratory rate variability monitoring in critically ill patients: a pilot study. Crit Care Med. 2013;41(2):433–44 [Research Support, Non-U.S. Gov't].
8. Menon G, Boyle EM, Bergqvist LL, McIntosh N, Barton BA, Anand KJ. Morphine analgesia and gastrointestinal morbidity in preterm infants: secondary results from the NEOPAIN trial. Arch Dis Child Fetal Neonatal Ed. 2008;93(5):F362–7 [Multicenter Study Randomized Controlled Trial].
9. Shehabi Y, Bellomo R, Reade MC, Bailey M, Bass F, Howe B, et al. Early intensive care sedation predicts long-term mortality in ventilated critically ill patients. Am J Respir Crit Care Med. 2012;186(8):724–31 [Multicenter Study Research Support, Non-U.S. Gov't].
10. Shehabi Y, Chan L, Kadiman S, Alias A, Ismail WN, Tan MA, et al. Sedation depth and long-term mortality in mechanically ventilated critically ill adults: a prospective longitudinal multicentre cohort study. Intensive Care Med. 2013;39(5):910–8 [Research Support, Non-U.S. Gov't].
11. Hill S. Pharmacokinetics of drug infusions. Cont Educ Anaesth Crit Care Pain. 2004;4(3):76–80.
12. Jenkins IA, Playfor SD, Bevan C, Davies G, Wolf AR. Current United Kingdom sedation practice in pediatric intensive care. Paediatr Anaesth. 2007;17(7):675–83.
13. Hemstapat K, Le L, Edwards SR, Smith MT. Comparative studies of the neuro-excitatory behavioural effects of morphine-3-glucuronide and dynorphin a(2-17) following spinal and supraspinal routes of administration. Pharmacol Biochem Behav. 2009;93(4):498–505 [Comparative Study Research Support, Non-U.S. Gov't].
14. Hemstapat K, Monteith GR, Smith D, Smith MT. Morphine-3-glucuronide's neuro-excitatory effects are mediated via indirect activation of n-methyl-d-aspartic acid receptors: mechanistic studies in embryonic cultured hippocampal neurones. Anesth Analg. 2003;97(2):494–505, table of contents [Research Support, Non-U.S. Gov't].
15. Spina SP, Ensom MH. Clinical pharmacokinetic monitoring of midazolam in critically ill patients. Pharmacotherapy. 2007;27(3):389–98 [Review].
16. Segredo V, Caldwell JE, Wright PM, Sharma ML, Gruenke LD, Miller RD. Do the pharmacokinetics of vecuronium change during prolonged administration in critically ill patients? Br J Anaesth. 1998;80(6):715–9 [Research Support, U.S. Gov't, P.H.S.].
17. Durrmeyer X, Vutskits L, Anand KJ, Rimensberger PC. Use of analgesic and sedative drugs in the NICU: Integrating clinical trials and laboratory data. Pediatr Res. 2010;67(2):117–27.
18. Anand KJ, Anderson BJ, Holford NH, Hall RW, Young T, Shephard B, et al. Morphine pharmacokinetics and pharmacodynamics in preterm and term neonates: secondary results from the NEOPAIN trial. Br J Anaesth. 2008;101(5):680–9 [Multicenter Study Randomized Controlled Trial Research Support, N.I.H., Extramural Research Support, Non-U.S. Gov't].
19. Rhodin MM, Anderson BJ, Peters AM, Coulthard MG, Wilkins B, Cole M, et al. Human renal function maturation: a quantitative description using weight and postmenstrual age. Pediatr Nephrol. 2009;24(1):67–76.
20. Kress JP, Pohlman AS, O'Connor MF, Hall JB. Daily interruption of sedative infusions in critically ill patients undergoing mechanical ventilation. N Engl J Med. 2000;342(20):1471–7 [Clinical Trial Randomized Controlled Trial].
21. Gupta K, Gupta VK, Jayashree M, Singhi S. Randomized controlled trial of interrupted versus continuous sedative infusions in

ventilated children. Pediatr Crit Care Med. 2012;13(2):131–5 [Randomized Controlled Trial].
22. Kress JP, Hall JB. The changing landscape of ICU sedation. JAMA. 2012;308(19):2030–1 [Comment Editorial].
23. Dale CR, Bryson CL, Fan VS, Maynard C, Yanez 3rd ND, Treggiari MM. A greater analgesia, sedation, delirium order set quality score is associated with a decreased duration of mechanical ventilation in cardiovascular surgery patients. Crit Care Med. 2013;41(11):2610–7.
24. Deindl P, Unterasinger L, Kappler G, Werther T, Czaba C, Giordano V, et al. Successful implementation of a neonatal pain and sedation protocol at 2 NICUs. Pediatrics. 2013;132(1):e211–8.
25. Le Guen M, Liu N, Bourgeois E, Chazot T, Sessler DI, Rouby JJ, et al. Automated sedation outperforms manual administration of propofol and remifentanil in critically ill patients with deep sedation: a randomized phase ii trial. Intensive Care Med. 2013; 39(3):454–62.
26. Kosarac B, Fox AA, Collard CD. Effect of genetic factors on opioid action. Curr Opin Anaesthesiol. 2009;22(4):476–82 [Review].
27. Borgland SL. Acute opioid receptor desensitization and tolerance: is there a link? Clin Exp Pharmacol Physiol. 2001;28(3):147–54.
28. Anand KJ, Willson DF, Berger J, Harrison R, Meert KL, Zimmerman J, et al. Tolerance and withdrawal from prolonged opioid use in critically ill children. Pediatrics. 2010;125(5):e1208–25 [Research Support, N.I.H., Extramural Review].
29. Crawford MW, Hickey C, Zaarour C, Howard A, Naser B. Development of acute opioid tolerance during infusion of remifentanil for pediatric scoliosis surgery. Anesth Analg. 2006; 102(6):1662–7.
30. Vinik HR, Kissin I. Rapid development of tolerance to analgesia during remifentanil infusion in humans. Anesth Analg. 1998; 86(6):1307–11 [Comparative Study Research Support, U.S. Gov't, P.H.S.].
31. Engelhardt T, Zaarour C, Naser B, Pehora C, de Ruiter J, Howard A, et al. Intraoperative low-dose ketamine does not prevent a remifentanil-induced increase in morphine requirement after pediatric scoliosis surgery. Anesth Analg. 2008; 107(4):1170–5.
32. Fraser GL, Devlin JW, Worby CP, Alhazzani W, Barr J, Dasta JF, et al. Benzodiazepine versus nonbenzodiazepine-based sedation for mechanically ventilated, critically ill adults: a systematic review and meta-analysis of randomized trials. Crit Care Med. 2013;41(9 Suppl 1):S30–8.
33. Jarman A, Duke G, Reade M, Casamento A. The association between sedation practices and duration of mechanical ventilation in intensive care. Anaesth Intensive Care. 2013;41(3):311–5.
34. Hatch DJ. Propofol in paediatric intensive care. Br J Anaesth. 1997;79(3):274–5 [Comment Editorial].
35. Martin PH, Murthy BV, Petros AJ. Metabolic, biochemical and haemodynamic effects of infusion of propofol for long-term sedation of children undergoing intensive care. Br J Anaesth. 1997;79(3):276–9 [Clinical Trial].
36. Parke TJ, Stevens JE, Rice AS, Greenaway CL, Bray RJ, Smith PJ, et al. Metabolic acidosis and fatal myocardial failure after propofol infusion in children: Five case reports. BMJ. 1992;305(6854):613–6 [Case Reports].
37. Trotter C, Serpell MG. Neurological sequelae in children after prolonged propofol infusion. Anaesthesia. 1992;47(4):340–2.
38. Wolf A, Weir P, Segar P, Stone J, Shield J. Impaired fatty acid oxidation in propofol infusion syndrome. Lancet. 2001;357(9256): 606–7 [Case Reports Letter].
39. Rowe K, Fletcher S. Sedation in the intensive care unit. Contin Educ Anaesth Crit Care Pain. 2008;8(2):50–5.
40. Pandharipande P, Shintani A, Peterson J, Pun BT, Wilkinson GR, Dittus RS, et al. Lorazepam is an independent risk factor for transitioning to delirium in intensive care unit patients. Anesthesiology. 2006;104(1):21–6.
41. Smith HA, Boyd J, Fuchs DC, Melvin K, Berry P, Shintani A, et al. Diagnosing delirium in critically ill children: validity and reliability of the pediatric confusion assessment method for the intensive care unit. Crit Care Med. 2011;39(1):150–7.
42. Fonsmark L, Rasmussen YH, Carl P. Occurrence of withdrawal in critically ill sedated children. Crit Care Med. 1999;27(1):196–9.
43. Koinig H, Marhofer P. S(+)-ketamine in paediatric anaesthesia. Paediatr Anaesth. 2003;13(3):185–7 [Editorial].
44. Turner CP, Gutierrez S, Liu C, Miller L, Chou J, Finucane B, et al. Strategies to defeat ketamine-induced neonatal brain injury. Neuroscience. 2012;210:384–92 [Research Support, N.I.H., Extramural Research Support, Non-U.S. Gov't].
45. Bhutta AT, Schmitz ML, Swearingen C, James LP, Wardbegnoche WL, Lindquist DM, et al. Ketamine as a neuroprotective and anti-inflammatory agent in children undergoing surgery on cardiopulmonary bypass: a pilot randomized, double-blind, placebo-controlled trial. Pediatr Crit Care Med. 2012;13(3): 328–37 [Randomized Controlled Trial Research Support, Non-U.S. Gov't].
46. Lahtinen P, Kokki H, Hakala T, Hynynen M. S(+)-ketamine as an analgesic adjunct reduces opioid consumption after cardiac surgery. Anesth Analg. 2004;99(5):1295–301, table of contents [Clinical Trial Randomized Controlled Trial].
47. Laulin JP, Maurette P, Corcuff JB, Rivat C, Chauvin M, Simonnet G. The role of ketamine in preventing fentanyl-induced hyperalgesia and subsequent acute morphine tolerance. Anesth Analg. 2002;94(5):1263–9.
48. Filanovsky Y, Miller P, Kao J. Myth: ketamine should not be used as an induction agent for intubation in patients with head injury. CJEM. 2010;12(2):154–7 [Review].
49. Sehdev RS, Symmons DA, Kindl K. Ketamine for rapid sequence induction in patients with head injury in the emergency department. Emerg Med Australas. 2006;18(1):37–44 [Review].
50. Albanese J, Arnaud S, Rey M, Thomachot L, Alliez B, Martin C. Ketamine decreases intracranial pressure and electroencephalographic activity in traumatic brain injury patients during propofol sedation. Anesthesiology. 1997;87(6):1328–34.
51. Chang LC, Raty SR, Ortiz J, Bailard NS, Mathew SJ. The emerging use of ketamine for anesthesia and sedation in traumatic brain injuries. CNS Neurosci Ther. 2013;19(6):390–5.
52. Denmark TK, Crane HA, Brown L. Ketamine to avoid mechanical ventilation in severe pediatric asthma. J Emerg Med. 2006; 30(2):163–6 [Case Reports].
53. Jat KR, Chawla D. Ketamine for management of acute exacerbations of asthma in children. Cochrane Database Syst Rev. 2012;11:CD009293 [Review].
54. Allen JY, Macias CG. The efficacy of ketamine in pediatric emergency department patients who present with acute severe asthma. Ann Emerg Med. 2005;46(1):43–50 [Randomized Controlled Trial Research Support, Non-U.S. Gov't].
55. Williams GD, Philip BM, Chu LF, Boltz MG, Kamra K, Terwey H, et al. Ketamine does not increase pulmonary vascular resistance in children with pulmonary hypertension undergoing sevoflurane anesthesia and spontaneous ventilation. Anesth Analg. 2007;105(6):1578–84, table of contents [Comparative Study Research Support, N.I.H., Extramural].
56. Sheth RD, Gidal BE. Refractory status epilepticus: response to ketamine. Neurology. 1998;51(6):1765–6 [Case Reports].
57. Gaspard N, Foreman B, Judd LM, Brenton JN, Nathan BR, McCoy BM, et al. Intravenous ketamine for the treatment of refractory status epilepticus: a retrospective multicenter study. Epilepsia. 2013;54(8):1498–503.
58. Wheeler DS, Clapp CR, Ponaman ML, Bsn HM, Poss WB. Isoflurane therapy for status asthmaticus in children: a case series and protocol. Pediatr Crit Care Med. 2000;1(1):55–9.
59. Sackey PV, Martling CR, Nise G, Radell PJ. Ambient isoflurane pollution and isoflurane consumption during intensive care unit

sedation with the anesthetic conserving device. Crit Care Med. 2005;33(3):585–90.

60. Eifinger F, Hunseler C, Roth B, Vierzig A, Oberthuer A, Mehler K, et al. Observations on the effects of inhaled isoflurane in long-term sedation of critically ill children using a modified AnaConDa©-system. Klin Padiatr. 2013;225(4):206–11.
61. Arnold JH, Truog RD, Molengraft JA. Tolerance to isoflurane during prolonged administration. Anesthesiology. 1993;78(5):985–8.
62. Sackey PV, Martling CR, Radell PJ. Three cases of PICU sedation with isoflurane delivered by the 'AnaConDa'. Paediatr Anaesth. 2005;15(10):879–85.
63. Jung C, Granados M, Marsol P, Murat I, Gall O. Use of sevoflurane sedation by the AnaConDa device as an adjunct to extubation in a pediatric burn patient. Burns. 2008;34(1):136–8.
64. Soukup J, Scharff K, Kubosch K, Pohl C, Bomplitz M, Kompardt J. State of the art: sedation concepts with volatile anesthetics in critically ill patients. J Crit Care. 2009;24(4):535–44 [Review].
65. Kirkland LL. Protecting both heart and brain: a noble goal for a noble gas. Crit Care Med. 2013;41(9):2228–9.
66. Goto T, Nakata Y, Morita S. Will xenon be a stranger or a friend?: the cost, benefit, and future of xenon anesthesia. Anesthesiology. 2003;98(1):1–2.
67. Rossaint R, Reyle-Hahn M, Schulte Am Esch J, Scholz J, Scherpereel P, Vallet B, et al. Multicenter randomized comparison of the efficacy and safety of xenon and isoflurane in patients undergoing elective surgery. Anesthesiology. 2003;98(1):6–13.
68. Bedi A, Murray JM, Dingley J, Stevenson MA, Fee JP. Use of xenon as a sedative for patients receiving critical care. Crit Care Med. 2003;31(10):2470–7 [Clinical Trial Randomized Controlled Trial Research Support, Non-U.S. Gov't].
69. Hanss R, Bein B, Turowski P, Cavus E, Bauer M, Andretzke M, et al. The influence of xenon on regulation of the autonomic nervous system in patients at high risk of perioperative cardiac complications. Br J Anaesth. 2006;96(4):427–36.
70. Dingley J, Tooley J, Porter H, Thoresen M. Xenon provides short-term neuroprotection in neonatal rats when administered after hypoxia-ischemia. Stroke. 2006;37(2):501–6.
71. Hobbs C, Thoresen M, Tucker A, Aquilina K, Chakkarapani E, Dingley J. Xenon and hypothermia combine additively, offering long-term functional and histopathologic neuroprotection after neonatal hypoxia/ischemia. Stroke. 2008;39(4):1307–13.
72. Banks P, Franks NP, Dickinson R. Competitive inhibition at the glycine site of the N-methyl-D-aspartate receptor mediates xenon neuroprotection against hypoxia-ischemia. Anesthesiology. 2010; 112(3):614–22.
73. Arola OJ, Laitio RM, Roine RO, Gronlund J, Saraste A, Pietila M, et al. Feasibility and cardiac safety of inhaled xenon in combination with therapeutic hypothermia following out-of-hospital cardiac arrest. Crit Care Med. 2013;41(9):2116–24.
74. Lockwood GG, Franks NP, Downie NA, Taylor KM, Maze M. Feasibility and safety of delivering xenon to patients undergoing coronary artery bypass graft surgery while on cardiopulmonary bypass: phase I study. Anesthesiology. 2006;104(3):458–65.
75. Jungwirth B, Gordan ML, Blobner M, Schmehl W, Kochs EF, Mackensen GB. Xenon impairs neurocognitive and histologic outcome after cardiopulmonary bypass combined with cerebral air embolism in rats. Anesthesiology. 2006;104(4):770–6.
76. Kamibayashi T, Maze M. Clinical uses of alpha2 -adrenergic agonists. Anesthesiology. 2000;93(5):1345–9 [Review].
77. Gertler R, Brown HC, Mitchell DH, Silvius EN. Dexmedetomidine: a novel sedative-analgesic agent. Proc (Bayl Univ Med Cent). 2001;14(1):13–21.
78. Fleetwood-Walker SM, Mitchell R, Hope PJ, Molony V, Iggo A. An alpha 2 receptor mediates the selective inhibition by noradrenaline of nociceptive responses of identified dorsal horn neurones. Brain Res. 1985;334(2):243–54 [Research Support, Non-U.S. Gov't].
79. Kuraishi Y, Hirota N, Sato Y, Kaneko S, Satoh M, Takagi H. Noradrenergic inhibition of the release of substance p from the primary afferents in the rabbit spinal dorsal horn. Brain Res. 1985;359(1–2):177–82 [Research Support, Non-U.S. Gov't].
80. Correa-Sales C, Rabin BC, Maze M. A hypnotic response to dexmedetomidine, an alpha 2 agonist, is mediated in the locus coeruleus in rats. Anesthesiology. 1992;76(6):948–52 [Research Support, U.S. Gov't, Non-P.H.S. Research Support, U.S. Gov't, P.H.S.].
81. Tobias JD, Chrysostomou C. Dexmedetomidine: antiarrhythmic effects in the pediatric cardiac patient. Pediatr Cardiol. 2013;34(4):779–85 [Review].
82. Bhana N, Goa KL, McClellan KJ. Dexmedetomidine. Drugs. 2000;59(2):263–8; discussion 269–270.
83. Iirola T, Aantaa R, Laitio R, Kentala E, Lahtinen M, Wighton A, et al. Pharmacokinetics of prolonged infusion of high-dose dexmedetomidine in critically ill patients. Crit Care. 2011;15(5):R257 [Clinical Trial Research Support, Non-U.S. Gov't].
84. Iirola T, Ihmsen H, Laitio R, Kentala E, Aantaa R, Kurvinen JP, et al. Population pharmacokinetics of dexmedetomidine during long-term sedation in intensive care patients. Br J Anaesth. 2012;108(3):460–8 [Clinical Trial Research Support, Non-U.S. Gov't].
85. Potts AL, Larsson P, Eksborg S, Warman G, Lonnqvist PA, Anderson BJ. Clonidine disposition in children; a population analysis. Paediatr Anaesth. 2007;17(10):924–33 [Research Support, Non-U.S. Gov't].
86. Ambrose C, Sale S, Howells R, Bevan C, Jenkins I, Weir P, et al. Intravenous clonidine infusion in critically ill children: dose-dependent sedative effects and cardiovascular stability. Br J Anaesth. 2000;84(6):794–6.
87. Arenas-Lopez S, Riphagen S, Tibby SM, Durward A, Tomlin S, Davies G, et al. Use of oral clonidine for sedation in ventilated paediatric intensive care patients. Intensive Care Med. 2004;30(8):1625–9 [Research Support, Non-U.S. Gov't].
88. Gamble C, Wolf A, Sinha I, Spowart C, Williamson P. The role of systematic reviews in pharmacovigilance planning and Clinical Trials Authorisation application: example from the SLEEPS trial. PLoS One. 2013;8(3):e51787 [Research Support, Non-U.S. Gov't].
89. Pandharipande PP, Pun BT, Herr DL, Maze M, Girard TD, Miller RR, et al. Effect of sedation with dexmedetomidine vs lorazepam on acute brain dysfunction in mechanically ventilated patients: the mends randomized controlled trial. JAMA. 2007;298(22): 2644–53.
90. Riker RR, Shehabi Y, Bokesch PM, Ceraso D, Wisemandle W, Koura F, et al. Dexmedetomidine vs midazolam for sedation of critically ill patients: a randomized trial. JAMA. 2009;301(5):489–99 [Comparative Study Multicenter Study Randomized Controlled Trial Research Support, Non-U.S. Gov't].
91. Goodwin HE, Gill RS, Murakami PN, Thompson CB, Lewin JJ III, Mirski MA. Dexmedetomidine preserves attention/calculation when used for cooperative and short-term intensive care unit sedation. J Crit Care. 2013;28(6):1113.e7–e10.
92. Devabhakthuni S, Pajoumand M, Williams C, Kufera JA, Watson K, Stein DM. Evaluation of dexmedetomidine: safety and clinical outcomes in critically ill trauma patients. J Trauma. 2011;71(5): 1164–71.
93. Gerlach AT, Dasta JF, Steinberg S, Martin LC, Cook CH. A new dosing protocol reduces dexmedetomidine-associated hypotension in critically ill surgical patients. J Crit Care. 2009;24(4): 568–74.
94. Mann NS, Shinkle JM. Effect of clonidine on gastrointestinal transit time. Hepatogastroenterology. 1998;45(22):1023–5.
95. Memis D, Dokmeci D, Karamanlioglu B, Turan A, Ture M. A comparison of the effect on gastric emptying of propofol or

dexmedetomidine in critically ill patients: preliminary study. Eur J Anaesthesiol. 2006;23(8):700–4.

96. Iirola T, Vilo S, Aantaa R, Wendelin-Saarenhovi M, Neuvonen PJ, Scheinin M, et al. Dexmedetomidine inhibits gastric emptying and oro-caecal transit in healthy volunteers. Br J Anaesth. 2011;106(4):522–7 [Randomized Controlled Trial Research Support, Non-U.S. Gov't].
97. Jakob SM, Ruokonen E, Grounds RM, Sarapohja T, Garratt C, Pocock SJ, et al. Dexmedetomidine vs midazolam or propofol for sedation during prolonged mechanical ventilation: two randomized controlled trials. JAMA. 2012;307(11):1151–60 [Comparative Study Multicenter Study Randomized Controlled Trial Research Support, Non-U.S. Gov't].
98. Tobias JD, Berkenbosch JW. Sedation during mechanical ventilation in infants and children: dexmedetomidine versus midazolam. South Med J. 2004;97(5):451–5 [Clinical Trial Comparative Study Randomized Controlled Trial].
99. Buck ML, Willson DF. Use of dexmedetomidine in the pediatric intensive care unit. Pharmacotherapy. 2008;28(1):51–7.
100. Hosokawa K, Shime N, Kato Y, et al. Dexmedetomidine sedation in children after cardiac surgery. Pediatr Crit Care Med. 2010;11(1):39–43.
101. Su F, Nicolson SC, Zuppa AF. A dose-response study of dexmedetomidine administered as the primary sedative in infants following open heart surgery. Pediatr Crit Care Med. 2013;14(5):499–507.
102. Malviya S, Voepel-Lewis T, Tait AR, Merkel S, Tremper K, Naughton N. Depth of sedation in children undergoing computed tomography: validity and reliability of the University of Michigan Sedation Scale (UMSS). Br J Anaesth. 2002;88(2):241–5.
103. Su F, Nicolson SC, Gastonguay MR, Barrett JS, Adamson PC, Kang DS, et al. Population pharmacokinetics of dexmedetomidine in infants after open heart surgery. Anesth Analg. 2010;110(5): 1383–92.
104. Darnell C, Steiner J, Szmuk P, Sheeran P. Withdrawal from multiple sedative agent therapy in an infant: is dexmedetomidine the cause or the cure? Pediatr Crit Care Med. 2010;11(1):e1–3.
105. Burbano NH, Otero AV, Berry DE, Orr RA, Munoz RA. Discontinuation of prolonged infusions of dexmedetomidine in critically ill children with heart disease. Intensive Care Med. 2012;38(2):300–7 [Research Support, N.I.H., Extramural].
106. Shehabi Y, Ruettimann U, Adamson H, Innes R, Ickeringill M. Dexmedetomidine infusion for more than 24 hours in critically ill patients: sedative and cardiovascular effects. Intensive Care Med. 2004;30(12):2188–96.
107. Walker J, Maccallum M, Fischer C, Kopcha R, Saylors R, McCall J. Sedation using dexmedetomidine in pediatric burn patients. J Burn Care Res. 2006;27(2):206–10.
108. Hammer GB, Philip BM, Schroeder AR, Rosen FS, Koltai PJ. Prolonged infusion of dexmedetomidine for sedation following tracheal resection. Paediatr Anaesth. 2005;15(7):616–20.
109. Tobias JD. Dexmedetomidine: are tolerance and withdrawal going to be an issue with long-term infusions? Pediatr Crit Care Med. 2010;11(1):158–60.
110. Tobias JD. Subcutaneous dexmedetomidine infusions to treat or prevent drug withdrawal in infants and children. J Opioid Manag. 2008;4(4):187–91.
111. Farling PA, Johnston JR, Coppel DL. Propofol infusion for sedation of patients with head injury in intensive care. A preliminary report. Anaesthesia. 1989;44(3):222–6.
112. Marik PE. Propofol: therapeutic indications and side-effects. Curr Pharm Des. 2004;10(29):3639–49.
113. Bray RJ. Propofol infusion syndrome in children. Paediatr Anaesth. 1998;8(6):491–9.
114. Reed MD, Blumer JL. Propofol bashing: the time to stop is now! Crit Care Med. 1996;24(1):175–6.
115. Reed MD, Yamashita TS, Marx CM, Myers CM, Blumer JL. A pharmacokinetically based propofol dosing strategy for sedation of the critically ill, mechanically ventilated pediatric patient. Crit Care Med. 1996;24(9):1473–81.
116. Cornfield DN, Tegtmeyer K, Nelson MD, Milla CE, Sweeney M. Continuous propofol infusion in 142 critically ill children. Pediatrics. 2002;110(6):1177–81.
117. Withington DE, Decell MK, Al Ayed T. A case of propofol toxicity: further evidence for a causal mechanism. Paediatr Anaesth. 2004;14(6):505–8.
118. Wolf AR, Potter F. Propofol infusion in children: when does an anesthetic tool become an intensive care liability? Paediatr Anaesth. 2004;14(6):435–8.
119. Vanlander AV, Jorens PG, Smet J, De Paepe B, Verbrugghe W, Van den Eynden GG, et al. Inborn oxidative phosphorylation defect as risk factor for propofol infusion syndrome. Acta Anaesthesiol Scand. 2012;56(4):520–5 [Case Reports].
120. Anonymous. Propofol (Diprivan) infusion: sedation in children aged 16 years or younger contraindicated. Curr Probl Pharmacovigil. 2001;27:10.
121. Wooltorton E. Propofol: contraindicated for sedation of pediatric intensive care patients. CMAJ. 2002;167(5):507.
122. Svensson ML, Lindberg L. The use of propofol sedation in a paediatric intensive care unit. Nurs Crit Care. 2012;17(4):198–203.
123. Kumar MA, Urrutia VC, Thomas CE, Abou-Khaled KJ, Schwartzman RJ. The syndrome of irreversible acidosis after prolonged propofol infusion. Neurocrit Care. 2005;3(3):257–9.
124. Eriksen J, Povey HM. A case of suspected non-neurosurgical adult fatal propofol infusion syndrome. Acta Anaesthesiol Scand. 2006;50(1):117–9.
125. Fudickar A, Bein B, Tonner PH. Propofol infusion syndrome in anaesthesia and intensive care medicine. Curr Opin Anaesthesiol. 2006;19(4):404–10.
126. Liolios A, Guerit JM, Scholtes JL, Raftopoulos C, Hantson P. Propofol infusion syndrome associated with short-term large-dose infusion during surgical anesthesia in an adult. Anesth Analg. 2005;100(6):1804–6.
127. Cremer OL, Moons KG, Bouman EA, Kruijswijk JE, de Smet AM, Kalkman CJ. Long-term propofol infusion and cardiac failure in adult head-injured patients. Lancet. 2001;357(9250): 117–8.
128. Vernooy K, Delhaas T, Cremer OL, Di Diego JM, Oliva A, Timmermans C, et al. Electrocardiographic changes predicting sudden death in propofol-related infusion syndrome. Heart Rhythm. 2006;3(2):131–7.
129. Ernest D, French C. Propofol infusion syndrome—report of an adult fatality. Anaesth Intensive Care. 2003;31(3):316–9.
130. Kang TM. Propofol infusion syndrome in critically ill patients. Ann Pharmacother. 2002;36(9):1453–6.
131. Mijzen EJ, Jacobs B, Aslan A, Rodgers MG. Propofol infusion syndrome heralded by ECG changes. Neurocrit Care. 2012; 17(2):260–4 [Case Reports].
132. Murray DM, Thorne GC, Rigby-Jones AE, Tonucci D, Grimes S, Tooley MA, et al. Electroencephalograph variables, drug concentrations and sedation scores in children emerging from propofol infusion anaesthesia. Paediatr Anaesth. 2004;14(2):143–51.
133. Al-Hashimi M, Scott SW, Thompson JP, Lambert DG. Opioids and immune modulation: more questions than answers. Br J Anaesth. 2013;111(1):80–8.
134. Bidri M, Royer B, Averlant G, Bismuth G, Guillosson JJ, Arock M. Inhibition of mouse mast cell proliferation and proinflammatory mediator release by benzodiazepines. Immunopharmacology. 1999;43(1):75–86.
135. Webster NR. Opioids and the immune system. Br J Anaesth. 1998;81(6):835–6.

136. Platt M, Platt S, Royston D. Lymphocyte proliferation: dichotomy of effect of related anaesthetic agents. Br J Anaesth. 1986; 58(1):132P.
137. Helmy SA, Al-Attiyah RJ. The immunomodulatory effects of prolonged intravenous infusion of propofol versus midazolam in critically ill surgical patients. Anaesthesia. 2001;56(1):4–8.
138. Massoco C, Palermo-Neto J. Effects of midazolam on equine innate immune response: a flow cytometric study. Vet Immunol Immunopathol. 2003;95(1–2):11–9 [Research Support, Non-U.S. Gov't].
139. Mikawa K, Akamatsu H, Nishina K, Shiga M, Maekawa N, Obara H, et al. Propofol inhibits human neutrophil functions. Anesth Analg. 1998;87(3):695–700.
140. Nishina K, Akamatsu H, Mikawa K, Shiga M, Maekawa N, Obara H, et al. The inhibitory effects of thiopental, midazolam, and ketamine on human neutrophil functions. Anesth Analg. 1998;86(1): 159–65.
141. Nishina K, Akamatsu H, Mikawa K, Shiga M, Maekawa N, Obara H, et al. The effects of clonidine and dexmedetomidine on human neutrophil functions. Anesth Analg. 1999;88(2):452–8.
142. Sanders RD, Ma D, Brooks P, Maze M. Balancing paediatric anaesthesia: preclinical insights into analgesia, hypnosis, neuroprotection, and neurotoxicity. Br J Anaesth. 2008;101(5):597–609 [Review].
143. Roze JC, Denizot S, Carbajal R, Ancel PY, Kaminski M, Arnaud C, et al. Prolonged sedation and/or analgesia and 5-year neurodevelopment outcome in very preterm infants: results from the EPIPAGE cohort. Arch Pediatr Adolesc Med. 2008;162(8):728–33.
144. Anand KJ, Garg S, Rovnaghi CR, Narsinghani U, Bhutta AT, Hall RW. Ketamine reduces the cell death following inflammatory pain in newborn rat brain. Pediatr Res. 2007;62(3):283–90 [Research Support, N.I.H., Extramural Research Support, Non-U.S. Gov't].
145. Batt J, dos Santos CC, Cameron JI, Herridge MS. Intensive care unit-acquired weakness: clinical phenotypes and molecular mechanisms. Am J Respir Crit Care Med. 2013;187(3):238–46 [Research Support, Non-U.S. Gov't Review].
146. Hund E. Neurological complications of sepsis: critical illness polyneuropathy and myopathy. J Neurol. 2001;248(11):929–34 [Review].
147. Tabarki B, Coffinieres A, Van Den Bergh P, Huault G, Landrieu P, Sebire G. Critical illness neuromuscular disease: clinical, electrophysiological, and prognostic aspects. Arch Dis Child. 2002;86(2):103–7 [Case Reports Review].
148. Bolton CF, Young GB. Critical illness polyneuropathy. Curr Treat Options Neurol. 2000;2(6):489–98.
149. Robinson BR, Berube M, Barr J, Riker R, Gelinas C. Psychometric analysis of subjective sedation scales in critically ill adults. Crit Care Med. 2013;41(9 Suppl 1):S16–29.
150. Ely EW, Truman B, Shintani A, Thomason JW, Wheeler AP, Gordon S, et al. Monitoring sedation status over time in ICU patients: reliability and validity of the Richmond Agitation-Sedation Scale (RASS). JAMA. 2003;289(22):2983–91.
151. Riker RR, Fraser GL, Cox PM. Continuous infusion of haloperidol controls agitation in critically ill patients. Crit Care Med. 1994;22(3):433–40.
152. Riker RR, Picard JT, Fraser GL. Prospective evaluation of the sedation-agitation scale for adult critically ill patients. Crit Care Med. 1999;27(7):1325–9.
153. Ambuel B, Hamlett KW, Marx CM, Blumer JL. Assessing distress in pediatric intensive care environments: the comfort scale. J Pediatr Psychol. 1992;17(1):95–109.
154. Marx CM, Smith PG, Lowrie LH, Hamlett KW, Ambuel B, Yamashita TS, et al. Optimal sedation of mechanically ventilated pediatric critical care patients. Crit Care Med. 1994;22(1): 163–70.
155. van Dijk M, de Boer JB, Koot HM, Tibboel D, Passchier J, Duivenvoorden HJ. The reliability and validity of the comfort scale as a postoperative pain instrument in 0 to 3-year-old infants. Pain. 2000;84(2–3):367–77.
156. Carnevale FA, Razack S. An item analysis of the comfort scale in a pediatric intensive care unit. Pediatr Crit Care Med. 2002; 3(2):177–80.
157. Ista E, van Dijk M, Tibboel D, de Hoog M. Assessment of sedation levels in pediatric intensive care patients can be improved by using the comfort "behavior" scale. Pediatr Crit Care Med. 2005; 6(1):58–63.
158. Hartwig S, Roth B, Theisohn M. Clinical experience with continuous intravenous sedation using midazolam and fentanyl in the paediatric intensive care unit. Eur J Pediatr. 1991;150(11):784–8.
159. Hunseler C, Merkt V, Gerloff M, Eifinger F, Kribs A, Roth B. Assessing pain in ventilated newborns and infants: validation of the Hartwig score. Eur J Pediatr. 2011;170(7):837–43.
160. Shields CH, Styadi-Park G, McCown MY, Creamer KM. Clinical utility of the bispectral index score when compared to the University of Michigan Sedation Scale in assessing the depth of outpatient pediatric sedation. Clin Pediatr. 2005;44(3):229–36 [Clinical Trial Comparative Study].
161. Aneja R, Heard AM, Fletcher JE, Heard CM. Sedation monitoring of children by the Bispectral Index in the pediatric intensive care unit. Pediatr Crit Care Med. 2003;4(1):60–4 [Comparative Study].
162. Davidson AJ, McCann ME, Devavaram P, Auble SA, Sullivan LJ, Gillis JM, et al. The differences in the bispectral index between infants and children during emergence from anesthesia after circumcision surgery. Anesth Analg. 2001;93(2):326–30, 2nd contents page [Clinical Trial Research Support, Non-U.S. Gov't].
163. Playfor SD. The use of bispectral index monitors in paediatric intensive care. Crit Care. 2005;9(1):25–6 [Comment].
164. Triltsch AE, Nestmann G, Orawa H, Moshirzadeh M, Sander M, Grosse J, et al. Bispectral index versus COMFORT score to determine the level of sedation in paediatric intensive care unit patients: a prospective study. Crit Care. 2005;9(1):R9–17 [Clinical Trial].
165. Amigoni A, Mozzo E, Brugnaro L, Gentilomo C, Stritoni V, Michelin E, et al. Assessing sedation in a pediatric intensive care unit using comfort behavioural scale and bispectral index: these tools are different. Minerva Anestesiol. 2012;78(3):322–9.
166. Berkenbosch JW, Fichter CR, Tobias JD. The correlation of the bispectral index monitor with clinical sedation scores during mechanical ventilation in the pediatric intensive care unit. Anesth Analg. 2002;94(3):506–11, table of contents.
167. Courtman SP, Wardurgh A, Petros AJ. Comparison of the bispectral index monitor with the COMFORT score in assessing level of sedation of critically ill children. Intensive Care Med. 2003; 29(12):2239–46.
168. Messner M, Beese U, Romstock J, Dinkel M, Tschaikowsky K. The bispectral index declines during neuromuscular block in fully awake persons. Anesth Analg. 2003;97(2):488–91, table of contents.
169. LeBlanc JM, Dasta JF, Pruchnicki MC, Gerlach A, Cook C. Bispectral index values, sedation-agitation scores, and plasma lorazepam concentrations in critically ill surgical patients. Am J Crit Care. 2012;21(2):99–105 [Research Support, Non-U.S. Gov't].
170. Froom SR, Malan CA, Mecklenburgh JS, Price M, Chawathe MS, Hall JE, et al. Bispectral index asymmetry and COMFORT score in paediatric intensive care patients. Br J Anaesth. 2008;100(5): 690–6.
171. Fernandez Nievas IF, Spentzas T, Bogue CW. Snap II index: an alternative to the COMFORT scale in assessing the level of sedation in mechanically ventilated pediatric patients. J Intensive Care Med. 2013;29(4):225–8.
172. Ely EW, Inouye SK, Bernard GR, Gordon S, Francis J, May L, et al. Delirium in mechanically ventilated patients: validity and

reliability of the confusion assessment method for the intensive care unit (CAM-ICU). JAMA. 2001;286(21):2703–10.
173. Morandi A, Pandharipande P, Trabucchi M, Rozzini R, Mistraletti G, Trompeo AC, et al. Understanding international differences in terminology for delirium and other types of acute brain dysfunction in critically ill patients. Intensive Care Med. 2008;34(10): 1907–15.
174. Abelha F, Luis C, Veiga D, Parente D, Fernandes V, Santos P, et al. Outcome and quality of life in patients with postoperative delirium during an ICU stay following major surgery. Crit Care [Serial on the Internet]. 2013;17(5):R257. http://ccforum.com/content/17/5/R257
175. Gehlbach BK, Chapotot F, Leproult R, Whitmore H, Poston J, Pohlman M, et al. Temporal disorganization of circadian rhythmicity and sleep-wake regulation in mechanically ventilated patients receiving continuous intravenous sedation. Sleep. 2012;35(8):1105–14 [Research Support, N.I.H., Extramural Research Support, Non-U.S. Gov't].
176. Yoshitaka S, Egi M, Morimatsu H, Kanazawa T, Toda Y, Morita K. Perioperative plasma melatonin concentration in postoperative critically ill patients: its association with delirium. J Crit Care. 2013;28(3):236–42 [Research Support, Non-U.S. Gov't].
177. Gunther ML, Jackson JC, Ely EW. Loss of IQ in the ICU brain injury without the insult. Med Hypotheses. 2007;69(6):1179–82.
178. Svenningsen H, Egerod I, Videbech P, Christensen D, Frydenberg M, Tonnesen EK. Fluctuations in sedation levels may contribute to delirium in ICU patients. Acta Anaesthesiol Scand. 2013;57(3):288–93 [Research Support, Non-U.S. Gov't].
179. Ely EW, Margolin R, Francis J, May L, Truman B, Dittus R, et al. Evaluation of delirium in critically ill patients: validation of the confusion assessment method for the intensive care unit (CAM-ICU). Crit Care Med. 2001;29(7):1370–9.
180. Mac Sweeney R, Barber V, Page V, Ely EW, Perkins GD, Young JD, et al. A national survey of the management of delirium in UK intensive care units. QJM. 2010;103(4):243–51.
181. Routsi C, Stamataki E, Nanas S, Psachoulia C, Stathopoulos A, Koroneos A, et al. Increased levels of serum S100B protein in critically ill patients without brain injury. Shock. 2006;26(1): 20–4.
182. Cotton BA, Girard TD, Ely EW. Increased levels of serum S100B protein in critically ill patients without brain injury. Shock. 2006;26(1):20–4. Shock. United States 2007. p. 338; author reply 339.
183. Pandharipande PP, Morandi A, Adams JR, Girard TD, Thompson JL, Shintani AK, et al. Plasma tryptophan and tyrosine levels are independent risk factors for delirium in critically ill patients. Intensive Care Med. 2009;35(11):1886–92.
184. Pandharipande PP, Sanders RD, Girard TD, McGrane S, Thompson JL, Shintani AK, et al. Effect of dexmedetomidine versus lorazepam on outcome in patients with sepsis: an a priori-designed analysis of the MENDS randomized controlled trial. Crit Care. 2010;14(2):R38.
185. Sikich N, Lerman J. Development and psychometric evaluation of the pediatric anesthesia emergence delirium scale. Anesthesiology. 2004;100(5):1138–45 [Validation Studies].
186. Turkel SB, Trzepacz PT, Tavare CJ. Comparing symptoms of delirium in adults and children. Psychosomatics. 2006;47(4):320–4 [Comparative Study].
187. Schieveld JN, Leroy PL, van Os J, Nicolai J, Vos GD, Leentjens AF. Pediatric delirium in critical illness: phenomenology, clinical correlates and treatment response in 40 cases in the pediatric intensive care unit. Intensive Care Med. 2007;33(6):1033–40.
188. Turkel SB, Jacobson JR, Tavare CJ. The diagnosis and management of delirium in infancy. J Child Adolesc Psychopharmacol. 2013;23(5):352–6.
189. Barr J, Fraser GL, Puntillo K, Ely EW, Gelinas C, Dasta JF, et al. Clinical practice guidelines for the management of pain, agitation, and delirium in adult patients in the intensive care unit. Crit Care Med. 2013;41(1):263–306 [Consensus Development Conference Practice Guideline Research Support, Non-U.S. Gov't Review].
190. Page V, Ely E, Gates S, Xiao B, Alce T, Shintani A, et al. Effect of intravenous haloperidol on the duration of delirium and coma in critically ill patients (Hope-ICU): a randomised, double-blind, placebo-controlled trial. Lancet Respir Med. 2013;1(7):515–23.
191. van Eijk MM, Roes KC, Honing ML, Kuiper MA, Karakus A, van der Jagt M, et al. Effect of rivastigmine as an adjunct to usual care with haloperidol on duration of delirium and mortality in critically ill patients: a multicentre, double-blind, placebo-controlled randomised trial. Lancet. 2010;376(9755):1829–37 [Multicenter Study Randomized Controlled Trial Research Support, Non-U.S. Gov't].
192. Arnold JH, Truog RD, Orav EJ, Scavone JM, Hershenson MB. Tolerance and dependence in neonates sedated with fentanyl during extracorporeal membrane oxygenation. Anesthesiology. 1990;73(6):1136–40.
193. Jenkins IA. Tolerance and addiction; the patient, the parent or the clinician? Paediatr Anaesth. 2011;21(7):794–9 [Review].
194. Tobias JD. Tolerance, withdrawal, and physical dependency after long-term sedation and analgesia of children in the pediatric intensive care unit. Crit Care Med. 2000;28(6):2122–32.
195. Ypsilantis P, Mikroulis D, Politou M, Tsoukali H, Pitiakoudis M, Didilis V, et al. Tolerance to propofol's sedative effect in mechanically ventilated rabbits. Anesth Analg. 2006;103(2):359–65.
196. Cunliffe M, McArthur L, Dooley F. Managing sedation withdrawal in children who undergo prolonged PICU admission after discharge to the ward. Paediatr Anaesth. 2004;14(4):293–8 [Case Reports Review].
197. Ista E, van Dijk M, Gischler S, de Leeuw M, Poley MJ, Tibboel D. Weaning of opioids and benzodiazepines at home after critical illness in infants: a cost-effective approach. J Opioid Manag. 2010;6(1):55–62 [Comparative Study].
198. Greenberg M, Sauberan J. Clonidine withdrawal in a 3 month old premature male infant. Internet J Pediatr Neonatol. 2009. http://ispub.com/IJPN/10/1/8312.
199. Bachiocco V, Lorenzini L, Baroncini S. Severe withdrawal syndrome in three newborns subjected to continuous opioid infusion and seizure activity dependent on brain hypoxia—ischemia. A possible link. Paediatr Anaesth. 2006;16(10):1057–62.
200. Guignard B, Bossard AE, Coste C, Sessler DI, Lebrault C, Alfonsi P, et al. Acute opioid tolerance: intraoperative remifentanil increases postoperative pain and morphine requirement. Anesthesiology. 2000;93(2):409–17.
201. Katz R, Kelly HW, Hsi A. Prospective study on the occurrence of withdrawal in critically ill children who receive fentanyl by continuous infusion. Crit Care Med. 1994;22(5):763–7 [Research Support, U.S. Gov't, P.H.S.].
202. Smith HA, Fuchs DC, Pandharipande PP, Barr FE, Ely EW. Delirium: an emerging frontier in the management of critically ill children. Anesthesiol Clin. 2011;29(4):729–50.
203. Finnegan LP, Connaughton Jr JF, Kron RE, Emich JP. Neonatal abstinence syndrome: assessment and management. Addict Dis. 1975;2(1–2):141–58.
204. Ista E, van Dijk M, Gamel C, Tibboel D, de Hoog M. Withdrawal symptoms in critically ill children after long-term administration of sedatives and/or analgesics: a first evaluation. Crit Care Med. 2008;36(8):2427–32.
205. Ista E, van Dijk M, de Hoog M, Tibboel D, Duivenvoorden HJ. Construction of the Sophia Observation withdrawal Symptoms-scale (SOS) for critically ill children. Intensive Care Med. 2009;35(6):1075–81.

206. Franck LS, Scoppettuolo LA, Wypij D, Curley MA. Validity and generalizability of the Withdrawal Assessment Tool-1 (WAT-1) for monitoring iatrogenic withdrawal syndrome in pediatric patients. Pain. 2012;153(1):142–8 [Validation Studies].
207. Ista E, de Hoog M, Tibboel D, Duivenvoorden HJ, van Dijk M. Psychometric evaluation of the Sophia observation withdrawal symptoms scale in critically ill children. Pediatr Crit Care Med. 2013;14(8):761–9.
208. Mazurier E, Cambonie G, Barbotte E, Grare A, Pinzani V, Picaud JC. Comparison of chlorpromazine versus morphine hydrochloride for treatment of neonatal abstinence syndrome. Acta Paediatr. 2008;97(10):1358–61.
209. Wischmeyer PE, Johnson BR, Wilson JE, Dingmann C, Bachman HM, Roller E, et al. A survey of propofol abuse in academic anesthesia programs. Anesth Analg. 2007;105(4):1066–71, table of contents.
210. Wilson C, Canning P, Caravati EM. The abuse potential of propofol. Clin Toxicol. 2010;48(3):165–70.
211. Zacny JP, Lichtor JL, Thompson W, Apfelbaum JL. Propofol at a subanesthetic dose may have abuse potential in healthy volunteers. Anesth Analg. 1993;77(3):544–52.
212. Berge KH, Seppala MD, Lanier WL. The anesthesiology community's approach to opioid- and anesthetic-abusing personnel: time to change course. Anesthesiology. 2008;109(5):762–4.
213. McAuliffe PF, Gold MS, Bajpai L, Merves ML, Frost-Pineda K, Pomm RM, et al. Second-hand exposure to aerosolized intravenous anesthetics propofol and fentanyl may cause sensitization and subsequent opiate addiction among anesthesiologists and surgeons. Med Hypotheses. 2006;66(5):874–82.
214. Li KY, Xiao C, Xiong M, Delphin E, Ye JH. Nanomolar propofol stimulates glutamate transmission to dopamine neurons: a possible mechanism of abuse potential? J Pharmacol Exp Ther. 2008;325(1):165–74.
215. Joshi ST, editor. H.L. Mencken on religion. Amherst: Prometheus Books; 2002.

Sedation for Pediatric Gastrointestinal Procedures

18

Jenifer R. Lightdale

Abstract

Providing sedation to ensure safe and successful performance of gastrointestinal endoscopy is fundamental to the diagnosis and treatment of digestive diseases of childhood. Nevertheless, no single sedative or combined sedation regimen has yet been established as ideal. General anesthesia and moderate sedation remain the two primary options for endoscopy in both children and adults. General anesthesia requires the presence and expertise of an anesthesiologist or Certified Registered Nurse Anesthetist, and may involve inhalational or intravenous anesthetics. Moderate sedation, aimed at maintaining the child's ability to breathe spontaneously with intact protective airway reflexes, almost always utilizes intravenous sedatives and may be administered by a physician or nurse, in the absence of an anesthesiologist. In general, either moderate sedation or anesthesia is necessary for children to remain comfortable and cooperative during gastrointestinal procedures. However, complications attributed to the sedation occur more commonly than do technical complications, such as bleeding or perforation, from endoscopy. Improving efficacy and safety for the sedation of gastrointestinal procedures has, in turn, been a topic of great interest among pediatric gastroenterologists (GI) since its inception in the 1970s.

Keywords

Pediatric • Sedation • Gastrointestinal (GI) • Endoscopy • Endoscopic retrograde cholangiopancreatography (ERCP) • Endoscopic mucosal resection (EMR) • Submucosal dissection (ESD) • Magnetic resonance enterography (MRE) • Meperidine • Fentanyl • Diazepam • Midazolam • Reversal agents • Ketamine • Nitrous oxide • Propofol • Dexmedetomidine • Pulse oximetry • Precordial stethoscope • Capnography • North American Society of Pediatric Gastroenterology, Hepatology and Nutrition (NASPGHAN) • American Society of Anesthesiologists (ASA) • Body mass index (BMI) • Non-anesthesiologist-administered propofol sedation (NAAPS) • Nurse-administered propofol sedation (NAPS) • Bispectral index (BIS) • Patient-controlled sedation • American Society of Gastrointestinal Endoscopy (ASGE) • American Gastroenterological Association (AGA) • American College of Gastroenterology • Food and Drug Administration (FDA) • Computer-assisted personalized sedation (CAPS)

J.R. Lightdale, M.D., M.P.H. (✉)
Division of Pediatric Gastroenterology and Nutrition, Department of Pediatrics, UMass Memorial Children's Medical Center, 55 Lake Avenue North, Worcester, MA 01655, USA
e-mail: jenifer.lightdale@umassmemorial.org; Jenifer.Lightdale@childrens.harvard.edu

K.P. Mason (ed.), *Pediatric Sedation Outside of the Operating Room: A Multispecialty International Collaboration*,
DOI 10.1007/978-1-4939-1390-9_18, © Springer Science+Business Media New York 2015

Introduction

Providing sedation to ensure safe and successful performance of gastrointestinal endoscopy is fundamental to the diagnosis and treatment of digestive diseases of childhood. Nevertheless, no single sedative or combined sedation regimen has yet been established as ideal [1, 2]. General anesthesia and moderate sedation remain the two primary options for endoscopy in both children and adults [3, 4]. General anesthesia requires the presence and expertise of an anesthesiologist or Certified Registered Nurse Anesthetist, and may involve inhalational or intravenous anesthetics. Moderate sedation, aimed at maintaining the child's ability to breathe spontaneously with intact protective airway reflexes, almost always utilizes intravenous sedatives and may be administered by a physician or nurse, in the absence of an anesthesiologist.

In general, either moderate sedation or anesthesia is necessary for children to remain comfortable and cooperative during gastrointestinal procedures. However, complications attributed to the sedation occur more commonly than do technical complications, such as bleeding or perforation, from endoscopy [5–9]. Improving efficacy and safety for the sedation of gastrointestinal procedures has, in turn, been a topic of great interest among pediatric gastroenterologists (GI) since its inception in the 1970s [3, 5]. Predicting which patients are better candidates for general anesthesia rather than moderate sedation, in order to avoid complications related to undersedation, remains an elusive goal [10, 11].

In recent years, a considerable change in the landscape of sedation practices has occurred worldwide. As is often surprisingly under-recognized, endoscopists around the world vary greatly in determining which procedures warrant sedation, who should administer it, which drugs should be used, in what doses, and to what effect [12]. These variations appear to be based in part upon cultural norms and endoscopic training, but are also increasingly reflective of diverse institutional, third-party payor and governmental policies. A number of regions, especially those of developing countries, are increasingly reporting the use of sedation for pediatric GI procedures [13–15]. Although to a great extent this may reflect a greater interest in establishing patient satisfaction while prioritizing patient safety [16], cost has nonetheless remained a central consideration for healthcare systems worldwide [4].

Cost is particularly a concern in the more developed countries that use anesthesia procedures for endoscopy [4, 17]. While a 2005 survey of members of the North American Society of Pediatric Gastroenterology, Hepatology and Nutrition (NASPGHAN) reported wide practice variation in sedation delivery for pediatric procedures [18], current data suggests that anesthesiologist-administered propofol sedation has become the more common experience [1]. Additionally, although many gastrointestinal procedures may be performed in hospital operating rooms, this is almost always considered more costly and inconvenient from a scheduling perspective as compared with performing procedures in dedicated endoscopy units [18]. As such, there have been growing numbers of these procedures occurring outside of the operating room, and anesthesiologists are increasingly being asked to provide sedation in nontraditional settings [1].

This chapter will review the range of sedation approaches and techniques for pediatric gastrointestinal endoscopy, with a focus on method of delivery in addition to benefits, limitations, and pitfalls of various regimens. We will also explore trends in sedation for GI procedures in adult patients that may portend future trends for pediatrics. Both "traditional" and innovative sedative regimens for all ages will be discussed, as well as opportunities for minimizing patient risk, while optimizing procedural efficiency.

Goals and Optimal Levels of Sedation to Minimize Complications for Pediatric GI Procedures

The primary purpose of sedation for children undergoing upper and lower endoscopies is to perform procedures safely, with minimal emotional and physical discomfort. Secondary goals may include amnesia for the procedure, procedural efficiency, and cost-effectiveness.

Optimal levels of sedation may vary depending upon the procedure [19]. For upper endoscopy, a combination of topical local anesthetic with orally administered anxiolysis prior to intravenous line insertion has been shown to improve pediatric patient tolerance and satisfaction [20]. Important sedation goals of upper endoscopy are to avoid gagging and to increase patient cooperation. For colonoscopy, the goal of sedation is often to avoid visceral pain as the endoscope loops through the colon.

Many advanced therapeutic procedures require longer treatment times, and may be associated with increased patient discomfort caused by rotation of the endoscope, prolonged air insufflation, and heat-induced pain during application of coagulation. For example, endoscopic retrograde cholangiopancreatography (ERCP) is an invasive procedure increasingly performed in children that is highly associated with intra- and post-procedural patient pain and discomfort [21]. Along with other gastrointestinal procedures, such as endoscopic mucosal resection (EMR), submucosal dissection (ESD), and magnetic resonance enterography (MRE), immobility is particularly important to improve success and safety [22–24]. Achieving deep levels of sedation, with or without endotracheal intubation, may therefore be key to performing these procedures in both children and adults [25].

Table 18.1 Parameters that can be used to assess sedation regimens for pediatric endoscopy

Sedation measures
• Adverse events related to sedation
• Adverse events related to procedure
• Procedure completion rate
• Procedure times
• Patient recovery times
• Patient satisfaction
• Parent satisfaction
• Provider satisfaction
• Cost
• Speed of recovery of cognition
• Speed of recovery of locomotion

The risk of achieving moderate to light sedation must be balanced against the potential to become deeply sedated [26]. As previously mentioned, relative immobility may be the primary objective in some clinical situations, as opposed to achieving a particular level of sedation [3]. Neither societal nor regulatory guidelines to date have succeeded in reconciling assessments of depth of sedation with likelihood of immobility [27]. This may contribute to varying definitions of ideal patient outcomes of sedation.

Sedation outcomes during gastrointestinal procedures have been measured using a number of different benchmarks (Table 18.1). To some extent, the definitions of sedation success are defined by the individual sedation provider. Vargo et al. propose that the development and psychometric evaluations of both a patient satisfaction measure and a clinician satisfaction measure should be used together to provide a global measure of sedation effectiveness [28]. However, each clinician may differ in his/her assessment of procedural sedation. For example, nurses may be more inclined to rate procedural quality in terms of patient comfort, while physicians may be more likely to consider the technical success of the procedure [29]. The variation in outcomes has limited the potential to compare sedation regimens between published studies, and suggests that it may be preferable to design controlled trials that utilize independent observers and standardized scales [30, 31].

Pre-procedure Preparation and Patient Assessment

Sedation for pediatric gastrointestinal procedures should be tailored to a patient's physical status. This is most typically done in accordance with guidelines from the American Society of Anesthesiologists (ASA) [32–35]. Increased use of electronic medical records has improved the potential for providers to identify and manage patients with complex medical histories before procedures are performed [36]. In pediatrics and in adults, consideration of the patient's age, medical condition (ASA level), and developmental status is often critical. Data suggests that the smallest and youngest pediatric patients with the highest ASA classifications are at greatest risk for complications during gastrointestinal procedures [1, 37].

When working with children undergoing gastrointestinal procedures, it has been noted that personality and psychosocial development stages may vary widely and impact a child's response to sedatives, both in terms of the rapidity of effect and the depth achieved [38, 39]. Patients can be roughly divided into four different age groups: less than 6 months, greater than 6 months, school aged (4–11 years), and adolescents. Infants under 6 months of age may have little anxiety and tend to sedate easily. Infants greater than 6 months who have developed "stranger anxiety" may respond best if parents remain next to them during the induction of sedation. School-aged children manifest "concrete thinking" and may be surprisingly difficult to sedate, as they tend to conceal high anxiety levels [10]. Adolescents also may appear composed during pre-procedure preparations, and then become disinhibited and anxious after initial doses of sedatives.

Especially in school-aged children, a relaxed, detailed, and reassuring discussion of what to expect during the procedure, including the insertion of an intravenous catheter (IV) may decrease patient anxiety levels [39]. The use of topical anesthetics for IV insertion such as topical lidocaine cream, or oral anxiolytics, such as midazolam, may be warranted [20, 40]. Children who exhibit greater distress during the IV insertion have been shown to experience significantly greater distress and pain throughout the rest of the procedure [40].

Regardless of sedation regimens employed, it is essential to perform airway assessments at every step of the endoscopic process, beginning with the pre-procedure evaluation and concluding in the recovery room. All providers who care for children with gastrointestinal disorders should be schooled in airway assessment, including anesthesiologists, gastroenterologists, and nurses [3]. There is increasing interest among gastroenterologists in understanding how best to assess a patient airway using standardized methods, such as the Mallampati score [41] (Table 18.2, Fig. 18.1).

It also may be particularly important to identify patients at risk for obstructive sleep apnea, as they are considered at high risk for sedation-related complications [42]. Many such

Table 18.2 Mallampati score for airway assessment [41]

Mallampati score
• Class I: Uvula is completely visible
• Class II: Partially visible uvula
• Class III: Soft palate visible but not uvula
• Class IV: Hard palate visible only, not soft or uvula

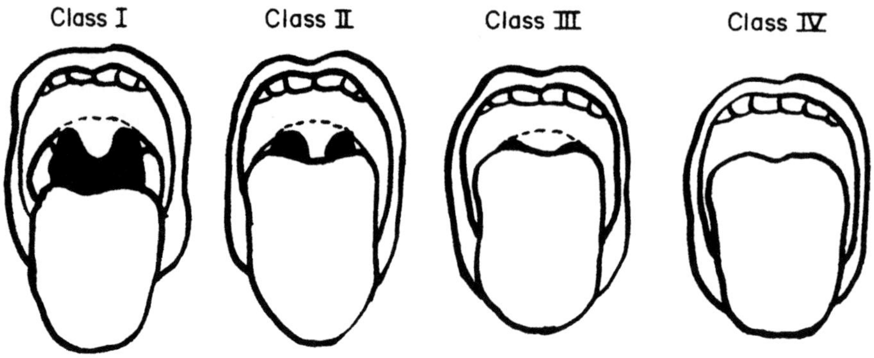

Fig. 18.1 Mallampati classification of pharyngeal structures (Reprinted with permission from Figs. 1 and 2, page 488. Samsoon GL, Young JR. Difficult tracheal intubation: A retrospective study. Anaesthesia. 1987 May;42(5):487-490.)

Table 18.3 STOP-BANG scoring model[a]

S	Snoring: Do you snore loudly (louder than talking or loud enough to be heard through closed doors)?	Yes	No
T	Tired: Do you often feel tired, fatigued, or sleepy during the daytime?	Yes	No
O	Observed: Has anyone observed you stop breathing during your sleep?	Yes	No
P	Blood pressure: Do you have or are you being treated for high blood pressure?	Yes	No
B	BMI: BMI more than 35 kg/m^2	Yes	No
A	Age: Age over 50 years	Yes	No
N	Neck circumference: Neck circumference greater than 40 cm	Yes	No
G	Gender: Male	Yes	No

Reprinted with permission from Mehta PP, Kochhar G, Kalra S, Maurer W, Tetzlaff J, Singh G, et al. Can a validated sleep apnea scoring system predict cardiopulmonary events using propofol sedation for routine EGD or colonoscopy? A prospective cohort study. Gastrointestinal Endoscopy. 9 November 2013 [Epub ahead of print]

[a]High risk of obstructive sleep apnea: yes to ≥3 questions; low risk of obstructive sleep apnea: yes to <3 questions

patients are obese, which along with hypertension, diabetes, and heart disease may function as independent risk factors for hypoxemia and other complications during gastrointestinal procedures [43]. “STOP-BANG” is a validated bedside screening instrument that has been used by anesthesiologists to predict the risk of unrecognized obstructive sleep apnea in adults [44, 45] (Table 18.3). In one prospective study, Cote et al. demonstrated that more than 40 % of adults presenting for screening colonoscopies at a US academic medical center meet criteria for a positive STOP-BANG score [44]. (Refer to Chaps. 4 and 7.) To date, there is no literature to support the validity of the STOP-BANG tool for pediatrics and modifications would need to be made to adapt it for use in children. Obese patients at risk for obstructive sleep apnea may specifically benefit from advanced monitoring or from tailored sedation regimens. One such regimen known as “Target-Controlled Infusions” (TCI) utilizes computers to achieve goal drug concentrations and modifies dosages using physiologic feedback [46, 47]. (Refer to Chap. 31.) It is unknown whether application of the STOP-BANG tool is appropriate in children. Nevertheless, it is an irrefutable fact that obesity and associated comorbidities, such as obstructive sleep apnea, are increasingly common in pediatric populations, and it may be reasonable to assume that obese children have similar risk profiles to obese adults.

Beyond airway assessment, a careful review of patient gastrointestinal conditions, past medical history, as well as prior experiences with sedation and procedures guides the triage of a child undergoing a gastrointestinal procedure. Some gastrointestinal disorders increase the riskiness of the procedure [48]. In particular, upper gastrointestinal bleeds, anatomic or physiologic obstruction of the upper gastrointestinal tract, recent ingestion of blood or food, and septic patients who need common bile duct clearance all will place a patient at higher risk for complications both from the procedures and from the sedation [49]. Premature infants as well as older children with body mass indices (BMI) for age greater than the 85th percentile may also be at increased risk [50, 51]. In addition, patients with significant liver disease or cirrhosis may be at increased risk of sedation-related complications, including respiratory compromise and delayed recovery, as well as psychometric deterioration and even encephalopathy, due to altered drug clearance [52, 53].

Patient Positioning

All patients undergoing diagnostic upper and lower endoscopic procedures with sedation should be placed in the left lateral decubitus position [35]. This is because patients who are placed in the supine position are more susceptible to pooling of secretions in oral pharynx, and risk upper airway obstruction or laryngospasm. Patients undergoing ERCP may require a prone or prone-oblique position [48]. Obviously, airway monitoring and management is more challenging for patients in prone positions and they may require advanced monitoring.

Common IV Sedation Regimens for Pediatric Gastrointestinal Procedures

Table 18.4 lists commonly used sedative regimens for pediatric gastrointestinal procedures. In general, the most common moderate sedation regimens used for pediatric endoscopy combine a narcotic analgesic (e.g., meperidine or fentanyl) with a benzodiazepine (e.g., diazepam or midazolam) [18]. A brief review of the important pharmacokinetic, pharmacodynamic, and clinical properties of those medications most commonly used for GI sedation, directed to the GI concerns, will follow. Chapter 9: *Pharmacology and Clinical Application of Sedatives, Analgesics, and Adjuncts* provides a more thorough and detailed review of all sedative agents and adjuncts.

Fentanyl

As a fat-soluble narcotic that rapidly penetrates the blood–brain barrier, fentanyl is considerably more potent and fast acting than both morphine and meperidine. Its onset of action is about 30 s after IV administration, and its opioid effects last about 30–45 min. Intravenous fentanyl should always be administered slowly, as it has been associated with the dangerous side effects of chest wall and glottic rigidity after rapid administration [54].

Fentanyl is variably metabolized by the liver, especially in young children. Delayed fentanyl excretion has been reported in neonates with compromised hepatic blood flow [55].

Table 18.4 Recommendations for dosages of drugs commonly used for IV sedation for pediatric gastrointestinal procedures*

Drug	Route	Maximum dose (mg/kg)	Time to onset (min)	Duration of action (min)
Benzodiazepines				
Diazepam	IV	0.1–0.3	1–3	15–30
	Rectal	0.2–0.3	2–10	15–30
Midazolam	Oral	0.5–0.75	15–30	60–90
	IV	0.05–0.15	2–3	45–60
	Rectal	0.5–0.75	10–30	60–90
Opioids				
Meperidine	IV	1–3	<5	120–240
	IM	1–3	10–15	120–180
Fentanyl	IV	0.001–0.005 (1–5 μg/kg in 0.5–1.0 μg/kg increments)	2–3	30–60
Ketamine	IV	1–3	1	15–60
	IM	2–10	3–5	15–150

*This table reflects common dosings and sedation considerations but must be interpreted and applied with caution. The table reflects the views of the author

Several studies have suggested that fentanyl may not represent an ideal sedative for infants. In particular, it has been associated with significant apnea in infants less than 3 months of age [56]. These unique pharmacokinetics of fentanyl are certainly relevant to the performance of pediatric endoscopy. In particular, fentanyl's termination of action occurs with redistribution of drug metabolites from the plasma, rather than from metabolism, causing its potential respiratory depressive effects to outlast its opioid effects. Fentanyl should be administered to children in small increments, allowing for a minimum of several minutes between doses.

Midazolam

Midazolam is a benzodiazepine that is 3–6 times more potent than diazepam. It may be administered by many routes: IV, oral, rectal, intramuscular, and intranasal. When administered IV, the onset of action is 1–5 min, with peak effect achieved at 30 min to 1 h. Several early pharmacokinetic studies have bolstered evidence that midazolam may be metabolized and excreted more rapidly in children than adults [20, 57, 58]. Midazolam is relatively unique among benzodiazepines in that its clearance appears to be dose-related, with increased clearance at escalating dosage [59]. Pediatric gastroenterologists have reported the need to require larger weight-adjusted doses for pediatric versus adult patients in order to achieve similar doses and duration of sedation [60].

Reversal Agents for Narcotics and Benzodiazepines

Reversal agents are available only for benzodiazepines and narcotics. Table 18.5 lists reversal agents and their recommended dosages for children. Although reversal agents have been used in adults to expedite recovery, it is important to recognize that there may be resedation as the effect of sedative outlasts that of the reversal agent [33]. Most endoscopy and pediatric sedation guidelines stipulate that patients who receive a dose of a reversal agent should be monitored for an extended period and administered repeat doses if necessary [35, 61].

Ketamine

Ketamine is a dissociative agent that largely spares upper airway muscular tone and laryngeal reflexes, and may represent an alternative to narcotics and benzodiazepines for sedating children for gastrointestinal procedures [62–66].

Table 18.5 Reversal agents for benzodiazepines and opioids and recommended dosages*

Drug	Class	Route	Dose (mg/kg)	Time to onset (min) action (min)	Duration of antagonist
Flumazenil	Benzodiazepines	IV (max 3 mg/h)	0.01	1–2	<60
Naloxone	Narcotics	IV/IM	0.1	2–5	20–60

*This table reflects common dosings and sedation considerations but must be interpreted and applied with caution. The table reflects the views of the author

Ketamine may also be useful for sedating patients who are opioid tolerant [67]. As a derivative of phencyclidine, ketamine binds to opiate receptors, and rapidly induces a trance-like cataleptic condition with significant analgesia. Routes of administration include oral or rectal, although intravenous or intramuscular is a more common route of administration during endoscopy.

Unlike most sedatives, ketamine is almost always effective at significantly immobilizing patients with minimal cardiac and respiratory effects, and is considered to have a broad margin of safety. It should be used with caution in patients less than 3 months of age, as well as those with histories of airway instability, tracheal abnormalities, active pulmonary disease, cardiovascular disease, head injury, central nervous system masses, hydrocephalus, porphyria, and thyroid disease [68–70].

Ketamine is considered by many to be contraindicated in patients with a history of psychosis [69, 70]. To date, its main drawback has been its association with hallucinogenic emergence reactions in some children [71, 72]. Its administration may be partnered with that of a short-acting benzodiazepine, such as midazolam. Brecelj et al. demonstrated in a single-blind randomized controlled trial that premedication with 0.1 mg of midazolam IV (2.5 mg maximum dose midazolam) prior to ketamine may reduce the frequency of emergence reactions [73]. However, outcomes of this approach have not been consistent, and some data suggest that midazolam may actually increase agitation in postpubertal children [74, 75]. Ketamine has also been recently reported to be successfully combined with other agents, including analgesics, such as fentanyl and tramadol [76], remifentanil [77], and even dexmedetomidine [78], to provide excellent regimens for a variety of endoscopic procedures.

Ketamine has been associated with increased airway secretions and an increased incidence of postoperative nausea and vomiting. During upper endoscopy, ketamine has been associated with a potential for laryngospasm [30, 63, 79]. Attempts to minimize this risk by administering anticholinergics may not be successful. Indeed, matched case–control analysis of 8,282 ketamine procedures in the emergency department revealed no association between age, dose, procedure, medical status, route of delivery, and the administration of anticholinergics with the occurrence of laryngospasm [64].

Nevertheless, the question remains whether ketamine is superior enough to replace the traditional moderate sedation regimens for pediatric endoscopy (opioids and benzodiazepines). A retrospective review of 402 endoscopic procedures with different sedation combinations reported that a combination of midazolam and ketamine was both safe and superior (by physician report) to such traditional sedation regimens [79]. However, more recent data collected by independent observers suggests that ketamine is associated with a comparably higher rate of laryngospasm and similar incidence of patient movement and need for restraint than do those sedated with midazolam and fentanyl [30]. These findings may substantiate those who have suggested that ketamine may be most appropriately used for liver biopsy, a very brief procedure with minimal upper airway stimulation [69].

Nitrous Oxide

Nitrous oxide is an inhalational gaseous mixture that has analgesic, sedative, and amnestic properties. It is generally prepared as 50 % nitrous oxide in oxygen, and is a short-acting agent with rapid onset of action (3–5 min) and short duration of effects after withdrawal (3–5 min). Several studies have suggested that nitrous oxide may provide rapid and effective sedation for children undergoing gastrointestinal procedures, without inducing deep sedation [80, 81]. Nitrous oxide may be adequate for procedures that do not induce pain, such as upper gastrointestinal endoscopy and flexible sigmoidoscopy. Comparisons of nitrous oxide with opioid and benzodiazepine regimens for more uncomfortable procedures have had conflicting results: Forbes et al. have found that nitrous oxide may not provide enough analgesia for colonoscopy [81], while Mcculloch et al. have reported that nitrous oxide is as effective as IV midazolam and pethidine at relieving pain and bloating, while minimizing cardiopulmonary risks in elderly patients [82].

Propofol

Propofol is an ultra-short-acting anesthetic that features both a rapid onset of action and a short recovery time. It can be used to induce and maintain a spectrum of sedation levels, as well as to achieve anesthesia. Investigation with Functional Near-Infrared Spectroscopy (fNIRS) has shown that drug-related effects on cerebral hemodynamic activity are dose dependent, with decreased oxygenation of the dorsolateral prefrontal cortex during bolus infusions and deeper levels of sedation [83]. Studies of propofol in healthy volunteers have found that sedation with propofol alone allows esophageal intubation at the beginning of a procedure, and that recovery from both induced loss of consciousness and respiratory compromise occurs within 3–4 min of stopping an infusion [84].

Propofol may be administered during pediatric endoscopy either as a total intravenous anesthetic or in combination with other sedatives, including inhalational agents [24, 85]. Propofol, alone or in combination with other agents, has been shown in multiple studies to be highly effective at inducing sedation in children who are undergoing both upper and lower endoscopy, and provides excellent amnesia for the procedure [86–90]. Several recent studies have also suggested it may be a preferable agent in patients with significant liver disease or cirrhosis [52, 53].

Currently, many pediatric gastroenterologists, both in the United States and abroad, use anesthesiologist-administered propofol as a primary means of sedation [1]. This trend has paralleled the performance of pediatric GI procedures in dedicated endoscopy units as a means of decreasing the need for operating room time [89, 91, 92]. Although the use of propofol by anesthesiologists in dedicated endoscopy units may offer scheduling advantages, it is not clear that this practice changes day-to-day efficiency. Indeed, while children who receive propofol have shorter induction times than children who received midazolam and fentanyl, use of propofol compared with more traditional intravenous regimens has not been shown to improve unit throughput times [85].

A main pharmacologic disadvantage of propofol is its relatively narrow therapeutic range. Pharmacokinetic studies of children who received propofol demonstrate that average total propofol doses per kilogram of body weight to achieve targeted plasma propofol concentrations are higher in younger children [93, 94]. Propofol also has a high propensity to cause hypotension. One recent study has suggested that use of diluted propofol may significantly reduce sedation-related hypotension and other adverse events, without affecting its potential to provide deep sedation [95].

Propofol can be given alone or in combination with other sedatives. Elitsur et al. reviewed propofol sedation for endoscopic procedures in children and found that a lower propofol dosage was needed when propofol was given in combination with midazolam and fentanyl than when propofol was given alone [96]. Propofol was also found to confer amnestic effects, independently of those conferred by midazolam.

Titrating propofol to achieve sedation without inducing general anesthesia requires clinical expertise and, even when administered by anesthesiologists, carries the risk of inducing anesthesia rather than sedation. Kaddu et al. reported transient apnea in 20 % of pediatric patients receiving anesthesiologist-administered propofol for upper endoscopy [89]. A retrospective review of 176 children in Thailand, 175 of whom received propofol delivered by anesthesia personnel or an anesthesiologists, reported one patient who required an unanticipated endotracheal intubation [97]. Slow (not rapid) administration of propofol (over 3 min) may confer less respiratory depression [98].

Non-anesthesiologist-Administered Propofol Sedation

Non-anesthesiologist-administered propofol sedation (NAAPS) is an acronym used to describe the administration of propofol under the direction of a physician by an appropriately qualified registered nurse or physician who has not been trained as an anesthesiologist [99–101]. Multiple NAAPS protocols have been developed, and all have stressed a curriculum of drug knowledge, as well as specific practical skills in airway management [101, 102]. Nurse-administered propofol sedation (NAPS) involves administration of propofol by dedicated nurses in the endoscopy unit, and has been described as successful by groups in many countries across the world, after implementation of special training programs [103].

Although there is little reported data of either NAAPS in children, one prospective study described a protocol of 1–2 mg/kg of propofol induction dose followed by 0.5–1.0 mg/kg supplements that was administered by pediatric residents [104]. The sedation providers had been specifically trained in cardiopulmonary resuscitation via a 4-week training period during which they had performed bag-mask ventilation and endotracheal intubation a minimum of 20 times. Patients were limited to ASA I and ASA II. Those with any indication of airway obstruction (existing or potential), respiratory disease, seizures, or risk of aspiration were excluded. Overall there was a 0.7 % (6/811) incidence of positive pressure ventilation, brief oxygen desaturation in 12 %, and no occurrence of endotracheal intubation. Although this study was too small to adequately demonstrate the safety of NAAPS in children, it does substantiate the need for training and airway management skills.

NAAPS has been a controversial topic since its inception [105]. Generally speaking, gastroenterologists and their representative medical societies across the United States and Europe have repeatedly noted that in adults the administration of propofol and standard sedation regimens have been found to be comparable with respect to efficacy and reported rates of complications [106–108]. Nevertheless, a guideline

Table 18.6 Continuum of depth of sedation. Definition of general anesthesia and levels of sedation/analgesia[a,*]

	Minimal sedation anxiolysis	Moderate sedation/analgesia ("conscious sedation")	Deep sedation/analgesia	General anesthesia
Responsiveness	Normal response to verbal stimulation	Purposeful[b] response to verbal or tactile stimulation	Purposeful[b] response following repeated or painful stimulation	Unarousable even with painful stimulus
Airway	Unaffected	No intervention required	Intervention may be required	Intervention often required
Spontaneous ventilation	Unaffected	Adequate	May be inadequate	Frequently inadequate
Cardiovascular function	Unaffected	Usually maintained	Usually maintained	May be impaired

Reprinted with permission of the American Society of Anesthesiologists from Committee of Origin: Quality Management and Departmental Administration (Approved by the ASA House of Delegates on October 27, 2004, and amended on October 21, 2009) http://www.asahq.org/For-Members/Standards-Guidelines-and-Statements.aspx

[a]Monitored anesthesia care does not describe the continuum of depth of sedation, rather it describes "a specific anesthesia service in which an anesthesiologist has been requested to participate in the care of a patient undergoing a diagnostic or therapeutic procedure"

[b]Reflex withdrawal from a painful stimulus is NOT considered a purposeful response

[*]Rescue of a patient from a deeper level of sedation than intended is an intervention by a practitioner proficient in airway management and advanced life support. The qualified practitioner corrects adverse physiologic consequences of the deeper-than-intended level of sedation (such as hypoventilation, hypoxia, and hypotension) and returns the patient to the originally intended level of sedation. It is not appropriate to continue the procedure at an unintended level of sedation

in 2010 from the Center for Medicare and Medicaid Services (CMS) restricted the administration of deep sedation with propofol, in particular, without the presence of a clinician trained in anesthesia [109]. A major factor in this policy decision was the fact that non-anesthesiologists, such as gastroenterologists, are not specifically trained in the comprehensive skills required to care for patients along the entire continuum of sedation (Table 18.6). In 2011, 21 European National Societies of Anesthesia published a consensus statement that upheld the CMS statement that propofol should be administered only by those trained in the administration of general anesthesia [110]. At this time, propofol in children is recognized to have high potential to induce respiratory depression and cardiovascular instability and is essentially universally administered by anesthesiologists for pediatric endoscopy [1, 2].

Dexmedetomidine

Dexmedetomidine is a highly selective alpha2-adrenoreceptor agonist with sedative, analgesic, and antisialagogue effects. In many ways, the drug profile of dexmedetomidine suggests it may be a good drug for pediatric endoscopic sedation, as it offers hemodynamic stability, and has minimal effects on respiration and cognitive function. Nevertheless, to date there has been little to no investigation of the efficacy, safety, or cost of this sedative for gastrointestinal procedures. A small prospective study used independent observers to evaluate the sedation of 50 patients in terms of vital signs, as well as patient and endoscopist satisfaction during upper endoscopy with either dexmedetomidine or midazolam [111]. Patients were not randomized, and only the independent observer was blinded, which limited the study's conclusions. The results suggested that dexmedetomidine was superior as a sole sedation agent to midazolam. Another recent abstract publication prospectively randomized 231 adults to receive either propofol or dexmedetomidine and found both regimens comparably safe [112]. Future studies may help to identify clinical situations where use of dexmedetomidine may be preferable during endoscopic sedation.

Training in Sedation Administration

Regardless of sedative regimen used, performance of sedated gastrointestinal endoscopy in children requires a carefully coordinated team of physicians and nurses [35, 113]. Optimization of team performance may be enhanced through routine drills that involve high fidelity simulation, and allow a chance for teams to practice high-stakes patient management in a safe environment [114]. Generally speaking, GI clinicians find simulation to be enjoyable, valuable, and realistic to their practice. A multisociety sedation curriculum for gastrointestinal endoscopy was published in 2012 and recognizes the basic competencies in knowledge and performance that must be achieved by non-anesthesiology trainees [35]. Anesthesiologists who are involved with the administration of sedation for gastrointestinal procedures can benefit from developing specific skill sets, as well as a good understanding of the range and goals of endoscopic procedures [115–117].

Monitoring of Children Undergoing Endoscopic Procedures with Sedation

Generally speaking, the emphasis of patient monitoring during GI procedures is on ventilation—either by visual assessment or from physiologic monitors (pulse oximetry, precordial stethoscope, capnography). All team members need to work together to identify suboptimal ventilation and to employ appropriate timely interventions.

Pulse Oximetry

Although visual assessments are considered to be as important as electronic monitoring for ensuring patient safety, oxygen desaturation represents a particularly objective means of detecting poor respiratory effort in sedated children undergoing gastrointestinal procedures. (Refer to Chap. 2.) If a provider fails to detect suboptimal ventilation by clinical assessment, he/she will often intervene to stimulate patient respiration if a pulse oximeter detects minor desaturation. On the other hand, it is important to recognize that oxygen desaturation is a relatively late sign of suboptimal ventilation [50]. Furthermore, while supplemental oxygen during upper GI endoscopy has been shown to decrease the incidence of desaturation and increase the likelihood of achieving 100 % arterial oxygen saturation [118], it is critical to understand that even patients with supplemental oxygen may be poorly ventilating [3].

Capnography

The dilemma posed by relying on pulse oximetry for monitoring children during endoscopy is that patients may be well saturated despite having significant carbon dioxide retention. In the past decade, improved compact microstream capnographs with aspiration flow technology have allowed the accurate real-time graphic display of ventilatory waveforms in non-intubated patients [119]. (Refer to Chap. 6.) Employing capnography in the pediatric endoscopy setting may reveal that abnormal ventilation is occurring during procedures in children at rates higher than expected [120]. The ASA in 2009 released a statement entitled *Statement on Respiratory Monitoring During Endoscopic Procedures*, which suggests that capnography "be considered" [121]. (Refer to Chap. 2.)

One randomized controlled trial of children undergoing endoscopic procedures demonstrated capnography to be more effective than direct visualization at identifying patient hypoventilation [120]. Endoscopy staff documented poor ventilation in three percent of all procedures and no apnea, while capnography indicated alveolar hypoventilation in more than half and apnea during a quarter of procedures. Integrating capnography into patient monitoring protocols both in adult and pediatric endoscopy settings may ultimately improve the safety of non-intubated patients receiving moderate sedation [50]. Recent multisociety guidelines published by the American Gastroenterological Association (AGA) Institute, the American Society of Gastrointestinal Endoscopy (ASGE), and the American College of Gastroenterology suggest that capnography may become a standard for patient monitoring [35]. The ASA recommends capnography for moderate sedation [121].

Bispectral Index Monitoring

Bispectral index (BIS) monitoring is an EEG-based method of assessing a patient's level of consciousness using a complex algorithm to generate a weighted index [122]. (Refer to Chap. 6.) In two studies of NAPS for colonoscopy in adults, BIS monitoring was not found to predict adverse respiratory events [123, 124]. However, EEG-based systems used to guide propofol administration during ERCP have been shown to result in lower propofol doses [122], as well as improved patient tolerance and shorter recovery times [125, 126]. The use of EEG monitoring has been investigated in children undergoing procedures in the emergency department and critical care settings, and may have a role in the future for delivery of sedation for pediatric endoscopy [127–129].

Future Sedation Strategies for Endoscopy in Children

Patient-controlled sedation and analgesia (PCS) represents a sedation strategy that has been reported in adults with inhalational anesthetics and propofol. A randomized multicenter trial recently compared the feasibility and effectiveness of PCS with inhaled methoxyflurane to the traditional regimens of clinician-administered midazolam and fentanyl [130]. In this strategy, the drug administration with PCS is essentially controlled by the patient, via frequency and depth of inhalation. The inhaled methoxyflurane had a rapid onset of action (noted after 3–6 breaths), with 3 mL of solution providing analgesic effect for approximately 30 min.

In a study of PCS with propofol, Kulling et al. randomized 150 adults to three sedation arms: PCS with propofol/alfentanil (Group I), continuous propofol/alfentanil infusion (Group II), and nurse-administered midazolam/meperidine (Group III) [131]. Group I exhibited a high degree of patient satisfaction and more complete recovery at 45 min when compared with conventional sedation and analgesia. In a similar study, Ng et al. randomized 88 patients undergoing colonoscopy to PCS with propofol alone or midazolam alone [132]. Patients receiving propofol PCS exhibited significantly shorter mean recovery times (43 min versus 61 min) and improved comfort. A pilot study of PCS for ERCP used a software system to deliver a targeted plasma propofol concentration; 80 % of patients received safe and fully effective sedation [133]. There are a number of "smart infusion" strategies, which combined with developing technologies may also improve the potential for safe and successful sedation for pediatric endoscopy in the foreseeable future [47, 100, 132, 134]. For example, computer-assisted personalized sedation (CAPS) is a sedation strategy that utilizes multiple physiologic feedback parameters including electrocardiography, capnography, and automated response monitoring to target moderate levels of sedation during procedures by periodically assessing patient responses to otic and vibratory stimuli [134]. (Refer to Chap. 31.) CAPS introduces a computer-generated voice to demand (via headphones) that the patient press a button at regular intervals, while at the same time a hand piece with a built-in vibrator delivers the tactile stimulus. If no response is elicited, the verbal and tactile stimuli are increased in intensity until the patient responds. If the patient still does not respond, the patient is considered oversedated and no further drug is administered. In one small multicenter open label trial, Pambianco and colleagues demonstrated the feasibility of CAPS in 48 patients undergoing colonoscopy, leading the investigators to suggest that CAPS may provide endoscopists with a safe and effective means to deliver propofol without anesthesiologist assistance [134].

One specific example of a CAPS system that was recently approved by the FDA is the SEDASYS® system. SEDASYS® is designed to enable physician-led teams to administer minimal-to-moderate propofol sedation by integrating patient monitoring and drug delivery. (Refer to Chaps. 31 and 38.) The FDA has indicated the SEDASYS® system can be used for the initiation and maintenance of minimal-to-moderate sedation in ASA physical status I and II patients ≥18 years old undergoing colonoscopy and upper endoscopic procedures, but should only be offered in facilities where an anesthesia professional is immediately available to the user for assistance or consultation as needed. To date, there are no pediatric studies demonstrating feasibility or effectiveness of SEDASYS® in children. Nevertheless, it represents an important intersection of improving care through technology and a scientific understanding of the physiology of sedation.

Conclusion

In conclusion, sedation for pediatric endoscopy is currently considered integral to the successful performance of the procedure. Best practices for sedating children for gastrointestinal endoscopy involve tailoring the regimen in consideration of both patient and procedural factors. While maintaining patient safety during pediatric gastrointestinal procedures remains paramount, it is also becoming increasingly important to consider efficiency and costs when choosing location and type of sedation. In turn, both pediatric endoscopists and anesthesiologists should work together to assess benefits and risks associated with various sedation regimens if they are to optimize the performance of gastrointestinal endoscopy in children.

Case Studies

Case 1

A 5-year-old, 17 kg previously healthy child (ASA I) with new onset weight loss of 2 kg, is determined to have elevated serological tests consistent with celiac disease. She is scheduled to undergo upper endoscopy with biopsies in a dedicated endoscopy unit, with sedation to be administered by a nurse anesthetist, and supervised by an anesthesiologist. After arriving at the unit on the day of the procedure, the patient is brought awake and alert to the procedure room accompanied by her parents, the nurse anesthetist, the staff anesthesiologist, a circulating nurse, and the gastroenterologist. The lights are dimmed and sevoflurane is administered. Once the patient becomes sleepy, the parents are escorted to a waiting area and an intravenous line is established in the right antecubital vein by the anesthesiologist, while the nurse anesthetist provides airway management and administers the inhalational agent. Subsequently, the sevoflurane is discontinued and IV propofol is administered. The patient is placed in the left lateral decubitus position, and a dual-purpose nasal cannula is placed in the nares to allow a baseline 2 L NCO_2 to be administered and capnography to be monitored. Once the patient is determined to be moderately to deeply sedated, the anesthesiologist leaves the room to prepare the next patient, and the procedure begins with endoscopic intubation of the esophagus. The endoscope is then advanced to the third part of the duodenum, where multiple tissue biopsies are obtained. The procedure takes a total of 6 min. After the endoscope is withdrawn, the propofol is discontinued by the nurse anesthetist and the patient is brought immediately to a post-anesthesia care area for recovery.

Considerations

Performance of pediatric endoscopic procedures with deep sedation in dedicated endoscopy units is becoming a standard in many institutions, and is generally safe [135]. However, as illustrated by this case, it may require significant staffing considerations. If more than one procedure room will be operating at the same time, it may

(continued)

be preferable to use one supervising anesthesiologist and multiple physician extenders. Recovery units must also be staffed appropriately to monitor patients who are emerging from deep levels of sedation.

This case also illustrates the need to tailor the level of sedation achieved and the regimen used appropriately to the procedure. In this case, the patient is healthy and has no known risk factors for airway compromise. The planned procedure of diagnostic upper endoscopy with biopsies is brief and not painful. The patient is young and at risk for distress with placement of an intravenous line. If she is allowed to stay with her parents until she is sedated, and if line placement is reserved until after her parents leave the room, she is able to remain calm. It may also be helpful to create a calming environment by dimming the lights, as well as playing quiet music. By opting to perform the sedation without endotracheal intubation, the anesthesiologists have essentially committed to maintaining a level of sedation that is deep enough to allow the procedure, while maintaining spontaneous patient ventilation. In turn, unit throughput efficiency is not compromised by a sedative regimen that involves long induction and recovery periods. Use of dual-purpose nasal cannula allows for the administration of supplemental oxygen, as well as electronic monitoring of ventilation in the absence of endotracheal intubation.

Case 2

A 17-year-old male with known ulcerative colitis presents to the emergency room with frequent bloody stools despite recent treatment with IV steroids for a flare of his inflammatory bowel disease. A decision is made to readmit and restage his colitis by performing colonoscopy the following day prior to pursuing further medical therapy, such as the use of cyclosporine as a rescue agent. The medical team opts to schedule the urgent procedure in a dedicated procedure unit and plans to use endoscopist-administered moderate sedation. Upon admission to the floor, the patient undergoes an intravenous line placement and is administered maintenance fluids. He receives a bowel preparation by mouth up until midnight and then is maintained NPO until the time of the procedure. Once in the endoscopy unit, the patient is brought to the procedure room by two nurses and the endoscopist. One nurse stays at the head and monitors the airway. The second acts as circulator and documents medications. Serial doses of midazolam and fentanyl are administered by protocol using the established intravenous line until the patient is determined to be comfortable and responding to light tactile stimulation. At that point, he is encouraged to turn on his side in the left lateral decubitus position and lidocaine jelly is administered to the anal canal. The endoscope is inserted into the anus, where severe mucosal inflammatory disease is noted. The endoscope is then advanced past the splenic flexure, where the mucosa abruptly becomes more normal appearing, and all the way to the cecum. The procedure takes a total of 25 min. Throughout, the patient is occasionally administered further doses of fentanyl and midazolam, and his airway is continually monitored. In addition, pulse oximetry readings and capnograms are monitored and recorded. Evidence of hypoventilation on capnograms is managed by rubbing the patient's back and verbally encouraging him to take deep breaths. Upon withdrawal of the endoscope, the patient is brought to the recovery area.

Considerations

In most institutions, gastroenterology teams may find it more efficient and preferable to schedule urgent procedures in a dedicated endoscopy unit with endoscopist-administered moderate sedation [136]. Older children and teenagers may be particularly appropriate candidates for this option. In this case, the patient sedated easily and safely with a typical regimen of midazolam and fentanyl. Midazolam is a highly potent benzodiazepine with water-soluble properties that greatly diminishes the pain associated with intravenous administration. It also has a short beta elimination half-life, which is particularly advantageous for brief procedures.

One of midazolam's most desirable side effects is its retrograde and anterograde amnesia for procedures. According to the Versed brand package insert (Roche laboratories), 71 % of patients sedated with midazolam were shown to have no recall of introduction of the endoscope, and 82 % had no recall of withdrawal of the endoscope. This drug generally produces a calm, compliant patient who is receptive to nonthreatening procedures. The opioid fentanyl (Sublimaze) is approximately 100 times more potent than morphine due to a high degree of fat solubility that allows rapid penetration of the blood–brain barrier. The resulting onset of opioid effect is therefore much faster for fentanyl than for meperidine (onset of action is 30 s–5 min versus 5–10 min).

Of course, sedatives likely instigate desaturation either by central respiratory depression with resulting hypoxemia and CO_2 retention or by blunting ventilatory reflexes that are driven by hypercarbia. In addition,

(continued)

looping of the colonoscope has been associated with respiratory splinting and transient hypoxemia. As this case illustrates, it is routine to administer supplemental oxygen by intranasal cannulation, at a generally recommended rate of 2 L per minute. This approach is considered low cost and high benefit, but does not negate the need for ventilatory monitoring for desaturation. As is illustrated by this case, monitoring with capnography may reveal transient periods of suboptimal ventilation, which can be treated with minimal but effective interventions. A randomized controlled trial in pediatric patients suggests transient apnea and hypoventilation may not be recognized by clinical staff, despite a dedicated airway nurse, but may be detected by patient monitoring that uses capnography [137]. Acting on capnographic evidence of suboptimal ventilation may lead to decreased incidence of arterial oxygen desaturation.

This case also illustrates that timely performance of endoscopy can be invaluable at guiding therapy. The limited extent of disease detected during this procedure may be amenable to medical therapy, and can allow the team to defer surgical options.

Case 3

A 2-year-old 10 kg male with nonspecific atypical facial features, pervasive developmental delay, and feeding difficulties is referred to the gastroenterology consult service for percutaneous endoscopic gastrostomy (PEG) placement. The procedure is planned for general anesthesia to be administered by the anesthesiology team in the endoscopy unit. The patient has no unifying diagnosis, but is otherwise medically stable, and a standardized assessment by the unit nursing team performed via telephone confirms the scheduling gastroenterologist's assessment that he is an ASA II patient, eligible to have the procedure performed in the unit. However, on the day of the procedure, a focused physical exam suggests his airway is best scored as Mallampati IV, with neither his soft palate nor his uvula visible when he is in a sitting position with his mouth open. A decision is made to reschedule the case for the main operating room the following day.

Considerations

Decisions around procedural location and type should be tailored to the patient and the procedure. Although there has been no formal study to help guide the decisions of which patients are safe for deep sedation or general anesthesia in the endoscopy unit, the American Society of Anesthesiologists' (ASA) classification scheme may be of use in institutional policies. Generally speaking, ASA I and II patients are considered good candidates for moderate sedation, and are generally considered safe for the endoscopy unit. ASA III patients with a severe systemic disease should be evaluated carefully, but have been described to be safe for sedation in the endoscopy suite, rather than an operating room [91]. ASA IV and V patients with either a severe systemic disease that is a threat to their life or who are moribund, respectively, should receive general anesthesia in an operating room setting. Nevertheless, this case illustrates the limitations of relying on ASA alone in guiding the decision for procedural location. Indeed, as with deciding appropriate levels and types of sedation, it is important to recognize that the ASA classification system provides crude patient categories to serve a multidisciplinary purpose, and does not adequately capture complex clinical scenarios.

Instead, all medical societies of gastroenterology, endoscopy, and anesthesia emphasize in their guidelines that a careful history must be obtained before sedation is administered. Much of this history can be acquired in a phone call prior to the procedure [138] or by reviewing the medical chart [36]. Inquiries must include a history of all current medications, untoward or allergic reactions, alcohol or other substance abuse, chronic use of sedatives or analgesics, and past endoscopic experiences. Risk assessments will also include the patient's age, comorbid illnesses or organ dysfunction, and obesity. A history of cardiopulmonary disease, neurological concerns, liver disease, and surgical history, as well any condition that might affect access to the patient's airway, should also be obtained. Had this assessment identified any other risk factors, presumably this patient would have triaged to the main operating room.

As this case also illustrates, risk factors were not identified until a focused physical exam prior to the procedure revealed the patient to have a difficult airway. A relevant physical exam to sedation plans involves careful evaluation of the heart, circulation, lungs, head, neck, and airway. Patients with limited neck extension, decreased hyoid-mental distance, nonvisible uvula, mandibular disease, or other disorders of the head and neck may be difficult to intubate in an unlikely emergency. In terms of an airway assessment, the standardized Mallampati score may be of use for identifying patients at high risk for airway issues. Anesthesiology teams may better serve these patients in the main operating room, where resources, such as fiberoptic laryngoscopes and anesthesiology staff backup, are more readily available.

References

1. van Beek EJ, Leroy PL. Safe and effective procedural sedation for gastrointestinal endoscopy in children. J Pediatr Gastroenterol Nutr. 2012;54(2):171–85.
2. Friedt M, Welsch S. An update on pediatric endoscopy. Eur J Med Res. 2013;18(1):24.
3. Lightdale JR. Sedation for pediatric endoscopy. Tech Gastrointest Endosc. 2013;15(1):3–8.
4. Liu H, Waxman DA, Main R, Mattke S. Utilization of anesthesia services during outpatient endoscopies and colonoscopies and associated spending in 2003-2009. JAMA. 2012;307(11):1178–84.
5. Ament ME, Christie DL. Upper gastrointestinal fiberoptic endoscopy in pediatric patients. Gastroenterology. 1977;72(6):1244–8.
6. Gilger MA, Jeiven SD, Barrish JO, McCarroll LR. Oxygen desaturation and cardiac arrhythmias in children during esophagogastroduodenoscopy using conscious sedation. Gastrointest Endosc. 1993;39(3):392–5.
7. Mamula P, Markowitz JE, Neiswender K, Zimmerman A, Wood S, Garofolo M, et al. Safety of intravenous midazolam and fentanyl for pediatric GI endoscopy: prospective study of 1578 endoscopies. Gastrointest Endosc. 2007;65(2):203–10.
8. Choi CH. Safety and prevention of complications in endoscopic sedation. Dig Dis Sci. 2012;57(7):1745–7.
9. Dietrich CG, Kottmann T, Diedrich A, Drouven FM. Sedation-associated complications in endoscopy are not reduced significantly by implementation of the German S-3-guideline and occur in a severe manner only in patients with ASA class III and higher. Scand J Gastroenterol. 2013;48(9):1082–7.
10. Lightdale JR, Valim C, Mahoney LB, Sharon W, DiNardo J, Goldmann DA. Agitation during procedural sedation and analgesia in children. Clin Pediatr (Phila). 2010;49(1):35–42.
11. Hazeldine S, Fritschi L, Forbes G. Predicting patient tolerance of endoscopy with conscious sedation. Scand J Gastroenterol. 2010;45(10):1248–54.
12. Amornyotin S. Sedation and monitoring for gastrointestinal endoscopy. World J Gastrointest Endosc. 2013;5(2):47–55.
13. Pradhan B, Pandey N. Colonoscopy in patients without sedation: an experience from Nepal. Health Renaiss. 2012;10(1):27–9.
14. Chen PH, Wu TC, Chiu CY. Pediatric gastrointestinal endoscopic sedation: a 2010 nationwide survey in Taiwan. Pediatr Neonatol. 2012;53(3):188–92.
15. Nwokediuko SC, Obienu O. Sedation practices for routine diagnostic upper gastrointestinal endoscopy in Nigeria. World J Gastrointest Endosc. 2012;4(6):260–5.
16. Amornyotin S, Lertakayamanee N, Wongyingsinn M, Pimukmanuskit P, Chalayonnavin V. The effectiveness of intravenous sedation in diagnostic upper gastrointestinal endoscopy. J Med Assoc Thai. 2007;90(2):301–6.
17. Behrens A, Kainzinger FA, Nolling T, Wienke A, Pech O, Ell C. [S3 guideline on "sedation in gastrointestinal endoscopy": how much does the new guideline cost in everyday hospital work? A calculation model and analysis of implementation in 2011 among ALGK members]. Z Gastroenterol. 2012;50(9):1002–7.
18. Lightdale JR, Mahoney LB, Schwarz SM, Liacouras CA. Methods of sedation in pediatric endoscopy: a survey of NASPGHAN members. J Pediatr Gastroenterol Nutr. 2007;45(4):500–2.
19. Zakeri N, Webster S, Coda S, Humphries S, Thillainayagam A. Safe sedation in endoscopy: time for a new approach? Gut. 2013;62:A159.
20. Liacouras CA, Mascarenhas M, Poon C, Wenner WJ. Placebo-controlled trial assessing the use of oral midazolam as a premedication to conscious sedation for pediatric endoscopy. Gastrointest Endosc. 1998;47(6):455–60.
21. Jeurnink SM, Steyerberg E, Kuipers E, Siersema P. The burden of endoscopic retrograde cholangiopancreatography (ERCP) performed with the patient under conscious sedation. Surg Endosc. 2012;26(8):2213–9.
22. Sasaki T, Tanabe S, Ishido K, Azuma M, Katada C, Higuchi K, et al. Recommended sedation and intraprocedural monitoring for gastric endoscopic submucosal dissection. Dig Endosc. 2013;25 Suppl 1:79–85.
23. Absah I, Bruining DH, Matsumoto JM, Weisbrod AJ, Fletcher JG, Fidler JL, et al. Mr enterography in pediatric inflammatory bowel disease: retrospective assessment of patient tolerance, image quality, and initial performance estimates. AJR Am J Roentgenol. 2012;199(3):W367–75.
24. Chun SY, Kim KO, Park DS, Kim SY, Park JW, Baek IH, et al. Safety and efficacy of deep sedation with propofol alone or combined with midazolam administrated by nonanesthesiologist for gastric endoscopic submucosal dissection. Gut Liver. 2012;6(4):464–70.
25. Barnett SR, Berzin T, Sanaka S, Pleskow D, Sawhney M, Chuttani R. Deep sedation without intubation for ERCP is appropriate in healthier, non-obese patients. Dig Dis Sci. 2013;58(11):3287–92.
26. American Society of Anesthesiology. Distinguishing monitored anesthesia care ("MAC" from moderate sedation/analgesia (conscious sedation) (approved by the ASA House of delegates on October 27, 2004). 2004. http://www.asahq.org/publicationsAndServices/standards/35.pdf. Accessed 1 Mar 2005.
27. Dial S, Silver P, Bock K, Sagy M. Pediatric sedation for procedures titrated to a desired degree of immobility results in unpredictable depth of sedation. Pediatr Emerg Care. 2001;17(6):414–20.
28. Vargo J, Howard K, Petrillo J, Scott J, Revicki DA. Development and validation of the patient and clinician sedation satisfaction index for colonoscopy and upper endoscopy. Clin Gastroenterol Hepatol. 2009;7(2):156–62.
29. Rostom A, Ross ED, Dube C, Rutter MD, Lee T, Valori R, et al. Development and validation of a nurse-assessed patient comfort score for colonoscopy. Gastrointest Endosc. 2013;77(2):255–61.
30. Lightdale JR, Mitchell PD, Fredette ME, et al. A pilot study of ketamine versus Midazolam/Fentanyl sedation in children undergoing GI endoscopy. International Journal of Pediatrics. Article ID 623710, 2011 p 6. doi:10.1155/2011/623710.
31. Trummel JM, Surgenor SD, Cravero JP, Gordon SR, Blike GT. Comparison of differing sedation practice for upper endoscopic ultrasound using expert observational analysis of the procedural sedation. J Patient Saf. 2009;5(3):153–9.
32. Anonymous. Practice guidelines for sedation and analgesia by non-anesthesiologists. A report by the American Society of Anesthesiologists Task Force on Sedation and Analgesia by Non-Anesthesiologists. Anesthesiology. 1996;84(2):459–71.
33. Cote CJ, Wilson S. Guidelines for monitoring and management of pediatric patients during and after sedation for diagnostic and therapeutic procedures: an update. Pediatrics. 2006;118(6):2587–602.
34. Cote CJ. American academy of pediatrics sedation guidelines: are we there yet? Arch Pediatr Adolesc Med. 2012;166(11):1067–9.
35. Vargo JJ, DeLegge MH, Feld AD, Gerstenberger PD, Kwo PY, Lightdale JR, et al. Multisociety sedation curriculum for gastrointestinal endoscopy. Gastroenterology. 2012;143(1):e18–41 [Practice Guideline].
36. Campbell EJ, Krishnaraj A, Harris M, Saini S, Richter JM. Automated before-procedure electronic health record screening to assess appropriateness for GI endoscopy and sedation. Gastrointest Endosc. 2012;76(4):786–92.
37. Thakkar K, El-Serag HB, Mattek N, Gilger MA. Complications of pediatric EGD: a 4-year experience in PEDS-CORI. Gastrointest Endosc. 2007;65(2):213–21.

38. Kupietzky A. Treating very young patients with conscious sedation and medical immobilization: a Jewish perspective. Alpha Omegan. 2005;98(4):33–7.
39. Gilger MA. Conscious sedation for endoscopy in the pediatric patient. Gastroenterol Nurs. 1993;16(2):75–9; discussion 80.
40. Lewis Claar R, Walker LS, Barnard JA. Children's knowledge, anticipatory anxiety, procedural distress, and recall of esophagogastroduodenoscopy. J Pediatr Gastroenterol Nutr. 2002;34(1):68–72.
41. Mallampati SR, Gatt SP, Gugino LD, Desai SP, Waraksa B, Freiberger D, et al. A clinical sign to predict difficult tracheal intubation: a prospective study. Can Anaesth Soc J. 1985;32(4):429–34.
42. Cha JM, Jeun JW, Pack KM, Lee JI, Joo KR, Shin HP, et al. Risk of sedation for diagnostic esophagogastroduodenoscopy in obstructive sleep apnea patients. World J Gastroenterol. 2013;19(29):4745–51.
43. Long Y, Liu HH, Yu C, Tian X, Yang YR, Wang C, et al. Pre-existing diseases of patients increase susceptibility to hypoxemia during gastrointestinal endoscopy. PLoS One. 2012;7(5):e37614.
44. Cote GA, Hovis CE, Hovis RM, Waldbaum L, Early DS, Edmundowicz SA, et al. A screening instrument for sleep apnea predicts airway maneuvers in patients undergoing advanced endoscopic procedures. Clin Gastroenterol Hepatol. 2010;8(8):660–5.e1.
45. Corso RM, Piraccini E, Agnoletti V, Lippi M, Buccioli M, Negro A, et al. Clinical use of the stop-bang questionnaire in patients undergoing sedation for endoscopic procedures. Minerva Anestesiol. 2012;78(1):109–10.
46. Kumar N, Prasad P. Procedural sedation in the obese patient. In: Thompson CC, editor. Bariatric endoscopy. New York: Springer Science + Business Media; 2013. p. 215–20.
47. Lin HC, Friedman M. Target-controlled infusion of propofol-induced sleep endoscopy for patients with obstructive sleep apnea. Otolaryngol Head Neck Surg. 2013;149:272.
48. Garewal D, Vele L, Waikar P. Anaesthetic considerations for endoscopic retrograde cholangio-pancreatography procedures. Curr Opin Anaesthesiol. 2013;26(4):475–80.
49. Lichtenstein DR, Jagannath S, Baron TH, Anderson MA, Banerjee S, Dominitz JA, et al. Sedation and anesthesia in GI endoscopy. Gastrointest Endosc. 2008;68(2):205–16.
50. Qadeer MA, Vargo JJ, Dumot JA, Lopez R, Trolli PA, Stevens T, et al. Capnographic monitoring of respiratory activity improves safety of sedation for endoscopic cholangiopancreatography and ultrasonography. Gastroenterology. 2009;136(5):1568–76. quiz 1819–520.
51. Thakkar K, El-Serag HB, Mattek N, Gilger MA. Immediate complications of upper endoscopy in children. Gastrointest Endosc. 2006;63(5):AB95.
52. Agrawal A, Sharma BC, Sharma P, Uppal R, Sarin SK. Randomized controlled trial for endoscopy with propofol versus midazolam on psychometric tests and critical flicker frequency in people with cirrhosis. J Gastroenterol Hepatol. 2012;27(11):1726–32.
53. Tanaka N, Horiuchi A, Nakayama Y, Katsuyama Y, Isobe M, Aoyama T, et al. Safety and effectiveness of low-dose propofol sedation during and after esophagogastroduodenoscopy in child A and B cirrhotic patients. Dig Dis Sci. 2013;58(5):1383–9.
54. Arandia HY, Patil VU. Glottic closure following large doses of fentanyl. Anesthesiology. 1987;66(4):574–5.
55. Koehntop DE, Rodman JH, Brundage DM, Hegland MG, Buckley JJ. Pharmacokinetics of fentanyl in neonates. Anesth Analg. 1986;65(3):227–32.
56. Balsells F, Wyllie R, Kay M, Steffen R. Use of conscious sedation for lower and upper gastrointestinal endoscopic examinations in children, adolescents, and young adults: a twelve-year review. Gastrointest Endosc. 1997;45(5):375–80.
57. Tolia V, Brennan S, Aravind MK, Kauffman RE. Pharmacokinetic and pharmacodynamic study of midazolam in children during esophagogastroduodenoscopy. J Pediatr. 1991;119(3):467–71.
58. Salonen M, Kanto J, Iisalo E, Himberg JJ. Midazolam as an induction agent in children: a pharmacokinetic and clinical study. Anesth Analg. 1987;66(7):625–8.
59. Jacobsen J, Flachs H, Dich-Nielsen JO, Rosen J, Larsen AB, Hvidberg EF. Comparative plasma concentration profiles after i.v., i.m. And rectal administration of pethidine in children. Br J Anaesth. 1988;60(6):623–6.
60. Gremse DA, Kumar S, Sacks AI. Conscious sedation with high-dose midazolam for pediatric gastrointestinal endoscopy. South Med J. 1997;90(8):821–5.
61. Fredette ME, Lightdale JR. Endoscopic sedation in pediatric practice. Gastrointest Endosc Clin N Am. 2008;18(4):739–51, ix.
62. Shemesh E, Bat L, Yahav J, Niv Y, Jonas A, Rozen P. Ketamine anesthesia for pediatric gastrointestinal procedures. Isr J Med Sci. 1982;18(7):760–2.
63. Aggarwal A, Ganguly S, Anand VK, Patwari AK. Efficacy and safety of intravenous ketamine for sedation and analgesia during pediatric endoscopic procedures. Indian Pediatr. 1998;35(12):1211–4.
64. Green SM, Klooster M, Harris T, Lynch EL, Rothrock SG. Ketamine sedation for pediatric gastroenterology procedures. J Pediatr Gastroenterol Nutr. 2001;32(1):26–33.
65. Miqdady MI, Hayajneh WA, Abdelhadi R, Gilger MA. Ketamine and midazolam sedation for pediatric gastrointestinal endoscopy in the Arab world. World J Gastroenterol. 2011;17(31):3630–5.
66. Motamed F, Aminpour Y, Hashemian H, Soltani AE, Najafi M, Farahmand F. Midazolam-ketamine combination for moderate sedation in upper GI endoscopy. J Pediatr Gastroenterol Nutr. 2012;54(3):422–6.
67. Gharaei B, Jafari A, Aghamohammadi H, Kamranmanesh M, Poorzamani M, Elyassi H, et al. Opioid-sparing effect of preemptive bolus low-dose ketamine for moderate sedation in opioid abusers undergoing extracorporeal shock wave lithotripsy: a randomized clinical trial. Anesth Analg. 2013;116(1):75–80.
68. Green SM, Nakamura R, Johnson NE. Ketamine sedation for pediatric procedures: part 1, a prospective series. Ann Emerg Med. 1990;19(9):1024–32.
69. Mason KP, Padua H, Fontaine PJ, Zurakowski D. Radiologist-supervised ketamine sedation for solid organ biopsies in children and adolescents. AJR Am J Roentgenol. 2009;192(5):1261–5.
70. Mason KP, Michna E, DiNardo JA, Zurakowski D, Karian VE, Connor L, et al. Evolution of a protocol for ketamine-induced sedation as an alternative to general anesthesia for interventional radiologic procedures in pediatric patients. Radiology. 2002;225(2):457–65.
71. Green SM, Sherwin TS. Incidence and severity of recovery agitation after ketamine sedation in young adults. Am J Emerg Med. 2005;23(2):142–4.
72. Spearman RS, Spearman G, Wilsey MJ Jr., Gilger M. Is Ketamine a safe sedative agent for pediatric endoscopy? Journal of Pediatric Gastroenterology and Nutrition. 2000;31 p. S29.
73. Brecelj J, Trop TK, Orel R. Ketamine with and without midazolam for gastrointestinal endoscopies in children. J Pediatr Gastroenterol Nutr. 2012;54(6):748–52.
74. Wathen JE, Roback MG, Mackenzie T, Bothner JP. Does midazolam alter the clinical effects of intravenous ketamine sedation in children? A double-blind, randomized, controlled, emergency department trial. Ann Emerg Med. 2000;36(6):579–88.
75. Sherwin TS, Green SM, Khan A, Chapman DS, Dannenberg B. Does adjunctive midazolam reduce recovery agitation after ketamine sedation for pediatric procedures? A randomized, double-blind, placebo-controlled trial. Ann Emerg Med. 2000;35(3):229–38.

76. Bedirli N, Egritas O, Cosarcan K, Bozkirli F. A comparison of fentanyl with tramadol during propofol-based deep sedation for pediatric upper endoscopy. Paediatr Anaesth. 2012;22(2): 150–5.
77. Fabbri LP, Nucera M, Marsili M, Al Malyan M, Becchi C. Ketamine, propofol and low dose remifentanil versus propofol and remifentanil for ERCP outside the operating room: is ketamine not only a "rescue drug"? Med Sci Monit. 2012;18(9): CR575–80.
78. Goyal R, Singh S, Shukla RN, Patra AK, Bhargava DV. Ketodex, a combination of dexmedetomidine and ketamine for upper gastrointestinal endoscopy in children: a preliminary report. J Anesth. 2013;27(3):461–3.
79. Gilger MA, Spearman RS, Dietrich CL, Spearman G, Wilsey Jr MJ, Zayat MN. Safety and effectiveness of ketamine as a sedative agent for pediatric GI endoscopy. Gastrointest Endosc. 2004; 59(6):659–63.
80. Michaud L, Gottrand F, Ganga-Zandzou PS, Ouali M, Vetter-Laffargue A, Lambilliotte A, et al. Nitrous oxide sedation in pediatric patients undergoing gastrointestinal endoscopy. J Pediatr Gastroenterol Nutr. 1999;28(3):310–4.
81. Forbes GM, Collins BJ. Nitrous oxide for colonoscopy: a randomized controlled study. Gastrointest Endosc. 2000;51(3):271–7.
82. Mcculloch A, Muthlagappan S, Harrison E, Mannath J, Nwokolo C, Arasaradnam R. Entonox vs. sedation in colonoscopy: a prospective cohort study. Gut. 2013;62:A48.
83. Curtin A, Izzetoglu K, Reynolds J, Menon R, Izzetoglu M, Osbakken M, et al. Functional near-infrared spectroscopy for the measurement of propofol effects in conscious sedation during outpatient elective colonoscopy. Neuroimage. 2014;85(Pt 1): 626–36.
84. LaPierre CD, Johnson KB, Randall BR, Egan TD. A simulation study of common propofol and propofol-opioid dosing regimens for upper endoscopy: implications on the time course of recovery. Anesthesiology. 2012;117(2):252–62.
85. Lightdale JR, Valim C, Newburg AR, Mahoney LB, Zgleszewski S, Fox VL. Efficiency of propofol versus midazolam and fentanyl sedation at a pediatric teaching hospital: a prospective study. Gastrointest Endosc. 2008;67(7):1067–75.
86. Larsen R, Galloway D, Wadera S, Kjar D, Hardy D, Mirkes C, et al. Safety of propofol sedation for pediatric outpatient procedures. Clin Pediatr (Phila). 2009;48(8):819–23.
87. Cravero JP. Pediatric sedation with propofol-continuing evolution of procedural sedation practice. J Pediatr. 2012;160(5):714–6.
88. Khoshoo V, Thoppil D, Landry L, Brown S, Ross G. Propofol versus midazolam plus meperidine for sedation during ambulatory esophagogastroduodenoscopy. J Pediatr Gastroenterol Nutr. 2003;37(2):146–9.
89. Kaddu R, Bhattacharya D, Metriyakool K, Thomas R, Tolia V. Propofol compared with general anesthesia for pediatric GI endoscopy: is propofol better? Gastrointest Endosc. 2002;55(1): 27–32.
90. Cohen S, Glatstein MM, Scolnik D, Rom L, Yaron A, Otremski S, et al. Propofol for pediatric colonoscopy: the experience of a large, tertiary care pediatric hospital. Am J Ther. 2013 Apr 5.
91. Wengrower D, Gozal D, Gozal Y, Meiri C, Golan I, Granot E, et al. Complicated endoscopic pediatric procedures using deep sedation and general anesthesia are safe in the endoscopy suite. Scand J Gastroenterol. 2004;39(3):283–6.
92. Barbi E, Gerarduzzi T, Marchetti F, Neri E, Verucci E, Bruno I, et al. Deep sedation with propofol by nonanesthesiologists: a prospective pediatric experience. Arch Pediatr Adolesc Med. 2003; 157(11):1097–103.
93. Schuttler J, Ihmsen H. Population pharmacokinetics of propofol: a multicenter study. Anesthesiology. 2000;92(3):727–38.
94. Eyres R. Update on TIVA. Paediatr Anaesth. 2004;14(5):374–9.
95. Amornyotin S, Srikureja W, Chalayonnavin W, Kongphlay S. Dose requirement and complications of diluted and undiluted propofol for deep sedation in endoscopic retrograde cholangiopancreatography. Hepatobiliary Pancreat Dis Int. 2011;10(3):313–8.
96. Elitsur Y, Blankenship P, Lawrence Z. Propofol sedation for endoscopic procedures in children. Endoscopy. 2000;32(10):788–91.
97. Amornyotin S, Aanpreung P, Prakarnrattana U, Chalayonnavin W, Chatchawankitkul S, Srikureja W. Experience of intravenous sedation for pediatric gastrointestinal endoscopy in a large tertiary referral center in a developing country. Paediatr Anaesth. 2009; 19(8):784–91.
98. Dosani M, McCormack J, Reimer E, Brant R, Dumont G, Lim J, et al. Slower administration of propofol preserves adequate respiration in children. Paediatr Anaesth. 2010;20(11):1001–8.
99. Rex DK, Deenadayalu VP, Eid E, Imperiale TF, Walker JA, Sandhu K, et al. Endoscopist-directed administration of propofol: a worldwide safety experience. Gastroenterology. 2009;137(4): 1229–37. quiz 1518–229.
100. Luginbuhl M, Vuilleumier P, Schumacher P, Stuber F. Anesthesia or sedation for gastroenterologic endoscopies. Curr Opin Anaesthesiol. 2009;22(4):524–31.
101. Parkinson I. Non-anaesthetist administration of propofol for sedation: caught 'NAAP'ing? Br J Hosp Med (Lond). 2012;73(12): 666–7.
102. Molina-Infante J, Duenas-Sadornil C, Mateos-Rodriguez JM, Perez-Gallardo B, Vinagre-Rodriguez G, Hernandez-Alonso M, et al. Nonanesthesiologist-administered propofol versus midazolam and propofol, titrated to moderate sedation, for colonoscopy: a randomized controlled trial. Dig Dis Sci. 2012;57(9):2385–93.
103. Slagelse C, Vilmann P, Hornslet P, Hammering A, Mantoni T. Nurse-administered propofol sedation for gastrointestinal endoscopic procedures: first Nordic results from implementation of a structured training program. Scand J Gastroenterol. 2011;46(12): 1503–9.
104. Barbi E, Petaros P, Badina L, Pahor T, Giuseppin I, Biasotto E, et al. Deep sedation with propofol for upper gastrointestinal endoscopy in children, administered by specially trained pediatricians: a prospective case series with emphasis on side effects. Endoscopy. 2006;38(4):368–75.
105. Lee SH. Non-anesthesiologist administered propofol with or without midazolam for moderate sedation-the problem is not "which regimen" but "who's regimen". Dig Dis Sci. 2012; 57(9):2243–5.
106. Vargo JJ, Cohen LB, Rex DK, Kwo PY. Position statement: non-anesthesiologist administration of propofol for GI endoscopy. Gastrointest Endosc. 2009;70(6):1053–9.
107. Dumonceau JM, Riphaus A, Aparicio JR, Beilenhoff U, Knape JT, Ortmann M, et al. European society of gastrointestinal endoscopy, European Society of Gastroenterology and Endoscopy Nurses and Associates, and the European Society of Anaesthesiology Guideline: non-anesthesiologist administration of propofol for GI endoscopy. Endoscopy. 2010;42(11):960–74.
108. Heuss LT, Froehlich F, Beglinger C. Nonanesthesiologist-administered propofol sedation: from the exception to standard practice. Sedation and monitoring trends over 20 years. Endoscopy. 2012;44(5):504–11.
109. DHHS, CMS. Clarification of the interpretative guidelines for the anesthesia services condition of participation. 2010. https://www.cms.gov/Regulations-and-Guidance/Guidance/Transmittals/downloads/R74SOMA.pdf
110. Perel A. Non-anaesthesiologists should not be allowed to administer propofol for procedural sedation: a Consensus Statement of 21 European National Societies of Anaesthesia. Eur J Anaesthesiol. 2011;28(8):580–4.
111. Demiraran Y, Korkut E, Tamer A, Yorulmaz I, Kocaman B, Sezen G, et al. The comparison of dexmedetomidine and midazolam

used for sedation of patients during upper endoscopy: a prospective, randomized study. Can J Gastroenterol. 2007;21(1):25–9.

112. Sula H, Domi R, Ohri I, Broqi I, Beqiri A, Gani H. Propofol versus dexmedetomidine for sedation in colonoscopy: a prospective, randomized study. Eur J Anaesthesiol. 2012;29 p 32.
113. Heard L. Taking care of the little things: preparation of the pediatric endoscopy patient. Gastroenterol Nurs. 2008;31(2):108–12.
114. Heard LA, Fredette ME, Atmadja ML, Weinstock P, Lightdale JR. Perceptions of simulation-based training in crisis resource management in the endoscopy unit. Gastroenterol Nurs. 2011; 34(1):42–8.
115. Amornyotin S, Aanpreung P. Clinical effectiveness of an anesthesiologist-administered intravenous sedation outside of the main operating room for pediatric upper gastrointestinal endoscopy in Thailand. Int J Pediatr. 2010;2010:748564.
116. Chawla S, Katz A, Attar BM, Go B. Endoscopic retrograde cholangiopancreatography under moderate sedation and factors predicting need for anesthesiologist directed sedation: a county hospital experience. World J Gastrointest Endosc. 2013;5(4):160–4.
117. Bergese SD, Dalal P, Vandse R, Satlin A, Lin Z, Candiotti K, et al. A double-blind, randomized, multicenter, dose-ranging study to evaluate the safety and efficacy of fospropofol disodium as an intravenous sedative for colonoscopy in high-risk populations. Am J Ther. 2013;20(2):163–71.
118. Wang CY, Ling LC, Cardosa MS, Wong AK, Wong NW. Hypoxia during upper gastrointestinal endoscopy with and without sedation and the effect of pre-oxygenation on oxygen saturation. Anaesthesia. 2000;55(7):654–8.
119. Gerstenberger PD. Capnography and patient safety for endoscopy. GI & Hepatology News. 2011
120. Lightdale JR, Goldmann DA, Feldman HA, Newburg AR, Dinardo JA, Fox VL. Microstream capnography improves patient monitoring during moderate sedation: a randomized, controlled trial. Pediatrics. 2006;117(6):1170–8.
121. American Society of Anesthesiologists statement on respiratory monitoring during endoscopic procedures. 2009. http://www.asahq.org/For-Members/Standards-Guidelines-and-Statements.aspx
122. Jang SY, Park HG, Jung MK, Cho CM, Park SY, Jeon SW, et al. Bispectral index monitoring as an adjunct to nurse-administered combined sedation during endoscopic retrograde cholangiopancreatography. World J Gastroenterol. 2012;18(43):6284–9.
123. Drake LM, Chen SC, Rex DK. Efficacy of bispectral monitoring as an adjunct to nurse-administered propofol sedation for colonoscopy: a randomized controlled trial. Am J Gastroenterol. 2006;101(9):2003–7.
124. Chen SC, Rex DK. An initial investigation of bispectral monitoring as an adjunct to nurse-administered propofol sedation for colonoscopy. Am J Gastroenterol. 2004;99(6):1081–6.
125. Krugliak P, Ziff B, Rusabrov Y, Rosenthal A, Fich A, Gurman GM. Propofol versus midazolam for conscious sedation guided by processed EEG during endoscopic retrograde cholangiopancreatography: a prospective, randomized, double-blind study. Endoscopy. 2000;32(9):677–82.
126. Wehrmann T, Grotkamp J, Stergiou N, Riphaus A, Kluge A, Lembcke B, et al. Electroencephalogram monitoring facilitates sedation with propofol for routine ERCP: a randomized, controlled trial. Gastrointest Endosc. 2002;56(6):817–24.
127. Agrawal D, Feldman HA, Krauss B, Waltzman ML. Bispectral index monitoring quantifies depth of sedation during emergency department procedural sedation and analgesia in children. Ann Emerg Med. 2004;43(2):247–55.
128. Powers KS, Nazarian EB, Tapyrik SA, Kohli SM, Yin H, van der Jagt EW, et al. Bispectral index as a guide for titration of propofol during procedural sedation among children. Pediatrics. 2005; 115(6):1666–74.
129. McDermott NB, VanSickle T, Motas D, Friesen RH. Validation of the bispectral index monitor during conscious and deep sedation in children. Anesth Analg. 2003;97(1):39–43, table of contents.
130. Nguyen NQ, Toscano L, Lawrence M, Moore J, Holloway RH, Bartholomeusz D, et al. Patient-controlled analgesia with inhaled methoxyflurane versus conventional endoscopist-provided sedation for colonoscopy: a randomized multicenter trial. Gastrointest Endosc. 2013;78(6):892–901.
131. Kulling D, Fantin AC, Biro P, Bauerfeind P, Fried M. Safer colonoscopy with patient-controlled analgesia and sedation with propofol and alfentanil. Gastrointest Endosc. 2001;54(1):1–7.
132. Ng JM, Kong CF, Nyam D. Patient-controlled sedation with propofol for colonoscopy. Gastrointest Endosc. 2001;54(1):8–13.
133. Gillham MJ, Hutchinson RC, Carter R, Kenny GN. Patient-maintained sedation for ERCP with a target-controlled infusion of propofol: a pilot study. Gastrointest Endosc. 2001; 54(1):14–7.
134. Pambianco DJ, Whitten CJ, Moerman A, Struys MM, Martin JF. An assessment of computer-assisted personalized sedation: a sedation delivery system to administer propofol for gastrointestinal endoscopy. Gastrointest Endosc. 2008;68(3):542–7.
135. Agostoni M, Fanti L, Gemma M, Pasculli N, Beretta L, Testoni PA. Adverse events during monitored anesthesia care for GI endoscopy: an 8-year experience. Gastrointest Endosc. 2011; 74(2):266–75.
136. Lightdale J, Valim C, Newburg A, Zgleszewski S, Donovan K, Heard L, et al. Efficiency of propofol sedation versus conscious sedation with midazolam and fentanyl in a pediatric endoscopy unit. Gastrointest Endosc. 2005;61(5):AB92.
137. Lightdale J, Feldman H, Newburg A, Turbini V, Heard L, Donovan K, et al. A randomized double-blind controlled trial of microstream capnography to reduce oxygen desaturation during gastrointestinal procedures with conscious sedation. Gastrointest Endosc. 2005;61(5):AB81.
138. Vargo JJ, DeLegge MH, Feld AD, Gerstenberger PD, Kwo PY, Lightdale JR, et al. Multisociety sedation curriculum for gastrointestinal endoscopy. Gastrointest Endosc. 2012;76(1): e1–25.

Sedation in the Emergency Department: A Complex and Multifactorial Challenge

19

Robert M. Kennedy

The Wand is only as good as the Wizard.

Abstract

Safe and effective management of procedure-related pain and anxiety in the emergency department (ED) has become expected. It facilitates controlled accomplishment of therapeutic and diagnostic procedures, reduces psychological trauma and its sequelae, reduces healthcare provider and parental distress, and improves parental acceptance of rendered care. Many advances in procedural sedation and analgesia (PSA) for nonelective procedures in non-fasted patients in the ED have occurred over the past 20 years as a result of intense interest in this concept and the development of general and pediatric emergency medicine specialties, for whom PSA is now considered core training. This chapter reviews some of the PSA techniques shown to safely and effectively decrease children's pain and anxiety associated with procedures in the ED. Since pain and anxiety are frequently indistinguishable, the combination will often be referred to as distress.

Keywords

Emergency department • Procedural sedation and analgesia (PSA) • Local anesthesia • Psychological intervention • Pain • Anxiety • Motion • Adverse events • Upper airway obstruction • Laryngospasm • Emesis • Pulmonary aspiration • Eutectic Mixture of Local Anesthetics (EMLA) • Nil per os (NPO) • American Society of Anesthesiologists (ASA) • American College of Emergency Physicians • Capnography • Moderate sedation • Deep sedation • Naloxone (Narcan) • Flumazenil • Atropine • Succinylcholine • Ketamine • Ondansetron (Zofran) • Gamma-aminobutyric acid (GABA) • Chloral hydrate • Barbiturates • Diazepam • Etomidate • Fentanyl • Fospropofol • Ketamine • Ketofol • Lorazepam • Meperidine (Demerol) • Methohexital (Brevital) • Midazolam (Versed) • Morphine • Nitrous oxide • Pentobarbital (Nembutal) • Propofol • Remifentanil • S-ketamine • Sufentanil • Flumazenil • Naloxone (Narcan) • Lidocaine • Ondansetron (Zofran) • Metoclopramide (Reglan) • Scopolamine • Diphenhydramine (Benadryl) • Dexamethasone (Decadron) • Codeine • Oxycodone • Glycopyrrolate • Mallampati

R.M. Kennedy, M.D. (✉)
Department of Pediatrics, St. Louis Children's Hospital, 1 Children's Place, 9103 Northwest Tower, St. Louis, MO 63110, USA
e-mail: Kennedy@kids.wustl.edu

Introduction

Why Procedural Sedation and Analgesia (PSA)?

Painful therapeutic procedures are frequently necessary during emergency care of children, many of whom already have a painful and frightening injury or illness. Immobility for diagnostic radiological procedures in young children is

K.P. Mason (ed.), *Pediatric Sedation Outside of the Operating Room: A Multispecialty International Collaboration*, DOI 10.1007/978-1-4939-1390-9_19, © Springer Science+Business Media New York 2015

also often required. These procedures are distressful for the children, their parents, and their healthcare providers. Inadequately relieved procedure-related pain and distress produces physiological and psychological reactions that have acute and long-term consequences [1–6].

Safe and effective management of procedure-related pain and anxiety in the emergency department (ED) has become expected [7]. It facilitates controlled accomplishment of therapeutic and diagnostic procedures [3, 8, 9], reduces psychological trauma and its sequelae [3, 5, 8, 10], reduces healthcare provider and parental distress, and improves parental acceptance of rendered care [11]. Many advances in PSA for nonelective procedures in non-fasted patients in the ED have occurred over the past 20 years as a result of intense interest in this concept and the development of general and pediatric emergency medicine specialties, for which PSA is now considered core training [12]. Family and third-party payer's desire for definitive management of acute injuries during initial ED visits also seems to be increasing. This chapter reviews some of the PSA techniques shown to safely and effectively decrease children's pain and anxiety associated with procedures in the ED. Since pain and anxiety are frequently indistinguishable, the combination will often be referred to as distress.

Long-Term Negative Impact of Painful Procedures

Elimination or relief of pain and suffering, whenever possible, is an important responsibility of physicians caring for children [13], as unmanaged pain can result in a variety of negative long-term consequences [14]. Accumulating evidence indicates that by the middle of the third trimester of human gestation, ascending pain fibers fully connect to the primary somatosensory cortex of the brain [15, 16]. Descending inhibitory pain pathways, on the other hand, appear to require postnatal development. Rather than being less sensitive to pain, young infants may actually experience pain more intensely than older children [17]. As the brain rapidly matures during the first weeks to months after birth, recurrent painful stimuli may alter the formation of new neuronal circuits, resulting in children's hypersensitivity and increased behavioral response to noxious stimuli [15, 18–23].

Inadequately controlled procedure-related pain has been correlated to increased distress and maladaptive behaviors during subsequent healthcare interactions. Boys circumcised at birth without effective anesthesia had increased distress at their 4- and 6-month routine vaccinations compared to uncircumcised controls [24]. Similarly, toddlers who had painful postoperative care during the first 3 months of life demonstrated greater pain responses at their 14-month immunizations compared with controls [25]. In older children, painful therapeutic procedures have been associated with negative memory and greater pain during similar future procedures [26–28], even when those future procedures are performed with adequate analgesia [5]. Although the mechanisms underlying these observations have yet to be fully elucidated, these studies show that painful episodes can be encoded into children's implicit and explicit memories [23]. While praising a child following a painful procedure, in an effort to modify negative memories, may lessen these memories and reduce distress during subsequent procedures [29], prevention of negative memories by employing effective sedation–analgesia for intensely painful procedures is likely a crucial part of preventing the negative feedback loop that can then cause greater anxiety and pain during future procedures and healthcare interactions [30, 31].

When May PSA Not Be Needed?

PSA requires substantial and frequently scarce healthcare resources in a busy ED and has significant, albeit rare, risks. Emergency healthcare providers therefore increasingly are employing strategies that provide effective minimally painful techniques for local anesthesia or systemic analgesia. Combined with psychological or behavioral approaches to reduce patient anxiety, these strategies may greatly reduce the need for PSA as well as diminish the need for deeper sedation [32].

Nearly Painless Local Anesthesia

Topical Anesthetics

Use of topical anesthesia for children's lacerations has become standard in many EDs. Locally compounded solutions or gels containing 4 % lidocaine, 0.1 % epinephrine (adrenaline), and 0.5 % tetracaine (LET or LAT) provide local anesthesia when instilled for 20–30 min into an open wound or abscess [33–35]. These solutions are more effective in scalp and facial lacerations than those on extremities or the trunk, but their initial use markedly reduces the pain of subsequent injection of lidocaine, if such is needed. Careful application of limited amounts of these solutions onto lip or mucous membrane lacerations (e.g., using a cotton-tip swab) has been shown safe and can be quite effective [36]. Caution must be used, especially in small children, as rapid absorption of the anesthetics could cause toxicity. A recent study also found use of LET on finger lacerations safe and effective [37].

Buffering Injected Lidocaine

Pain associated with injection of lidocaine can be markedly reduced by buffering the anesthetic, injecting slowly through fine needles (e.g., 30 gauge) subcutaneously instead of intradermally, and warming the anesthetic to body temperature [38–42]. Buffering lidocaine, with or without epinephrine, to pH 7.0–7.2 by mixing 1 part of 1 mEq/mL sodium bicarbonate with 9–10 parts of 1 % lidocaine markedly decreases the pain of injection [43, 44]. Buffering also decreases onset time for anesthesia [44] without affecting efficacy or duration [44–46]. The buffered mixture is stable for at least 3 weeks when stored at room temperature [45] and longer when refrigerated [47].

Psychological Interventions Reduce Distress and Need for PSA

Acute injury or illness causes significant anxiety and stress for most children and their parents. Lack of understanding of ED routines for care, ongoing pain, prolonged waits, preconceived notions about emergency care, and numerous other known and unknown factors interfere with effective preparation of the child and use of the child's and parents' coping mechanisms [48]. Consequently, many young children are frightened and unwilling to cooperate with necessary procedures, even when little or no pain is involved. A warm smile and a slow respectful and sometimes playful approach may reduce the frightened child's perception of the provider as a threat and increase the likelihood of cooperation without need for sedation. Addressing parental concerns and providing them with an explanation of the plan for care, along with age-specific suggestions on how they can allay some of their child's fears and anxieties, allows them to prepare their child as well as themselves.

Having their parent at their side during painful procedures in the ED is of utmost importance for school-aged and younger children, despite realizing their parent can do little to alleviate procedural pain [49]. Parents likewise believe their presence during procedures is important and beneficial to their children [50–52]. EDs increasingly are enacting policies to give parents the option of staying with their child during all procedures and resuscitations, usually with a staff member dedicated to explain the care provided and to monitor the parent for signs of extreme distress, syncope, etc. [53–55]. When suggestions are given to parents on how to help their child (e.g., touching, distracting with stories, reciting the alphabet, counting, etc.), parents can provide significant assistance in accomplishing anxiety-provoking procedures without sedation [56, 57]. In addition, nonthreatening language should be used to characterize anticipated sensations, e.g., "freezing, poking, or squeezing" instead of "burning, bee sting, or hurting." Simply allowing young children to sit in their willing parent's lap, with parents providing distraction and hugs for mild restraint, markedly reduces the child's distress during minor procedures [58]. Combining this technique with LET for topical wound anesthesia, supplemented as needed with buffered lidocaine injected via a 30-gauge needle, the author rarely finds it necessary to employ PSA for suturing lacerations in young children.

What Makes PSA in the Emergency Department Different?

Children often exhibit significant distress when faced with emergency department (ED) procedures despite administration of analgesic medications and psychological interventions. They may be anxious about sounds and sights they do not understand, fearful because of prior experience or hearsay, or in pain because of incomplete analgesia or local anesthesia. Furthermore, their usual coping mechanisms may be in disarray because of the unexpected nature of their illness or injury and their perception that they have no control over the impending treatment. When children refuse or are unable to cooperate with necessary procedures or if effective local anesthesia is not possible, safe and effective pharmacologic sedation can avert detrimental patient, parent, and practitioner sequelae and facilitate accomplishment of the procedure [5, 59, 60].

ED PSA in children, however, has greater inherent risks when contrasted to elective sedation. Patients frequently have not fasted for traditional periods and consequently may have "full stomachs" [61–63]. Postponement of procedures to allow fasting in the ED may be impractical due to limited resources. More importantly, postponement to allow gastric emptying is likely ineffective because painful injuries and serious illnesses unpredictably delay emptying of stomach contents; moreover, necessary administration of opioids for pain management likely exacerbates this problem. Compounding these issues, children undergoing painful or anxiety-provoking procedures typically require deeper levels of sedation than adults or teenagers who may be able to better control their behavior [1]. Unanticipated arrival or deterioration of other ED patients and overextended ED staff may result in the sedating physician unpredictably being pulled away or distracted by other patients' emergencies. Finally, therapeutic procedures performed by trainees in academic EDs frequently are more prolonged and require longer periods of sedation.

Deciding Whether to Perform PSA

The first and foremost goal of pediatric PSA is assurance of the patient's safety and welfare during the sedation and recovery. With this in mind and the limitations noted earlier, the clinician considering PSA must carefully consider the following:

1. *Is the procedure necessary*? Some procedures that would require PSA in many children may be unnecessary. For example, it is likely that, as in adults, many lacerations of the hand and feet heal as well with bandaging as with suturing [64]. Similarly, virtually all tongue lacerations heal well without suturing [65].
2. *Do I have the resources and skills to rescue if rare but serious adverse events occur*? For example, would I be able to administer a paralytic drug for severe laryngospasm or secure the airway by intubation?
3. *What if an unexpected patient with a critical emergency arrives*? Do I have the resources to continue the PSA and procedure? Or, if I had to leave the patient, do I have the resources to safely recover the patient?

Systematic Approach to Safe ED PSA

Knowledge of Clinical Policies Specific to Emergency Department

Although each facility and institution may have their own specific policies, procedures, and guidelines, it is important that the sedation provider in the emergency department is familiar with the clinical policies of their specialty. In February 2014, the American College of Emergency Physicians released the most recent clinical policy to date. Entitled *Clinical Policy*: *Procedural Sedation and Analgesia in the Emergency Department*, it updates the 2005 policy [66]. The clinical policy was based on literature review, with recommendations identified as Levels A, B, and C. The levels were determined from the degree of clinical certainty after review of the literature. High certainty, moderate certainty, and inadequate/absence evidence corresponded to Level A, B, and C recommendation, respectively. The importance of NPO was a Level B recommendation, advising that there was no evidence to support preprocedural fasting of children for procedural sedation in the emergency department. The routine use of capnography was assigned a Level B recommendation, recognizing that as an adjunct to pulse oximetry it may detect hypoventilation and apnea earlier than pulse oximetry or clinical assessment. The recommendation for the number of personnel necessary to manage sedation-related complications was a Level C—without supporting evidence; the recommendation was that in addition to the provider performing the procedure, a nurse or other qualified individual needed to be continuously present. The final recommendations with respect to sedatives were Levels A, B, and C. Ketamine and propofol were based on Level A recommendations, deemed safe for pediatric sedation in the emergency department. Etomidate for children was considered Level C, supported with expert consensus, despite absent/inadequate supporting published literature. The combination of ketamine and propofol was considered Level B for safe pediatric sedation in the emergency department. No recommendations could be made for dexmedetomidine, as there is only one case report of its use in the emergency department. This 2014 Clinical Policy of the American College of Emergency Physicians highlights the value of designing studies to specifically examine patient-specific outcomes. It also recognizes that unique patient-care environments and high-risk patient populations may pose unique challenges, which may require modification of the Clinical Policy. Reviewing the literature, the College of Emergency Physicians Clinical Policies Committee made evidence-based recommendations for important clinical questions. The following questions were addressed [66]:

1. Is preprocedural (nil per os, NPO) fasting necessary to decrease risk of emesis and aspiration during sedation in the emergency department?
2. Does capnography decrease risk of adverse events?
3. How many personnel are necessary to manage sedation-related complications?
4. Are ketamine, propofol, etomidate, dexmedetomidine, alfentanil, and remifentanil appropriate sedatives for the emergency department?

Goals of PSA

Pediatric PSA by experienced providers has inevitable risks of adverse events including respiratory depression, apnea, airway obstruction, vomiting, hypotension, and dysphoria [67]. The first and foremost goal of pediatric PSA is assurance of the patient's safety and welfare during the sedation and recovery [59, 68]. Within this context, additional goals include control of behavior (muscle relaxation or relative immobility) and minimization of procedure-related pain, anxiety, memory, and negative psychological responses [59]. Safe attainment of these goals requires careful patient screening for factors associated with increased sedation-related risk of adverse events or difficult airway management, preparation for management of possible adverse events, and meticulous assurance of effective patient cardiopulmonary and other vital functions during and after the procedural sedation.

By developing a routine or systematic approach for ED PSA, the emergency physician reduces risks for the patient by identifying children at increased risk of adverse events and increasing preparedness for safe and effective management of adverse events should they occur [69]. The systematic approach should include the following steps:

1. Pre-sedation patient assessment
2. Informed consent
3. Plan for sedation
4. Documentation/sedation record
5. Recovery/discharge
6. Quality improvement

Pre-sedation Patient Evaluation and Risk Assessment

Children should be screened for factors that may be associated with increased risk of adverse events or difficult management of these events during sedation. Identification of these risks allows for better preparation for management of untoward events or development of alternative plans to reduce the likelihood of undesired effects. In addition to general sedation screening in preparation for an ED procedure, a focused physical exam immediately prior to sedation should be repeated to detect any acute changes in the child's physiological status such as acute onset of wheezing or fever.

Pre-sedation *history and physical examination* should focus upon the patient's cardiorespiratory status and airway to determine the sedator's ability to rescue breathe for this individual, if necessary [59, 70, 71]. A focused history may be guided by the mnemonic *AMPLE*:

(*A*) Allergies to medications, latex, CT contrast, and food (e.g., egg allergy prohibits use of propofol; shellfish allergies are associated with CT contrast reactions).

(*M*) Current medications or illicit drugs that might interact with PSA medications; these often reveal concurrent diagnoses that may impact PSA choices, e.g., psychiatric medications.

(*P*) Past medical history, including any complications with sedation or anesthesia and chronic illnesses; history of snoring/stridor, recent URI/respiratory infections or asthma exacerbations, GERD, cardiac history, prematurity, any neuromuscular disease (may contraindicate succinylcholine), and history of airway surgery/tumors/malformations.

(*L*) Last meal/fluid intake.

(*E*) Events leading to a need for procedure, e.g., associated injuries:

(a) *ASA physical status classification*

The patient physical status classification endorsed by the American Society of Anesthesiologists (ASA) [72] to predict risk for adverse events during general anesthesia [73, 74] is helpful in assessing sedation risks and is summarized in Table 19.1. ASA Class I and II children are at low risk for serious adverse events when carefully monitored. Events that are initially minor, such as upper airway obstruction during deep sedation, usually can be easily addressed with simple interventions and catastrophic sequelae prevented. However, children with underlying illnesses often have less cardiopulmonary reserve and thus a greater risk for adverse responses to sedative and analgesic medications, and their rescues often are more difficult and complex. Therefore, when possible, it is suggested an experienced sedation provider or anesthesiologist be consulted for planning sedation of ASA Class III patients and an anesthesiologist consulted for Class IV or V patients.

Table 19.1 ASA physical status-E classification [72]

Status	Disease state
I	No organic, physiologic, biochemical, or psychiatric disturbance
II	Mild to moderate systemic disturbance that may or may not be related to the reason for procedure, e.g., *mild asthma, well-controlled diabetes, controlled seizure disorder, and anemia*
III[a]	Severe systemic disturbance that may or may not be related to the reason for procedure, e.g., *heart disease that limits activity, poorly controlled essential hypertension, diabetes mellitus with complications, chronic pulmonary disease that limits activity, and poorly controlled seizure disorder*
IV[b]	Severe systemic disturbance that is life threatening with or without procedure, e.g., *advanced cardiac, pulmonary, renal, endocrine, or hepatic dysfunction*, e.g., *severe bronchopulmonary dysplasia* and *sepsis*
V[b]	Moribund patient who has little chance of survival but is submitted to procedure as a last resort (resuscitative effort), e.g., *septic shock, cerebral trauma, and pulmonary embolus*

"E" is added to indicate a nonelective or emergent procedure, e.g., ASA I–E

[a]Consultation with experienced sedation provider or anesthesiologist encouraged

[b]Consultation with anesthesiologist strongly encouraged

(b) *Airway assessment*: *comorbid risk factors, Mallampati classification*

Factors associated with difficulty in airway management include those that make it hard to visualize the larynx or partially or completely obstruct the upper airway. Examples include: history of previous problems with anesthesia or sedation including prolonged intubation or unplanned hospitalization; stridor, snoring, or sleep apnea; chromosomal abnormality (e.g., trisomy 21); history of prematurity with prolonged intubation; significant obesity; short neck or limited neck mobility; receding mandible (small lower jaw) or decreased hyoid-mental distance; dysmorphic facial features (e.g., Pierre–Robin syndrome); small mouth opening; protruding incisors; loose teeth; dental appliances; high, arched, and narrow palate or history of cleft palate repair; large tongue; tonsillar hypertrophy; or no visible uvula (Fig. 19.1; Mallampati airway classification III, IV) [70, 71].

Problems associated with increased risk of adverse events and for which consultation with an experienced sedation practitioner or anesthesiologist is suggested include [76]:

- ASA physical status Class III or IV
- Current upper respiratory illness (URI)[1]

[1]Note: Upper respiratory illness (URI) may increase the risk of laryngospasm, bronchospasm, and hypoxia during sedation. Mild URI symptoms alone (non-purulent rhinitis, afebrile, cough that clears) may not be an indication to cancel PSA, but management should reflect anticipation of above potential complications. Severe URI (febrile, purulent discharge, wet cough) should prompt consideration of cancellation of non-emergent or urgent procedures.

Samsoon and Young modification: Mallampati Classification

Increasing difficulty with intubation or mask ventilation -----►

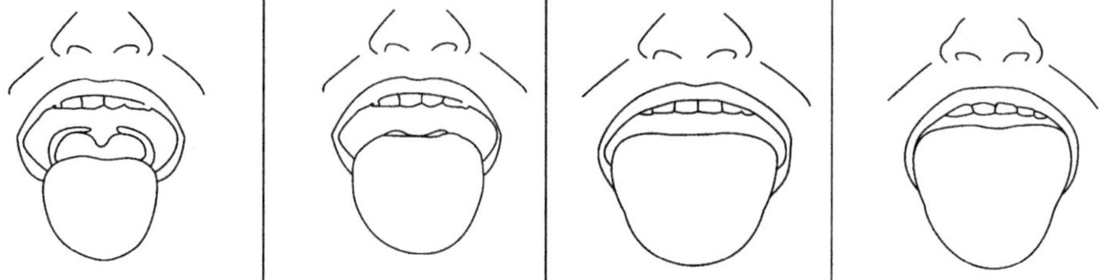

I	II	III	IV
Visible Structures when patient opens mouth, protrudes tongue without help			
-soft palate -fauces -uvula -tonsillar pillars	-soft palate -fauces -uvula	-soft palate -fauces -uvula	-None of the previous structures

Fig. 19.1 Mallampati airway classification (adapted with permission from Mallampati SR. Recognition of the difficult airway. In: Benumof JL (ed) Airway management: principles and practice. St. Louis: Mosby-Yearbook; 1996. p. 132 [75])

- Pulmonary: wheezing not cleared by a bronchodilator, obstructive sleep apnea
- Morbid obesity (>2 × ideal body weight)
- Cardiovascular conditions: cyanosis, congestive heart failure
- Neurological conditions: poorly controlled seizures, central apnea
- Gastrointestinal conditions: uncontrolled gastroesophageal reflux
- Prematurity with residual pulmonary, cardiovascular, gastrointestinal, and neurological problems
- Age <3 months
- Pregnancy or suspected pregnancy
- Neuromuscular disease
- Severe developmental delay
- Patients who are difficult to control
- History of failed sedation, oversedation, or paradoxical response to sedatives

Screening for acute illness: Patients should be screened for acute illnesses that may increase their risk for sedation-related adverse effects. When acute illness is detected, the sedation provider must weigh the increased risk against the need for the diagnostic or therapeutic procedure.

(c) *Fasting status and risk of aspiration*

To decrease the risk of pulmonary aspiration of gastric contents in healthy children undergoing general anesthesia for elective procedures, fasting from clear liquids a minimum of 2 h and from milk or solid food 6–8 h is a well-established consensus-based practice [77]. However, as noted in these guidelines, "Published evidence is silent on the relationship between fasting times, gastric volume, or gastric acidity and the risk of emesis/reflux or pulmonary aspiration in humans." In two more recent reviews of the literature examining whether children should undergo fasting prior to ED PSA [78, 79], it is noted that little clinical data has been published to help answer this question. It is difficult to extrapolate directly to PSA from the long experience with safe general anesthesia. It is likely that risk of aspiration is less during ED PSA compared to general anesthesia in the operating room for several reasons. First, protective airway reflexes are generally preserved at the depth of moderate sedation [70, 80]. Second, airway reflexes are also relatively intact during sedation with the commonly used dissociative agent ketamine during deep sedation or even light general anesthesia [81]. Of concern, however, these reflexes are likely blunted during deep sedation with opioids, benzodiazepines, barbiturates, propofol, and etomidate, especially if sedation is deep enough to cause apnea [79]. Third, intubation of the trachea, rarely performed in children undergoing ED PSA, likely increases the risk of pulmonary aspiration due to pharmacological abolition of protective reflexes to facilitate intubation and mechanical interference with these reflexes during passage of the endotracheal tube into the trachea [73, 74, 82].

Fourth, the great majority of children receiving ED PSA meet ASA physical status Class I or II criteria [9, 61–63, 80, 83] and, compared to those in ASA physical status Classes III and IV, are associated with less risk of adverse events during anesthesia [73, 74]. It is the combination of these differences—i.e., moderate sedation, common use of dissociative ketamine for deep sedation, lack of manipulation of the larynx, and healthy patients—that likely results in ED PSA having lower risk of aspiration compared to general anesthesia.

A more robust literature on identification of risk factors for aspiration in children undergoing general anesthesia has found no benefit from routine preoperative administration of antacids or pharmacological agents to increase gastric motility [77, 84]. Gastric fluid volume or pH were not different with NPO periods of 2, 4, and 12 h after drinking apple juice in one study [85] or after 30 min to 3 h, 3–8 h, or more than 8 h after clear liquid ingestion in another trial [86]. No studies have examined gastric emptying in children after solid intake, but one small study of adult women after a light breakfast found 3 of 8 had emptied their stomachs by 2 h and all by 6 h [87].

The incidence of pulmonary aspiration during ED PSA is uncertain but appears to be very low. In a literature review of adverse events during ED PSA [78], after combining studies with a total of 4,814 children, clinically apparent aspiration during PSA was reported in only one account of two children, both of whom had fasted standard NPO periods and did not appear to be ED patients. These patients were deeply sedated with opioid–barbiturate combinations (which blunt airway reflexes), one for a radiological procedure and the other for bronchoscopy. Both required only supplemental oxygen and observation [69]. In nearly 50,000 elective propofol-based sedations, 4 children were noted to have aspirated; all recovered without sequelae after positive-pressure ventilation and supplemental oxygen and were discharged the day of or day after the procedure [88]. The incidence of aspiration in more than 100,000 children undergoing general anesthesia has been reported to be 1:978 and 1:2,632 patients by Warner [73] and Borland [74]. During emergency surgery, aspiration occurred as frequently as 1:373 patients in the Warner study [73]. Although only a rough estimate, pooling of the available data in the literature suggests the incidence of clinically apparent pulmonary aspiration during ED PSA is no more frequent than 1:2,000 pediatric patient encounters [78]. Because of the rarity of its occurrence, much larger studies are needed to accurately estimate the incidence of aspiration, and any relationship with fasting, during ED PSA. For now, given the many variables present, clinical judgment has to weigh the risk and benefits for each patient [78, 79].

Vomiting, although not likely to result in aspiration when protective airway reflexes are intact, is a common adverse event during ED PSA in children, occurring in as much as 25 % of patients, especially when opioids are coadministered prior to sedation [89, 90]. As supported by literature reviews [78, 79, 91], recent series of children receiving ketamine or nitrous oxide for ED PSA suggest there is poor correlation between the length of time of preprocedural fasting and vomiting [62, 63, 92]. No significant difference in frequency of vomiting was found between children that fasted between 0, 2, 4, 6, 8, and greater than 8 h. This may be because the vomiting is medication induced and gastric contents have little effect on likelihood of vomiting.

Gastric emptying may also be unpredictably delayed in ill or injured patients due to development of ileus [93]. ED management of pain with opioids likely exacerbates this problem. Whether brief delay (1–6 h) of PSA decreases vomiting is undetermined. Coadministration of ondansetron has been found to reduce vomiting associated with ketamine-based ED PSA but only from 12.6 to 4.7 % with 13 patients needing to be treated to prevent one episode of vomiting [94]. This and other strategies need further investigation. It is the practice of the author to consider all sedated ED patients to have "full stomachs" and to manage them with vigilance and preparation for assisting them in clearing their oropharynx by rolling them to their side or assisting them in leaning forward. Suctioning of the mouth is then used, if needed, to "mop up."

Pregnancy: Since many medications administered for ED PSA have the potential for causing harm to a fetus, it is recommended that the menstrual status be reviewed with post-menarchal girls and a urine pregnancy test performed prior to sedation. The US Food and Drug Administration (FDA) has categorized medications based upon known or possible risk to a developing fetus as listed in Table 19.2. Increasing uterine size, greater tendency for vomiting, and many other changes also increase the complexity of PSA during pregnancy.

Informed Consent

The physician responsible for the sedation should provide to the patient and/or parents' information concerning the objectives of the sedation, behavioral changes associated with the sedative regimen (especially important when the parent/guardian plans to remain with the patient during the sedation/procedure), and potential adverse effects during and after the sedation [59, 70, 95]. Parents should understand that, albeit rare, there is a risk of pulmonary aspiration, cardiopulmonary compromise, hypoxic brain injury, and/or death. *It is also recommended to discuss with them the*

Table 19.2 United States FDA pharmaceutical pregnancy categories

Category A	Adequate studies have failed to demonstrate a risk to the fetus in the first trimester of pregnancy and there is no evidence of risk in later trimesters
Category B	Animal reproduction studies have failed to demonstrate a risk to the fetus, and there are no adequate and well-controlled studies in pregnant women. Animal studies have shown an adverse effect, but adequate and well-controlled studies in pregnant women have failed to demonstrate a risk to the fetus in any trimester
Category C	Animal reproduction studies have shown an adverse effect on the fetus and there are no adequate and well-controlled studies in humans, but potential benefits may warrant use of the drug in pregnant women despite potential risks
Category D	There is a positive evidence of human fetal risk based on adverse reaction data from investigational or marketing experience or studies in humans, but potential benefits may warrant use of the drug in pregnant women despite potential risks
Category X	Studies in animals or humans have demonstrated fetal abnormalities and/or there is positive evidence of human fetal risk based on adverse reaction data from investigational or marketing experience, and the risks involved in use of the drug in pregnant women clearly outweigh potential benefits

possible need for muscle relaxation, intubation, hospitalization, and unsuccessful sedation with inability to perform the procedure. These issues that have been discussed with the parent/guardian (and patient when appropriate) and that they have given their informed consent to proceed with the sedation should be documented on the sedation record.

Adverse effects/events generally discussed include:

- Incomplete analgesia and/or amnesia
- Respiratory depression/apnea
- Pulmonary aspiration
- Psychosis and recovery dysphoria
- Catatonia/nystagmus
- Dysrhythmias

Plan for Sedation

(a) Selection of a medication plan

Selection of medications and dosages should be guided by the desired key effect(s). An ideal regimen would provide acceptable analgesia, sedation, and amnesia for residual awareness of procedure-related pain or anxiety, cause minimal adverse effects, and work reliably with a wide therapeutic index; i.e., small differences in dose would not cause oversedation or adverse events, have rapid onset and recovery, and be easy to titrate to effect. No single agent or combination of agents fully achieves these goals. Selection of procedural sedation medications therefore is based upon balancing desired effects with the potential for adverse effects. For procedures that are very painful (e.g., fracture reduction), control of the pain will be paramount. For procedures that require the child to be motionless—e.g., computerized tomography (CT) or magnetic resonance imaging (MRI) scans—immobility may be most important. Most procedures in children require some combination of analgesia and immobility along with anxiolysis; therefore, sedation planning can be broadly organized into categories of these parameters.

Analgesia, hypnosis, anxiolysis, or amnesia? Balanced sedation: Medication selection and dose can be organized by anticipation of whether the procedure is (1) nonpainful/noninvasive or associated with (2) low level of pain and high anxiety or (3) high level of pain, high anxiety, or both, (4) whether local anesthesia can be used, and (5) whether the patient needs to be motionless; i.e., for some procedures, some motion is acceptable during painful and/or invasive procedures to the extent that the motion neither causes risk to the patient nor hinders the successful performance of the procedure, whereas in others (e.g., MRI), any movement prevents completing the procedure (see Table 19.3) [61, 96, 97].

Principle and secondary effects of sedative–analgesic medications are summarized in Table 19.4. Although combining sedative–analgesic medications generally increases the risks of adverse effects [98, 99], the actual depth of sedation is likely to be a better predictor of these risks [96, 100]. Thoughtful "balanced sedation" with anxiolytic and analgesic drugs, carefully titrated to effect, can achieve very satisfactory sedation and typically results in smaller effective doses of individual drugs than if a single drug is used. For example, fentanyl is a potent analgesic but has little or no anxiolytic or amnestic effect, whereas midazolam is a potent anxiolytic and amnestic agent with no analgesic effect. Combining fentanyl and midazolam results in effective procedural sedation, but the combination causes significantly greater respiratory depression than either fentanyl or midazolam alone [98].

Depth of sedation: Since increasing depth of sedation is associated with increasing frequency of adverse events [96, 101], use of the lightest effective sedation is usually preferred. However, frequently the depth of sedation required for a particular procedure cannot be accurately predicted in a specific patient [96]. Incompletely appreciated anxiety and lack of comprehension in younger children or those with developmental delay often cause need for deeper-than-anticipated sedation for procedures in which local anesthesia or mild sedation would suffice in a self-controlled adolescent or adult. For intensely painful procedures, deep sedation is typically required. Clinicians providing sedation, therefore, ideally should be trained and prepared to administer increasingly deeper

Table 19.3 Indications and strategies for procedural sedation and analgesia [96, 97]

Pain	Anxiety	Motion	Clinical examples	Suggestion sedation strategies
No	Moderate	Some acceptable	Echo, EEG, infant PFTs (sedation rarely needed)	Comforting, distraction
				Chloral hydrate PO (in patients <2 years of age)
				Midazolam PO
		Motionless	Computed tomography	Chloral hydrate PO (in patients <6 months of age)
			Magnetic resonance	Pentobarbital ± midazolam IV
				Propofol IV
Low or local anesthesia can be used	Moderate to high	Relatively motionless	Abscess incision and drainage	Topical or local anesthesia
		But some acceptable	Dental procedures, lumbar puncture	Comforting, distraction
			Flexible fiber-optic laryngoscopy	Oxycodone PO
			Ocular irrigation	Nitrous oxide
			Foreign-body removal	Midazolam PO, PR, IN, IV
			Phlebotomy, IV cannulation	
			Laceration repair, simple	
			Fracture reduction with hematoma block	
			Paraphimosis reduction	
			Sexual-assault examination	
High	Moderate to high	Relatively motionless	Abscess incision and drainage	Midazolam and fentanyl IV
		But some acceptable	Arthrocentesis	Ketamine IM or IV
			Bone marrow aspiration	Nitrous oxide and oxycodone PO
			Burn debridement	Propofol and ketamine or fentanyl IV
			Cardioversion	
			Foreign-body removal	
			Complicated	
			Fracture or dislocation reduction	
			Hernia reduction	
			Laceration repair, complex	
			Paracentesis	
			Thoracentesis	
			Thoracostomy-tube placement	

Table 19.4 Procedural sedation medication effects

Medication	Sedation	Analgesia	Amnesia	Anxiolysis	Emetogenic
Barbiturates	+++	–	–	–	
Benzodiazepines	+++	–	+++	+++	Antiemetogenic
Fentanyl	+	+++	–		++
Ketamine	+++	+++	++		+
Propofol	+++	–	+	+	Antiemetogenic
Chloral hydrate	++	–	–		
Nitrous oxide	++	++	+–++	+++	++

sedation as guided by the patient's response to the procedure. It is important, too, for the clinician to realize that many sedative analgesic agents also induce varying degrees of amnesia. When midazolam, ketamine, or propofol, and to a lesser extent nitrous oxide, are administered, the patient is unlikely to recall clearly procedure-related pain despite occasional moaning or crying out during intensely painful parts of the procedure [9]. However, it is unwise to promise complete amnesia during the informed consent process. The extent of procedural amnesia can be assessed in part by asking the patient if he/she "recalls anything hurting" after they have recovered; a negative answer is reassuring to parents who have remained with the patient during the procedure. Because of amnesia for procedure-related pain, lighter and presumably safer levels of sedation may be acceptable when patient motion does not interfere with accomplishment of the procedure.

For this reason, the amnestic agent midazolam is combined with fentanyl for PSA because completely effective analgesia cannot be achieved with fentanyl without marked respiratory depression. Of note, deeper sedation with ketamine is usually much less associated with adverse cardiopulmonary effects in comparison to other agents and, in addition, ketamine induces moderate amnesia.Some older children may prefer not to be deeply sedated; in the same way many adults fear general anesthesia. As an example, a 13-year-old boy sedated by the author with nitrous oxide in conjunction with a lidocaine fracture hematoma block recalled the next day the details of the reduction of his displaced distal radius and ulnar fractures. Yet, he was adamant that he would not have preferred to have been "put to sleep" and unaware of the reduction. Since the hematoma block was very effective and he recalled no pain, he was very satisfied with his experience of altered awareness during the fracture reduction. When local anesthesia or other analgesic technique can be achieved, some children may prefer lighter levels of sedation without loss of awareness, a concept that needs further investigation.

(b) Staffing

For moderate sedation, a sedation provider trained in the sedation protocol and skilled in pediatric advanced life-support techniques is responsible for the procedural sedation–analgesia, including monitoring of the patient's status. In the ED, this is typically the emergency physician. If, after induction of adequate sedation, that individual then performs the procedure for which sedation is provided, a second individual, typically a registered nurse, with sedation training and knowledgeable in pediatric basic life support must be at the bedside and responsible for monitoring the patient's cardiopulmonary status and the need for interventions to manage adverse events. This second individual often is responsible for recording the patient's status on the sedation record and may assist with minor, interruptible tasks once the patient's level of sedation and cardiopulmonary functions have stabilized, provided that adequate monitoring of the patient is maintained [59, 68, 70, 102].

For deep sedation in the ED, a sedation provider, again, typically the emergency physician, with training in the pharmacology of the agents to be administered and skilled in pediatric advanced life support must be in the procedure room and is responsible for the procedural sedation–analgesia, including monitoring of the patient's status. At least one clinician must be assigned to monitor and record the patient's airway patency and cardiorespiratory status and, in contrast to moderate sedation planning, should have no other responsibilities during induction of sedation, the procedure, and the early post-procedure period when the patient is at greatest risk for respiratory depression, partial upper airway obstruction, and aspiration. If an experienced sedation provider has induced adequate sedation and will then perform the procedure, primary responsibility for monitoring the patient's cardiopulmonary status may be designated to a second sedation-trained clinician, typically a registered nurse, if the responsible provider can easily interrupt performance of the procedure to assist with or assume management of adverse events. It should not be planned that the clinician monitoring the patient would assist with the procedure as that may distract this clinician from monitoring the patient's vital signs and clinical status or interfere with rapid intervention [59, 68, 70, 102, 103]. Brief, interruptible assistance with the procedure may be provided by this person but with caution and with assured concurrent attention to the patient's vital functions. Safe use of deep sedation is dependent upon this clinician's meticulous attention to the patient's airway and breathing and anticipation and early recognition of adverse events. Threats to ventilation and oxygenation usually are easily managed when rapidly recognized and interventions immediately implemented. Experience with deep sedation has shown that some patients (~5–25 %) will develop oxygen desaturation of <90 % and partial upper airway obstruction, both of which are usually easily managed when rapidly recognized.

Since deeper-than-intended sedation may occur or be necessary in any patient, it is recommended that all but the lightest sedations (e.g., use of nitrous oxide) be staffed and monitored as if deep sedation may occur, particularly when gaining initial experience with sedation protocols or using agents with narrow therapeutic indices (e.g., propofol, midazolam + fentanyl, or etomidate). This usually means a third provider is needed if assistance will be necessary in performing the procedure. In addition, at least one provider should be present who is intimately familiar with location of resuscitation and other necessary medical equipment.

In most hospitals, physician sedation providers and nurses must be credentialed to administer PSA. Credentialing typically includes didactic sessions on use of specific PSA medications, demonstration of safe and effective administration of PSA, and competency in skills needed for rescue from adverse events [95].

(c) Monitoring and equipment

Direct patient observation: In addition to electrophysiological monitoring, airway patency, rate and depth of respiration, and the child's color (nail beds, mucosa) should be checked frequently by vigilant direct observation, especially after each medication administration and in the early postprocedure period when painful procedural stimuli have ended. This enables essential immediate interventions for adverse events such as marked respiratory depression, positional obstruction of the upper airway as muscle relaxation occurs (snoring, paradoxical chest wall motion without exhaled breaths may be noted), or vomiting. Opening of the airway by realignment or jaw thrust, applying painful stimulation to awaken and induce breathing, administering supplemental oxygen, or turning and suctioning to clear vomit often are usually all that is needed to correct problems that can otherwise rapidly deteriorate to life-threatening situations.

Direct monitoring during recovery should continue by a designated healthcare provider until the patient emerges to a level of moderate sedation; thereafter direct monitoring can be designated to the child's parent or another responsible adult with the healthcare provider immediately available until the patient returns to the pre-sedation level of responsiveness [59, 68, 102, 103].

Patients undergoing sedation should wear a loose-fitting top or hospital gown to ensure easy direct observation of the chest. The patient's mouth and nose should not be obscured and skin should be visible for monitoring of color. A stethoscope should be immediately available.

For *moderate sedation*, in addition to direct observation, measurement of oxygen saturation by pulse oximetry is strongly recommended [59, 68, 102, 103]. Additional continuous electrophysiological monitoring throughout sedation and recovery of ECG-based heart rates, respiratory rates, and noninvasive automated blood pressures measured after each medication bolus and/or every 5 min add further measures of safety.

For *deep sedation*, in addition to direct observation, routine use of noninvasive physiologic monitoring should include continuously measured oxygen saturation, heart rate, and respiratory rate, and, in addition, noninvasive automated blood pressure measurements after each medication bolus and/or every 5 min throughout sedation and recovery [59, 68, 102, 103].

Pulse oximetry has been demonstrated to detect hypoxemia well before cyanosis occurs and is therefore critical for monitoring for respiratory compromise. In one study of infants, O_2 saturations were ≤83 % before perioral cyanosis was detected by experienced emergency pediatricians [104]. Monitoring of oxygen saturation with pulse oximetry has been suggested as the most important means of reducing sedation-related injury and should be used for all but minimal sedations [59, 68, 70, 100, 102, 103]. The *pulse oximeter audible tone should be activated* to alert providers to changes without the need to frequently read the monitor instead of observing the patient.

End-tidal CO_2 capnography provides breath-to-breath information on the effectiveness of ventilation and is increasingly being investigated in patients undergoing ED PSA. Assessment of ventilation by continuous end-tidal CO_2 capnography has been found more sensitive than either direct observation or decreases in oxygen saturation in detecting respiratory depression or airway obstruction. Changes in capnographic waveform and/or changes in end-tidal CO_2 are frequently noted well before changes in oxygen saturation, including in patients' breathing room air [105–111]. Of note, no changes in end-tidal CO_2 were found in children sedated with ketamine alone [112, 113]. Changes in end-tidal CO_2 capnography can aid in early recognition of respiratory depression and/or airway obstruction and allow initial interventions that may avert the need to administer positive-pressure ventilations, e.g., limitation of further administration of sedative medications or opening of the airway. Assisted ventilation during oxygen desaturation due to apnea or periods of respiratory depression should be administered as needed. However, positive-pressure ventilation increases gastric pressures due to insufflation of air into the stomach. At a depth of sedation that induces apnea or significant respiratory depression, there is likely concurrent relaxation of esophageal muscle tone and significant blunting of protective airway reflexes. Thus, there is likely increased risk of pulmonary aspiration associated with positive-pressure ventilation due to gastroesophageal reflux into the oropharynx.

Routine administration of supplemental oxygen has been recommended to prevent hypoxemia during deep and moderate sedation [103]. However, sedation providers should recognize that administration of supplemental oxygen may delay oxygen desaturation for several minutes during respiratory depression or apnea [114]. Therefore, use of supplemental oxygen may delay recognition of these adverse events with their likely concurrent depression of protective airway reflexes, unless the patient is also monitored by end-tidal CO_2 with capnography [115]. Similarly, recognition of airway obstruction is likely delayed [105–109, 112, 116]. When capnography is unavailable, consideration should be given to monitoring patients by pulse oximetry as they breathe room air. Although an indirect and less-sensitive measure of ventilation than capnography, decreases in oxygen saturation alert the clinician to decreases in ventilation and facilitate interventions before hypoxemia and a need for positive-pressure ventilation occurs. With this strategy, administration of supplemental oxygen may be reserved for patients whose oxygen saturations drop below 90 % without rapid rise in response to airway maneuvers such as head tilt/jaw thrust and/or stimulation. Respiratory depression is sufficiently commonplace during sedation with propofol that many providers recommend as routine administration of supplemental oxygen during propofol PSA [107, 108, 117].

Equipment

Resuscitation equipment must be immediately available. A self-inflating (Ambu-type) bag–mask positive-pressure device with a PEEP attachment and appropriately sized mask, continuous oxygen supply, and an airway suctioning device with a large rigid suction tip should be prepared for each sedation. Anesthesia-style CPAP bags, endotracheal intubation equipment, and resuscitation medications, with a dosing guide, including reversal agents such as naloxone and flumazenil, a paralytic agent such as succinylcholine, and antiepileptic and antiarrhythmic medications for drug-induced seizures and dysrhythmias should be immediately available for all sedations [59, 68, 70, 102, 103].

No suction apparatus can clear the oropharynx during active vomiting. The patient must be helped to turn or roll to the side or to sit upright to clear his airway. The suction device is used to clear residual emesis from the mouth after active vomiting has stopped. If the patient is unresponsive and emesis is noticed in the posterior pharynx or mouth, the patient should be rapidly rolled to the side to allow emesis to passively flow out as suctioning of the posterior pharynx is performed; there is significant risk for pulmonary aspiration in this situation.

Intravenous access adds an additional invasive procedure to the patient's treatment, but it enables easily controlled and rapid titration of medications and provides an increased margin of safety by enabling rapid administration of reversal and resuscitation agents, if needed. When medications are administered intravenously, the intravenous access should be maintained throughout sedation and recovery. When medications are administered by a non-intravenous route (e.g., by intramuscular injection), whether to establish intravenous access should be decided on an individual basis. If vascular access is not established, the ability to immediately accomplish such must exist for all sedations, especially when a multiple drug sedation regimen is used. For agents that frequently cause hypotension (e.g., propofol), it is recommended that intravenous access be established with an indwelling catheter and maintained with a resuscitation fluid (lactated Ringer's solution or normal saline). Patients who have been NPO for an extended period may benefit from an infusion of 10–20 mL/kg of LR or NS to counter any hypotensive effects of sedation medications. A stopcock near the hub of the IV catheter (e.g., on the tail of a T-connector inserted into the hub of the catheter and in-line with the IV fluids) facilitates controlled and complete administration of sedation medications. This setup allows a syringe containing the sedative to be connected to the stopcock and the medication injected near the hub as the IV fluids infuse. This reduces the possibility of uncertain medication infusion amount and rate that might occur if the medication is added considerably upstream of the catheter hub. For agents such as ketamine that do not frequently cause hypotension, an indwelling "saline lock" is typically sufficient; the ketamine can be flushed into the bloodstream with 5–10 mL boluses of saline following ketamine administration.

A mnemonic some find helpful in preparing equipment is MS MAID: Machine Suction – Monitors Airway (oral airway, bag-mask, ETT, blade) IV Drugs.

Preparation for and Management of Adverse Events

Anticipation

The rarity of serious adverse events in ED PSA can lull the provider into complacency [118, 119]. It is suggested that the possibility of a life-threatening event during PSA should be thought of as inevitable, as a matter of "when" rather than "if." Since these events are so infrequent and variations in individuals' responses to a medication are not always predictable, the provider must always be prepared.

Effective management of adverse events begins first and foremost with preparation for the planned sedation. Thorough pre-sedation evaluation to identify patients at increased risk for adverse events or difficult airway management, monitoring and staffing based upon intended sedation depth, and immediate availability of resuscitation equipment and medications are critical. Factors associated with serious adverse outcomes include late recognition of hypoxemia and inadequate resuscitation, thus emphasizing the importance of preparation and continual monitoring during the sedation and recovery periods [100]. If recognized early, most adverse effects can be addressed effectively with relatively minor interventions. Stimulation, airway realignment, jaw thrust, and supplemental oxygen are usually all that is needed to avoid further deterioration to life-threatening events [119].

Management of Respiratory Depression and Apnea

Respiratory depression is one of the most common potentially serious effects of pediatric PSA [67, 118, 119]. A critical incident analysis of serious adverse outcomes in pediatric sedation found 80 % initially presented with respiratory depression [100]. Widespread use of pulse oximetry has since dramatically improved early recognition of respiratory depression. Agents commonly associated with respiratory depression include the sedative–hypnotics (barbiturates, benzodiazepines, chloral hydrate, propofol), particularly when used in conjunction with opioids [101, 120].

Apnea has also been rarely reported with administration of ketamine [121–123].

Avoiding respiratory depression (see also Basic Pharmacokinetics): Most sedative medications variably blunt brainstem receptor response to increases in plasma levels of CO_2. Since response to rising levels of CO_2 determines breathing rate and depth, significant increases in sedative concentrations in the brainstem quickly lead to respiratory depression or apnea. The more rapidly a sedative drug is infused, the higher its initial brainstem concentration and the greater the respiratory depression. A primary strategy for reducing respiratory depression and maintaining adequate ventilation (and, in association, oxygenation) is slow administration of PSA drugs, often achieved by repeatedly infusing half or less of the total expected dose until the desired effect is achieved (titration). Ketamine can be an exception to the recommended slow administration approach because of its unique relative lack of respiratory depression. Taking advantage of first-pass kinetics, experienced sedators may choose to administer smaller doses rapidly for very brief procedures (see "Ketamine" section).

At-risk periods: Patients may experience respiratory depression at any time during the sedation, but the greatest risks are immediately after medication administration and again after cessation of painful procedural stimuli [124].

Recognition of ineffective ventilation: As detailed previously, direction observation of the patient including general color and chest wall movement continues to be one of the most important means of recognizing respiratory depression and/or airway obstruction. The patient's oropharynx and chest wall should be directly visible at all times to facilitate observation for lack of respiratory effort or respiratory effort without air exchange. In addition, *pulse oximetry with audible tone* and *end-tidal capnography* facilitate detection of ventilatory changes before they are clinically apparent.

Airway and Ventilation Maintenance

Initial management of hypoventilation may simply require *verbal encouragement* to the patient *to breathe* as their sensitivity to rising CO_2 has been blunted by the sedation medications. Patients who have received opioids such as fentanyl may be awake but "forget" to breathe. *Stimulation*, painful if necessary, to arouse the patient may improve muscle tone and prompt breathing. If oxygen saturations are falling despite these maneuvers, supplemental oxygen administration and airway-opening maneuvers and/or positive-pressure ventilation may be necessary. See section below for management of "Upper Airway Obstruction."

Treatment: Respiratory Depression and Apnea

When monitors alarm (e.g., indicating dropping oxygen saturation), ASSESS THE PATIENT. DO NOT presume the pulse oximeter probe has slipped off, monitor malfunction, etc. Evaluate equipment later!

First Line (in Rapid Succession, if Needed)

1. Verbally encourage or stimulate patient to breathe deeply (patients may require intensely painful stimuli, e.g., squeezing the fracture site or a hard sternal rub with knuckles); if insufficient, then do number 2.
2. Support airway (chin lift/jaw thrust); if insufficient, then do number 3.
3. Administer supplemental oxygen.
4. If spontaneous ventilation continues to be inadequate, administer positive-pressure ventilation via bag–mask.
5. If patient is on a continuous infusion (e.g., propofol)—slow down or stop medication infusion, and then do number 6.
6. Call for help, if needed.

Second Line: Reversal Medications for Opioids and Benzodiazepines

If respiratory depression occurs after administration of an opioid or benzodiazepine and does not readily resolve after the above supportive measures, or requires continued positive-pressure ventilation, consider use of reversal agents. *Slow, titrated reversal* is preferred if positive-pressure ventilation is effective. The desired endpoint is lessening of the respiratory depression with slightly lighter sedation. Rapid, full reversal may lead to severe pain, hypertension, and agitation or seizure [125]. Reversal agents are rarely needed by experienced sedation providers.

Naloxone (Narcan®)

Indications: opioid-induced apnea, respiratory depression, or "wooden/rigid chest syndrome" not responding to stimulation, airway-opening maneuvers, supplemental oxygen, and/or positive-pressure ventilations.

Dose: 1–2 mg/kg (0.001–0.002 mg/kg) *IV push* repeated every 1–3 min until the patient begins to have spontaneous respirations. Doses of 1–2 mg/kg are recommended to "gently" reverse opioid-induced respiratory depression yet maintain analgesia. Larger doses, such as 10–100 mg/kg, may awaken the patient and reverse the analgesic effects resulting in significant pain, hypertension, pulmonary edema, vomiting, or seizures [125].

During the interval of apnea, the patient is supported with assisted ventilations until adequate spontaneous respirations are restored. Thereafter, the patient is observed closely as the reversal effects of naloxone may be briefer than the opioid-induced respiratory depression. For "wooden chest syndrome," if the patient cannot be ventilated and oxygen saturations are dropping rapidly, naloxone may be given in 1 or 2 mg boluses for convenience. Alternatively, succinylcholine 1–2 mg/kg may be used to paralyze the patient.

Caution: Opioid-induced respiratory effects may outlast the duration of naloxone, and patients must be closely monitored for recurrence of respiratory depression, typically at least 2 h after naloxone administration [126].

Flumazenil (Romazicon®)

Indications: Benzodiazepine (e.g., midazolam)-induced apnea or respiratory depression not responding to stimulation, airway-opening maneuvers, supplemental oxygen, and/or positive-pressure ventilation.

Dose: 0.01–0.04 mg/kg (maximum 0.5 mg) IV over 30 s. Repeat every 60 s to desired response. A cumulative dose of 3 mg may be necessary. Flumazenil may reverse midazolam-induced hypnotic and amnestic effects but may not reverse ventilatory depression [127]. When appropriate, naloxone should be used as the first line in reversal therapy. Drug therapy does not obviate the need to protect the airway and support ventilation.

Caution: Flumazenil may cause seizures in patients chronically on benzodiazepine medications and should be used cautiously in patients on medications that can lower seizure threshold. Also, benzodiazepine-induced respiratory effects may outlast the duration of flumazenil, and patients must be closely monitored for recurrence of respiratory depression, typically at least 2 h after flumazenil administration [128, 129]. Recurrence of sedation has been reported in up to 7 % of cases, most commonly in children under 5 years of age [128] (Table 19.5).

Upper Airway Obstruction

The pediatric airway is particularly prone to dynamic obstruction due to the relatively large size of the tongue and tonsillar tissues. As sedation depth increases, the muscles of the tongue, jaw, and oropharynx lose tone in a manner similar to deep sleep. Sedation-induced "obstructive sleep apnea" may result in partial or complete airway obstruction, exacerbated by the supine position and nasal passage obstruction. A history of snoring or obstructive sleep apnea alerts the clinician to the increased likelihood of this occurrence. Placement of a shoulder roll in infants and a head roll in older children and adolescents to align the oropharynx, posterior pharynx, and trachea may help align the patient's airway and relieve this obstruction. Markedly, obese patients also may benefit from a large head or shoulder roll to compensate for their large trunk.

A jaw thrust or chin lift may be necessary to open the upper airway by pulling the tongue and related muscles away from the posterior pharynx. Patients who are very deeply sedated or have inadvertently reached the depth of general anesthesia may benefit from placement of an oro- or nasopharyngeal airway, but because oropharyngeal airways may induce a gag reflex and vomiting, these devices should be used with caution. Laryngospasm is a special type of upper airway obstruction and is addressed later in this chapter.

At-risk periods: Positional airway obstruction may occur at any time during sedation but, in association with respiratory depression, it may more likely be shortly after medication administration or after the painful procedural stimulus has ended. Ketamine-related laryngospasm may occur in settings of current URI, unsuctioned secretions/vomitus, or stimulation of the hyperactive gag reflex during a procedure.

Recognition of upper airway obstruction: Signs of partial upper airway obstruction include stridor or noisy breathing. Paradoxical chest wall movement (sucking in of the chest and distention of the abdomen with inspiration) may be seen with partial or complete obstruction. Hypoxemia is a late sign. An obstructive pattern is seen on capnography well before changes in oxygen saturation and allows early detection of airway obstruction (or apnea).

Table 19.5 Naloxone and flumazenil for reversal of respiratory depression [129]

Agent	Route	Dose	Frequency	Maximum dose (mg)	Onset	Duration (min)
Naloxone	IV, IM, or SC	1–2 μg/kg for respiratory depression 100 μg/kg (0.1 mg/kg) if unable to ventilate or *wooden chest*	Q 2–3 min as needed	2	1–2 min (IV) 15 min (IM/SC)	30–60
Flumazenil	IV	10 μg/kg (0.01 mg/kg)	Q 1 min as needed	1[a]	1–2 min, maximum effect 6–10 min	20–60

[a]If resedation after response to flumazenil, additional doses of up to 1 mg/dose may be given Q 20 min to a maximum total dose of 3 mg

Treatment

1. Align airway and open with chin lift or jaw thrust; provide supplemental oxygen as needed.
2. Suction airway if excessive secretions are present.
3. If not responding to repositioning, consider continuous positive airway pressure (CPAP) with bag–mask (CPAP or anesthesia-type bag is preferable to self-inflating-type bag as CPAP can be delivered more effectively to open the airway by distending the posterior pharynx).
4. If having difficulty maintaining an open airway, consider an oral airway (unconscious patient) or nasal airway.
5. If unable to ventilate with CPAP, rapidly consider treatment for laryngospasm with *succinylcholine*.

Laryngospasm

Laryngospasm is an uncommon but *potentially life-threatening* sedation-related adverse event. It is a partial or complete upper airway obstruction, with oxygen desaturation, caused by involuntary and sustained closure of the vocal cords and is not relieved by routine airway repositioning maneuvers, suctioning, or insertion of a nasal or oral airway. Laryngospasm may be intermittent or sustained and brief or prolonged [130, 131].

The incidence of laryngospasm during pediatric ED PSA is difficult to determine as it is a rare event and large sedation databases are not available for estimation. Relative preservation of upper airway protective reflexes during ketamine-based sedation reduces the risk of pulmonary aspiration and thus makes ketamine one of the safest agents for ED PSA in unfasted children, yet, paradoxically, ketamine PSA may have increased risk for laryngospasm [132–134]. A meta-analysis of pediatric ketamine-based ED PSA found an incidence of laryngospasm of 0.3 %; the only identifiable association with increased risk of laryngospasm was an initial intravenous dose of greater than 2.5 mg/kg, but data was unable to be analyzed for associations with URI, wheezing, or other risk factors found to be associated with increased risk during general anesthesia [135]. Of particular interest, young age and oropharyngeal procedures (excluding endoscopy) were not associated with increased risk, but prospective larger data sets are needed to better clarify these risks.

Laryngospasm in almost 50,000 non-intubated children undergoing elective propofol sedation/anesthesia was noted to occur at a rate of 21/10,000 (0.2 %) [88]. Laryngospasm associated with general anesthesia has been estimated as high as 14 % in younger children and as low as 0.1 %, with lower likelihood reported in non-intubated children [136, 137]. The wide variability may be due to differences in definition and study design, patient populations, anesthetic techniques, and airway manipulation [138]. However, consistently noted risk factors for laryngospasm include young age, upper respiratory infection, asthma, manipulation of the airway, and exposure to smoking in the home [139, 140].

It is unclear whether prophylactic administration of atropine or glycopyrrolate with ketamine to reduce hypersalivation reduces the risk of laryngospasm [141, 142]. The meta-analysis of pediatric ketamine-based ED PSA, noted earlier, found that overall airway and respiratory adverse events (but not laryngospasm) were actually increased in children who received concurrent anticholinergics [135]; this unexpected association needs further investigation.

At-risk periods: Laryngospasm may occur at any time during sedation, including recovery. In one report of non-intubated children undergoing sedation/general anesthesia, laryngospasm occurred most frequently during emergence (48 %) but was also seen during induction (29 %) and maintenance (24 %) phases [137]. Increased risk for ketamine-related laryngospasm may occur in children with current URI, especially if febrile, if secretions/emeses pool in the posterior pharynx, or if a procedure such as endoscopy stimulates the gag reflex [140, 143, 144].

Recognition of laryngospasm: Early signs of laryngospasm may include coughing. A characteristic stridulous noise can be heard with partial laryngospasm. Chest wall movement is noted, but there is a mismatch between the patients' respiratory effort and the small amount of air exchange. If complete laryngospasm occurs, no stridulous noise will be heard and no air exchange or breath sounds will be noted despite chest wall movement. No ventilation with a bag–mask device will be possible.

Oxygen saturations will drop rapidly if the patient is breathing room air, typically within 30–60 s. If the patient has been preoxygenated, saturations may remain above 90 % for 1–5+ min, dropping more rapidly in younger children and infants [114]. Capnographic changes are a very sensitive means of diagnosing laryngospasm. During partial laryngospasm, turbulence affects expiratory flow, but the amplitude of the capnogram will correlate with the extent of hypoventilation. During complete laryngospasm the CO_2 waveform will be lost despite chest wall movement [110].

Treatment (Fig. 19.2) [134]

If the patient develops stridor during sedation:

1. *Remove stimulus* to posterior oropharynx; consider gentle suction of excessive secretions and emesis.
2. *Reposition airway* with jaw thrust; vigorous, painful intrusion of the thumbs in the *laryngospasm notch*[2] may help.

[2]The laryngospasm notch is behind the lobule of each ear, between the ascending ramus of the mandible and the mastoid process and the base of the skull. Painful pressure at this point over the styloid process is thought to cause afferent input that causes relaxation of the cords by a poorly defined mechanism. This maneuver may also be a modified jaw thrust.

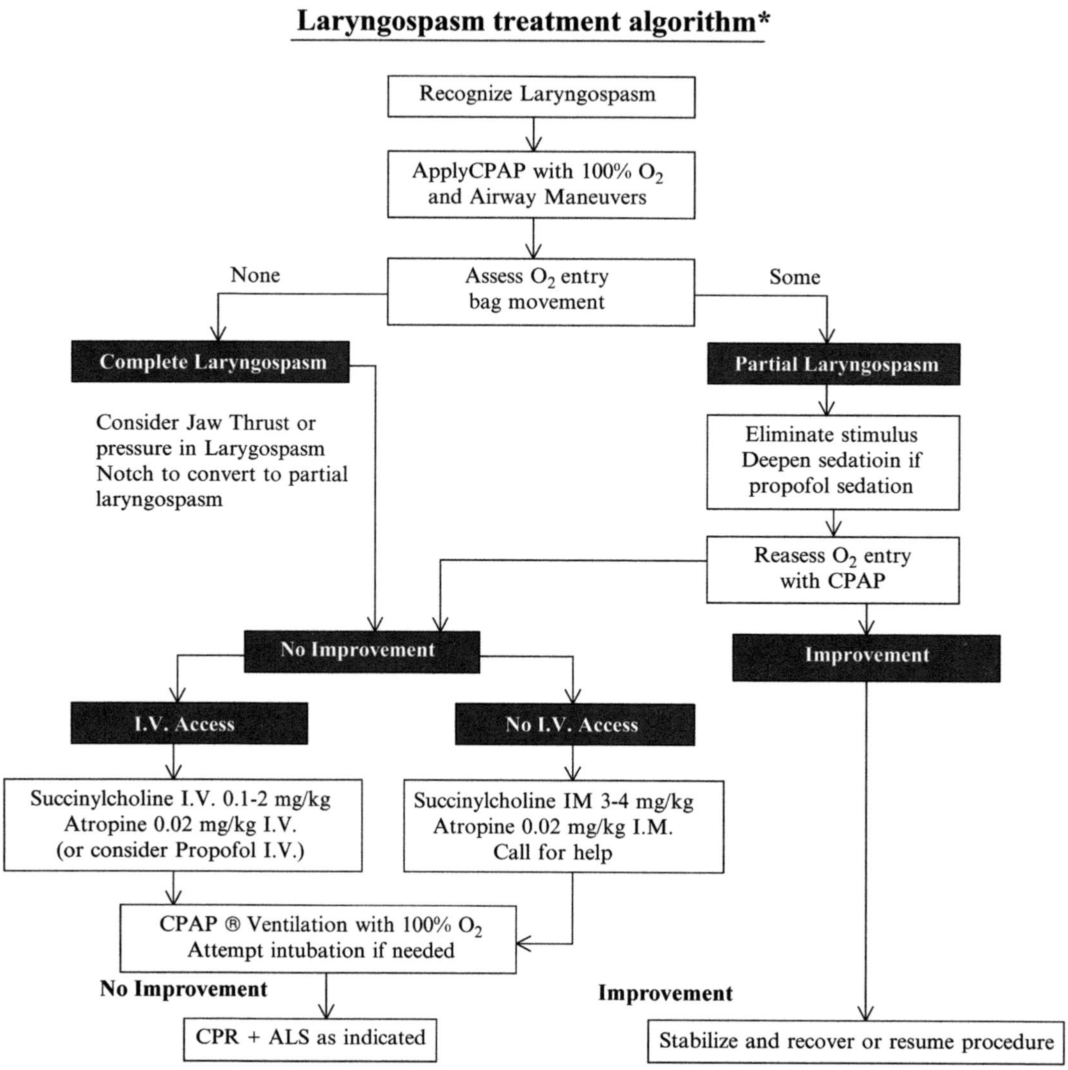

Fig. 19.2 Laryngospasm treatment algorithm (Modified for sedation from Hompson-Evans et al. [145])

3. *Apply CPAP* (continuous positive airway pressure) with *100% O_2* with anesthesia-type bag–mask; CPAP may reduce partial obstruction by distending the posterior pharynx, which exerts pull to open the partially closed larynx and vocal cords.
4. *Assess air movement*, if unable to oxygenate with CPAP.
5. Rapidly consider *atropine 0.02 mg/kg IV followed by low-dose succinylcholine (0.1–0.25 mg/kg IV)* with ventilatory support as needed [146]; consider an additional dose of *propofol* if propofol sedation is underway.
6. If still unable to oxygenate, administer *full-dose succinylcholine (1–2 mg/kg IV or 3–4 mg/kg IM)* followed by intubation.

Attempts to provide intermittent positive-pressure ventilation with a face mask may distend the stomach and make subsequent ventilation more difficult. In complete laryngospasm CPAP may worsen the obstruction by forcing the area just above the false cords closed. Therefore, if complete spasm cannot be broken, early IV agents should be considered [134].

When laryngospasm occurs in the midst of propofol PSA, deepening the sedation with administration of an additional 0.5 mg/kg of propofol has been shown to be an effective treatment for laryngospasm [147]. Transient apnea with this technique should be anticipated.

Low-dose succinylcholine (0.1 mg/kg IV) may be effective in relaxing laryngospasm [146]. Onset of neuromuscular blockade is generally more rapid at the larynx compared with the peripheral muscles [148]. Relaxation of the larynx induced with this small dose will be brief but may allow the patient to be oxygenated by CPAP and intubation avoided. Alternatively, administration of a fully paralyzing dose (1–3 mg/kg IV) followed by intubation should be considered if the patient is rapidly becoming severely hypoxic [134]. The intravenous route is preferred for administration of succinylcholine, but if there is no vascular access, it can be administered intramuscularly at a dose of 3–4 mg/kg. Although full effect may take about 4 min, onset of relaxation of the larynx occurs earlier than maximum suppression of the muscle twitch response and enables ventilation [149].

Succinylcholine administration following hypoxia may be associated with severe bradycardia and even cardiac arrest. *Atropine 0.02 mg/kg IV* administered prior to succinylcholine is recommended [150].

Emesis

Nausea and vomiting occur in 5–25 % of children during or after ED PSA. Use of opioids before or during sedation increases the likelihood of vomiting [90, 151], whereas concurrent use of midazolam with an opioid [9], ketamine [89], or nitrous oxide [10] reduces the incidence of PSA-related vomiting. Propofol appears to be less emetogenic and may not benefit from addition of midazolam to the regimen. Coadministration of ondansetron (Zofran®) with ketamine reduces vomiting both in the ED and after discharge [94]. Children with a history of prior postoperative nausea and vomiting or with a history of motion sickness are at increased risk for vomiting [152]. Further investigations are needed to better predict sedation-associated nausea and vomiting and to determine strategies to significantly reduce this relatively minor but very undesirable adverse effect.

At-risk periods: Emesis may occur at any point during procedural sedation but most commonly is seen during the postprocedure recovery period [9, 10, 90]. Since emesis can occur at any point and with every systemic agent used for procedural sedation, the provider responsible for monitoring the patient's airway should always be vigilant for signs of impending retching and prepared to turn the patient to the side to clear the airway. Suction equipment should be prepared and immediately available during and after all sedations. This equipment is used to finish clearing the emesis from the mouth after the patient stops vomiting. It is also advisable to have a large emesis basin at the bedside during each ED PSA.

Treatment: Emesis During Procedural Sedation

- Position patient's head to side, allow patient to clear own mouth during active vomiting, and suction oropharynx with rigid large bore Yankauer-type suction tip.
- If using nitrous oxide, immediately remove the mask to allow clearing of emesis and discontinue nitrous use, at least temporarily. It is preferred to allow the patient to hold the face mask during sedation with nitrous oxide so that they can immediately remove the mask if they feel nauseated.

Ondansetron (Zofran®)

An anti-serotonin agent, ondansetron is not routinely administered to prevent emesis during ED PSA. However, one study of children receiving ketamine for ED PSA showed that vomiting in the ED or after discharge was less frequent with ondansetron coadministration: 8 % versus 19 %, with 9 patients needing to be treated to prevent one episode of vomiting [94]. Ondansetron also may be considered in a child with significant prior history of postoperative nausea and vomiting. Further evaluation of the effectiveness of this antiemetic agent during ED PSA is needed. Other antiemetic agents such as prochlorperazine (Compazine®) and promethazine (Phenergan®) usually are not used because of sedating effects and increased risk for causing dystonic reactions.

Dose: IV, PO; 0.1–0.15 mg/kg, maximum dose 4 mg. Rapidly dissolving 4 mg oral tabs (ODT) are available and can be split in half for easy administration to young children. Dosing can be simplified by administering ondansetron ODT 2 mg to children 3 years of age and younger and 4 mg to children 4 years of age and older.

Cautions: may rarely cause bronchospasm, tachycardia, headaches, and lightheadedness.

Not requiring patients to drink fluids prior to discharge also may reduce vomiting. Historically, assuring patients can drink prior to discharge has been done to prevent postoperative "dehydration." Given shortened fasting times and the common practice of administration of IV fluids during sedation, the risk of dehydration is low compared to the risk of inducing vomiting [151].

Pulmonary Aspiration

Clinically significant or life-threatening pulmonary aspiration of gastric contents during pediatric procedural sedation is extremely rare. Aspiration occurs in approximately 0.1 % of cases under general anesthesia and was noted to have occurred in 4 of 49,836 children undergoing elective propofol sedation/anesthesia, but it has not been reported in association with ED PSA [73, 74, 80, 88]. Patients with ASA physical status Class III or higher and those requiring intubation are likely at higher risk. Risk for aspiration is likely greater, too, in patients who experience brief periods of apnea or significant respiratory depression as esophageal tone and protective airway reflexes may be absent during these periods and gastric contents may reflux into the trachea with little or no initial patient response. Because of the potential gravity of this adverse event, it is suggested clinicians consider using ketamine or nitrous oxide that better preserves protective airway reflexes or, when possible, lighter sedation combined with local anesthesia for non-fasted emergency patients [153].

Recognition: Clinical symptoms of pulmonary aspiration may include cough, crackles/rales, decreased breath sounds, tachypnea, wheeze, rhonchi, and respiratory distress that were not present before the sedation and present before the end of the ED recovery phase. These are usually accompanied by a decrease in oxygen saturation from baseline, requiring supplemental oxygen, and, if obtained, focal infiltrate, consolidation, or atelectasis on chest radiograph [80, 130]. As noted previously, clinically significant pulmonary aspiration may more likely occur in the unresponsive patient when gastric contents passively flow out of the stomach to the larynx. As the aspiration occurs, there may be little or no immediate signs due to the depth of sedation/anesthesia. The aspiration may become evident as the patient emerges from sedation.

Treatment: If emesis is seen, turn patient to side, allow to retch, and suction posterior pharynx as needed. Administer supplemental oxygen by nasal cannula or mask as needed. Many cases of transient hypoxia will resolve with this simple maneuver. CPAP may improve oxygenation in cases of severe aspiration with alveolar collapse. The majority of children who experience pulmonary aspiration require only close observation and simple supportive care with supplemental oxygen with or without CPAP and recover without sequelae [73, 74, 84, 88]. Endotracheal intubation should be considered if definitive protection of the airway or tracheal suctioning is required; RSI (rapid sequence induction) may be necessary. Uncommonly, severely symptomatic patients may need to be taken to the OR for emergent bronchoscopy with bronchial lavage of particulate matter. Arrange for appropriate continued monitoring, support, and work-up as needed including chest radiograph. For symptomatic patients, this usually means inpatient admission to an intensive care unit.

Medications

Basic Pharmacokinetics: Simplified

Parenteral drugs effective for PSA are small, hydrophobic lipophilic compounds that rapidly diffuse out of the bloodstream into the lipophilic tissues of the brain and spinal cord where they cause sedation/anesthesia.

Since the brain receives a disproportionately high percentage of the cardiac output (15–25 %) [154], a large portion of a sedative drug injected into the bloodstream circulates on first-pass out of the heart into the brain's circulation and quickly crosses the blood–brain barrier to exert its clinical effects within a single circulation time (first-pass or "one arm–brain" kinetics). As the drug circulates throughout the body and diffuses into muscle, bone, and, at a slower rate, into poorly perfused fat, the blood plasma concentration falls. The concentration gradient between the brain and the blood then favors drug diffusion out of the brain. As the brain's drug concentration falls, the drug effect lessens. This secondary reequilibration ("biphasic redistribution") causes the patient to awaken or respiratory depression to lessen. These effects are relatively independent of metabolic clearance of the drug from the body. PSA drugs' metabolic half-lives tend to be on the order of hours, whereas their sedative effect half-lives or "wake-up times" are on the order of minutes [155].

The duration of action of a single intravenous dose is similar for all these anesthetic/hypnotic drugs and is determined by redistribution of the drugs out of the brain. However, after repeated doses or prolonged infusions, a drug's duration of action is determined by complex interactions between the rate of redistribution of the drug, the amount of drug accumulated in fat, and the drug's metabolic clearance. The wake-up time of some drugs such as etomidate, propofol, and ketamine increases only modestly with prolonged infusions while others such as diazepam and thiopental increase dramatically and midazolam less so [155].

A rapidly injected drug travels as a more concentrated bolus on the first-pass out of the heart into the brain circulation than a slowly injected drug that is diluted by the passing blood. Thus, with rapid infusion, the initial concentration gradient between the plasma and the brain is greater. Consequently, the brain's concentration of the drug rises more rapidly and a greater portion of the administered dose enters the brain with resultant deeper sedation than when the same drug dose is slowly infused.

Thus, small doses of medications can have significant clinical effect if administered rapidly. Since the blood–brain concentration gradient also reverses more rapidly with these smaller doses, "wake-up" time may be shorter, making this strategy beneficial for brief procedures. Importantly, however, clinicians must be aware that rapid changes in the brainstem's concentration of opioid and sedative drugs markedly increase the potential for respiratory depression and apnea. As a practical point, this technique can be used only for ketamine administration because it causes markedly less respiratory depression than opioid and GABAergic drugs. This technique needs further study to delineate its safety and effectiveness and is suggested for consideration only by clinicians with extensive experience in ED PSA (Fig. 19.3).

A drug's *therapeutic window* is used to describe the difference between the dose of that drug that results in the

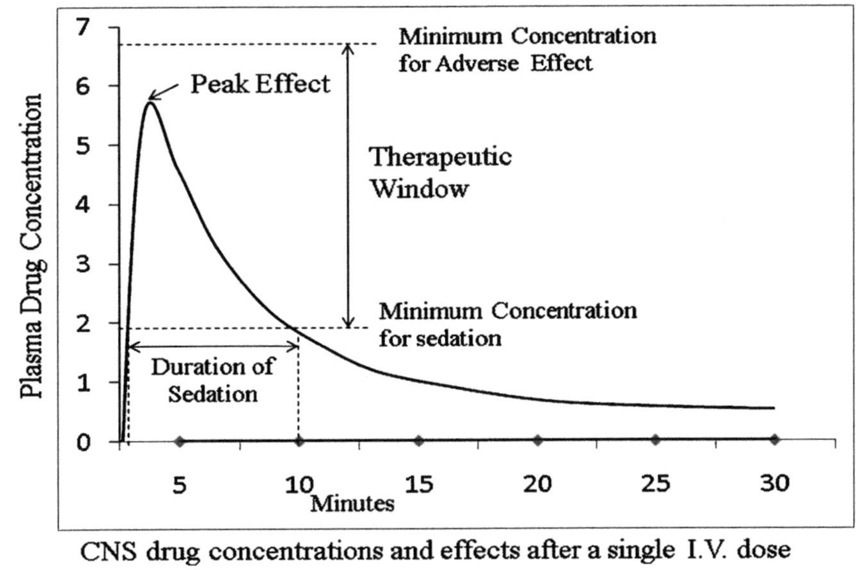

Fig. 19.3 Plasma drug concentration and CNS drug concentrations and effects after a single IV dose

desired sedative or analgesic effect and the dose that results in adverse effects. A drug with a wide therapeutic window has a greater margin of safety for use for ED PSA. For example, accidental administration of a tenfold greater-than-intended dose of ketamine will likely result in prolonged recovery but relatively little cardiopulmonary depression [156], whereas the same error with propofol will result in apnea and hypotension [157].

Many reasonable medication options exist for ED PSA [78, 158]. Use of analgesic medication when pain is the primary cause of distress is the key, and balancing analgesia with anxiolysis makes sedations more pleasant for patients. For nonpainful procedures when immobility is the primary objective, sedative–hypnotic medications may be chosen. It is recommended that the clinician initially become familiar with a few specific agents or combination of agents that provide the desired effects of analgesia, sedation, and/or anxiolysis. Limiting one's experience to a few agents better enables one to anticipate and manage adverse effects and events associated with those agents. One's pharmacologic armamentarium then can be gradually increased and refined with tailoring of regimens to a specific patient's characteristics. The following section summarizes medication effects and pharmacology in healthy children. Abnormalities in renal and hepatic function can significantly alter these parameters, particularly the duration of effects. In addition, significant variability in effect may occur between individuals due to genetically determined factors such as differences in drug receptor sites, metabolic activation, or clearance. Patients with ASA physical status Class III and higher also have less physiological reserves and therefore are more likely to have adverse effects with smaller doses.

Dosing Details

Titration to Desired Effect

Careful intravenous "titration" of medications using repeatedly administered small doses to achieve the desired clinical effect enables the practitioner to use the smallest effective dose and reduce the peril of oversedation with its increasing risks of respiratory depression and aspiration, and, furthermore, hasten recovery [70, 98, 103, 159]. Individual variation in sensitivity to the medication can also be detected; thus a smaller-than-expected dose may be found adequate for a given individual.

Knowledge of the time to peak effect of the specific medication is necessary to avoid "stacking" of doses when first gaining experience with titration. That is, if, to achieve deeper sedation, a subsequent dose is administered before the peak effect of the preceding dose has occurred, deeper-than-intended sedation can easily occur. For example, morphine has a peak effect of approximately 10 min. If an additional dose of morphine is administered after 5 min because the patient is still in significant pain, by 15 min after the original dose, when both the first and second doses are near peak effects, the patient may have significant respiratory depression due to an excessive accumulative dose. For this reason, titration is difficult with drugs that have longer than 1–3 min to peak effect time.

When a "typical" total dose for a specific procedure is known, that total dose may be divided and the increments administered at intervals shorter than "the time to peak effect" without likely overshoot. This strategy of repeated administration of fractional doses for fixed dose protocols—e.g., half of the anticipated total dose administered twice with administration separated by a short interval—reduces the risk for significant respiratory depression induced by some agents such as the combined technique using fentanyl and midazolam. This approach is suggested for providers who have less experience with a specific medication.

Intravenous Administration at the Hub

Injecting medications at or near the hub of the indwelling venous catheter allows one to know more precisely when the drug enters circulation and when the entire dose has been administered. This can avoid unintended continued infusion of residual drug in the intravenous tubing when adverse effects are occurring.

Intramuscular Administration

While IM administration avoids the need for placement of an IV catheter, it still requires a feared needlestick and makes titration to effect difficult. More importantly, if a serious adverse event occurs (e.g., severe laryngospasm), an emergent IV for resuscitation medications or fluids may be difficult to place. Specifically, ketamine-administered IM has been shown to be effective in achieving sedation. However, the IM route requires either use of a dose large enough to sedate all children—e.g., 4 mg/kg, which will oversedate some and result in greater frequency of adverse events [135]—or painful repeat administration of a smaller dose if the original dose is insufficient. Since the onset of IM ketamine is 5–15 min, titration without oversedation is difficult. Due to the large dose typically administered IM, recovery is prolonged [160].

Sedative–Hypnotic Agents

Commonly used sedative–hypnotic medications for procedural sedation include barbiturates, chloral hydrate, propofol, and etomidate. These drugs induce general depression of the central nervous system (CNS) by stimulation of inhibitory gamma-aminobutyric acid (GABA) receptors or other mechanisms that are not yet fully elucidated. None of these drugs have an analgesic effect. While deeply induced sedation (e.g., with propofol) may enable painful procedures to be accomplished, lighter sedation with less respiratory depression may be facilitated by the addition of an analgesic agent as described in subsequent sections. This chapter will review the common sedatives used in the ED with particular focus on their clinical applications and supporting literature from the speciality. (Refer to Chap. 9.)

Chloral Hydrate [78]

Indications: Chloral hydrate may be used to provide effective ED PSA in children less than 2 years of age, including those with congenital cardiac anomalies, who are undergoing painless diagnostic studies such as CT and MRI scans. Sedation is achieved in >80 % of young children. Chloral hydrate should not be considered a first-line agent in children older than 48 months because of decreased efficacy as compared with younger children. The drug may be administered orally or rectally. The oral preparation has a bitter taste that frequently requires administration in a flavored vehicle to disguise its taste; approximately a third of children may vomit soon after oral administration.

Contraindications/cautions/adverse effects: Children receiving chloral hydrate should be properly monitored and managed by appropriately trained personnel due to the risk of respiratory depression and hypoxia. Chloral hydrate should not be used in children with neurodevelopmental disorders due to an increased incidence of adverse effects and decreased efficacy as compared with healthy children. Chloral hydrate has the potential for resedation and may produce residual effects up to 24 h after administration. The elimination half-life is age dependent, with much longer effects in infants. These effects may occur long after the procedure is finished; reports describe infant deaths due to slumping in car seats with obstruction of the airway after discharge. Many infants may have unsteady gait, hyperactivity, or irritability the day after sedation. Other adverse effects include respiratory depression, hypotension, paradoxical excitement (0–15 %), vomiting (10–30 %), and, rarely, hepatic failure, areflexia, jaundice, gastrointestinal hemorrhage, and esophageal stricture [78, 161, 162]. These disadvantages along with its highly variable effects on older children and inherent difficulty with titration of oral medications make this agent less than ideal for children older than 1–2 years of age. Interestingly, children who have been fasted may have increased PSA failure rates. See Mace et al. for further details on dosing and adverse effects [78].

Pregnancy Category C

Dose: PO or PR; 50–125 mg/kg; typical initial dose 75 mg/kg. A second dose may be given, if needed, to a maximum of 2 g or 100–125 mg/kg total dose.

Onset/duration: sedation within 30–60 min, recovery by 60–120 min.

Mechanism of action: halogenated hydrocarbon with sedative–hypnotic but no analgesic effects.

Metabolization: rapidly metabolized by hepatic alcohol dehydrogenase to its active compound trichloroethanol and subsequently excreted in the urine [155]. The elimination half-life is age dependent: 40 h in preterm infant, 28 h in term infant, and 6–8 h in toddler.

Barbiturates

Barbiturates are pure sedatives with no analgesic effect. They potentiate the effect of GABA, the principal inhibitory neurotransmitter in the CNS, by binding to the $GABA_A$ receptor and prolonging the open time of the membrane chloride ion channel. In addition, barbiturates block the excitatory AMPA receptor [155].

Methohexital (Brevital®)

Indications: Methohexital administered by either the intravenous, intramuscular, or rectal route can provide effective sedation for children undergoing painless diagnostic studies such as CT or MRI scans. However, because of the readily induced respiratory depression associated with this medication, methohexital has not been used or studied extensively for procedural sedation in children, and thus its use should be considered only by experienced and knowledgeable clinicians.

Adverse effects: Respiratory depression and apnea are dose- and infusion rate dependent and are readily induced with intravenous administration but may occur with any route of administration. Hangover-like residual effects may last for 24 h.

Pregnancy Category B

Dosages: 1 mg/kg IV, 10 mg/kg IM, 25 mg/kg P.R.

Onset/duration: IV, sedation within 30 s; recovery by 20–30 min [163]

PR: sedation within 6–9 min, recovery by 40–60 min [164, 165]

Mechanism of action: ultrashort-acting, highly lipid-soluble barbiturate with rapid CNS uptake and redistribution. It has marked sedative–hypnotic but no analgesic effects.

Metabolization: Hepatic degradation with renal excretion results in an elimination half-life of 3.5 h and less accumulation of drug in body tissues compared to other barbiturates.

Pentobarbital (Nembutal®)

Indications: Pentobarbital is a short-acting barbiturate that induces relative immobility and can be safely used to sedate children to facilitate nonpainful diagnostic studies such as CT and MRI scans; redundant but supportive measures may include head positioning, supplemental oxygen, and occasional bag–valve–mask ventilatory support [158]. Pentobarbital successfully sedates >97 % of children for CT or MRI scans with higher success rates in children younger than 8 years of age [166–168]. Pentobarbital is more effective in providing sedation than midazolam [169] or etomidate [170] and causes fewer adverse respiratory events than propofol [171]. The addition of midazolam with pentobarbital does not appear to increase success rates and prolongs time to discharge [167].

Oral pentobarbital (4 mg/kg) has been found similar to oral chloral hydrate (50 mg/kg) in time to sedation and length of sedation; overall adverse event rate, including oxygen desaturation, was slightly lower with pentobarbital (0.5 %) than with chloral hydrate (2.7 %) [172, 173]. Of note, a database review found infants younger than 12 months of age sedated for elective CT or MRI with PO pentobarbital (4–8 mg/kg) had comparable effectiveness and fewer respiratory complications compared with IV pentobarbital (2–6 mg/kg); time to sedation was slightly longer with PO than with IV pentobarbital (18 versus 7 min), but time to discharge (~1 h 45 min) was similar. Total adverse event rate was similar (0.8 % [PO] versus 1.3 % [IV]), but oxygen desaturation was slightly more frequent for IV (0.2 % [PO] versus 0.9 % [IV]). Sedation effectiveness was comparable (99.5 % [PO] versus 99.7 % [IV]), leading the authors to recommend consideration of PO administration for this age group, even when an IV is in place [174]. In a randomized comparison of IV pentobarbital (maximum 5 mg/kg in incremental doses) or oral chloral hydrate (75 mg/kg) prior to MRI, children who received pentobarbital had a higher incidence of paradoxical reaction (14 % versus 9 %) and prolonged recovery with a similar failure rate [173].

Adverse effects: Respiratory depression is dose- and infusion rate dependent and is generally less than that seen with equivalently sedating doses of opioids or chloral hydrate [172, 173, 175]. Mild respiratory depression is usually seen at doses required for hypnotic effect. The following adverse events and frequencies have been reported: transient respiratory depression with oxygen desaturation of ≥10 % below the baseline in 1–8 %; vomiting in ≤1 % [167, 176, 177]; increased airway secretions, airway obstruction, coughing, and bronchospasm [166–168, 172, 176–178]; emergence reactions (hyperactivity in 5–7 %) [176, 178] of 8.4 % in children older than 8 years [178]; and paradoxical reaction (sustained inconsolability and severe irritability and combativeness for more than 30 min) in 0.01 % with oral pentobarbital [172] and in 1.5 % with intravenous pentobarbital [167]. Up to 35 % of children will have increased sleeping or hangover-like effects in the 24 h following pentobarbital sedation [172, 178]. Pentobarbital should be avoided in children with porphyria.

Pregnancy Category D

Dosages: *IV* (protocol used by author)—first dose, 2.5 mg/kg; if needed, subsequent doses, 1.25 mg/kg, may repeat × 3 to maximum of 7.5 mg/kg or 200 mg maximum.

IM: 2–6 mg/kg, to a maximum of 100 mg.

PO or PR (<4 *years*): 3–6 mg/kg, to a maximum of 100 mg.
PO or PR (>4 *years*): 1.5–3 mg/kg, to a maximum of 100 mg.
Onset/duration: The onset of action is related to the route of administration and subsequent absorption. The duration of hypnotic effect is dependent upon redistribution with recovery occurring within 50–75 min after IV or IM administration, even though the biologic half-life in plasma is 15–20 h [175].
After IV administration: sedation by 1–10 min (peak by 5–10 min), recovery by 1–4 h; most patients awakening within 30–60 min. [167, 169]
After IM administration: sedation by 10–30 min, recovery by 2–4 h.
After PO administration: sedation by 15–60 min, recovery by 2–4 h.
Mechanism of action: short-acting barbiturate with sedative–hypnotic but no analgesic effects; it induces relative immobility through nonselective depression of the CNS via facilitation of GABA receptors.
Metabolization: hepatic degradation with elimination half-life 15–20 h [175]. This may explain why many parents note it may take their children up to a day to return to normal behavior.

Anxiolytic–Amnestic–Sedative Agents

Benzodiazepines

Benzodiazepines produce a range of hypnotic (sedative), anxiolytic, amnestic, anticonvulsant, and muscle relaxant effects via modulation of the $GABA_A$ receptor, the most common inhibitory receptor within the brain. The $GABA_A$ receptor is composed of five subunits, each of which has multiple subtypes. The varying combinations of subunit subtypes result in different pharmacological and clinical effects (Table 19.6). When benzodiazepine binds to its site on the GABA receptor, it causes the receptor to have a much higher affinity for the GABA neurotransmitter. This results in the associated chloride ion channel opening more frequently, causing the neuronal membrane to become hyperpolarized [155]. Benzodiazepines have no analgesic effect. Benzodiazepines administered without other medications rarely cause severe adverse effects [179]. However, when benzodiazepines are combined with other drugs such as opiates, marked respiratory depression and apnea can readily occur [98]. Midazolam (Versed®) and diazepam (Valium®) are commonly used benzodiazepines for procedural sedation because of their shorter duration and potent anxiolytic and amnestic effects.

Table 19.6 Comparison of benzodiazepines

Drug	Dose (mg/kg)	Onset (min)	Peak effect (min)	Duration (h)
Midazolam	0.05–0.15	1–3	3–5	0.5–1
Diazepam	0.1–0.2	1.5–3	1–2	2–6
Lorazepam	0.03–0.05	1–5		3–4

Paradoxical Reactions

Severe behavioral changes, typically during recovery, resulting from benzodiazepines as well as barbiturates have been reported including mania, anger, and impulsivity. Individuals with borderline personality disorder appear to have a greater risk of experiencing severe behavioral or psychiatric disturbances from benzodiazepines. Paradoxical rage reactions from benzodiazepines are thought to be due to partial deterioration from consciousness, generating automatic behaviors, fixation amnesia, and aggressiveness from disinhibition with a possible serotonergic mechanism playing a role [180, 181]. In the context of ED PSA, parents should be forewarned about the possibility of excitability, increased anxiety, and agitation in response to midazolam. Recommendations for management of this adverse effect include protecting patients from self-harm while allowing further recovery, deepening sedation with fentanyl or diphenhydramine or administration of caffeine [180, 182].

Midazolam (Versed®)

Indications: Midazolam is a water-soluble benzodiazepine that induces anxiolysis and mild sedation. Most children will not fall asleep with midazolam alone, even at higher doses. Consider another agent or combine with another agent (e.g., pentobarbital) if procedure requires patient to remain motionless (e.g., MRI scan). Midazolam has more potent amnestic effects, quicker onset, and shorter duration of action compared to diazepam [183–186]. Since it is water soluble, midazolam can be administered intramuscularly, as well as PO, IV, or intranasally (IN). Midazolam may be used for seizure control but longer-lasting agents such as lorazepam are typically used. Midazolam also has antiemetic effects, an additional benefit when coadministered with opioids or ketamine [187].

Contraindications/cautions/adverse effects: Midazolam causes minimal hemodynamic effects (mild hypotension with compensatory tachycardia) but dose- and infusion rate-dependent respiratory depression and apnea occur when midazolam is administered in concert with opioids [98]. An important adverse reaction to benzodiazepines in children is the disinhibitory reaction, possibly mediated by central cholinergic mechanisms [180]. Paradoxical excitement or dysphoria during recovery may be increased in older children when midazolam is coadministered with ketamine [89].

Pregnancy Category D

Dosages: IV/IM, anxiolysis, 0.05 mg/kg IV with maximum of 2 mg; sedation, 0.1 mg/kg IV with maximum of 5–10 mg. If titrating to effect, administer doses at 3 min or greater intervals to avoid stacking effects. However, the anticipated dose (e.g., 0.1 mg/kg) may be divided and administered at 1–2 min intervals to reduce respiratory depression.

PO: 0.2–0.75 mg/kg.

IN: 0.2–0.4 mg/kg (use 5 mg/mL IV solution to reduce volume, use atomizer, or drip slowly); more rapid onset and shorter duration than oral. When administered with an atomizer device, this technique is well tolerated and effective to achieve mild to moderate sedation [188]. If the intravenous solution is dripped into the nares without atomization, most children complain of a burning sensation [189–191].

PR: 0.3–0.5 mg/kg may not be preferred by older children [192, 193].

Onset/duration:

IV: sedation within 1 min, peak effect by 2–6 min, recovery by 30–60 min. [194]

IM: sedation within 5–15 min, peaks by 30 min, recovery by 30–60 min. [195]

PO: anxiolysis and mild sedation peak within 15–20 min, recovery by 60–90 min. [189]

IN: effect within 5–10 min, duration 45–60 min. Use of atomizer results in faster onset.

PR: sedation within 5–10 min, recovery 60 min. [192, 193]

Mechanism of action: See benzodiazepine introduction.

Metabolization: Midazolam is degraded almost completely by cytochrome P450-3A4 in the liver and excreted in the urine. Midazolam metabolites have little CNS activity, unlike those of diazepam.

Reversal: Midazolam-induced apnea or respiratory depression may be counteracted by administration of *flumazenil 0.01–0.04 mg/kg (maximum 0.5 mg) IV over 30 s* and repeated every 60 s to desired response. A cumulative dose of 3 mg may be necessary. Flumazenil may reverse midazolam-induced hypnotic and amnestic effects but not ventilatory depression [127]. The patient must be closely monitored, typically for 2 h after flumazenil administration, for resedation and respiratory depression. Recurrence of sedation has been reported in up to 7 % of cases, most commonly in children under 5 years of age [128]. Flumazenil may cause seizures in patients chronically on benzodiazepine medications and should be used cautiously in patients on medications that can lower seizure threshold.

Diazepam (Valium®)

Indications: Diazepam has excellent antianxiety, skeletal muscle relaxation, and amnestic properties, but because its duration of effect is longer than that of midazolam, diazepam is seldom used for ED PSA or preprocedure anxiolysis. It is considered 2–4 times less potent than midazolam.

Contraindications/cautions/adverse effects: Drowsiness may last 2–6 h with resedation occurring at 6–8 h due to enterohepatic recirculation and formation of active metabolites. Like other benzodiazepines, diazepam readily causes respiratory depression with rapid administration.

Diazepam's propylene glycol carrier causes burning sensations on intramuscular and intravenous injection and erratic absorption with intramuscular administration. Administer with caution in patients with liver and kidney dysfunction.

Pregnancy Category D

Dosages: IV, 0.04–0.2 mg/kg/dose q 2–4 h. PR: 0.5 mg/kg/dose.

PO: 0.12–0.8 mg/kg.

Onset/duration: IV, within 1.5–3 min. PR: 7–15 min.

PO: 30–60 min.

Mechanism of action: See benzodiazepine introduction.

Metabolization: Diazepam undergoes hepatic microsomal oxidation with renal excretion. Liver and kidney dysfunction, as well as active metabolites including desmethyldiazepam and oxazepam, may prolong effects.

Other Non-analgesic Sedative Agents

Propofol (Diprivan®)

Propofol is a sedative hypnotic agent with no analgesic properties [155]. It is the most commonly used parenteral agent for induction and maintenance of general anesthesia in the United States, due in large part to rapid and pleasant recovery from anesthesia induced by this potent agent [155]. Little or no nausea is associated with propofol and its amnestic effect is similar to that from midazolam [196]. Many adults and older children remark on awakening that they feel as if they have just had a good nap. These characteristics have resulted in propofol's rapid increase in popularity as an agent for scheduled [88, 197] and ED PSA for children [158, 198].

Propofol, however, has a narrow therapeutic window, which makes PSA titration to desired effect without oversedation more difficult than with many other agents. Significant respiratory depression and hypotension are relatively common (see "Adverse Effects" section) [88, 199]. Propofol can be used alone for painless procedures such as MRI or CT scans, or, at greater doses, for painful procedures. However, because significant respiratory depression or apnea is associated with doses necessary for painful procedures, smaller doses of propofol have been combined with analgesic opiates or ketamine for ED PSA [199–201]. Although combining ketamine with propofol may have theoretical benefit by using lower doses of each agent to reduce the undesirable adverse effects of both agents, a 2007 review of published studies in adults and children found the combination had not demonstrated superior clinical efficacy compared with propofol alone. Studies conflicted regarding reduced hemodynamic and respiratory adverse effects with the combination compared with propofol monotherapy [202]. A comparison of propofol + ketamine to propofol + fentanyl for PSA in toddlers undergoing burn dressing changes found similar minimal impact on blood pressure and respiratory rate but less restlessness with the addition of ketamine [203].

Use of propofol for ED PSA should be preceded by specific training and supervised experience. It is recommended that when propofol is administered, an experienced provider with advanced airway skills be dedicated to administering the sedation and managing the airway and cardiorespiratory status of the patient. In-depth knowledge of adverse effects and advanced airway skills are essential for safe use of this drug.

Pharmacology

The exact mechanism(s) by which propofol exerts global CNS depression has not been fully elucidated. However, there is evidence that propofol potentiates $GABA_A$ receptor activity by slowing the channel-closing time, with lesser effects on $GABA_B$ receptors, modestly inhibits the *N-methyl-d*-aspartate (NMDA) receptor, modulates calcium influx through slow calcium-ion channels, and locks sodium channels [204].

Pharmacokinetics [157]

Propofol is highly lipophilic and rapidly diffuses from plasma into body tissues, particularly the highly perfused brain. The onset of action of propofol as determined by time to unconsciousness (i.e., loss of response to voice command) is within 1 arm–brain circulation time (the time required for the drug to travel from the site of injection to the site of action in the brain) and can be as brief as 15–30 s, but is more typically 40–60 s, dependent upon the rate of administration. Since propofol is rapidly distributed from CNS to inactive storage sites such as muscle and fat, recovery from anesthesia is rapid with duration of action about 5–10 min. The short duration of sedation after repeated doses can be explained by rapid metabolic clearance from blood and slow redistribution of the drug from the peripheral tissues. Thus, the pharmacokinetics of propofol after IV administration are best described by a 3-compartment model with rapid distribution of the drug from blood into the brain and other tissues, rapid metabolic clearance from blood, and slow redistribution of the drug from the peripheral compartment back into the blood stream, resulting in sub-hypnotic plasma levels of drug.

Propofol is rapidly and extensively metabolized in the liver to less active conjugates, which are excreted mainly in the urine. Since plasma clearance exceeds hepatic blood flow, it appears that the drug also is metabolized at extrahepatic sites. Mean total body clearance of propofol appears to be proportional to body weight; obese patients have a substantially higher body clearance than leaner individuals.

Indications: Propofol sedation of children in the ED has been reported primarily for fracture reduction with fentanyl, morphine, or ketamine coadministered [199–201, 205]. Sedation or distress scores were low during fracture reduction with propofol + morphine or fentanyl and similar to ketamine + midazolam or morphine + midazolam [200, 201]. Mean recovery times after propofol for these studies were 15–23 min. Unlike other PSA techniques, with the exception of nitrous oxide, repeated or continuous dosing of propofol causes little prolongation of recovery when administered for less than 1–2 h. Thus, after longer procedures, such as complex laceration repair or emergent MRI scans during which either repeated doses or continuous infusion of propofol is required, recovery typically is still within 15–30 min. [206]

Contraindications/Cautions/Adverse Effects: Transient respiratory depression, apnea, upper airway obstruction, or laryngospasm may occur in many patients, especially during induction of sedation [88, 199, 207]. A recent study suggests that the administration of induction dosages of propofol slowly over 3 min decreases the incidence of respiratory depression [208]. Increasing upper airway narrowing due to muscle relaxation, especially at the level of the epiglottis, has been shown with increasing depth of propofol sedation/anesthesia [209]. Loss of protective airway reflexes during apneic periods may place patients at increased risk of pulmonary aspiration as the ensuing bag–mask positive-pressure ventilation increases gastric pressure and risk of passive regurgitation [88]. Therefore, candidates for propofol sedation must be carefully screened for risks of "full stomachs," URIs, and difficult airways [210]. These events are frequent enough when sedating with propofol that many providers routinely administer supplemental oxygen and monitor with end-tidal capnography, in addition to having a functioning anesthesia or CPAP ventilation bag at the bedside [107, 108, 117].

The main adverse cardiovascular effect of propofol is hypotension, in part related to decreases in peripheral vascular resistance [157, 211]. In spontaneously breathing patients, as much as a 30 % decrease in blood pressure may be seen with little or no changes in heart rate [205, 212]. The decrease in blood pressure is dose- and infusion rate dependent and is potentiated by coadministration of opioids such as fentanyl [211, 213]. Propofol may rarely induce profound bradycardia and cardiac arrest in hypovolemic patients or in those at risk for hypotension or with cardiac dysfunction [88, 214]. Administration of additional fluids and a cautious rate of IV infusion may help reduce the risk of propofol-induced hypotension.

Because of the increased risk of apnea and hypotension compared to other agents for PSA, many providers avoid use of propofol in ED patients determined to have difficult airways, cardiac dysfunction, brief fasting, or ASA physical status Class 3, 4, or 5 [117, 199].

Propofol is formulated as an emulsion in soybean oil, glycerol, and purified egg products because it is essentially insoluble in aqueous solutions. Propofol therefore cannot be administered to patients with allergies to eggs or soy. In addition, to inhibit bacterial growth, some preparations contain sodium metabisulfite, which may cause allergic-type reactions in susceptible individuals, including anaphylaxis and life-threatening or less severe asthmatic episodes [157].

Despite the addition of disodium EDTA or sodium metabisulfite to inhibit bacterial growth, significant bacterial contamination of open containers has been associated with serious patient infection. Using aseptic technique, propofol should be administered shortly after removal from sterile packaging [155].

Injection site pain is common with propofol but often may not be recalled due to propofol's amnestic effects. In ED PSA, coadministration of morphine or fentanyl for procedural analgesia may reduce this effect [117]. Lidocaine 0.5 mg/kg administered intravenously immediately prior to propofol infusion and use of large antecubital veins also may help ameliorate this minor adverse effect [157, 200].

Involuntary movement (myoclonus) has been reported in 15–20 % of pediatric patients undergoing propofol anesthesia, typically during induction [157]. Myoclonus significant enough to interrupt the procedure, the majority of which were radiological, however, occurred only at a rate of 2/10,000 in elective sedations with propofol [88].

Pregnancy Category B

Dosages: Propofol can be administered intravenously in doses of 1–2 mg/kg to achieve sedation. Note, however, administration of 2–3.5 mg/kg followed by continuous infusion of 100–300 mg/kg/min is commonly used for induction of general anesthesia [117, 199–201, 205, 215, 216].

Published studies of pediatric ED PSA for fracture reduction used an initial bolus of 1 mg/kg propofol administered over 1–2 min followed by additional doses of 0.5 mg/kg every 1–3 min based on patient response [199, 201, 205]. Mean total propofol doses in these studies were 2.5–4.5 mg/kg. Alternatively, one study followed the initial 1 mg/kg bolus immediately with a propofol infusion at 67–100 mg/kg/min until cast completion; most children required an additional bolus of propofol during the infusion to achieve the desired level of sedation [200]. In each of these studies, propofol was administered shortly after morphine or fentanyl administration.

Administration [157]: Commercially available 1 % propofol injectable emulsion (10 mg/mL) may be used without dilution. If dilution is necessary, the drug may be diluted with 5 % dextrose injection to a concentration of not less than 0.2 % (2 mg/mL) in order to maintain the emulsion. Propofol should be discarded if there is evidence of separation of the emulsion. The emulsion should be shaken well just prior to administration.

Using aseptic technique, contents of a vial may be transferred into a sterile, single-use syringe and administered shortly after removal from sterile packaging. The manufacturers state that propofol is compatible with several IV fluids (e.g., 5 % dextrose, 5 % dextrose and lactated Ringer's, 5 % dextrose, and 0.2 or 0.45 % sodium chloride) when a Y-type administration set is used.

Etomidate

Indications: Etomidate has potent hypnotic (sedative) and amnestic but no analgesic effects. It is in an aqueous solution of propylene glycol; therefore, burning on injection is a common complaint. Since etomidate rapidly induces unconsciousness with little hemodynamic effect and clinical recovery occurs within minutes, it is frequently used in the emergency setting to induce unconsciousness prior to neuromuscular blockade during endotracheal intubation [217–219].

Recent reports suggest etomidate may be safe and effective for brief nonpainful procedures such as CT scans and can be combined with fentanyl for fracture reductions. Early reports were inconclusive about the safety and effectiveness of etomidate for ED PSA in children [158, 220–223]. However, a small study of ED pediatric patients sedated for head and neck CT found successful completion of the CT in 57 % with etomidate doses up to 0.3 mg/kg and 76 % with doses up to 0.4 mg/kg, in contrast to a success rate of 97 % for pentobarbital [170]. Etomidate 0.2 mg/kg IV was infused over 30 s, with additional doses, if needed, of 0.1 mg/kg IV over 30 s at 1 min intervals, to a maximum total dose of 0.4 mg/kg. Duration of sedation was 13 min and parents felt their children returned to normal behavior much earlier than with pentobarbital. A more rapid infusion technique in another study reported a 99 % successful completion of CT scans with etomidate in 446 fasted ASA-PS Class I and II children; duration of sedation was 34 min [224]. With a proximal tourniquet in place, 0.5 mg/kg lidocaine (maximum dose 25 mg) was first administered through the intravenous catheter to mitigate burning from the subsequent etomidate infusion, a "mini-Bier block" technique. After 1 min, the tourniquet was removed and etomidate 0.3 mg/kg was infused over 2–3 s. If sedation was not adequate, an additional 0.15 mg/kg bolus was administered within 1 min of the initial dose. If needed, an additional 0.15 mg/kg bolus was given during scans requiring multiple views or repositioning. Median total etomidate dose was 3.3 mg/kg. With this technique, 1 patient had apnea and the CT scan was not completed; otherwise significant respiratory depression did not occur. Although most of these children were not ED patients, it suggests this agent may be used successfully for this purpose.

For fracture reduction, etomidate 0.2 mg/kg infused intravenously over 60–90 s resulted in effective sedation in 92 % of children compared to 36 % with midazolam 0.1 mg/kg IV [225]. Both were combined with fentanyl 1 mg/kg IV. Median recovery time in those reaching adequate sedation was 12 min with etomidate and 24 min with midazolam. Desaturation occurred in 22 % of children in both groups; all responded quickly to free flow oxygen administration or head repositioning; no patient experienced apnea or required positive-pressure ventilation. Myoclonus occurred in 22 % of patients who received etomidate, but it was described as mild and brief and did not interfere with the fracture reduction. Pain on injection of etomidate was noted in 46 % of children. Further studies of etomidate are needed to define better safety and efficacy parameters for PSA, particularly in unfasted emergency patients.

Contraindications/cautions/adverse effects: Similar to midazolam, transient apnea with rapid infusion may rarely occur when etomidate is administered alone [224], but respiratory depression may occur in 20 % or more of children receiving etomidate coadministered with fentanyl or morphine [225]. Pain with injection in 2–20 % and myoclonus in 8–40 % of patients are associated with etomidate infusion [221, 226, 227]. When present, myoclonus that can resemble seizures usually lasts less than 1 min and can be decreased by the coadministration redundant of other drugs. These tremors are benign and not epileptiform activity [226, 228].

Although trials investigating etomidate-induced adrenal suppression associated with PSA in noncritically ill children are not available, studies in adults and children have demonstrated cortisol depression for up to 24 h with as little as a single dose of etomidate. This suppression may be clinically significant in patients with hemorrhagic or septic shock, leading some to suggest consideration of alternative agents or to combine etomidate with glucocorticoids for induction of unconsciousness for tracheal intubation or PSA in these patients [229–232].

Pregnancy Category D

Dosages: 0.2–0.3 mg/kg IV.

Onset/duration: onset of sedation within 30–60 s, with duration of deep sedation 3–12 min when using a dose of 0.2–0.3 mg/kg [71]. Sufficient recovery for discharge may take 30–45 min. [224]

Mechanism of action: Etomidate, like propofol, is structurally unrelated to other anesthetics. It is an imidazole derivative that is thought to induce sedation through enhanced gamma-aminobutyric acid (GABA) neurotransmission [155].

Metabolization: Etomidate is highly protein bound in blood and is degraded by hepatic and plasma esterases to inactive products. It exhibits a bi-exponential decline, with a redistribution half-life of 2–5 min and an elimination half-life of 68–75 min [155].

Sedative–Analgesic Agents

The following are primary analgesic agents. Sedation generally requires higher doses of opioids or addition of sedative–hypnotic agents, both of which significantly increase respiratory depression. Ketamine induces sedation and amnesia but opioid agents cause little amnesia.

Opiates (Narcotics) (Table 19.7): Fentanyl (Sublimaze®)

Indications: Fentanyl is a high-potency synthetic opiate with minimal hemodynamic effects. Due to its lipophilic nature and rapid biphasic redistribution, onset of analgesia and sedation occur rapidly with intravenous administration but are of short duration, making it a favorable agent for ED PSA. Fentanyl, by weight, is 80–100 times more potent than morphine. It provides significant analgesia and mild sedation for painful procedures but is not recommended for anxiety control or for control of spontaneous movement. Since fentanyl, unlike morphine, does not cause clinically significant histamine release, it is the opiate of choice in patients who have increased potential for hypotension, e.g., trauma or sepsis [233].

Table 19.7 Comparison of opioid medications

Opioid	IV dose (mg/kg)	Peak	Duration
Fentanyl	0.001–0.002 (1–2 μg/kg)	30–60 s	30 min
Morphine	0.1	10 min	4–5 h
Meperidine	1	10 min	2–4 h

Fentanyl has been administered in oral lozenges (oral transmucosal fentanyl citrate (OTFC)) for ED PSA for laceration repair. However, titration to effect is difficult with this technique and it has been associated with frequent nausea, vomiting (20–50 %), and pruritus [234–237]. OTFC has also been used for rapid (30 min) analgesia in children with fractures [238].

Of note, atomized intranasal administration of fentanyl in children in acute pain in the ED has been shown to provide significant pain relief by 5–10 min [239, 240]. One small study of children 1–4 years old undergoing suturing in the ED found intranasal sufentanil, a more potent analog of fentanyl, plus midazolam provided sedation by 20 min without vomiting or other significant adverse events [241]. Further study is needed to clarify safety and efficacy of atomized intranasal techniques for ED PSA.

Fentanyl plus midazolam: A primary goal with most painful ED PSA is attenuated or blocked unpleasant recall of the procedure. Since fentanyl induces minimal amnesia and cannot completely block procedure-related pain without extreme respiratory depression, it is typically combined with midazolam to induce amnesia for residual procedural pain. Although the combination of fentanyl and midazolam can cause significant respiratory depression [98], both agents have competitive antagonists that readily reverse undesirable effects. If titrated carefully, a small dose of naloxone of 1 mg/kg will reverse respiratory depression but retain much of the analgesia effect. This reversibility makes this combined technique an optimum and frequently used approach for ED PSA [158].

The dose of midazolam that maximizes amnestic effect is not well established. Furthermore, while the onset of peak amnestic effect is indistinct, the duration of action appears to be fairly long, hence a broad window within which to administer the analgesic agent, fentanyl. Thus, it is recommended to maximize the capability to administer sufficient amnestic agent by infusing the midazolam before the fentanyl is given, since the synergistic respiratory depressant effects of the two medications may limit the ability to administer sufficient amnestic agent if it is given after the fentanyl.

Adequate analgesia for painful procedures always requires sufficient narcotic to cause some degree of respiratory depression (assuming narcotic naive patients). Use of local anesthesia for the procedure (e.g., a hematoma block for fracture reduction) can significantly reduce the amount of systemic analgesic agent needed and thus reduce respiratory depression. It is important to time the "peak analgesia effect" (peak brain concentration) with "maximal analgesia need" (at time of the maximally painful part of the procedure); hence the analgesic agent is administered after the amnestic agent. The respiratory depression is typically counteracted by the pain of the procedure. Particular attention to ventilatory sufficiency should occur after the painful procedural stimulus ends, since respiratory depressant effects will persist for minutes to hours after the last dose of medication [124]. This adverse effect may be exacerbated by oral or parenteral opioid analgesics administered prior to the PSA.

Contraindications/cautions/adverse effects: Fentanyl, like other opioid analgesics, causes dose- and infusion rate-dependent respiratory depression characterized by decreases in respiratory rate, tidal volume, minute ventilation, and ventilatory response to carbon dioxide. Hypotension and bradycardia may also occur with rapid infusion or larger doses. Although return to relative alertness typically occurs within 20–30 min after IV administration, respiratory depressant effects may last several hours. Patients may be awake but need to be reminded to breathe due to the drug's depression of the brainstem response to rising plasma CO [120, 124, 242].

Respiratory depression can be lessened by administering the expected total dose in divided amounts, e.g., 0.5 mg/kg/dose, and infusing each dose over 30–60 s at 1–2 min intervals. Respiratory depression is markedly increased by coadministration of sedative–hypnotic medications such as midazolam or barbiturates [9, 98]. At the level of deep sedation, many children will have respiratory depression or partial upper airway obstruction due to muscle relaxation and may require airway-opening maneuvers, supplemental oxygen, or painful stimulation [9].

Respiratory depression is readily reversed by the competitive antagonist naloxone. Titration of naloxone in small doses of 1 µg/kg stopping at the endpoint of reversal of respiratory depression will retain much of the analgesia effect. Repeated doses may be necessary as respiratory effects may outlast the reversal effects of naloxone. Administration of a "full" dose of naloxone may cause significant pain, hypertension, tachycardia, vomiting, and other undesirable adverse effects.

Chest wall rigidity may occur with rapid infusion of large doses (usually >5 mg/kg), especially in infants. This life-threatening adverse effect will manifest by lack of spontaneous chest wall movement, dropping oxygen saturations, and an inability to ventilate the patient with positive pressure by bag and mask. Reversal with naloxone or paralysis with succinylcholine may be needed to manage this adverse event.

Pregnancy Category C

Dosages: *for analgesia*; 1–2 µg/kg, intravenously. Titrate to effect by administering doses of 0.5 µg/kg over 15–30 s, repeated every 1–2 min. A total dose of 1–2 µg/kg usually can be administered without causing significant respiratory depression, unless coadministered with midazolam. For significantly painful injuries, an initial dose of 1 µg/kg usually may be administered safely over 30 s.

For ED PSA: *fentanyl + midazolam*; midazolam, 0.05–0.1 mg/kg intravenously over 1–2 min, is administered first, titrated to an endpoint of drooping eyelids and slurred speech. A total dose of 10 mg likely is sufficient for amnesia in large adolescents. Then fentanyl, 0.5 μg/kg intravenously over 30 s, is repeated to an endpoint of decreased patient responsiveness to a relevant painful stimulus such as squeezing the fracture site or palpating the abscess. If local anesthesia is used for the procedure, approximately 1 μg/kg fentanyl may be sufficient. For intensely painful procedures, such as fracture reduction without a hematoma block, up to 2 μg/kg may be necessary [9]. Respiratory depression is likely at this dose; therefore, time the end titration of fentanyl as the painful part of the procedure is begun; the procedure-related pain will stimulate the patient and counteract some of the respiratory depression. Additional doses of fentanyl may be administered after about 10 min if the patient becomes agitated or manifests significant pain during longer procedures.

Fentanyl comes in 2 mL vials of 50 μg/mL. Titration is easier and safer if the concentrated fentanyl is diluted to 10 μg/mL by adding 2 mL of fentanyl to 8 mL of normal saline, resulting in 10 mL of 10 μg/mL.

Onset/duration: Analgesia with mild sedation after IV administration of fentanyl is within 30–60 s, with greatest sedative–analgesic effects lasting 5–10 min. Although return to relative alertness typically occurs within 20–30 min after IV administration, respiratory depressant effects may last several hours. Patients may be awake but "forget to breathe" due to the drug's depression of the brainstem response to rising plasma CO_2 [120, 124, 242].

Mechanism of action: Fentanyl is a high-potency mu agonist opiate 50–100 times more potent than morphine [233].

Metabolization: Fentanyl is metabolized in the liver and excreted in the urine. There are no active metabolites [233].

Morphine

Indications: While the "standard" for analgesia, morphine is typically not used for procedural sedation because its slow onset of peak analgesic effect (~10 min) makes titration difficult. Repeating a dose before 10 min leads to "stacking"; i.e., administering a second dose before the peak effect of the first dose results in unnecessary excess medication administration, overshooting the intended level of analgesia, and is associated with excess adverse effects such as respiratory depression. Morphine is commonly administered to provide baseline analgesia if the patient is in pain from an injury, abscess, etc. Additional analgesia, typically with a different agent such as fentanyl or ketamine, is then administered for the procedure.

Contraindications/cautions/adverse effects: Additional administration of a benzodiazepine for anxiolysis increases the respiratory depression associated with morphine administration. Morphine induces histamine release and may result in hypotension, nausea/vomiting, dizziness, and pruritus; histamine release may exacerbate asthma. Pruritus can be treated with diphenhydramine.

Pregnancy Category C

Dosages: IV; 0.05–0.1 mg/kg, titrated to the effect of pain relief. Opioid naive patients may experience less nausea if the expected dose is divided. For example, an 80 kg teenager will likely better tolerate two 4 mg doses administered 10–15 min apart.

Onset/duration: 1–3 min, peak 10–20 min; duration of significant analgesia 1–2 h.

Mechanism of action: mu agonist (analgesia) and weak kappa agonist (respiratory depression).

Metabolization: glucuronidated in the liver and excreted in the urine; 10 % metabolized to active metabolite, which can accumulate in children with renal failure.

Meperidine (Demerol®)

Indications: Although a potent opioid, meperidine, like morphine, is seldom used for procedural sedation because its long time to peak effect (~10 min) makes it difficult to titrate without overshooting (stacking) the intended level of analgesia and sedation. In addition, meperidine causes histamine release at a greater frequency than do other opioids and its atropine-like effects may cause tachycardia and euphoria.

Contraindications/cautions/adverse effects: Interaction with MAO inhibitors may be catastrophic resulting in hypertension, excitation, tachycardia, seizure, and hyperpyrexia. Biodegradation to the active metabolite normeperidine (elimination half-life of 15–40 h) results in prolongation of effects. With large or repeated doses, accumulation of normeperidine may cause nervous system excitation with tremors, muscle twitches, and seizures.

Pregnancy Category C

Dosages: IV/IM; 1 mg/kg.

Onset/duration: IV; 1–5 min, peak by 10 min; duration of 1–2 h.

IM: peak effect by 10 min, duration 1–2 h.

Mechanism of action: a phenylpiperidine opioid with potent analgesic effects.

Metabolization: Hepatic degradation forms active metabolite normeperidine (elimination half-life of 15–40 h), which results in prolongation of effects and has adverse effects as noted earlier.

Codeine

Codeine is well absorbed after oral administration, but the drug must be metabolized by the liver to morphine to have an analgesic effect. Since up to 35 % or more of people are slow or non-metabolizers, codeine is an ineffective analgesic agent for many [243, 244]. Conversely, ultrarapid metabolizers may experience reduced analgesic effect but increased adverse effects from relatively small doses [245]. For these reasons, oxycodone is the oral analgesic of choice in the author's ED.

Oxycodone

Indications: Oxycodone, an opioid analgesic medication originally synthesized from opium-derived compounds, is readily absorbed by oral route and is often administered for painful conditions when no IV access is established, e.g., at triage for possible fractures or burns [246]. It can also be used to augment sedation for painful procedures, e.g., with nitrous oxide for abscess I&D or fracture reduction [90]. Oxycodone is preferred because, unlike codeine, it does not require metabolism to an active form. Oxycodone may cause less nausea than codeine [2], but one comparison found no difference in vomiting or other adverse effects at analgesically similar doses [246].

Contraindications/cautions/adverse effects: Oxycodone, as do other opiates, significantly increases frequency of vomiting when combined with other analgesic regimens, e.g., with ketamine or nitrous oxide. Vomiting prior to ED discharge after PSA increased from approximately 10 % with ketamine + midazolam [9] or nitrous oxide [10] to 25 % when oxycodone had been administered in triage [90]. Oxycodone also causes dose-dependent respiratory depression by blunting the brainstem response to increasing levels of carbon dioxide. A dose of 0.2 mg/kg administered to children with painful injuries caused tiredness but no clinically apparent changes in ventilation or oxygenation [246]. At a dose of 0.3 mg/kg administered to young children in preparation for painful abscess I&D, we have observed many patients become sleepy but are easily aroused with verbal stimuli and oxygen saturations usually remain within normal ranges as they breathe room air; however, these children should routinely be monitored for respiratory depression after this larger dose.

Pregnancy Category B (D for Prolonged Use)

Dosages: 0.05–0.15 mg/kg for out of hospital analgesia; *for procedural analgesia, 0.2–0.3 mg/kg*, with the larger end of the range for younger children for fracture reduction, burn debridement, or abscess management. Since absorption after gastric administration has large interindividual variation in the rate and extent of absorption [247], the higher dose is not recommended for home use due to the potential for oversedation. Similarly, oxycodone should be used with caution in infants younger than 6 months of age due to marked variation in clearance [248].

Onset/duration: Analgesia begins within 30 min and peaks at ~1 h; duration 2–3 h.

Mechanism of action: mu agonist (analgesia) and weak kappa agonist (respiratory depression).

Metabolization: Oxycodone is metabolized by the cytochrome P450 enzyme system in the liver with up to 20 % excreted unchanged in the urine. Thus, patients with poor renal function may accumulate higher plasma levels.

NMDA Antagonists

Ketamine (Ketalar®)

Ketamine is a phencyclidine-derived lipophilic dissociative agent with rapid biphasic redistribution. Potent analgesic and amnestic effects with relative lack of cardiopulmonary depression make ketamine quite likely the most widely used and appropriate agent for ED PSA [158, 249]. The American College of Emergency Physicians (ACEP) has recently published a Clinical Practice Guideline for Emergency Department Ketamine Dissociative Sedation: 2011 Update [250]. The major changes in these guidelines as compared to the former of 2004 are summarized in Table 19.8 [81, 250]. During fracture reduction, children receiving ketamine demonstrated significantly less distress and less respiratory depression than those receiving fentanyl or propofol coadministered with midazolam [9, 201]. Ketamine also induces significant amnesia and effective PSA for other intensely

Table 19.8 Major changes in the American College of Emergency Physicians (ACEP) Clinical Practice Guideline for Emergency Department Ketamine Dissociative Sedation: 2011 Update (modified from [250])

General changes
• Expansion of guideline to include adults
No longer contraindications
• Administration for ages 3–12 months
• Minor oropharyngeal procedures
• Head trauma
Route of administration
• Emphasis on IV over IM route when feasible
Coadministered medications
• Route prophylactic anticholinergics no longer recommended
• Route prophylactic benzodiazepines may benefit adults, but not children
• Prophylactic ondansetron can slightly reduce vomiting

painful ED procedures such as burn debridement and abscess incision and drainage, as well as relative immobility for procedures during which occasional spontaneous movement is tolerated, such as complex laceration repair, and brief radiological procedures such as CT scans or joint aspiration [81, 158].

Ketamine has unique and diverse mechanisms of action with beneficial and potentially adverse effects. Ketamine interacts with multiple binding sites including NMDA and non-NMDA glutamate receptors, nicotinic and muscarinic cholinergic and opioid receptors, and less so, peripheral neuronal sodium channels [251]. Ketamine's primary site of anesthetic action is in the CNS in thalamocortical pathways and the limbic system where it binds to a site on postsynaptic NMDA channels that regulate transmembrane calcium, sodium, and potassium flux. This binding inhibits glutamate activation of the channel in a noncompetitive manner and is time and concentration dependent [121, 251, 252].

Circulatory Effects

In contrast to other sedative and analgesic agents, cardiac output, including heart rate and blood pressure, is usually well maintained with ketamine administration, even at deeper levels of sedation or anesthesia. Ketamine causes 10–30 % increases in blood pressure and heart rate by blocking reuptake of catecholaminergic hormones norepinephrine, epinephrine, dopamine, and serotonin. These effects may increase intracranial pressure, and caution has been suggested with its use in patients with known intracranial pathology causing increased intracranial pressure. However, use of ketamine in ventilated patients with head trauma has been shown safe and not to impact intracranial pressure differently from opioids [253, 254]. Use of ketamine in the ED for rapid sequence intubation of patients with head trauma has also been advocated as safe [255]. Of note, ketamine also has a direct negative inotropic effect on the heart that is usually clinically inapparent due to the sympathetic stimulation [256]. In critically ill patients whose catecholamines are depleted due to maximal compensation for hypovolemia, hypoxemia, fluid–electrolyte, acid–base, and other physiologic insults, administration of ketamine may cause marked hypotension and bradycardia [257].

Ventilatory Effects

In marked contradistinction to other sedative–analgesic agents, doses of ketamine typically used for ED PSA rarely cause depression of pulmonary gas exchange or relaxation of upper airway muscles [258]. Intravenous infusion of 2 mg/kg of ketamine over 1 min characteristically causes no significant effect on respiratory rate, tidal volume, minute ventilation, or end-tidal CO_2, thus maintaining adequate gas exchange during unobstructed spontaneous room air breathing [259]. Furthermore, ketamine does not significantly decrease thoracic or airway muscle activity [258, 260, 261], or impair lung ventilation distribution, functional residual capacity, or minute ventilation with intravenous doses of 2 or 4 mg/kg [132]. These effects and maintenance of positive end-expiratory pressure (PEEP) [262] result in lack of peripheral alveolar collapse and regional hypoventilation seen with propofol and opioid agents. Interestingly, relatively low-dose ketamine (1 mg/kg administered intravenously over 5 min, i.e., 0.2 mg/kg/min) to adults caused respiratory stimulant effects with three distinct phases: Increased tidal volumes (deep breathing) were followed by increased respiratory rates and then large tidal volumes with low respiratory rates and occasional brief apnea, possibly compensating for hypocarbia due to the preceding hyperventilation [263]. These findings are consistent with the mild increase in respiratory rate with maintenance of normal oxygen saturation and end-tidal CO_2 noted in children receiving intravenous ketamine 1.5 mg/kg over 1 min for ED PSA [113].

Reduced responsiveness to increased CO_2 and hypoxemia, however, have been demonstrated during the initial period after a bolus of ketamine when plasma levels are high and resolving as levels decrease [259, 264, 265]. This suggests the possibility of apnea in sensitive individuals or a delayed response to hypercarbia if airway obstruction occurs during induction of sedation and may explain the case reports of brief respiratory arrest after administration of intramuscular ketamine for ED PSA [122, 266, 267]. A case series of 18 children who inadvertently received 5–100-fold larger-than-intended doses of ketamine described respiratory depression and prolonged recovery but no residual effects except for one critically ill infant who died [156]. A meta-analysis of more than 8,000 children who received ketamine for ED PSA found that the overall incidence of airway and respiratory adverse events (upper airway obstruction, apnea, oxygen desaturation ≤90 %, or laryngospasm) was 4 %. Increased risk was found in younger children and teenagers, those receiving more than 2.5 mg/kg initial or 5 mg/kg total doses, and those receiving coadministered anticholinergic or benzodiazepine medications [135]. Airway and respiratory adverse events occurred at twice the overall rate in children younger than 2 years, except for laryngospasm or apnea, which were not increased. The overall frequency of airway and respiratory adverse events in adolescents 13 years or older was almost 3 times greater with more apnea but less laryngospasm. The overall frequency of apnea was 0.8 % in this series. Coadministration of other sedative–analgesic agents such as midazolam or morphine and young age also have been found by others to be associated with greater respiratory depression [89, 268].

Protective Airway Reflexes

Preservation of upper airway protective reflexes, even at deeper levels of sedation or anesthesia, reduces the risk of pulmonary aspiration and thus makes ketamine one of the safest agents for ED PSA in unfasted children, yet, paradoxically, it may increase the risk for one of the most significant life-threatening sedation-related adverse events: laryngospasm [132–134]. The incidence of laryngospasm in ketamine-based pediatric ED PSA is difficult to determine as it is a rare event and large sedation databases are not available for estimation. The meta-analysis of pediatric ketamine-based ED PSA found an incidence of laryngospasm of 0.3 %; the only identifiable association with greater risk was an initial intravenous dose of greater than 2.5 mg/kg, but data was unable to be analyzed for URI, wheezing, or other risk factors noted with general anesthesia. Young age and oropharyngeal procedures (excluding endoscopy) were not associated with increased risk [135]. Although in the past, the prophylactic administration of anticholinergics was believed to reduce the incidence of secretions, laryngospasm, and respiratory complication, this is no longer held true. Rather, a recent matched case–control analysis of 8,282 ketamine procedures in the emergency department revealed no association between age, dose, procedure, medical status, route of delivery, and the administration of anticholinergics with the occurrence of laryngospasm [269]. This data is important because it identifies the occurrence of laryngospasm as an unpredictable and idiosyncratic reaction. All practitioners, thus, who administer ketamine should be prepared to identify and treat laryngospasm.

Initial management of laryngospasm should include airway-opening maneuvers (straightening, jaw thrust) and administration of supplemental oxygen, preferably by CPAP. If these are insufficient to maintain oxygenation, low-dose succinylcholine should be considered (~0.1–0.2 mg/kg IV); if this low dose does not improve oxygenation, a full paralytic dose of 1–3 mg/kg succinylcholine should be administered. Laryngospasm induced by ketamine may be brief or it may be recurrent and it may occur during emergence as well as induction or mid-procedure [131]. Please see section on "Management of Laryngospasm."

Sedative–Analgesic Effects

Sedation and dissociation induced by ketamine likely occur primarily from blockade of the excitatory effects of glutamate, the most prevalent CNS excitatory neurotransmitter. By binding to the neuronal membrane's NMDA glutamate receptor complex associated with transmembrane calcium channels, ketamine prevents or reduces neurotransmission of pain and other stimuli by interfering with the calcium influx necessary for electrical propagation [251].

Dissociative Effects

Ketamine is classified as a dissociative general anesthetic agent because EEG and functional MRI (fMRI) recordings demonstrate electrical activity of the thalamus that is no longer synchronized with or is "dissociated" from the limbic system after ketamine administration [270]. The thalamus is believed to process and relay sensory information selectively to specific areas of the cerebral cortex and plays a major role in regulating arousal, the level of awareness, and activity as well as processing auditory, somatic, visceral, and visual sensory input [133]. It is thought this dissociative effect is the primary mechanism for preventing patients' response to pain or other sensory stimuli after ketamine administration. More precise understandings of the mechanisms are under investigation. The patient who has received ketamine without an adjunctive sedative agent may have his/her eyes open but be unresponsive to the environment, described by some as if "the lights are on but nobody's home." This catatonic stare may be frightening to unprepared observers such as family members.

Prolonged Analgesic Effects

A relatively unexplored potential analgesic benefit of ketamine use for ED PSA is reduction of windup and central sensitization [271]. Brief noxious stimulation of peripheral tissue receptors initiates rapid neural transmission along myelinated and unmyelinated axons to the nerve's central terminus located within the dorsal horn of the spinal cord and induces release of excitatory neurotransmitters, primarily glutamate, into the dorsal horn synapse. The glutamate initiates rapid firing of postsynaptic AMPA and kainate receptors, resulting in sharp "first" pain and reflex withdrawal from the stimulus, soon followed by dull, aching, burning, and poorly localized "second" pain. Persistent noxious stimulation of these peripheral nerves induces pre- and postsynaptic neurons in the dorsal horn to undergo changes in function, chemical profile, and structure that result in propagation of neural impulses at lower-than-normal thresholds, prolonged discharge, and widening of receptive fields. These changes have been termed "windup" and "central sensitization" hyperalgesia wherein successive similar stimuli cause increasing pain or normally subthreshold stimuli, such as light touch, produce intense pain at and adjacent to the site of original injury. Windup and central sensitization occur primarily by greater and more prolonged opening of postsynaptic NMDA channels to allow Ca^{2+} influx, which reduces transmembrane potential and facilitates postsynaptic depolarization [272]. This central facilitation manifests within seconds of a nociceptive stimulus and can outlast the stimulus for hours, days, or longer if the stimulus is maintained, even at low levels [273, 274]. Experimental and clinical studies in adults have demonstrated that a single small dose of ketamine reduces the magnitude of hyperalgesia and windup-like pain [275–278]. Adults undergoing elective orthopedic or abdominal operations, for example, had reduced postoperative pain and marked reduction of opiate medication use for hours to days when as little as 50 mg of ketamine was added to their general anesthetic regimen [133, 279, 280]. Continued low-dose infusion of ketamine has also been shown to markedly augment morphine for analgesia after musculoskeletal injury in adults [281].

Paradoxically, opiates have been found to induce short-lasting analgesia and long-lasting hyperalgesia [282]. This opiate-induced hyperalgesia is also under the influence of excitatory neurotransmission and is similarly reduced by ketamine blockade of the NMDA glutamate receptor [283–285]. Whether these prolonged beneficial effects occur with ketamine administration for ED PSA after an acute traumatic injury has yet to be explored.

Neurotoxicity

Concern has been raised about use of ketamine in children due to evidence of neurotoxicity in animals after high doses. Toxicity manifested as neuronal vacuolization has been found within specific areas of the midbrain of rats after administration of 40 mg/kg ketamine, but not after doses of 5, 10, or 20 mg/kg [286]. Other investigators found no evidence of neuronal injury (apoptosis) in 7-day-old rat pups after single doses of 25, 50, or 75 mg/kg; only with repeated injections of ketamine 25 mg/kg every 90 min for 9 h was any evidence of toxicity noted [287]. Of possible pediatric relevance, neuronal vacuolization was not found even with large doses of a potent ketamine-like drug (MK-801) in animals prior to puberty [288]. In addition, GABAergic drugs (e.g., diazepam) and alpha agonists (e.g., clonidine) markedly reduce the excitotoxic effects of ketamine-like drugs; it has been suggested these should be coadministered with ketamine as a neuroprotective strategy [289].

A marked increase in normal CNS apoptosis or programmed cell death and some evidence of subsequent learning disabilities in association with administration of ketamine, ethanol, benzodiazepines, propofol, and volatile anesthetics also has been found in rodent animal models [290–292]. Of potential importance, the brain area most affected may vary by species. In rodents, key regions for learning are targeted, whereas in the monkey perhaps less-essential cortical redundant cells are more affected [293]. While it is difficult to compare the effect of specific dosages across species, doses that achieve similar clinical effects as PSA have been shown to increase CNS apoptosis in infant mice [294]. Although ketamine has been used extensively in children without apparent ill effect, these studies raise serious concerns that are the targets of ongoing investigations.

Psychotomimetic Effects

Transient ketamine-induced schizophrenia-like symptoms including hallucinations, delusions, illogical thinking, poverty of speech and thought, agitation, disturbances of emotion and affect, withdrawal, decreased motivation, decreases in memory, and dissociation are well described in adults and a major constraint to use of the drug [295–298]. These symptoms occur when plasma levels of ketamine are relatively low and thus are seen during recovery from sedation. Similar to onset of schizophrenia, these symptoms are thought to be more common in adults and adolescents than in prepubertal children, but this has not been confirmed in children or in association with ED PSA [89, 252, 256, 299–301]. Dependent upon definitions, overall emergence phenomena are well tolerated and occur in approximately 5–25 % of children recovering from ED PSA with ketamine, as well as with other drug regimens, and in similar frequency at home within days of discharge [9, 89, 300, 302]. However, significantly unpleasant and disturbing phenomena (i.e., nightmares, hallucinations, and severe agitation) occur unpredictably in approximately 5 % or fewer children and are also seen with other drug regimens such as fentanyl plus midazolam [9, 89]. Midazolam routinely administered after ketamine or mixed within the same syringe does not appear to reduce significant recovery dysphoria and may increase agitation in postpubertal children [89, 303]. Of interest, preinduction anxiety and agitation have been correlated with emergence delirium for both ED PSA and general anesthesia [303, 304]. Whether pre-sedation midazolam for anxiolysis may reduce recovery dysphoria in significantly anxious children undergoing ED PSA, as has been shown with general anesthesia, is unclear [302, 305].

A potentially effective strategy to reduce emergence delirium, and one regularly employed by the author and others, is to inform the patient to expect transient funny dreams, diplopia, blindness, etc., and to have pleasant thoughts during induction of sedation [306].

Other Adverse Effects

Ketamine administration occasionally causes an evanescent erythematous rash shortly after infusion, and more commonly, double vision and dizziness during emergence from sedation; hypersalivation, typically with repeated or larger doses; and vomiting [9]. Vomiting in children who receive ketamine without adjunctive medications for ED PSA has been reported in 10–20 % of children [89, 94]. Fortunately, vomiting almost always occurs during the recovery period and after discharge from the ED [9, 307].

Coadministration of opioids such as morphine or oxycodone increases emesis whereas coadministration of midazolam with ketamine significantly reduces the likelihood of vomiting (19 % versus 10 %) [89] as does ondansetron (13 % versus 5 %) [94]. Since vomiting may be more likely to occur in older children, ondansetron should be especially considered in children older than 5 years [94]. Vomiting does not appear to be linked to the length of pre-sedation fasting or the dose of ketamine administered [63, 92, 308].

Ketamine-associated hypersalivation is thought to be mediated via cholinergic effects [133]. Because of concern that excess saliva may trigger laryngospasm and other adverse airway events, anticholinergic antisialagogues such as atropine or glycopyrrolate have traditionally been coadministered with ketamine [121, 252]. However, an unblinded observational study of approximately 1,000 children receiving intravenous ketamine without an antisialagogue for ED PSA, mean dose 2 mg/kg, found no significant hypersalivation or adverse airway effects [142]. In contrast, a randomized blinded trial of intramuscular ketamine, 4 mg/kg, with or without atropine, found increased salivation but no adverse airway events in those receiving ketamine [141]. These studies suggest hypersalivation may be dose related. Importantly, a meta-analysis found an increased occurrence of respiratory adverse events associated with antisialagogues [135]. Because of these studies and that "dry mouth" is a common complaint after atropine or glycopyrrolate, the author no longer routinely administers an antisialagogue when a single intravenous ketamine dose or total doses of 2 mg/kg or less are used for ED PSA.

Contraindications/cautions/adverse effects: Please see specific effects.

While much less common than with other ED PSA regimens, respiratory depression, apnea, and upper airway obstruction may occur with ketamine administration [267]. When identified by close monitoring and direct observation, these adverse effects are usually easily managed with simple maneuvers such as jaw thrust and airway straightening [307]. Ketamine preserves cardiac output in healthy patients but should be used with caution in patients manifesting shock as it may cause cardiac depression and profound hypotension [257].

Psychotomimetic effects—e.g., hallucinations, paranoia, and other schizophrenia-like symptoms—occur unpredictably and usually become manifested as dysphoria during recovery. Some believe these symptoms may occur more frequently in postpubertal children and in children with psychiatric disorders. Since the pathologic mechanisms of schizophrenia appear to be similar to ketamine-induced effects, it is recommended to avoid use of ketamine in patients with psychiatric disorders and those whose close relatives carry these disorders. Although not well studied, children with attention deficit and hyperactivity disorders (ADHD) do not appear to have increased susceptibility to psychotomimetic effects. Ketamine is used routinely with and without midazolam in the author's ED for intensely painful procedures in adolescents; all verbal children are informed prior to sedation of what they might experience during recovery and given the suggestion to think of pleasant circumstances as sedation is induced. Midazolam routinely administered after ketamine or mixed within the same syringe does not appear to reduce dysphoria during recovery from ketamine sedation and may increase dysphoria in teenagers [89, 303]. Highly anxious children may benefit from receiving anxiolytic doses of midazolam well before ketamine, as has been shown with general anesthesia [305, 309, 310].

Ketamine is available in concentrations of 10, 50, or 100 mg/mL. For intravenous sedation, it is recommended only the 10 mg/mL concentration be used in order to reduce the risk of overdose and to facilitate titration to desired effect. It is also recommended that only one concentration be routinely available in the ED to reduce the likelihood that a more concentrated solution and thus, larger dose than intended, be inadvertently administered.

Pharmacokinetics

In unpremedicated children and adults, approximate ketamine distribution half-life is 24 s, redistribution half-life 4.7 min, and elimination half-life 2.2 h [311, 312]. The redistribution half-life of 5 min is consistent with the typical deepest sedation period of 5–10 min observed with single-dose ketamine for ED PSA. Midazolam or diazepam coadministration with ketamine may delay hepatic metabolism, yet it does not seem to prolong recovery although the midazolam sedative effects may prolong discharge [89, 313].

To reliably achieve the dissociated state for ED PSA, a minimum dose of ketamine 1.5–2 mg/kg administered intravenously over 30–60 s or 4–5 mg/kg administered intramuscularly is generally recommended [81, 250]. However, studies have found smaller intravenous or intramuscular doses to be effective, particularly when coadministered with midazolam [9, 90, 160, 314, 315]. Recent pharmacokinetic studies of ketamine ED PSA in children have helped elucidate why these different dosing strategies can be effective.

Age-specific ketamine pharmacokinetic profiles based upon measurement of plasma concentrations of ketamine in children 1.5–14 years of age who were undergoing ketamine ED PSA have been determined [316]. These profiles were then used to simulate several dosing strategies and recovery periods designed to achieve 15 min of very deep sedation/anesthesia (unresponsive or arouses, but not to consciousness, with painful stimulus) [159]. They predict a typical

Table 19.9 Ketamine dosing schedules to maintain very deep sedation levels for 15 min [159]

Age	Single dose (recovery ~70 min)	Intermittent dosing (recovery ~30 min)	Initial dose with 15 min infusion (recovery ~20 min)
Adult	1.5 mg/kg	1 mg/kg + 0.5 mg/kg at 10 min	0.25 mg/kg + 2.5 mg/kg/h
12 years	1.75 mg/kg	1 mg/kg + 0.5 mg/kg at 8 min	0.275 mg/kg + 2.75 mg/kg/h
6 years	2 mg/kg	1.25 mg/kg + 0.625 mg/kg at 8 min	0.3 mg/kg + 3 mg/kg/h
2 years	2.125 mg/kg	1.5 mg/kg + 0.75 mg/kg at 8 min	0.35 mg/kg + 3.5 mg/kg/h
		or	
		1 mg/kg + 0.5 mg/kg at 6 min + 0.5 mg/kg at 10 min	

6-year-old child would recover (drowsy, eyes open or closed but easily arouses to consciousness with verbal stimulus) by 70 min after a 2 mg/kg infusion over 30–60 s. An alternative strategy of an initial bolus of 1.25 mg/kg with a subsequent half dose (0.625 mg/kg) "top-up" at 8 min would achieve recovery by 30 min. Finally, an initial dose of 0.3 mg/kg followed by an infusion of 3 mg/kg/h for 15 min would result in recovery by 20 min after the infusion was stopped. These and doses for other ages are listed in Table 19.9.

As with most drugs, between-subject variability has been found in ketamine effect and clearance. The mean target ketamine plasma concentration of 0.65 mg/L would only be effective in 50 % of children; a concentration of 1.59 mg/L would be required to achieve a similar effect, with longer recovery, in 95 % of children [159]. The rate of plasma clearance in children is similar to that in adults and correlates with hepatic blood flow. Clearance increases in a nonlinear function with decreasing age and is reflected by higher dose requirements (mg/kg) to maintain the desired effect in younger children. Size accounts for only about half of the clearance variability; it is unknown what impact pharmacogenomics add. In an individual child, titration to the desired depth of sedation must be gauged clinically.

Concern has been raised that very rapid intravenous administration of ketamine may increase the risk for apnea or marked respiratory depression, presumably due to rapid changes in brain ketamine concentrations [81, 250]. However, in the author's practice, small intravenous doses of 0.25–0.5 mg/kg administered over less than 5 s have not been associated with adverse respiratory effects and can provide effective PSA for procedures lasting for less than 5 min, such as simple fracture reductions or abscess incision and drainage (I&D).

Indications: Ketamine is particularly effective as PSA for intensely painful procedures such as fracture reduction, dislocated joint reduction, burn debridement, or abscess I&D [9, 158]. Ketamine is also an effective PSA technique for brief painful radiological procedures such as guided joint aspiration or nonpainful CT scans and repair of complex lacerations. Procedures that involve the oropharynx, such as peritonsillar abscess I&D or endoscopy, may be performed with light ketamine sedation (see case examples), but the sedating physicians must be prepared for an increased risk of laryngospasm [144, 317, 318].

Pregnancy Category B

Dosages: When administered in doses greater than 2 mg/kg, ketamine readily induces general anesthesia with unresponsiveness to painful stimuli yet with continued spontaneous respirations and good cardiac output. However, initial intravenous doses ≥2.5 mg/kg or total dose ≥5.0 mg/kg after repeated dosing have been associated with increased risk of adverse respiratory events [135]. It is recommended that ketamine be titrated to the desired degree of blunted response to intense pain. Complete lack of responsiveness to painful stimuli is unnecessary with ketamine as it is a potent amnestic agent [9, 81]. Providers and parents can be reassured (but not guaranteed) that most patients will have little or no memory of the painful procedure, even if moans occur during the most painful parts. It helps parents if providers confirm procedural amnesia by asking the patient what is remembered after recovery, especially when the parents have remained in the room during the procedure.

IV: Total dose 1–2 mg/kg when used alone is sufficient for the most intensely painful procedures lasting less than 5–15 min (see "Pharmacokinetics" section). If coadministered with midazolam, 1–1.5 mg/kg is often sufficient. The total dose can safely be administered as a single dose over 30–60 s, but many sedators begin with an initial dose of 0.5 mg/kg administered over 15–30 s and repeated every minute until the desired blunted response to pain is achieved. For prolonged procedures, additional doses of 0.25–0.5 mg/kg may be administered as needed (about every 5–10 min), depending on individual patient response to stimulus [9, 314]. The smaller initial dose with additional doses as needed may shorten time for recovery [159]. Use of local anesthetics, when applicable, is highly encouraged to decrease the amount of ketamine needed. For an intensely painful but very brief procedure in which patient movement can be tolerated—e.g., moving a patient with a femur fracture off the spine board onto the ED bed—a small dose (0.2–0.3 mg/kg) administered rapidly by IV (over less than 5 s) can enable the patient to tolerate the procedure without losing consciousness;

patients should be warned of feeling "weird" and monitored for possible sedation with this technique.

IM: 2–4 mg/kg, with smaller dose used for brief procedures in which local anesthesia is also used, e.g., laceration repair [315, 319].

Onset/duration:

IV: sedation–analgesia within 15–30 s with initial deeper effects lasting 5–10 min and recovery by 60 min, depending upon dose administered.

IM: sedation–analgesia within 5–15 min, duration 30–150 min, depending upon dose administered.

Metabolization: Hepatic degradation of ketamine within the cytochrome systems results in norketamine, which has one-third the analgesic potency of ketamine. Norketamine has a shorter elimination half-life (1.13 h) than ketamine (2.1 h) [320].

Adjuncts: Glycopyrrolate (Robinul®)

Indication: Antisialagogue is used by some clinicians before initial dose of ketamine. Preferred by some over atropine because it does not cross the blood–brain barrier, thus not causing possible undesirable CNS effects. Antisialagogues prior to single doses of 1–2 mg/kg of ketamine are likely unnecessary [135, 141, 142, 250]. It is unclear whether use of antisialagogues is beneficial in children with active URIs. Many children complain of "cotton-mouth" for 6–8 h after glycopyrrolate administration [9].

Concentration: 200 μg/mL.

Dose: 5 μg/kg IV. Maximum dose is 200 mg. Administer at least 5–15 min before the initial dose of ketamine.

Atropine

Indication: Antisialagogue used by some clinicians in conjunction with initial dose of ketamine (instead of glycopyrrolate). Concern has been raised about potential CNS adverse effects with atropine (e.g., excitation), but this appears uncommon [141]. Antisialagogues prior to single doses of 1–2 mg/kg of ketamine are likely unnecessary [135, 141, 142, 250]. It is unclear whether the use of antisialagogues is beneficial in children with active URIs.

Dose: 0.01 mg/kg (minimum 0.1 mg, maximum 0.5 mg).

Ketamine plus Propofol (Ketofol)

Coadministering ketamine and propofol (ketofol) intravenously has been shown to be an effective and efficient technique for ED PSA with fewer adverse effects than when both drugs are used as single agents [321, 322]. Of note, the decreased respiratory depression with ketofol may be due to the smaller doses of propofol needed to achieve sedation when coadministered with ketamine [323]. Moreover, use of ketamine for analgesia reduces the need for opioid coadministration with propofol, a combination that potentiates respiratory depression. Less frequent vomiting is also reported in patients receiving ketofol, when compared to use of ketamine alone, an effect similar to ondansetron [323]. Three studies of children receiving ketofol for ED PSA, primarily for fracture reductions, have been published to date [324–326]. The optimum relative doses of ketamine and propofol are unclear.

A well-designed double-blinded randomized controlled trial compared ketofol to ketamine alone [324]. Children received either (1) an initial dose of ketamine followed by propofol ("ketofol"), 0.5 mg/kg each, and then propofol 0.5 mg/kg every 2 min as needed to achieve deep sedation or (2) an initial 1.0 mg/kg of ketamine followed by 0.25 mg/kg of ketamine every 2 min, as needed. Each agent was administered intravenously over 30 s.

One hundred and thirty-six children, median age 11 years, were studied. The median total doses of propofol and ketamine were 0.5 mg/kg for those receiving ketofol and 1.0 mg/kg of ketamine for those receiving ketamine alone. In the ketofol group, total sedation time was shorter by 3 min (13 versus 16 min), and fewer patients experienced vomiting (2 % versus 12 %). Unpleasant recovery (agitation, hallucinations, delirium) occurred in 8 % with ketofol and 13 % with ketamine alone. Other adverse events were similar between the two groups; no patients in either group required any airway intervention other than repositioning or increased oxygen.

A case series described use of intravenous ketofol (ketamine–propofol mixed 1:1 in a single syringe) titrated to deep sedation for ED PSA [324]. Two hundred nineteen children, median age 13 years, were studied. The median dose was 0.8 mg/kg each of ketamine and propofol. Median recovery time was 14 min. Two patients required brief vigorous stimulation for central apnea, and positive-pressure ventilation was needed to manage laryngospasm in an infant with croup who had undergone laryngoscopy to look for a foreign body.

An earlier small case series evaluated ketamine 0.5 mg/kg followed 1 min later by propofol 1 mg/kg, both administered over 30 s [326]. Second doses of ketamine, 0.25 mg/kg, and/or propofol, 0.5 mg/kg, were permitted if the level of sedation was deemed inadequate. Twenty patients were evaluated, average age 9.6 years. The median time from injection of ketamine to the first purposeful response was 10 min and to suitability for discharge was 38 min. Transient mild oxygen desaturation occurred in three patients (15 %) and responded easily to airway repositioning. No assisted ventilation or supplemental oxygen was needed. One patient vomited.

A blinded randomized trial compared ketofol to propofol for ED PSA in children and adults (median ages 20 and 22 years) [327]. All patients received 0.5–1 μg/kg fentanyl 5 min prior to sedation. Then either 0.5 mg/kg of ketamine or saline was infused over 1 min followed by propofol 1 mg/kg over 2 min. Repeated doses of propofol 0.5 mg/kg were then administered as needed to attain or maintain deep sedation. Of note, respiratory depression was similar between the groups (22 % versus 28 %). They found the combination of ketamine and propofol resulted in greater provider satisfaction and perhaps better sedation quality. Time to recovery was not reported.

These studies found similar results to trials in adults. A blinded trial randomized 284 adults to receive either ketofol or propofol alone, primarily for fracture reduction in the ED [328]. To achieve deep sedation, patients received either (1) propofol or (2) 0.375 mg/kg each of ketamine and propofol, with additional doses of each as needed. Adverse respiratory events were similar in both groups (30 % with ketofol versus 32 % with propofol). Three patients received bag–valve–mask ventilation with ketofol and 1 with propofol. Recovery agitation was seen in 6 with ketofol. Other secondary outcomes were similar between the groups. Patients and staff were highly satisfied with both agents.

A comparison of 0.3 mg/kg ketamine followed by propofol titrated to deep sedation was found to be more effective than 1.5 μg/kg fentanyl followed by propofol [329]. Patients receiving fentanyl required less additional propofol but had 5 times more serious intra-sedation events than patients receiving ketamine. Time to discharge readiness was 28 min for the ketamine group versus 37 min for the fentanyl group.

Finally, a comparison of ketofol to midazolam and ketamine for fracture reductions in adults found both provided satisfactory ED PSA, but perceived pain was greater in the midazolam–fentanyl group [330]. Adverse effects were similar except for emergence reaction (29 % with ketamine–propofol versus none with midazolam–fentanyl).

Although coadministration of ketamine with propofol enables use of smaller doses of both propofol and ketamine to achieve effective sedation, it is unclear that the slightly faster recovery with this more complex technique in children is clinically significant and needs further evaluation.

Ketamine plus Dexmedetomidine (Ketadex)

Coadministration of ketamine and dexmedetomidine has been found to reduce or prevent the tachycardia, hypertension, salivation, and emergence phenomena seen with ketamine and the bradycardia and hypotension/hypertension seen with dexmedetomidine in children undergoing cardiac procedures and lithotripsy [331]. However, no studies have been conducted to date evaluating this combination for ED PSA in children.

Nitrous Oxide (N_2O)

Nitrous oxide (N_2O) is a colorless, odorless, and tasteless gas that, in a linear dose–response pattern, induces dissociative euphoria, drowsiness, anxiolysis, and mild to moderate amnesia and analgesia with onset and offset of effects within 2–5 min [332, 333]. N_2O is blended with oxygen (N_2O/O_2) and typically is described by the N_2O component: "70 % N_2O" is 70 % N_2O = 30 % O_2 [334]. At a specific concentration of N_2O, however, depth of sedation can vary considerably. One study of N_2O for ED PSA found 90 % of children receiving 50–70 % N_2O were mildly sedated (drowsy, eyes open or closed, but easily aroused to consciousness with verbal stimulus), whereas moderate or deep sedation occurred in 3 % receiving 70 % N_2O and in none receiving 50 % [335]. Others report 2–10 % of children may be poorly sedated during ED PSA with N2O [10, 335, 336].

Since N_2O sedation and analgesia are usually mild to moderate, children are partially aware and strategies to enhance the gas's anxiolytic, dissociative, and euphoric effects are vital to successful use for PSA. Guided imagery significantly augments N_2O's efficacy and helps allay anxiety [333, 337]. Children naive to intoxication are frequently frightened by the floating or tingling sensations caused by the gas, but they readily accept these effects when incorporated into non-frightening scenarios. The author often encourages preschool and school-aged children to imagine flying to a favorite or imaginary place, "soaring with eagles, past clouds and stars to check out the moon," guiding the child during the sedation by detailed descriptions of what might be "seen" along the way. Alternatively, some children like describing their own imaginings, allowing the author to figuratively "tag along," as with a 5-year-old girl who portrayed in great detail her "chocolate ponies" as her radius fracture was being reduced. Finally, some older children and teenagers prefer the partial awareness with N_2O sedation as they, like many adults, fear loss of vigilance or control associated with potent sedation or anesthesia.

Effective pain reduction by concurrent use of local anesthesia and/or systemic analgesia for painful procedures is also crucial for successful N_2O ED PSA [338]. For examples, forearm fractures can be reduced with minimal distress when N_2O sedation is augmented by a lidocaine hematoma block [90, 339, 340] or lacerations repaired calmly in young children when they have also received topical anesthetic [10]. The lack of painful administration or need for venous access and the rapid onset and offset of effects make N_2O ED PSA an attractive option for many clinical situations.

N_2O can safely be administered by specially trained nurses to healthy children for ED PSA [62, 341, 342].

Indications: N_2O, along with local anesthesia and/or oral analgesics, primarily is used for anxiolysis, mild analgesia, and amnesia during brief (<5–10 min) procedures, such as laceration repair, abscess incision and drainage, lumbar puncture, IV placement, and some fracture reductions. Use of 60–70 % N_2O or coadministration of opioids or sedatives may deepen sedation and improve efficacy [343–345]. The author frequently administers oxycodone 0.2–0.3 mg/kg orally 30–60 min prior to N_2O sedation for I&D of an abscess in toddler and preschool children. Although seldom seen, these children are monitored for respiratory depression before, during, and after the sedation.

Many find the gas more effective in children old enough to cooperate and use imagination, but significant reduction of procedure-related distress has been observed in 2-year-old and younger children [10]. In the author's ED, N_2O sedation is regularly used effectively in infants of 3 months of age and older by administering with a continuous-flow system, described later.

Suturing-related distress in children can be reduced by N_2O [10, 336, 346–348]. We found 2- to 6-year-old children who had received topical anesthetic and were viewing cartoons with a parent at the bedside had less distress during wound cleaning, supplemental lidocaine injection, and suturing if receiving 50 % N_2O instead of oral midazolam. Children who received N_2O alone recovered rapidly without ataxia or dizziness, but did have more vomiting (10 %) [10]. Of note, 30 % N_2O was found insufficient in children younger than 8 years old in another study [346].

Mid to distal forearm fracture reduction can be effectively performed with N_2O sedation, particularly when combined with a local anesthetic hematoma block [90, 339, 340, 349–351]. We found N_2O plus 1 % lidocaine hematoma block (2.5 mg/kg, maximum 100 mg) as effective as intravenous ketamine in reducing distress during fracture reductions in children aged 5–17 years. This technique is often most effective in displaced mid to distal forearm fractures that have large fracture site hematomas that enable effective hematoma blocks, whereas torus or greenstick fractures that require reduction likely have small or no fracture hematomas making the lidocaine block less effective; an effective fracture hematoma block is the key for maximum success. For these incomplete fractures, hematoma blocks may provide partial pain relief and, combined with 70 % nitrous oxide along with prior oral oxycodone or another potent analgesic, enable many children to tolerate fracture reduction with acceptable distress. The child usually recalls less pain related to the fracture reduction performed with N_2O sedation than an observer would expect based upon the child's response during the procedure [339]. It is usually reassuring to ask the child after recovery, with the parent(s) present, what he or she recalls of the procedure, especially when the parent was present during the reduction and the child had manifested some distress. Recovery is markedly faster from N_2O compared to ketamine-based sedation for fracture reduction (16 versus 83 min) [90]. If the N_2O is turned off as soon as any painful molding of the cast at the fracture site after reduction is completed, the patient is typically recovered to near baseline before the casting or splinting is finished.

Children's distress during other painful ED and outpatient procedures such as lumbar puncture, abscess drainage, dressing change, and intravenous catheter placement likewise can be reduced by N_2O [335, 348, 352–357]. Recovery from N_2O sedation typically is very rapid, with the child able to sit alone within 5 min and ready for discharge within 15 min [78].

Technique: As described previously, successful N_2O sedators engage the child in imaginative stories throughout the procedure. Distraction, imagery, and storytelling significantly enhance desired effects by giving the child a nonthreatening construct in which to place the sensations caused by the gas. While breathing N_2O, children are able to follow commands, describe sensations of floating, frequently laugh, and occasionally chew or lick masks that have been scented with bubblegum spray or flavored lip-balm to enhance acceptance of the mask. Adolescent and school-aged children often begin giggling if it is suggested to them that this is expected, and their parents typically also begin laughing when this occurs, presumably easing their own anxiety. Coaxing children as young as 2 years of age to hold the mask on their face adds a measure of safety by allowing them to remove the mask quickly if vomiting occurs. Their ability to hold the mask also indicates their depth of sedation and may reduce anxiety related to the mask covering their mouth/nose. When the mask is held in place by a sedator, that person must be vigilant for evidence of vomiting and quickly remove the mask to allow the child to clear the emesis.

Titration of the gas beginning at 30 %, the anxiolytic dose, and increasing the concentration to 50–70 % over 2 min may reduce children's fear during induction. Others find when children have been prepared with explanations about what effects they are likely to feel, they tolerate beginning at 50–70 %. With either technique, the child should breathe the maximum concentration desired for 1–2 min, allowing full effect, before beginning the procedure.

Administration of 100 % oxygen after cessation of N_2O to prevent "diffusion hypoxia" is unnecessary unless the patient is emerging from deep sedation or general anesthesia. N_2O diffusing from the bloodstream into the alveoli and displacing oxygen is readily exhaled without causing hypoxia in patients recovering from sedation with N_2O alone [358–360]. As with any sedation technique, children should be monitored with pulse oximetry until alert, usually less than 3–5 min after ending N_2O administration.

Delivery system: Until recently, delivery of N_2O (fixed at 50 %) in the ED has been by demand-valve systems designed for adult use (Nitronox/Entonox®). Children have difficulty generating the negative inspiratory pressure required to initiate gas flow with these devices. Continuous-flow systems, such as those used by dentists, oral surgeons, and anesthesiologists, in contrast, provide free flow of gases with the ability to deliver up to 70 % N_2O. These systems allow normal respirations and are easily used by patients of all ages [334, 361]. Dental systems with nasal hoods can be adapted for use with a full face mask by adding into the expiratory limb an open gas interface designed for anesthesia machines. N_2O concentration is limited to a maximum of 70–75 % as concentrations exceeding 79 % (+21 % O_2) would cause hypoxia. Accidental administration of 100 % N_2O due to machine or system failure can be rapidly lethal [153, 362, 363]. Providers must be very familiar with the mechanisms of the N_2O delivery system used. A machine or systems check should be performed before each use of N_2O to assure proper function of the machine and monitors.

A scavenging device should be an integral part of the delivery system to minimize ambient levels of N_2O gas exposure to healthcare workers since chronic and repeated exposure to N_2O may cause abnormalities in hematologic, neurologic, and reproductive systems (see cautions). The N_2O delivery device and the treatment area in which it is used should be in compliance with National Institute of Occupational Safety and Health Standards and state safety guidelines and regulations [364]. It is beneficial to have room air exchanges of at least 10–20/h in treatment rooms to remove any N_2O that has escaped the scavenging process.

Monitoring: An in-line oxygen analyzer should be used to assure proper equipment functioning/adequate oxygen delivery during N_2O administration [153]. A gas analyzer that measures inspiratory and expiratory N_2O and end-tidal CO_2 concentrations adds additional assurance of patient safety and equipment function.

Administration of ≤50 % N_2O, without any other sedative, narcotic, or other respiratory depressant drug, to children ASA-PS Class I or II is considered minimal sedation, and the patient may be monitored by direct visualization and intermittent assessment of their level of sedation [153]. The child should be able to be verbally interactive throughout the sedation. If >50 % N_2O is administered or if the patient receives concurrent narcotic or other sedative drugs, the patient should be observed for moderate sedation and monitoring escalated accordingly if that should occur. Since oxygen is blended with N_2O, even mild hypoxemia is very unlikely and should cause immediate investigation to determine the cause.

Contraindications/cautions: At normal atmospheric pressure, N_2O cannot induce general anesthesia, unless combined with other agents. N_2O at 30–70 % has been safely used widely for more than a century to reduce distress in children during dental procedures [365]. Review of nearly 36,000 administrations of 50 % N_2O for nondental procedures, 82 % of which were in children, found 9 (0.03 %) serious adverse events (somnolence, vomiting, bradycardia, vertigo, headache, nightmares, sweating) that may have been attributed to the N_2O [366]. In healthy patients (ASA-PS I, II), N_2O has minimal cardiovascular or respiratory effects [78, 344, 359]. N_2O, however, may enhance the depressed response to hypoxia and hypercarbia induced by other agents [335, 343–345, 367].

N_2O diffuses rapidly into air-filled cavities causing volume and/or pressure increases proportional to concentration and duration of N_2O inhaled. Therefore, N_2O should not be administered to patients with areas of trapped gas such as pneumothorax, obstructive pulmonary disease, or bowel obstruction. Albeit seemingly rare, patients with acute otitis media may experience painful increase in middle ear pressure. Other relative contraindications include significant head injury (N_2O mildly increases intracranial blood flow), altered mental status, and psychiatric disorder (N_2O may cause dysphoric effects similar to ketamine).

Bone marrow suppression, liver, CNS, and testicular dysfunction, decreased fertility and increased spontaneous fetal loss, and peripheral neuropathy may possibly occur with repeated and chronic exposure [78, 334]. None of these adverse effects have been found when scavenging devices are integrated into the system. Therefore, use of a scavenging device is essential to minimize ambient levels of gas and exposure to healthcare workers.

Deaths associated with N_2O use have been due to inadvertent administration of 100 % nitrous oxide, with subsequent hypoxia [362, 363]. These occurrences primarily were in patients already sedated with other drugs as part of anesthetic regimens. These tragedies point out the essential need for clinicians to understand all aspects, including mechanical, of the gas delivery device being used.

Pregnancy Category C

Adverse effects: Vomiting occurs in approximately 10 % of children receiving 50 % N_2O, along with transient dizziness and headache in some [78]. These effects usually resolve within 5 min of cessation of N_2O administration. Vomiting frequency increases with opiate and decreases with midazolam coadministration [10, 90]. Some providers believe the risk of vomiting increases when the duration of administration exceeds 5–10 min, especially with greater than 50 % concentrations, but this is yet to be substantiated. Whether antiemetics such as ondansetron reduce N_2O-induced nausea and vomiting is unclear. Protective airway reflexes are largely intact when N_2O is used alone [368–370]. Whether combining N_2O with other sedatives or analgesics increases risk for aspiration and other adverse events is unknown, but the risk likely correlates with the patient's depth of sedation and effects of the coadministered drug.

Dosages: Concentrations of 30–50 %, blended with oxygen, achieve minimal to light moderate sedation in most children without adverse cardiopulmonary effects [78]. More recently, routine use of 60–70 % has been recommended and found safe in children undergoing sedation in the ED [335]. In the author's ED, 50–70 % concentrations are typically used with initial higher concentrations and then reduced as the most painful part of the procedure is accomplished.

Onset/duration: Patients experience the effects of N_2O within 1 min, but for optimum effect, they should inhale the gas for 2–3 min before beginning a procedure to allow brain concentrations to equilibrate with the delivered concentration of gas. Recovery occurs rapidly with children being able to sit alone by 3–5 min after cessation, but initially they should be assisted with walking as ataxia may occur for a bit longer.

Mechanism of action: N_2O has NMDA glutamate receptor antagonist, opioid agonist, and GABAergic effects [371–373].

Metabolization: N_2O is excreted unchanged by exhalation.

Ketamine + Midazolam or Fentanyl + Midazolam Techniques for Deep Sedation

Providers utilizing these regimens should be thoroughly familiar with these medications and sedation guidelines outlined in text. Sedation should be performed in an area fully equipped for resuscitation.

Pre-sedation Assessment and Preparation

1. Initial assessment: Determine patient's ASA classification, airway risks, and time of last oral intake, and obtain informed consent.
2. Establish indwelling venous access maintained with normal saline or Ringer's lactate.
3. Attach patient monitors to continuously measure patient's oxygen saturation (with variable pitch indicator), heart rate, and respiratory rate and intermittently measure blood pressure. Consider preoxygenation and supplemental oxygen delivery during the sedation if capnography is available and staff trained in use.
4. Prepare positive-pressure ventilation bag and mask; assure ability to deliver supplemental oxygen.
5. Prepare oral suctioning device with rigid tip.

During Sedation

1. Assign a provider whose sole responsibility is to monitor patient safety.
2. Continuously monitor patient by direct observation, oxygen saturation (with variable pitch indicator), HR, and RR, and monitor blood pressure after each medication infusion and at 5 min intervals. Patient monitoring and direct observation at increasing intervals is continued during recovery until discharge criteria are met.
3. Infuse medications near the hub of the catheter over 10–20 s, in small incremental doses to titrate to desired endpoint of analgesia, sedation. Use of dilute solutions and precalculated dosage tables based upon patient weight is recommended.
4. Administer medications when supportive staff is present and prepared to render support if necessary and provider prepared to begin and perform the procedure.

Fentanyl Technique

(a) Midazolam: 0.05–0.1 mg/kg (0.05–0.1 mL/kg) at 2–3 min intervals; endpoint (decreased patient anxiety, mildly slurred speech, drooping eyelids); typically effective dose, not more than 0.1 mg/kg to induce marked amnesia along with sedation.

(b) Fentanyl (10 mg/mL): 0.5 mg/kg (0.05 mL/kg) at 2–3 min intervals; endpoint, decreased patient responsiveness to painful stimulus or decreasing oxygen saturations; typically effective dose, 1–1.5 mg/kg.

Ketamine Technique

(a) Midazolam may be reserved for anxious patients undergoing ketamine sedation. For anxiolysis, dose, 0.05 mg/kg; maximum dose, 2 mg; single administration, 5–15 min prior to initiation of sedation.

(b) Ketamine (10 mg/mL): dose, 0.5–1 mg/kg (0.05–0.1 mL/kg) at 1 min intervals; end-point, decreased patient responsiveness to painful stimulus; typically effective dose, 1–2 mg/kg. Supplemental doses of 0.5 mg/kg may be administered as indicated by patient distress.

Consider using an antisialagogue (e.g., glycopyrrolate 5 mg/kg or atropine 0.01–0.02 mg/kg) prior to ketamine administration if it is an anticipated procedure that will require multiple supplemental doses of ketamine.

Caution: Suggested doses may readily result in oxygen saturation falling below 90 % in patient's breathing room air, particularly when fentanyl is used. Providers must be prepared to immediately turn the patient to his side if vomiting, reposition or suction patient's airway, and provide supplemental oxygen or positive-pressure ventilation until patient has returned to baseline physiologic status and recovered from sedation.

Conclusion: Final Thoughts

This chapter has presented the sedation provider with a range of sedation techniques and options for painful and nonpainful procedures that may need to be performed on an urgent basis. There is no doubt that sedation and analgesia are important components of the emergency department care and should be an integral component of the emergency medicine physician's practice. The training and credentialing process for sedation is an area of recent interest from the American College of Emergency Physicians. In July 2011, the American College of Emergency Physicians released a policy statement entitled *Procedural Sedation and Analgesia in the Emergency Department: Recommendations for Physician Credentialing, Privileging, and Practice* [374]. This policy iterated that the chief of the emergency medicine service at each institution will be responsible for establishing criteria for credentialing and recommending emergency physicians for sedation privileges. Sedation training should "focus on the unique ED environment." This policy is important, because it empowers the chief of emergency medicine with the responsibility of establishing sedation training and credentialing requirements for the emergency medicine specialty. Furthermore, the policy expands the role of the emergency physicians as well as emergency medicine nurses by condoning the capability of qualified ED nurses to "administer propofol, ketamine, and other sedatives under the direct supervision of a privileged emergency physician." The policy also recognizes that there may be occasions whereby the emergency medicine environment may not lend itself to having a separate physician administer the sedative and another to perform the procedure: For these situations, the policy states "Deep sedation may be accomplished…by the same emergency physician both administering sedation and performing the procedure."

As the practice of sedation evolves, one can anticipate that the American College of Emergency Physicians will continue to survey the landscape, evaluate the literature, and recommend policies and guidelines to promote the safe and efficacious delivery of sedation in the emergency medicine environment.

Case Studies

Case 1

A 12-year-old boy has closed *displaced metaphyseal fractures of his distal right radius and ulna* and numbness in his 3rd and 4th fingers. He fell 30 min ago running in gym class and has no other injury. He takes methylphenidate for attention deficit hyperactivity disorder (ADHD). He otherwise is healthy and has never received sedation or anesthesia. He ate lunch 2 h prior to arrival and was given ibuprofen by his mother on the way to the hospital. He is anxious and crying in triage.

Issues: pain relief now and during radiographs and exams; PSA for fracture reduction with consideration of his fasting status, anxiety, ADHD, and neurovascular status of his injury:

1. *Pain relief* will facilitate imaging of the fractures, accurate assessment of the injury, and preparation of the patient for PSA for fracture reduction. Options include:
   (a) *Splinting* the injured area to prevent movement of the fractured bones provides significant pain relief.
   (b) *Systemic analgesia*: Administer before radiographs, even if the child indicates less pain after splinting. Repositioning of the injured limb for radiographs and subsequent exams will be quite painful. Options include:
   - *Oxycodone orally*: In our ED, nurses follow standing orders to administer a first dose of oxycodone 0.2 mg/kg orally (maximum dose 10 mg) in triage to children with a potential isolated extremity fracture or another painful injury. This allows rapid and effective attention to the reduction of pain and high patient, family, and staff satisfaction. Noticeable analgesia occurs by 20–45 min with peak effect by an hour and with duration of 2–4 h. This dose is unlikely to cause sedation in children with painful injuries. Doses for home use are 0.05–0.15 mg/kg. Oxycodone is preferred over codeine because it does not require metabolic conversion for analgesic effect. Codeine is slowly or poorly converted to morphine in 2–40 % of patients and thus provides poor or no pain relief to such

(continued)

children. If codeine previously has been effective for a specific child, a first dose of codeine 2 mg/kg orally is effective for these painful injuries with subsequent or home doses of 1 mg/kg.

- *Fentanyl intranasally*, 1.5–2 mg/kg, achieves significant pain relief within 5–10 min with duration of 30–90 min. Use atomizer to spray small volumes of concentrated intravenous fentanyl solution (50 mg/mL) to improve absorption. Divide total dose into repeated sprays of ~0.1–0.2 mL/nostril. Use of small volumes reduces drainage of drug into posterior pharynx where it is less absorbed. If a wide margin of safety is determined after more extensive use of this technique, it might be performed by nurses in triage, but currently it is performed by a physician in a treatment room with patient monitoring for respiratory depression.
- *Opioids intravenously* titrated to effect will provide the greatest pain relief. Fentanyl 1–2 mg/kg IV will provide analgesia within 1–2 min, lasting 30–60 min, whereas morphine 0.1 mg/kg IV will provide initial analgesia within 5–10 min with peak effect at 10–20 min and lasting 2–3 h. This strategy requires IV insertion, typically in a treatment room after physician assessment and orders. Anxiety and pain associated with catheter insertion are significant for many children and are greatly reduced by use of local anesthesia such as buffered lidocaine injected subcutaneously via a 30-gauge needle at the site of insertion.
- *Nitrous oxide 50–70 %* provides rapid pain relief. However, because continued analgesia requires ongoing administration and N_2O scavenging systems are not mobile, a longer-acting systemic analgesic usually is needed. One strategy is to use N_2O to reduce the patient's pain and distress while an IV catheter is inserted for subsequent opioid administration. This strategy typically requires physician assessment and orders, access to N_2O, and IV catheter insertion in a treatment room.

2. *Fasting status*: This child ate lunch 2 h prior to his arrival. Pain from injury and opioid analgesics unpredictably slow intestinal motility. It is uncertain if delaying sedation for 2–4 h in these patients will allow significant additional gastric emptying. Vomiting with PSA does not correlate with the length of fasting. Furthermore, ED PSA does not involve tracheal intubation, a procedure that significantly increases risk of pulmonary aspiration during general anesthesia. Of note, pulmonary aspiration has not been reported in children undergoing ED PSA, despite most being incompletely fasted. As with general anesthesia, no studies have determined if pulmonary aspiration risk is reduced in non-fasted patients by pre-sedation administration of medications to enhance gastric emptying, inhibit gastric acid production, or decrease pH of gastric contents, and such strategies are not recommended. The author's practice is to use PSA techniques that preserve airway reflexes as described herein, to be prepared for vomiting in all patients, and to perform PSA when the full complement of providers is available to perform the procedure and monitor the patient.
3. *PSA techniques*: Since this non-fasted patient has potentially increased risk of pulmonary aspiration of gastric contents, a sedation technique that better preserves protective airway reflexes may increase patient safety. Ketamine and N_2O are NMDA receptor antagonists that blunt protective airway reflexes less than the opioid and GABAergic agents such as fentanyl, midazolam, and propofol:
   (a) *Nitrous oxide (50–70 %) plus lidocaine fracture hematoma block*, along with oxycodone administered at triage, is as effective in reducing distress associated with fracture reduction as intravenous ketamine, provided an effective hematoma block is placed. To reduce risk of nerve and vascular injury from injection, hematoma blocks are typically reserved for mid to distal forearm, and, occasionally, ankle fractures. We administer 50 % N_2O to the child as the orthopedic surgeon, using sterile technique and a dorsal approach, injects 1 % buffered lidocaine (2.5 mg/kg or 0.25 mL/kg, maximum dose 100 mg or 10 mL) into the fracture hematoma. N_2O 70 % is usually administered for the subsequent fracture reduction. Aspiration of hematoma blood into the lidocaine-containing syringe confirms proper location of the needle for injection. Perhaps counterintuitively, the worse the fracture, the more effective is fracture site anesthesia due to larger hematomas. The provider must be prepared for as yet unreported but potential seizure or dysrhythmia due to rapid intraosseous absorption of lidocaine. This theoretical risk is

(continued)

low since the injected lidocaine is within the drug's therapeutic dose range. Some orthopedic surgeons prefer not to use this technique if the fracture and swelling cause numbness in the hand, typically median nerve distribution, because of inability to reassess nerve function immediately postreduction. Use of lidocaine instead of longer-acting local anesthetics such as bupivacaine enables postreduction neurologic assessment within 1–2 h. Variable patient awareness is present with N_2O PSA; thus distraction and guided imagery are crucial to improve efficacy of this technique. Some older children and teenagers, as many adults, prefer not to be unconscious during a procedure if pain is sufficiently reduced.

(b) *Ketamine IV with or without midazolam* more effectively reduces patient distress during intensely painful procedures and causes less respiratory depression than fentanyl- or propofol-based techniques. Intravenous administration is preferred because multiple attempts likely will be needed to align both the radius and ulna, thus increasing potential need for additional doses of ketamine. Time of recovery is reduced by administering a smaller initial dose followed by a half dose. For a child of this age, an *initial ketamine dose 1 mg/kg followed by 0.5 mg/kg at 8 min* likely results in approximately 15 min of very deep sedation with recovery to drowsiness and easy arousal by verbal stimulation by about 30 min. If longer deep sedation is needed for repeated reduction attempts, additional dose of 0.5 mg/kg can be given as needed. Alternatively, an initial ketamine dose of 1.75 mg/kg will result in 15 min of deep sedation, but recovery likely will take 60–70 min.

Intramuscular ketamine 4 mg/kg provides effective PSA without vascular access, but additional doses, if necessary, will require 4–5 min to determine if sufficient. Recovery is significantly longer than with intravenous ketamine and vomiting is more frequent (26 % versus 12 %). Ability to obtain vascular access emergently (intraosseous, if necessary) must be present to manage life-threatening adverse events should they occur.

Midazolam 2 mg total dose may reduce the child's anxiety as preparations are made for PSA. Although yet unconfirmed with PSA, reduced anxiety at induction correlates with reduced dysphoria during recovery from general anesthesia. This small dose is not likely to cause respiratory depression or prolong recovery. Midazolam administered in the same syringe or immediately after ketamine does not appear to reduce recovery dysphoria.

Glycopyrrolate or atropine to reduce ketamine-associated increased salivation is recommended by some to reduce the low risk of laryngospasm. Hypersalivation is usually not significant with these doses of ketamine but may occur with repeated doses for prolonged procedures. The author no longer routinely administers an antisialagogue because these agents have been associated with increased likelihood of adverse respiratory events, and patients complain of dry mouth after recovery.

Vomiting: Administration of opioids such as morphine or oxycodone with ketamine increases emesis (10 % versus 25 %), whereas administration of midazolam decreases vomiting (19 % versus 10 %) as does ondansetron (13 % versus 5 %).

Cautions: Although unlikely to occur, providers must be prepared for hypoventilation, apnea, or laryngospasm with ketamine. As with all deep sedations, this child must be monitored for adverse effects by an experienced dedicated provider during induction, sedation, and recovery. If vomiting occurs, the procedure immediately is interrupted and the child turned to his side to assist his clearing emesis. Observers (e.g., parents) should be forewarned about nystagmus and catatonic stare during sedation and possible dysphoria during recovery. Similarly, patients should be prepared for possible diplopia, dizziness, hallucinations, and a brief period of blindness during recovery. Getting the child to focus on pleasant thoughts during induction and recovery may reduce some of these psychotomimetic effects. Most patients will have no memory of even intensely painful procedures, even if they occasionally moan, but some will have partial recall, usually quite vague. It may help reassure observers if the child indicates no recall when asked after recovery.

(continued)

(c) *Fentanyl+midazolam or propofol* provides effective PSA but blunts protective airway reflexes more than ketamine. This child's recent food intake makes these techniques less desirable. It is unknown whether delaying PSA will improve gastric emptying. Please see *Fasting Status* mentioned previously.

(d) *Reduction under general anesthesia* may be considered. However, reduction should not be delayed long because of the apparent median nerve impingement. Of interest, general anesthesia with endotracheal intubation in non-fasted children may have greater risk of pulmonary aspiration than ED PSA.

Case 2

A 5-year-old girl has a closed *distal radius fracture*, dorsally angulated 30° but hinged at the cortex. She gets "car sick" and had multiple episodes of vomiting after an operation last year.

Issues: pain management, history of motion sickness, and postanesthesia vomiting and optimum technique for a painful but brief fracture reduction. Of note, in young children, some orthopedic surgeons do not reduce metaphyseal fractures "minimally displaced" in the primary plane of motion because they will remodel to normal over the coming months. Standardized determination of how much displacement will successfully remodel remains to be developed:

1. *Pain relief*: Please see Case 1. Splinting and oral oxycodone likely are sufficient.
2. *PSA technique options*: Since this fracture reduction will take "one brief but painful push," effective local anesthesia or brief deep sedation with rapid recovery is desirable:

(a) *Nitrous oxide (50–70%) plus fracture hematoma lidocaine block*: This fracture may not have a significant hematoma, thus reducing the effectiveness of a hematoma block. Combining 70 % N_2O with oxycodone, 0.2 mg/kg orally without the hematoma block, may provide sufficient analgesia and partial amnesia for remaining pain. N_2O should be administered for at least 2 min prior to reduction to maximize the gas's effects. Balancing potentially incomplete PSA against the benefits of not needing vascular access and rapid recovery should be discussed with the parents. A downside to this technique is the 25 % likelihood of vomiting when N_2O is coadministered with an opioid. Coadministration of oral midazolam with N_2O (without oxycodone) reduces vomiting but prolongs recovery. It is unknown if oral ondansetron significantly reduces vomiting with N_2O and oxycodone.

(b) *Ketamine with or without midazolam intravenously*: Since this fracture reduction will likely be very brief, experienced providers may consider *rapid administration* of *ketamine 0.5–0.75 mg/kg* (pushed over 3–5 s) to induce about 5 min of deep sedation, with additional ketamine given if necessary. The performer of the fracture reduction should be ready as the ketamine is infused. With the single small rapid dose, deep sedation will occur within 1 min and recovery to being drowsy but responsive to verbal stimulation will occur by 10–15 min, often as casting is completed. Alternatively, administered over 30–60 s, ketamine 1.25 mg/kg provides deep sedation for 10–15 min with recovery by about 30 min or ketamine 2 mg/kg provides deep sedation for 15 min with recovery by an hour. *Vomiting* frequency after small dose ketamine is unknown. See Case 1 for additional information.

Intramuscular ketamine 4 mg/kg provides effective PSA but recovery is significantly longer than with intravenous ketamine. See Case 1 for additional information.

(c) *Fentanyl with propofol or midazolam* intravenously provides effective PSA for fracture reduction but with more respiratory depression than ketamine techniques (desaturation to less than 90 % in approximately 25 % FM versus 20 % FP versus 5 % KM). Since respiratory depression/apnea occur frequently, providers should be experienced with this technique and well prepared to provide ventilatory support. Vomiting is less frequent with propofol- than ketamine-based techniques. Recovery is faster with propofol/fentanyl- than with ketamine/midazolam-based PSA (23 versus 33 min in one study), especially if repeated doses are needed. Recovery is described as more pleasant after propofol sedation compared to ketamine. Time to discharge after fentanyl/midazolam is similar to that of ketamine/midazolam.

(continued)

Case 3

A 3-year-old boy has blistering *hot water burns* to his right face and much of his anterior chest and abdomen, sustained when he pulled a pot with boiled water off the stove top. He was transported to the ED by EMS who was unable to insert an IV catheter, in part due to the child's obesity (weight 23 kg). The child has a history of mild asthma without hospitalization, controlled with albuterol MDI as needed. He has had a runny nose and cough without fever for 1–2 days; his usual snoring while sleeping has worsened with the URI. The child is crying loudly and coughing as he is placed in a treatment room. Good air exchange with expiratory wheezes bilaterally is noted on auscultation.

Issues: rapid pain relief, difficult vascular access, obesity, history of snoring, asthma with current wheezing, and upper respiratory infection:

1. Rapid pain relief options:
   (a) *Fentanyl intranasally* 1.5–2 mg/kg achieves significant pain relief within 5–10 min. See Case 1 for additional information. Base dose on estimated lean body weight (~15 kg for 3 year old); initial 2 mg/kg dose for this child is 30 mg or 0.6 mL. Divide the 0.6 mL total dose into four sprays of ~0.15 mL/nostril. The impact of an acute URI upon transmucosal absorption is unclear.
   (b) *Nitrous oxide 50–70%* will provide rapid pain relief, but its analgesic effect is lost within minutes when the gas is stopped. N_2O can be administered while IV catheter insertion is attempted. Use of a continuous circuit or N_2O delivery system easily activated by a young child is necessary.
   (c) *Oxycodone orally*, or other potent oral analgesic, will provide pain relief, but onset is 20–40 min. For this young patient with a very painful injury, an initial oxycodone dose of 0.3 mg/kg is given orally; based on estimated lean body weight of 15 kg, it is 4–4.5 mg. This dose may result in mild sedation as pain relief is achieved. See Case 1 for additional information.
   (d) *Opioids intravenously* titrated to effect will provide the greatest pain relief, if vascular access can be achieved. Fentanyl 1–2 mg/kg will provide analgesia within 1–2 min, lasting 30–60 min, whereas morphine 0.1 mg/kg will provide initial analgesia within 5–10 min with peak effect at 10–20 min and lasting 2–3 h.
   (e) *Intramuscular ketamine* 4 mg/kg provides rapid and marked pain relief and PSA without vascular access. Please see Case 1(b) for further information. If providers are available to monitor the patient and begin debridement, this may be a reasonable option. The greatest risk with this technique is that emergent vascular access to manage a life-threatening adverse event such as laryngospasm would be difficult, but an intraosseous needle could be placed, if necessary. IV catheter insertion for ongoing care can be attempted concurrently with the burn debridement.
2. *Difficult vascular access*: *Buffered lidocaine injected subcutaneously* with a 30-gauge needle provides nearly painless rapid local anesthesia for IV insertion. Use of this or other local anesthetic technique in this obese child will be especially important because multiple attempts likely will be needed. Because of the prolonged onset, topical anesthetic creams are not an optimum choice for local anesthesia. If available, *N_2O 50–70%* will reduce IV insertion-related distress as well as provide systemic analgesia as described in (b).
3. *Obesity, snoring*: As noted earlier, determine medication doses upon estimated lean body weight. Since fat is less perfused than brain and muscle, doses based upon total weight will result in higher initial plasma and brain concentrations and greater risk of adverse effects and prolonged recovery. Obesity also reduces lung functional residual capacity, increasing his risk of hypoxia with respiratory depression, and increases likelihood of upper airway obstruction as indicated by his history of snoring. Use of supplemental oxygen during sedation of this patient will provide a greater margin of safety by prolonging the time to hypoxia if decreased ventilation occurs. Monitoring with end-tidal capnography, in addition to pulse oximetry, will facilitate early detection of ventilatory insufficiency and allow supportive interventions before adverse consequences occur.
4. *History of asthma, currently wheezing, acute URI*: If the patient's wheezing clears readily with a single albuterol nebulization treatment, the increased risk of sedation-related adverse respiratory events likely is low, but providers should be prepared to administer additional asthma care if needed. The acute URI may increase the risk of laryngospasm, especially if the patient is febrile. It is unclear whether administration of a drying agent such as glycopyrrolate or atropine reduces this risk.

(continued)

PSA Technique Options

(a) *Ketamine with or without midazolam*: If vascular access is successful, the intravenous route is preferred as it allows titration to effect and use of the smallest effective dose, with repeat small doses as needed, thus decreasing length of recovery. Please see Case 1 for further information on ketamine dosing. It is likely this patient will need multiple subsequent painful burn debridements. Therefore, effective analgesia and amnesia for this initial burn care are especially important to establish the patient's future expectations. A sedating dose of midazolam, 0.1 mg/kg, prior to ketamine infusion, may increase the probability of complete procedural amnesia. A potential additional benefit for this patient is ketamine-induced reduction of central sensitization and windup from continued burn pain. While the risk of laryngospasm associated with ketamine is quite low, the presence of an active URI may increase this risk, and the sedation providers should be prepared to manage this potentially life-threatening adverse event.

Intramuscular ketamine 4 mg/kg: Please see Case 1 for additional information.

(b) *Fentanyl + midazolam or propofol* provides effective PSA but requires vascular access. Please see Case 2 for additional information.

(c) *Nitrous oxide 50–70 %* is unlikely to provide sufficient PSA for vigorous burn debridement in this young child unless it is coadministered with a potent systemic analgesic such as fentanyl or ketamine. These combinations can readily induce deep sedation and general anesthesia and should be considered only by providers experienced in such techniques.

Case 4

A 2-year-old boy has a *complex forehead laceration* that requires suturing. Topical anesthetic gel was applied in triage. Despite best efforts to calm him as he sits in his mother's lap, he continues to cry and vigorously resists exam. His mother predicts he will not calm and indicates this is typical behavior during interactions with healthcare providers.

Issues: The laceration repair requires the patient's forehead to be still; physical restraint will likely reinforce similar behavior during future healthcare; there are other ED patients waiting more than 4 h to be seen.

PSA Options

(a) *Nitrous oxide 50–70 %* provides effective calming for laceration repair in young children. A continuous circuit or another N_2O delivery system with a standard mask that covers the patient's mouth and nose and is designed for use by children is necessary for effective PSA with N_2O. Dental-type nose masks are less effective since they allow mouth breathing that bypasses the N_2O. If the laceration is on the chin or in an area covered by the standard mask, a neonatal size mask may be used as a nose mask and the child's mouth gently held closed. If the mother is amenable, this technique can be enhanced by administering the N_2O and suturing as the child sits in her lap with his head rested on her chest and her singing favorite songs or telling stories for distraction. A helper will need to help steady the child's head and gently hold the mask in place over the patient's mouth and nose. All must be vigilant for vomiting, often forewarned by abdominal or chest heaving. The N_2O should be administered for about 2 min before attempting to provide additional anesthesia (buffered lidocaine injected with a half-inch 30-gauge needle recommended) or suturing.

(b) *Midazolam intranasally* 0.2–0.4 mg/kg administered with atomizer to spray small volumes of concentrated intravenous solution (5 mg/mL) to improve absorption. Suggested dose for this 12 kg child is 5 mg or 1 mL. Divide the 1 mL total dose into four sprays of ~0.25 mL; alternate nostrils allow about a minute between repeat sprays into a given nostril. Use of small volumes improves efficacy by reducing drainage of drug into posterior pharynx from which it is less well absorbed and causes an unpleasant taste. Onset of sedation occurs by 3–5 min with duration of 20–40 min. As with other routes of midazolam administration, some children become dysphoric instead of sedated. When administered with an atomizer, intranasal midazolam is well tolerated and achieves anxiolysis with mild sedation. If the intravenous solution is dripped into the nares without atomization, most children complain of a burning sensation.

(c) *Ketamine intramuscularly* 2–3 mg/kg provides effective PSA for suturing when local anesthesia is also used. Minor restraint may be needed in a few children with this dose. Onset of sedation usually occurs by 5 min and recovery by 60–80 min.

(continued)

(d) *Propofol, ketamine, or fentanyl/midazolam intravenously*: Titration of any of these techniques will provide maximum effectiveness but intravenous access is required. Placement of an IV catheter in this resistant child certainly will require physical restraint unless it is inserted after sedation with N_2O, intranasal midazolam, or IM ketamine. Such strategy might be logical for a very complex laceration repair expected to last more than 20–30 min or involve a critical step that requires the patient to be motionless, such as approximating a lacerated eyelid margin.

Case 5

An otherwise healthy febrile 10-month-old infant needs *incision and drainage of a large buttock abscess.*

PSA Options

1. Ketamine IV or IM: See Case 2 for additional information.
2. Fentanyl + propofol or midazolam: See Case 2 for additional information.
3. Nitrous oxide + oxycodone can provide acceptable PSA if effective local anesthesia of the abscess can be achieved. Field blocks with buffered lidocaine are variably effective for smaller abscesses but usually unsuccessful for large abscesses. For larger and deeper abscesses, the author has occasional success by partially draining the abscess through a small (~1 cm) incision through skin well anesthetized with subcutaneous lidocaine. The abscess cavity then is gently refilled with the topical anesthetic solution commonly used for anesthetizing lacerations (4 % lidocaine, 1:100,000 epinephrine, and 0.5 % tetracaine [L.E.T.]). After 30 min, the entire abscess cavity often is well anesthetized, and the patient tolerates widening the incision and debridement of the cavity under N_2O sedation.

Case 6

You are asked to provide sedation for *incision and drainage of a peritonsillar abscess* in a very anxious 5-year-old boy who vigorously resists oropharyngeal exams. He has had a runny nose and cough with low-grade fever for 2–3 days.

Issues: Mild to light moderate PSA can safely be administered for I&D of peritonsillar abscesses in older children and teens who will cooperate with the procedure in the emergency department. However, this child will require deep sedation to overcome his resistance. Deep sedation by any technique carries increased risk of pulmonary aspiration due to variable blunting of protective airway reflexes. This patient will have blood and pus draining upon his larynx during the procedure. This patient should be considered for abscess drainage in the OR under general anesthesia, likely with endotracheal intubation.

For light PSA for peritonsillar abscess I&D in cooperative children, 30–45 min prior to the procedure, we administer morphine for baseline pain management and glycopyrrolate to dry secretions. Five to ten minutes prior to the procedure, we administer 2 mg of midazolam for anxiolysis. If the patient has difficulty tolerating the mucosal injection of buffered lidocaine with epinephrine at the site of the abscess, we may infuse 0.1–0.2 mg/kg of ketamine immediately prior to the surgeon's incision, i.e., a small dose. The patient is able to follow commands but appears a bit dazed after the ketamine and usually is better able to tolerate the procedural pain. Laryngospasm has been found to occur more frequently during endoscopy with ketamine sedation, presumably due to direct stimulation of the larynx. Whether laryngospasm risk correlates directly with the dose of ketamine is unclear. Likewise, it is unclear whether risk of laryngospasm is increased with laryngeal stimulation by drainage from a peritonsillar abscess. Using this approach, none of our patients have developed laryngospasm during peritonsillar I&D in our ED.

Case 7

A 15-month-old boy has fallen through stair railings an hour ago and has a large hematoma on his left parietal area. He is irritable and restless. An emergent head CT scan to evaluate for intracranial injury has been ordered. The CT tech calls to state they cannot get the patient to lie still for the brief period of the scan and asks that the patient be sedated.

Issues: need for emergent CT scan that requires motionless patient for about 1 min to conduct scan, potentially increased intracranial pressure from hemorrhage.

PSA Options

1. Pentobarbital intravenously will sedate patient but a full dose may cause mild reduction in blood pressure, which impacts brain perfusion. The prolonged

(continued)

recovery from pentobarbital makes monitoring patient for neurologic deterioration difficult and may complicate plans for general anesthesia if emergent craniotomy is needed.
2. Ketamine intravenously 0.25–0.5 mg/kg, pushed rapidly, will provide brief sedation. Some restraint may be necessary. Blood pressure likely will be maintained and brief increase in intracranial pressure probably is not critical.
3. Propofol intravenously provides sedation but brief hypotension and respiratory depression may rapidly worsen patient condition.
4. Etomidate intravenously will provide sedation and recovery within 5–10 min with less risk of hypotension. Myoclonic jerks during induction of sedation tend to be brief but may interfere with scanning.
5. Midazolam intravenously may be insufficient for sedation.
6. Fentanyl intravenously for pain may be sufficient to coax patient to be still for the brief period, as needed.

References

1. Carr D, Jacox A; Acute Pain Management Guideline Panel. Acute pain management in infants, children, and adolescents: operative and medical procedures and trauma. Publication No. AHCPR 92-0020. Rockville: Agency for Health Care Policy and Research, Public Health Service, U.S. Department of Health and Human Services; 1992.
2. Schechter NL, Berde C, Yaster M, editors. Pain in infants, children and adolescents. 2nd ed. Philadelphia: Lippincott, Williams & Wilkins; 2003.
3. Terndrup TE. Pediatric pain control. Ann Emerg Med. 1996; 27(4):466–70.
4. Walco GA, Cassidy RC, Schechter NL. Pain, hurt, and harm. The ethics of pain control in infants and children. N Engl J Med. 1994; 331(8):541–4.
5. Weisman SJ, Bernstein B, Schechter NL. Consequences of inadequate analgesia during painful procedures in children. Arch Pediatr Adolesc Med. 1998;152(2):147–9.
6. Zeltzer LK, Altman A, Cohen D, LeBaron S, Munuksela EL, Schechter NL. American Academy of Pediatrics report of the subcommittee on the management of pain associated with procedures in children with cancer. Pediatrics. 1990;86(5 Pt 2): 826–31.
7. Fosnocht DE, Heaps ND, Swanson ER. Patient expectations for pain relief in the ED. Am J Emerg Med. 2004;22(4):286–8.
8. Committee on Drugs, American Academy of Pediatrics. Guidelines for monitoring and management of pediatric patients during and after sedation for diagnostic and therapeutic procedures: addendum. Pediatrics. 2002;110(4):836–8.
9. Kennedy RM, Porter FL, Miller JP, Jaffe DM. Comparison of fentanyl/midazolam with ketamine/midazolam for pediatric orthopedic emergencies. Pediatrics. 1998;102(4 Pt 1):956–63.
10. Luhmann JD, Kennedy RM, Porter FL, Miller JP, Jaffe DM. A randomized clinical trial of continuous-flow nitrous oxide and midazolam for sedation of young children during laceration repair. Ann Emerg Med. 2001;37(1):20–7.
11. Dollfus C, Annequin M, Adam M, et al. Analgesia with nitrous oxide for painful procedures in pediatric hematology-oncology. Ann Pediatr (Paris). 1995;42(2):115–21.
12. American College of Emergency Physicians. The use of pediatric sedation and analgesia. Ann Emerg Med. 2008;52(5):595–6.
13. American Academy of Pediatrics. Committee on Psychosocial Aspects of Child and Family Health; Task Force on Pain in Infants, Children, and Adolescents. The assessment and management of acute pain in infants, children, and adolescents. Pediatrics. 2001; 108(3):793–7.
14. Brennan F, Carr DB, Cousins M. Pain management: a fundamental human right. Anesth Analg. 2007;105(1):205–21.
15. Anand KJ, Scalzo FM. Can adverse neonatal experiences alter brain development and subsequent behavior? Biol Neonate. 2000;77(2):69–82.
16. Fitzgerald M, Anand KJS. Developmental neuroanatomy and neurophysiology of pain. In: Schechter NL, Berde C, Yaster M, editors. Pain in infants, children and adolescents. Baltimore: Williams & Wilikins; 1993. p. 11–31.
17. Teng CJ, Abbott FV. The formalin test: a dose-response analysis at three developmental stages. Pain. 1998;76(3):337–47.
18. Grunau RV, Whitfield MF, Petrie JH. Pain sensitivity and temperament in extremely low-birth-weight premature toddlers and preterm and full-term controls. Pain. 1994;58(3):341–6.
19. Grunau RE, Whitfield MF, Petrie J. Children's judgements about pain at age 8–10 years: do extremely low birthweight (<or = 1000 g) children differ from full birthweight peers? J Child Psychol Psychiatry. 1998;39(4):587–94.
20. Holsti L, Grunau RE, Oberlander TF, Whitfield MF. Prior pain induces heightened motor responses during clustered care in preterm infants in the NICU. Early Hum Dev. 2005;81(3):293–302.
21. Reynolds ML, Fitzgerald M. Long-term sensory hyperinnervation following neonatal skin wounds. J Comp Neurol. 1995;358(4): 487–98.
22. Ruda MA, Ling QD, Hohmann AG, Peng YB, Tachibana T. Altered nociceptive neuronal circuits after neonatal peripheral inflammation. Science. 2000;289(5479):628–31.
23. Taddio A, Katz J. The effects of early pain experience in neonates on pain responses in infancy and childhood. Paediatr Drugs. 2005;7(4):245–57.
24. Taddio A, Katz J, Ilersich AL, Koren G. Effect of neonatal circumcision on pain response during subsequent routine vaccination. Lancet. 1997;349(9052):599–603.
25. Peters JW, Koot HM, de Boer JB, et al. Major surgery within the first 3 months of life and subsequent biobehavioral pain responses to immunization at later age: a case comparison study. Pediatrics. 2003;111(1):129–35.
26. Chen E, Zeltzer LK, Craske MG, Katz ER. Children's memories for painful cancer treatment procedures: implications for distress. Child Dev. 2000;71(4):933–47.
27. Cohen LL, Francher A, MacLaren JE, Lim CS. Correlates of pediatric behavior and distress during intramuscular injections for invasive dental procedures. J Clin Pediatr Dent. 2006;31(1):44–7.
28. Okawa K, Ichinohe T, Kaneko Y. Anxiety may enhance pain during dental treatment. Bull Tokyo Dent Coll. 2005;46(3):51–8.
29. Chen E, Zeltzer LK, Craske MG, Katz ER. Alteration of memory in the reduction of children's distress during repeated aversive medical procedures. J Consult Clin Psychol. 1999;67(4):481–90.
30. Pate JT, Blount RL, Cohen LL, Smith AJ. Childhood medical experience and temperament as predictors of adult functioning in medical situations. Child Health Care. 1996;25(4):281–98.
31. Cohen LL, Blount RL, Cohen RJ, Ball CM, McClellan CB, Bernard RS. Children's expectations and memories of acute distress: short- and long-term efficacy of pain management interventions. J Pediatr Psychol. 2001;26(6):367–74.

32. Pierluisi GJ, Terndrup TE. Influence of topical anesthesia on the sedation of pediatric emergency department patients with lacerations. Pediatr Emerg Care. 1989;5(4):211–5.
33. Ernst AA, Marvez E, Nick TG, Chin E, Wood E, Gonzaba WT. Lidocaine adrenaline tetracaine gel versus tetracaine adrenaline cocaine gel for topical anesthesia in linear scalp and facial lacerations in children aged 5 to 17 years. Pediatrics. 1995; 95(2):255–8.
34. Ernst AA, Marvez-Valls E, Nick TG, Mills T, Minvielle L, Houry D. Topical lidocaine adrenaline tetracaine (LAT gel) versus injectable buffered lidocaine for local anesthesia in laceration repair. West J Med. 1997;167(2):79–81.
35. Schilling CG, Bank DE, Borchert BA, Klatzko MD, Uden DL. Tetracaine, epinephrine (adrenalin), and cocaine (TAC) versus lidocaine, epinephrine, and tetracaine (LET) for anesthesia of lacerations in children. Ann Emerg Med. 1995;25(2):203–8.
36. Bonadio WA. Safe and effective method for application of tetracaine, adrenaline, and cocaine to oral lacerations. Ann Emerg Med. 1996;28(4):396–8.
37. White NJ, Kim MK, Brousseau DC, Bergholte J, Hennes H. The anesthetic effectiveness of lidocaine-adrenaline-tetracaine gel on finger lacerations. Pediatr Emerg Care. 2004;20(12):812–5.
38. Arndt KA, Burton C, Noe JM. Minimizing the pain of local anesthesia. Plast Reconstr Surg. 1983;72(5):676–9.
39. Brogan Jr GX, Giarrusso E, Hollander JE, Cassara G, Maranga MC, Thode HC. Comparison of plain, warmed, and buffered lidocaine for anesthesia of traumatic wounds. Ann Emerg Med. 1995; 26(2):121–5.
40. Colaric KB, Overton DT, Moore K. Pain reduction in lidocaine administration through buffering and warming. Am J Emerg Med. 1998;16(4):353–6.
41. Krause RS, Moscati R, Filice M, Lerner EB, Hughes D. The effect of injection speed on the pain of lidocaine infiltration. Acad Emerg Med. 1997;4(11):1032–5.
42. Scarfone RJ, Jasani M, Gracely EJ. Pain of local anesthetics: rate of administration and buffering. Ann Emerg Med. 1998;31(1): 36–40.
43. Christoph RA, Buchanan L, Begalla K, Schwartz S. Pain reduction in local anesthetic administration through pH buffering. Ann Emerg Med. 1988;17(2):117–20.
44. McKay W, Morris R, Mushlin P. Sodium bicarbonate attenuates pain on skin infiltration with lidocaine, with or without epinephrine. Anesth Analg. 1987;66(6):572–4.
45. Bartfield JM, Homer PJ, Ford DT, Sternklar P. Buffered lidocaine as a local anesthetic: an investigation of shelf life. Ann Emerg Med. 1992;21(1):16–9.
46. Orlinsky M, Hudson C, Chan L, Deslauriers R. Pain comparison of unbuffered versus buffered lidocaine in local wound infiltration. J Emerg Med. 1992;10(4):411–5.
47. Larson PO, Ragi G, Swandby M, Darcey B, Polzin G, Carey P. Stability of buffered lidocaine and epinephrine used for local anesthesia. J Dermatol Surg Oncol. 1991;17(5):411–4.
48. Siegel L. Preparation of children for hospitalization: a selected review of the research literature. J Pediatr Psychol. 1976;1(4):26–30.
49. Ross DM, Ross SA. Childhood pain: the school-aged child's viewpoint. Pain. 1984;20(2):179–91.
50. Bauchner H, Waring C, Vinci R. Parental presence during procedures in an emergency room: results from 50 observations. Pediatrics. 1991;87(4):544–8.
51. Merritt KA, Sargent JR, Osborn LM. Attitudes regarding parental presence during medical procedures. Am J Dis Child. 1990;144(3): 270–1.
52. Sacchetti A, Lichenstein R, Carraccio CA, Harris RH. Family member presence during pediatric emergency department procedures. Pediatr Emerg Care. 1996;12(4):268–71.
53. Mangurten J, Scott SH, Guzzetta CE, et al. Effects of family presence during resuscitation and invasive procedures in a pediatric emergency department. J Emerg Nurs. 2006;32(3):225–33.
54. O'Malley P, Brown K, Mace SE. Patient- and family-centered care and the role of the emergency physician providing care to a child in the emergency department. Pediatrics. 2006;118(5):2242–4.
55. O'Malley PJ, Brown K, Krug SE. Patient- and family-centered care of children in the emergency department. Pediatrics. 2008; 122(2):e511–21.
56. Alcock DS, Feldman W, Goodman JT, McGrath PJ, Park JM. Evaluation of child life intervention in emergency department suturing. Pediatr Emerg Care. 1985;1(3):111–5.
57. Manne SL, Bakeman R, Jacobsen PB, Gorfinkle K, Redd WH. An analysis of a behavioral intervention for children undergoing venipuncture. Health Psychol. 1994;13(6):556–66.
58. Sparks LA, Setlik J, Luhman J. Parental holding and positioning to decrease IV distress in young children: a randomized controlled trial. J Pediatr Nurs. 2007;22(6):440–7.
59. American Academy of Pediatrics Committee on Drugs. Guidelines for monitoring and management of pediatric patients during and after sedation for diagnostic and therapeutic procedures. Pediatrics. 1992;89(6 Pt 1):1110–5.
60. Bijttebier P, Vertommen H. The impact of previous experience on children's reactions to venepunctures. J Health Psychol. 1998; 3(1):39–46.
61. Agrawal D, Manzi SF, Gupta R, Krauss B. Preprocedural fasting state and adverse events in children undergoing procedural sedation and analgesia in a pediatric emergency department. Ann Emerg Med. 2003;42(5):636–46.
62. Babl FE, Puspitadewi A, Barnett P, Oakley E, Spicer M. Preprocedural fasting state and adverse events in children receiving nitrous oxide for procedural sedation and analgesia. Pediatr Emerg Care. 2005;21(11):736–43.
63. Roback MG, Bajaj L, Wathen JE, Bothner J. Preprocedural fasting and adverse events in procedural sedation and analgesia in a pediatric emergency department: are they related? Ann Emerg Med. 2004;44(5):454–9.
64. Quinn J, Cummings S, Callaham M, Sellers K. Suturing versus conservative management of lacerations of the hand: randomised controlled trial. BMJ. 2002;325(7359):299.
65. Lamell CW, Fraone G, Casamassimo PS, Wilson S. Presenting characteristics and treatment outcomes for tongue lacerations in children. Pediatr Dent. 1999;21(1):34–8.
66. Godwin SA, Burton JH, Gerardo CJ, Hatten BW, Mace SE, Silvers SM, Fesmire FM; American College of Emergency Physicians. Clinical policy: procedural sedation and analgesia in the emergency department. Ann Emerg Med. 2014;63(2):247–58.e18.
67. Roback MG, Wathen JE, Bajaj L, Bothner JP. Adverse events associated with procedural sedation and analgesia in a pediatric emergency department: a comparison of common parenteral drugs. Acad Emerg Med. 2005;12(6):508–13.
68. American College of Emergency Physicians. Clinical policy for procedural sedation and analgesia in the emergency department. Ann Emerg Med. 1998;31(5):663–77.
69. Hoffman GM, Nowakowski R, Troshynski TJ, Berens RJ, Weisman SJ. Risk reduction in pediatric procedural sedation by application of an American Academy of Pediatrics/American Society of Anesthesiologists process model. Pediatrics. 2002;109(2):236–43.
70. American Society of Anesthesiologists Task Force on Sedation and Analgesia by Non-Anesthesiologists. Practice guidelines for sedation and analgesia by non-anesthesiologists. Anesthesiology. 2002;96(4):1004–17.
71. McAllister JD, Gnauck KA. Rapid sequence intubation of the pediatric patient. Fundamentals of practice. Pediatr Clin North Am. 1999;46(6):1249–84.

72. Owens WD, Felts JA, Spitznagel Jr EL. ASA physical status classifications: a study of consistency of ratings. Anesthesiology. 1978;49(4):239–43.
73. Warner MA, Warner ME, Warner DO, Warner LO, Warner EJ. Perioperative pulmonary aspiration in infants and children. Anesthesiology. 1999;90(1):66–71.
74. Borland LM, Sereika SM, Woelfel SK, et al. Pulmonary aspiration in pediatric patients during general anesthesia: incidence and outcome. J Clin Anesth. 1998;10(2):95–102.
75. Benumof JL, editor. Airway management: principles and practice. St. Louis: Mosby-Yearbook; 1996. p. 132.
76. Cote CJ, Todres ID, Ryan JF, et al., editors. A practice of anesthesia for infants and children. 3rd ed. Philadelphia: WB Saunders; 2001.
77. American Society of Anesthesiologist Task Force on Preoperative Fasting. Practice guidelines for preoperative fasting and the use of pharmacologic agents to reduce the risk of pulmonary aspiration: application to healthy patients undergoing elective procedures. Anesthesiology. 1999;90(3):896–905.
78. Mace SE, Brown LA, Francis L, et al. Clinical policy: critical issues in the sedation of pediatric patients in the emergency department. Ann Emerg Med. 2008;51(4):378–99; 399.e1–57.
79. Green SM, Roback MG, Miner JR, Burton JH, Krauss B. Fasting and emergency department procedural sedation and analgesia: a consensus-based clinical practice advisory. Ann Emerg Med. 2007;49(4):454–61.
80. Green SM, Krauss B. Pulmonary aspiration risk during emergency department procedural sedation—an examination of the role of fasting and sedation depth. Acad Emerg Med. 2002;9(1):35–42.
81. Green SM, Krauss B. Clinical practice guideline for emergency department ketamine dissociative sedation in children. Ann Emerg Med. 2004;44(5):460–71.
82. Warner MA, Warner ME, Weber JG. Clinical significance of pulmonary aspiration during the perioperative period. Anesthesiology. 1993;78(1):56–62.
83. Green SM, Rothrock SG, Lynch EL, et al. Intramuscular ketamine for pediatric sedation in the emergency department: safety profile in 1,022 cases. Ann Emerg Med. 1998;31(6):688–97.
84. Engelhardt T, Webster NR. Pulmonary aspiration of gastric contents in anaesthesia. Br J Anaesth. 1999;83(3):453–60.
85. Maekawa N, Mikawa K, Yaku H, Nishina K, Obara H. Effects of 2-, 4- and 12-hour fasting intervals on preoperative gastric fluid pH and volume, and plasma glucose and lipid homeostasis in children. Acta Anaesthesiol Scand. 1993;37(8):783–7.
86. Ingebo KR, Rayhorn NJ, Hecht RM, Shelton MT, Silber GH, Shub MD. Sedation in children: adequacy of two-hour fasting. J Pediatr. 1997;131(1 Pt 1):155–8.
87. Soreide E, Hausken T, Soreide JA, Steen PA. Gastric emptying of a light hospital breakfast. A study using real time ultrasonography. Acta Anaesthesiol Scand. 1996;40(5):549–53.
88. Cravero JP, Beach ML, Blike GT, Gallagher SM, Hertzog JH. The incidence and nature of adverse events during pediatric sedation/anesthesia with propofol for procedures outside the operating room: a report from the Pediatric Sedation Research Consortium. Anesth Analg. 2009;108(3):795–804.
89. Wathen JE, Roback MG, Mackenzie T, Bothner JP. Does midazolam alter the clinical effects of intravenous ketamine sedation in children? A double-blind, randomized, controlled, emergency department trial. Ann Emerg Med. 2000;36(6):579–88.
90. Luhmann JD, Schootman M, Luhmann SJ, Kennedy RM. A randomized comparison of nitrous oxide plus hematoma block versus ketamine plus midazolam for emergency department forearm fracture reduction in children. Pediatrics. 2006;118(4):e1078–86.
91. McGlone R, Carley S. Towards evidence based emergency medicine: best BETs from the Manchester Royal Infirmary. BET 3: does the time of fasting affect complication rates during ketamine sedation? Emerg Med J. 2008;25(6):367–9.
92. Treston G. Prolonged pre-procedure fasting time is unnecessary when using titrated intravenous ketamine for paediatric procedural sedation. Emerg Med Australas. 2004;16(2):145–50.
93. Schreiner MS. Preoperative and postoperative fasting in children. Pediatr Clin North Am. 1994;41(1):111–20.
94. Langston WT, Wathen JE, Roback MG, Bajaj L. Effect of ondansetron on the incidence of vomiting associated with ketamine sedation in children: a double-blind, randomized, placebo-controlled trial. Ann Emerg Med. 2008;52(1):30–4.
95. Joint Commission on Accreditation of Healthcare Organizations. Standards and intents for sedation and anesthesia care. Revisions to anesthesia care standards, comprehensive accreditation manual for hospitals. Oakbrook Terrace: Joint Commission on Accreditation of Healthcare Organizations; 2001. http://www.jcaho.org/standard/aneshap.html
96. Dial S, Silver P, Bock K, Sagy M. Pediatric sedation for procedures titrated to a desired degree of immobility results in unpredictable depth of sedation. Pediatr Emerg Care. 2001;17(6):414–20.
97. Krauss B, Green SM. Sedation and analgesia for procedures in children. N Engl J Med. 2000;342(13):938–45.
98. Yaster M, Nichols DG, Deshpande JK, Wetzel RC. Midazolam-fentanyl intravenous sedation in children: case report of respiratory arrest. Pediatrics. 1990;86(3):463–7.
99. Cote CJ, Karl HW, Notterman DA, Weinberg JA, McCloskey C. Adverse sedation events in pediatrics: analysis of medications used for sedation. Pediatrics. 2000;106(4):633–44.
100. Cote CJ, Notterman DA, Karl HW, Weinberg JA, McCloskey C. Adverse sedation events in pediatrics: a critical incident analysis of contributing factors. Pediatrics. 2000;105(4 Pt 1):805–14.
101. Maxwell LG, Yaster M. The myth of conscious sedation. Arch Pediatr Adolesc Med. 1996;150(7):665–7.
102. Godwin SA, Caro DA, Wolf SJ, et al. Clinical policy: procedural sedation and analgesia in the emergency department. Ann Emerg Med. 2005;45(2):177–96.
103. American Academy of Pediatrics. Committee on Drugs. Guidelines for monitoring and management of pediatric patients during and after sedation for diagnostic and therapeutic procedures: addendum. Pediatrics. 2002;110(4):836–8.
104. Shaw KN, Bell LM, Sherman NH. Outpatient assessment of infants with bronchiolitis. Am J Dis Child. 1991;145(2):151–5.
105. Hart LS, Berns SD, Houck CS, Boenning DA. The value of end-tidal CO_2 monitoring when comparing the three methods of conscious sedation for children undergoing painful procedures in the emergency department. Pediatr Emerg Care. 1997;13(3):189–93.
106. Miner JR, Heegaard W, Plummer D. End-tidal carbon dioxide monitoring during procedural sedation. Acad Emerg Med. 2002;9(4):275–80.
107. Anderson JL, Junkins E, Pribble C, Guenther E. Capnography and depth of sedation during propofol sedation in children. Ann Emerg Med. 2007;49(1):9–13.
108. Yldzdas D, Yapcoglu H, Ylmaz HL. The value of capnography during sedation or sedation/analgesia in pediatric minor procedures. Pediatr Emerg Care. 2004;20(3):162–5.
109. Burton JH, Harrah JD, Germann CA, Dillon DC. Does end-tidal carbon dioxide monitoring detect respiratory events prior to current sedation monitoring practices? Acad Emerg Med. 2006;13(5):500–4.
110. Krauss B, Hess DR. Capnography for procedural sedation and analgesia in the emergency department. Ann Emerg Med. 2007;50(2):172–81.
111. Kodali BS. www.capnography.com: an animated website. Anesth Analg. 2001;93(5):1364.
112. Tobias JD. End-tidal carbon dioxide monitoring during sedation with a combination of midazolam and ketamine for children undergoing painful, invasive procedures. Pediatr Emerg Care. 1999;15(3):173–5.

113. Kim G, Green SM, Denmark TK, Krauss B. Ventilatory response during dissociative sedation in children-a pilot study. Acad Emerg Med. 2003;10(2):140–5.
114. Patel R, Lenczyk M, Hannallah RS, McGill WA. Age and the onset of desaturation in apnoeic children. Can J Anaesth. 1994; 41(9):771–4.
115. Keidan I, Gravenstein D, Berkenstadt H, Ziv A, Shavit I, Sidi A. Supplemental oxygen compromises the use of pulse oximetry for detection of apnea and hypoventilation during sedation in simulated pediatric patients. Pediatrics. 2008;122(2):293–8.
116. Rubin DM, Eisig S, Freeman K, Kraut RA. Effect of supplemental gases on end-tidal CO_2 and oxygen saturation in patients undergoing fentanyl and midazolam outpatient sedation. Anesth Prog. 1997;44(1):1–4.
117. Miner JR, Burton JH. Clinical practice advisory: emergency department procedural sedation with propofol. Ann Emerg Med. 2007;50(2):182–7, 187.e181.
118. Pena BM, Krauss B. Adverse events of procedural sedation and analgesia in a pediatric emergency department. Ann Emerg Med. 1999;34(4 Pt 1):483–91.
119. Cravero JP, Blike GT, Beach M, et al. Incidence and nature of adverse events during pediatric sedation/anesthesia for procedures outside the operating room: report from the Pediatric Sedation Research Consortium. Pediatrics. 2006;118(3):1087–96.
120. Bailey PL, Pace NL, Ashburn MA, Moll JW, East KA, Stanley TH. Frequent hypoxemia and apnea after sedation with midazolam and fentanyl. Anesthesiology. 1990;73(5):826–30.
121. Green SM, Johnson NE. Ketamine sedation for pediatric procedures: part 2. Review and implications. Ann Emerg Med. 1990;19(9):1033–46.
122. Mitchell RK, Koury SI, Stone CK. Respiratory arrest after intramuscular ketamine in a 2-year-old child. Am J Emerg Med. 1996;14(6):580–1.
123. Litman RS. Apnea and oxyhemoglobin desaturation after intramuscular ketamine administration in a 2-year-old child. Am J Emerg Med. 1997;15(5):547–8.
124. Newman DH, Azer MM, Pitetti RD, Singh S. When is a patient safe for discharge after procedural sedation? The timing of adverse effect events in 1367 pediatric procedural sedations. Ann Emerg Med. 2003;42(5):627–35.
125. Neal JM, Owens BD. Hazards of antagonizing narcotic sedation with naloxone. Ann Emerg Med. 1993;22(1):145–6.
126. Chamberlain JM, Klein BL. A comprehensive review of naloxone for the emergency physician. Am J Emerg Med. 1994;12(6): 650–60.
127. Jones RD, Lawson AD, Andrew LJ, Gunawardene WM, Bacon-Shone J. Antagonism of the hypnotic effect of midazolam in children: a randomized, double-blind study of placebo and flumazenil administered after midazolam-induced anaesthesia. Br J Anaesth. 1991;66(6):660–6.
128. Ghouri AF, Ruiz MA, White PF. Effect of flumazenil on recovery after midazolam and propofol sedation. Anesthesiology. 1994; 81(2):333–9.
129. Shannon M, Albers G, Burkhart K, et al. Safety and efficacy of flumazenil in the reversal of benzodiazepine-induced conscious sedation. The Flumazenil Pediatric Study Group. J Pediatr. 1997; 131(4):582–6.
130. Bhatt M, Kennedy RM, Osmond MH, et al. Consensus-based recommendations for standardizing terminology and reporting adverse events for emergency department procedural sedation and analgesia in children. Ann Emerg Med. 2009;53(4): 426–35.e424.
131. Cohen VG, Krauss B. Recurrent episodes of intractable laryngospasm during dissociative sedation with intramuscular ketamine. Pediatr Emerg Care. 2006;22(4):247–9.
132. von Ungern-Sternberg BS, Regli A, Frei FJ, et al. A deeper level of ketamine anesthesia does not affect functional residual capacity and ventilation distribution in healthy preschool children. Paediatr Anaesth. 2007;17(12):1150–5.
133. Lois F, De Kock M. Something new about ketamine for pediatric anesthesia? Curr Opin Anaesthesiol. 2008;21(3):340–4.
134. Hampson-Evans D, Morgan P, Farrar M. Pediatric laryngospasm. Paediatr Anaesth. 2008;18(4):303–7.
135. Green SM, Roback MG, Krauss B, et al. Predictors of airway and respiratory adverse events with ketamine sedation in the emergency department: an individual-patient data meta-analysis of 8,282 children. Ann Emerg Med. 2009;54(2):158–68.e151–4.
136. Murat I, Constant I, Maud'huy H. Perioperative anaesthetic morbidity in children: a database of 24,165 anaesthetics over a 30-month period. Paediatr Anaesth. 2004;14(2):158–66.
137. Burgoyne LL, Anghelescu DL. Intervention steps for treating laryngospasm in pediatric patients. Paediatr Anaesth. 2008;18(4): 297–302.
138. Black AE. Laryngospasm in pediatric practice. Paediatr Anaesth. 2008;18(4):279–80.
139. Flick RP, Wilder RT, Pieper SF, et al. Risk factors for laryngospasm in children during general anesthesia. Paediatr Anaesth. 2008;18(4):289–96.
140. Olsson GL, Hallen B. Laryngospasm during anaesthesia. A computer-aided incidence study in 136,929 patients. Acta Anaesthesiol Scand. 1984;28(5):567–75.
141. Heinz P, Geelhoed GC, Wee C, Pascoe EM. Is atropine needed with ketamine sedation? A prospective, randomised, double blind study. Emerg Med J. 2006;23(3):206–9.
142. Brown L, Christian-Kopp S, Sherwin TS, et al. Adjunctive atropine is unnecessary during ketamine sedation in children. Acad Emerg Med. 2008;15(4):314–8.
143. Green SM, Klooster M, Harris T, Lynch EL, Rothrock SG. Ketamine sedation for pediatric gastroenterology procedures. J Pediatr Gastroenterol Nutr. 2001;32(1):26–33.
144. Novak H, Karlsland Akeson P, Akeson J. Sedation with ketamine and low-dose midazolam for short-term procedures requiring pharyngeal manipulation in young children. Paediatr Anaesth. 2008; 18(1):48–54.
145. Hompson-Evans D, Morgan P, Farrar M. Pediatric laryngospasm. Pediatr Anesth. 2008;18:303–7.
146. Chung DC, Rowbottom SJ. A very small dose of suxamethonium relieves laryngospasm. Anaesthesia. 1993;48(3):229–30.
147. Batra YK, Ivanova M, Ali SS, Shamsah M, Al Qattan AR, Belani KG. The efficacy of a subhypnotic dose of propofol in preventing laryngospasm following tonsillectomy and adenoidectomy in children. Paediatr Anaesth. 2005;15(12):1094–7.
148. Donati F, Meistelman C, Plaud B. Vecuronium neuromuscular blockade at the adductor muscles of the larynx and adductor pollicis. Anesthesiology. 1991;74(5):833–7.
149. Warner DO. Intramuscular succinylcholine and laryngospasm. Anesthesiology. 2001;95(4):1039–40.
150. Alalami AA, Ayoub CM, Baraka AS. Laryngospasm: review of different prevention and treatment modalities. Paediatr Anaesth. 2008;18(4):281–8.
151. Yaster M, Sola JE, Pegoli Jr W, Paidas CN. The night after surgery. Postoperative management of the pediatric outpatient—surgical and anesthetic aspects. Pediatr Clin North Am. 1994;41(1): 199–220.
152. Thomas M, Woodhead G, Masood N, Howard R. Motion sickness as a predictor of postoperative vomiting in children aged 1–16 years. Paediatr Anaesth. 2007;17(1):61–3.
153. American Academy of Pediatrics, American Academy of Pediatric Dentistry, Cote CJ, Wilson S, Work Group on Sedation. Guidelines for monitoring and management of pediatric patients during and

after sedation for diagnostic and therapeutic procedures: an update. Pediatrics. 2006;118(6):2587–602.

154. Holzman RS MT, Polaner DM, editors. A practical approach to pediatric anesthesia. Philadelphia: Lippincott, Williams & Wilkins; 2008.

155. Brunton LL, editor. Goodman & Gilman's the pharmacological basis of therapeutics. 11th ed. New York: McGraw-Hill; 2006.

156. Green SM, Clark R, Hostetler MA, Cohen M, Carlson D, Rothrock SG. Inadvertent ketamine overdose in children: clinical manifestations and outcome. Ann Emerg Med. 1999;34(4 Pt 1):492–7.

157. McEnvoy GK. AHFS (American Hospital Formulary Service) drug information. 2009. http://www.ahfsdruginformation.com. Accessed 20 Feb 2010.

158. Mace SE, Barata IA, Cravero JP, et al. Clinical policy: evidence-based approach to pharmacologic agents used in pediatric sedation and analgesia in the emergency department. Ann Emerg Med. 2004;44(4):342–77.

159. Dallimore D, Herd DW, Short T, Anderson BJ. Dosing ketamine for pediatric procedural sedation in the emergency department. Pediatr Emerg Care. 2008;24(8):529–33.

160. Roback MG, Wathen JE, MacKenzie T, Bajaj L. A randomized, controlled trial of i.v. versus i.m. ketamine for sedation of pediatric patients receiving emergency department orthopedic procedures. Ann Emerg Med. 2006;48(5):605–12.

161. Judisch GF, Anderson S, Bell WE. Chloral hydrate sedation as a substitute for examination under anesthesia in pediatric ophthalmology. Am J Ophthalmol. 1980;89(4):560–3.

162. Houpt MI, Sheskin RB, Koenigsberg SR, Desjardins PJ, Shey Z. Assessing chloral hydrate dosage for young children. ASDC J Dent Child. 1985;52(5):364–9.

163. Freyer DR, Schwanda AE, Sanfilippo DJ, Hackbarth RM, Hassan NE, Kopec JS, et al. Intravenous methohexital for brief sedation of pediatric oncology outpatients: physiologic and behavioral responses. Pediatrics. 1997;99(5):E8.

164. Audenaert SM, Montgomery CL, Thompson DE, Sutherland J. A prospective study of rectal methohexital: efficacy and side effects in 648 cases. Anesth Analg. 1995;81(5):957–61.

165. Manuli MA, Davies L. Rectal methohexital for sedation of children during imaging procedures. AJR Am J Roentgenol. 1993; 160(3):577–80.

166. Karian VE, Burrows PE, Zurakowski D, Connor L, Mason KP. Sedation for pediatric radiological procedures: analysis of potential causes of sedation failure and paradoxical reactions. Pediatr Radiol. 1999;29(11):869–73.

167. Mason KP, Zurakowski D, Karian VE, Connor L, Fontaine PJ, Burrows PE. Sedatives used in pediatric imaging: comparison of IV pentobarbital with IV pentobarbital with midazolam added. AJR Am J Roentgenol. 2001;177(2):427–30.

168. Strain JD, Campbell JB, Harvey LA, Foley LC. IV Nembutal: safe sedation for children undergoing CT. AJR Am J Roentgenol. 1988;151(5):975–9.

169. Moro-Sutherland DM, Algren JT, Louis PT, Kozinetz CA, Shook JE. Comparison of intravenous midazolam with pentobarbital for sedation for head computed tomography imaging. Acad Emerg Med. 2000;7(12):1370–5.

170. Kienstra AJ, Ward MA, Sasan F, Hunter J, Morriss MC, Macias CG. Etomidate versus pentobarbital for sedation of children for head and neck CT imaging. Pediatr Emerg Care. 2004;20(8): 499–506.

171. Zgleszewski SE, Zurakowski D, Fontaine PJ, D'Angelo M, Mason KP. Is propofol a safe alternative to pentobarbital for sedation during pediatric diagnostic CT? Radiology. 2008;247(2):528–34.

172. Rooks VJ, Chung T, Connor L, Zurakowski D, Hoffer FA, Mason KP, et al. Comparison of oral pentobarbital sodium (nembutal) and oral chloral hydrate for sedation of infants during radiologic imaging: preliminary results. AJR Am J Roentgenol. 2003;180(4):1125–8.

173. Malviya S, Voepel-Lewis T, Tait AR, Reynolds PI, Gujar SK, Gebarski SS, et al. Pentobarbital vs chloral hydrate for sedation of children undergoing MRI: efficacy and recovery characteristics. Paediatr Anaesth. 2004;14(7):589–95.

174. Mason KP, Zurakowski D, Connor L, Karian VE, Fontaine PJ, Sanborn PA, et al. Infant sedation for MR imaging and CT: oral versus intravenous pentobarbital. Radiology. 2004;233(3):723–8.

175. Strain JD, Harvey LA, Foley LC, Campbell JB. Intravenously administered pentobarbital sodium for sedation in pediatric CT. Radiology. 1986;161(1):105–8.

176. Greenberg SB, Adams RC, Aspinall CL. Initial experience with intravenous pentobarbital sedation for children undergoing MRI at a tertiary care pediatric hospital: the learning curve. Pediatr Radiol. 2000;30(10):689–91.

177. Egelhoff JC, Ball Jr WS, Koch BL, Parks TD. Safety and efficacy of sedation in children using a structured sedation program. AJR Am J Roentgenol. 1997;168(5):1259–62.

178. Slovis TL, Parks C, Reneau D, Becker CJ, Hersch J, Carver CD, et al. Pediatric sedation: short-term effects. Pediatr Radiol. 1993;23(5):345–8.

179. Gaudreault P, Guay J, Thivierge RL, Verdy I. Benzodiazepine poisoning. Clinical and pharmacological considerations and treatment. Drug Saf. 1991;6(4):247–65.

180. van der Bijl P, Roelofse JA. Disinhibitory reactions to benzodiazepines: a review. J Oral Maxillofac Surg. 1991;49(5):519–23.

181. Gillies D, Beck A, McCloud A, Rathbone J. Benzodiazepines alone or in combination with antipsychotic drugs for acute psychosis. Cochrane Database Syst Rev. 2005;(4):CD003079.

182. Rubin JT, Towbin RB, Bartko M, Baskin KM, Cahill AM, Kaye RD. Oral and intravenous caffeine for treatment of children with post-sedation paradoxical hyperactivity. Pediatr Radiol. 2004; 34(12):980–4.

183. Cole SG, Brozinsky S, Isenberg JI. Midazolam, a new more potent benzodiazepine, compared with diazepam: a randomized, double-blind study of preendoscopic sedatives. Gastrointest Endosc. 1983;29(3):219–22.

184. Ghoneim MM, Mewaldt SP. Benzodiazepines and human memory: a review. Anesthesiology. 1990;72(5):926–38.

185. Ramoska EA, Linkenheimer R, Glasgow C. Midazolam use in the emergency department. J Emerg Med. 1991;9(4):247–51.

186. Wright SW, Chudnofsky CR, Dronen SC, Kothari R, Birrer P, Blanton DM, et al. Comparison of midazolam and diazepam for conscious sedation in the emergency department. Ann Emerg Med. 1993;22(2):201–5.

187. Unlugenc H, Guler T, Gunes Y, Isik G. Comparative study of the antiemetic efficacy of ondansetron, propofol and midazolam in the early postoperative period. Eur J Anaesthesiol. 2004;21(1):60–5.

188. Lane RD, Schunk JE. Atomized intranasal midazolam use for minor procedures in the pediatric emergency department. Pediatr Emerg Care. 2008;24(5):300–3.

189. Connors K, Terndrup TE. Nasal versus oral midazolam for sedation of anxious children undergoing laceration repair. Ann Emerg Med. 1994;24(6):1074–9.

190. Theroux MC, West DW, Corddry DH, Hyde PM, Bachrach SJ, Cronan KM, et al. Efficacy of intranasal midazolam in facilitating suturing of lacerations in preschool children in the emergency department. Pediatrics. 1993;91(3):624–7.

191. Wilton NC, Leigh J, Rosen DR, Pandit UA. Preanesthetic sedation of preschool children using intranasal midazolam. Anesthesiology. 1988;69(6):972–5.

192. Saint-Maurice C, Meistelman C, Rey E, Esteve C, de Lauture D, Olive G. The pharmacokinetics of rectal midazolam for premedication in children. Anesthesiology. 1986;65(5):536–8.

193. Shane SA, Fuchs SM, Khine H. Efficacy of rectal midazolam for the sedation of preschool children undergoing laceration repair. Ann Emerg Med. 1994;24(6):1065–73.

194. Buhrer M, Maitre PO, Crevoisier C, Stanski DR. Electroencephalographic effects of benzodiazepines. II. Pharmacodynamic modeling of the electroencephalographic effects of midazolam and diazepam. Clin Pharmacol Ther. 1990; 48(5):555–67.
195. Krauss B, Shannon M, Damian FJ, Fleisher GR, editors. Guidelines for pediatric sedation. 2nd ed. Dallas: American College of Emergency Physicians; 1998.
196. Veselis RA, Reinsel RA, Feshchenko VA, Wronski M. The comparative amnestic effects of midazolam, propofol, thiopental, and fentanyl at equisedative concentrations. Anesthesiology. 1997; 87(4):749–64.
197. Lalwani K, Michel M. Pediatric sedation in North American children's hospitals: a survey of anesthesia providers. Paediatr Anaesth. 2005;15(3):209–13.
198. Sacchetti A, Stander E, Ferguson N, Maniar G, Valko P. Pediatric Procedural Sedation in the Community Emergency Department: results from the ProSCED registry. Pediatr Emerg Care. 2007; 23(4):218–22.
199. Bassett KE, Anderson JL, Pribble CG, Guenther E. Propofol for procedural sedation in children in the emergency department. Ann Emerg Med. 2003;42(6):773–82.
200. Havel Jr CJ, Strait RT, Hennes H. A clinical trial of propofol vs midazolam for procedural sedation in a pediatric emergency department. Acad Emerg Med. 1999;6(10):989–97.
201. Godambe SA, Elliot V, Matheny D, Pershad J. Comparison of propofol/fentanyl versus ketamine/midazolam for brief orthopedic procedural sedation in a pediatric emergency department. Pediatrics. 2003;112(1 Pt 1):116–23.
202. Slavik VC, Zed PJ. Combination ketamine and propofol for procedural sedation and analgesia. Pharmacotherapy. 2007;27(11): 1588–98.
203. Tosun Z, Esmaoglu A, Coruh A. Propofol-ketamine vs propofol-fentanyl combinations for deep sedation and analgesia in pediatric patients undergoing burn dressing changes. Paediatr Anaesth. 2008;18(1):43–7.
204. Kotani Y, Shimazawa M, Yoshimura S, Iwama T, Hara H. The experimental and clinical pharmacology of propofol, an anesthetic agent with neuroprotective properties. CNS Neurosci Ther. 2008;14(2):95–106.
205. Skokan EG, Pribble C, Bassett KE, Nelson DS. Use of propofol sedation in a pediatric emergency department: a prospective study. Clin Pediatr (Phila). 2001;40(12):663–71.
206. Mallory MD, Baxter AL, Kost SI. Propofol vs pentobarbital for sedation of children undergoing magnetic resonance imaging: results from the Pediatric Sedation Research Consortium. Paediatr Anaesth. 2009;19(6):601–11.
207. Bell A, Treston G, McNabb C, Monypenny K, Cardwell R. Profiling adverse respiratory events and vomiting when using propofol for emergency department procedural sedation. Emerg Med Australas. 2007;19(5):405–10.
208. Dosani M, McCormack J, Reimer E, Brant R, Dumont G, Lim J, et al. Slower administration of propofol preserves adequate respiration in children. Paediatr Anaesth. 2010;20(11):1001–8.
209. Evans RG, Crawford MW, Noseworthy MD, Yoo SJ. Effect of increasing depth of propofol anesthesia on upper airway configuration in children. Anesthesiology. 2003;99(3):596–602.
210. Green SM. Propofol for emergency department procedural sedation—not yet ready for prime time. Acad Emerg Med. 1999; 6(10):975–8.
211. Gan TJ. Pharmacokinetic and pharmacodynamic characteristics of medications used for moderate sedation. Clin Pharmacokinet. 2006;45(9):855–69.
212. Fulton B, Sorkin EM. Propofol. An overview of its pharmacology and a review of its clinical efficacy in intensive care sedation. Drugs. 1995;50(4):636–57.
213. Skues MA, Prys-Roberts C. The pharmacology of propofol. J Clin Anesth. 1989;1(5):387–400.
214. Tramer MR, Moore RA, McQuay HJ. Propofol and bradycardia: causation, frequency and severity. Br J Anaesth. 1997;78(6): 642–51.
215. Smith I, White PF, Nathanson M, Gouldson R. Propofol. An update on its clinical use. Anesthesiology. 1994;81(4):1005–43.
216. Bryson HM, Fulton BR, Faulds D. Propofol. An update of its use in anaesthesia and conscious sedation. Drugs. 1995;50(3): 513–59.
217. Zuckerbraun NS, Pitetti RD, Herr SM, Roth KR, Gaines BA, King C. Use of etomidate as an induction agent for rapid sequence intubation in a pediatric emergency department. Acad Emerg Med. 2006;13(6):602–9.
218. Guldner G, Schultz J, Sexton P, Fortner C, Richmond M. Etomidate for rapid-sequence intubation in young children: hemodynamic effects and adverse events. Acad Emerg Med. 2003;10(2):134–9.
219. Sokolove PE, Price DD, Okada P. The safety of etomidate for emergency rapid sequence intubation of pediatric patients. Pediatr Emerg Care. 2000;16(1):18–21.
220. Dickinson R, Singer AJ, Carrion W. Etomidate for pediatric sedation prior to fracture reduction. Acad Emerg Med. 2001;8(1):74–7.
221. Ruth WJ, Burton JH, Bock AJ. Intravenous etomidate for procedural sedation in emergency department patients. Acad Emerg Med. 2001;8(1):13–8.
222. Vinson DR, Bradbury DR. Etomidate for procedural sedation in emergency medicine. Ann Emerg Med. 2002;39(6):592–8.
223. Keim SM, Erstad BL, Sakles JC, Davis V. Etomidate for procedural sedation in the emergency department. Pharmacotherapy. 2002;22(5):586–92.
224. Baxter AL, Mallory MD, Spandorfer PR, Sharma S, Freilich SH, Cravero J. Etomidate versus pentobarbital for computed tomography sedations: report from the Pediatric Sedation Research Consortium. Pediatr Emerg Care. 2007;23(10):690–5.
225. Di Liddo L, D'Angelo A, Nguyen B, Bailey B, Amre D, Stanciu C. Etomidate versus midazolam for procedural sedation in pediatric outpatients: a randomized controlled trial. Ann Emerg Med. 2006;48(4):433–40, 440.e1.
226. Helmers JH, Adam AA, Giezen J. Pain and myoclonus during induction with etomidate. A double- blind, controlled evaluation of the influence of droperidol and fentanyl. Acta Anaesthesiol Belg. 1981;32(2):141–7.
227. McDowall RH, Scher CS, Barst SM. Total intravenous anesthesia for children undergoing brief diagnostic or therapeutic procedures. J Clin Anesth. 1995;7(4):273–80.
228. Modica PA, Tempelhoff R. Intracranial pressure during induction of anaesthesia and tracheal intubation with etomidate-induced EEG burst suppression. Can J Anaesth. 1992;39(3):236–41.
229. den Brinker M, Hokken-Koelega AC, Hazelzet JA, de Jong FH, Hop WC, Joosten KF. One single dose of etomidate negatively influences adrenocortical performance for at least 24h in children with meningococcal sepsis. Intensive Care Med. 2008;34(1):163–8.
230. den Brinker M, Joosten KF, Liem O, et al. Adrenal insufficiency in meningococcal sepsis: bioavailable cortisol levels and impact of interleukin-6 levels and intubation with etomidate on adrenal function and mortality. J Clin Endocrinol Metab. 2005;90(9): 5110–7.
231. Mohammad Z, Afessa B, Finkielman JD. The incidence of relative adrenal insufficiency in patients with septic shock after the administration of etomidate. Crit Care. 2006;10(4):R105.
232. Cotton BA, Guillamondegui OD, Fleming SB, Carpenter RO, Patel SH, Morris Jr JA, et al. Increased risk of adrenal insufficiency following etomidate exposure in critically injured patients. Arch Surg. 2008;143(1):62–7; discussion 67.
233. McClain DA, Hug Jr CC. Intravenous fentanyl kinetics. Clin Pharmacol Ther. 1980;28(1):106–14.

234. Klein EJ, Diekema DS, Paris CA, Quan L, Cohen M, Seidel KD. A randomized, clinical trial of oral midazolam plus placebo versus oral midazolam plus oral transmucosal fentanyl for sedation during laceration repair. Pediatrics. 2002;109(5):894–7.
235. Schutzman SA, Burg J, Liebelt E, Strafford M, Schechter N, Wisk M, et al. Oral transmucosal fentanyl citrate for premedication of children undergoing laceration repair. Ann Emerg Med. 1994; 24(6):1059–64.
236. Schutzman SA, Liebelt E, Wisk M, Burg J. Comparison of oral transmucosal fentanyl citrate and intramuscular meperidine, promethazine, and chlorpromazine for conscious sedation of children undergoing laceration repair. Ann Emerg Med. 1996;28(4):385–90.
237. Schechter NL, Weisman SJ, Rosenblum M, Bernstein B, Conard PL. The use of oral transmucosal fentanyl citrate for painful procedures in children. Pediatrics. 1995;95(3):335–9.
238. Mahar PJ, Rana JA, Kennedy CS, Christopher NC. A randomized clinical trial of oral transmucosal fentanyl citrate versus intravenous morphine sulfate for initial control of pain in children with extremity injuries. Pediatr Emerg Care. 2007;23(8):544–8.
239. Borland M, Jacobs I, King B, O'Brien D. A randomized controlled trial comparing intranasal fentanyl to intravenous morphine for managing acute pain in children in the emergency department. Ann Emerg Med. 2007;49(3):335–40.
240. Borland ML, Jacobs I, Geelhoed G. Intranasal fentanyl reduces acute pain in children in the emergency department: a safety and efficacy study. Emerg Med (Fremantle). 2002;14(3):275–80.
241. Bates BA, Schutzman SA, Fleisher GR. A comparison of intranasal sufentanil and midazolam to intramuscular meperidine, promethazine, and chlorpromazine for conscious sedation in children. Ann Emerg Med. 1994;24(4):646–51.
242. Caspi J, Klausner JM, Safadi T, Amar R, Rozin RR, Merin G. Delayed respiratory depression following fentanyl anesthesia for cardiac surgery. Crit Care Med. 1988;16(3):238–40.
243. Williams DG, Hatch DJ, Howard RF. Codeine phosphate in paediatric medicine. Br J Anaesth. 2001;86(3):413–21.
244. Williams DG, Patel A, Howard RF. Pharmacogenetics of codeine metabolism in an urban population of children and its implications for analgesic reliability. Br J Anaesth. 2002;89(6):839–45.
245. Gasche Y, Daali Y, Fathi M, Chiappe A, Cottini S, Dayer P, et al. Codeine intoxication associated with ultrarapid CYP2D6 metabolism. N Engl J Med. 2004;351(27):2827–31.
246. Charney RL, Yan Y, Schootman M, Kennedy RM, Luhmann JD. Oxycodone versus codeine for triage pain in children with suspected forearm fracture: a randomized controlled trial. Pediatr Emerg Care. 2008;24(9):595–600.
247. Kokki H, Rasanen I, Reinikainen M, Suhonen P, Vanamo K, Ojanpera I. Pharmacokinetics of oxycodone after intravenous, buccal, intramuscular and gastric administration in children. Clin Pharmacokinet. 2004;43(9):613–22.
248. Pokela ML, Anttila E, Seppala T, Olkkola KT. Marked variation in oxycodone pharmacokinetics in infants. Paediatr Anaesth. 2005; 15(7):560–5.
249. Bhargava R, Young KD. Procedural pain management patterns in academic pediatric emergency departments. Acad Emerg Med. 2007;14(5):479–82.
250. Green SM, Roback MG, Kennedy RM, Krauss B. Clinical practice guideline for emergency department ketamine dissociative sedation: 2011 update. Ann Emerg Med. 2011;57:449–61.
251. Sirinathsinghji D. NMDA antagonists as potential analgesic drugs. Basel: Birkhauser; 2002.
252. White PF, Way WL, Trevor AJ. Ketamine–its pharmacology and therapeutic uses. Anesthesiology. 1982;56(2):119–36.
253. Bourgoin A, Albanese J, Wereszczynski N, Charbit M, Vialet R, Martin C. Safety of sedation with ketamine in severe head injury patients: comparison with sufentanil. Crit Care Med. 2003;31(3):711–7.
254. Albanese J, Arnaud S, Rey M, Thomachot L, Alliez B, Martin C. Ketamine decreases intracranial pressure and electroencephalographic activity in traumatic brain injury patients during propofol sedation. Anesthesiology. 1997;87(6):1328–34.
255. Sehdev RS, Symmons DA, Kindl K. Ketamine for rapid sequence induction in patients with head injury in the emergency department. Emerg Med Australas. 2006;18(1):37–44.
256. Reich DL, Silvay G. Ketamine: an update on the first twenty-five years of clinical experience. Can J Anaesth. 1989;36(2):186–97.
257. Lippmann M, Appel PL, Mok MS, Shoemaker WC. Sequential cardiorespiratory patterns of anesthetic induction with ketamine in critically ill patients. Crit Care Med. 1983;11(9):730–4.
258. Drummond GB. Comparison of sedation with midazolam and ketamine: effects on airway muscle activity. Br J Anaesth. 1996;76(5): 663–7.
259. Hamza J, Ecoffey C, Gross JB. Ventilatory response to CO_2 following intravenous ketamine in children. Anesthesiology. 1989; 70(3):422–5.
260. Mankikian B, Cantineau JP, Sartene R, Clergue F, Viars P. Ventilatory pattern and chest wall mechanics during ketamine anesthesia in humans. Anesthesiology. 1986;65(5):492–9.
261. Tokics L, Strandberg A, Brismar B, Lundquist H, Hedenstierna G. Computerized tomography of the chest and gas exchange measurements during ketamine anaesthesia. Acta Anaesthesiol Scand. 1987;31(8):684–92.
262. Shulman DL, Bar-Yishay E, Godfrey S. Respiratory mechanics and intrinsic PEEP during ketamine and halothane anesthesia in young children. Anesth Analg. 1988;67(7):656–62.
263. Morel DR, Forster A, Gemperle M. Noninvasive evaluation of breathing pattern and thoraco-abdominal motion following the infusion of ketamine or droperidol in humans. Anesthesiology. 1986;65(4):392–8.
264. Joly LM, Benhamou D. Ventilation during total intravenous anaesthesia with ketamine. Can J Anaesth. 1994;41(3):227–31.
265. Zsigmond EK, Matsuki A, Kothary SP, Jallad M. Arterial hypoxemia caused by intravenous ketamine. Anesth Analg. 1976;55(3):311–4.
266. Smith JA, Santer LJ. Respiratory arrest following intramuscular ketamine injection in a 4-year-old child. Ann Emerg Med. 1993; 22(3):613–5.
267. Jonnavithula N, Kulkarni DK, Ramachandran G. Prolonged apnea with intramuscular ketamine: a case report. Paediatr Anaesth. 2008;18(4):330–1.
268. Bourke DL, Malit LA, Smith TC. Respiratory interactions of ketamine and morphine. Anesthesiology. 1987;66(2):153–6.
269. Green SM, Roback MG, Krauss B. Laryngospasm during emergency department ketamine sedation: a case-control study. Pediatr Emerg Care. 2010;26(11):798–802.
270. Rogers R, Wise RG, Painter DJ, Longe SE, Tracey I. An investigation to dissociate the analgesic and anesthetic properties of ketamine using functional magnetic resonance imaging. Anesthesiology. 2004;100(2):292–301.
271. Visser E, Schug SA. The role of ketamine in pain management. Biomed Pharmacother. 2006;60(7):341–8.
272. McMahon SB, Koltzenburg M, editors. Wall and Melzack's textbook of pain. 5th ed. Philadelphia: Elsevier/Churchill Livingstone; 2005.
273. Woolf CJ, Thompson SW. The induction and maintenance of central sensitization is dependent on N-methyl-D-aspartic acid receptor activation; implications for the treatment of post-injury pain hyper- sensitivity states. Pain. 1991;44(3):293–9.
274. Ji RR, Kohno T, Moore KA, Woolf CJ. Central sensitization and LTP: do pain and memory share similar mechanisms? Trends Neurosci. 2003;26(12):696–705.
275. Ilkjaer S, Petersen KL, Brennum J, Wernberg M, Dahl JB. Effect of systemic N-methyl-D-aspartate receptor antagonist (ketamine) on primary and secondary hyperalgesia in humans. Br J Anaesth. 1996;76(6):829–34.

276. Warncke T, Stubhaug A, Jorum E. Ketamine, an NMDA receptor antagonist, suppresses spatial and temporal properties of burn-induced secondary hyperalgesia in man: a double-blind, cross-over comparison with morphine and placebo. Pain. 1997;72(1–2): 99–106.
277. De Kock M, Lavand'homme P, Waterloos H. 'Balanced analgesia' in the perioperative period: is there a place for ketamine? Pain. 2001;92(3):373–80.
278. Willert RP, Woolf CJ, Hobson AR, Delaney C, Thompson DG, Aziz Q. The development and maintenance of human visceral pain hypersensitivity is dependent on the N-methyl-D-aspartate receptor. Gastroenterology. 2004;126(3):683–92.
279. Menigaux C, Fletcher D, Dupont X, Guignard B, Guirimand F, Chauvin M. The benefits of intraoperative small-dose ketamine on postoperative pain after anterior cruciate ligament repair. Anesth Analg. 2000;90(1):129–35.
280. Fu ES, Miguel R, Scharf JE. Preemptive ketamine decreases post-operative narcotic requirements in patients undergoing abdominal surgery. Anesth Analg. 1997;84(5):1086–90.
281. Gurnani A, Sharma PK, Rautela RS, Bhattacharya A. Analgesia for acute musculoskeletal trauma: low- dose subcutaneous infusion of ketamine. Anaesth Intensive Care. 1996;24(1):32–6.
282. Angst MS, Clark JD. Opioid-induced hyperalgesia: a qualitative systematic review. Anesthesiology. 2006;104(3):570–87.
283. Célèrier E, Rivat C, Jun Y, Laulin JP, Larcher A, Reynier P, et al. Long-lasting hyperalgesia induced by fentanyl in rats: preventive effect of ketamine. Anesthesiology. 2000;92(2):465–72.
284. Stubhaug A, Breivik H, Eide PK, Kreunen M, Foss A. Mapping of punctuate hyperalgesia around a surgical incision demonstrates that ketamine is a powerful suppressor of central sensitization to pain following surgery. Acta Anaesthesiol Scand. 1997;41(9): 1124–32.
285. Joly V, Richebe P, Guignard B, Fletcher D, Maurette P, Sessler DI, et al. Remifentanil-induced postoperative hyperalgesia and its prevention with small-dose ketamine. Anesthesiology. 2005;103(1): 147–55.
286. Olney JW, Labruyere J, Price MT. Pathological changes induced in cerebrocortical neurons by phencyclidine and related drugs. Science. 1989;244(4910):1360–2.
287. Hayashi H, Dikkes P, Soriano SG. Repeated administration of ketamine may lead to neuronal degeneration in the developing rat brain. Paediatr Anaesth. 2002;12(9):770–4.
288. Farber NB, Wozniak DF, Price MT, Labruyere J, Huss J, St Peter H, et al. Age-specific neurotoxicity in the rat associated with NMDA receptor blockade: potential relevance to schizophrenia? Biol Psychiatry. 1995;38(12):788–96.
289. Farber NB, Price MT, Labruyere J, Nemnich J, St Peter H, Wozniak DF, et al. Antipsychotic drugs block phencyclidine receptor-mediated neurotoxicity. Biol Psychiatry. 1993;34(1–2): 119–21.
290. Ikonomidou C, Bosch F, Miksa M, Bittigau P, Vöckler J, Dikranian K, et al. Blockade of NMDA receptors and apoptotic neurodegeneration in the developing brain. Science. 1999;283(5398):70–4.
291. Fredriksson A, Archer T, Alm H, Gordh T, Eriksson P. Neurofunctional deficits and potentiated apoptosis by neonatal NMDA antagonist administration. Behav Brain Res. 2004;153(2): 367–76.
292. Patel P, Sun L. Update on neonatal anesthetic neurotoxicity: insight into molecular mechanisms and relevance to humans. Anesthesiology. 2009;110(4):703–8.
293. Wang C, Sadovova N, Hotchkiss C, Fu X, Scallet AC, Patterson TA, et al. Blockade of N-methyl-D-aspartate receptors by ketamine produces loss of postnatal day 3 monkey frontal cortical neurons in culture. Toxicol Sci. 2006;91(1):192–201.
294. Young C, Jevtovic-Todorovic V, Qin YQ, Tenkova T, Wang H, Labruyere J, et al. Potential of ketamine and midazolam, individually or in combination, to induce apoptotic neurodegeneration in the infant mouse brain. Br J Pharmacol. 2005;146(2):189–97.
295. Krystal JH, Karper LP, Seibyl JP, Freeman GK, Delaney R, Bremner JD, et al. Subanesthetic effects of the noncompetitive NMDA antagonist, ketamine, in humans. Psychotomimetic, perceptual, cognitive, and neuroendocrine responses. Arch Gen Psychiatry. 1994;51(3):199–214.
296. Malhotra AK, Pinals DA, Weingartner H, Sirocco K, Missar CD, Pickar D, et al. NMDA receptor function and human cognition: the effects of ketamine in healthy volunteers. Neuropsychopharmacology. 1996;14(5):301–7.
297. Adler CM, Goldberg TE, Malhotra AK, Pickar D, Breier A. Effects of ketamine on thought disorder, working memory, and semantic memory in healthy volunteers. Biol Psychiatry. 1998;43(11):811–6.
298. Newcomer JW, Farber NB, Jevtovic-Todorovic V, Selke G, Melson AK, Hershey T, et al. Ketamine-induced NMDA receptor hypofunction as a model of memory impairment and psychosis. Neuropsychopharmacology. 1999;20(2):106–18.
299. Hollister GR, Burn JM. Side effects of ketamine in pediatric anesthesia. Anesth Analg. 1974;53(2):264–7.
300. Hostetler MA, Davis CO. Prospective age-based comparison of behavioral reactions occurring after ketamine sedation in the ED. Am J Emerg Med. 2002;20(5):463–8.
301. Lin C, Durieux ME. Ketamine and kids: an update. Paediatr Anaesth. 2005;15(2):91–7.
302. Kain ZN, Mayes LC, Wang SM, Hofstadter MB. Postoperative behavioral outcomes in children: effects of sedative premedication. Anesthesiology. 1999;90(3):758–65.
303. Sherwin TS, Green SM, Khan A, Chapman DS, Dannenberg B. Does adjunctive midazolam reduce recovery agitation after ketamine sedation for pediatric procedures? A randomized, double-blind, placebo-controlled trial. Ann Emerg Med. 2000;35(3): 229–38.
304. Kain ZN, Caldwell-Andrews AA, Maranets I, McClain B, Gaal D, Mayes LC, et al. Preoperative anxiety and emergence delirium and postoperative maladaptive behaviors. Anesth Analg. 2004; 99(6):1648–54, table of contents.
305. Kennedy RM, McAllister JD. Midazolam with ketamine: who benefits? Ann Emerg Med. 2000;35(3):297–9.
306. Gorelick M, Nagler J, Losek JD. Pediatric sedation pearls. Clin Pediatr Emerg Med. 2007;8(4):268–78.
307. Gloor A, Dillier C, Gerber A. Ketamine for short ambulatory procedures in children: an audit. Paediatr Anaesth. 2001;11(5):533–9.
308. Thorp AW, Brown L, Green SM. Ketamine-associated vomiting: is it dose-related? Pediatr Emerg Care. 2009;25(1):15–8.
309. Vlajkovic GP, Sindjelic RP. Emergence delirium in children: many questions, few answers. Anesth Analg. 2007;104(1):84–91.
310. Kain ZN, Mayes LC, O'Connor TZ, Cicchetti DV. Preoperative anxiety in children. Predictors and outcomes. Arch Pediatr Adolesc Med. 1996;150(12):1238–45.
311. Domino EF, Domino SE, Smith RE, Domino LE, Goulet JR, Domino KE, et al. Ketamine kinetics in unmedicated and diazepam-premedicated subjects. Clin Pharmacol Ther. 1984; 36(5):645–53.
312. Grant IS, Nimmo WS, McNicol LR, Clements JA. Ketamine disposition in children and adults. Br J Anaesth. 1983;55(11): 1107–11.
313. Atiba JO, Horai Y, White PF, Trevor AJ, Blaschke TF, Sung ML. Effect of etomidate on hepatic drug metabolism in humans. Anesthesiology. 1988;68(6):920–4.
314. Bleiberg AH, Salvaggio CA, Roy LC, Kassutto Z. Low-dose ketamine: efficacy in pediatric sedation. Pediatr Emerg Care. 2007; 23(3):158–62.
315. McGlone RG, Howes MC, Joshi M. The Lancaster experience of 2.0 to 2.5 mg/kg intramuscular ketamine for paediatric sedation: 501 cases and analysis. Emerg Med J. 2004;21(3):290–5.

316. Herd D, Anderson BJ. Ketamine disposition in children presenting for procedural sedation and analgesia in a children's emergency department. Paediatr Anaesth. 2007;17(7):622–9.
317. Luhmann JD, Kennedy RM, McAllister JD, Jaffe DM. Sedation for peritonsillar abscess drainage in the pediatric emergency department. Pediatr Emerg Care. 2002;18(1):1–3.
318. Bauer PW, Lieu JE, Suskind DL, Lusk RP. The safety of conscious sedation in peritonsillar abscess drainage. Arch Otolaryngol Head Neck Surg. 2001;127(12):1477–80.
319. Green SM, Hummel CB, Wittlake WA, Rothrock SG, Hopkins GA, Garrett W. What is the optimal dose of intramuscular ketamine for pediatric sedation? Acad Emerg Med. 1999;6(1):21–6.
320. Herd DW, Anderson BJ, Holford NH. Modeling the norketamine metabolite in children and the implications for analgesia. Paediatr Anaesth. 2007;17(9):831–40.
321. Thomas MC, Jennett-Reznek AM, Patanwala AE. Combination of ketamine and propofol versus either agent alone for procedural sedation in the emergency department. Am J Health Syst Pharm. 2011;68:2248–56.
322. Alletag MJ, Auerbach MA, Baum CR. Ketamine, propofol, and ketofol use for pediatric sedation. Pediatr Emerg Care. 2012; 28:1391–8.
323. Green SM, Andolfatto G, Krauss B. Ketofol for Procedural Sedation? Pro and Con. Ann Emerg Med. 2011;57(5):444–8.
324. Shah A, Mosdossy G, McLeod S, Lehnhardt K, Peddle M, Rieder M. A blinded, randomized controlled trial to evaluate ketamine/propofol versus ketamine alone for procedural sedation in children. Ann Emerg Med. 2011;57:425–33.
325. Andolfatto G, Willman E. A prospective case series of pediatric procedural sedation and analgesia in the emergency department using single-syringe ketamine-propofol combination (ketofol). Acad Emerg Med. 2010;17:194–201.
326. Sharieff GQ, Trocinski DR, Kanegaye JT, Fisher B, Harley JR. Ketamine-propofol combination sedation for fracture reduction in the pediatric emergency department. Pediatr Emerg Care. 2007;23(12):881–4.
327. David H, Shipp JA. Randomized controlled trial of ketamine/propofol versus propofol alone for emergency department procedural sedation. Ann Emerg Med. 2011;57:435–41.
328. Andolfatto G, Abu-Laban RB, Zed PJ, Staniforth SM, Stackhouse S, Moadebi S, Willman E. Ketamine-propofol combination (ketofol) versus propofol alone for emergency department procedural sedation and analgesia: a randomized double-blind trial. Ann Emerg Med. 2012;59:504–12.
329. Messenger DW, Murray HE, Dungey PE, van Vlymen J, Sivilotti ML. Subdissociative-dose ketamine versus fentanyl for analgesia during propofol procedural sedation: a randomized clinical trial. Acad Emerg Med. 2008;15:877–86.
330. Nejati A, Moharari RS, Ashraf H, Labaf A, Golshani K. Ketamine/propofol versus midazolam/fentanyl for procedural sedation and analgesia in the emergency department: a randomized, prospective, double-blind trial. Acad Emerg Med. 2011;18:800–6.
331. Tobias JD. Dexmedetomidine and ketamine: an effective alternative for procedural sedation? Pediatr Crit Care Med. 2012;13:423–7.
332. Parbrook GD. The levels of nitrous oxide analgesia. Br J Anaesth. 1967;39(12):974–82.
333. Benedetti C, Chapman CR, Colpitts YH, Chen AC. Effect of nitrous oxide concentration on event- related potentials during painful tooth stimulation. Anesthesiology. 1982;56(5):360–4.
334. Clark M, Brunick A. A handbook of nitrous oxide and oxygen sedation. 3rd ed. St. Louis: Mosby; 2008.
335. Babl FE, Oakley E, Seaman C, Barnett P, Sharwood LN. High-concentration nitrous oxide for procedural sedation in children: adverse events and depth of sedation. Pediatrics. 2008;121(3): e528–32.
336. Burton JH, Auble TE, Fuchs SM. Effectiveness of 50% nitrous oxide/50% oxygen during laceration repair in children. Acad Emerg Med. 1998;5(2):112–7.
337. Clark MS, Campbell SA, Clark AM. Technique for the administration of nitrous oxide/oxygen sedation to ensure psychotropic analgesic nitrous oxide (PAN) effects. Int J Neurosci. 2006;116(7):871–7.
338. Babl FE, Oakley E, Puspitadewi A, Sharwood LN. Limited analgesic efficacy of nitrous oxide for painful procedures in children. Emerg Med J. 2008;25(11):717–21.
339. Hennrikus WL, Simpson RB, Klingelberger CE, Reis MT. Self-administered nitrous oxide analgesia for pediatric fracture reductions. J Pediatr Orthop. 1994;14(4):538–42.
340. Hennrikus WL, Shin AY, Klingelberger CE. Self- administered nitrous oxide and a hematoma block for analgesia in the outpatient reduction of fractures in children. J Bone Joint Surg Am. 1995; 77(3):335–9.
341. Frampton A, Browne GJ, Lam LT, Cooper MG, Lane LG. Nurse administered relative analgesia using high concentration nitrous oxide to facilitate minor procedures in children in an emergency department. Emerg Med J. 2003;20(5):410–3.
342. Farrell MK, Drake GJ, Rucker D, Finkelstein M, Zier JL. Creation of a registered nurse-administered nitrous oxide sedation program for radiology and beyond. Pediatr Nurs. 2008;34(1):29–35; quiz 35–6.
343. Litman RS, Kottra JA, Berkowitz RJ, Ward DS. Breathing patterns and levels of consciousness in children during administration of nitrous oxide after oral midazolam premedication. J Oral Maxillofac Surg. 1997;55(12):1372–7; discussion 1378–9.
344. Litman RS, Berkowitz RJ, Ward DS. Levels of consciousness and ventilatory parameters in young children during sedation with oral midazolam and nitrous oxide. Arch Pediatr Adolesc Med. 1996; 150(7):671–5.
345. Litman RS, Kottra JA, Verga KA, Berkowitz RJ, Ward DS. Chloral hydrate sedation: the additive sedative and respiratory depressant effects of nitrous oxide. Anesth Analg. 1998;86(4):724–8.
346. Gamis AS, Knapp JF, Glenski JA. Nitrous oxide analgesia in a pediatric emergency department. Ann Emerg Med. 1989;18(2): 177–81.
347. Bar-Meir E, Zaslansky R, Regev E, Keidan I, Orenstein A, Winkler E. Nitrous oxide administered by the plastic surgeon for repair of facial lacerations in children in the emergency room. Plast Reconstr Surg. 2006;117(5):1571–5.
348. Keidan I, Zaslansky R, Yusim Y, Ben-Ackon M, Rubinstien M, Perel A, et al. Continuous flow 50:50 nitrous oxide:oxygen is effective for relief of procedural pain in the pediatric emergency department. Acute Pain. 2003;5(1):25–30.
349. Evans JK, Buckley SL, Alexander AH, Gilpin AT. Analgesia for the reduction of fractures in children: a comparison of nitrous oxide with intramuscular sedation. J Pediatr Orthop. 1995; 15(1):73–7.
350. Gregory PR, Sullivan JA. Nitrous oxide compared with intravenous regional anesthesia in pediatric forearm fracture manipulation. J Pediatr Orthop. 1996;16(2):187–91.
351. Wattenmaker I, Kasser JR, McGravey A. Self- administered nitrous oxide for fracture reduction in children in an emergency room setting. J Orthop Trauma. 1990;4(1):35–8.
352. Babl FE, Belousoff J, Deasy C, Hopper S, Theophilos T. Paediatric procedural sedation based on nitrous oxide and ketamine: sedation registry data from Australia. Emerg Med J. 2010;27:607–12.
353. Babl FE, Oakley E, Sharwood LN. The utility of nitrous oxide. Emerg Med J. 2009;26(7):544–5.
354. Burnweit C, Diana-Zerpa JA, Nahmad MH, Lankau CA, Weinberger M, Malvezzi L, et al. Nitrous oxide analgesia for minor pediatric surgical procedures: an effective alternative to conscious sedation? J Pediatr Surg. 2004;39(3):495–9; discussion 495–9.

355. Ekbom K, Jakobsson J, Marcus C. Nitrous oxide inhalation is a safe and effective way to facilitate procedures in paediatric outpatient departments. Arch Dis Child. 2005;90(10):1073–6.
356. Henderson JM, Spence DG, Komocar LM, Bonn GE, Stenstrom RJ. Administration of nitrous oxide to pediatric patients provides analgesia for venous cannulation. Anesthesiology. 1990;72(2):269–71.
357. Kanagasundaram SA, Lane LJ, Cavalletto BP, Keneally JP, Cooper MG. Efficacy and safety of nitrous oxide in alleviating pain and anxiety during painful procedures. Arch Dis Child. 2001;84(6):492–5.
358. Dunn-Russell T, Adair SM, Sams DR, Russell CM, Barenie JT. Oxygen saturation and diffusion hypoxia in children following nitrous oxide sedation. Pediatr Dent. 1993;15(2):88–92.
359. Stewart RD, Gorayeb MJ, Pelton GH. Arterial blood gases before, during, and after nitrous oxide:oxygen administration. Ann Emerg Med. 1986;15(10):1177–80.
360. Cheney FW. An early example of evidence-based medicine: hypoxemia due to nitrous oxide. Anesthesiology. 2007;106(1):186–8.
361. Luhmann JD, Kennedy RM, Jaffe DM, McAllister JD. Continuous-flow delivery of nitrous oxide and oxygen: a safe and cost-effective technique for inhalation analgesia and sedation of pediatric patients. Pediatr Emerg Care. 1999;15(6):388–92.
362. Duncan GH, Moore P. Nitrous oxide and the dental patient: a review of adverse reactions. J Am Dent Assoc. 1984;108(2):213–9.
363. Herff H, Paal P, von Goedecke A, Lindner KH, Keller C, Wenzel V. Fatal errors in nitrous oxide delivery. Anaesthesia. 2007;62(12):1202–6.
364. National Institute for Occupational Safety and Health (NIOSH). Criteria for a recommended standard: occupational exposure to waste anesthetic gases and vapors. Publication Number 77–140; 1977. http://www.cdc.gov/niosh/docs/1970/77-140.html
365. Ruben H. Nitrous oxide analgesia in dentistry. its use during 15 years in Denmark. Br Dent J. 1972;132(5):195–6.
366. Onody P, Gil P, Hennequin M. Safety of inhalation of a 50% nitrous oxide/oxygen premix: a prospective survey of 35,828 administrations. Drug Saf. 2006;29(7):633–40.
367. Everett GB, Allen GD. Simultaneous evaluation of cardiorespiratory and analgesic effects of nitrous oxide-oxygen inhalation analgesia. J Am Dent Assoc. 1971;83(1):129–33.
368. Cleaton-Jones P. The laryngeal-closure reflex and nitrous oxide-oxygen analgesia. Anesthesiology. 1976;45(5):569–70.
369. Roberts GJ, Wignall BK. Efficacy of the laryngeal reflex during oxygen-nitrous oxide sedation (relative analgesia). Br J Anaesth. 1982;54(12):1277–81.
370. Rubin J, Brock-Utne JG, Greenberg M, Bortz J, Downing JW. Laryngeal incompetence during experimental "relative analgesia" using 50% nitrous oxide in oxygen. A preliminary report. Br J Anaesth. 1977;49(10):1005–8.
371. Jevtović-Todorović V, Todorović SM, Mennerick S, Powell S, Dikranian K, Benshoff N, et al. Nitrous oxide (laughing gas) is an NMDA antagonist, neuroprotectant and neurotoxin. Nat Med. 1998;4(4):460–3.
372. Gillman MA. Analgesic (sub anesthetic) nitrous oxide interacts with the endogenous opioid system: a review of the evidence. Life Sci. 1986;39(14):1209–21.
373. Dzoljic M, Van Duijn B. Nitrous oxide-induced enhancement of gamma-aminobutyric acidA-mediated chloride currents in acutely dissociated hippocampal neurons. Anesthesiology. 1998;88(2):473–80.
374. O'Connor RE, Sama A, Burton JH, Callaham ML, House HR, Jaquis WP, et al. Procedural sedation and analgesia in the emergency department: recommendations for physician credentialing, privileging, and practice. Ann Emerg Med. 2011;58(4):365–70.

Sedation of Pediatric Patients for Dental Procedures: The United States, European, and South American Experience

20

Stephen Wilson, Marie Therese Hosey, and Luciane Rezende Costa

Abstract

The challenges of sedating a child for dental procedures are multifactorial: The patient's age, health, temperament and emotional status, parental concerns, clinician philosophy on patient management, extent and quality of clinician training and experiences with sedation, state dental board regulation of sedation, issues of third-party coverage or parental reimbursement, knowledge of and adherence by clinicians to sedation guidelines, facility preparedness, and support staff experiences are but a few of many important considerations. To overcome these challenges, a pediatric dentist has to be at the hub of the preventive, operative and behavioral treatment plan.

The first section of this chapter is devoted to sedation practices performed primarily in the United States. The second section of this chapter describes sedation practices associated with the United Kingdom and Europe. The closing section will provide an overview of the state of sedation for pediatric dental procedures in South America, as an example of different solutions to sedation management in underdeveloped/developing countries.

Keywords

Pediatric dentistry • Sedation • United States • United Kingdom • Europe • South America • Nitrous oxide • Local anesthesia • Chloral hydrate • Meperidine • Midazolam • American Dental Association (ADA) • American Academy of Pediatric Dentistry (AAPD) • Basic life support (BLS) • Pediatric advanced life support (PALS) • Fentanyl • Etomidate • Frankl Scale • American Academy of Pediatrics • Commission of Dental Accreditation • Cochrane review • European Union • United Kingdom • International Association of Pediatric Dentistry (IAPD) • European Academy of Pediatric Dentistry (EAPD) • General Dental Council • British Society of Pediatric Dentistry (BSPD) • National Institute for Clinical Excellence (NICE) • Minimal sedation • Moderate sedation • Deep sedation • Modified Child Dental Anxiety Scale (MCDAS) • Facial Image Scale • Propofol • Target-controlled infusion (TCI) • Children's Fear Survey Schedule-Dental Subscale (CFSS-DS)

S. Wilson, D.M.D., M.A., Ph.D. (✉)
Division of Pediatric Dentistry, Cincinnati Children's Hospital Medical Center, Cincinnati, OH, USA
e-mail: stephen.wilson1@cchmc.or

M.T. Hosey, D.D.S., M.Sc. B.D.S., F.D.S., R.C.P.S.
Department of Paediatric Dentistry, King's College Hospital, London, UK

L.R. Costa, D.D.S., M.S., Ph.D.
Division of Pediatric Dentistry, Federal University of Goiás, Goiania, Goias, Brazil

Introduction

The challenges of sedating a child for dental procedures are multifactorial [1]: The patient's age, health, temperament and emotional status, parental concerns, clinician philosophy on patient management, extent and quality of clinician training and experiences with sedation, state dental board regulation of sedation, issues of third-party coverage or parental reimbursement,

K.P. Mason (ed.), *Pediatric Sedation Outside of the Operating Room: A Multispecialty International Collaboration*, DOI 10.1007/978-1-4939-1390-9_20, © Springer Science+Business Media New York 2015

knowledge of and adherence by clinicians to sedation guidelines, facility preparedness, and support staff experiences are but a few of many important considerations. To overcome these challenges, a pediatric dentist has to be at the hub of the preventive, operative and behavioral treatment plan.

The extent of the dental disease, the absolute need for complete patient cooperation, good manual dexterity on behalf of the dentist, and the choice of dental materials that will best perform in the circumstances (e.g., salivary contamination versus tooth longevity) are paramount. Probably the most disconcerting issue is that dental disease, more specifically dental caries or cavities, is the single most common chronic disease of childhood and it is preventable [2].

The first section of this chapter is devoted to sedation practices performed primarily in the United States. Other countries perform sedation for dentistry on children and vary in respect to settings, sedative routes, personnel, guidelines and regulations from those performing similar procedures in the United States. The second section of this chapter, authored by Professor Hosey, describes sedation practices associated with the United Kingdom and Europe. The closing section, authored by Luciane Costa, will provide an overview of the state of sedation for pediatric dental procedures in South America, as an example of different solutions to sedation management in underdeveloped/developing countries.

Extent and Treatment of Dental Caries

Dental caries is the result of a process involving a bacterial infection wherein the metabolic, acidic by-products of certain bacteria over time slowly dissolve the mineralized portion of the enamel and dentin. The bacterial infection is usually transmitted by the mother, father, or others to the infant and bacteria may begin colonization as primary teeth begin erupting [3, 4]. Possible consequences of the destruction of enamel and dentin are pain and swelling due to pulpal involvement. A dental lesion or cavity may be isolated to a small portion of one tooth or affect all erupted teeth in an individual (see Fig. 20.1). Dental caries affecting the primary dentition may often continue with the same degree and severity when the permanent dentition erupts.

Definitive treatment of dental caries depends on the extent of destruction of the crown of a tooth. Small lesions can often be treated with tooth-colored composite materials. Dental treatment can require restorations or crowns as the carious lesions increase in size. Sometimes the extent of caries is sufficient to involve the pulp chamber that houses the nerve and blood supply to the tooth resulting in the need for pulpotomies, root canal therapy, or extraction.

When tooth decay involves the dentine, treatment usually requires local anesthetics for pain control associated with the operative tooth preparation (i.e., instrumentation) or tooth conditioning (e.g., etching and bonding). Administration of

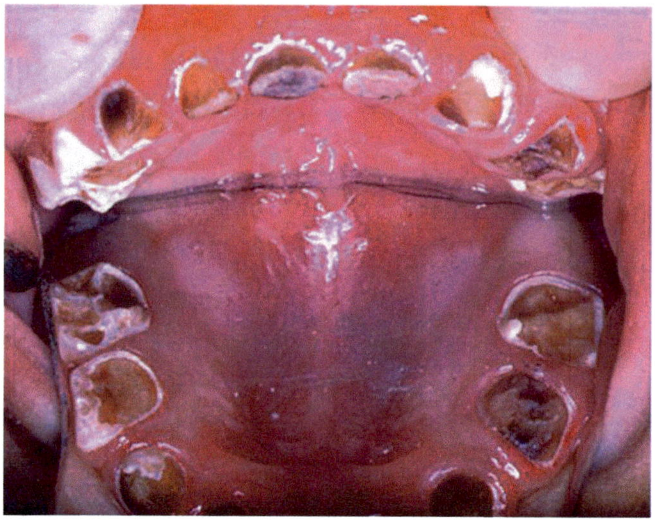

Fig. 20.1 Extensive dental caries

local anesthetics involves needles and syringes, which in and of themselves may cause patient anxiety and discomfort. This "intrusion" of the patient's personal space by a dentist during this procedure has been suggested as possibly the most difficult part of the patient–doctor relationship involving children [5].

Nerve blocks and infiltration with local anesthetics may not always result in profound anesthesia especially when the extent of caries has impacted the nerve chamber of the tooth or anesthesia administration (i.e., technique and/or amount) is inadequate. Simple classical conditioning that involves the pairing of dental instrumentation and pain including transmitted sounds and other sensations often result in patient discomfort, anxiety, and fear [6].

Children can learn to be dental phobics. They are susceptible at almost any age to such conditioning and may have limited psychological, emotional, and social resources to cope with its effects. Avoiding procedural pain in almost any situation or setting can have a strong element of positive reinforcement of the avoidance process. Pharmacological management of the patient's behaviors during dental treatment may then become necessary.

The number of children who require sedation for dental treatment is unknown. One can estimate, based on information in a report [7], that pediatric dentists who use sedative agents other than nitrous oxide alone may sedate at least 300,000 children per year. This rate apparently has been slowly increasing over a 15-year period. In reality this is probably a significant underestimate of children who are sedated as the report involved a sample survey of pediatric dentists focusing primarily on orally administered sedation; and there are significantly fewer pediatric dentists in the country compared to the number of general practitioners who may also be administering sedatives to children. Furthermore, another survey report involving approximately the same magnitude of respondents as the previous study [7] indicated that the majority of pediatric dentists use nitrous oxide inhalation sedation on a routine basis [8].

Guidelines, Training, and Protocols

In 2007, the American Dental Association (ADA) published Guidelines for Teaching Pain Control and Sedation to Dentists and Dental Students along with a separate set of Guidelines for the Use of Sedation and General Anesthesia by Dentists [9, 10]. The ADA guidelines for Teaching Pain Control and Sedation to Dentists and Dental Students encourage psychological and pharmacological modalities [9]. Local anesthesia is stressed as the foundation of dental analgesia. The administration of local anesthesia, mild and moderate sedation are considered as skills that should be acquired in predoctoral or continuing education programs.

The curriculum for minimal sedation, a 16 h minimum course, should include nitrous oxide and enteral techniques. Intravenous (IV) and intramuscular techniques, in addition to the enteral and inhalation component, are taught with the moderate sedation curriculum. The Moderate Enteral Sedation Course is a minimum of 24 h didactics with ten adult cases (includes a mandatory three live adult cases). This course is not intended for the sedation of anyone under the age of 12. The Moderate Parenteral Sedation Course is a minimum of 60 h didactics and requires the management of a minimum of 20 patients via parenteral route of administration. This also is not directed for the sedation of patients <12 years of age. The sedation of <12 years of age requires additional supervised clinical experience and should follow the American Academy of Pediatrics (AAP)/American Academy of Pediatric Dentists (AAPD) Guidelines for Monitoring and Management of Pediatric Patients During and After Sedation for Diagnostic and Therapeutic Procedures [10, 11]. The administration of deep sedation and/or General Anesthesia (GA) requires separate, directed education as approved by the ADA Commission on Dental Accreditation (CODA) as well as current Basic Life Support (BLS) and Advanced Cardiac Life Support (ACLS). The accompanying clinical staff(s) of the dentist(s) who provide deep sedation and/or GA all require current BLS certification [10]. The dentist providing the deep sedation or GA is permitted to perform the dental procedures as long as there are two BLS trained individuals present—one of which is designated to monitor the patient. All deep sedation or general anesthetics require a minimum of three individuals, including the dentist providing the sedation/anesthetic [10]. All deep sedation/GA requires IV access prior to initiating the sedation with the exception of brief procedures or the poorly cooperative child. In the latter case, the IV may be initiated after deep sedation/GA is initiated [10].

Many state dental boards issue permits that are necessary before a dentist can perform sedation during dental procedures. The training requisite for permits varies according to individual state board rules and regulations and the permitting process often may involve a system that is dependent on practitioner training and route of administration of the sedative. For example, a practitioner may be issued a permit limiting his/her sedations to oral administration only. A practitioner who is issued a parenteral IV permit can use any route of administration but not progress to a depth of GA. Only an individual who has a GA permit can administer any agent via any route of administration. These sedation providers are usually dental anesthesiologists or oral and maxillofacial surgeons.

The breadth and status of teaching received by dental students about pediatric sedation is minimal [12, 13]. Furthermore, it is likely that such experiences vary widely and are probably dependent primarily on faculty training, support services, and resources at each dental institution. It is no longer possible, since the introduction of sedation permits, to sedate a patient without prior experience or training.

Specialty training in pediatric dentistry requires a minimum of 2 years and includes required didactic and clinical experiences in pharmacological management of children, according to the CODA. The extent of those experiences in clinical context, quality, and quantity has varied in the past from program to program; and standardization of experiences among the 70 plus advanced training programs was relatively unregulated and minimal. However, as a result of a report from a taskforce commissioned by the American Academy of Pediatric Dentistry (AAPD), CODA changed its accreditation standards specifically related to sedation training. Now the CODA standard for all advanced training programs in Pediatric Dentistry indicates that every resident in every program must participate in 50 sedation experiences. Furthermore, they must be the operator in 25 of the 50 cases. This new standard should impact all programs and bring more consistency and standardization to training of pediatric dentists. The overwhelming majority of programs primarily teach the use of the oral route of sedation. Rarely, IV sedation is taught and if so, a dental anesthesiologist or oral and maxillofacial surgeon provides that aspect of care.

In the private practice setting of pediatric dentistry, typically a single dentist or small group utilizes an office remote from a hospital or surgical center to provide oral health care including sedation procedures. Local resources of dental/medical anesthesiologists or other personnel trained in IV sedation are relatively rare, but growing in popularity in certain regions of the US. Otherwise, the practitioner is left with little option but to provide minimal or moderate depths of sedation via the oral route, consistent with his/her training.

Five years ago, directors of pediatric dentistry training programs indicated that as compared to a decade prior, there was an increase in the volume of sedations as well as more didactic hours devoted to sedation, and the management of sedation-related emergencies [14]. More recently, the directors of these programs have the impression that there is a greater emphasis on sedation, likely reflective of the current influence of state board regulations, professional societies, litigation, and in particular, guidelines. Similar tendencies have been addressed in the medical community [15].

Children's Behavior

In 1991, the AAPD first published a Guideline on Behavior Guidance for the Pediatric Dental Patients. These guidelines have been updated six times, as recently as 2011 [16]. These guidelines are important because they reflect the role of the entire Sedation Team, inclusive of the parents, in caring for the dental patient. The guidelines present and reinforce the role of the parents in assessing and predicting how their child will respond to the procedure, taking into account past experiences with medical procedures (see Table 20.1) [17]. Tools at patient assessment are reviewed and detailed (see Table 20.2) [16]. It also provides specific recommendations on different approaches to communicating with and interacting with a child and parents: Tell-show-do, voice control, non-verbal communication, positive reinforcement, distraction, and parental presence/absence. Techniques of Advanced Behavior Guidance are described, which include protective stabilization, sedation, and general anesthesia.

Dental anxiety and fear are thought to affect 8–20 % of children. Some have emphasized that patients with dental anxiety and fear do not necessarily display disruptive behaviors. Furthermore, some patients who do react negatively in the dental setting may not have significant fear and/or anxiety toward dental procedures [18]. Older children generally can successfully cope with the experience of sitting cooperatively for routine dental procedures (including injections) and those who cannot tend to be preschoolers and toddlers. However, there are notable subsets of older children who tend to have greater fear and anxiety over dental treatment [19]. Age, cognitive and emotional development, maturational aspects of coping with challenging situations, and other characteristics of the child are well recognized as important discriminators for the clinician in recommending certain management techniques to the parent.

Another characteristic that has shown promise in discriminating how children may react to novel clinical situations is temperament. The temperament of a child may influence the outcome of sedations and other techniques used by pediatric dentists in managing child patients [20–22]. Generally, the more approachable a child, the more likely the clinician can effectively interact and deliver care. Also, children who score differently on temperamental dimensions than their peers and have higher dental fears tend to have more negative emotionality, shyness, and higher degrees of impulsivity [19].

Several scales have been used to describe children's behaviors during dental sedation procedures [23]. The Frankl scale

Table 20.1 Parent assessment of child behavior [17]

How do you think your child has reacted to past medical procedures?
1. Very poor
2. Moderately poor
3. Moderately good
4. Very good
How would you rate your child's anxiety (fear, nervousness) at this moment?
1. Very high
2. Moderately high
3. Moderately low
4. Low
How do you think your child will react to this procedure?
1. Very poor
2. Moderately poor
3. Moderately good
4. Very good
In the past 2 years my child experienced actual physical pain in connection with medical procedures:
1. Quite often (three or more times)
2. Occasionally (one or two times)
3. Never
How do you feel about the previous sedation experience?
1. Very poor
2. Moderately poor
3. Moderately good
4. Very good

Table 20.2 Patient assessment tools (American Academy of Pediatric Dentistry, 1990)

Tool	Format	Application
Toddler temperament scale	Parent questionnaire	Behavior of 12- to 36-month-old child
Behavioral style questionnaire (BSQ)	Parent questionnaire	Temperament of child 3–7 years old
Eyberg Child Behavior Inventory (ECBI)	Parent questionnaire	Frequency and intensity of 36 common behavioral problems
Facial Image Scale (FIS)	Drawings of faces, child chooses	Anxiety indicator suitable for preliterate children
Children's Dental Fear Picture Test (CDFP)	Three picture subtests, child chooses	Dental fear assessment for children >5 years old
Child Fear Survey Schedule-Dental Subscale (CFSS-DS)	Parent questionnaire	Dental fear assessment
Parent–child Relationship Inventory (PCRI)	Parent questionnaire	Parent attitudes and behaviors that may result in behavior problems in their child
Corah's Dental Anxiety Scale (DAS)	Parent questionnaire	Dental anxiety of parent

Modified from [16]

Table 20.3 Frankl Behavioral Rating Scale (American Academy of Pediatric Dentistry, 1990) [16]

Rating	Behavior
1	Definitely negative: • Refusal of treatment • Forceful crying • Fearfulness • Or any other overt evidence of extreme negativism
2	Negative: • Reluctance to accept treatment • Uncooperative • Some evidence of negative attitude but not pronounced (sullen, withdrawn)
3	Positive: • Acceptance of treatment • Cautious behavior at times • Willingness to comply with the dentist, at times with reservation, but patient follows the dentist's directions cooperatively
4	Definitely positive: • Good rapport with the dentist • Interest in the dental procedures • Laughter and enjoyment

Table 20.4 Houpt Sedation Rating Scale

Sleep	Score
Fully awake, alert	1
Drowsy, disoriented	2
Asleep	3
Movement	
Violent movement interrupting treatment	1
Continuous movement making treatment difficult	2
Controllable movement that does not interfere with treatment	3
No movement	4
Crying	
Hysterical crying that demands attention	1
Continuous, persistent crying that makes treatment difficult	2
Intermittent, mild crying that does not interfere with treatment	3
No crying	4
Overall behavior	
Aborted	1
Poor—treatment interrupted, only partially completed	2
Fair—treatment interrupted, but eventually all completed	3
Good—difficult, but all treatment performed	4
Very good—some limited crying or movement	5
Excellent—no crying or movement	6

is one of the more popular and widely used scales for categorizing children who may require sedation (Table 20.3) [16].

Probably the most popular scale for rating sedated children during dental procedures is the Houpt-modified scale, which relies on a categorical feature for a portion of the procedure (e.g., local anesthesia) or all portions of the entire procedure (e.g., "Fair" sedation) (see Table 20.4) [24].

Sedation Appointment Protocols

Typically, a sedation appointment in a dental office or clinic involves multiple steps, all of which follow a protocol. The protocol encompasses all the steps: the informed consent process, preoperative instructions, presedation history and physical examination including airway assessment, weighing the child, administering the agent orally, waiting for a latency period wherein the effects of sedation become noticeable, placement of the child in the dental chair and the nitrous oxide (N_2O) hood over the patient's nose, attaching monitors, proceeding with dental treatment, recovery, postoperative instructions, and discharge when appropriate criteria are attained (Fig. 20.2).

Sedative protocols used by pediatric dentists can be generally characterized as follows. The children selected for sedation are usually healthy ((American Society of Anesthesiologists) ASA I). Children who have medical conditions whose risk is more moderate to severe (greater than ASA II) are very likely to be sedated only in hospital-based settings. Most children are preschoolers although significant numbers of older children may be anxious or fearful and require sedation. Sedatives are administered almost exclusively in pediatric and general dentistry offices via the oral route consistent with the predominant type of training currently occurring in programs [14], and the behavior and physiology are recorded while the child receives routine restorative care [22, 25–37]. Usually, the behavior and physiology are documented on a time-based record by a dental assistant who performs interruptible tasks while working with the dentist. A standardized sedation recording sheet has been developed by the AAPD, Committee on Sedation and Anesthesia that conforms to the protocol portion of the AAPAAPD sedation guidelines (see Fig. 20.3).

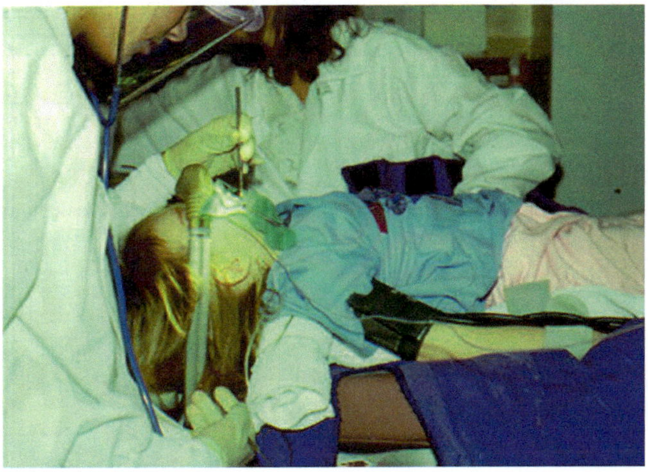

Fig. 20.2 Sedated dental patient with monitors

a

PATIENT SELECTION CRITERIA Date:________________

Patient: ________________________ ☐ M ☐ F Age:____yr____mo Weight:_______kg Physician: ________________

Indication for sedation:
- ☐ Fearful/anxious patient for whom basic behavior guidance techniques have not been successful
- ☐ Patient unable to cooperate due to lack of psychological or emotional maturity &/or mental, physical, or medical disability
- ☐ To protect patient's developing psyche
- ☐ To reduce patient's medical risk

Medical history / review of systems (ROS)	NONE	YES*	Describe positive findings:
Allergies &/or previous adverse drug reactions	☐	☐	________
Current medications (including OTC)	☐	☐	________
Relevant diseases, physical /neurologic impairment	☐	☐	________
Previous sedation/general anesthetics	☐	☐	________
Snoring, obstructive sleep apnea, mouthbreathing	☐	☐	________
Other significant findings (eg, family history)	☐	☐	________

Airway Assessment	NO	YES*
Obesity	☐	☐
Limited neck mobility	☐	☐
Micro/ retrognathia	☐	☐
Macroglossia	☐	☐
Tonsillar obstruction (___%)	☐	☐
Limited oral opening	☐	☐

ASA classification: ☐ I ☐ II ☐ III * ☐ IV* ☐ E *Medical consultation indicated? ☐ NO ☐ YES Date requested: ________

Comments: ________________________

Is this patient a candidate for in-office sedation? ☐ YES ☐ NO Doctor's signature: ________________ Date:________

PLAN	Name/relation to patient	Initials	Date	By
Informed consent obtained from	________	____	____	____
Pre-op instructions reviewed with	________	____	____	____
Post-op precautions reviewed with	________	____	____	____

ASSESSMENT ON DAY OF SEDATION Date ____________

Accompanied by: ________________ Relationship(s) to patient: __________

Medical Hx & ROS update	NO	YES	NPO status	Airway assessment	NO	YES	Check list
Change in medical hx /ROS	☐	☐	Clear liquids ____ hrs	Upper airway clear	☐	☐	☐ Appropriate transportation home
Change in medications	☐	☐	Foods ____ hrs	Lungs clear	☐	☐	☐ Monitors functioning
Recent respiratory illness	☐	☐	Medications ____ hrs	Tonsillar obstruction (____%)	☐	☐	☐ Emergency kit, suction, & O_2 available
Weight:_______kg							

Vital signs (If unable to obtain, check ☐ and document reason: ________________)

Blood pressure: _____/_____mmHg Resp: _____/min Pulse: _____/min Temp: _____°F SpO_2: ______%

Comments: ________________________

Presedation cooperation level: ☐ Unable/unwilling to cooperate ☐ Rarely follows requests ☐ Cooperates with prompting ☐ Cooperates freely

Behavioral interaction: ☐ Definitively shy and withdrawn ☐ Somewhat shy ☐ Approachable

Gurdian was provided an opportunity to ask questions, appeared to understand, and reaffirmed consent for sedation? ☐ YES ☐ NO

DRUG DOSAGE CALCULATIONS

Sedatives

Agent ________________ Route ______ ________mg/kg X _______kg = ________ mg ÷ ________mg/mL = ________mL

Agent ________________ Route ______ ________mg/kg X _______kg = ________ mg ÷ ________mg/mL = ________mL

Agent ________________ Route ______ ________mg/kg X _______kg = ________ mg ÷ ________mg/mL = ________mL

Reversal agent

For narcotic: NALOXONE IV, IM, or subQ Dose: 0.01 mg/kg X _____kg = _____mg (May repeat after 2-3 minutes)

For benzodiazepine: FLUMAZENIL IV Dose: 0.01 mg/kg X _____kg = _____mg (NOT to exceed 0.2 mg/min & total dose of 1mg)

Local anesthetics (maximum dosage based on weight)

Lidocaine 2% (36 mg/1.8mL cartridge) 4.4 mg/kg X _______kg = ________ mg (not to exceed 300 mg total dose)

Articaine 4% (72mg/1.8mL cartridge) 7 mg/kg X _______kg = ________ mg (not to exceed 500 mg total dose)

Mepivicaine 3% (54 mg/1.8 mL cartridge) 4. 4 mg/kg X _______kg = ________ mg (not to exceed 300 mg total dose)

Prilocaine 4% (72 mg/1.8mL cartridge) 6 mg/kg X _______kg = ________ mg (not to exceed 400 mg total dose)

Bupivicaine 0.5% (9mg/1.8mL cartridge) 1. 3 mg/kg X _______kg = ________ mg (not to exceed 500 mg total dose)

Fig. 20.3 (**a**, **b**) Sedation record consistent with American Academy of Pediatrics and American Academy of Pediatric Dentistry guidelines

b

INTRAOPERATIVE MANAGEMENT & POST-OPERATIVE MONITORING EMS telephone number: ______________ Monitors: ❑ Observation ❑ Pulse oximeter ❑ Precordial/pretracheal stethoscope ❑ Blood pressure cuff ❑ Capnograph ❑ EKG ❑ Thermometer

Protective stabilization/devices: ❑ Papoose ❑ Head positioner ❑ Manual hold ❑ Neck/shoulder roll ❑ Mouth prop ❑ Rubber dam ❑ ________

TIME	Baseline	:	:	:	:	:	:	:	:	:	:	:	:	:	:	:	:
Sedatives[1]																	
N_2O / O_2 (%)																	
Local[2] (mg)																	
O_2 sat																	
Pulse																	
BP																	
Resp																	
CO_2																	
Procedure[3]																	
Comments[4]																	
Sedation level*																	
Behavior*																	

1. Agent ____________ Route ________ Dose ______ Time ________ Administered by ____________
   Agent ____________ Route ________ Dose ______ Time ________ Administered by ____________
   Agent ____________ Route ________ Dose ______ Time ________ Administered by ____________
2. Local anesthetic agent ____________
3. Record dental procedure start and completion times, transfer to recovery area, etc.
4. Enter letter on chart and corresponding comments (eg, complications/side effects, airway intervention, reversal agent, analgesic) below
   A.____________ C. ____________
   B.____________ D. ____________

Sedation level*
- None (typical response/cooperation for this patient)
- Mild (anxiolysis)
- Moderate (purposeful response to verbal commands ± light tactile sensation)
- Deep (purposeful response after repeated verbal or painful stimulation)
- General Anesthesia (not arousable)

Behavior/responsiveness to treatment*
- Excellent: quiet and cooperative
- Good: mild objections &/or whimpering but treatment not interrupted
- Fair: crying with minimal disruption to treatment
- Poor: struggling that interfered with operative procedures
- Prohibitive: active resistance and crying; treatment cannot be rendered

Overall effectiveness: ❑ Ineffective ❑ Effective ❑ Very effective ❑ Overly sedated

Additional comments/treatment accomplished: ____________

DISCHARGE

Criteria for discharge
- ❑ Cardiovascular function is satisfactory and stable.
- ❑ Airway patency is satisfactory and stable.
- ❑ Patient is easily arousable.
- ❑ Responsiveness is at or very near presedation level (especially if very young or special needs child incapable of the usually expected responses).
- ❑ Protective reflexes are intact.
- ❑ Patient can talk (return to presedation level).
- ❑ Patient can sit up unaided (return to presedation level).
- ❑ State of hydration is adequate

Discharge vital signs
Pulse: _____/min
SpO_2: _____%
BP: ____/_____mmHg
Resp: _____/min
Temp: _____°F

Discharge process
❑ Post-operative instructions reviewed with ____________ by ____________
❑ Transportation ❑ Airway protection/observation ❑ Activity ❑ Diet ❑ Nausea/vomiting ❑ Fever ❑ Rx________
❑ Anesthetized tissues ❑ Dental treatment rendered ❑ Pain ❑ Bleeding ❑ ________ ❑ Emergency contact
❑ Next appointment on: ____________ for:________

I have received and understand these discharge instructions. The patient is discharged into my care at ________ ❑ AM ❑ PM

Signature: ____________ Relationship: ________ After hours phone number: ____________

Operator signature:____________ Chairside assistant: ____________ Monitoring personnel signature:____________

POST OP CALL Date: ________ Time: ________ By: ________ Spoke to: ________ Comments: ____________

Fig. 20.3 (continued)

Other incidental protocol events often include patient immobilization or stabilization (i.e., Papoose board®) [25, 37–47]. Pediatric dentistry views the use of restraint not as punishment but as an intervention to improve the outcome or success of the sedation and procedure [48]. Pulse oximeters, blood pressure cuffs, and pretracheal or precordial stethoscopes are standard. Occasionally, side stream capnography is used but electrocardiography is rarely followed.

The choice of monitors is somewhat dependent on the behaviors exhibited by sedated children, the depth of sedation, and sedation guidelines. Behaviors and physiological parameters are fluid during the sedation, affected by the child's reaction to the stimulation, the timing of the more intense procedural stimulation, and the dentist's talents in calming or distracting the patient (rarely a part of study designs). For instance, heart rate typically increases most significantly and predictably during the injection of local anesthetics compared to other times of the procedure [36]. Generally, pediatric dentists target minimal or moderate sedation. Older children who require adult molar extractions, especially those that are bony impacted, the uncovering of impacted teeth, and other orthognathic surgeries are usually seen by oral and maxillofacial surgeons. Typically, they use intravenous sedation and general anesthesia in performing the aforementioned procedures.

In most practices, a parent and child arrive at least 30 min prior to the sedation procedure for preoperative assessment, consent, and further review of the medical history. The time between oral administration of sedative(s) and initiation of treatment may vary from 10 min to an hour depending on the drug or drug combination used (e.g., midazolam versus chloral hydrate [CH], respectively). The length of time involved with dental treatment ranges from 20 min to 2 h, according to the patient's dental needs. Recovery is usually done in the dental chair or a quiet room of the dental office under direct parent and dental staff observation and monitoring. Discharge is consistent with the guidelines of the AAP and AAPD [49].

The oral route of administration remains the most popular route used by pediatric (and general) dentists in the US [7, 12–14, 50–53]. The most probable reason for this route of administration is historical and related to individual training and experience. The IV route of sedation is the most popular for oral surgeons, although their procedural need (e.g., frenectomies) to sedate preschoolers is probably much less than that of pediatric dentists. Some studies exist in which the IV route is used and managed by dental or medical anesthesiologists while the pediatric dentist performs restorative procedures in the office or outpatient care facility [54–58]. Essentially these usually involve general anesthesia administered by an individual with a GA permit or training. Various agents have been used including methohexital [58], propofol [56, 57, 59], and ketamine [59–61]. This type of care is generally limited across the US, but many pockets of the country use this protocol on a fairly frequent basis. This type of protocol seems more popular in countries outside of the US. The advantages and disadvantages of the oral route of administration compared to other routes are widely appreciated and understood even by parents.

The submucosal route is another fairly popular route of administration used by many pediatric dentists [22, 62–65]. This route of administration may limit the range and number of sedative agents that can be used (e.g., CH cannot be administered via this route), but affords a clinical onset time and sedative impact more closely resembling IV compared to the oral route in children. The clinical effects happen relatively rapidly because children usually have excellent blood supply in and around the maxillary vestibules. Caution is advised because inadvertent and rapid injection of sedatives directly into blood vessels or a venous plexus can result in a more profound effect than anticipated. The submucosal technique is relatively easy to perform, and similar to administering local anesthesia for dental procedures, hence its relative popularity among pediatric dentists.

Sedatives

Most of the pediatric dental studies reported in the literature focus on drugs or drug combinations involving CH, meperidine, and midazolam used in conjunction with other agents such as hydroxyzine [14, 21, 22, 24–34, 36, 37, 40, 42–44, 46, 63–114]. Occasional reports involve other benzodiazepines [41, 43, 108, 115–117] but their widespread use is not common. Rarely and usually in collaboration with a dental or medical anesthesiologist, other drugs such as ketamine are used and compared to other drugs or combinations [71, 73, 109, 118–125]. Other studies involve the IV or intramuscular routes usually done by or in collaboration with oral and maxillofacial surgeons or dental anesthesiologists for school-aged children [35, 42, 73, 89, 92, 126–135].

CH was once the most popular sedative agent in pediatric dentistry. It still remains very popular. Its dosage range when used in combination with hydroxyzine, a relatively popular regimen, is 30–50 mg/kg CH and 1–2 mg/kg of hydroxyzine. A truly effective regimen is CH, meperidine, and hydroxyzine. The dosage range in this combination varies from a "low" dose combination (15–30 mg/kg CH, 1–2 mg/kg each of meperidine and hydroxyzine) to a "high" dose combination wherein the CH is relatively high but the meperidine and hydroxyzine are low (50 mg/kg CH, 1 mg/kg meperidine, and 25 mg of hydroxyzine). There seems to be a slightly higher incidence of true desaturations and apnea episodes in the "high" compared to the "low" dose combination but further study is needed. Studies have shown this "triple combination" technique to be relatively effective and safe [26, 44, 79, 80, 84, 91]. Yet, some postoperative events may raise some concern, even if discharge criteria are met [30].

The concept behind this triple combination is that all three agents induce variable degrees of drowsiness in a dosage-dependent fashion. Meperidine also provides euphoria and analgesia, reducing the amount of local anesthetic needed. Hydroxyzine provides some protection against mucosal irritation and vomiting. The effective onset time is usually 45 min and provides procedural sedation for 60–90 min, sufficient time for significant restorative dentistry. Most patients meet discharge criteria within 30–60 min following the dental procedure [26, 44, 79, 80, 84, 91].

Table 20.5 Most commonly used sedative agents in pediatric dentistry[a]

Drug	Dose	Characteristics	Warnings	Sedation considerations (timing)	Reversibility
Chloral hydrate	20–50 mg/kg, max: 1 g	Oily Not-palatable Irritability Sleep/drowsiness	Airway blockage Mucosal irritant Laryngospasms Respiratory depressant Cardiac arrhythmias	Onset: 30–45 min Separation time: 45 min Work: 1–1.5 h[b]	No
Meperidine	1–2 mg/kg, max: 50 mg (pethidine)	Clear Non-palatable Analgesia Euphoria Dysphoria	Respiratory depression Hypotension	Onset: 30 min Separation time: 30 min Work: 1 h[b]	Yes (narcan)
Midazolam	0.3–1.0 mg/kg, max: 15 mg (young child) 20 mg (older child)	Clear Non-palatable Relaxation Anterograde amnesia	Angry child syndrome Paradoxical reduction Respiratory depression Loss of head righting reflex	Onset: 10 min Separation time: 10 min Work: 20 min[b]	Yes (flumazenil)

[a]This table reflects common dosing, warnings, and sedation considerations but must be interpreted and applied with caution. The table reflects the views of the author

[b]Work: the procedure duration usually tolerated following sedative effect

Midazolam in recent years has surpassed CH in popularity as the most often used sedative agent among pediatric dentists. It is most often administered orally, but the intranasal (IN) route is also used frequently [39, 75, 96, 97, 136–139]. One of the shortcomings of orally administered midazolam is its short working time that is limited to approximately 20 min of restorative care. Its advantage is that its onset of action when given by this route is 10 min or less. It is the sedative drug of choice for short restorative or extraction cases for children who require sedation. Midazolam frequently is combined with other sedatives and analgesics [31, 46, 67, 128, 140]. One of the primary purposes of combining these agents is to increase the restorative working time, take advantage of the properties of individual drugs (e.g., meperidine's analgesic property when used with midazolam, which has no analgesic properties) and utilizing additive or potentiation effects of multiple agents, each of which may be used in lower doses. The dose of orally administered midazolam when used alone varies from 0.3 to 1.0 mg/kg. When combined with other agents, the dose usually decreases to 0.3–0.5 mg/kg. Likewise, in combination therapy the dose of meperidine is reduced from 2 to 1 mg/kg. The oral dosages of drugs, patient findings and characteristics, and concerns of these sedative agents are shown in Table 20.5. Drugs such as etomidate are not frequently utilized in the private practice community.

A recent paper reviewed the efficacy and adverse event profile of midazolam with and without narcotics, both administered via different routes [141]. All patients received local anesthesia of lidocaine with epinephrine infiltrated into the gingiva. This was an important study because it evaluated the efficacy and safety of midazolam via the oral (PO) and the intranasal (IN) route and then examined the outcome when combined with oral transmucosal fentanyl citrate (OTFC) or IN sufentanil. There were four groups: PO midazolam (1 mg/kg), IN midazolam (0.7 mg/kg), IN midazolam (0.5 mg/kg)+OTFC (10–15 μ[mu]g/kg), IN midazolam (0.3 mg/kg)+IN sufentanil (1 μg/kg). IN midazolam had shortest time to onset (17 min) and similar efficacy to all the other groups. All groups were similarly efficacious (27 % of sedations were graded as ineffective). The OTFC was the poorest performer with a 37 min time to onset and 39 min recovery (other groups 26.5–30 min). This study suggests that IN midazolam may be an efficacious method of delivery, eliminating need for parenteral administration and supplemental narcotics [141]. Still, controversy over the best route remains, as some have shown better results with the intranasal route [142] while others favor the oral [143] or intramuscular route [42].

Nitrous oxide (N_2O) is the most frequently used anxiolytic and analgesic agent used in pediatric dentistry. Typically, a nasal hood delivers nitrous oxide in an open system, thus entraining a significant amount of room air (see Fig. 20.2). In fact, adults and some children can decrease the proportion of nitrous oxide entering the lungs by breathing through their mouth (e.g., purposeful behavior or crying). The amount of N_2O entering into the lungs of patients is 30–50 % less than the amount leaving the regulator portion of the dental N_2O delivery system. Thus, if the dentist sets the N_2O flow to 50 % at the regulator, only 25–35 % of N_2O actually enters into the patient's lung [144].

Nitrous oxide at concentrations of 30–50 % can be an excellent anxiolytic as well as a mild analgesic, via a mechanism that appears related to endogenous opioid systems [145]. For these reasons, N_2O is very frequently and effectively used with oral sedatives, primarily as the "titrating" agent for managing behavior. Another advantage to the nitrous oxide delivery system is that it provides supplemental oxygen. Nonetheless, caution must be used to consider that N_2O has been shown to inhibit the swallowing reflex [146]. There are limited studies that investigate an association between vomiting and N_2O during operative treatment in children and most suggest that vomiting is infrequent [147–149].

Morbidity and Mortality: Dental Sedation

The true number of adverse events that occur during sedation of children for dental treatment is unknown. Most "adverse" events that are reported in the literature do not involve cardiopulmonary stabilization nor unplanned admission to a hospital [25, 28, 74, 85, 87, 88, 100]. The adverse events usually include desaturations or apnea, usually associated with patient crying and behavioral posturing, vomiting, or paradoxical excitement. More significant adverse events such as laryngospasm, seizures, or coma are less common but have been reported [150, 151].

In 2000, the incidence of significant sedation-related adverse events in pediatric patients was reviewed and published [152]. One hundred-and-eighteen case reports were reviewed. Sixty resulted in death or permanent neurological injury. Twenty-nine of these critical events occurred in children sedated for dental procedures. The occurrence of death and permanent neurological injury was more likely with the administration of three or more sedatives. Nitrous oxide in combination with other sedatives was also associated with the negative outcome [93]. It is important to realize, however, that at the time this study was published, pulse oximetry was not being used routinely and capnography was not a Standard of Care for sedation. Today, these statistics and outcomes would most likely be different.

Recent studies specifically address morbidities and mortalities associated with dental treatment of children [153, 154]. One study was based on closed claims cases involving two dental insurance companies and another involved media reports identified in the LexisNexis® Academia search engine and a private foundation formed after the death of a young child (i.e., Raven Maria Blanco Foundation). A selection bias may have weakened the strength and objectivity of the reports [154]. The studies may have some overlap with the reports previously published in 2000 [93]. These studies indicated that the majority of children who received dental treatment were less than 6 years of age and cared for by general dentists. No single sedative was consistently implicated, and some cases involved excessive/overdose amounts of local anesthetics. This data raises many issues such as whether there was appropriate clinical judgment, knowledge of or compliance with applicable clinical guidelines, and training and skills in rescue skills. Since the number of sedations actually performed annually is unknown but estimated in the hundreds of thousands, it is likely these cases represent outliers in the provision of quality sedation for oral health care.

Reimbursement for Dental Sedation and Anesthesia

Financial considerations of sedation for dental care are noteworthy. Most insurance plans do not cover the cost of sedation (including nitrous oxide) or anesthesia for dental procedures. Therefore, the parent is left with the financial decision of whether to pay "out of pocket" for sedation during restorative care or exodontia. However, 32 of the states have mandatory general anesthesia (GA) legislation that will cover some costs associated with the medical fees incurred during a GA for pediatric dental care (see Fig. 20.4).

The fees for sedation procedures vary considerably among dentists but may range from $100 to several hundred dollars per sedation appointment. Some states have implemented legislation requiring some third-party payors to reimburse fees associated with GA for dental restorative care. Nonetheless, often stipulations such as the patient's age or mental or emotional status may preclude some patients from receiving care.

Alternatives to Sedation

The alternatives to pharmacological interventions (i.e., sedation and GA) in managing fearful or uncooperative children during dental restorative or exodontia appointments may include, among others, psychological distraction techniques,

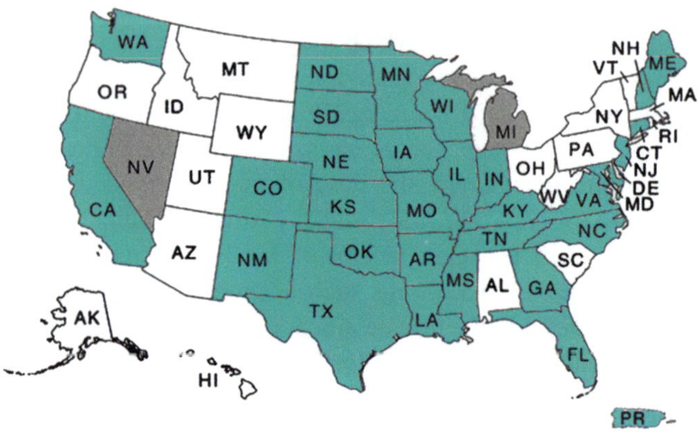

Fig. 20.4 States with general anesthesia coverage (*blue*) and those with negotiated regulatory coverage (*gray*)

hypnosis, protective stabilization (i.e., restraints such as Papoose Boards®) or no treatment. No study has assessed the cumulative outcome of these non-pharmacological techniques and often the degree of success is subject to interpretation [48]. Anecdotally, there are many concurrent factors that have an unknown impact and interaction: the family's cultural background, child rearing techniques, the child's coping abilities in defending against potential physical and emotional trauma, and the quality of the work provided. Some dentists and parents perceive that if the needed treatment was completed, it was a successful outcome, regardless of the non-pharmacological techniques applied and the child's response. This perception may be biased by the financial burden that would be incurred should pharmacological therapy be administered. Others refuse or reject these alternative means of treatment and elect not to seek care. This failure to seek treatment can have significant and event fatal consequences. Untreated dental disease does not regress and may progress to a localized abscessed condition or cellulitis. Cellulitis may be life threatening if it spreads to other organs (e.g., brain) and death may result.

Sedation Guidelines in the United States

Sedation guidelines for children have been followed by most pediatric dentists since they first were published in the United States in 1985 [155–157]. The first guidelines of the AAP were created as a response to deaths in dental patients who received meperidine [157–159]. The most recent joint guidelines of the AAP and AAPD emphasize, among other concepts, patient safety and rescue as well as practitioner education and training [49]. The impact of these latest guidelines (in terms of access to care, the number and types of sedations performed by pediatric dentists) remains to be seen. State dental boards regulate sedation performed by dentists. Most states require a licensed dentist also to have a special sedation permit. There are different classifications of sedation permits, such as permits for enteral versus parenteral routes of administration. Documentation of training, performance of sedation in the presence of a board consultant, and on-site inspection of offices are usually required for all permits.

Future of Sedation for Dental Procedures in the United States

In the future, sedation of children for dental procedures will continue to be influenced by societal demands, regulatory agencies, guidelines, financial implications, alternative options, and practitioner training. It has been proposed that pediatric patients will be assessed and then classified into one of three groups, depending on their ability to cope with dental procedures. The first group represents those who easily accept and adapt to dental procedures and thus would not require any pharmacological intervention. Those in the second group may be slightly anxious and benefit from mild sedation or pharmacological adjuncts (e.g., nitrous oxide or a benzodiazepine). The last group would constitute those who exhibit highly anxious or fearful behaviors and cannot cope with the routine dental environment. This group would benefit from deep sedation or general anesthesia. The first two groups could easily be managed by most pediatric dentists, even in an office-based setting. The latter group poses a challenge for many reasons, largely based on the limited resources (e.g., financial) in all geographic regions of the country.

Deep sedation and general anesthesia for dental procedures may best be offered by a team involving a dentist and another professional with advanced training in these techniques (e.g., dental anesthesiologist), along with other support personnel. Depending on the state dental board regulations, which vary from state to state, the location for the provision of services by such a team may be in-office, at a surgical center, or hospital. One of the advantages of in-office sedation is the elimination of expensive hospital fees associated with the operating room and recovery [160]. Other proposed advantages to an office-based setting are improved efficiency, efficacy, and safety [54, 161]. How this approach to sedation delivery progresses in the future remains to be seen.

The progression and evolution of safety in pediatric dental sedation must involve a change in the entire training process. Oral routes of sedation for mild and moderate levels are no longer considered as efficacious as other routes. New sedatives, different delivery routes and evolving techniques can only, however, be applied with careful training (didactic and clinical). Changes in training, with pediatric-focused specialty training programs are the most critical first step. Conceptually, more intense, prolonged periods of training with partial or full standardization of experiences across all training programs would be desirable. The extent and context of training would exceed that which currently occurs and must include well-defined and measurable competence. To this end, in 2013 the Commission of Dental Accreditation, the accrediting body of all dental school institutions and training programs in the US, increased the accreditation requirements: Each graduate student or resident in any advanced training programs in pediatric dentistry must complete 20 cases as the primary operator in which nitrous oxide is administered. Additionally, each graduate student or resident must have experiences in a minimum of 50 sedation cases with 25 as the primary operator and the remainder in a supportive role in various possible settings (e.g., dental trauma case involving IV sedation in the Emergency Department).

There are significant logistical and political hurdles to achieving the goal of seamless comprehensive training in sedation in educational institutions. Intense scrutiny, innovative approaches, funding considerations, and administrative support are needed to achieve success. A simple example would be a method to train or retrain a cadre of faculty that can be disseminated to training programs in order to institute mechanisms for standardizing sedation protocols. Who will do the training? Are special "centers" required initially? How many and where? How long will it take? What are the funding mechanisms?

Focused communication, collaboration, exchange of innovative ideas, remodeling of current training programs or creation of novel training centers are desirable and necessary to initiate a comprehensive and humane plan for oral health care of children. Many regulatory issues will remain as obstacles to be addressed. The first steps in staging such an initiative require the broad-based recognition and acceptance of change in sedation training and philosophy. This step must subsequently be followed by the identification of dedicated individuals from different disciplines who collaboratively desire to improve the treatment options for pediatric dental care in the future.

Sedation for Pediatric Dental Patients in the United Kingdom and Europe

Nitrous oxide inhalation sedation is the commonest method for pharmacological management of the child for dental treatment in the United Kingdom (UK). The technique and training and the suitability for usage in general dental practice was affirmed by a Directive of the European Council of Dentists in May 2012 [162].

The European Union (EU) is a culturally diverse group of countries and cultures, each with discrete laws, recommendations, and frameworks for delivery of dental services. Despite this, each member state is subject to EU law. One such law relates to specialty training: it has to be 3 years. Whilst each member state does not necessarily recognize pediatric dentistry as a specialty per se, they are surprisingly unanimous in their agreement on pediatric dental sedation and recognition of guidelines. Key in this has been the role of the International Association of Paediatric Dentistry (IAPD), and the European Academy of Paediatric Dentistry (EAPD). In a nutshell, sedation for pediatric dentistry is "conscious." This means the child remains in verbal contact with the clinician throughout the procedure. Popularity of method and sedative varies. In Greece, oral sedatives, especially chloral hydrate have been popular; in Scandinavia rectal benzodiazepines are used; and inhalation sedation was first used in the UK in 1889 for dental cavity preparation in the Liverpool Dental School. Many countries have environmental concerns about nitrous oxide pollution; in fact, in Scandinavia amalgam filling materials are no longer used for this same reason. This is why the Directive confirming the safety and efficacy of the titrated nitrous oxide inhalation sedation technique from the Directive from the European Council of Dentists was so important. All countries have tackled the issue of the dental operator-sedationist in different ways but are generally agreed that nitrous oxide inhalation sedation, titrated to effect using dedicated dental machines, is well within a dentist's remit and is suitable for use in high street general practice settings.

The British Commonwealth countries largely follow the UK practice and ethos relating to pediatric dental sedation; and now Middle Eastern countries are recognizing the value of titrated nitrous oxide inhalation sedation.

The Evidence for Conscious Sedation in Pediatric Dentistry: Cochrane

In the UK in particular, evidence-based practice is important. The importance of literature critique and meta-analysis has come to the fore nowadays in all aspects of medical and dental practice. This strength of evidence is critiqued and evaluated and informs guidelines. To summarize the Cochrane review relating to pediatric dental sedation: the method of randomization in studies was unclear; there were inappropriate statistical tests; cross-over type studies did not consider the carry-over effect; only 32 % of studies reported baseline anxiety—even fewer reported anxiety at the end and there was little information regarding the actual treatment; repeatability was not mentioned, especially when there was multiple operators or assessors; interpretation of outcome data relating to behavior was difficult; over 50 % of studies used scales that recorded behavior in different ways and many relied on bodily movement even when sometimes the subjects were papoosed. Finally, for many studies, all participants—even the controls—complete treatment! [163]. It isn't easy to carry out pediatric dental sedation research, and one could argue that placebo-controlled randomized trials are unethical. Therefore, the value of the review is to serve as a reminder that caution should be applied in the interpretation of sedation studies.

A series of useful papers was published after the review that merits a mention here. These studies compared midazolam given intravenously (IV), orally and transmucosally (buccal) against nitrous oxide inhalation sedation. They are flawed in that the IV paper mainly focuses on children undergoing orthodontic premolar extraction, so the participants were older and this was not necessarily an "anxious" sample; also, overall the carry-over effect was ignored. The researcher is a community dentist in a community dental clinic and was a keen supporter of midazolam. The results can be summarized as follows: all midazolam routes appeared to have minimal effect on the patients' vital signs; the IV route produced the fastest onset of sedation and therefore may be the most efficient; there were more withdrawals from the buccal route owing to the difficulty with the taste. However, these studies are of interest because they confirmed the efficacy of nitrous oxide IS—this provided the fastest onset of sedation and the fastest recovery—compared to midazolam [35, 164, 165].

UK Pediatric Dentistry

Background

All dentists must be registered with the General Dental Council (GDC). It is the GDC that investigates and disciplines malpractice. Only dentists can legally perform dental procedures. Children's dentistry is free of charge in the UK. The families pay nothing; irrespective of the level, complexity, or extent of dental and sedation/anesthesia service provided. There are only a handful of private practices (not part of the public health care system—practices that operate for profit) and the majority of care is delivered by general dental practitioners. The general dentists refer anxious children or complex cases into the community or hospital pediatric specialty services. The community dental services are at non-hospital sites and usually provide nitrous oxide inhalation sedation but refer into hospital units for oral and intravenous sedation and for general anesthesia. Therefore, whilst UK pediatric dentists have to sometimes "make a case" for their services, they are unfettered and unburdened by private insurance or a family's inability to pay. Treatment is based on evidence, clinical judgment, and hospital service delivery capability. The Department of Health sets targets for waiting times and activity and penalizes poor performance.

Over 40 % of 5-year-olds have tooth decay into dentin [166, 167]. Caries management is similar to the USA but has had a greater emphasis on stabilization of the caries lesion rather than complete removal. In other words: a "biological" rather than a "surgical" approach [168, 169]. The advantage of this approach is that it is non-invasive; and so, local anesthetic injection, or even the use of a drill is not required. So, it is less traumatizing for the child. In this way, sedation and general anesthesia can be avoided altogether in some cases. Therefore, general anesthesia is seen as a treatment of last resort. There are approximately 240 pediatric dental specialists registered with the GDC; the majority are 5-year-trained, hospital-based "consultants" (pediatric dentists who have trained for 5 years) at the Children's Hospital and Dental School. The designation of being on an "acute site" is important; it indicates that there are pediatric emergency care services available on the premises, i.e., pediatric medical intensive care. General anesthetic services are located on acute care sites; those few that are not have an emergency transfer protocol. Therefore, the settings in which oral and intravenous sedation are delivered to children generally follow the same pattern. As such, if a sedation emergency occurs, medical support and "crash team" services and pediatric life support are very close at hand.

UK: Local Anesthesia

The UK standard of measurement is metric, e.g., Kilograms (kg) and milliliters (mL) not imperial. This is common throughout the EU. The most common local anesthetic agent is usually 2 % lignocaine (xylocaine) with 1:80,000 adrenaline and is usually delivered in 2.2 mL cartridges. Maximum dosage can be calculated easily by a rough rule of thumb as "a tenth of a cartridge per kg body weight." Infiltration injections usually suffice, though once the first permanent molars are in occlusion a dental block is generally used in the mandible—especially for extractions and permanent tooth restoration. In some instances (e.g., patients with clotting disorders) intraligamentary techniques are used in preference to a block and the use of Articaine may be of special benefit in this regard. The anesthetic injection is coupled to behavioral management skill and technique, and topical anesthetics such as benzocaine are also utilized. New delivery systems such as the "Wand" are also gaining in popularity; though excellent behavioral management techniques and experience are still key to success. Readers are referred to the many pediatric dentistry textbooks for further advice and information.

United Kingdom Pediatric Dental Sedation Training

The GDC is the authority that registers all dentists, dental nurses, therapists, and technicians in the UK; it requires that all dentists undertake continued professional development. BLS, safe-guarding, and handling of medical emergencies are mandatory annual requirements.

The GDC does not set specific standards; instead, it takes the view that any dentist has to be able to prove themselves "competent" to provide the treatment that they offer. This test of competency is based on national training standards, knowledge, training, audit, and continued experience, and is subject to employee appraisal and peer review.

Therefore, whatever the type of conscious sedation training that is undertaken, proof of continued development and practice is essential. Specialties such as pediatric dentistry are recognized but the role of a sedationist is not. Instead, sedation is seen as part of the armamentarium that a dentist might provide for their patients; in the same way that they provide local anesthesia and other techniques such as hypnosis. Therefore, there is no nationally agreed upon training standard.

UK pediatric dentistry consultants train for 5 years and the scope of practice is broader than the US, and many parts of the EU, and includes inpatient and outpatient hospital care and minor oral surgery. The training is excusive to government-regulated and salaried trainees, and competition for these posts is fierce. Self-funding is almost impossible. Training is provided largely in hospital units and the examinations—set at year 3 for specialist and year 5 for consultant—are via the Royal Colleges of Surgeons. UK pediatric dentists perform their own surgery, e.g., on impacted teeth and exposure and bonding of orthodontic brackets for misplaced unerupted teeth, as well as permanent tooth extractions. They also perform any endodontic and aesthetic restorative procedures so long as these are in children aged below 16–18 years. Therefore, the training focus is not high street practice orientated but directed instead toward hospital practice and multi-disciplinary team working, e.g., cleft cases or hypodontia. Therefore, many units offer intravenous sedation to adolescents and do not need to refer to oral surgery. UK pediatric dentists work alongside oral and maxillofacial surgeons but only refer to them in difficult cases, e.g., an impacted canine in the floor of the nose or a large cyst or tumor. The complexity of these case means that general anesthesia is the management of choice.

The titrated nitrous oxide inhalation sedation technique is part of the UK dental undergraduate curriculum and this is further augmented, documented, and examined within pediatric dentistry specialist training. Intravenous sedation training is also within specialist's training but is usually augmented by further courses should the dentist require these to reach or to maintain "competency." The basic exposure to intravenous techniques has been recommended as: five assessments, five observations, and five sedations, but this is then followed by a period of mentoring before fully independent practice [170, 171].

Pediatric Dental Sedation and General Anesthesia in the United Kingdom

Today, general anesthesia for dentistry is the most common reason for day surgery and inpatient admissions; approximately 60,000–100,000 a year. It is a last resort treatment, usually confined to high caries risk children. Typically, 5- to 6-year-olds, needing extractions in three quadrants or more, an average of seven teeth are removed. This is also the method of choice for 8- to 10-year-olds who require removal of all four first permanent molars. These are quick general anesthetic procedures, usually lasting only 15 min or so. No endotracheal intubation is performed; inhalation/volatile anesthetic induction via a mask is common and a nasal or laryngeal mask is used; pediatric anesthetists work hand in hand with the dental surgeon to maintain "the shared airway" [172]. The author requests an endotracheal tube for removal of first permanent molars since these can be more difficult, especially when access is limited. She normally operates on 10 children during an "afternoon" session: 1:30 to 5:30 PM in theatre; then the last children remain until approximately 6:30 PM in the day surgery ward before discharge. A child requiring removal of all four first permanent molars will take up a "double slot" to enable time for endotracheal intubation.

Link Between "Conscious Sedation" and General Anesthesia

In the past, general anesthesia was commonly and widely practiced in general dental practices (in high streets) but this ceased in the 1990s following safety concerns. Department of Health recommendations and national guidelines led to general aesthetic services moving into acute care sites. At the same time, "conscious sedation" was recommended in favor of general anesthesia (GA) whenever clinically appropriate [173, 174]. In the United Kingdom and some of the European countries, the term "conscious sedation" is still utilized to indicate care that does not fall under the definition of anesthesia. In the United States and many other countries, "conscious sedation" is a term that is no longer utilized because it is felt that sedation is a continuum, and thereby patients cannot be "conscious" [175]. This led to various cohort studies seeking to define the suitable patient groups [176–179]. At that time many private GA services in general dental practices (non-acute—"high street" sites) lost income, so they switched to polypharmacy sedation, with the anesthetist providing the "deep" sedation and the general dentist providing the operative care. The UK pediatric dentists were against this and were united in their view that this polypharmacy deep sedation in high street settings was no safer than GA and that, equally importantly, the general dentist was underqualified to provide the standard of treatment planning and dental operative care needed for these children. This was the background to the production of the British Society of Paediatric Dentistry (BSPD) sedation guideline [180]. The guideline pre-dated the Cochrane Review and errs on the side of safety against a background of poor evidence and difficulties in the changes surrounding the move of GA services into acute hospital sites at that time, but it is still relevant today since a few "rogue" practices remain. BSPD guidelines are reviewed and updated as necessary every 5 years.

Premedication (Sedation) Prior to General Anesthesia

Children who need general anesthesia for dentistry usually require treatment in multiple teeth and in different parts of the mouth. For those who are already dentally anxious, they show increased distress at anesthetic induction and increased postoperative morbidity [181]. Indeed, psychological morbidity such as attention-seeking, tantrums, bed-wetting, separation anxiety, crying, and nightmares is well reported in those who are younger, have pre-existing behavioral problems, or dental anxiety [182–186].

Psychological preparation of children for GA is highly effective in reducing pre- and postoperative distress and complications [187]. This might be better than premedication. Indeed, facilitating the development of coping skills, modeling, play therapy, operating room tour, and parental involvement may be best [188, 189]. Interestingly, a recent Cochrane review suggested that the presence of parents during induction of GA does not reduce the child's anxiety and that parental acupuncture, clown doctors, hypnotherapy, low sensory simulation, and handheld video games need to be investigated further [190]. Surprisingly, even the use of a premedication such as midazolam has met with limited success by comparison [191].

Midazolam is a common premedicant at anesthetic induction and it has been suggested that post-anesthesia behavior disturbance is reduced. The drug is not registered for pediatric usage—few drugs are—and it has been common for the IV preparation to be used for oral usage, though this has a bitter taste. To overcome the taste, the preparation can be mixed with fruit-flavored cordials, sometimes including an analgesic such as paracetamol. However, the evidence for efficacy varies and there is a balance between optimal therapeutic effect, the need for fasting before general anesthesia, and delayed recovery even when doses as small as 0.2 mg/kg are used [192–194].

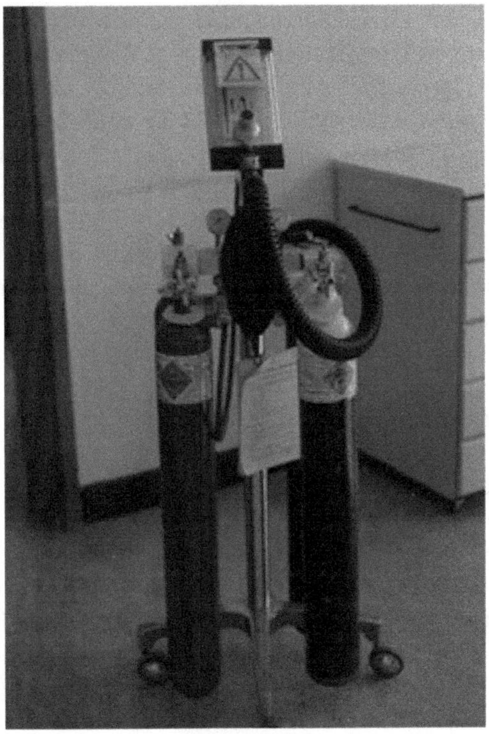

Fig. 20.5 Example of a portable dedicated titratable nitrous oxide machine (*note*: Oxygen cylinders are black in the UK and blue in the United States)

The UK Definition of Conscious Sedation

The National Institute for Clinical Excellence (NICE) guideline sets the UK definition of conscious sedation for dentistry. This is covered later in this chapter under guidelines.

There is no "deep sedation" definition for dentistry in the UK. If it is not "conscious" it is considered to be general anesthesia; as such, regulations relating to the site, facilities, and level of staff training apply. In summary, a drug or drugs can be used, the patient should be awake and communicating at all times, and IV is confined to emotionally mature adolescents. Importantly, the dentist is responsible for compliance of the anesthetist if they are working together on a sedated patient to ensure consciousness is maintained.

Titrated Nitrous Oxide Inhalation Sedation

Only dedicated dental machines are used (Fig. 20.5) and active scavenging is recommended. The typical child patient is moderately anxious and willing to co-operate by breathing in and out through the nose. There is no defined age limit, but a child is typically around 7 years old and needs only three or four visits to complete treatment. The treatment is usually for fillings or one or two extractions at any one appointment. Using a rubber dam to isolate the tooth for a filling helps the sedation by reminding the child to nose breath whilst limiting operator and environmental exposure. The operator gradually increases the concentration of nitrous oxide delivered to the patient in 5 % increments every few minutes, observes the effect, and as appropriate, increases (or sometimes decreases) the concentration to obtain optimum sedation in each individual patient. Although it is effective, it is important that it is used in combination with behavioral therapy and incorporated into the treatment plan. Nitrous oxide sedation should not be used as a "one-off." Local anesthesia is still required for dental procedures. Only a dedicated dental delivery system should be used since only this will allow titration of the dose. A nitrous oxide scavenging system is also needed to combat chronic environmental exposure to dental staff [195, 196].

Intravenous Sedation

Intravenous midazolam sedation is considered to be suitable only for "emotionally mature" adolescents. Sedation training ranges from a few days "intensive" to Diploma courses, but all practitioners should keep a portfolio to show continued practice and experience in both the assessment and delivery.

The patient is expected to maintain their own airway and to engage verbally; therefore, the use of a mouth prop is frowned upon. The operating pediatric dental sedationist generally uses titrated midazolam as the single sedative. The maximum dose is usually 7–10 mg but delivered in 1 mg then 0.5 mg increments. The term "emotionally mature adolescent" is difficult to define but fits in with the understanding of the UK law of the right and competency of adolescents. The parents still sign the consent, but the patient has to be clearly engaged with the treatment plan.

Oral Sedation

Oral sedation is not in common usage in the UK and is confined to midazolam, usually 0.5 mg/kg. The author's unit at King's College Hospital—an acute care site—is one of the largest UK providers of this service. The children need to be 30 kg or less in weight to be eligible so that the dose does not exceed 15 mg. A heavier child has more unpredictable onset of sedation and longer recovery. The treatment is confined to relatively quick procedures—commonly, extraction of a few traumatized primary incisors in a toddler. Paradoxical reactions are not uncommon, and although, theoretically the child has amnesia, it can be upsetting for the parent, who is present in the operatory, to witness. Pulse oximetry is used throughout and a dedicated recovery area is close-by. The pediatric dentists all have diplomas in sedation in addition to their specialty training, and the supporting dental nurse has an additional sedation qualification.

Sedation and Dental-Specific Guidelines of the United Kingdom and European Union

British Society of Paediatric Dentistry

The BSPD guideline supports the use on nitrous oxide inhalation sedation in non-acute sites and without monitors or fasting. Other types of sedation require monitoring and levels of staff training and facilities closer to those available on hospital departments. Therefore, it does not rule out the usage or research into other sedatives provided these are delivered by suitably trained staff and in appropriate facilities—for poorly evidence-based sedatives this means an acute care facility [180].

European Association of Paediatric Dentistry

The EAPD guideline encompasses diverse practice but its recommendations not only confirm the role of inhalation sedation but also maintain the definition of sedation.

Table 20.6 An example of the implementation of the NICE guideline for pediatric dentistry inhalation sedation in respect to emergency life support training and fasting

Moderate sedation	Conscious sedation	Deep sedation
Intermediate Life Support required	Intermediate Life Support required	Advanced Life Support required
No fasting if verbal contact is maintained	ILS = no fasting	Apply 2-4-6 rule

National Institute for Clinical Excellence

The NICE guidelines were developed to guide pediatric sedation practice for those in the National Health Service in England and Wales. This clinical guideline does not just cover dentistry but all sedation carried out for all medical or dental procedures for children aged up to 18 years. The guideline recommends that nitrous oxide inhalation sedation is the most common and also the safest sedative agent for use in children's dentistry and that this is considered to be the "standard technique" [197].

It states that sedation may be considered when a procedure is too frightening, too painful, or needs to be carried out in a child who is ill, in pain or who has behavioral problems. The recommendations include the following:

- Children and young people undergoing sedation and their parents and caregivers should have the opportunity to make informed decisions.
- Treatment and care and information should be culturally appropriate and pre-sedation assessment and documentation is required.
- The levels of expertise in sedation techniques as well as drug choice, fasting requirements, and level of life support training and monitoring are set out.
- The importance of psychological preparation is acknowledged.

An example of how the NICE guideline can be used is shown in Table 20.6.

NICE Levels of Sedation Definitions

- *Minimal sedation*: A drug-induced state during which patients are awake and calm and respond normally to verbal commands. Although cognitive function and coordination may be impaired, ventilatory and cardiovascular functions are unaffected.
- *Moderate sedation*: Drug-induced depression of consciousness during which patients are sleepy but respond purposefully to verbal commands (known as conscious sedation in dentistry) or light tactile stimulation. No interventions are required to maintain a patent airway. Spontaneous ventilation is adequate. Cardiovascular function is usually maintained.
- *Conscious sedation*: Drug-induced depression of consciousness, similar to moderate sedation, except that

verbal contact is always maintained. *This term is used commonly in dentistry.*

- *Deep sedation*: Drug-induced depression of consciousness during which patients are asleep and cannot be easily aroused but do respond purposefully to repeated or painful stimulation. The ability to maintain ventilatory function independently may be impaired. Patients may require assistance to maintain a patent airway. Spontaneous ventilation may be inadequate. Cardiovascular function is usually maintained.

Measuring the Effectiveness of Sedation in Children

Children may not have sufficient maturity, capability, or reading ability to report the physiological and cognitive manifestations of anxiety. Therefore, dental anxiety scales used for them tend to concentrate on the behavioral component of anxiety and seldom follow the questionnaire format commonly used for adults. Methods of administration of the scales vary but can be broadly summarized as: (1) parental reporting of child's anxiety, (2) child (self)-reporting, and (3) dental operator or observer reporting. To improve validity, multiple scales and methods are usually recommended to report research outcomes.

There are many different scales. A selection of those most commonly found in the literature are as follows: Children's Fear Survey Schedule-Dental Subscale (CFSS-DS) [198]; Modified Child Dental Anxiety Scale (MCDAS) [199]; Visual Analogue Scale (VAS) [200]; Frankl Scale [201]; Venham Picture Scale [202]; Venham Anxiety and Behavior Rating Scales [203]; Behavior Profile Rating Scale [204]; Children's Dental Fear Picture Test [205]; Facial Image Scale (FIS) [206, 207]; and the Global Rating Scale [79]. It is this lack of standardization of scales that has led to difficulty in reporting high quality evidence in pediatric sedation studies, though the challenge actually lies in the difficulty in reporting a child's thoughts, comprehension, and feelings in an age-specific and clinically meaningful way that is sensitive, valid and reproducible.

The Frankl scale is a common tool used for rating the behavior and patient selection in pediatric sedation studies (see Table 20.3). However, it is not sufficiently sensitive to use as a research tool; instead it is a useful as a screening tool to select participants and as an adjunct to the clinical record [79, 201, 208]. Aartman et al., 1998, reported that the CFSS-DS covered more aspects of the dental situation, measured dental fear more precisely, produced normative data, and had slightly superior psychometric properties compared to other scales. It consists of 15 items rated on a five-point scale, ranging from 1 (not afraid) to 5 (very afraid). The total score is calculated by summing item scores; giving a possible range of 15–75. Scores above 38 indicate significant

Table 20.7 Corah's Dental Anxiety Scale [210]

1. If you had to go to the dentist tomorrow for a check-up, how would you feel about it?
(a) I would look forward to it as a reasonably enjoyable experience
(b) I would not care one way or the other
(c) I would be a little uneasy about it
(d) I would be afraid that it would be unpleasant and painful
(e) I would be very frightened of what the dentist might do
2. When you are waiting in the dentist's office for your turn in the chair, how do you feel?
(a) Relaxed
(b) A little uneasy
(c) Tense
(d) Anxious
(e) So anxious that I sometimes break out in a sweat or almost feel physically ill
3. When you are in the dentist's chair waiting while the dentist gets the drill ready to begin working on your teeth, how do you feel?
(a) Relaxed
(b) A little uneasy
(c) Tense
(d) Anxious
(e) So anxious that I sometimes break out in a sweat or almost feel physically ill
4. Imagine you are in the dentist's chair about to have your teeth cleaned. While you are waiting and the dentist or hygienist is getting out the instruments which will be used to scrape your teeth around the gums, how do you feel?
(a) Relaxed
(b) A little uneasy
(c) Tense
(d) Anxious
(e) So anxious that I sometimes break out in a sweat or almost feel physically ill

dental fear. Scores from 32 to 38 indicate moderate dental anxiety and scores below 32 are considered to be low fearful [209]. Through a series of amendments to the original "Corah" scale (Table 20.7) [210], the MCDAS (Fig. 20.6) has been produced and has published UK norms [199, 211, 212]. It has eight dental anxiety items: the score in each question is from 1 (relaxed) to 5 (extremely worried), giving a total of 5–40. Scores more than 19 are considered to indicate a child is anxious and scores of more than 31 are considered to indicate a child is highly fearful. The sensitivity of the VAS has been previously confirmed for use as a measurement of state-anxiety in children and lends itself well to statistical analyses [200, 208]. Many of the other scales using pictures, such as Venham, are mainly used for very young children. However, the Venham picture scale looks very old fashioned to the eye of a modern child; the most-up-to-date and best validated scale nowadays is probably the FIS (Fig. 20.7). This is basically a five-point Likert type scale with faces rather than numbers. It is sometimes used in combination with the MCDAS [202, 205, 206].

Modified Child Dental Anxiety Scale (MCDAS)

For the next 8 questions I would like you to show me how relaxed or worried you get about the dentist and what happens at the dentist. To show me how relaxed or worried you feel, please use the simple scale below.

The scale is just like a ruler going from 1, which would show that you are relaxed, to 5, which would show that you are very worried.

1 would mean: relaxed/not worried
2 would mean: very slightly worried
3 would mean: fairly worried
4 would mean: worried a lot
5 would mean: very worried

How do you feel about …					
…going to the dentist generally?	1	2	3	4	5
…having your teeth looked at?	1	2	3	4	5
…having your teeth scraped and polished?	1	2	3	4	5
…having an injection in the gum?	1	2	3	4	5
…having a filling?	1	2	3	4	5
…having a tooth taken out?	1	2	3	4	5
…being put to sleep to have treatment?	1	2	3	4	5
…having a mixture of "gas and air" which will help you feel comfortable for treatment but cannot put you to sleep?	1	2	3	4	5

Fig. 20.6 Modified Child Dental Anxiety Scale (MCDAS)

Fig. 20.7 Facial Image Scale

Facial Image Scale

How do you feel right now?

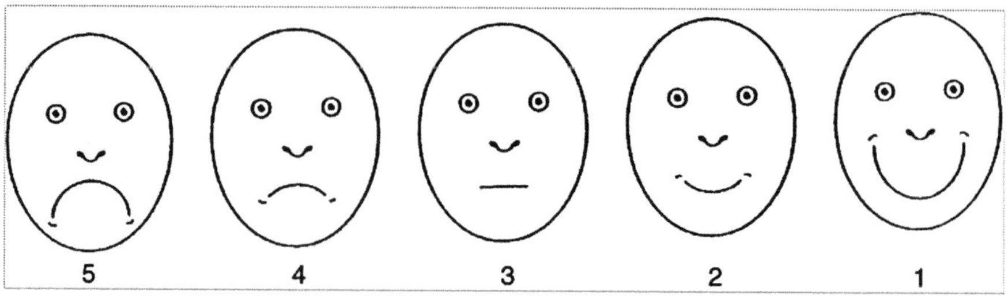

Off the Beaten Track—Ideas for the Future Sedation of Adolescents

Propofol

Propofol is a sedative hypnotic agent, used to induce and maintain general anesthesia but it can be used for conscious sedation when used in sub-anesthetic dosages. When propofol is administered in the UK and European Union, it is usually with a Target-Controlled Infusion (TCI) delivery system (for further information, see Chap. 31). TCI applies a pharmacokinetic model to predict and deliver the initial bolus dose and infusion rates of propofol in order to achieve and maintain a targeted sedation level. The "target" is generally a steady-state serum concentration of the sedative at the level of the brain [213–215].

Propofol (diprivan: 2,6 di-isopropophenol) is a lipid-based oil-in-water emulsion of egg lecithin, glycerol, and soybean oil. It is generally avoided when there is a history of allergy to these and is best avoided in epileptics as there is a theoretical epileptogenic effect (see Chap. 9, for further information).

The therapeutic margin between general anesthesia and sedation is small; as little as 2–10 μg/mL [216]. Therefore, the sedationist is usually an anesthetist and, in the UK, usage is recommended to be confined to pediatric dentistry units located on hospital sites. Moreover, intravenous sedation is only recommended for "emotionally mature" adolescents irrespective of drug choice [180].

A benefit of propofol conscious sedation is that dental treatment can usually be performed very soon after the onset of the infusion [217, 218] and the predicted concentration can be easily adjusted as clinically required during the procedure. Recovery is also very quick with full wakefulness occurring within minutes of discontinuation.

Pediatric dentists commonly undertake "quadrant dentistry," this means they give a local anesthetic injection in one area of the mouth (quadrant) then treat all the teeth in the anesthetized field, whatever treatment each tooth might need. Restorations (fillings) usually need to be placed in a dry field, this means that extractions are best performed at the end of the treatment visit; but this timing is at odds with the properties of other sedative agents that start to "wear off" toward the end of the visit. Thus more sedative is needed toward the end of the visit to facilitate extractions but this can then lead to a lengthier time in recovery. As such, propofol conscious sedation is ideal for those dental phobic, high caries risk adolescents who need multiple restorations as well as extraction of permanent teeth. The reader is reminded that, in the UK, pediatric dentists perform all restorations, root canal therapies and minor oral surgery procedures, including permanent tooth extraction, sometime beyond 16 years of age. So, it is not inconceivable for a dentally phobic British adolescent to have each of these treatments performed at the same sedative visit, but treatment is in a hospital setting with an anesthetist present.

Hosey et al. reported a mean infusion rate (maintenance rate) of 2.5 mg/kg/h (range 0.2–5.4 mg/kg) in their report of propofol IV sedation in dentally anxious adolescents in a hospital-based pediatric dental unit [219]. The children were awake and responsive throughout and neither mouth props nor laryngeal or pharyngeal airways were used. The patients also remembered aspects of the treatment and this lack of amnesia might even benefit them by facilitating coping skills for future visits [219].

Interestingly, in a case-controlled study of dentally anxious children comparing 36 undergoing inhalation sedation (mean age 11 years, range 6–16 years) with 40 undergoing propofol intravenous sedation (mean age 14 years, range 10–16 years), both sedative methods were found to be similarly efficacious at anxiety reduction. The propofol TCI was administered via an Alaris 2700 pump using the adult "Marsh" model. Blood levels are used as a guide and titrated to clinical endpoints. The two cohorts were closely matched in respect to preoperative anxiety as measured by the MCDAS and CFSS-DS scales and there were significant anxiety reductions afterwards within each cohort. Subjects undergoing propofol IVS were older than those undergoing IS, reflecting the adherence to the UK BSPD guideline regarding the use of intravenous sedation for mature adolescents only [219, 220].

Minor side effects of propofol include: pain on injection; a raised libido, "itchy nose," and increased "talkativeness." The increased talkativeness is of benefit since it assists the operator in ensuring that the sedation level has remained within the definition of "conscious"; it is for this reason that mouth props are discouraged. It is believed that it is the drug itself that causes the injection pain rather than other ingredients in the formulation. It has been suggested that lidocaine should be given intravenously with a rubber tourniquet before the propofol injection or mixed with the propofol sedative [134, 221–227].

"Propofol infusion syndrome" is characterized by acidosis, bradyarrhythmia, and rhabdomyolysis. This complication is rare but frequently fatal and has been reported in some 21 children and 14 adults sedated for more than 48 h. There are cases of metabolic acidosis, hyperlipidemia, and hepatomegaly in children in intensive care units sedated with propofol for prolonged time periods [228, 229] (for further information, see Chap. 9).

Propofol has no reversal agent. In cases of overdose, the patient has to be stabilized and ventilated until spontaneous respiration is regained. Some studies have reported respiratory depression, hypotension, bradycardia, and hypoxia [135, 219, 230]. This is why conscious sedation with propofol is considered safe only when administered by an anesthetist and in a hospital setting [180].

Pediatric Dental Sedation in South America

The use of sedation for dental procedures by pediatric dentists in South America is not common. Although children have significant dental treatment needs, most of the need is related to dental caries, and the management of their behavior has been primarily achieved via non-pharmacological techniques, including physical restraint.

Recent surveys of South American populations have shown encouraging outcomes regarding parental perception of pharmacological techniques. For instance, in Colombia, parental acceptance of nitrous oxide sedation is 89.1, 35.9 % general anesthesia, 53.5 % physical restraint by individuals, and 38.7 % using physical restraint involving a device (e.g., papoose board) [231]. Also, Colombian parents believe that 92.0 % of children aged 4–12 years liked nitrous oxide sedation [232].

Some South American countries have rules that guide the practice of sedation by dentists. In pediatric dentistry, a few reports about sedation suggest that dentists have been responsible for administering inhalation sedation with nitrous oxide, while other forms of sedation have been used in dental offices in conjunction with anesthesiologists.

There is little information on the offer of sedation in public services, but it is clear that private practices have sought to meet the demand of parents for more comfortable dental consultations involving children.

So, the aim of this section is to answer the following questions:

1. What are the ethical and legal aspects of performing dental sedation in the pediatric dental office?
2. What sedation guidelines do pediatric dentists follow?
3. What sedation regimens have being used and/or investigated?

What is the Regulatory Language Related to Performing Dental Sedation in the Pediatric Dental Office?

In South America, physicians and dentists can prescribe and administer medicaments. There are regulations in some countries stating the conditions for a dentist to provide dental sedation (Table 20.8). Usually, dentists are not required to have formal training before providing oral sedation to dental patients according to the institutions that regulate the practice of dentistry in South American (i.e., *Salon Dental Chile* in Chile, *Círculo Argentino de Odontología* in Argentina, and *Conselho Federal de Odontologia* in Brazil).

Even with the regulation of training to perform inhalation sedation with nitrous oxide, Brazilian dentists do not routinely use the technique. One reason for little use of sedation among Brazilian dentists is the controversy of sedation interacting with dentistry and medicine [233]. In one study, Brazilian dentists certified in nitrous oxide sedation were surveyed for their use of nitrous oxide. The majority of respondents were female (64.6 %). Of the 136 respondents, most of whom were located in the south and southeastern portion of Brazil, 77.0 % used this sedation method in clinical practice; however, most reported using the method "sometimes" (53.5 %), and focused more on adult patients [234]. Some evidence suggests Brazilian dentists do not use

Table 20.8 Examples of regulations regarding the use of sedatives by South American dentists

Country	Legal document	Recommendations
Brazil	Federal Law 5081, on August 24, 1966	Article 6. It is up to the dentist: (..) VI—to employ analgesia and hypnosis when they constitute effective methods for dental treatment
	College of Dental Surgeons, Resolution 51, on April 30, 2004	Establishes standards for enabling the dentist in the application of relative analgesia or conscious sedation with nitrous oxide. Dentists should complete a 96-h course about the topic
Chile	Ministry of Health, Guidelines for the management of anxiety in dental care 2005 (first edition) and 2007 (second edition)	Regulates nitrous oxide inhalation sedation in dentistry
Colombia	Ministry of Health, Resolution 1441 of May 6, 2013	Dentists can do minimal (level I) and moderate (level II) sedation in the dental office if s/he is not the same doing the dental procedure, is certified in Basic Life Support (BLS, renewed every 2 years) and in sedation; nurses can help in monitoring the patient
		Deep (level III) sedation requires more sophisticated training and apparatus, including advanced life support courses, SpO_2, PANI, EKG and $EtCO_2$ sometimes
		Level IV (general anesthesia) can be administered by anesthesiologists only
		Dentists should have theoretical and clinical training to use nitrous oxide in the dental office
Peru	Dental Ethics Code, December 2009	Dentists can prescribe medications containing narcotic substances, psychotropic drugs or other controlled substances. General anesthesia for dental treatment must be performed by an anesthesiologist

sedation in pediatric dentistry because little formal education and training on the subject occurs in dental schools [233].

In Peru, the use of oral sedation for dental purposes is restricted, as there are not many dentists who use these procedures. Most are done in hospital centers that have the resources necessary to perform and overcome any complications that arise, but most of them have not published their results [235].

What Sedation Guidelines do Pediatric Dentists Follow in South America?

As there have been relatively few guidelines created in South America to focus on pediatric behavior management in the dental office, pediatric dental sedation protocols are routinely based on recommendations from American and/or European institutions such as the AAPD, AAP, ASA, ADA, and NICE (for further information, see Chap. 2).

However, there are cultural differences affecting the application of these guidelines with regard to the indication of pharmacological methods for dental treatment. The paradigm that prevails in South America, when it comes to the management of child behavior in the dental chair, is based on the idea that sedation or general anesthesia would be indicated only if and when all other non-pharmacological techniques fail [236]. In another survey it was reported that South America favors non-pharmacological techniques [237].

The Brazilian Ministry of Health, Oral Health Department, recommends that children who do not cooperate with dental treatment in primary care services should be categorized as "special needs patients." Under this designation they should be referred to specialized public centers where they receive dental treatment in an outpatient level or under general anesthesia in the hospital. However, very few specialized dental public services in Brazil offer nitrous oxide sedation and none of them provide other methods of sedation.

In Chile, the recommendations of the Ministry of Health in controlling anxiety during dental care, aimed at adults and children, should include non-pharmacological and pharmacological features. Under those guidelines, children who need dental treatment and cannot cooperate due to cognitive impairment, anxiety and fear, or require extensive treatment are indicated for sedation during dental visits. On an outpatient basis, nitrous oxide and oxygen is recommended for children ASA 1 or 2. For other cases, sedation is indicated in specialized environments of critical care [238].

In Colombia, a multi-institutional work group[1] coordinated by the Colombian Society of Anesthesiology and Reanimation published two consensus statements related to pediatric sedation and analgesia by dentists and non-anesthesiologist physicians: one focused on children up to 12 years of age and the other on children older than 12 years.

Accordingly, children under 12 years old can have anxiolysis or minimal sedation outside the operating room if they need elective procedures as long as they are painless or cause minimal pain. Also, the children should be older than 2 years of age, ASA 1 or 2, have parental consent for the procedure, no history of the upper airway infection in the last week, are seen by the same sedationist professional in a pre-anesthetic consultation, and have proper fasting time. In this case, competent dentists would be able to administer nitrous oxide sedation in enabled certified dental office. They also recommended the use of only one sedative by oral route [239].

For children older than 12 years, sedation should always be performed by a trained physician, dentist, or a certified registered nurse or nurse assistant, provided that another person different from the sedationist perform the dental procedure. For minimal or moderate sedation, the recommended medications are midazolam, nitrous oxide, or propofol. They warned that "as propofol can produce general anesthesia, it can only be used by non-anesthesiologists when there is periodical certification of training and deep sedation and general anesthesia is avoided." These guidelines also consider that certain types of patients (e.g., non-cooperative patients or the very young) should be sedated by anesthesiologists to minimize the risk of preventable morbidity [240].

What Sedation Regimens are Being Used and/or Investigated in South America?

Reports of sedation regimens, albeit rare, have varied in the last 10 years (see Table 20.9 [101, 105, 235, 241–248]). Alternative medicines—substances such as *Melissa officinalis* (lemon balm) that have some sedative action have been used with apparent good results during less invasive dental procedures in children—are also being investigated [249].

The Dental Sedation Center (in Portuguese: Núcleo de Estudos em Sedação Odontológica or NESO) at the Federal University of Goias, in Brazil, has an extension developed in 1998 that aims to provide dental treatment under sedation or general anesthesia for children and adults. NESO is run by a multi-professional team, involving pediatric dentists, dentists from other specialties, pediatricians, anesthesiologists, psychologists, oral therapists, that follow most of the AAPD, AAP and ASA guidelines for outpatient sedation. Several protocols have been investigated in NESO, and in 2007 members of the NESO team published the book (in Portuguese): "Sedation in dentistry: Demythologizing its practice" [244]. Today NESO recommends oral midazolam with or without ketamine for pediatric dental sedation, which are provided by the anesthesiologist. Nitrous oxide sedation is provided by certified dentists.

[1]Sociedad Colombiana de Anestesiología y Reanimación (SCARE), Sociedade Colombiana de Pediatría, Asociación Colombiana de Gastroenterología, Asociación Colombiana de Endoscopia Digestiva, Secretaría Distrital de Salud, Colegio Colombiano de Odontólogos, Academia Colombiana de Odontología Pediátrica.

Table 20.9 Publications about pediatric dental sedation regimens investigated in South American institutions, 2003–2013

Citation	Institution	Sedative regimen
[105]	Dental Sedation Center ("Núcleo de Estudos em Sedação Odontológica," NESO), Federal University of Goias, Goiania, Brazil	Oral midazolam 1.0 mg/kg: 77.0 % effective
		Oral midazolam 0.75 mg/kg associated with hydroxyzine 2.0 mg/kg: 30.8 % effective
[241]	Dental School, Peruvian University Cayetano Heredia, Lima, Peru	Oral midazolam (0.5 mg/kg) as effective as intranasal midazolam (0.2 mg/kg) administered with syringe without atomizer
[242]	NESO Dental Sedation Center, Federal University of Goias, Goiania, Brazil	81.0 % of moderate sedation appointments needed physical restraint (active or passive) for dental treatment completion. Sedatives were oral midazolam or chloral hydrate associated or not with hydroxyzine
[243]	Dental School, Federal University of Santa Catarina, Florianopolis, Brazil	Oral midazolam in three distinct doses (0.2–0.25; 0.3–0.35 and 0.4 mg/kg) better than placebo
[244]	NESO Dental Sedation Center, Federal University of Goias, Goiania, Brazil	Oral chloral hydrate (75 mg/kg): 62.5 % effectiveness
		Oral chloral hydrate 50 mg/kg plus hydroxyzine 2.0 mg/kg: 61.5 % effectiveness
[101]	Dental School, University of Campinas, São Paulo, Brazil	Oral diazepam 5 mg better or oral chloral hydrate 40 mg/kg were ineffective
[235]	Pediatric Dentistry Department, Naval Medical Center, Lima, Peru	Oral midazolam (0.75 mg/kg): effectiveness 58.3 % very good to excellent, 33.3 % good to regular and 8.3 % poor
		Oral midazolam (0.75 mg/kg) associated with hydroxyzine (1.0 mg/kg): 91.7 % very good to excellent, 8.3 % good to regular
[245]	NESO Dental Sedation Center, Federal University of Goias, Goiania, Brazil	Case report: Oral chloral hydrate (100 mg/kg) caused extreme excitement and struggling in a young child
[246]	Dental Clinic, University of Valparaiso, Chile	Nitrous oxide (average 30 %)/oxygen: effective in 62.0 % of 129 visits, 8.8 % crying, 12 % restlessness; no adverse reactions
[247]	NESO Dental Sedation Center, Federal University of Goias, Goiania, Brazil	Oral midazolam (1.0–1.5 mg/kg) or chloral hydrate (70.0–100.0 mg/kg)
		The most common intraoperative and post-discharge adverse events were hallucination (3.9 %) and excessive sleep (41.9 %), respectively
		The chance of the occurrence of an adverse event following oral pediatric sedation was lesser among the children who received midazolam than those who received chloral hydrate (OR: 0.09; 95 % CI: 0.01–0.88)
[248]	NESO Dental Sedation Center, Federal University of Goias, Goiania, Brazil	Oral midazolam (0.5 mg/kg) and ketamine (3 mg/kg): more cooperative behavior and longer sessions
		Oral midazolam (1.0 mg/kg)

In summary, sedation for dental procedures involving children in South America occurs on a less frequent basis than that of North America and primarily in centers where certified dentists and other medical personnel are available.

Closing Thoughts on Sedation in South America

In South America, pediatric dental sedation is moving at a slow pace. In general, although dentists are authorized to practice inhalation sedation with nitrous oxide/oxygen, they rarely apply that technique because their skills and comfort level are limited: Their training and formal education are focused on the use of non-pharmacological methods and not pharmacological delivery. Sedation with parenteral agents and inhalational anesthetics (not including nitrous oxide) is even more rarely practiced in pediatric dental care and limited to delivery by an anesthesiologist. Because of the limited skills, training and sedative availability offered to the pediatric dentists, many younger children would benefit from a general anesthetic for extensive, painful procedures. As South America moves into twenty-first century, both the dentists and the patients are seeking and demanding that the sedation care progress in parallel with the developed nations. In the future it is hoped that the South American dentist will be better prepared to offer, when appropriate, the use of pharmacological agents to improve sedation care of the child.

Conclusion

The Future

The authors of this chapter firmly believe that pediatric dental sedation is a tool that can only be successfully used in the hands of a dentist. It is only in this way that the operative treatment planning, behavioral management expertise, pain-free procedure, and sedation can be encapsulated. Pain-free and stress-free dental care is the right of every child. The diversity of views and techniques reflect not only the paucity of evidence but also cultural diversity and expectation. This diversity in techniques, sedatives, and facilities will benefit the child population that is served and will fuel thought, exchange of ideas, and future study.

Case Studies

Case 1 (from South America)

Child is a healthy boy (ASA 1), aged 3 years old and 7 months, 15.7 kg weight, 98 cm height, Mallampati II, showing the following vital signs in the medical assessment: 120 beats per minute (heart rate), 99 % (oxygen saturation), 20 breaths per minute (respiratory rate), and 80×50 (blood pressure). He was referred to NESO to have a dental treatment done under sedation, because he did not cooperate with two attempts of conventional treatment without a sedative. During the dental exam, he remained calm, no restraint was needed, and asymptomatic carious lesions were detected in the four upper incisors and the two lower first primary molars. The pediatric dentist, pediatrician and anesthesiologist considered giving him an oral sedation with midazolam. His mother was informed about the whole sedation procedure and consented. Next, the mother was instructed about the NPO requirements and asked to bring a sheet from home for wrapping this child during dental treatment. The sedation session was scheduled for the next week. During the sedation session, the child's health status was reassessed to confirm no respiratory infections and he received oral midazolam (1.0 mg/kg). In Brazil, midazolam is available in oral syrup containing 2 mg of midazolam per mL; so the child received 7.5 mL using a needleless syringe. The child and mother stayed in a quiet room continuously observed by a trained professional for 20 min. Then, the child was taken to the dental office together with his mother. In the dental chair, the child was placed supine and his body was loosely wrapped in a sheet stabilized with tape; his mother sat with the child's legs over hers. A pulse oximeter probe was adapted on the child's toe. The child was quiet when positioned in the dental chair and remained that way during the use of topical anesthetic (Fig. 20.8).

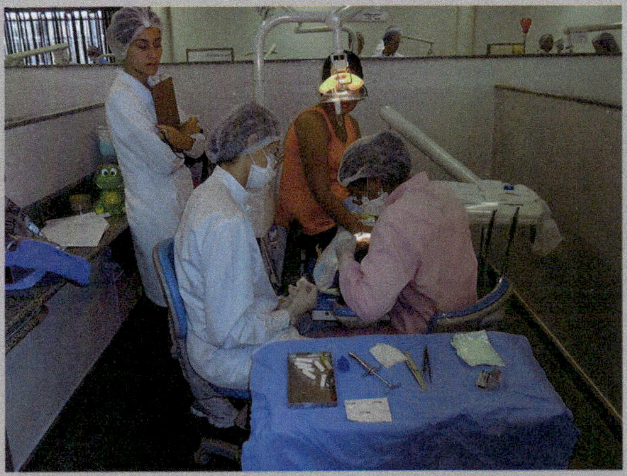

Fig. 20.8 Child during the beginning of the dental treatment. He is quiet, wrapped in a sheet stabilized with tape. His mother sits together in the dental chair. Pediatric dentist is using the topical anesthetic, a dental assistant is helping, and a trained observer is monitoring

The treatment planned was a composite restoration for the lower left primary first molar. When the pediatric dentist inserted the mouth prop and started injecting the local anesthetic for the inferior alveolar block (2 % lidocaine with 1:100,000 epinephrine, one carpule), the child started crying and moving, and struggled until the end of the dental treatment. Beside the protective stabilization with a sheet, the mother had to hold the child's legs to avoid movement, and the dental assistant had to hold the child's head to avoid injury during the performance of dental procedures. Non-pharmacological techniques were also used (e.g., distraction). The dentist used high and low speed hand pieces, rubber dam isolation and restored the tooth as planned, but with a child struggling. The child's vital signs (heart rate and oxygen saturation) did not change beyond accepted limits (Fig. 20.9).

During the dental treatment, as the child was uncooperative, the mother was asked if she preferred to have the session aborted or the restoration completion, and she chose the second option. The dental session was finished after 32 min. The child was taken to a recovery room, where he was monitored with pulse oximeter by a trained observer. The child slept for 40 min while in the recovery; discharge criteria were met after 55 min with no adverse events reported.

(continued)

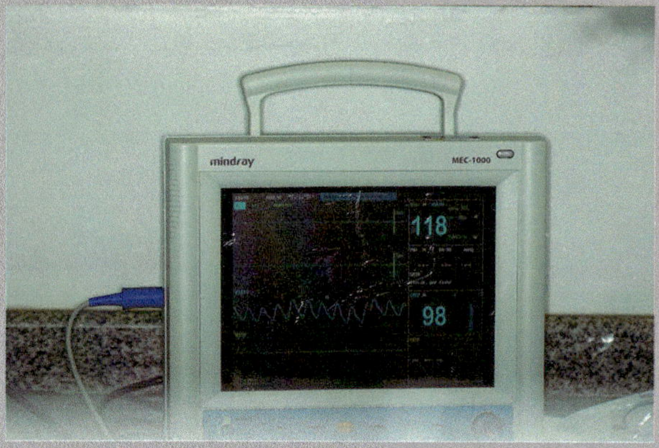

Fig. 20.9 Pulse oximeter showing normal heart rate and oxygen saturation

The sedation team (pediatric dentist, pediatrician, and anesthesiologist) asked the mother if she would like her son to have another sedation session with a different medication—ketamine would be added to reduce the chance of pain during the anesthesia. Other options would be: no sedation, midazolam sedation, or general anesthesia. Mother chose the ketamine/midazolam regimen for the next session. The next day, a member of the NESO team called the mother to ask about any postoperative adverse events at home, and mother answered that her child was fine, slept a lot after arriving home, but did not remember the dental treatment.

The second sedation session occurred 1 week later. A composite restoration for the other first primary molar was planned. The child entered quietly into the dental clinic holding his mother's hand. Medical and dental procedures were the same as before, during and after the dental treatment. After the routine preoperative assessment, the child orally received the mixture of oral midazolam (0.5 mg/kg) and ketamine (3 mg/kg) via a needleless syringe (Fig. 20.10).

Ketamine intravenous solution was mixed with the oral syrup of midazolam, which the child accepted well. After 20 min, the child was placed in the dental chair the same way as the other session. He was quiet and drowsy, a little bit dissociated from the context, but vital signs were normal. Dental procedures were the same as in the previous appointment, and the child did not complain. The tooth was restored and the whole dental procedure lasted 28 min. The child slept for 33 min in the recovery area; discharge criteria were met after 40 min with no adverse events reported, except episodes of hallucinations. The mother did not report adverse reactions at home in the next 24 h after the sedation session.

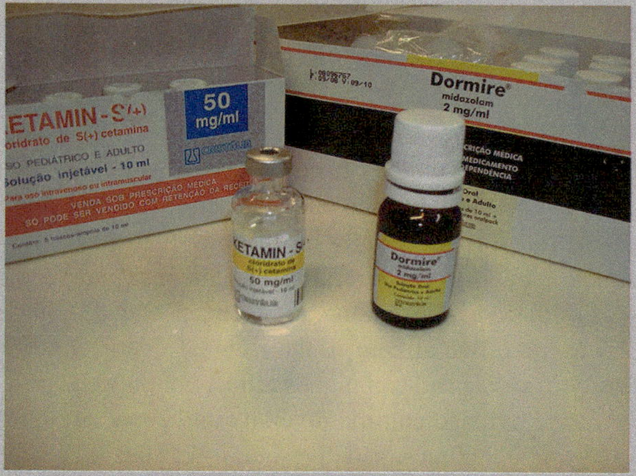

Fig. 20.10 Ketamine ampoule (*left*) and midazolam oral syrup (*right*)

Case 2 (from South America)

The child is a healthy girl with controlled asthma (ASA 2), aged 8.5 years old, 24.1 kg weight, 117 cm height, Mallampati II, showing the following vital signs in the medical assessment: 105 beats per minute (heart rate), 100 % (oxygen saturation), 18 breaths per minute (respiratory rate), and 80×50 (blood pressure). She was referred to NESO to have an oral biopsy under sedation, because she and her parents were very anxious about the procedure. The pediatric dentist suggested nitrous oxide/oxygen as the elective sedation method, as the child was pre-cooperative. The child and parent agreed. In that first consultation, the pediatric dentist performed a briefing session so the child would be familiarized with that kind of sedation; this potentially would diminish her anxiety toward the sedation method. The child felt good with 30 % of nitrous oxide in the mixture, and a pediatric size small mask was selected. The surgical procedure was scheduled for another week. The child was instructed to have a light breakfast in the morning before the sedation. At the day of the sedation, the child and her father entered the dental clinic. The child sat down in the dental chair without any restraint and the father also sat with the child's legs over his. Initially, the child received 100 % oxygen for 3 min (Fig. 20.11), while the dentist properly adapted the nitrous oxide nasal hood on her nose and the pulse oximeter probe on her toe (Fig. 20.12).

Then the level of nitrous oxide was set to 50 % so that the child could receive local anesthesia infiltration in the sublingual area with no pain, using 2 % lidocaine with 100,000 epinephrine without previous topi-

(continued)

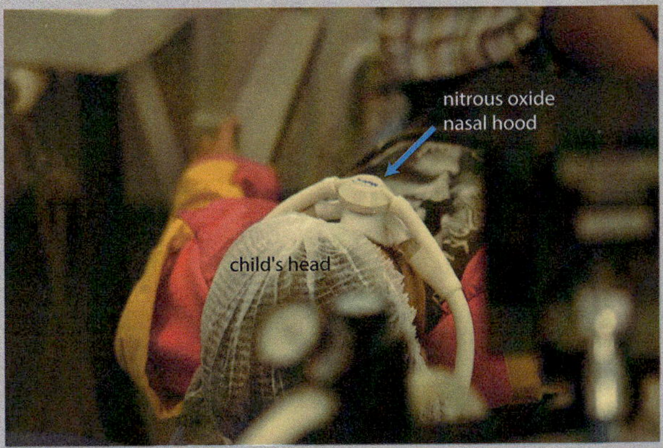

Fig. 20.11 After positioned with her father in the dental chair, child receives 100 % oxygen until nitrous oxide nasal hood is properly adapted to her nose

cal anesthetic. After anesthetic infiltration, nitrous oxide was set to 30 % and the lesion was removed. The wound was sutured and the child had 100 % oxygen at the end of the session, for 5 min, to wash out the nitrous oxide. Vital signs were stable during the procedure. The child stayed calm throughout the procedure. As she was feeling well as soon as the dental session was over, she did not need a recovery room and was immediately dismissed.

Case 3

Patient is a healthy (ASA I) 3-year-old boy with no known allergies and parent seeks care for the child because of cavities noticed on the front teeth (chief complaint). The cavities recently have been causing odontogenic pain during eating and occasionally wake the patient at night. Examination reveals 20 primary teeth, normal anatomy, and no soft tissue pathology. Of the 20 primary teeth, 13 involve frank carious lesions (four maxillary incisors, two maxillary canines, and seven molars). It is questionable as to whether the incisors can be saved. This presentation is referred to as early childhood caries, which is currently defined by the AAPD as "the presence of one or more decayed (non-cavitated or cavitated lesions), missing (due to caries), or tooth-filled surfaces in any primary tooth in a child 71 months of age or younger" [250]. The tonsils at the time occupied approximately 30 % of the airway and the parent denied the child snored. The head and neck were symmetrical in shape and the jaws and occlusion were normal in development for a child of his age. The child weighed 16 kg.

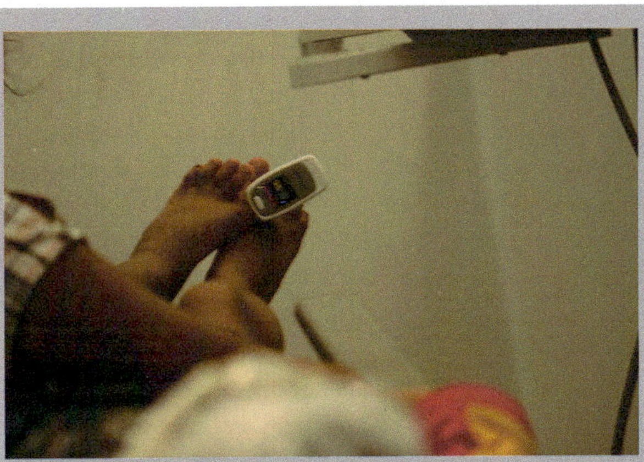

Fig. 20.12 Child is monitored with a portable pulse oximeter, which is placed on the toe

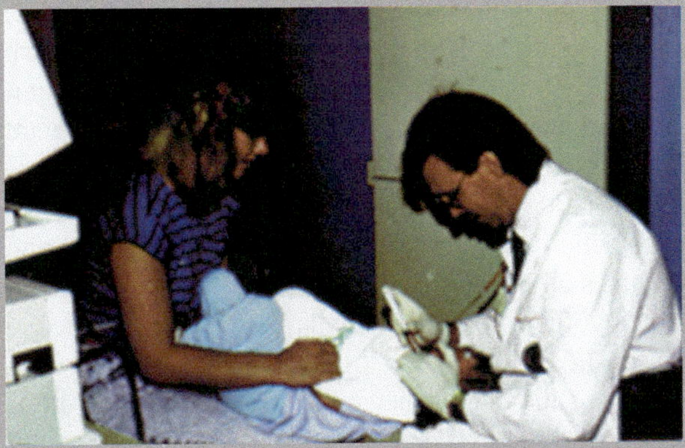

Fig. 20.13 Photo showing knee-to-knee position often used in pediatric dentistry

When the child first saw the dentist, he demonstrated shy, withdrawn behaviors and sought comfort from his mother. Oral examination was difficult as the child was uncooperative, crying, and required the mother of the child to stabilize and hold the arms and legs in a knee-to-knee examination position with the dentist (Fig. 20.13).

Dental radiographs were not possible to attain due to behavior. A discussion of the child's oral condition and the scope of treatment modalities occurred with the mother. The mother does not have dental insurance that will cover sedation or GA and has to pay out of pocket should she elect to consent to sedation or GA. GA costs are too expensive for the family and she elects to pay for sedation using a payment plan. The child is scheduled for two sedation appointments; however, the mother is advised that depending on the child's response to the drugs selected, including local anesthesia, the number of appointments may be altered. The parent consents.

(continued)

On the day of sedation, another oral examination including airway assessment is completed. The child has been NPO for 9 h. The dentist decides, based on the number and type of procedures to be completed, to use a combination of sedatives that have been shown in the literature to be effective. CH (20 mg/kg), meperidine (2 mg/kg), and hydroxyzine (1 mg/kg) will be administered orally with a latency period of 45 min. Should the child spit out the medication or vomit before any dentistry is done, no further administration of sedative agents occurs. This combination of agents and doses is based on the expected amount of dentistry to be completed and the child's temperament and personality (i.e., clinically shy, uncooperative, and difficult). Latency period refers to the time from administration of the oral agents to when the child is taken to the dental operatory to begin delivery of care. Local anesthesia is limited to 64 mg (4 mg/kg), which is slightly less than two carpules. A carpule is the unit of local anesthesia that fits into a standard dental syringe, which is typically 1.7 mL of 2 % lidocaine with 1:100,000 epinephrine. This amount of local anesthetic can be distributed over two quadrants and includes an inferior alveolar block and buccal infiltration involving approximately half of the care needed to be finished.

At the end of a latency period of 45 min, the child is placed supine in the dental chair. The child is awake, but drowsy and slightly less apprehensive of the doctor. An oxisensor of a pulse oximeter is attached to the second toe, a blood pressure cuff to the upper left extremity, a pretrachial stethoscope is placed over the upper airway above the manubrum, and plastic tubing from a capnography is readied should the child go into deeper levels of sedation. Nitrous oxide is initially administered using a nasal hood with the initial setting of 50 % concentration; however, the child begins to fuss, struggle, and cry. The concentration of nitrous is raised to 70 % (the maximum concentration attainable by a dental nitrous delivery system) and the hood held slightly above and over the nose and mouth of the patient. Within 5 min of distracting the child and administering the nitrous oxide, the child settles down and demonstrates slight ptosis of the eyelids. The nitrous concentration is immediately lowered to 50 % and the hood placed lightly over the nose. This process of using the nitrous to calm the child is called "settling." (If settling does not work within 10 min of nitrous administration, two options are available and presented to the parent for consent. One option is that the nitrous is no longer used—i.e., the hood is aggravating the child and interferes with the process—and a simple and relatively fast procedure, if available, is completed using local anesthesia and a papoose board; e.g., extraction of a tooth that has been causing odontogenic pain and brought the patient to the office. The second option is to reschedule the patient for another appointment during which a slightly different drug regimen is used or altering the dose of the current regimen. The child is kept in the dental clinic until they have recovered enough to meet discharge criteria.) The child is now comfortable and cooperative.

A small dollop of topical anesthetic (20 % benzocaine) is applied to the soft tissues where the injection will occur. The local anesthetic is slowly administered using an aspirating dental syringe and this elicits crying and new struggling on the part of the child. Once again, the "settling" procedure is done after the anesthetic has been administered. The child settles. A rubber dam is applied to prevent aerosol spray, tooth debris, and water from the dental hand piece from going into the child's airway. High speed suction to remove the debris and water is also done by the dental assistant. The child is reactive and has low intensity crying, minor movements, and no tears. Toward the end of the procedure the child becomes quiet and the eyes close. Besides the auscultation of the airway sounds, the plastic tubing from the capnography is taped under nostril orifice of the child and the side-stream end-tital CO_2 excursions monitored by the dentist and assistant. The dentist asks the child if they are "doing OK" and the child responds with a slight nodding of the head to which the dentist replies that we are "almost done." The work is completed. Seven teeth are restored with the restorations involving stainless steel crowns and white composite restorations. The child is stimulated by the dentist lightly tapping the child on the shoulders and declaring that "we are all finished." The child is slowly raised to a sitting position and reunited with the parent. The parent is informed of the procedures that were completed, how much remains, and the patient's responsiveness during the procedure. It turns out that this child exhibited "quiet" behaviors (no crying, but either eyes open or eyes temporarily closed) approximately 70 % of the time with the remainder of the operative time involving crying and mild struggling behaviors. This is "typical" of this particular regimen and younger children. The child is kept until discharge criteria is met (usually this occurs within 30 min after the dental procedure is completed). Another sedation appointment is booked and the plans are to use the same drugs and dosages as this appointment.

(continued)

Case 4

Patient is healthy (ASA I) and 2.5 years of age with no known allergies. The parent seeks care for the child because of cavities noticed on the front teeth by the parent and the child is complaining of sensitivity to cold (chief complaint). Examination reveals 20 primary teeth, normal anatomy, and no soft tissue pathology. Of the 20 primary teeth, the four maxillary incisors are grossly carious and a draining fistula is noted above the right central maxillary incisor. The indicated treatment is extraction of these four incisors due to non-restorability and periapical abscess. The tonsils are approximately 60 % of the airway and the parent indicated the child snored occasionally during sleep. The head and neck were symmetrical in shape and the jaws and occlusion were normal in development for a child of this age. The child weighed 14 kg. Vital signs are within normal limits. The patient has been NPO since 10 PM the previous evening.

The patient had an approachable temperament and interacted with the dentist but was age-specific hesitant and exhibited facial expressions suggestive of mild apprehension and anxiety for his age. He is classified temperamentally as "slow to warm up" and typical of a patient of his age. It was possible to obtain a maxillary dental radiograph confirming the abscess as well as caries encroaching on the pulp chamber of the remaining incisors. The sedation plan is to use midazolam (0.75 mg/kg) administered orally.

The midazolam is drawn up, flavored with FlavoRx®, and administered by cup. Due to the rapid onset and short duration of working time, it is planned to begin the procedure at 10 min after administration. The child is brought to the dental chair 10 min after drug administration and is placed on 50 % nitrous oxide using a nasal hood. The patient is loosely wrapped in a papoose board (with parental consent gained previously along with that for the sedation). The patient is somewhat uncooperative initially but finally accepts the mask after the dentist explained that it is a "pilot's mask." A pulse oximeter and blood pressure cuff are applied with a precordial handy on the assistant tray.

A small dollop of topical anesthetic (20 % benzocaine) in the form of a gel is swabbed over the mucosa in the maxillary vestibule overlying the four incisors, which had been thoroughly dried with a 2×2 gauze. The gel is left in place for 2 min as is the nitrous oxide. Stories are told to distract the patient. The patient is interactive and makes appropriate comments or questions in response to the stories. Next, a carpule (1.7 mL of 2 % lidocaine with epinephrine 1:100,000) is slowly administered by way of a dental syringe. This causes some minor movement with vocalization, especially when the palatal tissues are anesthetized. The child is consoled and distracted. A period of 10 min passes. The heart rate and oxygen saturation are monitored and recorded. The child's behavior is generally one of quietness but cries intermittently; nonetheless, distraction techniques are effective.

The four maxillary incisors are extracted using a curette and forceps without incident. The heart rate rose slightly, the child was interactive and struggled mildly, but expressed little discomfort indicating that the local anesthetic was effective. Pressure and gelfoam were used to obtain hemostasis. The child is losing tolerance for the procedure and is becoming more vocal with his crying and movement and expressing a desire to see his mother.

The mother is reunited with the child and postoperative instructions are given. The child initially begins to settle down. The parent and patient are kept in the dental room but now the child is becoming agitated, nonconsolable, and crying intensely. The child rips the oxisensor off the toe. The child, although relaxed, tries to escape from the parent's grasp. The child is now exhibiting the "angry child syndrome" that is often seen (20 % of the time) during dental procedures in which midazolam is used as the primary sedative agent. The parent had been forewarned of the possibility. A decision of whether to reverse the emotional condition with flumazenil is considered, but its shorter duration of action compared to the midazolam is a potential problem as explained to the parent. The patient is kept another 30 min and can now ambulate with assistance but continues to be disruptive and angry. After 15 more minutes, the child is discharged into the care of the two parents as they are becoming tired of the dental setting and feel they can better manage the child's behavior at home. The family is called 2 h later and the child has now settled down, is consuming clear liquids and soup.

Case 5

A 10-year-old female is referred to the office by a general practitioner who was unable to talk the child into receiving local anesthesia due to extreme apprehension and needle phobia for the extraction of a carious, nonrestorable first permanent molar and three other restorations. The patient is fearful and guarded but is complaining that the pain from the molar increases and ibuprofen is not helping anymore.

(continued)

A clinical examination is done with a great deal of tell-show-do, distraction, and coaxing necessary. The dentist and assistant attempted to behaviorally walk the child through intra-dental radiographs, but failed. Extra-oral radiographs are obtained with difficulty and confirm the molar is non-restorable. Vital signs and an airway examination are completed. They are within normal limits. The patient has not eaten since 7 PM the previous night. She weighs 37 kg.

The dentist decides to use diazepam (7 mg) and meperidine (2 mg/kg, but limits the dose to 50 mg). The patient reluctantly drinks the flavored medications in a vehicle of ibuprofen (100 mg) elixir. The patient becomes more relaxed 30 min after drug administration but still guarded. At 45 min after drug administration, the patient is introduced to the nitrous oxide hood but refuses to accept it and becomes more anxious with inconsolable crying. Attempts are made to calm the patient with some success. Topical anesthesia administration (20 % benzocaine) is done but the patient limits mouth opening despite encouragement. A mouth prop is inserted and this agitates the patient. Although the usual distraction and "out of sight" passing of the syringe is done, the patient's eyes follows the hand exchanges between dental assistant and dentist. The patient begins to scream and makes concerted efforts to escape from the chair despite being uncoordinated. The syringe is replaced on the dental tray and efforts are made to calm the patient again. The sequence of events is repeated but is not successful in overcoming the patient's will and lack of cooperation. The child is inconsolable and wants to go home. It is decided to cancel the session and perform the dentistry under general anesthesia (GA) in an outpatient care setting. The patient is duly monitored with a pulse oximeter until discharge criteria are met almost 1.5 h after the drug administration.

The parent's insurance does not cover sedation or GA for dental procedures. The parent wishes to wait and research possible financial resources. Two weeks pass and the patient returns to the office in chronic, moderate to severe pain, moderate trismus, and some localized swelling, which is affecting daily home functions. The patient is referred to an oral surgeon who reluctantly accepts a payment plan with the parents, uses intramuscular ketamine injection to achieve deep sedation, uses appropriate monitors, and starts an IV prior to removing the offending molar. The patient never returns to the office for follow-up on the three remaining carious lesions.

Case 6

A 5-year-old female was seen in the dental office with a chief complaint of a "dark spot" on her back molar. A review of the medical history indicates that the patient is healthy, was a full-term baby, has no allergies to medications or environmental factors, and has been developing normally. During the dental examination the patient was noted to be interactive but was nervous and talked incessantly in an effort to delay oral examination procedures. When it was time for a dental prophylaxis (cleaning up the teeth), the patient responded by occasionally raising her hands toward the dentist's arms but responded to "please place your hands on your belly button." The patient had 20 primary teeth. Three molars had incipient decay and a normally developing occlusal plane. The mother of the child indicated that she does very well during a physicians well patient visit but she does tend to be "a nervous kid." After discussing with the parent various options of approach in terms of behavior management for this child, it was decided with the parents' consent, to schedule a restorative dental visit and use a combination of nitrous oxide and liquid hydroxyzine sedation.

The mother and patient arrived at the office on time for the sedation appointment. A visit with the parent indicated that there had been no changes in the health history of the child and she has been healthy since the last visit. No new allergies have developed. A dental examination to confirm some curious lesions was done along with an oral airway assessment. The tonsils were noted to occupy approximately 30 % of the width of the posterior pharyngeal opening. The patient was again noted to be slightly nervous during the examination. The patient had been NPO for 10 h. The patient weighed 18 kg. The parent consented to oral sedation as a means of managing the patient's behavior.

An elixir containing 36 mg of hydroxyzine in a flavoring solution was prepared. The solution was brought to the operatory and the patient was asked to drink the solution. She complied and readily consumed the fluid. She was given some crayons and a coloring book. A latency period of 30 min occurred before the dentist returned to begin the procedure. During the latency period the patient was continually clinically monitored by the dental assistant. The child who was sitting in the dental chair was exhibiting more relaxation than when she had entered into the dental setting. She was told that the chair was going to recline and that she would receive some "happy gas" through a "pilot's mask."

(continued)

Once reclined the nitrous hood was placed over her nose, which she received without incident. The nitrous oxide was titrated in steps over 2 min to a concentration of 40 % nitrous oxide with 60 % oxygen. The patient was relaxed, appropriately communicative, and exhibited appropriate signs of nitrous oxide analgesia (e.g., open, warm palms, slight smile, and distant stare). An oxisensor probe was placed on the child's middle finger to monitor oxygen saturation and heart rate.

The patient was asked to open her mouth and was told that the dentist was placing a tooth chair (mouth prop) in her mouth to help keep her mouth open. Topical anesthesia was applied to the mucosa adjacent to the teeth to be restored. Local anesthesia consisting of 1.8 mL of 2 % lidocaine with epinephrine 1:100,000 was administered by way of a syringe and needle. During the administration of the local anesthesia, the patient at one time localized a quiet "ooh" but was otherwise quiet and did not move. The patient was told that she did a very good job of helping during the little "pinch." The dentist distracted the patient and carried on a two-way conversation with the patient over the next 10 min while the local anesthetic was producing profound anesthesia. Next, a rubber dam was placed on the teeth to be restored and white composite restorations were completed without incident. The heart rate remained at a normal and regular rhythm for the patient's age and there were no incidences of oxygen desaturation. Following the procedure the nitrous oxide was decreased to 0 % and the patient was given 100 % oxygen for the next 5 min. Then the hood was removed from the patient's nose and the patient was returned to the upright position; the patient was asked to sit still for a few minutes. Postoperative instructions were given to the mother of the patient. Finally, the patient was asked to get out of the chair and walk a few paces down the hallway on her own. She was able to ambulate without incident. The patient was released into the care of the mother.

Case 7

A 9-year-old boy was diagnosed with caries, erosion, and molar incisor hypomineralization (MIH), moderate anxiety and delayed dental development. He is ASA 1. He had received no previous dental treatment. He was currently asymptomatic but mentioned that there had been a "gum boil" in the lower left quadrant.

The enamel in the first permanent molars and incisors forms from birth up to around 4 years of age. This child had chicken pox at age 3 years and this has led to defects in the enamel formation and mineralization. The teeth are vulnerable to tooth decay, wear, and acid erosion. Typically, the child is more dentally anxious, probably because their general dentist has attempted to seal over the enamel defects, but these teeth are exquisitely sensitive so that the least puff of air is painful. Therefore, the general dentist referred this boy due to caries and dental anxiety.

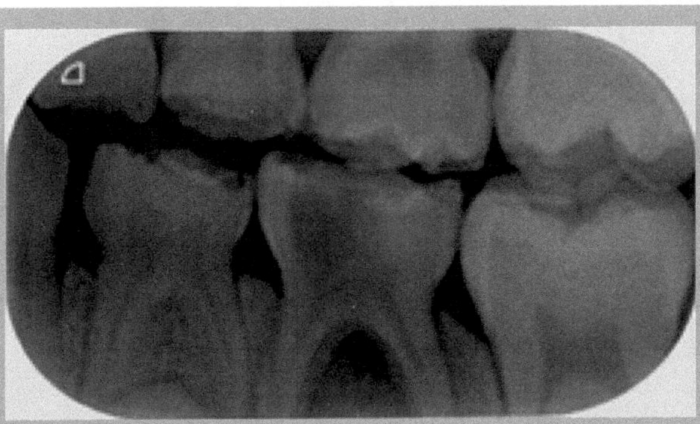

Fig. 20.14 Radiographically, the lower left second primary molar shows a radiolucency in the furcation extending down part of the root indicating it was non-vital

During the first examination, the child was happy to jump into the dental chair and to comply with the examination. He was chatty but clearly worried that the three-in-one "puffer" was going to be used. He asked for reassurance that "nothing will be done today—will it?" Clinical and radiographic examination confirmed that there was erosion of his retained primary incisors; caries in the lower right first permanent molar and both lower second primary molars; and radiographically, the lower left second primary molar had a radiolucency in the furcation extending down part of the root indicating it was non-vital (Fig. 20.14).

The various treatment options of (1) local anesthesia combined with behavior management; (2) augmenting these with inhalation sedation, and (3) general anesthesia were discussed with the parent and child. All agreed that use of inhalation sedation was the best option and written informed consent was obtained. The family was given an information sheet that repeated the verbal advice they had been given about the procedure, the sedation, and need for an escort. They were advised that there was no need to fast, but that a light meal only should be consumed in advice of the sedation appointment.

Three 1-h appointments were booked: (1) introduction to the inhalation technique and to apply fissure sealant to the three non-carious but sensitive first permanent molars; (2) restoration of the lower right first permanent molar and the second primary molar under

(continued)

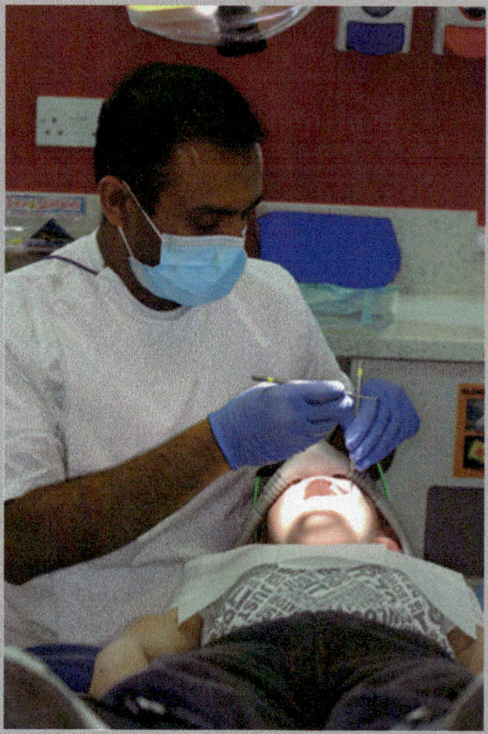

Fig. 20.15 Titrated nitrous oxide inhalation sedation—the first visit. (Acknowledgement to Mr. Sanjeev Sood)

rubber dam and using local anesthesia: 2.2 mL of 2 % xylocaine with 1:80,000 adrenaline (epinephrine) as in inferior dental block; (3) extraction of the non-vital and previously abscessed lower left second primary molar: 2.2 mL of 2 % xylocaine with 1:80,000 adrenaline (epinephrine) as an inferior dental block.

The retained primary incisors were monitored and seemed close to exfoliation; had the parent and child felt that he was too anxious to tolerate dental treatment under inhalation sedation, these teeth would have been removed at the time of the GA operation.

At each appointment only alert clinical monitoring was used. The nitrous oxide was titrated to effect; using 5 % increments every 3–5 min (Fig. 20.15).

Only 30–35 % nitrous oxide was required. Hypnotic suggestion was used throughout. The parent was present in the room and the dental nurse had undergone additional sedation training and qualification. She remained in the surgery at all times. A dedicated dental system was used; in this case an MDM Quantiflex head for gas delivery, installed on a hospital piped medical gas supply with active scavenging via a Porter-Brown scavenging nasal hood.

For many children with MIH, the first permanent molars are deemed to be of poor "lifelong" prognosis. Dependent on their orthodontic assessment, removal of these teeth, correctly timed to allow the second permanent molars to come into the space, is the treatment of choice. Therefore, some children between the ages of 8 and 10 years of age undergo removal of all four first permanent molar teeth. These children are otherwise similar to the case presented but in this circumstance, whilst the same treatment options are presented, general anesthesia is more forcefully recommended.

Case 8

A 14-year-old girl was referred by her general dentist due to her severe dental anxiety and high caries rate. She is ASA1, 60 kg, and accompanied by her mother.

She complained of recurrent pain and abscess in the lower right area and has had several courses of antibiotics. She does not like the appearance of a carious and discolored upper central incisor. She reported that she is a needle phobic. She was keen to have a nice smile and requests "to be put to sleep."

She is an irregular attender, presenting on an emergency basis only. The referring dentist has written that he placed a temporary dressing of antibiotic/steroid paste in a lower right second permanent molar and that this had deep caries through to the pulp.

Clinical and radiographic examination confirmed there is caries present in multiple permanent teeth; one or two of the molars need extraction and an upper incisor needs root canal treatment. Throughout the examination she is jumpy and does not look the dentist in the eye.

The treatment options were discussed kindly and with care but delivered firmly and honestly, they included: (1) local anesthesia and behavior management, (2) LA with inhalation sedation, and (3) LA with IV sedation. She is informed that general anesthetic is not an option—it is really only for medically compromised or learning disability patients at this age. Furthermore, the procedures that she needs are too lengthy for one GA event and that root canal therapy may need more than one visit to complete. She was shown that she has a role in her care and that prevention, excellent tooth brushing at the very least, needs to be in place to facilitate the operative treatment and prevent repeat visits due to new disease.

Treatment was predicted to take four or five appointments; at each visit a quadrant would be treated and so fillings and possibly extractions would be performed. However, these sedation visits were scheduled to occur after prevention visits to the dental therapist.

(continued)

The patient knew that root canal therapy will be started under the sedation but that there was an expectation that once the pulp was removed from this tooth that she would manage to accept the final root canal therapy visits normally, without need for sedation.

Written consent was obtained and the family were given an information sheet that repeats the verbal instructions to attend with an escort and to eat a light meal. (Patients who attend having fasted are given a glucose drink in advance of the procedure.) The child's veins were checked and the best site indicated and the family were given topical anesthetic skin cream and instructed to apply this an hour or so before the sedation visit.

For each sedation visit the following was prepared in advance: midazolam ampoules 5 mg/5 mL; venflon cannula; 5/10 mL syringes; midazolam syringe labels. At each visit the child's blood pressure is checked and consent and medical history confirmed.

The venflon was inserted in the antecubital fossa or the dorsum of the hand, is taped in place and remains until the treatment is complete. The standard regimen is to infuse midazolam slowly, in 1 mg increments to begin with, wait 2 min, then infuse at 0.5 mg (1 mL) increments every 2 min or so until the signs of sedation are reached and then maintained. Usually a total dose of 5–7 mg is all that is required. The appointments last an hour.

No reversal agent was needed—this is not used routinely—due to having a shorter half-life and because the reversed patient is often tearful on emergence.

Alert clinical monitoring was augmented with a pulse oximeter. No mouth prop was used. The child was constantly reminded to keep her mouth open. There is a sedation trained dental nurse in support and the surgery is in a busy area with help and support available within easy calling distance. As well as mandatory resuscitation equipment there is Flumazenil 500 μg/5 mL (reversal agent) at hand. The unit is on an acute care site.

In the case notes, the following is recorded: midazolam batch number and expiry date; pre- and post-sedation blood pressure; time of start and finish of administration; dosage delivered; oxygen saturation; site of cannulation; overall behavior; and time of discharge.

The child recovered uneventfully after each visit and sits in a separate recovery area with the pulse oximeter still in place and the sedation nurse and the rest of the team within line of sight. A proforma to ensure complete data capture was used, similar to that presented earlier in this chapter.

References

1. Wilson S. Pharmacological management of the pediatric dental patient. Pediatr Dent. 2004;26(2):131–6.
2. U.S. Department of Health and Human Services. Oral health in America: a report of the surgeon general. Rockville, MD: Department of Health and Human Services, National Institute of Dental and Craniofacial Research, National Institutes of Health; 2000 [cited 26 Nov 2013]. Available from: http://www2.nidcr.nih.gov/sgr/sgrohweb/welcome.htm.
3. Berkowitz RJ. Mutans streptococci: acquisition and transmission. Pediatr Dent. 2006;28(2):106–9; discussion 192–8.
4. Caufield PW, Griffen AL. Dental caries. An infectious and transmissible disease. Pediatr Clin North Am. 2000;47(5):1001–19; v.
5. Chapman HR, Kirby-Turner NC. Dental fear in children–a proposed model. Br Dent J. 1999;187(8):408–12.
6. Versloot J, Veerkamp JS, Hoogstraten J. Children's self-reported pain at the dentist. Pain. 2008;137(2):389–94.
7. Houpt M. Project USAP 2000—use of sedative agents by pediatric dentists: a 15-year follow-up survey. Pediatr Dent. 2002;24(4):289–94.
8. Wilson S. A survey of the American Academy of Pediatric Dentistry membership: nitrous oxide and sedation. Pediatr Dent. 1996;18(4):287–93.
9. American Dental Association. American Dentist Association guidelines for teaching pain control and sedation to dentists and dental students: as adopted by the October 2007 ADA house of delegates. Chicago: American Dental Association; [cited 26 Nov 2013]. Available from: http://www.ada.org/sections/about/pdfs/anxiety_guidelines.pdf.
10. American Dental Association. American Dentist Association guidelines for the use of sedation and general anesthesia by dentists as adopted by the October 2012 ADA house of delegates. Chicago: American Dental Association; 2013. Available from: http://www.ada.org/sections/educationAndCareers/pdfs/anesthesia_use_guidelines.pdf.
11. American Academy of Pediatric, American Academy of Pediatric Dentistry. Guideline for monitoring and management of pediatric patients during and after sedation for diagnostic and therapeutic procedures. Chicago: American Academy of Pediatric Dentistry; [cited 26 Nov 2013]. Available from: http://www.aapd.org/media/Policies_Guidelines/G_Sedation.pdf.
12. Adair SM, Schafer TE, Rockman RA, Waller JL. Survey of behavior management teaching in predoctoral pediatric dentistry programs. Pediatr Dent. 2004;26(2):143–50.
13. Waggoner WF. Conscious sedation in predoctoral pediatric dentistry programs. J Dent Educ. 1986;50(4):225–9.
14. Wilson S, Farrell K, Griffen A, Coury D. Conscious sedation experiences in graduate pediatric dentistry programs. Pediatr Dent. 2001;23(4):307–14.
15. Cravero JP, Blike GT. Review of pediatric sedation. Anesth Analg. 2004;99(5):1355–64.
16. American Association of Pediatric Dentistry. Guideline on behavior guidance for the pediatric dental patients. 1990 (revised 2011). Available from: http://www.aapd.org/media/Policies_Guidelines/G_BehavGuide.pdf.
17. Wright GZ, Alpern GD. Variables influencing children's cooperative behavior at the first dental visit. ASDC J Dent Child. 1971;38(2):124–8.
18. Klingberg G, Broberg AG. Dental fear/anxiety and dental behaviour management problems in children and adolescents: a review of prevalence and concomitant psychological factors. Int J Paediatr Dent. 2007;17(6):391–406.

19. Gustafsson A, Broberg A, Bodin L, Berggren U, Arnrup K. Dental behaviour management problems: the role of child personal characteristics. Int J Paediatr Dent. 2010;20(4):242–53.
20. Arnrup K, Broberg AG, Berggren U, Bodin L. Treatment outcome in subgroups of uncooperative child dental patients: an exploratory study. Int J Paediatr Dent. 2003;13(5):304–19.
21. Jensen B, Stjernqvist K. Temperament and acceptance of dental treatment under sedation in preschool children. Acta Odontol Scand. 2002;60(4):231–6.
22. Lochary ME. Temperament as a predictor of behavior for conscious sedation in dentistry. Pediatr Dent. 1993;15(5):348–52.
23. Wilson S. A review of important elements in sedation study methodology. Pediatr Dent. 1995;17(7):406–12.
24. Houpt MI, Weiss NJ, Koenigsberg SR, Desjardins PJ. Comparison of chloral hydrate with and without promethazine in the sedation of young children. Pediatr Dent. 1985;7(1):41–6.
25. Badalaty MM, Houpt MI, Koenigsberg SR, Maxwell KC, DesJardins PJ. A comparison of chloral hydrate and diazepam sedation in young children. Pediatr Dent. 1990;12(1):33–7.
26. Chowdhury J, Vargas KG. Comparison of chloral hydrate, meperidine, and hydroxyzine to midazolam regimens for oral sedation of pediatric dental patients. Pediatr Dent. 2005; 27(3):191–7.
27. Fishbaugh DF, Wilson S, Preisch JW, Weaver II JM. Relationship of tonsil size on an airway blockage maneuver in children during sedation. Pediatr Dent. 1997;19(4):277–81.
28. Leelataweedwud P, Vann Jr WF. Adverse events and outcomes of conscious sedation for pediatric patients: study of an oral sedation regimen. J Am Dent Assoc. 2001;132(11):1531–9; quiz 1596.
29. Marshall WR, Weaver BD, McCutcheon P. A study of the effectiveness of oral midazolam as a dental pre-operative sedative and hypnotic. Spec Care Dentist. 1999;19(6):259–66.
30. Martinez D, Wilson S. Children sedated for dental care: a pilot study of the 24-hour postsedation period. Pediatr Dent. 2006;28(3):260–4.
31. Musial KM, Wilson S, Preisch J, Weaver J. Comparison of the efficacy of oral midazolam alone versus midazolam and meperidine in the pediatric dental patient. Pediatr Dent. 2003;25(5): 468–74.
32. Religa ZC, Wilson S, Ganzberg SI, Casamassimo PS. Association between bispectral analysis and level of conscious sedation of pediatric dental patients. Pediatr Dent. 2002;24(3):221–6.
33. Sanders BJ, Potter RH, Avery DR. The effect of sleep on conscious sedation. J Clin Pediatr Dent. 1994;18(3):211–4.
34. Shapira J, Holan G, Botzer E, Kupietzky A, Kupieztky A, Tal E, et al. The effectiveness of midazolam and hydroxyzine as sedative agents for young pediatric dental patients. ASDC J Dent Child. 1996;63(6):421–5.
35. Wilson KE, Girdler NM, Welbury RR. Randomized, controlled, cross-over clinical trial comparing intravenous midazolam sedation with nitrous oxide sedation in children undergoing dental extractions. Br J Anaesth. 2003;91(6):850–6.
36. Wilson S. Chloral hydrate and its effects on multiple physiological parameters in young children: a dose-response study. Pediatr Dent. 1992;14(3):171–7.
37. Wilson S. Facial electromyography and chloral hydrate in the young dental patient. Pediatr Dent. 1993;15(5):343–7.
38. Brandes DA, Wilson S, Preisch JW, Casamassimo PS. A comparison of opinions from parents of disabled and non-disabled children on behavior management techniques used in dentistry. Spec Care Dentist. 1995;15(3):119–23.
39. Fuks AB, Kaufman E, Ram D, Hovav S, Shapira J. Assessment of two doses of intranasal midazolam for sedation of young pediatric dental patients. Pediatr Dent. 1994;16(4):301–5.
40. Houpt M, Manetas C, Joshi A, Desjardins P. Effects of chloral hydrate on nitrous oxide sedation of children. Pediatr Dent. 1989;11(1):26–9.
41. Houpt MI, Kupietzky A, Tofsky NS, Koenigsberg SR. Effects of nitrous oxide on diazepam sedation of young children. Pediatr Dent. 1996;18(3):236–41.
42. Lam C, Udin RD, Malamed SF, Good DL, Forrest JL. Midazolam premedication in children: a pilot study comparing intramuscular and intranasal administration. Anesth Prog. 2005;52(2):56–61.
43. Meyer ML, Mourino AP, Farrington FH. Comparison of triazolam to a chloral hydrate/hydroxyzine combination in the sedation of pediatric dental patients. Pediatr Dent. 1990;12(5):283–7.
44. Poorman TL, Farrington FH, Mourino AP. Comparison of a chloral hydrate/hydroxyzine combination with and without meperidine in the sedation of pediatric dental patients. Pediatr Dent. 1990;12(5):288–91.
45. Ram D, Mamber E, Chosack A, Fuks AB. The effect of metoclopramide and hydroxyzine in sedation of infants undergoing dental treatment. ASDC J Dent Child. 1999;66(1):49–52, 13.
46. Shapira J, Kupietzky A, Kadari A, Fuks AB, Holan G. Comparison of oral midazolam with and without hydroxyzine in the sedation of pediatric dental patients. Pediatr Dent. 2004;26(6):492–6.
47. Sharma RK, Pinto RR, Mirchandani NN. Use of sedation analgesia for pediatric dentistry. J Indian Soc Pedod Prev Dent. 1992;10(1):28–32.
48. Vargas KG, Nathan JE, Qian F, Kupietzky A. Use of restraint and management style as parameters for defining sedation success: a survey of pediatric dentists. Pediatr Dent. 2007;29(3):220–7.
49. Cote CJ, Wilson S. Guidelines for monitoring and management of pediatric patients during and after sedation for diagnostic and therapeutic procedures: an update. Pediatrics. 2006;118(6): 2587–602.
50. Acs G, Musson CA, Burke MJ. Current teaching of restraint and sedation in pediatric dentistry: a survey of program directors. Pediatr Dent. 1990;12(6):364–7.
51. Adair SM, Waller JL, Schafer TE, Rockman RA. A survey of members of the American Academy of Pediatric Dentistry on their use of behavior management techniques. Pediatr Dent. 2004;26(2):159–66.
52. Houpt M. Report of project USAP: the use of sedative agents in pediatric dentistry. ASDC J Dent Child. 1989;56(4):302–9.
53. Houpt M. Project USAP the use of sedative agents in pediatric dentistry: 1991 update. Pediatr Dent. 1993;15(1):36–40.
54. Tarver M, Guelmann M, Primosch R. Impact of office-based intravenous deep sedation providers upon traditional sedation practices employed in pediatric dentistry. Pediatr Dent. 2012;34(3):62–8.
55. Olabi NF, Jones JE, Saxen MA, Sanders BJ, Walker LA, Weddell JA, et al. The use of office-based sedation and general anesthesia by board certified pediatric dentists practicing in the United States. Anesth Prog. 2012;59(1):12–7.
56. Ozer L, Oktem ZB, Kucukyavuz Z. Effects of deep sedation on behaviors and side effects in children undergoing different dental procedures. Pediatr Dent. 2011;33(2):158–64.
57. Messieha Z, Cruz-Gonzalez W, Hakim MI. Retrospective outcomes evaluation of 100 parenteral moderate and deep sedations conducted in a general practice dental residency. Anesth Prog. 2008;55(4):116–20.
58. Lee JS, Gonzalez ML, Chuang SK, Perrott DH. Comparison of methohexital and propofol use in ambulatory procedures in oral and maxillofacial surgery. J Oral Maxillofac Surg. 2008;66(10):1996–2003.
59. Rai K, Hegde AM, Goel K. Sedation in uncooperative children undergoing dental procedures: a comparative evaluation of midazolam, propofol and ketamine. J Clin Pediatr Dent. 2007;32(1):1–4.
60. Wood M. The use of intravenous midazolam and ketamine in paediatric dental sedation. SAAD Dig. 2013;29:18–30.
61. Khattab AM, El-Seify ZA, Shaaban A, Radojevic D, Jankovic I. Sevoflurane-emergence agitation: effect of supplementary low-dose oral ketamine premedication in preschool children undergoing dental surgery. Eur J Anaesthesiol. 2010;27(4):353–8.

62. Cathers JW, Wilson CF, Webb MD, Alvarez ME, Schiffman T, Taylor S. A comparison of two meperidine/hydroxyzine sedation regimens for the uncooperative pediatric dental patient. Pediatr Dent. 2005;27(5):395–400.
63. Chen JW, Seybold SV, Yazdi H. Assessment of the effects of 2 sedation regimens on cardiopulmonary parameters in pediatric dental patients: a retrospective study. Pediatr Dent. 2006;28(4):350–6.
64. Roberts SM, Wilson CF, Seale NS, McWhorter AG. Evaluation of morphine as compared to meperidine when administered to the moderately anxious pediatric dental patient. Pediatr Dent. 1992;14(5):306–13.
65. Song YU, Webb MD. Comparison of the effect of orally versus submucosally administered meperidine on the behavior of pediatric dental patients: a retrospective study. Anesth Prog. 2003;50(3):129–33.
66. Bhatnagar S, Das UM, Bhatnagar G. Comparison of oral midazolam with oral tramadol, triclofos and zolpidem in the sedation of pediatric dental patients: an in vivo study. J Indian Soc Pedod Prev Dent. 2012;30(2):109–14.
67. Golpayegani MV, Dehghan F, Ansari G, Shayeghi S. Comparison of oral midazolam-ketamine and midazolam-promethazine as sedative agents in pediatric dentistry. Dent Res J. 2012;9(1):36–40.
68. Isik B, Baygin O, Kapci EG, Bodur H. The effects of temperament and behaviour problems on sedation failure in anxious children after midazolam premedication. Eur J Anaesthesiol. 2010;27(4):336–40.
69. Pandey RK, Padmanabhan MY, Saksena AK, Chandra G. Midazolam-fentanyl analgo-sedation in pediatric dental patients–a pilot study. J Clin Pediatr Dent. 2010;35(1):105–10.
70. Sams DR, Cook EW, Jackson JG, Roebuck BL. Behavioral assessments of two drug combinations for oral sedation. Pediatr Dent. 1993;15(3):186–90.
71. Alfonzo-Echever EC, et al. Oral ketamine for pediatric outpatient dental surgery sedation. Pediatr Dent. 1993;15(3):182–5.
72. Avalos-Arenas V, Moyao-Garcia D, Nava-Ocampo AA, Zayas-Carranza RE, Fragoso-Rios R. Is chloral hydrate/hydroxyzine a good option for paediatric dental outpatient sedation? Curr Med Res Opin. 1998;14(4):219–26.
73. Campbell RL, Ross GA, Campbell JR, Mourino AP. Comparison of oral chloral hydrate with intramuscular ketamine, meperidine, and promethazine for pediatric sedation–preliminary report. Anesth Prog. 1998;45(2):46–50.
74. Croswell RJ, Dilley DC, Lucas WJ, Vann Jr WF. A comparison of conventional versus electronic monitoring of sedated pediatric dental patients. Pediatr Dent. 1995;17(5):332–9.
75. Dallman JA, Ignelzi Jr MA, Briskie DM. Comparing the safety, efficacy and recovery of intranasal midazolam vs. oral chloral hydrate and promethazine. Pediatr Dent. 2001;23(5):424–30.
76. Duncan WK, De Ball S, Perkins TM. Chloral hydrate sedation: a simple technique. Compendium. 1994;15(7):884; 886–8; 890 passim; quiz 894.
77. Haas DA, Nenniger SA, Yacobi R, Magathan JG, Grad HA, Copp PE, et al. A pilot study of the efficacy of oral midazolam for sedation in pediatric dental patients. Anesth Prog. 1996;43(1):1–8.
78. Haney KL, McWhorter AG, Seale NS. An assessment of the success of meperidine and promethazine sedation in medically compromised children. ASDC J Dent Child. 1993;60(4–5):288–94.
79. Hasty MF, Vann Jr WF, Dilley DC, Anderson JA. Conscious sedation of pediatric dental patients: an investigation of chloral hydrate, hydroxyzine pamoate, and meperidine vs. chloral hydrate and hydroxyzine pamoate. Pediatr Dent. 1991;13(1):10–9.
80. Leelataweewud P, Vann WF, Dilley DC, Lucas WJ. The physiological effects of supplemental oxygen versus nitrous oxide/oxygen during conscious sedation of pediatric dental patients. Pediatr Dent. 2000;22(2):125–33.
81. McCann W, Wilson S, Larsen P, Stehle B. The effects of nitrous oxide on behavior and physiological parameters during conscious sedation with a moderate dose of chloral hydrate and hydroxyzine. Pediatr Dent. 1996;18(1):35–41.
82. Moody Jr EH, Mourino AP, Campbell RL. The therapeutic effectiveness of nitrous oxide and chloral hydrate administered orally, rectally, and combined with hydroxyzine for pediatric dentistry. ASDC J Dent Child. 1986;53(6):425–9.
83. Nathan JE, Vargas KG. Oral midazolam with and without meperidine for management of the difficult young pediatric dental patient: a retrospective study. Pediatr Dent. 2002;24(2):129–38.
84. Nathan JE, West MS. Comparison of chloral hydrate-hydroxyzine with and without meperidine for management of the difficult pediatric-patient. J Dent Child. 1987;54(6):437–44.
85. Needleman HL, Joshi A, Griffith DG. Conscious sedation of pediatric dental patients using chloral hydrate, hydroxyzine, and nitrous oxide—a retrospective study of 382 sedations. Pediatr Dent. 1995;17(7):424–31.
86. Reeves ST, Wiedenfeld KR, Wrobleski J, Hardin CL, Pinosky ML. A randomized double-blind trial of chloral hydrate/hydroxyzine versus midazolam/acetaminophen in the sedation of pediatric dental outpatients. ASDC J Dent Child. 1996;63(2):95–100.
87. Rohlfing GK, Dilley DC, Lucas WJ, Vann Jr WF. The effect of supplemental oxygen on apnea and oxygen saturation during pediatric conscious sedation. Pediatr Dent. 1998;20(1):8–16.
88. Sams DR, Thornton JB, Wright JT. The assessment of two oral sedation drug regimens in pediatric dental patients. ASDC J Dent Child. 1992;59(4):306–12.
89. Sanders BJ, Avery DR. The effect of sleep on conscious sedation: a follow-up study [published erratum appears in J Clin Pediatr Dent 1997 Summer;21(4):356]. J Clin Pediatr Dent. 1997;21(2):131–4.
90. Wilson S, Molina Lde L, Preisch J, Weaver J. The effect of electronic dental anesthesia on behavior during local anesthetic injection in the young, sedated dental patient. Pediatr Dent. 1999;21(1):12–7.
91. Wilson S, Easton J, Lamb K, Orchardson R, Casamassimo P. A retrospective study of chloral hydrate, meperidine, hydroxyzine, and midazolam regimens used to sedate children for dental care. Pediatr Dent. 2000;22(2):107–12.
92. Alhashemi JA, Daghistani MF. Effect of intraoperative intravenous acetaminophen vs. intramuscular meperidine on pain and discharge time after paediatric dental restoration. Eur J Anaesthesiol. 2007;24(2):128–33.
93. Cote CJ, Karl HW, Notterman DA, Weinberg JA, McCloskey C. Adverse sedation events in pediatrics: analysis of medications used for sedation. Pediatrics. 2000;106(4):633–44.
94. Davila JM, Herman HE, Proskin HM, Vitale D. Comparison of the sedative effectiveness of two pharmacological regimens. J Dent Child. 1994;61(4):276–81.
95. Erlandsson AL, Backman B, Stenstrom A, Stecksen-Blicks C. Conscious sedation by oral administration of midazolam in paediatric dental treatment. Swed Dent J. 2001;25(3):97–104.
96. Fukuta O, Braham RL, Yanase H, Atsumi N, Kurosu K. The sedative effect of intranasal midazolam administration in the dental treatment of patients with mental disabilities. Part 1. The effect of a 0.2 mg/kg dose. J Clin Pediatr Dent. 1993;17(4):231–7.
97. Fukuta O, Braham RL, Yanase H, Kurosu K. The sedative effects of intranasal midazolam administration in the dental treatment of patients with mental disabilities. Part 2: optimal concentration of intranasal midazolam. J Clin Pediatr Dent. 1994;18(4):259–65.
98. Hartgraves PM, Primosch RE. An evaluation of oral and nasal midazolam for pediatric dental sedation. ASDC J Dent Child. 1994;61(3):175–81.
99. Hulland SA, Freilich MM, Sandor GK. Nitrous oxide-oxygen or oral midazolam for pediatric outpatient sedation. Oral Surg Oral Med Oral Pathol Oral Radiol Endod. 2002;93(6):643–6.

100. Iwasaki J, Vann Jr WF, Dilley DC, Anderson JA. An investigation of capnography and pulse oximetry as monitors of pediatric patients sedated for dental treatment. Pediatr Dent. 1989;11(2):111–7.
101. Kantovitz KR, Puppin-Rontani RM, Gaviao MBD. Sedative effect of oral diazepam and chloral hydrate in the dental treatment of children. J Indian Soc Pedod Prev Dent. 2007;25(2):69–75.
102. Kil N, Zhu JF, VanWagnen C, Abdulhamid I. The effects of midazolam on pediatric patients with asthma. Pediatr Dent. 2003;25(2):137–42.
103. Krafft TC, Kramer N, Kunzelmann KH, Hickel R. Experience with midazolam as sedative in the dental treatment of uncooperative children. ASDC J Dent Child. 1993;60(4-5):295–9.
104. Kupietzky A, Holan G, Shapira J. Intranasal midazolam better at effecting amnesia after sedation than oral hydroxyzine: a pilot study. Pediatr Dent. 1996;18(1):32–4.
105. Lima AR, da Costa LR, da Costa PS. A randomized, controlled, crossover trial of oral midazolam and hydroxyzine for pediatric dental sedation. Pesqui Odontol Bras. 2003;17(3):206–11.
106. Lloyd CJ, Alredy T, Lowry JC. Intranasal midazolam as an alternative to general anaesthesia in the management of children with oral and maxillofacial trauma. Br J Oral Maxillofac Surg. 2000;38(6):593–5.
107. Myers GR, Maestrello CL, Mourino AP, Best AM. Effect of submucosal midazolam on behavior and physiologic response when combined with oral chloral hydrate and nitrous oxide sedation. Pediatr Dent. 2004;26(1):37–43.
108. Pisalchaiyong T, Trairatvorakul C, Jirakijja J, Yuktarnonda W. Comparison of the effectiveness of oral diazepam and midazolam for the sedation of autistic patients during dental treatment. Pediatr Dent. 2005;27(3):198–206.
109. Roelofse JA, Joubert JJ, Roelofse PG. A double-blind randomized comparison of midazolam alone and midazolam combined with ketamine for sedation of pediatric dental patients. J Oral Maxillofac Surg. 1996;54(7):838–44; discussion 845–6.
110. Silver T, Wilson C, Webb M. Evaluation of two dosages of oral midazolam as a conscious sedation for physically and neurologically compromised pediatric dental patients. Pediatr Dent. 1994;16(5):350–9.
111. Singh N, Pandey RK, Saksena AK, Jaiswal JN. A comparative evaluation of oral midazolam with other sedatives as premedication in pediatric dentistry. J Clin Pediatr Dent. 2002;26(2):161–4.
112. Tamura M, Nakamura K, Kitamura R, Kitagawa S, Mori N, Ueda Y. Oral premedication with fentanyl may be a safe and effective alternative to oral midazolam. Eur J Anaesth. 2003;20(6): 482–6.
113. Torres-Perez J, Tapia-Garcia I, Rosales-Berber MA, Hernandez-Sierra JF, Pozos-Guillen Ade J. Comparison of three conscious sedation regimens for pediatric dental patients. J Clin Pediatr Dent. 2007;31(3):183–6.
114. Wan K, Jing Q, Zhao J-Z. Evaluation of oral midazolam as conscious sedation for pediatric patients in oral restoration. Chin Med Sci J. 2006;21(3):163–6.
115. Karl HW, Milgrom P, Domoto P, Kharasch ED, Coldwell SE, Weinstein P, et al. Pharmacokinetics of oral triazolam in children. J Clin Psychopharmacol. 1997;17(3):169–72.
116. Quarnstrom FC, Milgrom P, Moore PA. Experience with triazolam in preschool children. Anesth Pain Control Dent. 1992;1(3): 157–9.
117. Smith BM, Cutilli BJ, Saunders W. Oral midazolam: pediatric conscious sedation. Compend Contin Educ Dent. 1998;19(6):586–88; 590; 592.
118. Abrams R, Morrison JE, Villasenor A, Hencmann D, Da Fonseca M, Mueller W. Safety and effectiveness of intranasal administration of sedative medications (ketamine, midazolam, or sufentanil) for urgent brief pediatric dental procedures. Anesth Prog. 1993;40(3):63–6.
119. Alderson PJ, Lerman J. Oral premedication for paediatric ambulatory anaesthesia: a comparison of midazolam and ketamine. Can J Anaesth. 1994;41(3):221–6.
120. Okamoto GU, Duperon DF, Jedrychowski JR. Clinical evaluation of the effects of ketamine sedation on pediatric dental patients. J Clin Pediatr Dent. 1992;16(4):253–7.
121. Reinemer HC, Wilson CF, Webb MD. A comparison of two oral ketamine-diazepam regimens for sedating anxious pediatric dental patients. Pediatr Dent. 1996;18(4):294–300.
122. Roelofse JA, Joubert JJ, Swart LC, Stander I, Roelofse PG. An evaluation of the effect of oral ketamine and standard oral premedication in the sedation of paediatric dental patients. J Dent Assoc S Afr. 1996;51(4):197–201.
123. Roelofse JA, Louw LR, Roelofse PG. A double blind randomized comparison of oral trimeprazine-methadone and ketamine-midazolam for sedation of pediatric dental patients for oral surgical procedures. Anesth Prog. 1998;45(1):3–11.
124. Sullivan DC, Wilson CF, Webb MD. A comparison of two oral ketamine-diazepam regimens for the sedation of anxious pediatric dental patients. Pediatr Dent. 2001;23(3):223–31.
125. van der Bijl P, Roelofse JA, Stander IA. Rectal ketamine and midazolam for premedication in pediatric dentistry. J Oral Maxillofac Surg. 1991;49(10):1050–4.
126. Bahetwar SK, Pandey RK, Saksena AK, Chandra G. A comparative evaluation of intranasal midazolam, ketamine and their combination for sedation of young uncooperative pediatric dental patients: a triple blind randomized crossover trial. J Clin Pediatr Dent. 2011;35(4):415–20.
127. Barr EB, Wynn RL. IV sedation in pediatric dentistry: an alternative to general anesthesia. Pediatr Dent. 1992;14(4):251–5.
128. Cagiran E, Eyigor C, Sipahi A, Koca H, Balcioglu T, Uyar M. Comparison of oral midazolam and midazolam-ketamine as sedative agents in paediatric dentistry. Eur J Paediatr Dent. 2010;11(1):19–22.
129. Downs AT, Dembo J, Ferretti G, Lyons TD, Pelphery A. A comparative study of midazolam to meperidine/promethazine as an IM sedative technique for the pediatric dental patient. J Dent Child. 1997;64(3):197–200.
130. Koroluk LD. Dental anxiety in adolescents with a history of childhood dental sedation. ASDC J Dent Child. 2000;67(3):200–205; 161.
131. Lu D, Lu G, Reed J III. Safety, efficacy, and acceptance of intramuscular sedation: assessment of 900 dental cases. Compendium. 1994;15(11):1348; 1350; 1352 passim; quiz 1362.
132. Milnes AR. Intravenous procedural sedation: an alternative to general anesthesia in the treatment of early childhood caries. J Can Dent Assoc. 2003;69(5):298–302.
133. Milnes AR, Maupome G, Cannon J. Intravenous sedation in pediatric dentistry using midazolam, nalbuphine and droperidol. Pediatr Dent. 2000;22(2):113–9.
134. Stephens AJ, Sapsford DJ, Curzon ME. Intravenous sedation for handicapped dental patients: a clinical trial of midazolam and propofol. Br Dent J. 1993;175(1):20–5.
135. Veerkamp JS, Porcelijn T, Gruythuysen RJ. Intravenous sedation for outpatient treatment of child dental patients: an exploratory study. ASDC J Dent Child. 1997;64(1):48–54.
136. al-Rakaf H, Bello LL, Turkustani A, Adenubi JO. Intra-nasal midazolam in conscious sedation of young paediatric dental patients. Int J Paediatr Dent. 2001;11(1):33–40.
137. Fukuta O, Braham RL, Yanase H, Kurosu K. Intranasal administration of midazolam: pharmacokinetic and pharmacodynamic properties and sedative potential. ASDC J Dent Child. 1997;64(2):89–98.
138. Lee-Kim SJ, Fadavi S, Punwani I, Koerber A. Nasal versus oral midazolam sedation for pediatric dental patients. J Dent Child (Chic). 2004;71(2):126–30.

139. Primosch RE, Bender F. Factors associated with administration route when using midazolam for pediatric conscious sedation. J Dent Child. 2001;68(4):233–8.
140. Al-Zahrani AM, Wyne AH, Sheta SA. Comparison of oral midazolam with a combination of oral midazolam and nitrous oxide-oxygen inhalation in the effectiveness of dental sedation for young children. J Indian Soc Pedod Prev Dent. 2009;27(1):9–16.
141. Heard C, Smith J, Creighton P, Joshi P, Feldman D, Lerman J. A comparison of four sedation techniques for pediatric dental surgery. Paediatr Anaesth. 2010;20(10):924–30.
142. Ozen B, Malamed SF, Cetiner S, Ozalp N, Ozer L, Altun C. Outcomes of moderate sedation in paediatric dental patients. Aust Dent J. 2012;57(2):144–50.
143. Johnson E, Briskie D, Majewski R, Edwards S, Reynolds P. The physiologic and behavioral effects of oral and intranasal midazolam in pediatric dental patients. Pediatr Dent. 2010;32(3):229–38.
144. Klein U, Bucklin BA, Poulton TJ, Bozinov D. Nitrous oxide concentrations in the posterior nasopharynx during administration by nasal mask. Pediatr Dent. 2004;26(5):410–6.
145. Guo TZ, Poree L, Golden W, Stein J, Fujinaga M, Maze M. Antinociceptive response to nitrous oxide is mediated by supraspinal opiate and spinal alpha(2) adrenergic receptors in the rat. Anesthesiology. 1996;85(4):846–52.
146. Roberts GJ, Wignall BK. Efficacy of the laryngeal reflex during oxygen-nitrous oxide sedation (relative analgesia). Br J Anaesth. 1982;54(12):1277–81.
147. Houck WR, Ripa LW. Vomiting frequency in children administered nitrous oxide-oxygen in analgesic doses. ASDC J Dent Child. 1971;28(6):404–6.
148. Kupietzky A, Tal E, Shapira J, Ram D. Fasting state and episodes of vomiting in children receiving nitrous oxide for dental treatment. Pediatr Dent. 2008;30(5):414–9.
149. Malamed SF. An update on pain and anxiety control in pediatric dentistry. Part II Inhalation sedation and local anesthesia. Alpha Omegan. 1979;72(2):29–33.
150. Houpt M. Death following oral sedation. ASDC J Dent Child. 1988;55(2):123–4.
151. Jastak JT, Pallasch T. Death after chloral hydrate sedation: report of case. J Am Dent Assoc. 1988;116(3):345–8.
152. Cote CJ, Notterman DA, Karl HW, Weinberg JA, McCloskey C. Adverse sedation events in pediatrics: a critical incident analysis of contributing factors. Pediatrics. 2000;105(4 Pt 1): 805–14.
153. Chicka MC, Dembo JB, Mathu-Muju KR, Nash DA, Bush HM. Adverse events during pediatric dental anesthesia and sedation: a review of closed malpractice insurance claims. Pediatr Dent. 2012;34(3):231–8.
154. Lee HH, Milgrom P, Starks H, Burke W. Trends in death associated with pediatric dental sedation and general anesthesia. Paediatr Anaesth. 2013;23(8):741–6.
155. Anonymous. Consensus development conference statement on anesthesia and sedation in the dental office. National Institutes of Health. J Am Dent Assoc. 1985;111(1):90–3.
156. Anonymous. Guidelines for the elective use of conscious sedation, deep sedation, and general anesthesia in pediatric patients. ASDC J Dent Child. 1986;53(1):21–2.
157. American Academy of Pediatric Dentistry. Guidelines for the elective use of conscious sedation, deep sedation, and general-anesthesia in pediatric-patients. Pediatrics. 1985;76(2):317–21.
158. Cote CJ. Sedation protocols–why so many variations? Pediatrics. 1994;94(3):281–3.
159. Cote CJ. Sedation for the pediatric patient. A review. Pediatr Clin North Am. 1994;41(1):31–58.
160. Yagiela JA. Making patients safe and comfortable for a lifetime of dentistry: frontiers in office-based sedation. J Dent Educ. 2001;65(12):1348–56.
161. Caputo AC. Providing deep sedation and general anesthesia for patients with special needs in the dental office-based setting. Spec Care Dentist. 2009;29(1):26–30.
162. Oulis C, Hosey MT, Martens L, Hammer D, Martínez J, Raya A. The use of nitrous oxide inhalation sedation in dentistry. CED RESOLUTION. 2012. Available from: https://www.omd.pt/noticias/2012/06/201205cedsedacaoconsciente.pdf.
163. Matharu L, Ashley PF. Sedation of anxious children undergoing dental treatment. Cochrane Database Syst Rev. 2006;(1): CD003877.
164. Wilson KE, Welbury RR, Girdler NM. A randomised, controlled, crossover trial of oral midazolam and nitrous oxide for paediatric dental sedation. Anaesthesia. 2002;57(9):860–7.
165. Wilson KE, Welbury RR, Girdler NM. Comparison of transmucosal midazolam with inhalation sedation for dental extractions in children. A randomized, cross-over, clinical trial. Acta Anaesthesiol Scand. 2007;51(8):1062–7.
166. Pitts N, Evans D, Nugent Z. The dental caries experience of 5-year-old children in Great Britain 1999/2000. Community Dent Health. 2001;18:49–55.
167. Steele J, Lader D. Social factors and oral health in children; children's dental health in the UK, 2003. London: Office of National Statistics; 2004.
168. Innes NP, Evans DJ, Stirrups DR. The hall technique; a randomized controlled clinical trial of a novel method of managing carious primary molars in general dental practice: acceptability of the technique and outcomes at 23 months. BMC Oral Health. 2007;7:18.
169. Ricketts DN, Kidd EA, Innes N, Clarkson J. Complete or ultraconservative removal of decayed tissue in unfilled teeth. Cochrane Database Syst Rev. 2006;(3):CD003808.
170. Cripps T, Debuse D, Girdler N, Hayward R, Holden C, Hosey M, et al. Standards for conscious sedation-report of an independent expert working group. London: SAAD; 2000.
171. Dental Sedation Teachers Group. Standards in conscious sedation for dentistry: dental sedation. 2000. Available from: www.dstg.co.uk.
172. Association of Pediatric Anesthetists of Great Britain and Ireland and Royal College of Anesthetists, Adewale L, Morton N, Blayney M. Guidelines for the management of children referred for dental extractions under general anesthesia. 2011. Available from: http://www.rcoa.ac.uk/system/files/PUB-DentalExtractions.pdf.
173. Poswillo D. General anaesthesia, sedation and resuscitation in Dentistry Advisory Committee March 1990 (AKA the Poswillo report). S.D.A.C.O.T. Department of Health. 1990.
174. Department of Health. A conscious decision: a review of the use of general anesthesia and conscious sedation in primary dental care. London: Department of Health; 2000. Available from: http://webarchive.nationalarchives.gov.uk/20130107105354/http://www.dh.gov.uk/prod_consum_dh/groups/dh_digitalassets/@dh/@en/documents/digitalasset/dh_4019200.pdf.
175. American Society of Anesthesiologists. Continuum of depth of sedation. Definition of general anesthesia and levels of sedation/analgesia. 2009.
176. Blain KM, Hill FJ. The use of inhalation sedation and local anaesthesia as an alternative to general anaesthesia for dental extractions in children. Br Dent J. 1998;184(12):608–11.
177. Hosey MT, Bryce J, Harris P, McHugh S, Campbell C. The behaviour, social status and number of teeth extracted in children under general anaesthesia: a referral centre revisited. Br Dent J. 2006;200(6):331–4; discussion 327.
178. Macpherson LM, Pine CM, Tochel C, Burnside G, Hosey MT, Adair P. Factors influencing referral of children for dental extractions under general and local anaesthesia. Community Dent Health. 2005;22(4):282–8.
179. Robb ND, Hosey MT, Leitch JA. Intravenous conscious sedation in patients under 16 years of age. Fact or fiction? Br Dent J. 2003;194(9):469–71.

180. Hosey MT. UK national clinical guidelines in paediatric dentistry. Managing anxious children: the use of conscious sedation in paediatric dentistry. Int J Paediatr Dent. 2002;12(5):359–72.
181. Hosey MT, Macpherson LMD, Adair P, Tochel C, Burnside G, Pine C. Dental anxiety, distress at induction and postoperative morbidity in children undergoing tooth extraction using general anaesthesia. Br Dent J. 2006;200(1):39–43.
182. Kain Z, Wang S, Mayes L, Caramico L, Hofstadter M. Sleeping characteristics of children undergoing outpatient elective surgery. Anesthiology. 2002;97(5):1093–101.
183. Kain ZN, Mayes LC, O'Connor TZ, Cicchetti DV. Preoperative anxiety in children. Predictors and outcomes. Arch Pediatr Adolesc Med. 1996;150(12):1238–45.
184. Kain ZN, Wang SM, Mayes LC, Caramico LA, Hofstadter MB. Distress during the induction of anesthesia and postoperative behavioral outcomes. Anesth Analg. 1999;88(5):1042–7.
185. Lumley MA, Melamed BG, Abeles LA. Predicting children's presurgical anxiety and subsequent behavior changes. J Pediatr Psychol. 1993;18(4):481–97.
186. Millar K, Asbury AJ, Bowman AW, Hosey MT, Musiello T, Welbury RR. The effects of brief sevoflurane-nitrous oxide anaesthesia upon children's postoperative cognition and behaviour. Anaesthesia. 2006;61(6):541–7.
187. Wright K, Stewart S, Finley G, Buffett-Jerrott S. Prevention and intervention strategies to alleviate preoperative anxiety in children: a critical review. Behav Modif. 2007;31(1):52–79.
188. Campbell C, Hosey MT, McHugh S. Facilitating coping behavior in children prior to dental general anesthesia: a randomized controlled trial. Pediatr Anesth. 2005;15(10):831–8.
189. O'Byrne KK, Peterson L, Saldana L. Survey of pediatric hospitals' preparation programs: evidence of the impact of health psychology research. Health Psychol. 1997;16(2):147–54.
190. Yip P, Middleton P, Cyna AM, Carlyle AV. Non-pharmacological interventions for assisting the induction of anaesthesia in children. Cochrane Database Syst Rev. 2009;(3):CD006447.
191. Hosey M, Asbury J, Bowman A, Millar K, Martin K, Musiello T, et al. The effect of trans mucosal 0.2 mg/kg midazolam premedication on dental anxiety, an aesthetic induction and psychological morbidity in children undergoing general anesthesia for tooth extraction. Br Dent J. 2009;1:E2.
192. Howell TK, Smith S, Rushman SC, Walker RW, Radivan F. A comparison of oral transmucosal fentanyl and oral midazolam for premedication in children. Anaesthesia. 2002;57(8):798–805.
193. Lonnqvist PA, Habre W. Midazolam as a premedication: is the emperor naked or just half dressed? Pediatr Aneasth. 2005;15:263–5.
194. Millar K, Asbury AJ, Bowman AW, Hosey MT, Martin K, Musiello T, et al. A randomised placebo-controlled trial of the effects of midazolam premedication on children's postoperative cognition. Anaesthesia. 2007;62(9):923–30.
195. Health Services Advisory Committee of the Health and Safety Commission. Anesthetic agents: controlling exposure under COSHH. London: HMSO: Health Services Advisory Committee of the Health and Safety Commission; 1995.
196. National Institute for Occupational Safety and Health. Control of nitrous oxide in dental operatories. Cincinnati: National Institute for Occupational Safety and Health (NIOSH); 1994. p. 94–129.
197. National Institute for Health and Clinical Excellence. Sedation in children and young people (CG112); sedation for diagnostic and therapeutic procedures in children and young people. 2010. Available from: http://guidance.nice.org.uk/CG112.
198. Cuthbert MI. A screening device. children at risk for dental fears and management problems. J Dent Child. 1982;49(6):432–6.
199. Wong HM, Humphris GM, Lee GT. Preliminary validation and reliability of the modified child dental anxiety scale. Psychol Rep. 1998;83(3 Pt 2):1179–86.
200. Aitken RC. Measurement of feelings using visual analogue scales. Proc R Soc Med. 1969;62(10):989–93.
201. Frankl S, Shiere F, Fogels H. Should the parent remain with the child in the operatory? J Dent Child. 1962;2:150–63.
202. Venham LL. The effect of mother's presence of child's response to dental treatment. ASDC J Dent Child. 1979;46(3):219–25.
203. Venham LL, Gaulin-Kremer E, Munster E, Bengston-Audia D, Cohan J. Interval rating scales for children's dental anxiety and uncooperative behavior. Pediatr Dent. 1980;2(3):195–202.
204. Melamed BG, Weinstein D, Katin-Borland M, Hawes R. Reduction of fear-related dental management problems with use of filmed modeling. J Am Dent Assoc. 1975;90(4):822–6.
205. Klingberg G. Children's dental fear picture test (CDFP): a projective test for the assessment of child dental fear. ASDC J Dent Child. 1994;61(2):89–96.
206. Buchanan H, Niven N. Validation of a Facial Image Scale to assess child dental anxiety. Int J Paediatr Dent. 2002;12(1):47–52.
207. Nazif M. Thioridazine and secobarbital as premedicating agents. ASDC J Dent Child. 1971;38(3):206–10.
208. Hosey MT, Blinkhorn AS. An evaluation of four methods of assessing the behaviour of anxious child dental patients. Int J Paediatr Dent. 1995;5(2):87–95.
209. Aartman IH, van Everdingen T, Hoogstraten J, Schuurs AH. Self-report measurements of dental anxiety and fear in children: a critical assessment. ASDC J Dent Child. 1998;65(4):252–8.
210. Corah NL, Gale EN, Illig SJ. Assessment of a dental anxiety scale. J Am Dent Assoc. 1978;97(5):816–9.
211. Arch LM, Humphris GM, Lee GT. Children choosing between general anaesthesia or inhalation sedation for dental extractions: the effect on dental anxiety. Int J Paediatr Dent. 2001; 11(1):41–8.
212. Humphris GM, Morrison T, Lindsay SJ. The modified dental anxiety scale: validation and United Kingdom norms. Community Dent Health. 1995;12(3):143–50.
213. Blayney MR, Ryan JD, Malins AF. Propofol target-controlled infusions for sedation—a safe technique for the non-anaesthetist? Br Dent J. 2003;194(8):450–2.
214. Marsh B, White M, Morton N, Kenny GN. Pharmacokinetic model driven infusion of propofol in children. Br J Anaesth. 1991;67(1):41–8.
215. Skipsey IG, Colvin JR, Mackenzie N, Kenny GN. Sedation with propofol during surgery under local blockade. Assessment of a target-controlled infusion system. Anaesthesia. 1993;48(3): 210–3.
216. Taylor I, White M, Kenny GN. Assessment of the value and pattern of use of a target controlled propofol infusion system. Int J Clin Monit Comput. 1993;10(3):175–80.
217. Oei-Lim LB, Vermeulen-Cranch DM, Bouvy-Berends EC. Conscious sedation with propofol in dentistry. Br Dent J. 1991;170(9):340–2.
218. Oei-Lim VL, Kalkman CJ, Makkes PC, Ooms WG, Hoogstraten J. Computer controlled infusion of propofol for conscious sedation in dental treatment. Br Dent J. 1997;183(6):204–8.
219. Hosey MT, Makin A, Jones R, Gilchrist F, Carruthers M. Propofol intravenous conscious sedation for anxious children in a specialist paediatric dentistry unit. Int J Paediatr Dent. 2004;14(1):2–8.
220. Alexopoulos E, Hope A, Clark SL, McHugh S, Hosey MT. A report on dental anxiety levels in children undergoing nitrous oxide inhalation sedation and propofol target controlled infusion intravenous sedation. Eur Arch Paediatr Dent. 2007;8(2):82–6.
221. Tan CH, Onsiong MK. Pain on injection of propofol. Anaesthesia. 1998;53(5):468–76.
222. Thomas JS, Boheimer NO. Amorous behaviour and sexual fantasies following anaesthesia or sedation. Med Leg J. 1990;58(Pt 3):157.
223. Zacharias M, Bridgman J, Parkinson R. Two methods of administration of propofol for dental sedation. Br J Oral Maxillofac Surg. 1998;36(1):19–23.
224. Canaday BR. Amorous, disinhibited behavior associated with propofol. Clin Pharm. 1993;12(6):449–51.

225. Brandner B, Blagrove M, McCallum G, Bromley LM. Dreams, images and emotions associated with propofol anaesthesia. Anaesthesia. 1997;52(8):750–5.
226. Klement W, Arndt JO. Pain on injection of propofol: effects of concentration and diluent. Br J Anaesth. 1991;67(3):281–4.
227. Picard P, Tramer MR. Prevention of pain on injection with propofol: a quantitative systematic review. Anesth Analg. 2000;90(4):963–9.
228. Playfor SD, Venkatesh K. Current patterns of propofol use in PICU in the United Kingdom and North America. Paediatr Anaesth. 2004;14(6):501–4.
229. Vasile B, Rasulo F, Candiani A, Latronico N. The pathophysiology of propofol infusion syndrome: a simple name for a complex syndrome. Intensive Care Med. 2003;29(9):1417–25.
230. Vardi A, Salem Y, Padeh S, Paret G, Barzilay Z. Is propofol safe for procedural sedation in children? A prospective evaluation of propofol versus ketamine in pediatric critical care. Crit Care Med. 2002;30(6):1231–6.
231. Cordero N, Cárdenas JM, Alvarez LG. Parental acceptance of pharmacologic and non-pharmacologic behavior management techniques in pediatric dentistry. Rev CES Odontol. 2012;25(2):24–32.
232. Betancur E, Londoño S, Alvarez C, Cárdenas JM, Manrrique R. Evaluación de la aceptación de la técnica de sedación inhalada con oxido nitroso por parte de padres y niños entre los 4 y 12 años de edad. CES Odontol. 2006;19(1):33–7.
233. Costa LR, Dias AD, Pinheiro LS, Chaves ME, Ferreira Rde A, Almeida RB, et al. Perceptions of dentists, dentistry undergraduate students, and the lay public about dental sedation. J Appl Oral Sci. 2004;12(3):182–8.
234. Daher A, Hanna RP, Costa LR, Leles CR. Practices and opinions on nitrous oxide/oxygen sedation from dentists licensed to perform relative analgesia in Brazil. BMC Oral Health. 2012;12:21.
235. Llaja KA, Lizárraga MN. Sedación consciente en tratamiento odontológico: efectividad de dos medicaciones en niños; conscious sedation in dentistry: effectiveness of two medications in children. Odontol Sanmarquina. 2009;12(2):52–6.
236. Alvarez JA, Pinto KM, Rezende C, Bönecker M, Corrêa FNP. Propuestas no-farmacológicas de manejo del comportamiento en niños. Rev Estomatol Herediana. 2010;20(2):101–16.
237. Wilson S, Alcaino EA. Survey on sedation in paediatric dentistry: a global perspective. Int J Paediatr Dent. 2011;21(5):321–32.
238. Fernández Fredes O, Flores Barret MT, Mánquez Hatta E. Norma control de la ansiedad en la atención odontológica; standard control of the anxiety in dental care. Santiago de Chile, Chile: Ministerio de Salud; 2007.
239. Marín P, Ibarra P, Rubiano A, Zuluaga M, Gómez L, Rivera D, et al. [National consensus. Recommendations for sedation and analgesia by non-anesthesiologists (physicians and dentists) in patients less than 12 years]. Bogota: Sociedad Colombiana de Anestesia y Reanimación; 2011 [cited 26 Nov 2013]. Available from: http://en.calameo.com/read/001024357d0ac0445a32a.
240. Ibarra P, Galindo M, Molano A, Niño C, Rubiano A, Echeverry P, et al. Sedation and analgesia recommendations for non-anesthesiologist physicians and dentists in patients over 12 years old. Colomb J Anesthesiol. 2012;40(1):67–74.
241. Castro Jeri ES, Díaz Pizán ME, Valdivieso Vargas-Machuca MJ. Comparación de la efectividad del midazolam en niños: Vía oral y vía intranasal; effectivemness of oral and intranasal midazolam in pediatric dentistry. Rev Estomatol Hered. 2005;15(2):133–8.
242. Lima ARA, Kajita M, Costa LRRS. Uso de restrição física em sedação moderada na odontopediatria; use of physical restraint in moderate sedation in pediatric dentistry. JBP rev Ibero-am odontopediatr odontol bebê. 2005;8(43):225–9.
243. Azevedo ID. Controle do comportamento infantil; child behavior management [PhD thesis]. Florianópolis, SC: Universidade Federal de Santa Catarina; 2006 [cited 2014 July 28]. Available from: http://repositorio.ufsc.br/xmlui/handle/123456789/89307.
244. Costa L, da Costa PS, Lima AR. A randomized double-blinded trial of chloral hydrate with or without hydroxyzine versus placebo for pediatric dental sedation. Braz Dent J. 2007;18(4):334–40.
245. de Rezende GP, da Costa LR, da Costa PS. The use of chloral hydrate for pediatric dental sedation. Spec Care Dentist. 2007;27(3):85–6.
246. Flores M, Mezzano S, Carrasco M, Sirandoni G, Morán M, Onetto J. Sedación inhalatoria con óxido nitroso como medio de reducción de la ansiedad en tratamientos restauradores y exodoncias en niños. JE Rev Facultad Odontol Univ Valparaiso. 2008;4(6):1001–7.
247. Costa LR, Costa PS, Brasileiro SV, Bendo CB, Viegas CM, Paiva SM. Post-discharge adverse events following pediatric sedation with high doses of oral medication. J Pediatr. 2012;160(5):807–13.
248. Moreira TA, Costa PS, Costa LR, Jesus-FranÇA CM, Antunes DE, Gomes HSO, et al. Combined oral midazolam–ketamine better than midazolam alone for sedation of young children: a randomized controlled trial. Int J Paediatr Dent. 2013;23(3):207–15.
249. Pardo K, Díaz M, Villegas L, Bernabé E. [Effect of ethanolic of the melissa officinalis (lemon balm) in the modification of the behaviour of the anxious child]. Rev Estomatol Hered. 2009;19(2):91–5.
250. American Association of Pediatric Dentistry. Policy on early childhood caries (ECC): classifications, consequences, and preventive strategies. 1978 (revised 2008) [Feb. 19, 2014]. Available from: http://www.aapd.org/assets/1/7/P_ECCClassifications.pdf.

Pediatric Sedation: The European Experience and Approach

21

Piet L.J.M. Leroy and Michael R.J. Sury

Abstract

With 53 countries and as many national histories, Europe can hardly be considered as a solid set of common elements. Despite the increasing political, financial, economic, and administrative integration of a growing number of countries within the European Union (EU), European health-care systems remain highly diverse. In the last few years, European experts on pediatric sedation are increasingly exchanging insights and experiences, and a growing number of local and national initiatives intended to improve procedural sedation and analgesia (PSA) practice may be noticed.

This chapter avoids reiteration of what is commonly known in the United States and instead describes and contrasts what is different or new in Europe. In doing so, we have drawn upon our personal knowledge and experience in the Netherlands and United Kingdom, researched the European literature, and gathered some of our own data to describe what we believe to be the important and interesting European problems and perspectives with pediatric sedation.

Keywords

Pediatric sedation • Procedural sedation and analgesia (PSA) • Physical restraint • Europe • European Union • Guidelines • Training • Capnography • Bispectral index (BIS) • Electroencephalogram (EEG) • Conscious sedation • Nitrous oxide • Propofol • Ketamine • Chloral hydrate • Sevoflurane • Painless imaging • Interventional radiology • Cardiology • Gastroenterology • Endoscopy • Oncology • Emergency department (ED) • Dentistry • United Kingdom National Audit Project • National Institute for Clinical Excellence (NICE) • United Kingdom • Scottish Intercollegiate Guidelines Network (SIGN) • European Society of Anesthesiology (ESA) • European Society for Pediatric Anesthesia (ESPA) • European Pediatric Association (EPA) • Association of Paediatric Anaesthetists (APA) • European Society for Pediatric Research (ESPR) • Conscious sedation • Moderate sedation • Deep sedation • Dissociative sedation • Relative analgesia • Light anesthesia • Minimal anesthesia • Eutectic Mixture of Local Anesthetics (EMLA) • Chloral hydrate

P.L.J.M. Leroy, M.D., Ph.D. (✉)
Pediatric Procedural Sedation Unit, Division of Pediatric Critical Care, Department of Pediatrics, Maastricht University Medical Centre, Maastricht, The Netherlands
e-mail: p.leroy@mumc.nl

M.R.J. Sury, M.B. B.S., F.R.C.A., Ph.D.
Department of Anaesthestics, Great Ormond Street Hospital NHS Trust, London, UK

K.P. Mason (ed.), *Pediatric Sedation Outside of the Operating Room: A Multispecialty International Collaboration*, DOI 10.1007/978-1-4939-1390-9_21, © Springer Science+Business Media New York 2015

Introduction

With 53 countries and as many national histories, Europe can hardly be considered as a solid set of common elements. Despite the increasing political, financial, economic, and administrative integration of a growing number of countries within the European Union (EU), European health-care systems remain highly diverse. Each country organizes its health care in a different way and medical practice and standards are mainly determined by national policies and influenced by regional, historical, and cultural backgrounds. Although many European medical academies and societies have been set up recently, their impact on practice is unknown.

Within Europe the economical wealth of countries in general and health-care budgets differs substantially, leading to widely divergent resources and funding. An additional and relatively recent challenge within the European health-care settings is to sustain comprehensive public health systems while facing deindustrialization and, in some cases, economic decline. This challenge is exacerbated by a global financial crisis and demographic changes, including falling birth rates, increasing life expectancy, and migration. The pattern of diseases is changing and health and social services need to change to respond successfully [1].

For the management of children having diagnostic and therapeutic procedures, there remains considerable variation in practice. Nevertheless, health-care providers in Europe have been influenced by recommendations from within Europe and the United States, and this has led, and will continue to lead, to a general improvement in the quality of services available. In the last few years, European experts on pediatric sedation are increasingly exchanging insights and experiences, and a growing number of local and national initiatives intended to improve procedural sedation and analgesia (PSA) practice may be noticed.

This chapter avoids reiteration of what is commonly known in the United States and instead describes and contrasts what is different or new in Europe. In doing so, we have drawn upon our personal knowledge and experience in the Netherlands and United Kingdom, researched the European literature, and gathered some of our own data to describe what we believe to be the important and interesting European problems and perspectives with pediatric sedation.

General Problems and Challenges

Growing Demand for Optimal Procedural Sedation and Analgesia

The demand for PSA outside the operating room continues to increase. The absence of sufficient anesthetic support or availability has fuelled a need for untrained "non-anesthetists" to organize their own PSA practice. Five services are prominent and each is discussed in detail hereafter. Until recently sedationists had focused on patient comfort [2–4], but now more practitioners are learning the importance of professional competence and safety.

It is reasonable to state that, because of the characteristics of the procedures, each service requires a different sedation strategy and a set of techniques. Nevertheless, there are obvious similarities in terms of the facilities they need. In addition, a list of objectives that apply generally to a hospital may be useful to assess the standards of care. A basic but invaluable list of standards was created by the United Kingdom Children's National Service Framework.[1] Six essential components of a comprehensive high-quality service were identified:

- Early recognition and treatment of pain
- Procedural sedation/analgesia
- Rescue anesthesia
- Behavioral management (play therapy)
- Long-term venous access
- Symptom control

While there is debate around the pros and cons of sedation versus anesthesia, there is a growing consensus that safe and effective PSA is essential in modern medical care for children; it has become in fact a *condition sine qua non* [5]. The most important remaining questions follow the problem of "what happens when anesthesiologists are not available?"

1. What drugs are safe enough for non-anesthesiologists to use?
2. What minimal competencies and skills should non-anesthesiologists possess to ensure an optimal level of both safety and effectiveness?
3. How should PSA effectiveness be defined? Sedation effectiveness endpoints should focus on procedural success, time-effectiveness, optimal patient comfort, and adequate analgesia.

Cultural Aspects, Diversities, and Inconsistencies Within Europe

There are major cultural aspects affecting the demand for and the practice of sedation. A survey of practice in the United States and Europe highlighted major differences in the use of sedation and analgesia for oncology procedures [6] and although the replies may no longer apply, they could be taken as evidence of an acceptance by children, caregivers, and medical professionals in the United States that sedation and analgesia were not necessary for bone marrow aspiration and lumbar puncture. It is our impression that few children wish to remain conscious during painful or distressing procedures. That for these cases anesthesia cannot be

[1] http://www.ich.ucl.ac.uk/cypph/cnsf_audit_tool.pdf.

achieved or that this is not desirable is the essential driver to discuss PSA.

Cultural and religious variability throughout Europe, in patients as well as among health-care professionals, may have a huge impact on the assessment as well as the therapy of pain [7]. It has also been shown that personal expertise modulates the perception of pain in others [8]. Both observations may explain partially the wide variability in indications for and application of PSA, as well as individual determinations of optimal sedation end points.

Physical restraint is a taboo subject, although its application probably forms part of day-to-day pediatric care [9]. The literature suggests that the application of "straps" in precooperative small children was acceptable in some hospitals or situations in the United States [10–12]. However, the Scottish (2004) and Dutch (2012) guidelines on PSA in children both declare that restraint is unacceptable during a procedure that is not life-saving [13, 14]. A recent United Kingdom Royal College of Nursing guideline for nurses states that restraint must only be used to prevent serious injury to the child or to bystanders. According to this guideline, restraint must meet a number of basic principles, including the prevention of unnecessary procedures, setting a low threshold for using PSA, determining in advance the maximum number of attempts to perform the procedure, access to a training course and protocols, full informed consent from parents/caregivers, rigorous documentation of the procedure, and a subsequent evaluation of how the child, parents, and staff experienced it [15]. As far as we can ascertain, the British Society of Paediatric Dentistry is the only medical group to have published a policy document on the use of restraint. Based on ethical and legal considerations, the document recommends extreme reticence in applying restraint [16]. Several European authors have even postulated that procedural restraint is contrary to the Human Rights Act and the United Nations Convention on The Rights of the Child [17, 18]. The European Association for Children in Hospital states in their charter that the avoidance of restraint should be a fundamental part of any "comfort" policy.[2] Nevertheless, we believe restraint is still common practice within Europe. A recent survey among Danish emergency departments reported that physical restraint (or "Brutacaine" in the authors' words) was routinely applied during painful procedures in children by 80 % of the departments; PSA was available in only 33 %. A total of 73 % of the respondents believed that there was a need for better pain management and/or sedation of children in their emergency department (ED) [19].

Behavioral management embodies a holistic approach to optimize a child-friendly environment, reduce fear, and minimize the distress of a procedure [20, 21]. Behavioral management skills should be embedded in the training of everyone on the sedation team—not just play specialists and psychologists. This is already occurring in many training schemes and curricula within Europe. Behavioral management can reduce anxiety and the need for sedation drugs. Self-hypnosis and other coping strategies are useful for cooperative children [22, 23].

The early insertion of central venous catheters (CVC) avoids many painful peripheral intravenous "needles." In the major centers across Europe, interventional radiology and anesthesia services have radically reduced the time to achieve CVC access and therefore improved the quality of care. There is a wide and strong belief that if children undergo their first procedure without distress, subsequent procedures will be more easily managed and suffering reduced. The authors support this idea.

Parental presence or involvement during invasive procedures is another matter of debate. At many European institutions, parents are not consistently allowed to accompany their child during the induction of elective anesthesia for invasive procedures or surgery. There is no consistent approach to "parental presence" throughout Europe. A review of published literature demonstrated that parents also want to have the choice about whether they remain at their child's side during complex invasive procedures, even resuscitation, but they also revealed apprehensions and controversy abound among clinicians regarding this practice [24]. A recent Spanish multicenter study of pediatric emergency departments (PED) showed that the staff tends to prefer parents not to be present during invasive procedures. Parental presence is not common in Spanish PEDs [25]. In other countries, parents are encouraged to be present in many situations including resuscitation [26].

There are large variations in the choice of sedation drugs and PSA regimens within Europe: Chloral hydrate is used widely in the Netherlands and the United Kingdom because it is considered to have a high safety profile and success rate [27]. In France, however, it has been banned because of the suspicion of carcinogenicity [28]. In most Belgian hospitals, chloral hydrate has been replaced by general anesthesia because of dissatisfaction with its non-titratable and long-acting characteristics.

Nitrous oxide (N_2O) use and delivery is also inconsistent over Europe. For example, in France, many painful procedures are undertaken with nitrous oxide mixtures (50 % N_2O/O_2) alone [29, 30], and it is surprising that this practice has been transferred rather sparsely to other countries; probably it is not transferable because patients and parents expect and prefer anesthesia. Nitrous oxide is given without the need for special facilities or fasting—a clear advantage over anesthesia. Furthermore, there exists excellent evidence for the effectiveness and safety of nurse-administered N_2O/O_2, making this technique readily available at any time [31]. In the Netherlands, a group of midwives working with

[2] http://www.each-for-sick-children.org.

N_2O have birthed infants with major congenital defects. Nitrous oxide was blamed and therefore banned from many hospitals. A Dutch working group on pediatric procedural sedation has recently succeeded in reintroducing nitrous oxide for procedural sedation but there is still strong opposition to its use.

In some European countries any use of nitrous oxide remains an anesthesiologist's prerogative. The (theoretically based) recognition of potential problems of occupational exposure of N_2O has led internationally to the introduction of occupational exposure limits (OEL), expressed as 8-h time-weighted averages (in parts per million [ppm]). Strikingly, there is no clear consensus on which is an appropriate OEL for N_2O, resulting in time-weighted averages limits ranging from 25 ppm (e.g., New Zealand, Australia, the United States) to more than 50 ppm (Belgium, Norway, Denmark, Spain), 80 ppm (the Netherlands), and 100 ppm (Finland, Sweden, the United Kingdom, Switzerland). Canada has three different OELs (25 ppm (Ontario), 50 ppm (Quebec), and 100 ppm (Alberta)), whereas France has no specifically defined OELs. None of these limits have any scientific basis. At generally accepted OEL, there is no conclusive evidence for reproductive, genetic, hematologic, or neurologic toxicity from nitrous oxide exposure [32]. We believe that in many European institutions nitrous oxide inhalation is currently applied without meeting the statutory OEL. Limited financial resources may be the explanation for the absence of adequate scavenging systems.

There is inconsistent practice and beliefs regarding the delivery of ketamine, propofol, and dexmedetomidine. Ketamine (and in some European countries especially the *S*-ketamine enantiomer) is probably increasingly used for PSA in PEDs, mostly by non-anesthetists. Despite the growing evidence from recent European studies [33] that propofol can be safely used by appropriately trained non-anesthesiologists for PSA in selected children, its use still remains generally restricted to anesthesiologists in most European countries. The debate on this topic, however, continues [34–36]. We believe that non-anesthesiologist-administered propofol PSA will become a standard practice for European PSA-trained professionals in the future. The use of dexmedetomidine for PSA is still sparse but may increase as the drug only recently became available in Europe.

Finally, within Europe there are different attitudes among medical professionals and decision makers regarding professional behavior and self-criticism, multidisciplinary communication and collaboration, importance of professional title and hierarchy, credentialing, transparency, and the way medical errors and adverse effects are assessed and reported. There exist a wide variation of the extent in which nonmedical professionals—such as specialized nurses, nurse practitioners, or physician assistants—are involved in medical caring and acting. In a few countries, nurses have acquired competencies and responsibilities in organizing and performing pain control, procedural comfort, and PSA.

Anesthesia Services Are Limited in Europe

The delivery of anesthesia services in remote locations (i.e., outside the operating "theater") has been limited, but is now approximately 1/3 of the anesthesiologists' workload. Several reasons may explain this. In France, preoperative assessment by an anesthesiologist is compulsory, by law, at a minimum of 24 h before any routine procedure. This has restricted the involvement of anesthesia services and promoted alternative PSA techniques—especially the use of nitrous oxide. The demand for theater time has increased and therefore any procedure that can be transferred out of operating theaters is an advantage. In a recent Italian survey of 54 pediatric hemato-oncology departments comparing general anesthesia and PSA, it was concluded that PSA outside the operating room was preferred by patients because it entailed an earlier discharge and a more familiar environment and it allowed the parents to stay close to the child [37]. As hospitals grow in size, so has the availability of anesthesia delivery sites outside of/distant to the operating theater.

There has been a belief that once a sedation service was "given" to pediatricians, it would lead to a considerable increase in demand that would not be possible to satisfy. This perception is changing. With reports of unsafe or ineffective sedation practice, anesthesia services outside the operating theaters have flourished. Nevertheless, there are issues that retard this transition. We outline them below.

Mortality studies of surgery and anesthesia in the United Kingdom and elsewhere have identified that the sedation of the very young and the very old pose a high risk [38]. Consequently, this led to specialization and transfer of infants and small children to specialist centers. Some rural and suburban emergency departments have continued to accept pediatric trauma and medical problems that may need specialty anesthesia and intensive care services. This remains a common scenario around Europe. Fortunately, the links to larger centers are usually well established and transfer is not difficult, although there will be an inevitable delay in treatment. To avoid the need for transfer, some hospitals have developed sedation protocols, mainly ketamine, to help children with minor injuries. This is especially likely in remote rural towns.

The European Working Time Directive has limited the hours that doctors can work. This directive is a statute developed in the European Union to prevent excessive working hours and to encourage more equitable employment. For example, it may be fairer to employ two doctors to work 36 h per week rather than one for 72; night duty, even if the doctor is in-hospital and asleep, counts as work. Although this directive is not applied uniformly across the continent, in the United Kingdom it has severely limited the training experience for trainees. Since August 2009, this limit has been set to 48 h per week.

Non-anesthesia Practitioners in Europe

In the United Kingdom and much of Europe, anesthesia is a physician-led service. In Scandinavian countries and the Netherlands, nurses are employed to assist physicians; they look after patients during surgery but they are supervised by anesthesiologists and not by surgeons. This system has not developed in the United Kingdom probably because there are sufficient numbers of trained anesthesiologists. Almost all pediatric sedation services throughout Europe are physician led.

Because of the scarcity of pediatric anesthesiologists, several specialty groups have emerged with sedation practices. Dentists, emergency physicians, and intensivists have been prominent in this regard. Their journey, from inexperienced sedationist to skilled sedationist, has not reached its end. It is inevitable that they must continue in the venture to provide effective and safe services for their patients. Rigorous competencies, skills, and safety precautions have been developed, fulfillment of which has enabled some non-anesthesiologists in Europe to gain access to potent sedatives (e.g., propofol) [33, 39, 40]. However, this practice of sedation delivery by non-anesthesiologists remains controversial [34–36, 41].

Challenges and Setbacks in Europe

Safety issues, adherence to guidelines, and the training and skills of the sedation provider have been of recent concern in Europe. Three cases with disastrous outcomes have attracted widespread notoriety and press in Europe:

- A child's brain was damaged by 100 % nitrous oxide given from an anesthetic machine that did not have a hypoxic mixture alarm. The practitioner was untrained in its use.
- A child died after being suffocated by a team trying to use a breathing system to deliver a nitrous oxide/oxygen mixture because they failed to turn the gas flow on. They were untrained.
- A combination of midazolam, alfentanil, and ketamine was given to sedate a boy for dental extractions. He became apneic soon after arrival to the recovery area and neither the nurse nor the doctor reacted quickly enough to prevent permanent hypoxic brain damage [42].

Lack of sufficient training was the prominent issue with all of these cases. It is important to accept that every professional is vulnerable to human error. The doctor in the dental sedation disaster was an anesthesiologist. Strikingly, the outcomes of sedation delivery by non-anesthesiologists have been researched and presented by a very limited number of researchers [2, 43]. Despite recent publication of European sedation guidelines, the authors believe that unsafe practice is still prevalent.

In the Netherlands, there have been at least five severe accidents (between 1998 and 2008, two with a fatal outcome and one with permanent neurological damage) in children sedated for magnetic resonance imaging (MRI) scanning. In all cases, sedation was provided by non-anesthesiologists, using combinations of long-acting sedatives. Health Inspectorate's investigation clearly showed that the 1998 national safety PSA safety guidelines had not been implemented. Subsequently, adherence to the national guidelines was investigated in all hospitals in the Netherlands. Pediatricians from 88 of the 97 Dutch hospitals responded. Less than 25 % of respondents followed the guidelines [4].

In a pilot survey among European pediatric anesthesiologists, we have found that similar accidents have happened elsewhere although none have been published. A survey of 50 randomly selected Dutch pediatric residents revealed a high prevalence of unsafe practices, near accidents, and ineffective PSA (Table 21.1) [44]. There is hope, however, that the current nationwide project that supports the implementation of a new evidence-based guideline will improve PSA practices in Dutch pediatrics substantially.

Monitoring Practices in Europe Are Inconsistent

Capnography

Capnography is becoming more frequently used for PSA in specialist centers [45]. The United Kingdom National Audit Project 4[3] was a survey of individual reports of major complications of airway management related to anesthesia, intensive care, and emergency medicine. The project found many examples of airway complications that could have been avoided or better managed if capnography had been used. This finding, albeit a professional opinion (rather than clear evidence of benefit), supports the widespread use of capnography in the management of intubated patients. It is logical to extend the use of capnography to monitor all patients who are either unconscious or at risk of becoming unconscious. A study from Turkey promotes its value in maintaining safety [46], and also elsewhere in Europe capnography is increasingly considered as an essential tool during PSA [47]. The Dutch guidelines on pediatric PSA (2012) recommend that capnography should be considered whenever PSA is performed with a (possibility of) moderate or

[3] http://www.rcoa.ac.uk/nap4.

Table 21.1 Selection of PSA experiences commonly reported by Dutch pediatric residents [44]

Reported practices	Associated potentially serious consequences
• Unmonitored PSA during magnetic resonance imaging (MRI)	• Not discovering in time potentially dangerous side effects (respiratory depression, hypoxia or bradycardia)
• No formal monitoring, observation, or assessment during recovery following the procedure	• Not discovering in time potentially dangerous late side effects. Immediately after the procedure, procedural stress falls away while sedative effect is still present. This may cause suddenly and unexpectedly deep sedation and loss of control on vital functions
• Deeply sedated patients not accompanied by a professional competent in airway management	• Not discovering and/or managing in time potentially dangerous side effects
• Waking up or moving during MRI	• Incomplete and/or low-quality results, limiting diagnostic accuracy
• Being called for additional intravenous sedation in a child sedated with chloral hydrate for MRI	• Procedural delay • Risk of oversedation and undesirable deep sedation, associated with loss of control on vital functions
• Combination of preprocedural feeding, swaddling, and sedative drugs in infants undergoing MRI	• Risk of vomiting and aspiration
• Absence of age-specific resuscitation tools and drugs	• Not being able to start rescue interventions instantly
• Forced restraint during endoscopy procedures or oncology procedures (e.g., bone marrow puncture) because of ineffective PSA (mostly midazolam only)	• Extreme patient discomfort • Preprocedural anxiety for new procedure • Ineffective procedure
• Incomplete endoscopy procedures because of ineffective PSA	• Ineffective procedure leading to incomplete diagnosis and/or need for repeated endoscopy
• Nonapplication of topical anesthesia (e.g., EMLA®) in nonurgent vascular access	• Patient discomfort • Preprocedural anxiety for new procedure • Ineffective procedure

PSA procedural sedation and/or analgesia

deep sedation but that it is mandatory for any PSA during which continuous visual and auditory observation is impossible or unreliable (e.g., during an MRI investigation or during radiotherapy) [14]. Limited financial resources, however, have prevented widespread adoption of capnography.

Processed EEG

A recent advisory from the United Kingdom National Institute for Clinical Excellence (NICE) has stated that an EEG monitor should be considered for monitoring patients under anesthesia [48]. EEG monitoring is more common for total intravenous anesthesia because there are no monitors to follow the blood concentration of intravenous sedatives/anesthetics. Expired propofol measurement is possible, but not accurate enough to be a reliable tool [49, 50]. Although blood propofol assay machines are becoming available, they are not practical for standard short propofol PSA [51]. Bispectral index (BIS) monitoring and other electroencephalogram (EEG) monitors remain uncommon in European operating rooms.

Recommendations, Policy Statements, and Guidelines in Europe

Anesthesiologists throughout the world have been concerned about sedation by the *untrained* and have published guidelines to prevent patient harm. (Refer to Chap. 2.) Excluding dentistry, United Kingdom guidelines for doctors focused first on the radiology setting [52]. In 2001 the Academy of Medical Colleges responded to reports of unacceptable mortality in adult patients having esophagogastroscopy [53]. They stated clearly that "organizations should ensure that staff receives sedation training." To date, there are no universal guidelines to encompass all of Europe.

The Scottish Intercollegiate Guidelines Network (SIGN) [54] gathered a body of opinion from across many specialties and developed a clinical guideline that has been quoted and used widely. The SIGN guideline was limited to moderate sedation. In 2010 NICE issued a comprehensive guideline specifically for children and young people, and it incorporated guidance for all forms of sedation including deep sedation [55]. In Italy, a review and guideline was produced for pediatric neuroradiology [56]. A European guideline for PSA in adults has been published [57]. Evidence-based national guidelines are now available in the United Kingdom, the Netherlands, Germany, and France.

In a survey we recently performed among about 100 participants of symposia on procedural sedation during two recent European conferences (PREM, Ghent May 2013; ISSP, Stockholm June 2013), the vast majority was not aware of any national or European guidelines. The lack of an appropriate, well-tailored program for guideline awareness and implementation is likely to be an important factor in this ignorance. The European Society of Anesthesiology (ESA), the European Society for Pediatric Anesthesiology (ESPA), the Association of Paediatric Anaesthetists (APA), the Royal College of Paediatrics and Child Health, the European Academy of Pediatric Societies (EAPS), the European Pediatric Association (EPA), and the European Society for Pediatric Research (ESPR) are not involved in setting up, training, or implementing appropriate training for PSA by non-anesthesiologists.

We believe that had any of the available guidelines been applied, the aforementioned disasters would not have happened [58]. Although these guidelines may have already prevented many catastrophes, in the authors' opinion they would benefit from endorsement and dissemination by the national and European specialty organizations.

Ethical and Legal Aspects of Sedation Care in Europe

Ethical and legal considerations become increasingly important in European pediatric health care. In children undergoing a medical procedure, professionals must weigh the need to perform that procedure against the child's wishes to be left untouched. Most importantly, if the knowledge and technology to perform sedation/analgesia for this procedure easily and painlessly exists, one cannot justify merely restraining a terrified child for a painful procedure because of the cost or extra efforts involved.

Current European legislations usually hold that a young child (defined as <12 years in Dutch legislation; defined as below the developmental age of reasonable comprehension in most other European countries) is not autonomous—that is, he/she is not at liberty to refuse needed treatment, as long as informed consent is obtained from parents or caregivers. This reasoning is probably unhelpful and may be a misreading of the law. It has been postulated that only if society ultimately considers physical restraint to accomplish a medical procedure a violation of a child's civil liberty—which is, for example, the case in Scotland—we will all become more committed to alternative solutions such as PSA [59]. Medical professionals should help parents and children understand the nature of a given procedure and the possible options for altering perception of that procedure—be they emotional support, hypnosis, distraction techniques, anxiolytic/analgesic medications, or general anesthesia. Perhaps most importantly, the consideration of these ethical principles requires providers to reconsider alternative plans for sedation of each child: Physical immobilization or restraint cannot be a surrogate to sedation. Fear of potentially unsafe deep sedation is important but must be counterbalanced with the risk of unwanted emotional and psychological injury. Horrific accounts of painful procedures without effective PSA have been linked to post-traumatic stress disorder [6, 59–61].

Recent jurisprudence in the Netherlands shows that a care provider who does not allow sufficient time and effort to adopt a suitable approach to a resisting child may have to face negative consequences: Courts may rule that a defensive (panic) response from children resulting in injuries to the care provider is not unlawful. In these cases, any claim for damages against the parent(s) would fail [62]. Seen from the child's perspective, it could furthermore be argued that the child has a right to oppose a medical treatment, at least within certain specific boundaries.

Alternatively, the ethical principle "first do no harm" and the basic right for optimal care require the PSA practice to be optimally safe at all occasions. The potential toxicity of PSA drugs needs to be excluded. To this end, the recent concerns on the possible neurotoxicity of anesthetics on the developing brain may be relevant [63]. Although clinical relevance has not been substantiated, results to date indicate that exposure of animals to general anesthesia during active synaptogenesis is most detrimental [64]. Given the recent trend to administer ketamine and propofol for PSA, these observations may be relevant. Currently it is not known whether the experimental findings in animals can be simply extrapolated to human beings *in general* and to PSA in children *in particular*. Furthermore, the eventual (neuro)toxicity of non-anesthetics such as barbiturates, benzodiazepines, and chloral hydrate has never been subject of systematic research. The potential toxicity of potent PSA drugs must be counterbalanced with the potential biological and psychological consequences of ineffective sedation and repeatedly painful or distressing experiences during childhood [65]. Additional research is needed and in progress in order to clarify this dilemma.

Definitions Particular to Europe

Conscious sedation was an accepted endpoint or landmark in the continuum of conscious level. *Conscious*, meaning "able to respond to the spoken word," has been replaced by the term *moderate sedation* in the current literature because it does not assume consciousness but rather that the patient is easily roused—usually by communication but also by other similar appropriate light stimulus [66]. Nevertheless, conscious sedation remains a common term in Europe [52, 67]. In the United Kingdom, dentists prefer the term conscious sedation, referring to a level of sedation at which the patient responds easily to commands.

The term *deep sedation* is not approved [52] in some European professional groups, because it is possibly indistinguishable from anesthesia. This has led to the recommendation that both deep sedation and anesthesia should be managed with the same standard of care with respect to monitoring, equipment, facilities—and trained personnel. The definition therefore is more a description of the intended level of consciousness rather than a threshold identifying resources or risk. In a similar desire, two other descriptions of deep sedation/anesthesia have been used: *Light anesthesia* [68] and *minimal anesthesia* [69] are terms that describe a patient who is arousable with any appreciable stimulation. Techniques involving minimal anesthesia with propofol or sevoflurane have been used [70] for painless imaging.

Dissociative sedation is not a term in common use, but it is understood. Ketamine sedation or anesthesia is preferred generally.

Relative analgesia (RA) is a term intended to describe the analgesia and mild euphoria and calming properties of 30 % nitrous oxide. Dentists have become expert in its use [71].

The more relevant question is whether these definitions are useful. Although they may help identify sedation depths with drugs that are titratable, what is their value for non-titratable drugs? Motas et al. showed that common drugs (e.g., chloral hydrate, midazolam, pentobarbital) in average doses cause wide variations in depth of sedation [72]. The goal of achieving conscious or deep sedation was unable to be achieved in a significant number of children. With these findings in mind, the Dutch working group on procedural sedation decided to recommend the same safety precautions for all levels beyond light sedation.

Training and Credentialing Is Inconsistent in Europe

With the exception of dental sedation, there are no European training programs or specific qualifications for administering sedation. An Italian multicenter research group has reported the successful outcome of a strict training program for non-anesthesiologists who deliver propofol sedation to children [33, 39]. In the Netherlands, a national multidisciplinary training program (including the involvement of pediatric anesthesiologists) is currently being set up as to implement the PSA guidelines. In a first phase, participants will learn to *perform* light sedation (transmucosal midazolam, 50 % nitrous oxide inhalation), topical anesthesia, and hypnosis-like techniques. They will then progress to organize or manage procedures that require deep sedation (e.g., by setting up centralization or referral to anesthetists). The second phase is intended to give sedation providers sufficient exposure to become fully trained in deep sedation.

In the United Kingdom, an independent expert group has made recommendations on the training for pediatric dental sedation [73]. A challenge, however, is how to provide trainees with sufficient exposure to different, rarely used sedation techniques.

It is difficult to design a universal training curriculum for the many different types of sedation, some of which will not be relevant for all specialists. Strategies for credentialing have been clearly identified by Krauss and Green [74]. The authors of this chapter favor the option of creating a safe and effective sedation service that is controlled by the institution under direction from national and professional guidelines. Such a system will develop efficient training programs that may evolve into national training curricula.

All sedationists should have skills in airway management and resuscitation. Access to live patients is a limiting factor and the development of life-like manikins is a potential solution. (Refer to Chap. 35.) European resuscitation courses are widespread but do not aim to teach the monitoring and proactive airway skills that are critical for sedation providers. These skills should be an integral component of specialty-specific sedation training courses.

Implementation of Practice Standards in Europe

European standards of practice are mainly enforced by professionals themselves, and, unlike the United States, there are no financial penalties imposed by insurance companies. In the United Kingdom, clinical governance is a term applied in the National Health Service (NHS) to force individuals to bear responsibility and accountability for their actions. This governance has helped to improve quality and safety. In the United Kingdom and in the Netherlands, compulsory annual appraisal, and revalidation every 5 years, should motivate doctors and dentists to maintain their practice, skills, and knowledge. Failure to revalidate removes their license to practice.

Guidelines are designed to improve professional performance, health-care process, outcomes, and costs. However, the designing, publishing, and dissemination of guidelines do not necessarily imply the intended positive change in daily practice [75]. Guideline recommendations can be directed at a heterogeneous population of professionals with different backgrounds, experience, knowledge, skills, opinions, and motivational beliefs (i.e., positive and negative perceptions, evaluations, and expectations). This bewildering heterogeneity of factors must be reconciled, as illustrated in a recent study [76]. Since all these factors separately may act as both facilitators and barriers for guideline implementation, a thorough assessment of their interactive effects is critical in the design and implementation strategy. In the Netherlands, and elsewhere, the implementation of guidelines on PSA has been encouraged by raising public awareness through media and charities.

Financial Aspects of Sedation Delivery in Europe

How willing are society, health-care authorities, and insurance companies to invest in improving PSA? Given the current global financial crisis, it will be essential to demonstrate that implementing a guideline saves money. Probably, the "burden" of necessary investments to achieve more effective PSA services (e.g., training, new professionals, accessibility of propofol and nitrous oxide, appropriate monitoring and recovery, timely availability on a 24-h basis) can be quite easily calculated and will create immediately strong barriers for change. Calculating the economic aspects of the benefits will be much harder, balancing the costs of the improvements against the costs of unsafe practice and ineffectiveness.

A few studies on pediatric PSA have identified economical costs as an outcome measure. In the 1990s, Kain et al. compared propofol-based procedural sedation with intravenous thiopental/pentobarbital sedation for children undergoing MRI. A preliminary cost analysis was applied to the clinical data obtained and to a theoretical model of a pediatric MRI center. Cost analysis of the propofol-based services revealed an added drug cost ($1,600.76 per year for the propofol group) but a significant savings in post-sedation care unit (PACU) nursing time ($5,086.67 per year) [77]. Ekbom et al. published a randomized controlled study in children with difficulties in establishing venous access or anxious children in need for an IV access. The patients were randomized to conventional treatment—i.e., cutaneous application of Eutectic Mixture of Local Anesthetics (EMLA)—or nitrous oxide treatment. They concluded "the pre-treatment with nitrous oxide is a time effective and safe method to reduce pain, facilitate venous cannulation, and thereby reduce the number of costly cancellations of planned procedures" [78].

In 2013 the Dutch Association of Hospitals ordered a business-impact analysis and cost calculation on the implementation of the new Dutch PSA guideline. Their study showed that the implementation of deep sedation services for children undergoing major procedures (e.g., MRI, endoscopy, extensive wound care) in each of the 98 Dutch hospitals (on a total population of 16 million inhabitants) would not be financially effective. Centralization of these services to about 20 institutions would be financially more prudent. However, the same study demonstrated that setting up a 24-h sedation service to provide "light sedation" (e.g., application of nitrous oxide) for minor painful procedures would be cost-effective in all of the 98 Dutch hospitals.

The United Kingdom NICE guideline compared the costs of various sedation techniques and approaches [55]. (Refer to Chap. 2.) The most significant cost involved the salary for staff. This evaluation, however, was limited in its scope and applicability. For example, the comparison was based on a single procedure and did not consider the advantages of improved efficiency if, indeed, anesthesiologists were able to create "turnover" time.

Common European Sedation Practice for Selected Procedures

Painless Imaging

Both continents have tried to maximize the use of sedation for painless imaging. Nurse-led services for example were promoted as a practical alternative to anesthesia [79, 80]. Chloral hydrate [81] and Triclofos (Triclonam, Tricloryl, Nucloryl, Pedicloryl) [82] have been the mainstay for children under 15 kg and have very good safety and success records (safety depends upon the user more than the drug); 95 % of children fall asleep within 1 h and remain asleep for approximately 45 min. In older children, few drugs are as effective, leading most hospitals to abandon sedation in this group [83]. Pentobarbital was withdrawn in the United Kingdom in the 1960s due to its potential for abuse. Secobarbital has been used but causes paradoxical reactions (as in pentobarbital). Dexmedetomidine has recently become available but it is too early to know whether it will be widely used. It has been trialed extensively in Turkey [84, 85].

The unreliable nature of sedation has caused many, if not most, hospitals to develop anesthesia-led services [86] because there is a general belief that anesthesia is more efficient [87] and may be safer [88]. Certainly propofol [89] and sevoflurane [70] are standard drugs that are compatible with rapid recovery to street fitness. Propofol may need to be combined with other drugs to maintain immobility, and recently a combination of midazolam, nalbuphine, and low-dose propofol has been found to be reliable [90]. The centralization of nonurgent imaging in (mainly academic) pediatric anesthesia-led services has resulted, however, in progressively expanding waiting lists, making the need for non-anesthesiology involvement more prominent [91].

Interventional Radiology and Cardiology

Many intravenous lines can be inserted with a combination of local/topical anesthesia, moderate sedation, and behavioral techniques. There remain a large number of children who cannot remain immobile enough with deep sedation or anesthesia. Ketamine may be an alternative drugs but we believe that interventional radiology is more readily managed by an anesthesia service because of its flexibility and the ability to overcome almost any problem. For cardiology some countries have managed to maintain an effective sedation service using a range of techniques involving combinations of propofol [92], ketamine [93], and remifentanil [94], but our view is that the practice of controlled ventilation using tracheal intubation and standard anesthesia techniques is more reliable and creates optimal conditions for imaging and measurements [95, 96].

Gastroenterology

We believe that many hospitals in Europe use sedation for endoscopy with midazolam alone or a combination of benzodiazepines and opioids [97]. If there have been few problems, this is a credit to the judgment of gastroenterologists because the literature suggests that sedation is difficult especially for esophagoscopy [98]. Nevertheless, it is likely that most practitioners prefer anesthesia [99] and that propofol-based techniques are becoming more widespread. Propofol can cause sufficient sedation and suppression of gag reflex to allow insertion of an endoscope without the need for tracheal intubation or respiratory support [83]. Many anesthesiologists are confident that this is a safe approach [39, 83, 100, 101]. Colonoscopy needs much less propofol except when the ascending colon, the cecum, and the terminal ileum are entered (a small dose of opioid may be useful at these times). Not only is this technique a reliable and safe alternative to benzodiazepine-based sedation, but it radically increases the patient comfort as well as throughput [102]. In financial terms, there may be appreciable savings with efficiency.

Target-controlled infusion (TCI) of propofol has an application during endoscopy [103]. (Refer to Chap. 31.) The author (Sury), from personal experience, recommends a target of 6 μg/mL. It is important to appreciate that the effect site concentration is unknown and may take a few minutes to "catch up" with the blood concentration. A background infusion of remifentanil counters the discomfort of the procedure (usually less than 0.1 μg/kg/h). Nasal prongs delivering oxygen and monitoring breathing by capnography are essential to safety: Capnography is as important as pulse oximetry in this scenario. Respiratory depression and airway obstruction are uncommon complications, usually managed easily and not needing tracheal intubation.

Oncology

Many techniques are possible for children who need repeated painful oncology procedures. With practice, nitrous oxide combined with optimal topical/local anesthesia is potentially useful. In most countries we believe that intravenous anesthesia or deep sedation is preferred [104]. Without anesthesia services, ketamine is a reliable technique. The addition of a short-acting opioid to propofol is probably a common technique because it reduces the dose of propofol. In the Maastricht sedation unit, we recently found that children who had experienced both ketamine and propofol-based PSA for oncology procedures always select propofol-based PSA when they are given the choice. Unpleasant psychological experiences during recovery, double vision, the longer recovery time, and the relatively high incidence of nausea are the most important arguments for refusing ketamine. Propofol with remifentanil has the potential to provide the most rapid technique. It almost always causes apnea and assisted ventilation will be necessary; that it does cause apnea indicates that the child will remain immobile during the procedure [105]. The doses usually required to cause sleep and immobility for a 3-min-long painful procedure are propofol 2–3 mg/kg and remifentanil 1 mg/kg. TCI propofol may have an application for longer procedures.

Emergency Medical Care

There seems to be a gradual but steady progress by emergency physicians to develop their own standards and protocols, such that in Europe and in the United States hospitals support the use of ketamine [106], opioids, and propofol to manage children for minor procedures. There may be a trend for emergency departments (ED) becoming focused on quality and safety. However, PSA is currently not incorporated in European training programs. A recent European study showed that in most PEDs, PSA is practiced to the level of mild to moderate sedation. In about 20 % of the PEDs deep sedation is not provided by the staff, while 7.5 % of departments had no PSA available [107]. As a consequence, unnecessary or avoidable procedural pain and distress seems to be common [19, 108, 109].

Within most European countries, pediatric emergency care is not yet considered as a separate specialty and is performed by a mixed group of professionals from diverse disciplines. We hope that further professionalization and training will lead to the implementation of safe and effective PSA services in the ED. Some hospitals have made extra efforts to provide anesthesia services, usually at fixed times of the day, to meet maximum demand [110].

In the United Kingdom, a ketamine protocol has been produced by the College of Emergency Physicians.[4] It is a clear and explicit guideline that seems to have provided a good safety record. It is generally appreciated that ketamine alone is a more effective reliable and safer technique than the combination of midazolam and fentanyl [111].

[4] http://www.collemergencymed.ac.uk/CEC/cec_ketamine.pdf.

Dentistry

Dentists have been pioneers of sedation and many are expert. They know that during conscious sedation the patient should be rousable by verbal command and, in addition, they have observed that the mouth closes during deeper sedation.

Nitrous oxide relative analgesia (RA) has been popular because it is remarkably safe and surprisingly well tolerated by children [112]. In children who tolerate nitrous oxide, gas mixtures with less than 30 % nitrous oxide are almost always effective. More than this causes dysphoria, dizziness, and nausea [37]. Hypoxia is so unlikely that pulse oximetry and fasting are considered unnecessary (large meals beforehand are discouraged however) [113]. Nitrous oxide given in a 1:1 mix with oxygen has been used in many children for a variety of procedures [21]. Hypoxia was rare, as was any airway obstruction, and these problems only occurred when the patient had a cerebral disorder or was having another sedative drug [22].

Standard sedation for children is limited to nitrous oxide relative analgesia (RA) in most parts of Europe [114]. When nitrous oxide is insufficient to calm a patient, other drugs have been added. These may *tip* the patient into deep sedation, which is an obvious hazard, even though the risk may be small. In a study comparing RA with a combination of RA and 0.1–0.3 % sevoflurane, the dental treatment was completed in 52 % and 89 %, respectively. The same team, in another study, found that sevoflurane (0.3 %) added to nitrous oxide (40 %) and intravenous midazolam was effective in 93 % (249/267) of anxious children who would have been given general anesthesia otherwise [115]. All children remained rousable and none required airway management or oxygen—nevertheless, all children were fasted and monitored and these techniques were delivered by trained anesthesia personnel in a specialist dental clinic.

Other dentists have tried oral drugs. Oral and rectal benzodiazepines are commonplace in Sweden [116]. Midazolam is often useful to calm children [117] but treatment may have to be limited to minor restorations only [118]. In uncooperative toddlers (2–4 years old) an oral mixture of chloral hydrate, meperidine, and hydroxyzine was effective in only 72 %, and adverse conditions including vomiting, desaturation, prolonged sedation, and an apneic event occurred in 3 % of all sedations [119]. Nasal midazolam also has a place [120].

Intravenous midazolam alone is recommended in the United Kingdom for anxiolysis in children over 16 [114] and may be appropriate and effective in younger adolescents [121]. Propofol has been used alone as a sedation technique but lacks the analgesic component to enable insertion of local anesthesia [122]. Consequently, intravenous oral mixtures containing midazolam, alfentanil, ketamine, and propofol are being explored [123, 124]. A recent review of experience in 1,000 cases shows that these drugs can be combined safely [125]; loss of verbal contact occurred in approximately 0.05 % and nausea was a problem in 5 %. Whether this "alternative" technique can be called sedation is debatable if it is unknown whether it will cause accidental anesthesia. Some practitioners have become very experienced with combinations of drugs with ketamine [126, 127]. The danger of potent opioids causing apnea when the pain of dental treatment has subsided is a concern [42].

Many of these specialist techniques may not be applicable outside specialist centers, and there is some evidence to support the view that most dentists and anesthetists believe that uncooperative children should be managed with short-acting anesthesia in a hospital setting [128, 129].

Conclusion

New and Future Developments

The NICE guideline—*Sedation for diagnostic and therapeutic procedures in children and young people*—has been developed in the United Kingdom and published by NICE in December 2010 [55, 130] incorporates evidence of safety and efficacy of selected sedation drugs, consensus statements about patient management, and cost-effectiveness considerations. Important deviations in these guidelines from those of the United States are the recognition of propofol and sevoflurane as potentially useful techniques for pediatric sedation [130]. The crucial statement is that "healthcare professionals trained in the delivery of anesthesia may administer sevoflurane, propofol, or a combination of opioids with ketamine" [130]. A treatment pathway and sedation algorithm is detailed in Fig. 21.1. (Refer to Chap. 2.)

In the Netherlands, the Dutch Institute for Healthcare Improvement (CBO) commissioned pediatric guidelines for PSA at locations outside the operating theater from the Netherlands Society of Anesthesiologists and the Dutch Society of Pediatrics [14]. (Refer to Chap. 2.) Recently published in 2012, the guidelines were meant to represent five important cornerstones, notably including the optimal use of local or topical anesthesia, non-pharmacological techniques, and the prohibition of forced securing and restraint [14] (Table 21.2). These guidelines were noteworthy because they distinguished deep sedation from dissociative sedation [14] (Table 21.3). However, for the sake of achieving consistent safety standards, only two sedation levels were retained in the final implementation plan: Regarding monitoring, fasting status, and professional competences, the same safety precautions apply for all levels beyond light sedation/anxiolysis. Basically the safety standards for any PSA regimen that (potentially) causes deep sedation should be similar.

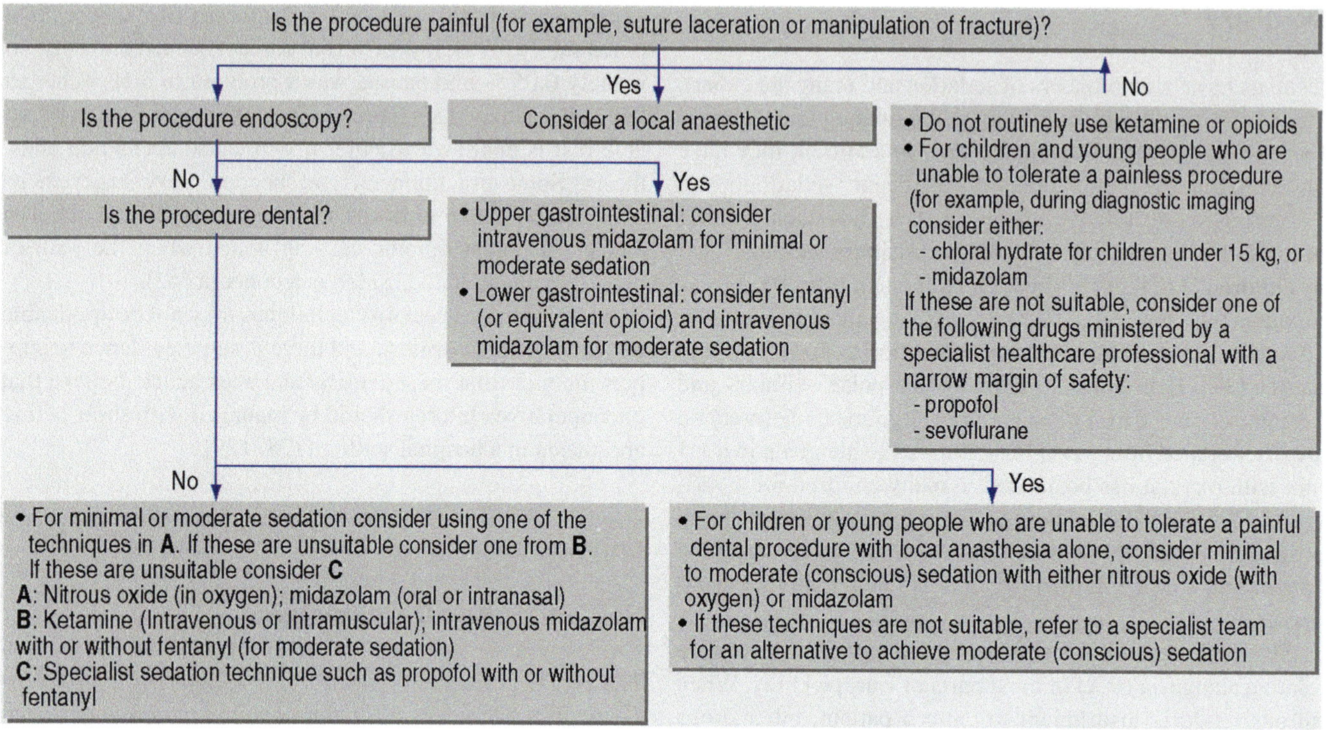

Fig. 21.1 Sedation algorithm and pathway (Reproduced from Sury M, Bullock I, Rabar S, Demott K. Sedation for diagnostic and therapeutic procedures in children and young people: summary of NICE guidelines. BMJ. 2010;341:c6819 with permission from BJM Publishing Group Ltd.)

Table 21.2 Cornerstones of a comprehensive policy toward optimal procedural comfort and the avoidance of forced immobilization (restraint) in children, Dutch Institute for Healthcare Improvement [14]

Strategy	Examples
Preventive measures	Avoid superfluous procedures
	Only allow an experienced professional to carry out procedures
	Agree on a maximum number of attempts at the procedure in advance
	Early insertion of a central venous line under general anesthesia (e.g., during long-term treatment with intravenous antibiotics)
Optimal local and topical anesthesia	Allow sufficient time for topical anesthesia to become effective (e.g., at least 60 min for EMLA®)
	Apply topical anesthesia to the correct location
	Implementation of new topical anesthetic techniques [14]
	For infiltration with lidocaine: buffer lidocaine with bicarbonate and use the smallest possible needle to significantly reduce the pain upon infiltration [15]
Non-pharmacological techniques	Optimal positioning of the child [16]
	Presence of the parent(s) or guardian(s)
	Preparation, game therapy
	Distraction techniques and hypnosis
Ready availability of effective procedural sedation and/or analgesia (PSA)	Light sedation for "small" procedures (e.g., blends of nitrous oxide and oxygen)
	Deep, titratable sedation for very painful procedures (e.g., propofol)
	Professionals trained in PSA
Rescue anesthesia	Availability of anesthesia if other techniques appear or turn out to be ineffective or unsafe

These Dutch guidelines discourage the delivery of sedation by non-anesthesiologists to American Society of Anesthesiologists (ASA) class III and IV patients. If performed, it should be after consultation with an anesthesiologist and delivered by a specially trained and credentialed practitioner. The fasting recommendation deviates from guidelines of other specialty societies in that light sedation does not need any special fasting. However, an emergency with a child who does not have an empty stomach is not an absolute contradiction for PSA [14] (Table 21.4).

Propofol, in the Dutch guidelines, although preferably administered by an anesthesiologist, may be delivered by an experienced non-anesthesiologist to ASA class I and II patients. Patients of ASA class III status and higher can only

Table 21.3 Definitions of different levels of sedation, Dutch Institute for Healthcare Improvement

1. Light sedation/anxiolysis	Two states that are difficult to tell apart, in which the anxiety and stress level of the patient have been lowered while the patient remains basically fully conscious. The patient responds adequately and consistently to verbal stimuli, and verbal communication therefore remains possible. This state is associated with few risks in patients without significant comorbidity. Although cognitive functions and coordination are reduced, ventilatory and cardiovascular functions remain unaffected. Light sedation/anxiolysis is typically a state of mind that occurs after one standard dose of midazolam (0.1 mg/kg intravenously *or* 0.2–0.5 mg/kg transmucosally) and with nitrous oxide sedation (inhalation concentration up to 50 %). Higher doses, other medicines, and combinations with other analgesics will virtually always lead to a deeper sedation level
2. Moderate sedation	Pharmaceutically induced reduction in awareness, during which the patient still responds purposefully when spoken to, or to light tactile stimuli. In this stage, no interventions are needed to keep the airway open, airway reflexes are intact, and ventilation is adequate. If the response is not clearly adequate and purposeful but more of a withdrawal reflex, we speak of deep sedation
3. Deep sedation	This is a pharmaceutically induced decline in awareness, during which the patient does not respond to being spoken to, but reacts purposefully to repeated or painful stimuli. Airway reflexes and ventilation may be reduced and it may be necessary to keep the airway open. The concept of "deep sedation" is a contested term because the distinction with anesthesia becomes less clear. A typical example is the deep sedation caused by propofol, during which it is possible, with the necessary expertise, to keep spontaneous respiration going and the airway open. The risk of reduced breathing is more or less a linear function of the dose and depth of sedation
4. Dissociative sedation	Also called a trance-like cataleptic sedation, it is typically the result of sedation with ketamine. As far as the depth of sedation, analgesia, and response level is concerned, ketamine causes a state that primarily corresponds to anesthesia. However, contrary to anesthesia, the airway reflexes, respiration, and hemodynamics largely remain intact, even at comparatively high doses. It makes ketamine attractive for use in PSA, particularly for painful procedures
5. General anesthesia	A pharmaceutically induced state of unconsciousness, in which the patient is unresponsive, even to painful stimuli. The ability to keep the airway open will often be reduced or absent, and ventilation will frequently be depressed, consequently requiring support. Cardiovascular functions may also be impaired. Can only be applied under the personal supervision of an anesthesiologist

Reproduced with permission from Leroy P, Schipper D, Knape J. Summary of the Dutch evidence-based guideline on procedural sedation and/or analgesia (PSA) in children at locations outside the operating theater. Dutch Institute for Health Care Improvement (Chapter 5 in Improving Procedural Sedation and/or Analgesia in Children. 2012; ISBN 978-94-6159-120-3. http://arno.unimaas.nl/show.cgi?fid=24183)
PSA procedural sedation and/or analgesia

Table 21.4 NPO fasting recommendations, Dutch Institute for Healthcare Improvement

1. Fasting is not needed for children undergoing light sedation
2. A child must *preferably have an empty stomach* for any (elective) PSA with moderate or deep sedation, in accordance with the same guidelines that apply to interventions taking place under general anesthesia (2 h for clear liquids, 4 h for breastfeeding, and 6 h for other meals)
3. A child in an acute condition without an empty stomach is in itself *no absolute contraindication* for PSA. This is important if postponing the procedure would pose health risks and/or discomfort. However, in that case the choking risks must always be carefully considered, taking into account the choice of sedative, the depth of sedation, and any protection of the airway. In practice, this amounts to the following recommendations:
(a) With PSA in an acute situation (without an empty stomach), deep sedation must be avoided as much as possible, since the protective airway reflexes may be disturbed or there is a high risk of respiratory impairment
(b) If a procedure requires a form of *deep* sedation, the patient must have an empty stomach
(c) If a procedure requiring a form of deep sedation is urgently needed and an empty stomach can therefore not be guaranteed, deep sedation must be performed under the supervision of an anesthesiologist in order to ensure optimal protection of the airway
4. Not having an empty stomach must be no reason or excuse for performing a procedure with an ineffective form of light or moderate sedation

Reproduced with permission from Leroy P, Schipper D, Knape J. Summary of the Dutch evidence-based guideline on procedural sedation and/or analgesia (PSA) in children at locations outside the operating theater. Dutch Institute for Health Care Improvement (Chapter 5 in Improving Procedural Sedation and/or Analgesia in Children. 2012; ISBN 978-94-6159-120-3. http://arno.unimaas.nl/show.cgi?fid=24183)
PSA procedural sedation and/or analgesia

Table 21.5 Propofol recommendations, Dutch Institute for Healthcare Improvement

Propofol is suitable for application in (urgent) painful procedures in children. Propofol causes deep sedation to anesthesia. The preconditions on patient selection, skills, competencies, monitoring, and the other preconditions set out in part I of this guideline must therefore be complied with. Since propofol is a fast-acting, very potent medicine that can quickly lead to oversedation and respiratory depression in untrained hands, the working group also has the following recommendations:
1. The person who performs the PSA must never be the same person as the one carrying out the procedure or intervention
2. The PSA is preferably carried out by an anesthesiologist
3. If the PSA with propofol is carried out by a non-anesthesiologist, it must be performed by a physician who has already been working with the medicine for a longer period of time and who is able to assess and deal with any respiratory complications
4. PSA with propofol in patients of ASA class III or higher must be performed by an anesthesiologist
5. Preoxygenation and monitoring through capnography with PSA using propofol is strongly encouraged in order to restrict the comparatively high risk of respiratory complications

Reproduced with permission from Leroy P, Schipper D, Knape J. Summary of the Dutch evidence-based guideline on procedural sedation and/or analgesia (PSA) in children at locations outside the operating theater. Dutch Institute for Health Care Improvement (Chapter 5 in Improving Procedural Sedation and/or Analgesia in Children. 2012; ISBN 978-94-6159-120-3. http://arno.unimaas.nl/show.cgi?fid=24183)
PSA procedural sedation and/or analgesia

Table 21.6 Sedation recommendations for GI procedures, Dutch Institute for Healthcare Improvement

1. A gastrointestinal (GI) endoscopic examination in a child must be carried out in principle under general anesthesia or deep sedation. If it is decided to opt for deep sedation, then titratable medicines must be used that are certain to lead to an effective level of deep sedation. Of all the medicines studied, propofol is the most effective—if necessary in combination with midazolam or an opiate
2. The working group advises against the following forms of PSA for GI endoscopic examinations:
• Using ketamine for endoscopic examinations of the esophagus, stomach, and duodenum, since there is an increased risk of laryngospasm
• Using a benzodiazepine on its own or the combination of benzodiazepine with an opiate. Both forms of PSA are substantially less effective than anesthesia or deep sedation with propofol
• Benzodiazepines must not be considered as suitable medicines to generate a reliable level of amnesia for endoscopic procedures
3. As far as rectoscopies are concerned, it is worth contemplating whether the investigation could be carried out without PSA insofar as informed consent has been obtained and provided the child is not scared or opposed to the examination
4. If general anesthesia or the support of an anesthesiologist is not feasible, an endoscopic department must have access to the logistic possibilities as well as trained professionals in order to provide safe and effective deep sedation that fulfills the preconditions of these guidelines
5. Premedication with midazolam taken orally can be considered prior to deep sedation. It reduces stress levels for inserting the drip at the start of the procedure and may therefore result in a smaller dose of propofol being required

Reproduced with permission from Leroy P, Schipper D, Knape J. Summary of the Dutch evidence-based guideline on procedural sedation and/or analgesia (PSA) in children at locations outside the operating theater. Dutch Institute for Health Care Improvement (Chapter 5 in Improving Procedural Sedation and/or Analgesia in Children. 2012; ISBN 978-94-6159-120-3. http://arno.unimaas.nl/show.cgi?fid=24183)
PSA procedural sedation and/or analgesia

receive propofol from an anesthesiologist [14] (Table 21.5). These guidelines are unique in that they have specific recommendations that are procedure based: Gastrointestinal procedures in particular should favor propofol, if necessary in combination with midazolam or an opioid [14] (Table 21.6).

Finally, the Dutch guideline contains a chapter with evidence-based recommendations on essential competences for PSA providers. Essential competences and skills depend on the intended sedation level (light versus deeper). These recommendations, which have been published separately, may become the foundation for future training development and accreditation [131].

It is hoped both the United Kingdom NICE and Dutch initiatives will encourage an improvement in the services available to children in Europe and beyond.

In the last decade a growing attention for PSA can be seen in European health-care providers, as demonstrated by a modest but increasing number of publications, symposia, and guidelines. However, a clear policy-driven European strategy toward full professionalization, supported by the relevant specialties and their professional bodies, is still missing. The vast majority of recent progresses are still the result of the work of a limited (but also growing!) number of "local heroes."

Training and accreditation will be the most important objectives for sedation providers around the world. Ideally, in Europe, these skills need to focus on the type of sedation needed and protocols to ensure safety. We believe that airway management and monitoring skills will become a crucial component to future sedation training and development in Europe.

Case Studies

The first three cases were managed by the sedation team of the Pediatric Procedural Sedation Unit of the Maastricht University Medical Centre (the Netherlands). Sedation strategy is based on an evidence-based protocol. The last three cases (Cases 4–6) were developed at Great Ormond Street Hospital, London, England.

Case 1 (the Netherlands)

A 6-year-old girl, previously healthy, ASA 1, weight 25 kg, presented with a right-sided distal forearm fracture 5 weeks ago. The fracture was corrected surgically under general anesthesia with 2K-wires. She presents for removal of the wires, which are in her forearm. She is not NPO.

The Sedation

The sedation goal for this child who has not been fasted is to achieve light sedation and analgesia. The stepwise approach to her sedation is outlined below:

Please note: The negative (−) minutes indicate the time course prior to start (time 0) of the procedure.

1. *Preparation phase*: During a 15-min play-therapy session, the child gets instructions on facemask and nitrous oxide inhalation. An individual distraction technique is determined. In addition, play therapy is used to achieve optimal facemask sealing and to minimize ambient N_2O pollution.
2. *Time schedule and drug regimen*:
   - *T*=−10 min: Fentanyl 2 μg/kg nasally administered divided in two doses, one for each nostril. Administration via the Mucosal Atomization Device (MAD®).
   - *T*=−5 min: Start inhalation of 50 % N_2O/O_2 equimolar mixture (Livopan®, Linde Healthcare), by anesthetic facemask (QuadraLite, Intersurgical), on-demand valve, and mobile scavenging and destruction unit (Excidio®, Linde Healthcare).
   - *T*=0: Start procedure. During the procedure, light and noise are tempered. The sedationist and parents are at the left side of the child, keeping the child in a hypnosis-based distraction. The surgeon enters the room after full nitrous oxide sedation is achieved, by approaching the patient from the right side and without entering the "distraction zone." The procedure is performed in silence.
   - Continuous visual and verbal contact is maintained with the child throughout the sedation until the child meets discharge criteria in the recovery room.

Summary Points

- Comfortable light sedation; eyes opened.
- Minor painful reaction at the time of K-wire removal, but no obvious emotions. No resistance; no restraint needed.
- Procedure time: 3 min; at the end of the procedure N_2O mixture is replaced by 100 % oxygen, while scavenging of exhaled air is continued for another 5 min.
- Recovery time: 7 min.
- No memory of procedural pain; no adverse events.

Case 2 (the Netherlands)

A 23-month-old girl, recently diagnosed with neurodevelopmental delay, ASA 1, weight 9 kg, is scheduled for a venous puncture and lumbar puncture for extensive metabolic and genetic testing on blood and cerebrospinal fluid. A previous attempt was unsuccessful due to heavy resistance by the child. The child is not NPO and has not been fasted.

The Sedation

The sedation goal for this child is light sedation and local/topical analgesia. The stepwise approach to her sedation is outlined as follows:

1. *Preparation phase*: 90 min before procedure: application of EMLA® (Eutectic Mixture of Local Anesthetics Prilocaine and Lidocaine; AstraZeneca), covered with transparent film dressing (Tegaderm®, 3M) on three different visible vein sites and one on the lumbar puncture site.
2. *Time schedule and drug regimen*:
   - *T*=−15 min: Topical anesthesia of the nasal mucosa with lidocaine 2 %, 0.3 mL nasally administered in each nostril. Administration via the MAD®.
   - *T*=−10 min: Midazolam 0.2 mg/kg nasally administered in each nostril. Administration via the MAD®. Total midazolam dose=0.4 mg/kg=3.6 mg=0.72 mL of a 5 mg/mL solution for IV use.
   - *T*=0: Start procedure. During the procedure light and noise are tempered. The sedationist and parents are at the left side of the child, keeping the child in a hypnosis-based distraction. The procedure-performing professional and material

(continued)

enter the room after adequate light sedation is achieved, by approaching the patient without entering the "distraction zone." The procedure is performed in silence.
- Pulse oximetry and continuous visual and verbal contact are maintained throughout the sedation until discharge criteria in the recovery room is met.

Summary Points

- Child becomes mildly agitated but is well controlled by tempering ambient stimuli. Child is smiling during the puncture and is behaving in a drunken-like manner. The sedationist follows slowly the child's waving behavior without challenging any reaction.
- No painful reaction at the time of both punctures. No resistance; no restraint needed. During lumbar punctures, the child's head is kept in a mild extension in order to prevent airway obstruction.
- Procedure time: 16 min.
- Recovery time: 35 min.
- No obvious procedural distress, no desaturations, no adverse events.

Case 3 (the Netherlands)

A 7-year-old girl is hospitalized for long-term IV antibiotic therapy for acute osteomyelitis (ASA 1; weight 29 kg; antibiotic therapy, flucloxacillin). She is scheduled for ultrasonography-aided insertion of a peripherally inserted central catheter (PICC) in the right elbow. The child is fully fasted according to ASA guidelines.

The Sedation

The sedation goal is deep sedation and local/topical analgesia. The stepwise approach is detailed as follows:

1. *Preparation phase*: 90 min before procedure: application of EMLA® (Eutectic Mixture of Local Anesthetics Prilocaine and Lidocaine; AstraZeneca), covered with transparent film dressing (Tegaderm®, 3M) on multiple, ultrasonographically determined puncture sites.
2. *Time schedule and drug regimen*:
   - $T=-10$ min: Fentanyl 1 μg/kg slowly intravenously.
   - $T=-5$ min: Prevention of propofol infusion pain: lidocaine 1 % 1 mL slowly intravenously for local anesthesia of the vein; during lidocaine infusion the vein is compressed proximally of the infusion site.
   - $T=0$: Start propofol induction: 1 mg/kg slow bolus (120 s). At the same time a propofol perfusion is started at a dose of 6 mg/kg/h. During induction, light and noise are tempered. The sedationist and parents are at the left side of the child. Capnography signal is used to optimize head position and to maintain an open airway. The procedure-performing professional and material enter the room after deep sedation is achieved. The procedure is performed in silence.
   - Based on the patient's reactions on stimuli, the propofol dose is adjusted up to 9 mg/kg/h. After successful catheter insertion, the propofol dose is immediately lowered to 3 mg/kg/h. Propofol is stopped once the procedure is fully terminated.
   - Capnography (combined with 2 L/min O_2; FilterLine® $etCO_2$ sampling line; Covidien), pulse oximetry, ECG, and blood pressure are documented every 5 min until discharge criteria from recovery room are met.

Summary Points

- During induction the child becomes mildly agitated (smiling, talking inconsistently), but is well controlled by tempering ambient stimuli. Sedation provider acknowledges and follows slowly the child's behavior without challenges or reaction. Deep sedation is achieved within 3 min.
- Difficult procedure. No painful reaction on multiple punctures. No resistance; no restraint needed.
- Procedure time: 47 min.
- Recovery time: 27 min
- No obvious procedural distress; no desaturations; no adverse events. Minimal blood pressure immediately after induction is 75/35 mmHg.

Case 4 (the United Kingdom) [81]

Magnetic Response Imaging (MRI) in a 10-Month-Old

An infant of 10 months of age, body weight 9 kg, needed an MRI scan of the brain for investigation of recurrent febrile convulsions and mild hypotonia. She had no other medical problems. Her grandmother had died recently during major surgery. The parents were offered the choice between anesthesia and sedation. They were told that sedation was probably as safe as anesthesia and that it would be supervised by a team

(continued)

of specially trained nurses. They were also told that sedation occasionally failed to keep infants sleeping throughout the scan (success rate over 95 %). The alternative was anesthesia, which was almost always successful. The parents requested sedation.

The Sedation

The patient was admitted direct to the MRI department. The radiographers and nurses met for a team brief. All members of the team were reminded of metallic safety. The radiographer performed a metal check on the patient and the mother. Nurses assessed the patient, performed all "medical" processes, and prescribed and administered 100 mg/kg oral chloral hydrate. Chloral hydrate has been in use for a long time. Triclofos (a phosphorylated version of chloral) would be better tolerated, but it is no longer manufactured.

The patient was cuddled by the mother in a quiet darkened room under the supervision of a nurse. The child fell asleep in 10 min and a pulse oximeter was applied. In 10 more minutes the patient was taken to the scanner and positioned. She stirred a little but remained asleep. Electrocardiogram, noninvasive blood pressure cuff, and nasal capnography were applied. A nurse and the mother remained in the scanning room. The patient was put into the center of the scanner. The nurse could not see the patient but could watch the patient monitor. The scan took 30 min.

At the end of the scan the infant was removed. She stirred a little but did not rouse. She was taken to the recovery room where she awoke spontaneously 50 min later. She remained sleepy for another 2 h and thereafter she was fed and remained awake without intervention. She was discharged with the advice that if there was sleepiness or inability to take fluids orally, she should return to the hospital.

Case 5 (the United Kingdom)

A 13-Year-Old Boy with Down Syndrome and Leukemia

Michael, a 13-year-old boy with Down syndrome, developed leukemia and needed a series of intrathecal chemotherapy injections. He was uncooperative and would not tolerate any procedure awake. (Only a few patients with leukemia request their procedures to be performed awake or under sedation. Virtually all parents in the authors unit request anesthesia for their children.) A CVC was inserted by the interventional radiology team under anesthesia. (The early insertion of a CVC is one of the most important factors in the delivery of high-quality care in children.) He was scheduled to receive intrathecal methotrexate and intravenous vincristine under sedation.

The Sedation

On the day of treatment, Michael was admitted direct to a "day admission" oncology unit. He had been fasted for 6 h. Like all such patients, he was fasted before anesthesia. However, ensuring that patients are not excessively fasted (e.g., fasted from the previous day) remains a challenge. Simple, consistent instructions and good communication will help. Fasting for fixed procedure times may help but will reduce flexibility of the procedure list order. Fasting in uncooperative children is an important problem on the day of treatment; nevertheless, the safety of the anesthetic and the delivery of chemotherapy are higher priorities.

He was planned to be first in a list of patients having procedures that morning. He was accompanied by his adoptive parents. (Parents are almost always helpful and should be encouraged to help their child remain calm.) Nurses "checked him in" and weighed him. A trainee doctor performed a clerking and physical examination. The report of an echocardiogram, performed the previous week, was checked, and cardiac function was within normal limits. Blood was sampled from the central venous line and sent for standard pre-lumbar puncture tests (Hb, platelet, white cell counts, and clotting function).

The oncologist met Michael and his parents and reviewed the results and treatment plan. The parents were told that Michael would receive only the methotrexate by lumbar puncture that day. The intravenous vincristine would be administered via the central venous line at his local hospital on another day. The parents signed the consent form. An anesthetist met Michael, reviewed the notes, and explained what the anesthesia entailed.

Throughout this process, Michael was occupied with toys and kept amused by a play specialist. (It is useful to have a team member dedicated only to delivering a calm caring approach. A play specialist will know what patients need; some want explanations and reassurance, and others need distraction. These things can be achieved by nurses if they have time.) Michael was passed to the procedure team, but the play specialist remained with him throughout.

Before the procedure list began, the sedation and procedure team met for a team brief. (A "minimum" procedure team consists of the "proceduralists" [a specialist doctor and a nurse] and the "anesthetists" [a specialist doctor and a nurse/technician]. A play

(continued)

specialist, pharmacist, and coordinator may also be part of the team.) All patients were discussed. The methotrexate for Michael was checked by a pharmacist.

Michael was thought to be manageable without any preprocedure sedation or anxiolysis. He walked into the procedure room with his parents and play specialist. His clinical record, methotrexate prescription, and consent form were all checked against his identification bracelet. (In some areas of the authors hospital, the "sign-in" and the "surgical pause" parts of the World Health Organization [WHO] Surgical Safety list are combined for short procedures where all members of the procedure team are present.) He refused to sit on the bed. Usually, a patient of his size and age would accept the application of monitoring and lie on their side ready for the lumbar puncture to begin as soon as anesthesia was induced. The team sensed that this was not achievable for Michael that day.

The anesthetist prepared the central venous line with antiseptic. Propofol 3 mg/kg[5] was injected by hand and followed by remifentanil 1 μg/kg,[6] and the line was flushed with 20 mL normal saline. (Later on the ward the oncology nurses flush the CVC line with heparinized saline before the patient is discharged as an extra precaution against residual anesthesia drugs.) As Michael became sleepy, the team positioned him to lie on his side ready for the lumbar puncture. A pillow was placed under his head. An anesthesia nurse/technician was ready at the "head end" to apply an anesthesia face mask to Michael. His breathing stopped and his lungs were inflated.[7]

[5]For most patients the following formula is used: 5 mg/kg of propofol is prepared in a 20 mL syringe and diluted to a total volume of 20 mL. The first bolus will always, therefore, be 12 mL (=3 mg/kg). If the procedure lasts longer than the anesthesia time given by this bolus, second or third boluses (each of 1 mg/kg=4 mL) can be given. If the procedure lasts longer than the anesthesia by these doses, the technique is converted to inhalation of sevoflurane.

[6]For most patients the following formula can be used: 2 μg/kg of remifentanil is prepared in a 20 mL syringe and diluted to a total volume of 20 mL. The first bolus will always, therefore, be 10 mL (=1 μg/kg). If the procedure lasts longer than the analgesia time given by this bolus, second or third boluses (each of 0.5 μg/kg=5 mL) can be given. If the procedure outlasts these doses, the technique is converted to inhalation of sevoflurane.

[7]Apnea is intended with this technique. Apnea is evidence of opioid effect and means that movement in response to lumbar puncture is extremely unlikely. The lumbar puncture has to be performed promptly for this technique to be advantageous. Longer procedures should be managed by an infusion or inhalation technique.

The doctor assigned to the procedure list was already prepared to perform the lumbar puncture (the methotrexate was also ready). Michael's back was prepped and curved as much as possible. (Lumbar puncture in large or obese children can be difficult.) The lumbar puncture was successful, the methotrexate was injected, and the adhesive skin dressing was applied. Within 60 s Michael began to breathe.[8] A simple oxygen mask was applied and he was sent to the recovery room next door. His oxygen saturations, heart rate, and blood pressure (one measurement only) had remained normal throughout. He was awake, talking, and ready to eat and drink 10 min later (see Glaisyer and Sury [105]). Therefore, he was discharged 2 h later. His parents were given advice about headache.

Key Points

1. Interventional radiology is a growing specialty in the United Kingdom and, in the authors hospital, the interventional radiology team is responsible for the insertion of almost all long-term CVCs. Anesthesia ensures immobility and therefore optimal conditions for safe and accurate venipuncture in children.
2. Cardiac defects are common in Down syndrome patients. Chemotherapy can cause cardiomyopathy.
3. Intrathecal vincristine is lethal. This distressing mistake has happened too frequently. The design and distribution of lumbar puncture needles that have special connectors to make the accidental injection of intravenous drugs impossible has yet to be achieved. The current strategy is to separate the administration of intravenous (IV) vincristine and intrathecal (IT) methotrexate to separate "place," "time," and "person," i.e., different hospital, day, and team. The procedure team never administers vincristine in the authors hospital. Occasionally, IV vincristine is administered on the ward to "in-patients" but only with a patient-specific request by an oncologist.
4. The WHO Surgical Safety list process should be applied to all procedures under anesthesia or sedation. The brief is an opportunity for the team to hear and discuss the details of the patients and procedure "once." This is a time-efficient method of communication that can improve safety and efficiency and

[8]The half-life of remifentanil is approximately 5–10 min and is not context dependent. If postoperative pain is expected, another analgesic is necessary. Almost no patients complain of backache or headache within the first hour after lumbar puncture under this technique. Postoperative nausea is rare.

(continued)

an also aid teaching and morale. The "busy" lists may need more than one team brief as the conditions and details of the patients change. A team leader or coordinator may need to be elected.

5. The management of CVCs by anesthetists should follow an agreed protocol. In the authors hospital this includes preparation of drugs in a clean plastic tray by gloved hands. The CVC should be prepared with 2 % alcoholic chlorhexidine for 30 s and allowed to dry before injecting of the drug. The CVC is flushed with 20 mL normal saline afterwards. Later on the ward, the oncology nurses flush the CVC line with heparinized saline before the patient is discharged as an extra precaution against residual anesthesia drugs.

Case 6 (the United Kingdom)

Gastrointestinal Endoscopy in an Anxious 15-Year-Old Girl

The patient has a 2-year history of constipation, diarrhea, and abdominal pain. Her weight is 35 kg; she has lost weight steadily over the past year. She is quiet and does not speak to health-care professionals much. This behavior could be related to being unwell from gastrointestinal disease but may also be related to physical or mental abuse. Child protection problems are common in this patient group. Her parents are with her and her mother does most of the talking. The patient has taken bowel preparation.[9] An intravenous cannula has been inserted and intravenous fluids are being administered to maintain her hydration. (Siting an intravenous cannula outside the endoscopy suite and by nurses may be better for anxious children. Experienced nurses can spend time reassuring the child—time that may not be available during an endoscopy session.)

At the *team brief*,[10] the anesthesia plan is made for her to receive anesthesia by an intravenous propofol infusion and for her to breathe spontaneously without an airway device or support.[11] The endoscopy staff perceives that she is anxious and that she should be first on the list of patients for that session. (This is a common scenario. The order of the patients may have to change and the team brief will enable full discussion and safe planning.) She is sent for but refuses to enter the endoscopy room; persuasion fails. She is persuaded however to accept buccal midazolam (10 mg). Fifteen minutes later, she is less anxious and is wheeled into the endoscopy suite on a trolley. She is in tears. Her parents are with her and try to calm her.

The notes and consent form are checked (these checks are important to avoid mistakes). She refuses to allow monitoring to be placed. The IV fluids are disconnected and 20 mg of lidocaine are injected slowly into the cannula.[12] A propofol TCI has been prepared (50 mL 10 % propofol) and the syringe driver is programmed using the Paedfusor algorithm. (This TCI model/algorithm is in common use in the UK and Europe. It delivers propofol to achieve a target blood level. The dose delivered follows the algorithm based on published data collected in children. Refer to Chaps. 11 and 31.) The target level is set at 6 μg/mL. The patient is not fully cooperative but will allow her parents to hold her hands while the propofol infusion line is connected to the cannula. She is crying.

The infusion begins. She is asleep within 60 s and the parents leave the room. The endoscopy team (anesthetists, endoscopist, and nurses) help to turn her on her side and apply the monitoring. Nasal cannulae incorporating an oxygen delivery portal and a capnography sampling tube is applied first. The breathing is continuously monitored by capnography. The pulse oximeter is applied next followed by the blood pressure cuff and ECG.

The patient's position and comfort is checked. A bite block is inserted into the mouth (the bite block protects the endoscope and prolongs its useful life). Five minutes after the start of the TCI a suction catheter

[9]Bowel preparation should achieve a clean colon and evidence of its effect will be the passing of watery stools. Dehydration is a common problem and therefore intravenous fluid replacement will be necessary in some children.

[10]The team brief should involve all members of the team. Communication of the details of the procedures and the expected problems can be discussed in order to minimize problems and delays. Essential safety and quality checks can be carried out at this stage.

[11]This method will not be appropriate for all children. Small children and those with cardiorespiratory problems may be more safely managed by tracheal intubation. Propofol infusion provides a recovery profile that has minimal side effects. Occasionally this method is not successful because of airway obstruction—prompt airway rescue/support including tracheal intubation will be necessary in some children.

[12]The lidocaine injection is for two reasons: to test the patency of the cannula and to help reduce any pain from the propofol.

(continued)

is inserted into the pharynx to aspirate secretions.[13] She moves and gags on the suction catheter. Another minute passes and the suction is applied again. There is little if any movement. The breathing is steady at approximately 20 breaths per minute. The capnograph number is low and the waveform is not "full," but it is sufficient to prove that she is breathing and that the airway is not obstructed.

The esophagus is intubated with the endoscope. Secretions in the pharynx are aspirated by the anesthetist who remains at the head of the patient throughout. (Secretions can cause laryngospasm. The lateral position and continuous suction may reduce this problem.) From this position the anesthetist can see the capnograph and support the airway by whatever is needed (suction, chin lift, jaw thrust, or other airway device). The endoscopy proceeds uneventfully until the duodenum is intubated. There is some retching and more secretions are aspirated. (Retching and other autonomic reflexes [bradycardia] can be triggered by duodenal intubation.)

The upper endoscopy ends and she (on the trolley) is turned around to receive the colonoscopy. The TCI is turned down to 3 μg/mL.[14] The colonoscopy proceeds uneventfully until the cecum is reached. The patient moves and the heart rate and breathing rate increase. The TCI is increased to 6 μg/mL and 1 min is awaited before the endoscopy proceeds. The ileum is biopsied and the colonoscope is gradually removed while biopsying all the parts of the colon. The TCI is reduced to 3 μg/mL. As the rectum is biopsied, the TCI is set to 0 μg/mL. (Setting the target to 0, rather than turning the infusion off, allows the possibility of restarting the infusion of anesthesia if it needs to be prolonged for any reason.)

The procedure ends. The infusion is disconnected. The staff checks that they have completed all the intended tasks. The cannula is flushed with saline and the patient is wheeled into the recovery area. She begins to rouse within 10 min and is sitting up, talking, and drinking water with 30 min. She is able to walk and is ready for discharge from the hospital 2 h later.

Key Points

1. Several anxiolytics are effective but buccal midazolam is one of the quickest and often the most easily tolerated. Some of the midazolam is likely to be spit out or swallowed in uncooperative patients.
2. Parents are generally helpful in reducing anxiety and helping to achieve cooperation.
3. The anesthetists and endoscopist must be prepared to abandon the procedure and remove the endoscope if airway obstruction cannot be resolved. An absent capnograph signal is a serious warning of impending hypoxia. The patient will look cyanosed before the pulse oximeter registers desaturation.
4. In the authors experience with this sedation technique, almost no children needed analgesia or antiemetics.

[13]The suction catheter stimulates the gag reflex and tests the "depth" of anesthesia to help predict whether or not the endoscope will be tolerated. If the patient does not tolerate the endoscope, the anesthetist needs to decide if the target propofol blood level should be increased or not. Often the patient will settle if extra time is allowed and this may be because the mechanism of action of propofol (i.e., its pharmacodynamics) takes more time than expected.

[14]Insertion of the colonoscope is not very stimulating. The first part of the colonoscopy is not stimulating until the colon is stretched by looping of the colonoscope. Some patients show signs of discomfort. A background infusion of remifentanil (0.1–0.5 μg/kg/min) is effective and, provided it is adjusted to the respiratory rate, appreciable respiratory depression is unlikely.

References

1. Mackenbach JP, Karanikolos M, McKee M. The unequal health of Europeans: successes and failures of policies. Lancet. 2013; 381:1125–34.
2. Coté CJ, Karl HW, Notterman DA, Weinberg JA, McCloskey C. Adverse sedation events in pediatrics: analysis of medications used for sedation. Pediatrics. 2000;106:633–44.
3. Coté CJ, Notterman DA, Karl HW, Weinberg JA, McCloskey C. Adverse sedation events in pediatrics: a critical incident analysis of contributing factors. Pediatrics. 2000;105:805–14.
4. Leroy PL, Nieman FH, Blokland-Loggers HE, Schipper DM, Zimmermann LJ, Knape JT. Adherence to safety guidelines on paediatric procedural sedation: the results of a nationwide survey under general pediatricians in The Netherlands. Arch Dis Child. 2010;95(12):1027–30.
5. Leroy P. Improving procedural sedation and/or analgesia in children. 2012. p. 23–43. ISBN:978-94-6159-120-3. http://arno.unimaas.nl/show.cgi?fid=24183.
6. Hain RD, Campbell C. Invasive procedures carried out in conscious children: contrast between North American and European paediatric oncology centres. Arch Dis Child. 2001;85(1):12–5.
7. Wiener L, McConnell DG, Latella L, Ludi E. Cultural and religious considerations in pediatric palliative care. Palliat Support Care. 2013;11:47–67.
8. Cheng Y, Lin CP, Hsu YY, Lim KE, Hung D, Decety J. Expertise modulates the perception of pain in others. Curr Biol. 2007; 17.1708–13.
9. Leroy P. Improving procedural sedation and/or analgesia in children. 2012. p. 148–55. ISBN:978-94-6159-120-3. http://arno.unimaas.nl/show.cgi?fid=24183.
10. Frankel RI. The Papoose Board and mothers' attitudes following its use. Pediatr Dent. 1991;13(5):284–8.

11. Carr KR, Wilson S, Nimer S, Thornton Jr JB. Behavior management techniques among pediatric dentists practicing in the southeastern United States. Pediatr Dent. 1999;21(6):347–53.
12. Cote CJ, Wilson S. Guidelines for monitoring and management of pediatric patients during and after sedation for diagnostic and therapeutic procedures: an update. Pediatrics. 2006;118(6):2587–602.
13. Morton N, et al. SIGN. Safe sedation of children undergoing diagnostic and therapeutic procedures. A national clinical guideline. Edinburgh: Scottish Intercollegiate Guidelines Network; 2004.
14. Leroy P, Schipper D, Knape J. Summary of the Dutch evidence based guideline on procedural sedation and/or analgesia (PSA) in children at locations outside the operating theater (Chapter 5 in Improving Procedural Sedation and/or Analgesia in Children). Dutch Institute for Health Care Improvement. 2012. ISBN:978-94-6159-120-3. http://arno.unimaas.nl/show.cgi?fid=24183.
15. Royal College of Nursing. Restrictive physical intervention and therapeutic holding for children and young people. Guidance for nursing staff. 2010. http://www.rcn.org.uk/__data/assets/pdf_file/0016/312613/003573.pdf.
16. Nunn J, Foster M, Master S, Greening S. British Society of Paediatric Dentistry: a policy document on consent and the use of physical intervention in the dental care of children. Int J Paediatr Dent. 2008;18 Suppl 1:39–46.
17. Folkes K. Is restraint a form of abuse? Paediatr Nurs. 2005; 17(6):41–4.
18. Hardy M, Armitage G. The child's right to consent to x-ray and imaging investigations: issues of restraint and immobilization from a multidisciplinary perspective. J Child Health Care. 2002; 6(2):107–19.
19. Sønderskov ML, Hallas P. The use of 'brutacaine' in Danish emergency departments. Eur J Emerg Med. 2013;20:370–2.
20. Pressdee D, May L, Eastman E, Grier D. The use of play therapy in the preparation of children undergoing MR imaging. Clin Radiol. 1997;52(12):945–7.
21. Armstrong TS, Aitken HL. The developing role of play preparation in paediatric anaesthesia. Paediatr Anaesth. 2000;10(1):1–4.
22. Liossi C, White P, Hatira P. Randomized clinical trial of local anesthetic versus a combination of local anesthetic with self-hypnosis in the management of pediatric procedure-related pain. Health Psychol. 2006;25(3):307–15.
23. Liossi C, Hatira P. Clinical hypnosis in the alleviation of procedure-related pain in pediatric oncology patients. Int J Clin Exp Hypn. 2003;51(1):4–28.
24. Dingeman RS, Mitcell EA, Meyer EC, Curley MA. Parent presence during complex invasive procedures and cardiopulmonary resuscitation: a systematic review of the literature. Pediatrics. 2007;120:842–54.
25. Corniero P, Gamell A, Cotanda CP, Trenchs V, Cubells CL. Family presence during invasive procedures at the emergency department. What is the opinion of Spanish Medical Staff? Pediatr Emerg Care. 2011;27:86–91.
26. Maxton FJ. Parental presence during resuscitation in the PICU: the parents' experience. Sharing and surviving the resuscitation: a phenomenological study. J Clin Nurs. 2008;17(23):3168–76.
27. Leroy P, Verbeke J, Nieman F, Blokland-Loggers H. Safe and effective procedural sedation for magnetic resonance imaging in children: daily practice in The Netherlands compared with the results of a systematic literature review. Dutch J Pediatr. 2011; 79:42–54.
28. Gauillard J, Cheref S, Vacherontrystram MN, Martin JC. Chloral hydrate: a hypnotic best forgotten? Encéphale. 2002;28(3 Pt 1):200–4.
29. Annequin D, Carbajal R, Chauvin P, Gall O, Tourniaire B, Murat I. Fixed 50% nitrous oxide oxygen mixture for painful procedures: a French survey. Pediatrics. 2000;105(4):E47.
30. Gall O, Annequin D, Benoit G, Glabeke E, Vrancea F, Murat I. Adverse events of premixed nitrous oxide and oxygen for procedural sedation in children. Lancet. 2001;358(9292):1514–5.
31. Zier JL, Drake GJ, McCormick PC, Clinch KM, Cornfield DN. Case-series of nurse-administered nitrous oxide for urinary catheterization in children. Anesth Analg. 2007;104(4):876–9.
32. Sanders RD, Weimann J, Maze M. Biologic effects of nitrous oxide: a mechanistic and toxicologic review. Anesthesiology. 2008;109:707–22.
33. Chiaretti A, Benini F, Pierri F, Vecchiato K, Ronfani L, Agosto C, Ventura A, Genovese O, Barbi E. Safety and efficacy of propofol administered by paediatricians during procedural sedation in children. Acta Paediatr. 2014;103:182–7.
34. Perel A. Non-anaesthesiologists should not be allowed to administer propofol for procedural sedation: a Consensus Statement of 21 European National Societies of Anaesthesia. Eur J Anesthesiol. 2011;28:580–4.
35. Delaunay L, Gentili M, Cittanova ML, Delbos A, Lile A. Anaesthesia by non-anaesthesiologists: the Pandora Box is open! Eur J Anaesthesiol. 2012;29:50–1.
36. Knape J. Procedural sedation and analgesia and the propofol affair: a unique opportunity for anaesthesiology. Eur J Anaesthesiol. 2012;29:51–2.
37. Po C, Benini F, Sainati L, Farina M, Cesaro S, Agosto C. Procedural pain management in Italy: learning from a nationwide survey involving centers of the Italian Association of Pediatric Hematology-Oncology. Pediatr Rep. 2011;3(4):e34.
38. NCEPOD. Extremes of age. The national confidential enquiry into perioperative deaths. 1999. http://www.ncepod.org.uk/.
39. Barbi E, Petaros P, Badina L, Pahor T, Giuseppin I, Biasotto E, et al. Deep sedation with propofol for upper gastrointestinal endoscopy in children, administered by specially trained pediatricians: a prospective case series with emphasis on side effects. Endoscopy. 2006;38(4):368–75.
40. Rex DK, Deenadayalu VP, Eid E, Imperiale TF, Walker JA, Sandhu K, et al. Endoscopist-directed administration of propofol: a worldwide safety experience. Gastroenterology. 2009;137(4): 1229–37; quiz.
41. Green SM, Krauss B. Barriers to propofol use in emergency medicine. Ann Emerg Med. 2008;52:392–8.
42. Strunin L. Intravenous conscious sedation for dental treatment: am I my brother's keeper? Anaesthesia. 2007;62(7):645–7.
43. Babl F, Munro FJ, Kainey G, Palmer GM, Iser A. Scope for improvement: hospital wide sedation practice at a children's hospital. Arch Dis Child. 2006;91(8):716–7.
44. Leroy P. Improving procedural sedation and/or analgesia in children. 2012. p. 16. ISBN:978-94-6159-120-3. http://arno.unimaas.nl/show.cgi?fid=24183.
45. Kannikeswaran N, Chen X, Sethuraman U. Utility of endtidal carbon dioxide monitoring in detection of hypoxia during sedation for brain magnetic resonance imaging in children with developmental disabilities. Paediatr Anaesth. 2011;21(12):1241–6.
46. Yldzdas D, Yapcoglu H, Ylmaz HL. The value of capnography during sedation or sedation/analgesia in pediatric minor procedures. Pediatr Emerg Care. 2004;20(3):162–5.
47. Burton F. Towards evidence based emergency medicine: best BETs from the Manchester Royal Infirmary. BET 2: should capnography be routinely used during procedural sedation in the Emergency Department? Emerg Med J. 2012;29:164–6.
48. Smith D, Andrzejowski J, Smith A. Certainty and uncertainty: NICE guidance on 'depth of anaesthesia' monitoring. Anaesthesia. 2013;68(10):1000–5.
49. Harrison GR, Critchley AD, Mayhew CA, Thompson JM. Real-time breath monitoring of propofol and its volatile metabolites during surgery using a novel mass spectrometric technique: a feasibility study. Br J Anaesth. 2003;91(6):797–9.
50. Perl T, Carstens E, Hirn A, Quintel M, Vautz W, Nolte J, et al. Determination of serum propofol concentrations by breath analysis using ion mobility spectrometry. Br J Anaesth. 2009; 103(6):822–7.

51. Cowley NJ, Laitenberger P, Liu B, Jarvis J, Clutton-Brock TH. Evaluation of a new analyser for rapid measurement of blood propofol concentration during cardiac surgery. Anaesthesia. 2012;67(8):870–4.
52. Royal College of Anaesthetists and Royal College of Radiologists. Sedation and anaesthesia in radiology. Report of a joint working party. London: Royal College of Anaesthetists; 1992.
53. Academy of Medical Royal Colleges. Safe sedation practice for healthcare procedures in adults. Report of an intercollegiate working party chaired by the Royal College of Anaesthetists. London: Academy of Medical Royal Colleges; 2001.
54. SIGN. Safe sedation of children undergoing diagnostic and therapeutic procedures. A national clinical guideline. Edinburgh: Scottish Intercollegiate Guidelines Network; 2004.
55. NICE. Sedation in children and young people (CG112). NICE. 2011. http://www.nice.org.uk/cg112.
56. Levati A, Paccagnella F, Pietrini D, Buscalferri A, Calamandrei M, Grossetti R, et al. SIAARTI-SARNePI guidelines for sedation in pediatric neuro-radiology. Minerva Anestesiol. 2004; 70(10):675–97.
57. Knape JT, Adriaensen H, van Aken H, Blunnie WP, Carlsson C, Dupont M, et al. Guidelines for sedation and/or analgesia by non-anaesthesiology doctors. Eur J Anaesthesiol. 2007;24(7):563–7.
58. Hoffman GM, Nowakowski R, Troshynski TJ, Berens RJ, Weisman SJ. Risk reduction in pediatric procedural sedation by application of an American Academy of Pediatrics/American Society of Anesthesiologists process model. Pediatrics. 2002; 109(2):236–43.
59. Cravero JP, Blike GT. Pride, prejudice, and pediatric sedation: a multispecialty evaluation of the state of the art. Report from a Dartmouth Summit on Pediatric Sedation. Boston, MA: National Patient Safety Foundation; 2001.
60. Daviss WB, Mooney D, Racusin R, Ford JD, Fleischer A, McHugo GJ. Predicting posttraumatic stress after hospitalization for pediatric injury. J Am Acad Child Adolesc Psychiatry. 2000;39(5):576–83.
61. Daviss WB, Racusin R, Fleischer A, Mooney D, Ford JD, McHugo GJ. Acute stress disorder symptomatology during hospitalization for pediatric injury. J Am Acad Child Adolesc Psychiatry. 2000;39(5):569–75.
62. Leroy P, ten Hoopen R. Forced immobilization ('restraint') during medical procedures in young children. An ethical and legal investigation of a common practice. (Chapter 4 in Improving Procedural Sedation and/or Analgesia in Children). 2012. ISBN:978-94-6159-120-3. http://arno.unimaas.nl/show.cgi?fid=24183.
63. Davidson AJ. Anesthesia and neurotoxicity to the developing brain: the clinical relevance. Paediatr Anaesth. 2011;21(7):716–21. doi:10.1111/j.1460-9592.2010.03506.x. Epub 2011 Apr 6.
64. Jevtovic-Todorovic V. Anesthesia and the developing brain: are we getting closer to understanding the truth? Curr Opin Anaesthesiol. 2011;24(24):395–9.
65. Green SM, Cote CJ. Ketamine and neurotoxicity: clinical perspectives and implications for emergency medicine. Ann Emerg Med. 2009;54(2):181–90.
66. Cote CJ. Round and round we go: sedation—what is it, who does it, and have we made things safer for children? Paediatr Anaesth. 2008;18(1):3–8.
67. Department of Health/Faculty of General Dental Practice (UK). Guidelines for the appointment of dentists with a special interest (DwSI) in conscious sedation. London: Department of Health; 2008.
68. Vangerven M, Van Hemelrijck J, Wouters P, Vandermeersch E, Van Aken H. Light anaesthesia with propofol for paediatric MRI. Anaesthesia. 1992;47:706–7.
69. Sury M, Harker H, Thomas M. Sedation for MRI using sevoflurane. Paediatr Anaesth. 2005;15(11):1025.
70. De Sanctis Briggs V. Magnetic resonance imaging under sedation in newborns and infants: a study of 640 cases using sevoflurane. Paediatr Anaesth. 2005;15:9–15.
71. Holroyd I. Conscious sedation in pediatric dentistry. A short review of the current UK guidelines and the technique of inhalational sedation with nitrous oxide. Pediatr Anesth. 2008;18:13–7.
72. Motas D, McDermott NB, VanSickle T, Friesen RH. Depth of consciousness and deep sedation attained in children as administered by nonanaesthesiologists in a children's hospital. Paediatr Anaesth. 2004;14(3):256–60.
73. Craig D. Safe and effective sedation. Br Dent J. 2011;211(8):343.
74. Krauss B, Green SM. Training and credentialing in procedural sedation and analgesia in children: lessons from the United States model. Paediatr Anaesth. 2008;18(1):30–5.
75. Sheldon TA, Cullum N, Dawson D, Lankshear A, Lowson K, Watt I, et al. What's the evidence that NICE guidance has been implemented? Results from a national evaluation using time series analysis, audit of patients' notes, and interviews. BMJ. 2004; 329(7473):999.
76. Leroy P, ten Hoopen R. Forced providing procedural sedation/analgesia in children. How satisfied are Dutch general paediatricians with their personal performance? (Chapter 2.4 in Improving Procedural Sedation and/or Analgesia in Children). 2012. ISBN: 978-94-6159-120-3. http://arno.unimaas.nl/show.cgi?fid=24183
77. Kain ZN, Gaal DJ, Kain TS, Jaeger DD, Rimar S. A first-pass cost analysis of propofol versus barbiturates for children undergoing magnetic resonance imaging. Anesth Analg. 1994;79(6):1102–10.
78. Ekbom K, Jakobsson J, Marcus C. Nitrous oxide inhalation is a safe and effective way to facilitate procedures in paediatric outpatient departments. Arch Dis Child. 2005;90(10):1073–6.
79. Sury MRJ, Hatch DJ, Deeley T, Dicks-Mireaux C, Chong WK. Development of a nurse-led sedation service for paediatric magnetic resonance imaging. Lancet. 1999;353:1667–71.
80. Keengwe IN, Hegde S, Dearlove O, Wilson B, Yates RW, Sharples A. Structured sedation programme for magnetic resonance imaging examination in children. Anaesthesia. 1999;54(11):1069–72.
81. Woodthorpe C, Trigg A, Alison G, Sury M. Nurse led sedation for paediatric MRI: progress and issues. Paediatr Nurs. 2007; 19(2):14–8.
82. Jackson EA, Rabbette PS, Dezateux C, Hatch DJ, Stocks J. The effect of triclofos sodium sedation on respiratory rate, oxygen saturation, and heart rate in infants and young children. Pediatr Pulmonol. 1991;10(1):40–5.
83. Sury MR, Smith JH. Deep sedation and minimal anesthesia. Paediatr Anaesth. 2008;18(1):18–24.
84. Koroglu A, Teksan H, Sagir O, Yucel A, Toprak HI, Ersoy OM. A comparison of the sedative, hemodynamic, and respiratory effects of dexmedetomidine and propofol in children undergoing magnetic resonance imaging (see comment). Anesth Analg. 2006;103(1):63–7.
85. Koroglu A, Demirbilek S, Teksan H, Sagir O, But AK, Ersoy MO. Sedative, haemodynamic and respiratory effects of dexmedetomidine in children undergoing magnetic resonance imaging examination: preliminary results. Br J Anaesth. 2005;94(6):821–4.
86. The Association of Anaesthetists of Great Britain and Ireland. Provision of anaesthetic services in magnetic resonance units. 2002.
87. Sammons HM, Edwards J, Rushby R, Picton C, Collier J, Whitehouse WP. General anaesthesia or sedation for paediatric neuroimaging: current practice in a teaching hospital. Arch Dis Child. 2011;96(1):114.
88. Zorab JS. A general anaesthesia service for magnetic resonance imaging. Eur J Anaesthesiol. 1995;12(4):387–95.
89. Levati A, Colombo N, Arosio EM, Savoia G, Tommasino C, Scialfa G, et al. Propofol anaesthesia in spontaneously breathing paediatric patients during magnetic resonance imaging. Acta Anaesthesiol Scand. 1996;40(5):561–5.
90. Machata AM, Willschke H, Kabon B, Kettner SC, Marhofer P. Propofol-based sedation regimen for infants and children undergoing ambulatory magnetic resonance imaging. Br J Anaesth. 2008;101(2):239–43.

91. Burijnen CJ, Halbertsma FJ, Mohns T, van Ooyen F, Dijkman KP. [Procedural sedation with propofol in non-painful interventions in children]. Ned Tijdschr Geneeskd. 2011;155(26):A2523. Dutch.
92. Akin A, Esmaoglu A, Guler G, Demircioglu R, Narin N, Boyaci A. Propofol and propofol-ketamine in pediatric patients undergoing cardiac catheterization. Pediatr Cardiol. 2005;26(5):553–7.
93. Rautiainen P, Meretoja OA. Ketamine boluses with continuous low-dose fentanyl for paediatric sedation during diagnostic cardiac catheterization. Paediatr Anaesth. 1993;3:345–51.
94. Donmez A, Kizilkan A, Berksun H, Varan B, Tokel K. One center's experience with remifentanil infusions for pediatric cardiac catheterization. J Cardiothorac Vasc Anesth. 2001;15(6):736–9.
95. Taylor CJ, Derrick G, McEwan A, Haworth SG, Sury MR. Risk of cardiac catheterization under anaesthesia in children with pulmonary hypertension. Br J Anaesth. 2007;98(5):657–61.
96. Bennett D, Marcus R, Stokes M. Incidents and complications during pediatric cardiac catheterization. Paediatr Anaesth. 2005; 15(12):1083–8.
97. Michaud L. Sedation for diagnostic upper gastrointestinal endoscopy: a survey of the Francophone Pediatric Hepatology, Gastroenterology, and Nutrition Group. Endoscopy. 2005; 37(2):167–70.
98. Stringer MD, McHugh PJM. Paediatric endoscopy should be carried out under general anaesthesia. Br Med J. 1995;311:452–3.
99. Lamireau T, Dubreuil M, Daconceicao M. Oxygen saturation during esophagogastroduodenoscopy in children: general anesthesia versus intravenous sedation [see comments]. J Pediatr Gastroenterol Nutr. 1998;27(2):172–5.
100. Barbi E, Gerarduzzi T, Marchetti F, Neri E, Verucci E, Bruno I, et al. Deep sedation with propofol by nonanesthesiologists: a prospective pediatric experience. Arch Pediatr Adolesc Med. 2003;157(11):1097–103.
101. Perera C, Strandvik GF, Malik M, Sen S. Propofol anesthesia is an effective and safe strategy for pediatric endoscopy. Pediatr Anesth. 2006;16(2A):220–1.
102. van Beek EJ, Leroy PL. Safe and effective procedural sedation for gastrointestinal endoscopy in children. J Pediatr Gastroenterol Nutr. 2012;54(2):171–85.
103. Mani V, Morton NS. Overview of total intravenous anesthesia in children. Paediatr Anaesth. 2010;20(3):211–22.
104. Culshaw V, Yule M, Lawson R. Considerations for anaesthesia in children with haematological malignancy undergoing short procedures. Paediatr Anaesth. 2003;13:375–83.
105. Glaisyer HR, Sury MR. Recovery after anesthesia for short pediatric oncology procedures: propofol and remifentanil compared with propofol, nitrous oxide, and sevoflurane. Anesth Analg. 2005;100(4):959–63.
106. McGlone RG, Howes MC, Joshi M. The Lancaster experience of 2.0 to 2.5 mg/kg intramuscular ketamine for paediatric sedation: 501 cases and analysis. Emerg Med J. 2004;21(3):290–5.
107. Mintegi S, Shavit I, Benito J. Pediatric emergency care in Europe: a descriptive survey of 53 tertiary medical centers. Pediatr Emerg Care. 2008;24(6):359–63.
108. Loryman B, Davies F, Chavada G, Coats T. Consigning "brutacaine" to history: a survey of pharmacological techniques to facilitate painful procedures in children in emergency departments in the UK. Emerg Med J. 2006;23(11):838–40.
109. MacLean S, Obispo J, Young KD. The gap between pediatric emergency department procedural pain management treatments available and actual practice. Pediatr Emerg Care. 2007; 23(2):87–93.
110. Morton NS. Ketamine for procedural sedation and analgesia in pediatric emergency medicine: a UK perspective. Paediatr Anaesth. 2008;18(1):25–9.
111. Kennedy RM, Porter FL, Miller JP, Jaffe DM. Comparison of fentanyl/midazolam with ketamine/midazolam for pediatric orthopedic emergencies. Pediatrics. 1998;102(4 Pt 1):956–63.
112. Foley J. Nitrous oxide inhalation sedation: what do patients, carers and dentists think about it? Eur J Paediatr Dent. 2005;6(1):23–9.
113. Department of Health UK. Conscious sedation in the provision of dental care: report of an Expert Group on Sedation for Dentistry, Standing Dental Advisory Committee. 2003. [cited 15 Mar 2006]. Available from: www.doh.gov.uk/dental.
114. Department of Health UK. Report by a Group chaired by the Chief Medical Officer and Chief Dental Officer. A conscious decision: a review of the use of general anaesthesia and conscious sedation in primary dental care. 2000. http://www.dh.gov.uk/en/Publications andstatistics/Publications/PublicationsPolicyAndGuidance/DH_ 40747022000.
115. Averley PA, Girdler NM, Bond S, Steen N, Steele J. A randomised controlled trial of paediatric conscious sedation for dental treatment using intravenous midazolam combined with inhaled nitrous oxide or nitrous oxide/sevoflurane. Anaesthesia. 2004;59(9):844–52.
116. Klingberg G. Pharmacological approach to the management of dental anxiety in children–comments from a Scandinavian point of view. Int J Paediatr Dent. 2002;12(5):357–8.
117. Wilson KE, Welbury RR, Girdler NM. A study of the effectiveness of oral midazolam sedation for orthodontic extraction of permanent teeth in children: a prospective, randomised, controlled, crossover trial. Br Dent J. 2002;192:457–62.
118. Day PF, Power AM, Hibbert SA, Paterson SA. Effectiveness of oral midazolam for paediatric dental care: a retrospective study in two specialist centres. Eur Arch Paediatr Dent. 2006;7(4):228–35.
119. Leelataweedwud P, Vann Jr WF. Adverse events and outcomes of conscious sedation for pediatric patients: study of an oral sedation regimen. J Am Dent Assoc. 2001;132(11):1531–9.
120. Wood M. The safety and efficacy of using a concentrated intranasal midazolam formulation for paediatric dental sedation. SAAD Dig. 2011;27:16–23.
121. Wilson KE, Girdler NM, Welbury RR. Randomized, controlled, cross-over clinical trial comparing intravenous midazolam sedation with nitrous oxide sedation in children undergoing dental extractions. Br J Anaesth. 2003;91(6):850–6.
122. Rodrigo MR, Jonsson E. Conscious sedation with propofol. Br Dent J. 1989;166(3):75–80.
123. The Royal College of Anaesthetists and the Faculty of Dental Surgery of the Royal College of Surgeons. Standards for conscious sedation in dentistry: alternative techniques. A report from the Standing Committee on Sedation for Dentistry. 2007. http:// www.rcoa.ac.uk/docs/SCSDAT.pdf.
124. Faculty of Dental Surgery, The Royal College of Surgeons of England. The Royal College of Anaesthetists. Standards for conscious sedation in dentistry: alternative techniques. Report from the Standing Committee on sedation for dentistry. London: Faculty of Dental Surgery, The Royal College of Surgeons of England; 2007.
125. Mikhael MS, Wray S, Robb ND. Intravenous conscious sedation in children for outpatient dentistry. Br Dent J. 2007;203(6):323–31.
126. Wood M. Intravenous ketamine and propofol in paediatric dental sedation: safe and effective? SAAD Dig. 2013;29:31–9.
127. Wood M. The use of intravenous midazolam and ketamine in paediatric dental sedation. SAAD Dig. 2013;29:18–30.
128. Davies MW, Nind D. Anaesthesia for exodontia in young children—a snapshot survey of European practice. Anaesthesia. 1996;51:713.
129. Worthington LM, Flynn PJ, Strunin L. Death in the dental chair: an avoidable catastrophe ? Br J Anaesth. 1998;80(2):131–2.
130. Sury M, Bullock I, Rabar S, Demott K. Sedation for diagnostic and therapeutic procedures in children and young people: summary of NICE guidelines. BMJ. 2010;341:c6819.
131. Leroy PL, Schipper DM, Knape HJ. Professional skills and competence for safe and effective procedural sedation in children: recommendations based on a systematic review of the literature. Int J Pediatr. 2010;2010:934298.

Pediatric Sedation: The South American Approach

22

Paulo Sérgio Sucasas da Costa
and Pablo Sepúlveda Voullième

Abstract

South America is comprised of 13 countries and a population of approximately 350 million people. It has an area of 6,890,000 mile^2 (17,840,000 km^2) and in 2005 its population was estimated at around 371,090,000. The languages of South America are mainly Castilian Spanish and Portuguese. A variety of social, political, and economic factors make this region very heterogeneous. In the medical field, specifically in the area of sedation, the heterogeneity continues. The diverse development of the varied region makes it possible to find profound backwardness adjacent to technological developments that are at the forefront of medicine. This incongruity is especially apparent in Brazil, Venezuela, Colombia, and Peru.

This chapter will explore the sedation practices within the various regions of South America.

Keywords

Pediatric sedation • Confederation of Latin American Societies of Anesthesiologists (CLASA) • South America • Brazil • Venezuela • Colombia • Peru • Anesthesiologist • Dentist • Nurse • Target-controlled infusion (TCI) • Propofol • Remifentanyl/remifentanil • Sufentanyl/sufentanil • Ketamine • Nitrous oxide • Fentanyl • Midazolam • Anestfusor • Ezfusor • Pharmacokinetics • Argentina • Chile

Introduction

South America is comprised of 13 countries and a population of approximately 350 million people. It has an area of 6,890,000 mile^2 (17,840,000 km^2) and in 2005 its population was estimated at around 371,090,000. The languages of South America are mainly Castilian Spanish and Portuguese. A variety of social, political, and economic factors make this region very heterogeneous [1].

P.S.S. da Costa, D.D.S., M.S., Ph.D.
Department of Pediatrics, Federal University of Goiás, Goiania, Goias, Brazil

P.S. Voullième, Dr. Med. (✉)
Servicio de Anestesia, Clinica Alemana Santiago Chile, Santiago, Chile
e-mail: pasevou@mi.cl

In the medical field, specifically in the area of sedation, the heterogeneity continues. The diverse development of the varied region makes it possible to find profound backwardness adjacent to technological developments that are at the forefront of medicine. This incongruity is especially apparent in Brazil, Venezuela, Colombia, and Peru.

This chapter will explore the sedation practices within the various regions of South America.

Pediatric Sedation in South America: A General Overview

In South America, a significant proportion of sedation is delivered by anesthesiologists. The anesthesia specialty in South America has evolved under the consolidation of the Confederation of Latin American Societies of Anesthesiologists

K.P. Mason (ed.), *Pediatric Sedation Outside of the Operating Room: A Multispecialty International Collaboration*,
DOI 10.1007/978-1-4939-1390-9_22, © Springer Science+Business Media New York 2015

(CLASA).[1] CLASA was established in 1963 following two decades of political and economic stability. CLASA has many working committees, including a Committee for Pediatric Anesthesia and Safety. Moreover, CLASA sponsors books that have been translated into Spanish, including *Understanding Pediatric Anesthesia* [2] as well as educational videos such as *Total Intravenous Anesthesia (TIVA) in Pediatric Anesthesia* [3]. The CLASA Committee on Pediatric Anesthesia has developed rules and guidelines that specifically address sedation outside the operating room: "Given the special characteristics of pediatric patients, which should be handled in most circumstances by deep sedation and/or anesthesia, operations outside the surgical area will have the same requirements for general equipment as the operating room, always under the supervision of the anesthesiologist."

The most significant difference between sedation practice in South America and North America is that in the South, it is rare for nurses to deliver sedation, even in isolated regions. Rather, sedation is delivered by physicians under the guidelines of their specialty societies. In general, the Ministries of Health in South America support this anesthesia delivery model, despite the paucity of anesthesiologists in some regions. As in many developing countries, the overwhelming proportion of anesthesiologists in South America is concentrated in large cities, fostering economic activity in the private sector. In spite of the irregular distribution of anesthesiologists, morbidity and mortality related to anesthesia are estimated to be very low.

The decrease in the acquisition costs of physiological monitors has enabled sedation services to meet the international standards. Today there is an almost universal implementation of hemodynamic and respiratory monitoring, which includes pulse oximetry and capnography.

There remain specific venues of sedation delivery in South America that need improvement: gastrointestinal endoscopy, dentistry, radiology, oncology, and urology. A lingering challenge is access to sedation in the remote forests and mountains where the indigenous peoples still live.

It is remarkable that in South America, the target-controlled infusion (TCI) delivery systems are available for anesthesiologists (TCI is not currently available in the United States). TCI is a computerized intravenous infusion device that delivers medication using pharmacokinetic (PK) models of propofol, remifentanil, and sufentanil. Currently, most TCI systems in South America include pediatric PK models, which were created in Chile (Ezfusor, Fig. 22.1). TCI intends to maintain a steady drug plasma concentration, prevent drug over accumulation, and achieve a targeted plasma serum concentration. TCI delivery systems are intended to replace the fixed-rate infusion delivery model, thereby avoiding the peaks and troughs in plasma levels. Avoiding these inconsistencies should reduce the risk of cardiorespiratory depression and episodes of awakening during sedation.

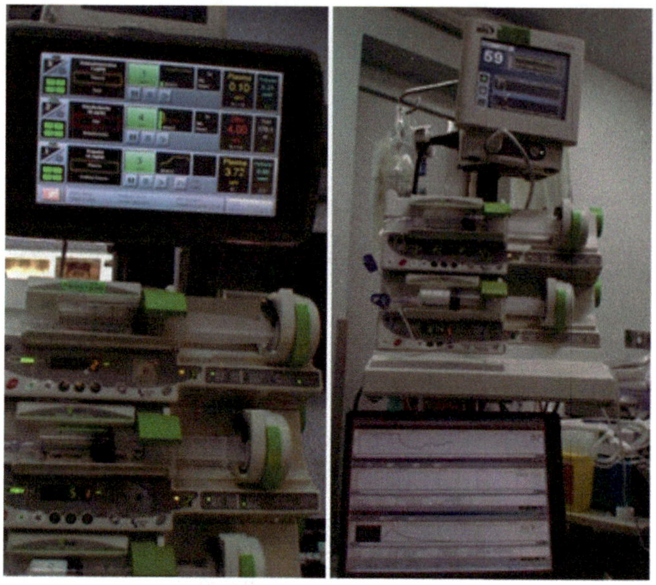

Figure 22.1 *Left*: Ezfusor. *Right*: Anestfusor. Both control infusion pumps (DPS, Fresenius Kabi)

Argentina

In Argentina tight control is exercised by the Federation of the Associations of Anesthesiology of Argentina[2] over the reimbursement for and practice of anesthesiology. This federation has a pediatric anesthesia subgroup, which follows the American Society of Anesthesiologists (ASA) guidelines and policies.

Brazil

In Brazil, there are approximately 9,000 anesthesiologists for a population of about 196 million people (estimated in 2011). There is a concentration of anesthesiologists in large urban areas and a paucity in the northern areas (which includes the Amazon rain forest). The Brazilian College of Physicians (Resolution 1670/2003) supports that deep sedation should only be performed by qualified doctors under conditions in which the procedure is performed by a second, separate professional (physician, dentist). The following should be immediately available: supplies to maintain a patient's airway, administer oxygen, resuscitate cardiovascular and respiratory complications, and document the sedation (medications, doses, effects, and the criteria for discharge).

[1] www.clasa-anestesia.org

[2] http://www.anestesia.org.ar/

Clear verbal and written instructions should be given to the patient and guardians upon discharge to detail the medications received, anticipated side effects, and procedure in the event of an emergency.

Brazilian law supports dentists to perform analgesia, sedation, and hypnosis. The Brazilian College of Dentists regulates the delivery of nitrous oxide: Dentists can administer nitrous oxide/oxygen inhalational sedation after attending an approved 96-h course. A recent survey of Brazilian anesthesiologists revealed that 92.8 % do not support the Brazilian College of Dentists statement that "dentists can administer sedation in the dental office" [4]. Rather, although 85.6 % of the anesthesia respondents had rarely or never provided sedation or anesthesia in the dental office, most were not favorable in their support of dentists providing sedation. Ironically, it was those anesthesiologists who had experience with dental sedation and anesthetics that were the most unsupportive of the dentist as a sedation provider [4]. A follow-up survey in 2012 revealed that 77 % of certified dentists in Brazil administer nitrous oxide. Adult patients with physical or mental disabilities were more likely to receive nitrous oxide [5]. To date, the surveys of dental sedation practice in Brazil are not specifically targeted to evaluate the pediatric population. Rather, they are directed to the adult patient population. It is difficult to thus fully ascertain the pediatric dental sedation practice in Brazil. A 2011 survey of pediatric dentists worldwide, however, supported the global popularity of nitrous oxide administration amongst pediatric dentists. Pediatric dentists cited general anesthesia, nitrous oxide, and oral sedation administration with a frequency of 52, 46, and 44 % consecutively [6]. These surveys suggest that the controversy of who is qualified and competent to administer dental sedation spans between countries and continents worldwide [7].

Physicians and dentists who perform outpatient sedation in Brazil usually follow the international guidelines of the American Academy of Pediatrics (AAP) and the American Academy of Pediatric Dentistry (AAPD). There are, however, documents from the Anesthesiology Societies of Rio de Janeiro and São Paulo (Table 22.1) that guide sedation [8, 9].

One limitation to the practice of safe dental sedation in Brazil is the lack of regulations regarding training, credentialing, and emergency resuscitation skills: Dentists and nurses are not required to have systematic training in medical emergencies (Basic Life Support, BLS; Advanced Cardiovascular Life Support, ACLS; Pediatric Advanced Life Support, PALS) during their formal education or continuing education. Ironically, certification courses for Advanced Life Support in Brazil are directed exclusively to doctors and nurses, forbidding enrollment of dentists.

Chile

In Chile, there are 1,100 anesthesiologists for 17 million people; the biggest challenge is their concentration in large cities. The current accreditation process for anesthesiologists in Chile mirrors those of the Joint International Commission. Pediatric anesthesia is a subspecialty, regulated by the well-established Chilean scientific society,[3] which includes clinical guidelines for sedation outside the operating room [10] with the strong recommendation that sedation in children be delivered by anesthesiologists. An exception to this model would be for dentists to administer oral midazolam and nitrous oxide and for radiologists to administer rectal chloral hydrate. The Chilean Dental Society has a pediatric branch that provides regular courses for sedation with nitrous oxide.

The University of Chile has also developed software (Anestfusor; www.smb.cl) to simulate and control the infusion of propofol using pharmacokinetic models (Paedfusor and Kataria), which have been validated in children [11, 12]. (Refer to Chaps. 11 and 31.) In 2011, a study performed in Chile examined the performance of eight propofol pharmacokinetic models in children (3–26 months of age). There was a tendency to underestimate propofol concentration 1 min after the bolus dose, suggesting that there is a risk of delivering a larger initial bolus than intended. Six models were validated in children: Short, Rigby-Jones, Coppens, Kataria, Paedfusor, and Saint-Maurice (Fig. 22.2). Details on TCI and the models are available in Chap. 31.

The Paedfusor (Glasgow, UK; pump: Arcomed ag—Swiss—Syramed uSP6000 premium) was developed in the early 1990s as a means to deliver propofol to children using pharmacokinetic models. Today the Paedfusor model is available in the Ezfusor (Anestfusor Serie II Pro software—Facultad de Medicina, Universidad de Chile; http://www.smb.cl/en/anestfusor_serie2_proen.html (Figure 22.1 and Figure 22.2), which has touch screen technology, capable of simultaneously controlling three different drugs in the TCI delivery system. This device is available in more than 20 pediatric hospitals in Chile.

In Chile, the difficulty lies in the complex, remote geography and the need to refer patients to tertiary centers from islands or isolated mountain villages. In many cases, the government supports transport costs in order to ensure the safety of the procedure.

[3] www.sachile.cl

Table 22.1 Comparison of different guidelines (AAP/AAPD + South America) related to pediatric sedation

Recommendations	AAP/AAPD [44]	São Paulo, Brazil [8]	Rio de Janeiro, Brazil [9]	Chile [10]	Colombia [13]
HEALTH CARE PROFESSIONAL					
Minimal sedation	Sufficiently skilled	Medical personnel	Sufficiently skilled	Anesthesiologist (strongly recommended)	Able to provide BLS
Moderate sedation	As above, plus personal to monitor	Medical personnel with PALS	Sufficiently skilled	Anesthesiologist (strongly recommended)	Basic airway competences
Deep sedation	As above, but training in PALS	Anesthesiologist	Sufficiently skilled	Anesthesiologist (strongly recommended)	Expert airway management skills (almost exclusively anesthesiologist)
FOODS BEFORE ELECTIVE SEDATION (HOURS)					
Water	–	–	–	1 (75 mL)	–
Clear liquids	2	3	–	2	–
Breast milk	4	2 (premature) 3 (0–6 mo) 4 (6–36 mo)	–	4	–
Infant formula	6	3 (premature) 4 (0–6 mo) 6 (6–36 mo)	–	6	–
Nonhuman milk	6	As above	–	6	–
Light meals	6	6	–	6	–
Heavy meals	8	–	–	8	–
MONITORING RECOMMENDATIONS					
SpO_2	Continuous	Continuous	Continuous	Continuous	Continuous
Respiratory rate	Intermittent	Continuous	Continuous	Continuous	Intermittent
Heart rate	Continuous	Continuous	Continuous	Continuous	Continuous
Blood pressure	Intermittent	Intermittent	Continuous	Continuous	Intermittent
Capnography	Encouraged	Encouraged	Encouraged	Encouraged	Encouraged

Other Countries

In Bolivia there are no clinical guidelines. In general, the first line plan for sedation is oral midazolam administered by a non-physician (radiology technologist). If the child fails to sedate with that protocol, the child is rescheduled for general anesthesia with halothane to be administered by an anesthesiologist. Propofol is not yet reimbursed by the government and is, thus, less favored to thiopental.

In Colombia, there are published guidelines for the sedation of children over 12 years of age by non-anesthesiologists [13]. These guidelines specify that the sedation must be delivered by a separate provider who performs the surgical procedure. Only one sedative is allowed.

In Peru there are no published sedation guidelines. There is some literature describing the Peruvian experience of administering intravenous midazolam, fentanyl, ketamine, and morphine for procedural sedation [14, 15]. There is also a published review describing the most common drugs used in pediatric dental sedation in Peru: midazolam, diazepam, and chloral hydrate [16].

Common Sedation Techniques and Strategies in South America

As a general rule, it is preferred that children (<than 8 years old) undergo procedures with general anesthesia. In all cases the informed consent, preoperative assessment, monitoring,

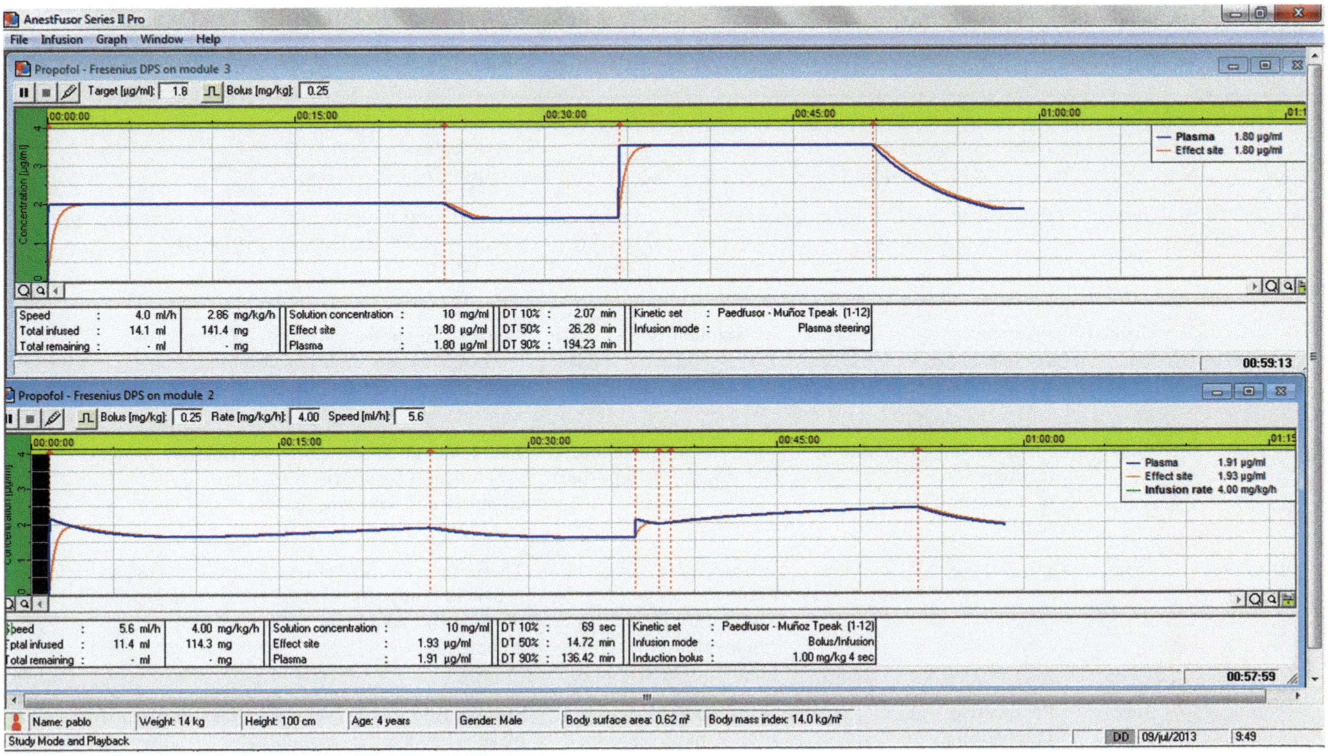

Figure 22.2 Display of Anestfusor simulator (Anestfusor Serie II Pro software—Facultad de Medicina, Universidad de Chile), which compares manual (*top*) versus target-controlled infusion (TCI) effect site of propofol delivery (*bottom*). Note that the proposed target maintains TCI infusion (*bottom*) despite the requirement for constant adjustment for stability. It is impossible to achieve these end points with manual titration (*top*). TCI uses specific parametric models with covariates of the treated population

and documentation mirror that of an anesthetic for a surgical procedure.

In children over 8 years of age, it is possible to use an intravenous sedative technique, ideally after applying a eutectic mixture of local anesthetic cream, which is limited in availability.

Premedications with oral or nasal <0.5 mg/kg midazolam are usually administered 30 min prior to the procedure. The child is then accompanied by a parent or a relative into the procedure room. The sedation may be supplemented with titrated doses of 1 mg/kg subcutaneous or intravenous ketamine and/or propofol TCI. Propofol is usually administered with a Paedfusor target model (1.5–3 µ[mu]g/mL) in progressive steps until the targeted depth of sedation is achieved. Supplemental oxygen is always with standard noninvasive monitoring that meets the ASA guidelines [17].

For painful procedures (lumbar puncture, bone marrow biopsy, fracture mobilization, local anesthetic injection for dental extraction, endoscopy), intravenous alfentanil (6–10 µg/kg) is often titrated at 1-min intervals prior to the stimulus. For colonoscopy and procedures in the emergency department, intravenous fentanyl (1 µg/kg) is preferred at 15-min intervals as required.

In South America there are few established protocols for pediatric sedation. The AAP and AAPD guidelines tend to be followed. The South American protocols are diverging slightly with respect to the qualifications for sedation providers and nil per os (NPO) recommendations (Table 22.1). For example, in the Chilean guidelines, there is a reference specifically to water: 75 mL of water is allowed for children (150 mL for adults) 1 h before sedation [10].

Review of Published Sedation Literature from South America

Over the past 20 years, a variety of sedation literature has been published in South America (Table 22.2) [18–43]. Most of the published studies used midazolam (24; 70.4 %). In 13 of those papers presented in Table 22.2 (68.4 %) midazolam was used as a single drug and its efficacy varied in different scenarios from 66.6 to 89.0 %. Dexmedetomidine, a more recently released drug, was only used in a single study. The most common indication for sedation was procedural sedation (nine papers), followed by its use in dental sedation (seven studies). It is important to highlight that the dental

Table 22.2 Data published (PubMed and Scielo) referring to pediatric sedation in South America (1993–2013)

Author	Country	Study design	Subjects	Sedative	Outcome	Scenario
Gallardo et al. 1994 [18]	Chile	Prospective Double-blind	32 uncooperative children	Midazolam (7.5 mg PO) × placebo	Midazolam provides fast and adequate sedation ($p < 0.001$)	Dental treatment
López et al. 1995 [19]	Chile	Prospective	92 children (0–4 y)	Midazolam (1mg/kg PO) × chloral hydrate (50mg/kg PO) (both rectal)	100% chloral hydrate fall asleep × 66.6% midazolam ($p < 0.01$)	Electroencephalography (EEG)
Riva et al. 1997 [20]	Uruguay	Prospective Double-blind Randomized	107 children (3–10 y)	Midazolam (0.75 mg/kg PO) × placebo	Midazolam showed a better level of sedation than placebo ($p < 0.05$)	Preoperative medication
Brunow de Carvalho et al. 1999 [21]	Brazil	Prospective (comparison of 2 sedating scales)	18 children (0–6 y)	Midazolam or fentanyl (IV doses, not reported)	There was no statistical difference in comparison of Comfort and Hartwig scales	ICU sedation
Ronco et al. 2003 [22]	Chile	Prospective	51 children (3mo–16 y)	Propofol 2–6 mg/kg IV alone (30) or in association (21) (midazolam, morphine, ketamine, or fentanyl)	There were no differences ($p = 0.4$) in comparison of propofol alone or in association	Procedures (endoscopy, bronchoscopy, biopsies, others)
Lima et al. 2003 [23]	Brazil	Prospective Double-blind Randomized	11 children (0–5 y; 37 dental sessions)	Midazolam (1 mg/kg PO) × midazolam (0.75 mg/kg PO) plus hydroxyzine (2.0 mg/kg PO) × placebo	Success rate was 7.7% placebo, 30.8% midazolam plus hydroxyzine, and 77.0% midazolam alone	Dental treatment
Saitua et al. 2003 [24]	Chile	Prospective	81 children (1 mo–12 y)	Midazolam 0.2 mg/kg IV plus fentanyl 2 μg/kg IV or General Anesthesia	No differences regarding sedation or general anesthesia. GA may be avoided in simple procedures	Percutaneous endoscopic gastrostomy
Matínez and Sossa 2003 [25]	Colombia	Retrospective	65 children (1 mo–18 y)	General anesthesia (halothane – 64 patients) and midazolam plus ketamine (IV, 1 patient)	The possibility of performing the procedure under sedation should be considered	Bronchoscopy
Sfoggia et al. 2003 [26]	Brazil	Prospective	124 children (1 mo–15 y)	Midazolam, ketamine, fentanyl and morphine (various doses IV continuous)	Sedative infusions in children submitted to mechanical ventilation were used to an average of 1.7 drugs/patient/day	ICU sedation (mechanical ventilation)
Gana et al. 2006 [27]	Chile	Prospective	123 children (2–10 y)	Midazolam and Dolantin (IV various doses)	No patient needed any antagonist or resuscitation maneuvers	Colonoscopy
Claro et al. 2006 [28]	Argentina	Retrospective	75 patients (6 mo–15 y; 150 procedures)	Midazolam 0.1 mg/kg IV and ketamine 1 mg/kg IV	A suitable level of sedation and pain relief was achieved in 80% of patients	Procedures (lumbar and bone marrow puncture, biopsy etc.)
Muñoz et al. 2006 [29]	Chile	Prospective	20 children (3–11 y) and 20 adults	Propofol (TCI) mean EC_{e50} 3.65 mg/ml	During propofol administration, the correlation between BIS and clinical sedation is similar in children and adults	Preoperative medication
da Silva et al. 2007 [30]	Brazil	Prospective Randomized	57 children (3 mo–14 y)	Midazolam (0.15–0.5 mg/kg IV) and fentanyl	The M/K sedation regimen was associated with a higher	Procedures (central venous catheter)

(continued)

Table 22.2 (continued)

				(1–3 μ[mu]/kg IV) or midazolam (0.15-0.5 mg/kg IV) and ketamine (0.5–5 mg/kg IV)	rate of minor complications (excessive secretion and desaturation)	
Schmidt et al. 2007 [31]	Brazil	Prospective Randomized	60 children (7–12 y)	Midazolam (0.5 mg/kg PO) or clonidine (4 μ[mu]g/kg PO) or dexmedetomidine transmucosal (1μ[mu]g/kg)	Children receiving clonidine or DEX preop have similar levels of anxiety as those receiving midazolam	Preoperative medication
Kantovitz et al. 2007 [32]	Brazil	Prospective Double-blind Randomized	20 children (3 –7 y; 40 dental sessions)	Chloral hydrate (40 mg/kg PO) or diazepam (5 mg PO) or placebo	Diazepam or CH alone had no influence on behavior management during dental treatment	Dental treatment
Costa et al. 2007 [33]	Brazil	Prospective Double-blind Randomized	12 children (0–5 y; 35 dental sessions)	Chloral hydrate (75 mg/kg PO) or chloral hydrate (50 mg/kg PO) plus hydroxyzine (2.0 mg/kg PO) or placebo	CH, CH plus hydroxyzine and placebo were effective in 62.5%, 61.5%, and 11.1% of cases, respectively	Dental treatment
Martinbiancho et al. 2009 [34]	Brazil	Prospective	343 children (0–18 y)	Chloral hydrate (median dose prescribed was 130 mg/kg/day, rectal)	CH may be an alternative during prolonged sedation in PICU	ICU sedation
Riera et al. 2010 [35]	Chile	Prospective	190 children (4–12 y)	Midazolam (0.13 mg/kg IV average) or Dolantin (0.82 mg/kg IV average)	Ambulatory endoscopic procedures can be performed safely on children, with moderate sedation	Endoscopy
Capp et al. 2010 [36]	Brazil	Prospective	40 children (0–5 y; 45 dental sessions)	Midazolam 0.2–0.3 mg/kg IM or 0.1mg/kg IV	Midazolam was effective in 89% of this sample for dental procedures in patients with neurological and behavioral disturbances	Dental treatment
Oliveira et al. 2011 [37]	Brazil	Case Report	1 child (7 y)	N_2O sedation	Dental procedure under N_2O sedation preferred in a cerebral palsy child considering short duration and safety	Dental treatment
da Silva et al. 2011 [38]	Brazil	Prospective	20 children (4–12 y)	Ketofol (1.25 mg/kg IV each of propofol and ketamine)	Ketofol provided effective sedation and analgesia for bone marrow aspiration	Procedures (bone marrow aspiration)
Sepulveda et al. 2011 [12]	Chile	Prospective	41 children (3–36 mo)	Propofol 2.5 mg/kg followed by 8 mg/kg/h IV (TCI)	Validation of the PK models; use for TCI might result in the administration of larger bolus doses than necessary in small child	Preoperative medication and GA
Costa et al. 2012 [39]	Brazil	Prospective	42 children (1–8 y)	Midazolam 1.0–1.5 mg/kg PO (max 20.0 mg) or chloral hydrate 70–100 mg/kg PO (max 2.0 g)	High oral doses of CH were more related to minor adverse events than was midazolam as the sole agent for moderate sedation	Dental treatment
Agudelo et al. 2012 [40]	Colombia	Retrospective	71 children (7 mo–6 y)	Propofol (2.1 ±1.3 mg/kg/h IV)	Propofol at a dose of 1–4 mg/kg/h is a safe alternative for sustained sedation in critically ill children	ICU sedation
Moreira et al. 2013 [41]	Brazil	Prospective Double-blind	41 children (0–36 mo)	Midazolam (0.5 mg/kg PO) and ketamine (3 mg/kg PO) or midazolam	The combination of oral midazolam and ketamine is efficacious for guiding the	Dental treatment

(continued)

Table 22.2 (continued)

		Randomized		(1.0 mg/kg PO) or placebo	behavior of children under 3 years old	
Godoy et al. 2013 [42]	Chile	Prospective	(1 mo–5 y)	Midazolam IV plus ketamine IV, propofol IV plus lidocaine SC, or midazolam IV plus propofol IV plus lidocaine (SC) (doses not shown)	Adequate deep sedation was obtained in 98% of cases, and that an adequate analgesia was achieved in 92% of patients; no differences in groups	Procedures (bronchoscopy, endoscopy, etc.)
Gómez et al. 2013 [43]	Colombia	Prospective	216 children (6 mo–8 y)	Midazolam (0.5 mg/kg PO) plus acetaminophen (12 mg/kg PO); named: "midazofén"	Premedication reduces anxiety and allows a good acceptance (92%) of GA	Preoperative medication

sedation studies used only oral or inhaled routes. In the intensive care units, intravenous sedatives are preferred (one study cites rectal chloral hydrate).

Summary

In South America, there is an enormous variability in sedation practice. The majority of sedation still continues to be administered by anesthesiologists with dentists limited only to nitrous oxide administration and emergency medicine physicians restricted to midazolam, ketamine, and narcotics. There is a huge variability in the culture of research and data collection between countries and regions, and grants for research vary between academic institutions. Although outcome data is scarce, there is now emerging literature on the use of TCI with propofol. With limited financial resources, TCI delivery devices have been created and adapted from existing equipment. Some data published in the literature over the past 20 years (PubMed and Scielo, 1993–2013) on issues associated with pediatric sedation in South America are shown in Table 22.2 and Figure 22.3. Although there is lack of uniform guidelines and recommendations, sedation guidelines for delivery and monitoring tend to follow ASA guidelines.

Case Studies

Case 1

IBS (2 years and 3 months old) was referred for dental treatment under sedation for the completion of three restorations. The patient's weight and height were on the 25th to 50th percentiles (National Center for Health Statistics; NCHS) and the vital signs were within normal limits. Then 1 mg/kg midazolam was administered orally and treatment started 15 min after drug administration. The patient struggled and showed a complete lack of cooperation. She was discharged without complications. In the next session, according to the local protocol [41], the patient received a combination of midazolam 0.5 and 3 mg/kg ketamine, both orally. After 15 min, the patient cooperated and was treated successfully (Ohio State University Behavior Rating Scale; OSUBRS Scale 2: *little crying*) and completed the proposed treatment. Only transient post-nystagmus was observed, with no other adverse events in the next 24 h after sedation.

Comments

Sedation without routine venous access is performed with several different medications alone or in association. In dental procedures this is a relatively common scenario. Options for this include oral (as used in association in this case), intranasal, transmucosal, and inhaled (mainly nitrous oxide) medications. Vein puncture is reserved for rare and severe adverse events.

Case 2

JBC (7 years old) was indicated for dental (endodontic) treatment. The patient was anxious and the parents refused to treat him without sedation. After discussion with the dentist and anesthesiologist, it was proposed to use a target model (Paedfusor) to infuse propofol (2.6 μg/mL) and alfentanil (8 μg/kg). These drugs were started before local anesthesia (Figure 22.4), which was performed without stress or even minor movements. The endodontic treatment was also finished successfully and no adverse events were observed. The patient was fully awake 2 min after the end of the infusion.

(continued)

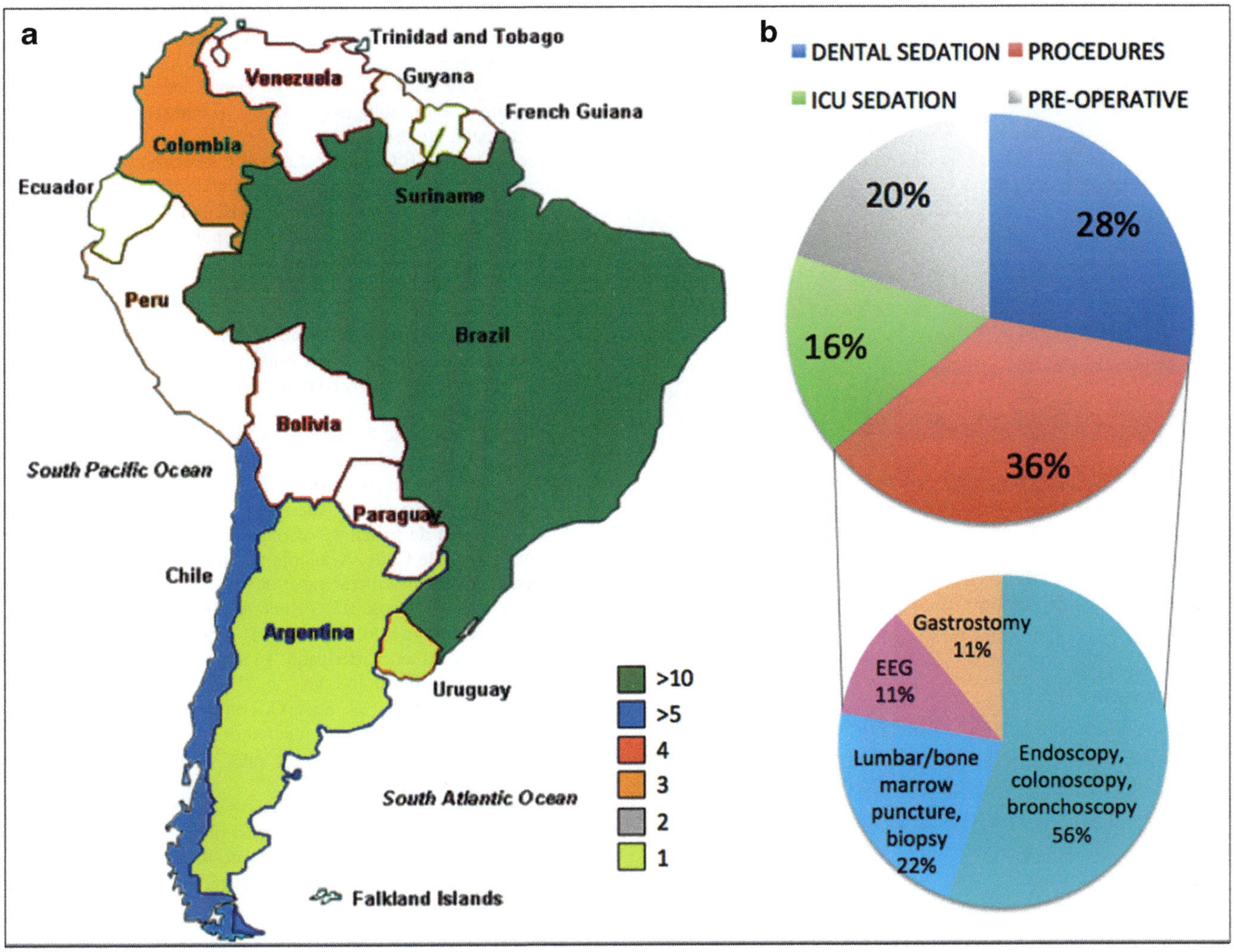

Figure 22.3 Publications related to sedation in children (27 papers) in the last 20 years (PubMed and Scielo) from South America: (**a**) number of papers published per country (1993–2013); (**b**) indications for sedation

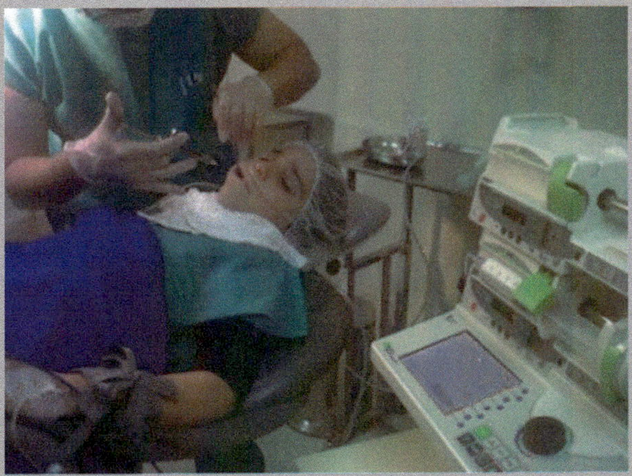

Figure 22.4 Sedation for oral surgery

Comments

Sedation with a target model allows the fine control of the drug plasma concentration, preventing deep sedation and cardiorespiratory depression on the one hand and arousal on the other. However, only trained anesthesiologists can use the target model.

Case 3

AOC (a 5-month-old boy) was burned (17 % of body surface) with hot liquids. Surgery for the healing procedure was proposed with a presumed duration of 75 min. Then it was decided to perform the healing process under sedation (Figure 22.5). A bolus of fentanyl 2 μg/kg was used, and a continuous propofol

(continued)

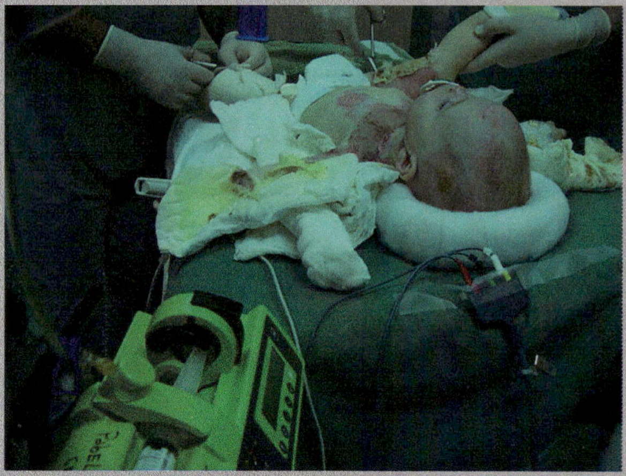

Figure 22.5 Sedation of a 5-month infant

infusion of 3 mg/kg/h. There was no desaturation (SpO_2>95 % throughout the time) under room air and no other adverse events were reported.

Comments

The association of propofol and fentanyl is common in sedation and is generally safe when used by qualified personnel. Even in infants, as in this case, it is a reasonable alternative to general anesthesia.

Conclusions

In summary, the subcontinent is a mosaic of complexities, with delayed progress in some areas, which contrasts with good innovations in others, but in general there is a broad use of technology and the emergence of more homogeneous processes. A lot of effort is needed to evaluate sedation outcomes in South America, but there appears to be low morbidity, as the majority of sedation is delivered by anesthesiologists and other medical specialists (pediatricians and, less frequently, dentists). There remains a critical need for sedation coverage in remote areas from which patients must be evacuated to urban centers for medical care.

References

1. Lester T. Putting America on the map. Smithsonian. 2009;40(9): 78–96.
2. Jacob R, Coté CJ, Thirlwell J, editors. Entendiendo la anestesia pediatrica. 2nd ed. New Delhi: B.I. publications. 2010. Available at: http://www.clasa-anestesia.org/site/version/index.php?pagina=libro.php
3. Campos G. Actualizando TIVA con expertos—TIVA en pediatria. Available at: http://www.ararosario.com.ar/ver.php?xlg=1&publicacion=292
4. Costa PS, Valadao Jr WJ, Costa LR. Dental sedation by dentists: a view from anesthesiologists working in central Western Brazil. Anesth Analg. 2010;110(1):110–4.
5. Daher A, Hanna RP, Costa LR, Leles CR. Practices and opinions on nitrous oxide/oxygen sedation from dentists licensed to perform relative analgesia in Brazil. BMC Oral Health. 2012;12:21.
6. Wilson S, Alcaino EA. Survey on sedation in paediatric dentistry: a global perspective. Int J Paediatr Dent. 2011;21(5):321–32.
7. Herlich A. How do we bridge the gap? Anesth Analg. 2010;110(1): 11–2.
8. Bastos Neto AS. [Policy for sedation by non-medical anesthesiologists]. Hospital Israelita Albert Einstein. 2009. Avaiable at: http://medsv1.einstein.br/diretrizes/anestesia/sedacao-para-nao-anestesiologistas.pdf
9. Silva MAD. Pediatric anesthesia—the outpatient limits—children are different. In: Cavalcanti IL, Cunha LBP, Abrão MA, Sarmento RFO, editors. Topics on anaesthesia and pain. Rio de Janeiro, Brazil: SAERJ—Society of Anesthesia; 2011. p. 492.
10. Anestesia fuera de pabellón: recomendaciones de la Sociedad de Anestesiología de Chile. Available at: http://www.sachile.cl/medicos/recomendaciones/fuera_pabellon/presentacion.php
11. Cortínez LI, Anderson BJ, Penna A, Olivares L, Muñoz HR, Holford NH, Struys MM, Sepulveda P. Influence of obesity on propofol pharmacokinetics: derivation of a pharmacokinetic model. Br J Anaesth. 2010;105(4):448–56.
12. Sepúlveda P, Cortínez LI, Sáez C, Penna A, Solari S, Guerra I, Absalom AR. Performance evaluation of paediatric propofol pharmacokinetic models in healthy young children. Br J Anaesth. 2011;107(4):593–600.
13. Ibarra P, Galindo M, Molano A, et al. Sedation and analgesia recommendations for non-anesthesiologist physicians and dentists in patients over 12 years old. Colomb J Anesth. 2012;40(1):67–74.
14. Navarro A, Llanos JP, Mendoza C, et al. Experience in flexible bronchoscopy in pediatric patients in two hospitals from Lima-Peru. Eur Respir J. 2005;26 Suppl 49:629s.
15. Navarro AAR. Bronchoscopy in children in South America. Paediatr Respir Rev. 2006;7(4):288–92.
16. Vargas-Machuca MV, Urbina SR. [Conscious sedation in pediatric dentistry]. Rev Estomatol Herediana. 2002;12(1–2):49–52.
17. Granting privileges for deep sedation to non-anesthesiologist sedation practitioners. (Approved by the ASA House of Delegates on 20 October 2010). http://www.asahq.org/For-Members/Standards-Guidelines-and-Statements.aspx
18. Gallardo F, Cornejo G, Borie R. Oral midazolam as premedication for the apprehensive child before dental treatment. J Clin Pediatr Dent. 1994;18(2):123–7.
19. Lopez MEB, Lopez IS, Troncoso LA, et al. [Chloral hydrate or midazolam to induce sleep for electroencephalographic records]. Rev Chil Pediatr. 1995;66(4):204–8.
20. Riva J, Lejbusiewicz G, Papa M, Lauber C, Kohn W, Da Fonte M, Burgstaller H, Comellas C, Ayala W. Oral premedication with midazolam in paediatric anaesthesia. Effects on sedation and gastric contents. Paediatr Anaesth. 1997;7(3):191–6.
21. Brunow de Carvalho W, Lucas da Silva PS, Paulo CS, Fonseca MM, Belli LA. Comparison between the Comfort and Hartwig sedation scales in pediatric patients undergoing mechanical lung ventilation. Sao Paulo Med J. 1999;117(5):192–6.
22. Ronco RM, Castillo AM, Carrasco J, et al. [Sedation and analgesia during procedures affecting children outside the operating room]. Rev Chil Pediatr. 2003;74(2):171–8.
23. Lima AR, Costa LR, Costa PS. A randomized, controlled, crossover trial of oral midazolam and hydroxyzine for pediatric dental sedation. Pesqui Odontol Bras. 2003;17(3):206–11.

24. Saitua F, Acuña R, Herrera P. Percutaneous endoscopic gastrostomy: the technique of choice? J Pediatr Surg. 2003;38(10):1512–5.
25. Martínez CR, Sossa MP. [Factors associated with complications caused by bronchoscopy in pediatric patients]. Arch Bronconeumol. 2003;39(11):501–6.
26. Sfoggia A, Fontela PS, Moraes A, da Silva F, Sober RB, Noer RB, Bruno F, Einloft P, Garcia PC, Piva JP. Sedation and analgesia in children submitted to mechanical ventilation could be overestimated? J Pediatr (Rio J). 2003;79(4):343–8.
27. Gana AJC, Glenz AC, Marchant AP, Vaca ZC, García RX, Larraín BF, Harris DP. Prospective evaluation of the safety and tolerance of colonoscopy in children. Rev Med Chil. 2006;134(5):613–22.
28. Claro MC, Podestá MC, Rosales A. [Sedation and analgesia for diagnostic and therapeutic procedures in the pediatric patient]. Arch Argent Pediatr. 2006;104(6):512–9.
29. Muñoz HR, Cortínez LI, Ibacache ME, León PJ. Effect site concentrations of propofol producing hypnosis in children and adults: comparison using the bispectral index. Acta Anaesthesiol Scand. 2006;50(7):882–7.
30. da Silva LPS, Iglesias OSB, Leão FV, Aguiar VE, Brunow de Carvalho W. Procedural sedation for insertion of central venous catheters in children: comparison of midazolam/fentanyl with midazolam/ketamine. Paediatr Anaesth. 2007;17(4):358–63.
31. Schmidt AP, Valinetti EA, Bandeira D, Bertacchi MF, Simões CM, Auler Jr JO. Effects of preanesthetic administration of midazolam, clonidine, or dexmedetomidine on postoperative pain and anxiety in children. Paediatr Anaesth. 2007;17(7):667–74.
32. Kantovitz KR, Puppin-Rontani RM, Gaviao MB. Sedative effect of oral diazepam and chloral hydrate in the dental treatment of children. J Indian Soc Pedod Prev Dent. 2007;25(2):69–75.
33. Costa LR, Costa PS, Lima AR. A randomized double-blinded trial of chloral hydrate with or without hydroxyzine versus placebo for pediatric dental sedation. Braz Dent J. 2007;18(4):334–40.
34. Martinbiancho JK, Carvalho PR, Trotta Ede A, Schweiger AP, Rau R, Moreira LB. Evidence of safety of chloral hydrate for prolonged sedation in PICU in a tertiary teaching hospital in southern Brazil. Eur J Clin Pharmacol. 2009;65(12):1253–8.
35. Riera FC, González CCF, Vaca CZ, et al. [Sedation, safety and usefulness of upper gastrointestinal endoscopy in pediatrics]. Rev Chil Pediatr. 2010;81(1):37–45.
36. Capp PL, de Faria ME, Siqueira SR, Cillo MT, Prado EG, de Siqueira JT. Special care dentistry: midazolam conscious sedation for patients with neurological diseases. Eur J Paediatr Dent. 2010;11(4):162–4.
37. Oliveira CA, de Paula VA, Portela MB, Primo LS, Castro GF. Bruxism control in a child with cerebral palsy. ISRN Dent. 2011;2011:146915.
38. da Silva PS, de Aguiar VE, Waisberg DR, Passos RM, Park MV. Use of ketofol for procedural sedation and analgesia in children with hematological diseases. Pediatr Int. 2011;53(1):62–7.
39. Costa LR, Costa PS, Brasileiro SV, Bendo CB, Viegas CM, Paiva SM. Post-discharge adverse events following pediatric sedation with high doses of oral medication. J Pediatr. 2012;160(5):807–13.
40. Agudelo SC, Mencía S, Faro A, Escudero V, Sanavia E, López-Herce J. Continuous propofol perfusion in critically ill children. Med Intensiva. 2012;36(6):410–5.
41. Moreira TA, Costa PS, Costa LR, Jesus-França CM, Antunes DE, Gomes HS, Neto OA. Combined oral midazolam-ketamine better than midazolam alone for sedation of young children: a randomized controlled trial. Int J Paediatr Dent. 2013;23(3):207–15.
42. Godoy LM, Pino PA, Córdova GL, et al. Sedation and analgesia in children undergoing invasive procedures. Arch Argent Pediatr. 2013;111(1):22–8.
43. Gómez LMB, Ocampo FA, Orozco JAA. Efficacy of anesthetic premedication in pediatric patients using oral midazolam and acetaminophen. Rev Colomb Anestesiol. 2013;41(1):4–9.
44. Coté CJ, Wilson S; American Academy of Pediatrics; American Academy of Pediatric Dentistry; Work Group on Sedation. Guidelines for monitoring and management of pediatric patients during and after sedation for diagnostic and therapeutic procedures: an update. Pediatrics. 2006;118(6):2587–602.

Pediatric Sedation: The Asian Approach—Current State of Sedation in China

23

Vivian Man-ying Yuen, Wang Ning ShangGuan, Bi-lian Li, Ying Xu, Xuan Chen, Chunyan Wang, and Michael G. Irwin

Abstract

In China, the need for sedation and analgesia for both diagnostic and therapeutic procedures performed outside the operating room has increased dramatically in recent years. In China there are currently no national guidelines on providing sedation to either children or adults. Hong Kong, although a Special Administrative Region of the Peoples Republic of China (PRC), has its own independent Academy of Medicine, which does issue guidelines. For the purpose of this chapter, the authors will consider Hong Kong as separate from China, since currently the two regions approach sedation in a vastly different manner. In order to understand the current state of pediatric sedation, a survey was sent to 41 hospitals, all members of the Pediatric Anesthesia Association in China. The size of hospitals ranged from 500 to 4,200 beds and the number of pediatric operations performed in these hospitals ranged from 3,000 to 60,000 in 2012. The response rate was 53.6 %. Of the 22 completed surveys, five hospitals responded that they had no sedation service (their surveys were not returned) and two indicated that anesthesiologists are not involved in their sedation services.

Keywords

Pediatric sedation • China • Sedation • Analgesia • Guidelines • Pediatric Anesthesia Association • Benzodiazepines • Diazepam • Midazolam • Local anesthetics • Restraint • Chloral hydrate • The Children's Hospital of Chongqing Medical University • The Guangzhou Women and Children's Hospital • Propofol • Sufentanil • Remifentanil • Dexmedetomidine • Acupuncture • Aldrete score • Joint Commission International • American Academy of Pediatrics (AAP) • American Society of Anesthesiologists (ASA) • University of Michigan Sedation Scale (UMSS)

V.M. Yuen, M.B.B.S., F.A.N.Z.C.A. (✉)
Department of Anesthesiology, University of Hong Kong Shenzhen Hospital, Shenzhen, Guangdong, China
e-mail: vtang131@hku.hk

W.N. ShangGuan, M.D., Ph.D.
Department of Anesthesiology, The 2nd Affiliated Hospital, Wenzhou Medical University, Wenzhou, Zhejiang, China
e-mail: sgwning@163.com

B.L. Li, M.D.
Department of Anesthesiology, Guangzhou Women and Children's Medical Centre, Guangzhou, Guangdong, China
e-mail: 13570226780@126.com

Y. Xu, Ph.D., M.D.
Department of Anesthesiology, Children's Hospital of Chongqing Medical University, Chongqing, China
e-mail: xuyingxy3066@gmail.com

X. Chen, M.Med. • C.Y. Wang, M.Med.
Department of Anesthesia, University of Hong Kong Shenzhen Hospital, Shenzhen, Guangdong, China
e-mail: mariechen789@gmail.com; wangcy@hku-szh.org

M.G. Irwin, M.D., F.R.C.A., F.H.K.A.M.
Department of Anesthesiology, Queen Mary Hospital, The University of Hong Kong, Hong Kong, China
e-mail: mgirwin@hku.hk

K.P. Mason (ed.), *Pediatric Sedation Outside of the Operating Room: A Multispecialty International Collaboration*, DOI 10.1007/978-1-4939-1390-9_23, © Springer Science+Business Media New York 2015

Introduction

In China, the need for sedation and analgesia for both diagnostic and therapeutic procedures performed outside the operating room has increased dramatically in recent years. In China there are currently no national guidelines on providing sedation to either children or adults. Hong Kong, although a Special Administrative Region of the Peoples Republic of China (PRC), has its own independent Academy of Medicine, which does issue guidelines. For the purpose of this chapter, the authors will consider Hong Kong as separate from China, since currently the two regions approach sedation in a vastly different manner.

Survey

In order to understand the current state of pediatric sedation, a survey was sent to 41 hospitals—all members of the Pediatric Anesthesia Association in China. The size of hospitals ranged from 500 to 4,200 beds and the number of pediatric operations performed in these hospitals ranged from 3,000 to 30,000 in 2012. The response rate was 53.6 %. Of the 22 completed surveys, five hospitals responded that they had no sedation service (their surveys were not returned) and two indicated that anesthesiologists are not involved in their sedation services. The distribution of hospitals involved in this survey is shown in Fig. 23.1.

In China, anesthesiologists are often involved in sedation for invasive and painful procedures, which include tracheobronchoscopy, gastrointestinal endoscopies, cardiac catheterization and interventional procedures. Anesthesiologists provide sedation to children undergoing tracheabronchoscopy in seven of the responding hospitals. At hospitals that perform these procedures without anesthesiologists, sedation is usually provided by pediatricians and nurses. Benzodiazepines (diazepam or midazolam) are the most common pharmacologic agents used in conjunction with local anesthetics. However, the sedative effect is reported as often unsatisfactory, necessitating restraint with parental

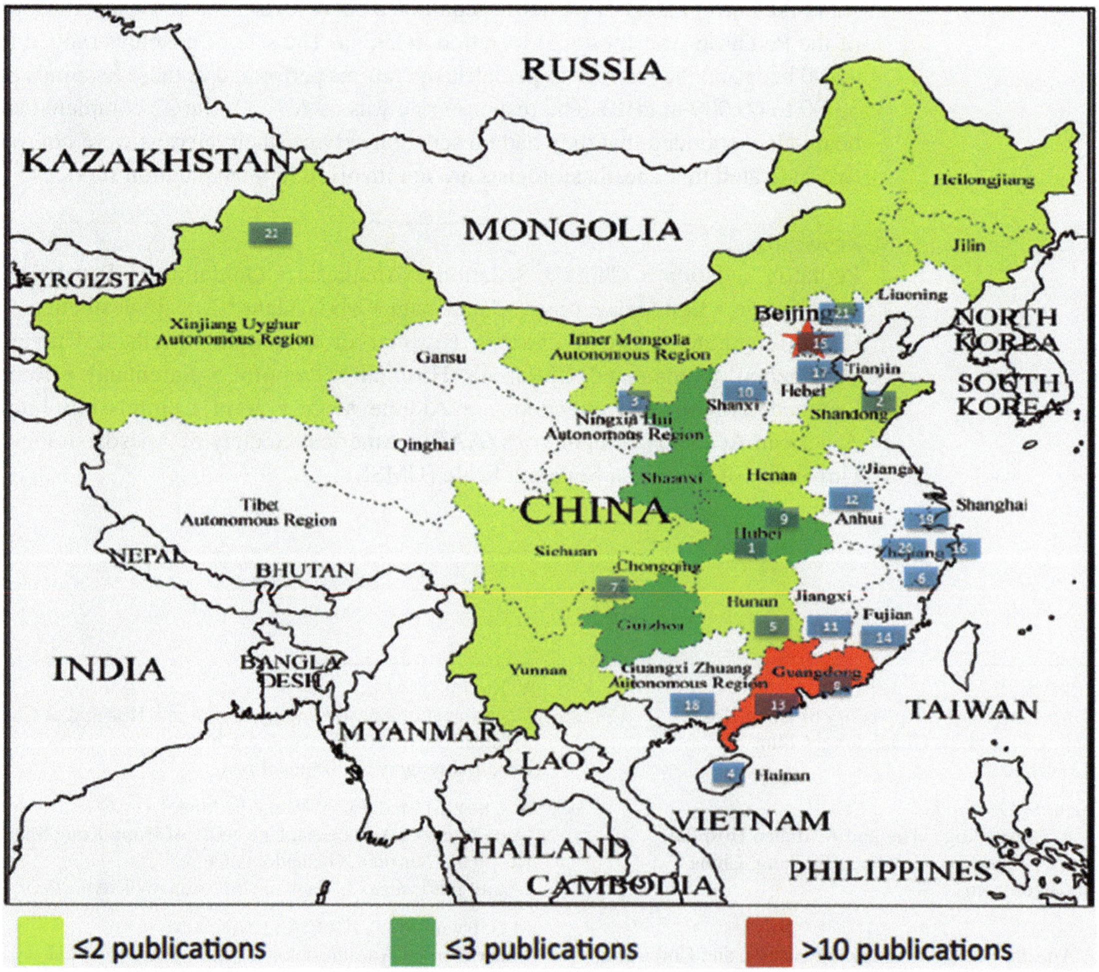

Fig. 23.1 Distribution of hospitals in the survey on sedation outside operating theater in China (number in *blue box* corresponds to the hospitals). Publications in sedation outside operating theater in children from China in year 2007–2013: number of papers published per province

assistance. Anesthesiologists staff a pediatric sedation service for gastroscopy and colonoscopy at 15, esophagoscopy at 5, and cardiac catheterization and intervention at 17 of the 22 respondent hospitals. In a few hospitals, anesthesiologists are also responsible for sedation for other invasive and painful procedures including cerebral angiography, bone marrow aspiration, lumbar puncture, liver biopsy, renal biopsy, enema reduction of intussusception, central line or dialysis catheter insertion, and suture removal.

A dedicated sedation service for children undergoing non-painful diagnostic procedures including computed tomography (CT), magnetic resonance imaging (MRI), and ultrasound is less common. Most commonly, the attending/staff emergency medicine physicians, pediatricians, intensive care medicine physicians or radiologists prescribe sedatives, which are administered by nursing staff. Oral or rectal chloral hydrate is commonly used. Children are commonly transported to recovery by their parents and recovered without monitoring. Anesthesiologists lead the sedation services for CT/MRI in five hospitals and ultrasound in eight hospitals. In one of these hospitals, anesthesiologists also lead the sedation service for auditory brainstem response (ABR), visual evoked potential (VEP) and minor surgery including tongue tie excision, oral mucoid cyst excision, circumcision, and dental extraction.

China is still evolving its allocation of resources to provide safe sedation: Only five out of the 22 hospitals are suitably equipped with physiological monitoring and seven hospitals identified their existing monitors as inadequate. Only ten hospitals, less than half of the respondents, feel that they have adequate resuscitation facilities. Seventeen hospitals have dedicated post-sedation recovery room facilities.

The Children's Hospital of Chongqing Medical University and the Guangzhou Women and Children's Hospital are two large centers in China that have an established sedation service for pediatric patients. Details of these renowned, organized sedation services will be reviewed in depth below.

Sedation Service in Chongqing Medical University

The Children's Hospital of Chongqing Medical University has approximately 1,400 beds and performs more than 30,000 operations annually. It is considered to be one of the top three childrens' hospitals in China and the largest center in southwest China. Anesthesiologists lead the sedation services for invasive procedures, which include bronchoscopy, gastroscopy, ultrasound-guided biopsies, renal, liver, cardiac catheterization and intervention, change of burn dressings, and other minor surgeries. Attending pediatricians, radiologists, and intensive care medicine physicians are responsible for sedation for non-painful procedures (CT/MRI, ultrasound, and echocardiography). There is an institutional guideline for providing sedation to children. These guidelines specify that only attending anesthesiologists (trained anesthesiologists who can work independently) who are trained in pediatric sedation have privileges to perform sedation outside the operating theater. All children must have pre-sedation assessment and evaluation. Patients with significant comorbidities and at high risk for sedation are identified, informed consent obtained from the legal guardian, and patients fasted (nil per os, NPO). Physiologic monitoring, resuscitation equipment and emergency medications, reversal agents for sedatives, and analgesia are available. Discharge criteria and recovery facilities are adopted to facilitate safe discharge. Commonly used sedatives by non-anesthesiologists include oral chloral hydrate and intramuscular phenobarbital. Anesthesiologists often use intravenous drugs, which include propofol, midazolam, sufentanil and remifentanil.

There are many challenges to providing a high standard of pediatric sedation. In the Children's Hospital of Chongqing Medical University, anesthesiologists provide sedation at four sedation centers. These centers are often remote and distant from the operating theater. Often, only one anesthesiologist is available for providing the sedation service in each center. The sedation volume is extremely high and it is, therefore, not unusual for one anesthesiologist to be responsible for 30 endoscopy sedations in a 2–3 h period: His responsibilities would include pre-sedation evaluation, sedative preparation and administration, physiological monitoring, and documentation. The specialty nurses are responsible for recovery and discharge. With such a large sedation volume in such a short time frame, the anesthesiologist may not have adequate time to perform or document a detailed pre-sedation evaluation, particularly on complicated inpatients, many of whom have significant comorbidities. This busy environment creates a significant potential for risk and errors as the workload and demand is high. This is especially hazardous when working alone in remote areas. With this high patient volume, there is significant potential should one wish to review sedation practice, outcomes, and clinical research. Unfortunately, however, data collection and review is virtually impossible due to insufficient manpower. Training provided to non-anesthesiologists who practice sedation is often inadequate. There is, in general, no formal training of these practitioners on emergency identification, management, and airway resuscitation skills.

Sedation Service in Guangzhou Women and Children's Medical Center

Guangzhou Women and Children's Medical Center is the largest pediatric hospital in south China. An anesthesiologist-led pediatric sedation service for moderate to deep sedation was established here in January 2012, following a recommendation by the Joint Commission International (JCI), which subsequently accredited them in 2013. This hospital has approximately 1,300 beds and 60,000 operations performed annually. More than 20,000 sedations were provided by the anesthesiology department in 2012. The sedation service includes sedation for CT, MRI, ultrasound, echocardiograph, ABR, VEP, endoscopies, interventional procedures, dental procedures, biopsies, and minor surgeries. There are a number of sedation units within the hospital that are responsible for providing sedation for different procedures. Each unit is led by one anesthesiologist and one nurse, both of whom are credentialed by the hospital to provide sedation. There is a comprehensive institutional guideline available for providing moderate to deep sedation. The guideline adopts recommendations that are similar to that of the American Academy of Pediatrics and includes pre-sedation evaluation, informed consent, fasting and preparation, monitoring and documentation, as well as equipment and drugs for both sedation and resuscitation. Similar to the Children's Hospital of Chongqing Medical University, the patient volume is very high and each anesthesiologist delivers sedation care for up to 50 patients per day. For invasive and painful procedures, intravenous analgesics and sedatives include sufentanil and propofol. For non-painful procedures, chloral hydrate is still the most commonly used sedative.

Even though a dedicated team and anesthesiologist-led sedation service is available in this center, the very high patient-to-anesthesiologist ratio makes it difficult to administer intravenous sedation to each patient for all non-painful procedures. Recently, dexmedetomidine has been introduced via the intranasal route in order to supplement or provide anxiolysis or sedation. Oral chloral hydrate with intranasal dexmedetomidine has been associated with a success rate of greater than 90 %, a combination that has become the primary mode of sedation [1]. After pre-sedation evaluation and informed consent, sedative(s) are prescribed by the attending/staff anesthesiologist. When the depth of sedation is assessed by the anesthesiologist to be adequate, the parent carries the child to the waiting area and waits with him until the procedure is ready to be performed. The success rate of chloral hydrate at 50 mg/kg is approximately 77–86 % for non-painful procedures in this center. Since chloral hydrate has an unpleasant taste, often children are encouraged to ingest it with other fluids such as fruit juice or a dairy drink. Therefore, children are, in fact, not fasted (not NPO) when chloral hydrate is used as the primary sedative. Subjectively, the author (Yuen) and anesthesiologists from this center observe that ingestion of chloral hydrate with a dairy drink tends to decrease irritability and hasten the onset of sedation. Nevertheless, this is only anecdotal experience and there are no such published reports to substantiate this. In this center, the anesthesiologist-led pediatric sedation service has been in operation for 2 years and to date there have been no cases of clinical aspiration nor aspiration-related events. In cases of failed chloral hydrate sedation after a first dosage, a repeat dose of 25 mg/kg is administered. The success rate after this repeat dose is 89–93 %. Only after a "failed" (unsuccessful at achieving adequate sedation conditions) oral sedation is intravenous sedation with propofol used for non-painful procedures. However, since these patients have consumed an oral drink with chloral hydrate, they are not meeting NPO guidelines for intravenous sedation, and the procedure is subsequently rescheduled or delayed until sufficient fasting time is achieved.

All sedated children are recovered in a post-sedation recovery room. Parents are encouraged to stimulate and wake up their children after sedation. Vital signs—which include SpO_2, blood pressure and respiratory rate—are monitored and recorded every 10 min. When the Aldrete score is greater than or equal to 9, the children would be discharged after parents are given post-discharge instruction (Table 23.1). (Refer to Chap. 5.) Inpatient and critically ill patients are often discharged to the inpatient ward or intensive care unit directly after the procedures with physiologic monitors for transport and escort by their attending medical officer.

Recently there has been an increasing interest in using intranasal dexmedetomidine as either a rescue sedative for failed chloral hydrate sedation or as a primary sedative for non-painful procedures. Intranasal dexmedetomidine is given by direct administration with a 1 mL tuberculin syringe. Atomizers are not yet available in China. The dose used for rescue ranges from 1 to 2 μg/kg. In a cohort of 194 children at Guangzhou Women and Children's Medical Center who had failed chloral hydrate sedation, the author [1] demonstrated that intranasal dexmedetomidine was successful for rescue in 83.6–96.8 %. The doses of intranasal dexmedetomidine used were 1, 1.5, and 2 μg/kg. By univariate logistic regression, higher rescue dosage was associated with an increased success rate with odds ratio of 4.116 (95 % CI 1.131–14.982), i.e., the estimated odds of success were increased by 4.116 with each 1 μg/kg increase in intranasal dexmedetomidine dose. The author (Yuen) believes that intranasal dexmedetomidine is often preferable to a second "rescue" dose of chloral hydrate because it avoids chloral hydrate's unpalatable flavor with accompanying negative response. Intranasal dexmedetomidine is also used as a primary sedative for non-painful procedures. The dose ranges from 2 to 3 μg/kg. The success rate with 2 and 3 μg/kg is about 90 % and 93 % respectively [2]. Chloral hydrate still remains the most popular primary sedative because it is inexpensive and, in general, produces consistent depths of moderate sedation with minimal significant adverse effects when dosed and monitored appropriately. In China, clinical research continues to evaluate whether intranasal dexmedetomidine is a feasible and cost-effective alternative to oral chloral hydrate for pediatric sedation, particularly in the challenging patients who tend not to be favorable candidates for chloral hydrate (older, autistic, or critically ill).

Table 23.1 The modified Aldrete scale

Domain	Response	Points
Activity	Able to move four extremities voluntarily or on command	2
	Able to move two extremities voluntarily or on command	1
	Unable to move extremities voluntarily or on command	0
Respiration	Able to breathe deeply and cough freely	2
	Dyspnea or limited breathing	1
	Apneic	0
Circulation	BP ± 20 % of pre-anesthetic level	2
	BP ± 20–49 % of pre-anesthetic level	1
	BP ± 50 % of pre-anesthetic level	0
Consciousness	Fully awake	2
	Arousable on calling	1
	Not responding	0
O_2 saturation	Able to maintain $SpO_2 > 92$ % on room air	2
	Needs O_2 inhalation to maintain $SpO_2 > 90$ %	1
	$SpO_2 < 90$ % even with O_2 supplement	0
Total		

Source: Aldrete JA. The post-anesthesia recovery score revisited. J Clin Anesth. 1995;7:89–91

Recent Publications on Pediatric Sedation in China

Between 2007 and April 2014, there were 40 publications [1–40] from China, at least 36 of which were published in Chinese and in Chinese medical journals (Figs. 23.1 and 23.2). The search engines used were http://oldweb.cqvip.com and http://www.wanfangdata.com. There were no double-blind investigations. One study was a single-blind randomized trial. Most studies were prospective observational studies and meta-analyses without a comparison group. Methodology of most investigations was unclear and without a clearly defined statistical analysis to determine sample size and data evaluation.

Approximately 50 % of the studies involved oral or rectal chloral hydrate (Fig. 23.2), a reflection of chloral hydrate as the most commonly used pediatric sedative in China. Propofol is the second most commonly studied drug, and is often described for endoscopic, dental and other invasive procedures. Only available in China for approximately 5 years, dexmedetomidine is emerging as the third most popular sedative under study. Early 2014 has shown emerging literature on dexmedetomidine from China [35–40].

The distribution of procedures that receive pediatric sedation in China is graphically presented in Fig. 23.3. Procedures currently involved in sedation investigations and publications include diagnostic imaging studies, endoscopies, other invasive procedures, and non-painful procedures such as

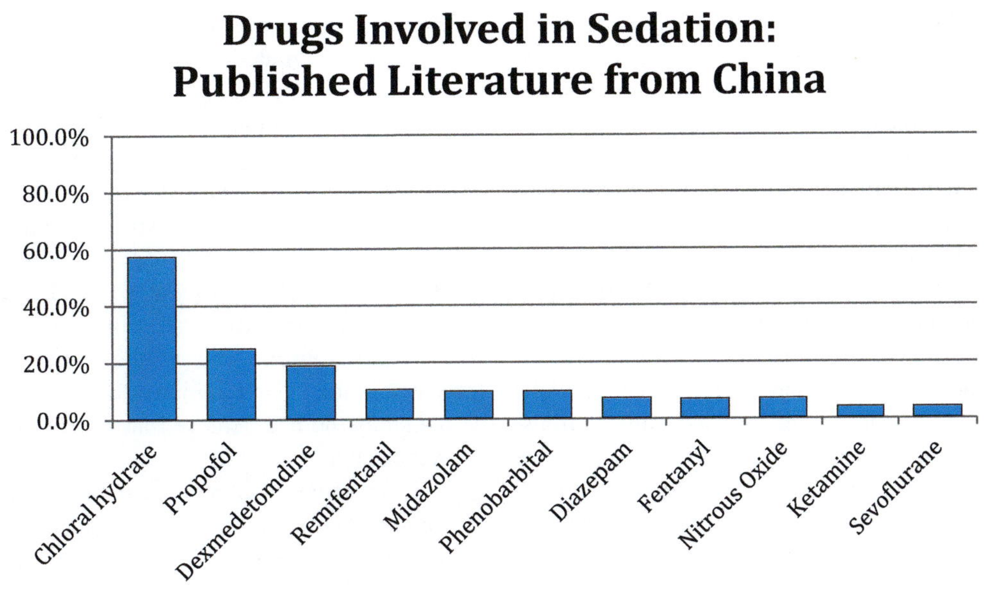

Fig. 23.2 Publications in sedation outside operating theater in children from China in year 2007–2013: sedative studied in these publications

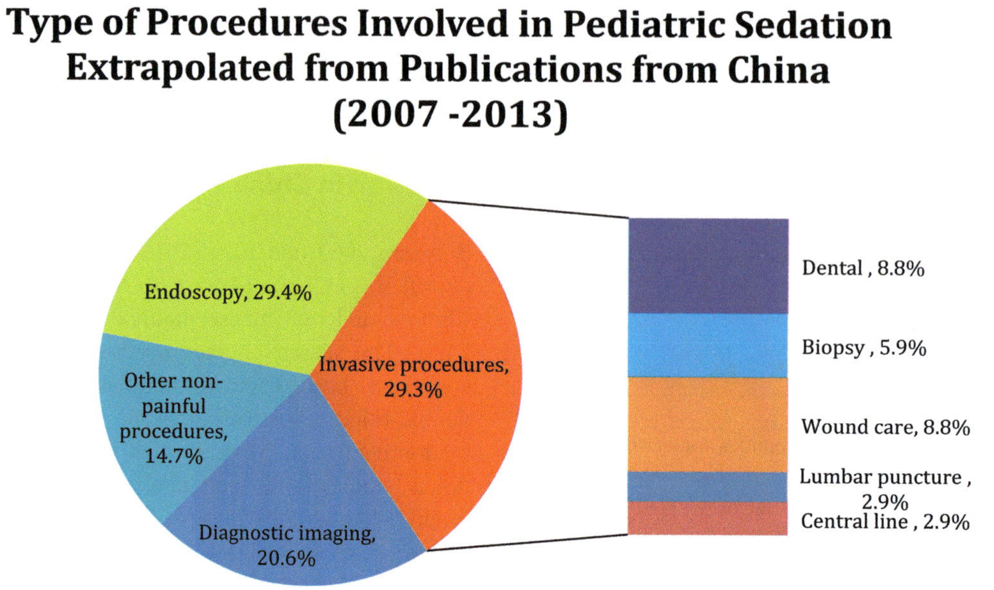

Fig. 23.3 Publications in sedation outside operating theater in children from China in year 2007–2013: indications for sedation

hearing tests. Many of these publications are published in nursing journals or journals of other medical specialties. Until 2013, there were few publications in anesthesia journals. This tendency to publish in non-anesthesia journals may reflect the common practice of sedation delivery by nurses and the physician performing the procedure.

Conclusion

China is a country of great contrasts. There is an overwhelming volume of pediatric sedation delivered, with limited resources to trained sedation care providers, sedatives, physiological monitors and sedation guidelines. With rare exception, there are no organized sedation services. Acupuncture is still being used as an adjunct or alternative to sedation in some of the rural and remote areas. The authors are not as familiar with this in their urban practice, and refer the reader to Chap. 32. This disparity between patient need and sedation provision is the current challenge for China. The next decade will, hopefully, improve the delivery of sedation in China with the organization of sedation services, development of sedation protocols, training of sedation providers, introduction of new sedatives and performance of well-designed, prospective, randomized, blinded clinical trials. Careful organization and harvesting of the impressive resources of patients, providers and intellectual capacity in China will surely lead the way for the country to become a sedation "powerhouse." This "powerhouse" contribution would be both in the field of sedation delivery and sedation research contributions in internationally recognized peer-reviewed journals, which can be shared with providers worldwide.

Case Studies

Case 1

This is a case from the Guangzhou Women and Children's Medical Center. A 3-year-old boy with autism presented for CT imaging with sedation. During pre-sedation evaluation, the boy was upset, crying, and agitated. The patient refused oral chloral hydrate, the most commonly used sedative for CT imaging. Intravenous sedation is not routinely administered and, subsequently, 3 μg/kg intranasal dexmedetomidine was administered. Adequate sedation conditions were achieved within 40 min with a sedation score (University of Michigan Sedation Scale, UMSS) of 2. (Refer to Chap. 5.) The CT study was completed uneventfully. At completion of the study, the child aroused as he was being lifted from the CT scanner table. Three minutes following completion of the study, he had achieved an Aldrete score of 9 and met discharge criteria.

It is often challenging to sedate children with autism. These children are frequently incompliant, may be aggressive, and non-amenable to common sedation delivery techniques (the oral route, in China).

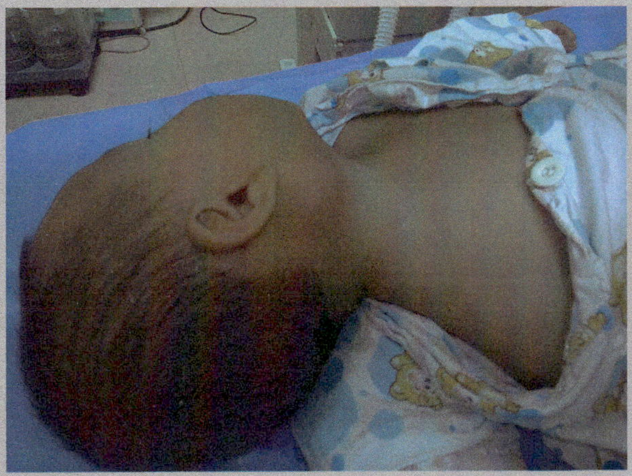

Fig. 23.4 The infant was induced after 3 μg/kg intranasal dexmedetomidine and followed by intravenous propofol and sufentanil

Dexmedetomidine offers an alternative route of delivery, which tends to be predictable, safe and effective for non-painful procedures. The success rate of using intranasal dexmedetomidine in these children is over 85 % in this center [35].

Case 2

A 7-year-old boy with hearing impairment was scheduled to undergo a sedated brainstem auditory evoked potential study. He was administered a single dose of 50 mg/kg oral chloral with no success: 30 min following administration he remained alert with a University of Michigan Sedation Score (UMSS) of 0; 2 μg/kg intranasal dexmedetomidine was administered as "rescue" and achieved successful sedation conditions within 10 min. The child's UMSS was 3 during the procedure. He was awake and meeting discharge criteria 55 min following completion of the procedure. (For the definition of UMSS refer to Chap. 5.)

Case 3

A 7-month-old boy presented with a parotid cystic lymphangioma and was to receive sedation for a needle aspiration and percutaneous sclerotherapy under fluoroscopic guidance in the interventional radiology suite. His UMSS was 2 at 18 min after 3 μg/kg intranasal dexmedetomidine (Figs. 23.4, 23.5, and 23.6). When he was adequately sedated,

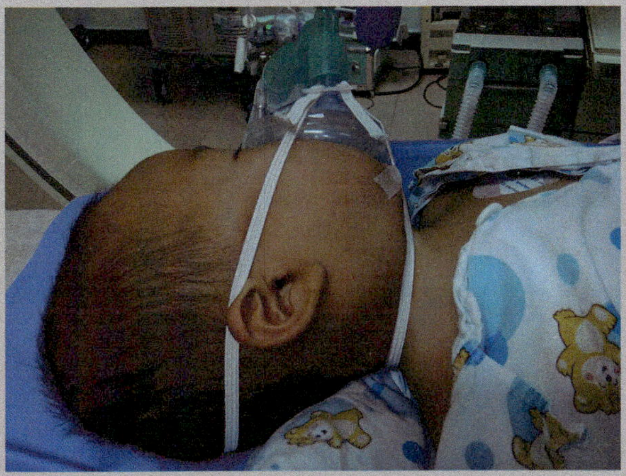

Fig. 23.5 A facemask was strapped to infant's face with elastic band and sedation was maintained with sevoflurane

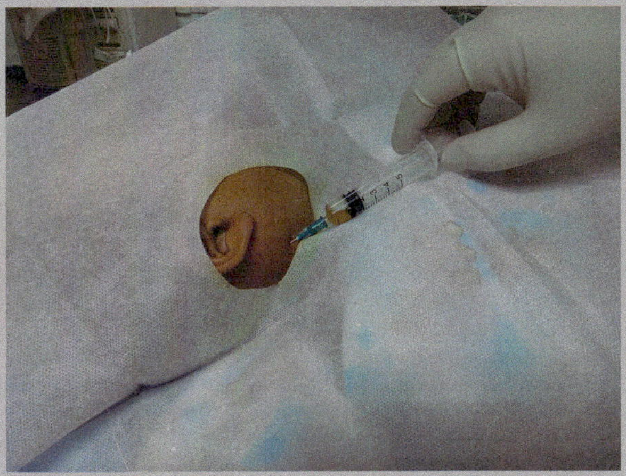

Fig. 23.6 The infant was satisfactorily sedated for needle aspiration of cystic fluid and percutaneous sclerotherapy of parotid cystic lymphangioma

he was transferred to the procedural room. Under the care of an anesthesiologist, he received intravenous propofol at 2 mg/kg and sufentanil at 0.1 μg/kg. Sedation was maintained with inhalation of sevoflurane, a general anesthetic, via a facemask at 3 % (Figs. 23.4 and 23.5). The child remained motionless throughout the 8-min procedure. He met discharge criteria 20 min after cessation of sevoflurane with an Aldrete score of 10. This case is an example of combining intranasal and intravenous sedatives with an inhalational anesthetic. In almost all areas of the world, sevoflurane administration is restricted to anesthesiologists for delivery.

References

1. Li BL, Yuen VM, Song XR, Ye J, Ni J, Huang JX, Irwin MG. Intranasal dexmedetomidine following failed chloral hydrate sedation in children. Anesthesia. 2014;69:240–4.
2. Li BL, Song XR, Li YQ, Li YM, Liu QX. The effectiveness and safety of intranasal dexmedetomidine and oral chloral hydrate for pediatric CT sedation. J Clin Anesthesiol. 2013;29(9):859–62.
3. Geng LL, Gong ST, Ou WJ, et al. Sedation effect of propofol injection in pediatric gastroscopy. J Clin Pediatr. 2007;7(22):500–1.
4. Lei SF. Use of 10% chloral hydrate sedation before pediatric CT examinations. J Qiqihaer Med School. 2007;5(28):549–50.
5. Luo XY, Luo LF, Huang YX, et al. Propofol for sedation in children undergoing gastroscopy. Int J Nurs. 2007;7(26):757–9.
6. Qi AH, Cao R, Chen GQ. Rectal chloral hydrate combined with intravenous midazolam for sedation in children undergoing renal biopsy. Mod Nurs. 2007;31(13):3019–20.
7. Qin LX. Comparison of sedative effect of two routes of administration of chloral hydrate in infants undergoing auditory brainstem response. J Med Forum. 2007;4(28):72.
8. Zhou YT, Xiao YF. Comparison of sedative effect of two routes of administration of chloral hydrate in Pediatric electroencephalograph study. Med Innov Res. 2007;4(12):86.
9. Zhang ZH, Su YJ, Wang PF, et al. Comparison of natural sleep and chloral hydrate for sedation in CT study in children. Cent Plains Med J. 2007;12(34):34–5.
10. Feng GQ. Chloral hydrate for auditory brainstem response in children. J Pract Med Technol. 2008;33(15):4819.
11. Yuan YZ, Zhai YX, Luo HF. Comparison of two administrative method of rectal chloral hydrate for sedation in children undergoing CT and MRI. Int J Nurs. 2008;1(27):61–2.
12. Xie GL, Zhang LR, Jiang LH. The use of propofol and remifentanil in children undergoing gastrointestinal endoscopy. Cent Plains Med J. 2008;14(35):43.
13. Zhang GL, Hou R, Qin RF, et al. Application of target controlled infusion of propofol in dental fear children for dental extraction. J Pract Stomatol. 2009;25(3):425–7.
14. Xiao DH, Wang F, Wang XY, et al. Propofol combined with midazolam for sedation in pediatric upper gastrointestinal endoscopy. J Cent South Univ Med Sci. 2009;34(7):595–8.
15. Huang F, Wei CF, Liu Y. The sedative effect of oral chloral hydrate for auditory brainstem response in children. J Audiol Speech Pathol. 2009;1(17):73–4.
16. Zhou JL. Comparison of oral chloral hydrate and intramuscular phenobarbitone for sedation in children with autism undergoing auditory brainstem response. J Audiol Speech Pathol. 2009; 17(1):72–3.
17. Dai YX. Comparison of different sedative regimen for children undergoing MRI. J Qilu Nurs. 2009;19(15):39–40.
18. Wang GH. Evaluation of the sedative effect of propofol combined with remifentanil in gastrointestinal endoscopy in children. Aerosp Med. 2010;3(21):335–6.
19. Huang XH, Li QY. Observational study in sedative effect of phenobarbitone and chloral hydrate for children undergoing lumbar puncture. Clin Med Eng. 2010;4(17):36–7.
20. Zhong WY, Ge S, Zhang SW, et al. Comparison of oral and rectal chloral hydrate for children undergoing dental procedure. J Oral Sci Res. 2010;4(26):560–2.
21. Rao ZW, Feng Y, Huang BJ, et al. Application of propofol infusion for sedation in pediatric gastrointestinal endoscopy. Med Chongqing. 2010;17(39):2371–2.
22. Shen JH, Tao GC. Application of sevoflurane for sedation in children undergoing central vein cannulation. Med Chongqing. 2010;23(39):3256–7.
23. Cai Y, Cai M, Xin D. The sedative effect of rectal chloral hydrate in children undergoing brainstem auditory evoked potentials. Jilin Med J. 2010;31(5):695.
24. Zhou J, Liu HF, Mei Y, et al. Application of diazepam in sigmoidoscopy in 136 Children. Her Med. 2011;1(30):61–2.
25. Ma XF, Liu XH, Hou CL, et al. Chloral hydrate enema as a sedative for removal of sutures after cleft lip repair in infants. J Oral Maxillofac Surg. 2011;3(21):195–6.
26. Cao MJ. Observation of the effect of background music combined with sedatives in children undergoing CT. J Qiqihar Univ Med. 2011;24(32):4114–5.
27. Zhang TX, Yu AY, Kou Z, et al. Comparison of oral and rectal chloral hydrate for pediatric emergence wound repair. Chin J Emerg Med. 2011;5(20):540–1.
28. Zhao J, Chen M. The application of chloral hydrate sedation in dental procedure of children. Chin Foreign Med Res. 2012;10(19):113.
29. Tian X, Yang YH, Zhang YH, et al. Propofol and fentanyl for sedation in children undergoing computer tomography-guided stereotactic biopsy of solid tumors. J Appl Clin Pediatr. 2012;21(27): 1961–2.
30. Chen SG, et al. Comparison of chloral hydrate and communication to children undergoing CT examination. Acta Med Sin. 2012;3(25):370–1.
31. Chen MH, Zhang Q, Hu G, et al. Effect of ketamine or ketamine combined with dexmedetomidine in change of dressing in pediatric burn patients. J Clin Anesthesiol. 2012;28(11):1055–7.
32. Yang CZ, Liang T, Liu Y. Anesthetic effects of dexmedetomidine during children colonoscopy. J Harbin Med Univ. 2012;46(5): 502–4.
33. Cheng B, Xu L. Clinical investigation of propofol combined with dexmedetomidine on analgesic effect in infants with enteroscopy. Sichuan Med J. 2013;1:37–9.
34. Song WF, Lin Q. The efficacy and safety of dexmedetomidine in enteroscopy in children. Contemp Med. 2013;19(15):314–5.
35. Xu YY, Song XR, Zhang GQ. The ED_{50} of intranasal dexmedetomidine in children undergoing computed tomography. Chin Med J. 2014, in press.
36. Chen KZ, Ye M, Hu CB, Shen X. Dexmedetomidine vs remifentanil intravenous anaesthesia and spontaneous ventilation for airway foreign body removal in children. Br J Anaesth. 2014;112:892–7.
37. Wu HH, Wang HT, Jin JJ, et al. Does dexmedetomidine as a neuraxial adjuvant facilitate better anesthesia and analgesia? A systematic review and meta-analysis. PLoS One. 2014;9(3):e93114.
38. Sun Y, Lu Y, Huang Y, Jiang H. Is dexmedetomidine superior to midazolam as a premedication in children? A meta-analysis of randomized controlled trials. Paediatr Anaesth. 2014;24(8):863–74.
39. Chen JJ, Yu YJ, Chu HJ, Han H, Cao Y, Dai ZP. Effects of dexmedetomidine on postoperative recovery profile after sevoflurane anesthesia in pediatric patients: a meta-analysis. J Anesth Clin Res. 2013;4(11).
40. Sun L, Guo R, Sun L. Dexmedetomidine for preventing sevoflurane-related emergence agitation in children: a meta-analysis of randomized controlled trials. Acta Anaesthesiol Scand. 2014;58:642–50.

Pediatric Sedation: The Approach in Australia and New Zealand

24

Franz E. Babl, Ian McKenzie, and Stuart R. Dalziel

Abstract

While two different countries in the Southern Hemisphere separated by a slice of the Pacific Ocean, sedation practice in Australia and New Zealand is similar and will be considered in a joint chapter. The two countries share related medical histories, practices, and conventions. Although medical registration bodies and medical regulatory agencies for drugs and devices are country-specific, many professional bodies cover both countries including key sedation relevant colleges. Where topics differ between countries, we will address this in relevant subsections. While distinctly local approaches have evolved, sedation practice in Australia and New Zealand also draws on overseas standards and experience.

Keywords

Australia • New Zealand • Pediatric • Sedation • Anesthesia • Guidelines • Australian and New Zealand College of Anaesthetists (ANZCA) • The Royal Australasian College of Surgeons (RACS) • The Australasian College of Emergency Medicine (ACEM) • The Royal Australasian College of Physicians (RACP) • Nitrous oxide • Methoxyflurane • Benzodiazepines • Midazolam • Opioids • Fentanyl • Propofol • Ketamine • Chloral hydrate • Distraction • Non-pharmacological

Introduction

While two different countries in the Southern Hemisphere separated by a slice of the Pacific Ocean, sedation practice in Australia and New Zealand is similar and will be considered in a joint chapter. The two countries share related medical histories, practices, and conventions. Although medical registration bodies and medical regulatory agencies for drugs and devices are country-specific, many professional bodies cover both countries including key sedation relevant colleges such as College of Anaesthetists (ANZCA), the Royal Australasian College of Surgeons (RACS), the Australasian College of Emergency Medicine (ACEM), and the Royal Australasian College of Physicians (RACP). The term Australasia is often used as a substitute for Australia and New Zealand, though other regions of Southeast Asia

F.E. Babl, M.D., M.P.H. (✉)
Emergency Department, Royal Children's Hospital, Melbourne, VIC, Australia
e-mail: franz.babl@rch.org.au

I. McKenzie, M.B.B.S., F.A.N.Z.C.A.
Department of Anaesthesia and Pain Management, The Royal Children's Hospital, Melbourne, VIC, Australia
e-mail: ian.mckenzie@rch.org.au

S.R. Dalziel, M.B.Ch.B., F.R.A.C.P., Ph.D.
Children's Emergency Department, Starship Children's Hospital, Auckland District Health Board, Auckland, New Zealand
e-mail: sdalziel@adhb.govt.nz

K.P. Mason (ed.), *Pediatric Sedation Outside of the Operating Room: A Multispecialty International Collaboration*, DOI 10.1007/978-1-4939-1390-9_24, © Springer Science+Business Media New York 2015

are also often included in this term. Where topics differ between countries, we will address this in relevant subsections.

Both Australia and New Zealand are large compared to the size of the population. In Australia, the majority of the population is concentrated in five large coastal metropolitan centers, often with only one or two major tertiary pediatric and academic centers in these major cities. New Zealand has one major tertiary pediatric hospital providing national services, with further extensive pediatric services found in five regional tertiary mixed pediatric and adult hospitals. In both countries, outside the major urban referral centers, pediatric services are provided in suburban and smaller regional centers with some specialist support, while vast remote areas that are thinly populated have limited access to specialist services and long transport times to definitive care. Thus for the region, transport over long distances through retrieval services is a fact of life. Distance from pediatric specialist services with access to pediatric anesthesiologists and other providers of pediatric sedation has an impact on the type of sedation care used remotely and during retrieval. While both countries have central government-funded national health-care services providing largely free health care to all citizens, health care in Australia is the responsibility of individual states. This has an impact on how health-care resources such as pain and sedation services are distributed and organized.

Sedation in children is provided by a range of providers including anesthesiologists, pediatricians, surgeons, dentists, emergency physicians, and accredited nursing staff. The key documents providing guidance for sedation in children are those developed by the ANZCA and the RACP. The *ANZCA Guidelines on Sedation and/or Analgesia for Diagnostic and Interventional Medical, Dental or Surgical Procedures* [1] has been endorsed by a number of additional key colleges and specialty societies, while the RACP guideline statements [2, 3] have not. However, neither country is providing mandatory national standards for sedation and anesthesia care such as the de facto national standard set by the Joint Commission (TJC), (formerly the Joint Commission on Accreditation of Healthcare Organizations [JCAHO]) in the United States [4]. The Australian Council on Healthcare Standards (ACHS) National Safety and Quality Health Service (NSQHS) Standards, and similar New Zealand equivalents, do not include management standards for the provision of sedation or anesthesia care. It is of note that the registration body for Australian medical and dental practitioners, the Australian Health Practitioner Regulation Agency (AHPRA), only provides formal endorsement rules for dentists wanting to practice "conscious sedation" through the Dental Board of Australia (DBA) [5, 6].

The Key Guiding Documents

The Australian and New Zealand College of Anaesthetists Guideline

The ANZCA *Guidelines on Sedation and/or Analgesia for Diagnostic and Interventional Medical, Dental or Surgical Procedures* [1] is intended to apply wherever procedural sedation and/or analgesia for diagnostic and interventional medical, dental, and surgical procedures is administered. The guidelines were initially developed by the ANZCA in 1984 and have had multiple reviews since. The latest revision in 2010 has been endorsed by the Faculty of Pain Medicine, the ANZCA, the Gastroenterological Society of Australia, the RACS, the Australasian College for Emergency Medicine, the College of Intensive Care Medicine of Australia and New Zealand, the Royal Australasian College of Dental Surgeons, and the Royal Australian and New Zealand College of Radiologists (RANZCR) [1]. Guidelines in this context are defined by ANZCA as "a document offering advice."

The ANZCA guideline sets out definitions, patient selection and preparation, staffing and equipment, monitoring and documentation, medication, discharge, and recovery and training recommendations.

The ANZCA definition of levels of sedation largely follows the definition of sedation depth set out by the American Society of Anesthesiologists (ASA) [7]. It uses the term *conscious sedation* rather than *moderate sedation*. It emphasizes that transition from complete consciousness through the various depths of sedation to general anesthesia is a continuum and not a set of discrete, well-defined stages.

In the text and an appendix, the ANZCA guideline sets out staffing requirements based on the depth of sedation targeted, the agents used, and the ASA classification of physical status (see Fig. 24.1). In any type of sedation, a medical or dental practitioner with airway and resuscitation skills must be available. For the majority of procedures, the guidelines state that there must be a minimum of three appropriately trained staff present: the proceduralist, the medical or dental practitioner administering sedation and monitoring the patient, and at least one additional staff member to provide assistance to the proceduralist and/or the practitioner providing sedation as required. Exceptions to the above staffing requirements are very light conscious sedation, and/or analgesic techniques such as inhaled nitrous oxide or low-dose oral sedation, where the proceduralist also provides the sedation and an assistant with training in monitoring sedation is also recommended. Techniques intended to produce deep sedation or general anesthesia must not be used unless an anesthesiologist or another appropriately

Personnel for procedural sedation and analgesia

Scenario 0: Two personnel – sedation by proceduralist

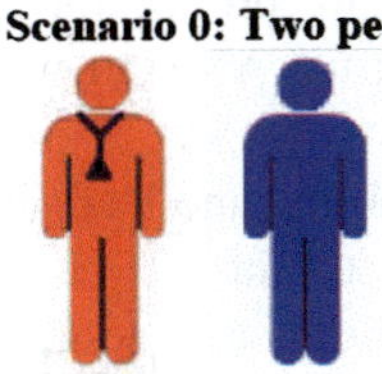

- Medical or dental practitioner proceduralist with airway and resuscitation skills, and training in nitrous oxide or low dose oral sedation techniques
- Assistant with training in monitoring sedation
- Conscious sedation using nitrous oxide alone and/or low dose oral sedation alone in ASA P 1-2 patients
- Heavy oral sedation and intramuscular or intravenous sedative/anaesthetic/analgesic agents must not be used

Scenario 1: Three personnel – sedation by proceduralist

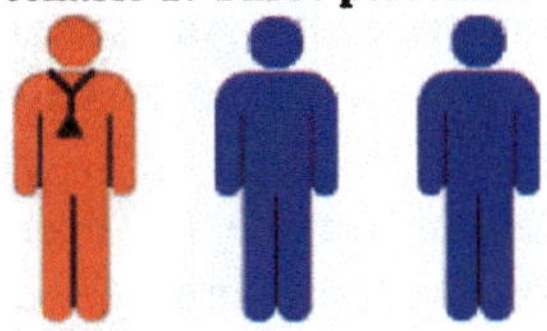

- Medical or dental practitioner proceduralist with airway and resuscitation skills, and training in sedation
- Assistant with training in monitoring sedation
- Assistant to assist both
- Conscious sedation in ASA P 1-2 patients
- Propofol, thiopentone and other intravenous anaesthetic agents must not be used

Scenario 2: Three personnel – sedation by medical or dental practitioner

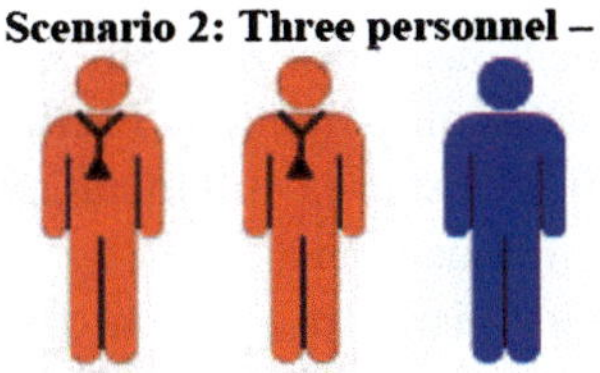

- Proceduralist
- Medical or dental practitioner with airway and resuscitation skills, and training in sedation
- Assistant to assist both
- Conscious sedation in ASA P 1-2 patients
- Propofol, thiopentone and other intravenous anaesthetic agents may only be used by a medical or dental practitioner trained in their use

Scenario 3: Four personnel – sedation by medical or dental practitioner

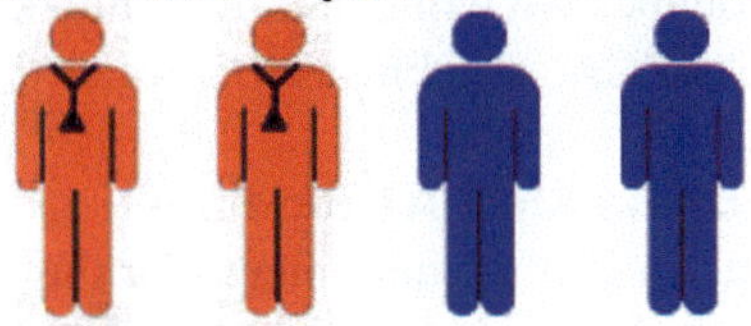

- Proceduralist
- Medical or dental practitioner with airway and resuscitation skills, and training in sedation
- Assistant to assist ***each****
- Conscious sedation in ASA P 1-3 patients [#]
- Propofol, thiopentone and other intravenous anaesthetic agents may only be used by a medical or dental practitioner trained in their use

Scenario 4: Three personnel – sedation by anaesthetist

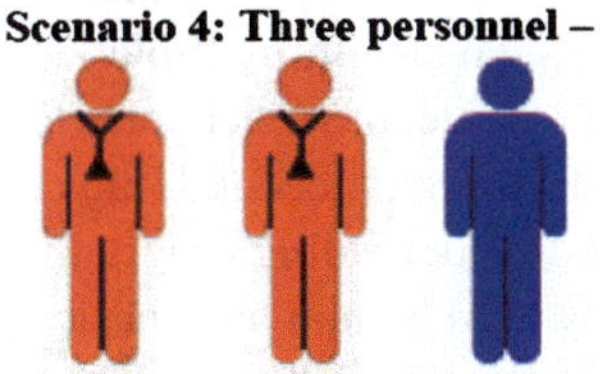

- Proceduralist
- Anaesthetist
- Assistant to assist both
- Conscious, deep sedation or general anaesthesia in all patients
- All approved anaesthetic drugs may be used

Scenario 5: Four personnel – sedation by anaesthetist

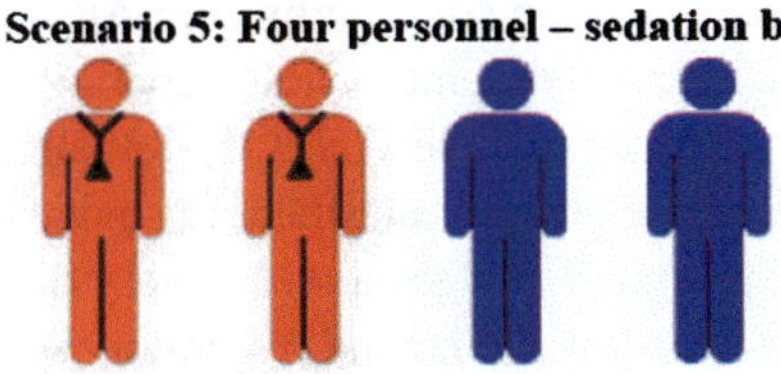

- Proceduralist
- Anaesthetist
- Assistant to assist ***each****
- Conscious sedation, deep sedation or general anaesthesia in all patients
- All approved anaesthetic drugs may be used

* ***Recommended if assistance is likely to be required for the majority of the case (e.g. complex or emergency patients)***

Fig. 24.1 Staffing requirements for procedural sedation and analgesia in Australia and New Zealand. Reprinted with permission from Australian and New Zealand College of Anaesthetists. Guidelines on Sedation and/or Analgesia for Diagnostic and Interventional Medical, Dental or Surgical Procedures. PS9. ANZCA (2010)

trained and credentialed medical specialist within his/her scope of practice is available.

Procedures must be performed in a location that is staffed and equipped to deal with cardiovascular and respiratory emergencies. This includes equipment for suctioning, equipment for advanced airway management, emergency drugs including reversal agents and adrenaline, equipment for monitoring including electrocardiogram (EKG) and pulse oximetry, and a defibrillator. Within the facility there should be access to devices for measuring expired carbon dioxide. When nitrous oxide or methoxyflurane is used, appropriate scavenging must be used to decrease chronic staff exposure. There must be the capacity to administer 100 % oxygen, and a low gas flow alarm must be established. For nitrous oxide delivery, a minimum of 3 L/min oxygen flow and a maximum of 10 L/min total flow are specified unless the device is designed to deliver a minimum of 30 % oxygen.

Reliable intravenous access should be in place for all procedures under procedural sedation, yet it is acknowledged that this may not be practical in those receiving non-intravenous sedation. Patients undergoing procedural sedation must be continuously monitored with pulse oximetry and pulse rate, with oxygen saturation and blood pressure regularly recorded. Oxygen administration is recommended for as much of the procedure as possible. Depending on clinical status, EKG monitoring and capnography may be required.

A variety of drugs and techniques are available for procedural sedation. The guidelines identify benzodiazepines (such as midazolam) and opioids (such as fentanyl) as the most commonly used intravenous agents. Because of the risk of unintentional loss of consciousness/respiratory effort, intravenous anesthetic agents such as propofol must not be administered by the proceduralist and may only be used by a second trained medical or dental practitioner.

The guidelines also include training recommendations for non-anesthesiologist medical or dental practitioners who provide procedural sedation and analgesia. They recommend a minimum of 3 months (full-time equivalent) supervised training in procedural sedation and/or analgesia and anesthesia or similar approved course, in addition to In-Training and Competency Assessment. Training should include completion of a crisis resource management simulation center course. Long-standing clinical experience may be deemed equivalent to a formal period of training. Credentialing, training, and clinical support of non-anesthesia sedation providers can be achieved with nominated local anesthesiologists. Rural practitioners, or those practicing in remote areas, may train with anesthesiologists in a major center, particularly when learning the skills of intravenous or intramuscular sedation. Maintenance of certification in cardiopulmonary resuscitation and evidence of relevant continuing professional development are required for credentialing.

A number of other ANZCA guidelines and statements are relevant to the provision of safe procedural sedation and analgesia; all are available via the ANZCA website.[1] They include:

- PS2 Statement on Credentialling and Defining the Scope of Clinical Practice in Anaesthesia
- PS4 Recommendations for the Post-Anaesthesia Recovery Room
- PS6 The Anaesthesia Record. Recommendations on the Recording of an Episode of Anaesthesia Care
- PS7 Recommendations for the Pre-Anaesthesia Consultation
- PS8 Recommendations on the Assistant for the Anaesthetist
- PS15 Recommendations for the Perioperative Care of Patients Selected for Day Care Surgery
- PS18 Recommendations on Monitoring During Anaesthesia
- PS26 Guidelines on Consent for Anaesthesia or Sedation
- T1 Recommendations on Minimum Facilities for Safe Administration of Anaesthesia in Operating Suites and Other Anaesthetising Locations
- TE3 Policy on Supervision of Clinical Experience for Vocational Trainees in Anaesthesia

While they are an excellent foundation for safe procedural sedation care, there are a number of issues with the ANZCA guideline. We will detail the limitations and omissions of the ANZCA guideline as follows:

Limitation of the ANZCA Guideline

The guideline's staffing requirements for the presence of at least one medical or dental practitioner during the sedation do not take into account the widespread use of nurse-led sedations using nitrous oxide in major centers and elsewhere in Australia and New Zealand. In multiple large Australian series [8–10], nitrous oxide has been provided safely by sedation-trained nurses when embedded into comprehensive sedation education and credentialing programs.

An agent frequently used by non-anesthesiologists for parenteral sedation is ketamine. Even though it is one of the most frequently used agents in some settings in Australia and New Zealand, particularly in emergency departments [11], the agent is not addressed in the ANZCA guideline. Ketamine, while technically a general anesthetic, provides dissociative sedation and profound analgesia with a very different profile of effect on the cardiovascular and respiratory systems as well as maintenance of muscle tone compared with other general anesthetic agents. Standard definitions of sedation depth such as used in the ANZCA guideline do not apply to ketamine sedation [12]. Furthermore, it has been shown to be a very safe agent in the hands of non-anesthesiologists [13, 14].

[1] www.anzca.edu.au/resources

Nitrous oxide in the guideline is listed as a method for providing "very light conscious sedation." This is very true of nitrous oxide titrated slowly from minimum concentrations, maintaining patient cooperation, as is done for minor procedures, especially dental procedures, commonly in association with local anesthesia. It is important to note that, based on the minimum oxygen concentration of 30 % noted in the ANZCA guideline, up to 70 % nitrous oxide can be administered. While generally very safe, nitrous oxide, especially at 70 %, can lead to deep sedation, and providers need to be aware of and be prepared for this [8, 15]. Combining other systemic sedatives or analgesics can be clinically useful but increases the likelihood of deeper sedation and some complications. Recently, nitrous oxide has been combined with intranasal fentanyl, improving the analgesic efficacy of nitrous oxide for non-parenteral sedation in painful procedures. This combination, while now widely used in some settings in Australia and New Zealand for painful procedures such as fracture reductions [16], may be associated with a much higher rate of emesis and a deeper level of sedation [17].

The ANZCA *Joint Guideline* recommends that medical and dental practitioners receive 3 months of anesthetic training in order to provide sedation. While there are no statistics available for non-anesthesiologists who fulfill these criteria, non-anesthesia colleges for dentistry, radiology, surgery, emergency medicine, and pediatrics do not require such training. Anecdotally, only a minority of trainees from colleges that endorse these guidelines will fulfill this recommendation.

Table 24.1 Minimizing pain and suffering in procedures

• Adopt a child-centered approach (listening to the needs of the child and family) rather than a procedure-focused "get-it-over-with" approach
• Make the child and their family active participants and members of the team, rather than passive recipients
• Use parents for positive assistance, not negative restraint
• Ensure that all procedures undertaken are necessary; that is, the benefit outweighs any negative impact caused by the procedure
• Ensure that all procedures are carried out in order to maximize safety for the child
• Perform procedures in a child-friendly environment, away from the bed
• Use pain assessment routinely
• Use the least invasive equipment where possible
• Ensure that the person performing the procedure has appropriate technical expertise or is closely supervised by someone who does
• Use appropriate combinations of non-pharmacological and pharmacological interventions to manage pain and anxiety. Sedation alone does not provide pain relief
• Optimize waiting time: too little time increases distress but too much time increases anticipatory anxiety. Time required for preparation is child-specific
• Ensure that the development of anticipatory anxiety is prevented as far as possible by maximizing the intervention to alleviate pain and distress for the first procedure (e.g., general anesthetic for bone marrow aspirate)

Reprinted with permission from Royal Australasian College of Physicians. Guideline statement: management of procedure-related pain in children and adolescents. J Paediatr Child Health. 2006 Feb;42 Suppl 1:S1-29

The Royal Australasian College of Physicians Guideline Statements

The RACP has published two evidence-based guidelines on the management of procedure-related pain in neonates [3] and in children and adolescents [2].

The RACP guideline statement *Management of Procedure-Related Pain in Neonates* addresses the following issues: consequences of newborn pain, responses of infants to pain, general principles for the prevention and management of pain in newborns, assessment of pain in neonates, and evidence and suggested techniques. The intent of the guideline was to encourage increased use of analgesia for newborn infants undergoing procedures, including those in neonatal intensive care units. While the guideline does not address procedural sedation in detail, procedural sedation/anesthesia is recommended for endotracheal intubation and for consideration in infants undergoing chest tube insertion and laser therapy for retinopathy of prematurity [3].

The RACP guideline statement *Management of Procedure-Related Pain in Children and Adolescents* [2] includes sections on sedation for procedures but provides a broader—where possible evidence-based—canvas to improve procedural care in an integrated approach of pharmacological and non-pharmacological techniques to address the problems of procedural pain, anxiety, and behavioral distress in children. An executive summary provides a list of key principles to minimize pain and suffering in procedures as listed in Table 24.1.

After a brief background, definitions and methodology for the literature review are undertaken. The RACP guideline addresses the following issues: pre-procedural preparation with evaluation of the patient, informed consent, and role of the parent; resources required including environment, personnel, equipment, monitoring, and documentation; and procedure, including suggested techniques for commonly performed procedures. Children with communication and behavior problems and those who require repeat procedures are addressed in separate sections. A unique section presents a consumer's perspective, such as from a mother of a 4-year-old girl who had undergone repeated painful procedures. Appendices address non-pharmacological techniques for procedural pain management, use of local anesthetics, and three sedatives: nitrous oxide, midazolam, and ketamine.

The definition of sedation lists three different definitions by the American Academy of Pediatrics [18, 19], the ASA [20],

Table 24.2 The total procedural process

Before	During	After
Non-pharmacological		
• Assessment of child's previous experience • Assessment of child's expectations • Find out child's likes and interests • Enlist parent's help • Start distraction immediately prior to procedure	• Distraction • Breathing techniques • Other coping-promoting behavior and techniques	• Correct any misconceptions • Reinforce coping behavior • Focus on positive • Instill sense of achievement
Pharmacological		
• Consent • Fasting • Pre-procedure assessment	• Appropriate technique used for procedure	• Post-procedure assessment • Ongoing analgesia
General		
• Personnel • Equipment	• Monitoring: pain and safety • Documentation • Management of complications	• Discharge advice • Preparation for next time nearer the time

Reprinted with permission from Royal Australasian College of Physicians. Guideline statement: management of procedure-related pain in children and adolescents. J Paediatr Child Health. 2006 Feb;42 Suppl 1:S1-29

and the American College of Emergency Physicians [21]. The ASA classification system is used as part of pre-procedural risk assessment. Pre-procedural fasting is discussed critically with a consideration of risk and benefit by weighing up the risk of vomiting and aspiration with the urgency of the procedure. No specific fasting times are recommended. The guideline recommends that informed consent is obtained and documented in the medical record. Without clear evidence regarding the appropriate number of staff required to perform safe procedural sedation, the guidelines make recommendations on staffing based on consensus opinion: "a number of international and local protocols recommend one medical staff member…" should be responsible for monitoring the airway and the patient's clinical status (the "sedationist") with an additional staff member performing the procedure. The guideline cites that similar to the ANZCA guideline, it is recognized that some situations may warrant additional staff members. While the RACP guideline does not recommend training or specialty of staff members undertaking sedation, it recommends that those undertaking sedation have knowledge and experience in the use of the techniques being utilized: an ability to monitor clinical effectiveness and possible deterioration, ability to manage adverse events, and to be skilled in advanced airway management.

Resuscitation equipment is recommended to be available where the sedation and procedure are occurring. Non-pharmacological techniques are also recommended to minimize pain and distress. Monitoring should include pulse oximetry (recognizing the limits of this modality to detect hypoventilation and hypercarbia) and capnography (particularly when the patient's respiratory efforts are not able to be visualized). When administering nitrous oxide, ketamine, and midazolam, it is recommended that the sedationist should be separate from the proceduralist. For nitrous oxide administration, an anesthesiologist is recommended for children under 12 months of age, in cases of preexisting airway problems, or for patients who have received adjuvant sedatives. As with the ANZCA guideline, when using nitrous oxide, a separate means of delivering 100 % oxygen and a system for scavenging of expired gas are recommended. For ketamine and midazolam, practitioners are recommended to be specifically trained in their administration and possess advanced airway management skills.

The RACP guideline emphasizes consideration of the total procedure process including non-pharmacological pain management at all stages of the procedure (Table 24.2) and the provision of a psychologically supportive environment including the use of appropriate language.

The guidelines are unique in that they present evidence and suggested techniques for 23 commonly undertaken procedures: capillary sampling, intramuscular injections, suprapubic aspiration, central venous port access, venepuncture, intravenous cannulation, arterial puncture, intra-arterial cannulation, central venous line insertion, nasogastric tube insertion, orogastric tube insertion, endotracheal intubation, endotracheal suction, chest tube insertion or removal, urethral catheterization, laceration repair, fracture manipulation, foreign body removal, burns and other wound dressing, lumbar puncture, bone marrow aspiration, joint aspiration and/or injection, renal biopsy, and radiological imaging.

For a number of procedures (bone marrow aspiration, joint aspiration, and renal biopsy) conscious sedation or general anesthesia is recommended as first choice in children less than 12 years of age and for adolescents, based on their psychological coping skills, preparation level, and patient/family choice. Nitrous oxide is suggested as a safe and efficacious technique for peripheral and central vascular access procedures, urethral catheterization, laceration repair, burn dressings, lumbar punctures, bone marrow aspiration and joint aspiration, and renal biopsy. Chloral hydrate is suggested for sedation for computed tomography (CT) and magnetic resonance imaging (MRI) scans in infants >3 months and toddlers. Sedation with midazolam or ketamine is recommended for consideration for central venous line insertion, complex laceration repair, fracture reduction, bone marrow and joint aspiration, and renal biopsy. Sedation or general anesthesia is recommended for consideration for CT or MRI scans in children with preexisting behavior problems, for procedures with breath-holding requirements, and in children unable to lie still or who are anxious. The guideline emphasizes that fracture manipulation is highly painful and in many settings manipulation is performed under anesthesia in the operating room. However, in centers with expertise in procedural sedation and analgesia, fracture manipulation is often performed outside the operating room. In such instances the RACP guideline recommends ketamine and ketamine/midazolam. Propofol/fentanyl is not recommended due to the much higher incidence of airway complications. In cooperative older children, with specialized equipment and experienced staff, intravenous regional anesthesia (Bier's block) is also recommended. Nitrous oxide is recommended for consideration in fracture manipulation in children with minimally displaced fractures.

The RACP guideline addresses the needs of children who require repeat procedures and for those with communication or behavior problems. The guideline groups the latter children into four categories and provides specific suggestions and recommendations for procedural interventions. For children with impaired cognition and inability to communicate, the key recommendations are to explore their means of communication, err on the side of over-treating, and integrate pharmacological and non-pharmacological techniques. The guideline recognizes that comorbidities may contraindicate conscious sedation by the non-anesthesiologist. For children with physical disability and preserved cognition, the key recommendation is to establish how best to communicate with the child. For children with behavioral problems related to preexisting disorders of inattention and hyperactivity, the recommendation is to have a low threshold for pharmacological intervention. For children with procedure-related behavior problems, the recommendations include systematic desensitization, cognitive behavioral therapy, and coping strategies.

The appendices of the RACP guideline include more detailed information on three sedative agents: nitrous oxide, midazolam, and ketamine. The use of demand valve fixed 50 % nitrous oxide and 50 % oxygen as well as continuous flow nitrous oxide up to 70 % is discussed, requiring a circuit for both to scavenge exhaled gas. A minimum 2 h NPO is recommended as a prerequisite if nitrous oxide above 50 % is used. After discontinuing nitrous oxide, 100 % oxygen is recommended for 2–3 min to avoid diffusion hypoxia. For those patients at risk of B_{12} inactivation (preexisting vitamin B_{12} or folate deficiency, preexisting bone marrow suppression, severe sepsis, and extensive tissue damage) who receive nitrous oxide frequently for 2 weeks or more, two protocols to minimize vitamin B_{12} deficiency due to the metabolic effects of nitrous oxide are recommended.

In summary, there is little overlap between the RACP guideline and the ANZCA guideline, although there are shared members of each college. Application of the RACP guidelines suggests appropriate use of non-pharmacological techniques and local analgesia for children. The ANZCA guideline addresses sedation in relation to procedures at any age group. There is no specific consideration of pediatric issues nor of overall procedural management. The ANZCA guideline focuses on the delivery of sedation compared to the RACP guidelines, which attempt to take a more holistic approach. A limitation of the RACP guidelines is that since 2006, when the guideline was published, a number of overseas guidelines referenced have been revised or updated and new evidence has become available.

Development of a Sedation Program

While major Australian and New Zealand procedural sedation guidelines [1, 2] are available, and key overseas guidelines are in use as well, there is limited knowledge in how far these guidelines and recommendations are used "on the shop floor." A review in 2004 of the spectrum and the quality of procedural sedation performed by non-anesthesiologist staff outside the intensive care unit at Royal Children's Hospital in Melbourne, a large Australian tertiary pediatric hospital, indicated some problematic practices [22]. Sedations were tracked prospectively twice daily through hospital walk-through by the authors. One hundred and twenty sedations took place over a 3-week period, for 24 indications, utilizing eight agents in 26 different locations. Neither medical nor nursing staff were present during 7 % of the sedation and during 23 % of the recovery periods. Formal monitoring of vital signs occurred in only 72 %. Fasting practice was highly variable, few sedations used non-pharmacological techniques, and some children were restrained.

A good overview of the challenges involved in minimizing pain and distress in children across initially a ward and then an entire hospital is well described in two papers outlining the experience of a single pediatric service in the United States [23, 24]. The 1997 paper describes the initial few years of a program designed for a pediatric ward in a general hospital. The key principles were to bring uniformity to pain management, sedation, and pain assessment (by the introduction of guidelines/protocols), with particular emphasis on the importance of appropriate topical anesthesia for procedures involving "needle sticks" and the need to involve the child's parents. The second paper, from 2008, reviews the progress of the program, which was then applied to an entire children's hospital and not confined to ward activities. The importance of ensuring that all areas of the hospital minimize distress and pain was clearly identified as the program was named "Comfort Central." The aims addressed the culture of the organization: the physical environment, education, governance, audit and quality processes, matching clinical services to need, collaborating across departments, and involving the patients and families in the process. These principles mirror the concepts summarized in the RACP 2006 Guidelines [2].

At Royal Children's Hospital, Melbourne, the findings of the audit described earlier in this chapter [22] have led to profound hospital-wide changes in sedation practice: the abolishment of unmonitored or technician-only sedation and the concentration of sedation in a few central locations away from low frequency or remote locations. Hospital-wide sedation guidelines, sedation education, and sedation documentation were implemented across the whole hospital.

Departmental and hospital-wide sedation guidelines have been implemented across many Australian and New Zealand institutions. Sedation care is still often highly variable between hospitals and between departments within the same institution. Regulatory authorities do not mandate a standard accreditation or training process for sedation providers. There is no requirement to standardize sedation care throughout an institution as has been mandated in the United States by the Joint Commission [4].

A number of relatively large series from Australia and New Zealand have shown that pediatric sedation by non-anesthesiologists can be performed safely when embedded in local sedation education programs [9, 10]. However, even among tertiary pediatric institutions, few have hospital-wide sedation education programs. While there are no national sedation education programs nor education conferences that exist in the United States, departments at larger pediatric tertiary hospitals often provide education or education materials for non-tertiary institutions who conduct pediatric sedation. For example, a validated sedation education program from Royal Children's Hospital and Sunshine Hospital in Melbourne [25, 26] has been adopted by the state health department and rolled out statewide in the state of Victoria [27]. This program includes central education sessions, sedation education materials, and a standardized sedation record.

Only one tertiary children's hospital in Australia provides a formal "sedation service" run by anesthesiology staff. At a few centers, nurse-led sedation with nitrous oxide is provided hospital-wide. At most centers, sedation is delivered by anesthesiologists, except for some subspecialties such as dentistry or emergency medicine.

Specific Locations and Services

Inpatient Wards

A wide range of interventions are carried out at inpatient wards. The role of sedation is important, but optimizing the use of other techniques to minimize distress is likely to decrease the number of patients who require sedation.

At the Royal Children's Hospital, Melbourne, Australia [28], the sedation guidelines for procedures on the wards (and outpatient areas) provide an example in Australia. These guidelines consider non-pharmacological techniques and non-sedative agents such as sucrose and topical local anesthetic. The Royal Children's Hospital guidelines assume that there is a continuous pediatric intensive care-based emergency response team available at all times, which may not be the case in all pediatric institutions.

At Royal Children's Hospital, according to the local guidelines, junior ward medical staff can prescribe oral midazolam for a child due to have a procedure, and the "sedationist" and "proceduralist" (who may both be nursing staff) can manage the patient on the ward according to the guidelines. If nitrous oxide or intravenous midazolam is to be used, the staff member performing the sedation and monitoring the patient must have been appropriately accredited (and may be nursing or medical staff). If the patient is found to have risk factors in the pre-procedure assessment process, consultation with more senior anesthesia staff is required to formulate an appropriate plan. In some specialized areas, such as the cardiac surgery ward (not an intensive care ward), local procedures have been developed that acknowledge specific scope of practice of specialized staff in that area. A key component of the guideline is that a "record of sedation" form be used to document all sedations.

These guidelines require that deep sedation be administered by a member of the critical care medical staff (anesthetist, intensivist, or ED physician).

A contentious issue for procedures on the ward is: "Is it best to preserve a child's hospital room as a 'safe place' and conduct procedures in a separate area, such as a treatment room?" "Pros" for not using the patient's bed/room include: the sense of security the child has about their "usual place" in the hospital, minimizing of impact on other patients in shared rooms, ensuring an appropriate specialized area with resuscitation and monitoring, and providing distraction equipment (audiovisual or age-appropriate toys) to optimize care.

"Cons" include having to move the patient, the potential impact on staffing, and the potential for child distrust if there is distress and pain in the treatment room.

Sedation in the Pediatric Intensive Care Units

A pediatric intensive care unit (PICU) provides a complex environment for minimization of pain and distress relating to procedures. In general, in Australia and New Zealand, PICU staff does not provide a "sedation service" for patients who are not in an intensive care unit setting. The central role of sedation and analgesia in PICU management is addressed in two of the eight items on the PICU "KIDS SAFE" checklist [29] recently developed at the Royal Children's Hospital in Brisbane. PICU management has evolved. In the 1980s there was recognition that the adverse effects of inadequately treated pain and anxiety could create short-term complications [30] such as marked sympathoadrenal activation and subsequently longer term complications such as allodynia and hyperalgesia and post-traumatic stress syndrome. More recently, there has been a focus on balancing analgesia and sedation with the risk of prolonged ventilation and withdrawal.

PICU patients in Australia and New Zealand require analgesia and sedation for a variety of procedures. Examples are listed below with common management techniques and strategies:

- *The presenting condition*, such as major surgery or trauma; treated with established acute pain management regimens.
- "Minor" *brief* but potentially very distressing interventions, such as tracheal intubation, suctioning of an endotracheal tube, vascular cannulation, insertion of chest drains or peritoneal dialysis catheters, and removal of drains; managed with intravenous boluses of systemic medications, which may be escalated to general anesthesia as appropriate. Local anesthesia may provide profound analgesia and minimize the need for systemic medications where it is applicable. Inhaled nitrous oxide is being used for brief "minor" procedures, in the absence of contraindications, in minimally sedated patients.
- *Formal surgical interventions* that may be performed urgently or planned to be done in the PICU. In many of these situations, anesthesia consultation is often sought. Most PICU units in this region will use intravenous agents and not integrate volatile anesthesia delivery. Pediatric intensivists and anesthetists will often collaborate in the care of these children.
- *Ongoing management* such as tolerating endotracheal tubes or intravenous cannulation for extracorporeal cardiovascular or respiratory support. The main pharmacological interventions for these scenarios remain opioid analgesia with benzodiazepine supplementation. The role of centrally acting alpha2-adrenergic agonists such as clonidine and dexmedetomidine is increasing in PICUs, to treat and minimize the side effects (tolerance and withdrawal) of benzodiazepines. The cardiovascular effects of dexmedetomidine, particularly bradycardia, and its expense on the Australian market have limited its widespread use.

The ongoing evolution of methods for synchronizing mechanical ventilation with patient effort and the use of less invasive respiratory support (without endotracheal intubation) have improved patient tolerance of ventilator support with less systemic sedation.

Although there are well-established sedation protocols for management, they must be tailored to the patient's circumstances. Examples of common issues that arise in PICU include:

- Patients with severe loss of cardiovascular reserve who may not tolerate "usual" acute boluses of analgesia or sedation drugs without compromising their circulation.
- Patients who have required long-term management who develop tolerance to standard dosing, who may require escalation of dose or changes of medication or combinations to provide adequate analgesia and sedation.
- Patients who develop symptoms of withdrawal when doses are decreased. Monitoring with assessment tools such as the Withdrawal Assessment Tool 1 (WAT-1) [31] and tailoring management accordingly is now standard in many Australian units.
- Other special circumstances such as development of opioid-induced hyperalgesia, which may require decreased dose, change of opioid, and alternative non-opioid agents.
- Recognition of the special needs of patients who require cardiorespiratory support with extracorporeal membrane oxygenation (ECMO) or ventricular assist devices (VAD). Protocols specific to this for different age groups have been developed (guidelines on RCH Melbourne intranet, for information: http://www.rch.org.au/picu/contact_us/Contact_ICU/#ECLS_contacts).
- Recent concerns regarding the potential adverse effects of drugs affecting the central nervous system on the developing brain, especially in the first months to years of life.

A "Procedural Pain Management Decision Tree" to assist PICU staff at Royal Children's Hospital, Melbourne, has recently been developed to supplement the hospital-wide Procedural Pain Management Guideline [28, 32].

Neonatal Intensive Care Units

In Australia, the majority of neonatal intensive care units are colocated with obstetric units. The non-tertiary care centers tend to have limited pediatric surgical services. These units focus on prematurity and conditions managed medically.

Inadequate procedural pain management in the neonatal period may be associated with profound physiological responses to procedural pain, such as tachycardia, hypertension, apnea, and hypoxia, with the potential to create significant adverse outcomes. Overall, appropriate care to avoid excessive or gratuitous use of centrally acting analgesics, anxiolytics, sedatives, and anesthesia in neonates has been adopted. The apparent lack of induction of apoptosis by the centrally acting alpha2-adrenergic agonists, clonidine and dexmedetomidine, has increased interest in their use, but the associated bradycardia is problematic in this age group [33]. For patients requiring long-term intensive care in the region, the alpha2-adrenergic agonists are already part of protocols for preventing and managing withdrawal syndromes for neonates. These patients are protected from the cardiovascular adverse effects by their underlying increased sympathetic drive.

Non-pharmacological management has become a key part of protocols in neonatal units. Non-pharmacological approaches include comforting, swaddling, the use of soothing speech and music, feeding, non-nutritive sucking, as well as the manipulation of lighting, sound, and other environmental factors [34].

For minor procedures, local anesthesia can minimize the need for adjuvant medications, which may act directly on the central nervous system. Care must be taken with total dosage and administration of local anesthesia due to the risk of high systemic levels especially from high concentrations injected in smaller patients. Prilocaine, a component of a proprietary eutectic mixture, EMLA cream, can cause methemoglobinemia in the newborn [35], and care with use or alternatives are recommended [36].

Sucrose for modifying the response to procedural interventions is now well established [37, 38]. Protocols for its use are virtually universal in NICUs in the region. There is good quality data supporting its efficacy and safety, including with repeated use. Although there may remain some concerns that the neurophysiological "fast" pain remains activated [39], the efficacy of sucrose in decreasing distressed behavioral overrides these concerns.

For premature NICU patients who require a surgical procedure, the risk benefit assessment of transport to an operating theater versus operating in situ in the NICU is complex. An individual risk assessment of the circumstances of the individual patient is required. Results of audits in this region support the strategy of operating on the sicker and smaller NICU patients in the NICU [40]. The anesthesia is usually based on muscle relaxation and high-dose fentanyl. This should certainly provide adequate analgesia and has been demonstrated to be associated with beneficial effects on the stress response. NICUs at obstetric hospitals have even brought in specified pediatric surgical teams from outside centers to perform interventions (ligation of a patent ductus arteriosus) that are not offered by their own staff.

Paracetamol, morphine, and fentanyl are the most commonly used analgesics in this region, with increasing use of tramadol [41, 42].

Assessment of pain management in NICUs is performed using a range of tools. The "PAT" (pain assesment tool) has been develped and is most commonly used in this region [43].

Emergency Departments

Over the last two decades, alongside the development of emergency medicine and pediatric emergency medicine as recognized medical specialties within both countries, pediatric sedation within emergency departments has become the expected standard. In smaller urban and rural settings, lack of trained, experienced sedation staff may result in transfer of the child to larger centers for definitive care [44]. Given the vast distances involved, this transfer can be inconvenient for children and families, as well as an expensive burden on the health-care system.

In both countries, procedural sedation within emergency departments commonly occurs for fracture manipulation, joint relocation, laceration repair, foreign body removal, urethral catheterization, lumbar puncture, abscess drainage, and neuroimaging [11]. A survey of pediatric emergency medicine specialists, mainly at the tertiary sites, indicates that agents commonly used include continuous nitrous oxide (100 % report some use), ketamine (96 %), benzodiazepines (91 %), and fentanyl (64 %), with limited use of propofol (24 %) and other agents (37 %) [11]. While the agents used tend to be consistent across the region, the use of specific agents for given indications shows considerable heterogeneity and is in part reflective of the practice of individual institutions [11].

Emergency medicine within Australia and New Zealand operates as a hybrid of North American and UK models. Senior staffing levels (consultants) are generally higher than those seen in the United Kingdom; however, the majority of service provision is still by physicians in training. "Time targets" (4 or 6 h) for provision of care within emergency departments have emerged. Both these issues, to some extent, affect agent choice and provision of procedural sedation within individual departments, although formal comparisons to other regions are lacking.

Issues for emergency department pediatric sedation in the region mirror those described in other parts of the world: lack of a recognized standard regarding staffing, lack of consensus regarding documentation and consent, lack of consensus regarding fasting, and lack of consistency regarding training and credentialing. For example, just over 50 % of clinicians use formal sedation records, and only one-third of sites have a formal staff education and competency program [11]. Although these issues are not unique to the region, they reflect the inherent problems with the two local guidelines: the ANZCA guideline is predominantly written as a guide for anesthesiologists and is not pediatric specific; the older RACP guideline lacks recent evidence. Both are guidelines rather than consensus standards of care.

As in North America, emergency departments in Australia and New Zealand have widely adopted the use of ketamine for procedural sedation [12–14], and, to a lesser degree, consensus-based recommendations for the reporting of intervention-based adverse events [45, 46].

Nitrous oxide (up to 70 %) is consistently widely used across the region for procedural sedation. A survey of pediatric emergency medicine specialists indicates that most would consider nitrous oxide as a possible agent for wound/burn management, fracture manipulation/plaster procedures, intravenous cannula insertion, and laceration repair [11, 16]. Single-center registries have reported that continuous nitrous oxide is relatively safe [8], with few serious adverse events [9].

The use of intranasal fentanyl (1.5 μg/kg) has emerged from Perth, Western Australia [47, 48], and has become widespread throughout the region, both in emergency department [11] and pre-hospital settings [49]. The combination of intranasal fentanyl with nitrous oxide is frequently used for procedural sedations that anticipate moderate rather than severe pain. For example, when surveyed, 42 % of pediatric emergency medicine specialists stated they would use a combination of intranasal fentanyl with nitrous oxide for a 10-year-old requiring manipulation of a distal forearm fracture with minor angulation. Only 1 % would consider this combination in the same patient with 100 % displacement of fracture fragments [16]. In this same survey, a small percentage (8 %) reported use of a Bier's block instead of procedural sedation.

Dental Sedation

The main document setting the clinical parameters for sedation in dentistry in Australia and New Zealand is the ANZCA guideline [1]. Pediatric dentists are also guided by overseas documents of the European Academy of Paediatric Dentistry [50], the American Academy of Pediatric Dentistry (AAPD), the Scottish Dental Clinical Effectiveness Programme [51], and the United Kingdom National Clinical Guidelines in Paediatric Dentistry [52], as well as the clinical guidelines on sedation of children and young people by the National Institute for Health and Clinical Excellence [53].

The DBA, a dental section of the AHPRA, has published a registration standard for sedation by dentists, setting a consistent set of requirements [5] and guidelines [6]. Sedation is defined in the documents as a drug-induced depression of consciousness during which patients respond purposefully to verbal commands. No interventions should be required to maintain respiratory and cardiovascular function. Dentists who seek endorsement for "conscious sedation" are required to have a minimum of 2 years of general dental experience. The minimum standard for endorsement is a graduate diploma in conscious sedation from the Westmead Hospital, University of Sydney, or training from an institution that is acceptable to the Dental Board. The dentist undertaking the sedation is to be assisted by a registered nurse trained in intensive care or anesthesia or by a registered dentist or medical practitioner who is trained in monitoring and resuscitation. The DBA guideline stipulates ongoing annual education with either a course at the Centre for Resuscitation Education and Simulation Training (Incorporated) (CREST) or the Medical Emergencies and the Sedated Dental Patient course offered by the Australian Society of Dental Anaesthesiology. The assistant to the endorsed dentist is recommended to attend and successfully participate in an advanced life support course in each 12-month period. The DBA sedation standard and guideline does not include the use of single-dose oral agents or nitrous oxide, neither of which requires endorsement under the standard.

The dental sedation course at the University of Sydney offers a graduate diploma on conscious sedation and pain control in clinical dentistry. This is the only such course offered in Australia and New Zealand. This course focuses mostly on intravenous sedation in adults but includes a pediatric section. It offers study in the practice of sedation and the recognition and management of crisis. To date, there is no course specifically intended for pediatric sedation.

The agents most frequently used for sedation in anxious or uncooperative pediatric patients in Australia and New Zealand are continuous flow nitrous oxide and oral midazolam [54]. In centers that treat more complex pediatric patients, there is ongoing debate as to whether dentists should use sedation or refer to anesthesia for management. A tool has been developed to assess if people with disabilities can be effectively allocated for treatment under sedation or general anesthesia [55], accounting for the medical, behavioral, and social factors as well as the complexity of the dental treatment. A limitation of this tool is that it was devised from a wide range of patients (age 4–75 years). In young children and those with developmental disability or complex medical needs, general anesthesia is generally applied, in part because of limited access to other options.

There are, however, publicly funded hospitals that offer sedation by anesthesiologists for dental care. There are also a small number of private dental clinics that provide IV sedation for children staffed by pediatric dentists and anesthesiologists.

Sedation for Medical Imaging

In general, specialized sedation services within pediatric teaching hospitals do not exist within Australia and New Zealand. The provision of analgesia and sedation is mainly led by emergency physicians for acute presentations, radiologists for simple analgesia and sedation, and anesthesiologists for complicated or prolonged sedation. In general pediatric imaging in Australia and New Zealand attempts to balance the sometimes competing interests of image quality, radiation exposure, and sedation need and risk.

The majority of children undergoing radiologic procedures in Australia and New Zealand are covered for non-pediatric hospitals in units attached to adult radiology departments. This situation has been recognized by the RANZCR who have produced recommendations for imaging of children in non-dedicated pediatric centers [56]. These guidelines provide clear recommendations for the use of anesthesia and sedation for various image modalities. In addition, the guidelines recognize a number of key principles, including: the need to gain the required information from pediatric imaging using the fewest images and the least radiation; that some movement artefact may be acceptable for the clinical question the study is addressing; if a child is not cooperating, the study should be quickly terminated rather than continuing with further distress and radiation exposure. Intravenous contrast should be administered only when absolutely necessary.

For CTs, the RANZCR prefers utilizing intravenous contrast if appropriate to both limit sedation need and radiation exposure. For contrast CT scans, the use of general anesthesia for children less than 3 years is recommended and should be considered in all other ages. Other recommendations are intended to minimize the need for sedation: the use of topical anesthetic creams prior to cannulation, use of a mock CT scanner to encourage non-sedation, use of explanation pamphlets and videos, tour of imaging facilities, and listening to favorite music during imaging. For non-contrast CT scans, immobilization and the aforementioned non-pharmacological techniques are encouraged. Individual units often "feed and wrap" infants aged 3 months or less. Chloral hydrate or oral midazolam is administered to those children with prolonged scan times or in children unable/unlikely to remain static enough for suitable image quality.

For MRI, the RANZCR recommends immobilization for infants less than 3 months, often using "feed and wrap" if possible. For children between 4 and 6 years of age, RANZCR recommends a general anesthetic. For older children, prior preparation and non-pharmacological techniques are encouraged. Furthermore, when performing MRIs, the RANZCR recommends that the most important sequences should be obtained first, so that if the scan is interrupted, enough images may be available to answer the clinical indication, minimizing the need for adjuvant sedation. Some hospitals have mock MRI scanners to introduce anxious children to the imaging setup and reduce sedation needs (see "Non-pharmacology" section below).

Over the last decade, the use of micturating cystourethrograms (MCUs) for diagnosis and management of vesicoureteric reflux following urinary tract infections has reduced dramatically within Australia and New Zealand. The RANZCR guidelines recognize this and recommend that radiologists discuss referrals with referring physicians to determine if a positive finding of vesicoureteric reflux on MCU will alter management, thus potentially avoiding a painful procedure and unnecessary radiation exposure. Individual units often use oral midazolam for infants older than 12 months [57].

Plain film X-rays for acute trauma are usually ordered via emergency departments with analgesia and sedation ordered by emergency clinicians, as detailed in the previous section. The RANZCR guidelines do not address these patients' sedation and analgesic concerns.

The RANZCR have a second position statement on the use of sedation and anesthesia for pediatric imaging in both pediatric and non-pediatric hospitals [58]. This statement reinforces the principle that whenever possible the use of sedation and anesthesia should be avoided. The statement recommends that Fellows follow the ANZCA guideline for sedation and anesthesia, and apply non-pharmacological techniques when possible. RANZCR principles cover the small number of specialized imaging procedures that occur within dedicated pediatric hospitals (angiograms, arthrograms, and solid organ biopsies).

Sedation of Children with Burns

Burn management in children in this region is focused on a small number of referral units based in major cities within each region, with only very minor pediatric burn injuries being managed outside these facilities.

The majority of burns represent scalding in younger children, but a small number of children have major burns over significant proportions of their body, which require prolonged management and repeat grafting, debridement, dressing changes, and cleansing. Compared with developing nations, there are few burn injuries related to heating and lighting sources in this region [59–61].

Scald injuries are commonest in "toddlers" and mostly involve small areas, so the management is usually straightforward with dressings, assessment and, if required, a single grafting procedure under anesthesia. Nitrous oxide inhalation has become a key supplement to non-pharmacological therapy for these patients.

Major burns require complex intensive care with multisystem disease and complications such as sepsis and respiratory infections. Areas of partial thickness skin damage are particularly painful, and analgesic requirements are often significant. Recurrent grafting and debridement is done under anesthesia. The period after the initial acute phase is particularly challenging for ward management. Repeated major dressing changes, often with "burn baths" in a ward treatment area, as well as physiotherapy mobilization require frequent and potentially very painful procedural interventions. This is often emotionally stressful with the potential for significant pre-procedural anxiety, especially if previous experiences have been unpleasant.

Children with major burns have significant issues with being moved and pressure care. Sophisticated pneumatic bed systems have greatly helped the pressure issues, but simple movement, whether active or passive, is frequently painful and a common part of daily management. Experienced staff to provide pharmacological and non-pharmacological support are key to minimizing such distress.

Most centers have evolved specialized responses to the aforementioned scenarios. Children's Hospital Westmead in Sydney has a separately funded "Burns Anaesthesia Fellow" to support these patients, while at Royal Children's Hospital, Melbourne, a mobile specialist anesthesia team anesthetizes these patients in a ward treatment room to allow baths and dressing changes during the early phase of burn management on the ward. They are the only elective patients in the hospital anesthetized outside of critical care areas. As the burn and donor sites heal and the dressings and cleansing become less painful, the patient is "weaned" from general anesthesia to conscious sedation to the point where ward staff can manage the dressings with oral agents, nitrous oxide, and non-pharmacological techniques.

Sedation for Oncologic Procedures

Similar to intensive care services, oncology services within Australia and New Zealand are centered on 14 units attached to pediatric or tertiary (mixed pediatric and adult) hospitals. Patients undergoing initial and intensive therapy tend to be based at these oncology units, often for many months. However, those undergoing maintenance treatment, who may reside a long distance from the oncology units, often receive shared care at regional pediatric units. The management of procedural sedation within oncology units is particularly focused on the repetitive painful procedures, specifically lumbar puncture and bone marrow aspirates. Procedural sedation management strategies for medical imaging, discussed previously, are also utilized within the radiology departments of these hospitals.

The importance of procedural sedation for oncologic patients has been well recognized within Australia and New Zealand for some time. In the early 2000s, sedation practices at 14 pediatric oncology units were surveyed [62]. Three-quarters of lumbar punctures and bone marrow aspirates were performed under general anesthesia with the remaining receiving sedation predominantly with benzodiazepines, opiates, nitrous oxide, and chloral hydrate. While sedation was being performed in the presence of a medical staff member in all cases, the adherence to monitoring, documentation, and staffing guidelines was inconsistent.

In oncology, there has been increased focus on the multidisciplinary nature of procedural pain management, consistent use of simple analgesic techniques (local anesthetic creams), and non-pharmacological cognitive behavioral techniques. This has resulted in formal multidisciplinary pain management strategies such as the Comfort First Program, used within the Children's Cancer Centre, Royal Children's Hospital, Melbourne [63]. The Comfort First Program aims to provide children and their caregivers with early support in procedural pain management via education and enhancement of existing coping strategies. Child life/occupational therapists meet with families within a month of diagnosis to assess the child's pain experiences and provide individualized strategies for managing painful procedures. These strategies are formally incorporated within the child's medical record for use by all members of the multidisciplinary team. Audit of this program has shown good adherence to current RACP procedural pain guidelines with >90 % of children receiving non-pharmacological strategies alongside pharmacological management [63].

Non-pharmacological Management

The principles of non-pharmacological management are highlighted in the introductory section of this chapter. Tables 24.1 and 24.2 provide an overview. Pediatric institutions in this region have recently introduced non-pharmacologic programs, which reflect the RACP guideline on procedural management in children:

- The importance of "procedural management" for every clinical interaction with a child has been recognized.

Even completely painless interactions, such as clinical examination, temperature measurement, or simple medical imaging, can distress a child. Children can rapidly develop fear of interacting with hospital staff if any interaction has been distressing. Procedures with local or systemic analgesia can be distressing if non-pharmacological management is inadequate. Thus, procedural management must include appropriate "non-pharmacological" management in every clinical interaction.

- All clinical interactions with the child should be aimed to minimize distress. Every clinical staff member (and probably other staff in a pediatric institution) should have training in developmentally appropriate techniques for minimizing distress during interactions with children.

Programs to improve the use of non-pharmacological techniques for procedural pain management require education of staff, children, and their families. The program should ensure that age-appropriate devices to engage a child (such as toys, screen-based devices, or bubble blowing) are available and that staff know how to appropriately use them. In this region, the role of educational play therapists has evolved and continues to evolve. The role is converging on that of the "child life specialist" in North America. The potential for this allied health group to have an increasing role in procedural management is clear. This includes being the support person for the child and applying specific techniques that will be appropriate to the child and the procedure. Tools such as the Child-Adult Medical Procedure Interaction Scale (CAMPIS) [64] and CAMPIS-R [65] (CAMPIS [ages 5–13], CAMPIS-R21 [ages 4–7]) and CAMPIS-SF (short form [66]) summarize the likelihood of various behaviors and language to have a positive effect.

The "Comfort Kids" section of the RCH Melbourne website has much material for both families and health professionals [67]. The concept of "Positioning for Comfort" where care to position the child in an appropriate way, often involving the parent, can provide reassurance, comfort, and appropriate ergonomics for the conduct of a procedure. Some suggestions for such positions are available on the Web at a number of sites including positions for infants [68] and older children [69]. Suggestions for age-appropriate distraction are also available [70] (Table 24.3). Other pediatric institutions in the region have also produced flow diagrams for procedural pain management in children [71].

The incorporation of non-pharmacological techniques into all clinical interactions with children and their families can lessen the distress of children, families, and staff. Education in these techniques should involve all these groups and be incorporated into routine daily practice. (Refer to Chap. 34.)

Table 24.3 Distraction ideas for children (Royal Children's Hospital, Melbourne [71])

Distraction ideas for infants under 6 months
• Rocking and stroking face • Gentle patting and family present • Rattles and/or other baby toys • Singing • Swaddle—expose areas of body for procedure; keep baby wrapped up and warm • Sucrose and breastfeeding
Distraction ideas for toddlers 6 months to 2 years
• Bubbles or blowing windmill • Sitting up when possible, hug-like hold • Toys and books that make noise when pushed or with buttons • Singing child's favorite song • Light-up toys • Reading a book
Distraction ideas for children
• Big belly breathing, blowing away scary feelings, or blowing away hurt. Hint: cue by saying breathe in through your nose and blow out of your toes • Blowing bubbles and windmills • Counting games • Reading a book: noise book, counting, or search-and-find book • Playing a favorite DVD, iPod, or electronic game • Mind pictures; e.g., think about a favorite sport, family vacation, school game, or activity. Let child tell a story or answer questions about what is pictured in their mind • Ask your child if they want to know what's happening or if they prefer to focus on an activity instead
Distraction ideas for adolescents
• Listen to music, iPod • Choice: parental presence—handheld • Mind pictures; e.g., think about a favorite sport, family vacation, school game or activity. Let child tell a story or answer questions about what is pictured in their mind • Relaxation and breathing—with or without cues • Use humor or non-procedure talk • Play a favorite DVD, iPod, or electronic game

Case Studies

Case 1

An 8-year-old boy ran across a road and was stuck by a car. He was thrown 15 ft and was found crying and complaining of leg pain. He had no loss of consciousness. When paramedics arrived they found a distressed boy lying on the sidewalk with an obviously angulated and swollen thigh with normal pedal pulses. His mother was in attendance. The rest of his examination was normal except for abrasions on his arms and chin. The paramedics assessed the child's pain as 10 out of

10 on a verbal numerical scale. After coaching the patient, the paramedics administered inhaled methoxyflurane via the Penthrox inhaler with rapid relief of pain. They splinted the leg and transported the patient to hospital; the patient continued to use methoxyflurane as needed with pain scores of 2–4.

In the emergency department, the patient was administered intranasal fentanyl 1.5 μ(mu)g/kg on arrival. Five minutes after fentanyl, his pain was assessed at 0. He was assessed according to Advanced Trauma Life Support protocol and was found to have an isolated lower limb injury. He was then administered nitrous oxide sedation at 70 % by continuous flow to administer an ultrasound-guided femoral nerve block. After orthopaedic review he was placed in traction while receiving nurse-administered nitrous oxide.

Key Points of Management

- Inhaled methoxyflurane, where licensed, such as in Australia and New Zealand, provides powerful analgesia and can be self-administered by children and adolescents. It can also be used to perform brief painful procedures in awake patients. It should only be administered once or twice in sequence to avoid dose-related renal problems.
- Intranasal fentanyl is a powerful analgesic that can be used in isolation or in combination with nitrous oxide. The combination is useful for relatively painful brief procedures.
- Nitrous oxide at 70 % (30 % oxygen) provides moderate sedation. The likelihood of deep sedation increases when combined with other agents.
- Nitrous oxide can be safely administered by credentialed nurses when embedded into a comprehensive sedation program.
- Nerve blocks provide long-lasting, profound regional anesthesia and can be supplemented with nitrous oxide sedation.

Case 2

A 10-year-old girl was admitted to the hospital with recent-onset ataxia and scheduled for a relatively urgent MRI. With worsening symptoms, both parents were anxious about the possible underlying diagnosis, and the patient was terrified of the MRI. The child was referred to the anesthesia team for assessment. The anesthetist noted the circumstances and referred the patient to the play therapy and medical imaging mock MRI team. The patient was familiarized with the process in the mock MRI scanner. Distraction and video goggles to watch a movie in the MRI scanner were discussed, and a successful mock scan was conducted. A plan was also made for intravenous access for administration of contrast during the scan. This involved use of local anesthesia cream and specific distraction. Subsequently, the actual MRI scan was conducted without sedation.

Key Points of Management

- MRIs often require sedation or anesthesia in young or anxious and uncooperative children. Non-pharmacological interventions such as distraction or desensitization in mock MRI scanners utilizing play therapists or other expert staff can reduce or eliminate the need for sedation. The sedation team should be in close cooperation with play therapy staff to achieve this.

Case 3

A 2-year-old sustained a partial thickness scald burn to a 30 % body surface area (chest, abdomen, and anterior thighs) when he pulled a large saucepan off the stove top. After initial pain control in the emergency department with intranasal fentanyl and oral oxycodone, he received ongoing pain control with IV morphine. In the emergency department, he was administered nitrous oxide to debride large blisters and apply burn dressings. While admitted to the hospital, he had initial debridements, skin grafting, and dressing changes under anesthesia in the operating theater. Dressing changes and cleansing were performed on the hospital ward with anesthesia-delivered intravenous agents (including ketamine) and weaned over several weeks to a combination of oral agents and inhaled nitrous oxide. Eventually a tailored sedation program supervised by ward medical and nursing staff was used for subsequent dressing changes and baths in the ward treatment room.

Key Points of Management

- Ketamine is frequently used for burn-dressing changes due to its powerful analgesic effect.
- Sedation completed anywhere outside the operating room should follow the same safety criteria as in the operating room. All safety and emergency equipment should be available, and a means to summon additional help quickly should be preestablished.

(continued)

- If parents are present during ketamine sedations, they need to be appropriately educated about what to expect. Patients may move and stare ahead with open eyes—"the lights are on but nobody is home" has been used as the term to describe the dissociate state they are in.
- Some situations may lend themselves to anesthesia management. Procedures that involve extreme pain and multimodal sedatives and analgesics may be better to cared for by an anesthesiologist.

References

1. Australian and New Zealand College of Anaesthetists. Guidelines on sedation and/or analgesia for diagnostic and interventional medical, dental or surgical procedures. PS9. ANZCA. 2010. Available at: http://www.anzca.edu.au/resources/professional-documents/documents/professional-standards/pdf-files/PS9-2010.pdf. Accessed 1 June 2013.
2. Royal Australasian College of Physicians. Guideline statement: management of procedure-related pain in children and adolescents. J Paediatr Child Health. 2006;42 Suppl 1:S1–29.
3. Royal Australasian College of Physicians. Guideline statement: management of procedure-related pain in neonates. J Paediatr Child Health. 2006;42 Suppl 1:S31–9.
4. Krauss B, Green SM. Training and credentialing in procedural sedation and analgesia in children: lessons from the United States model. Pediatr Anesth. 2008;18:30–5.
5. Dental Board of Australia. Australian Health Practitioner Regulation Agency (AHPRA) DBA. 2010. Available at: http://www.dentalboard.gov.au/Registration/Conscious-Sedation.aspx. Accessed 1 June 2013.
6. Dental Board of Australia. Australian Health Practitioner Regulation Agency (AHPRA) DBA. Conscious Sedation Area of Practice Endorsement. 2012. Available at: http://www.dentalboard.gov.au/Codes-Guidelines/Policies-Codes-Guidelines.aspx. Accessed 1 June 2013.
7. American Society of Anesthesiologists. Continuum of depth of sedation: definition of general anesthesia and levels of sedation/analgesia. 2009. Available at: http://www.asahq.org/For-Members/Standards-Guidelines-and-Statements.aspx. Accessed 1 June 2013.
8. Babl FE, Oakley E, Seaman C, Barnett P, Sharwood LN. High concentration nitrous oxide for procedural sedation: adverse events and depth of sedation. Pediatrics. 2008;121:e528–32.
9. Babl FE, Belousoff J, Theophilos T, Hopper S, Deasy C. Paediatric procedural sedation based on nitrous oxide and ketamine: data from an Australian Sedation Registry. Emerg Med J. 2010;27(8):607–12.
10. Frampton A, Browne GJ, Lam LT, Cooper MG, Lane LG. Nurse administered relative analgesia using high concentration nitrous oxide to facilitate minor procedures in children in an emergency department. Emerg Med J. 2003;20(5):410–3.
11. Borland M, Esson A, Babl FE, Krieser D. Procedural sedation in children in the emergency department: a PREDICT Study. Emerg Med Australas. 2009;21:71–9.
12. Green SM, Roback MG, Kennedy RM, Krauss B. Clinical practice guideline for emergency department ketamine dissociative sedation: 2011 update. Ann Emerg Med. 2011;57(5):449–61.
13. Green SM, Roback MG, Krauss B, Brown L, McGlone RG, Agrawal D, McKee M, Weiss M, Pitetti RD, Hostetler MA, Wathen JE, Treston G, Garcia Pena BM, Gerber AC, Losek JD; Emergency Department Ketamine Meta-Analysis Study Group. Predictors of emesis and recovery agitation with emergency department ketamine sedation: an individual-patient data meta-analysis of 8,282 children. Ann Emerg Med. 2009;54(2):171–80.e1-4.
14. Green SM, Roback MG, Krauss B, Brown L, McGlone RG, Agrawal D, McKee M, Weiss M, Pitetti RD, Hostetler MA, Wathen JE, Treston G, Garcia Pena BM, Gerber AC, Losek JD; Emergency Department Ketamine Meta-Analysis Study Group. Predictors of airway and respiratory adverse events with ketamine sedation in the emergency department: an individual-patient data meta-analysis of 8,282 children. Ann Emerg Med. 2009;54(2):158–68.e1-4.
15. Zier JL, Liu M. Safety of high-concentration nitrous oxide by nasal mask for pediatric procedural sedation: experience with 7802 cases. Pediatr Emerg Care. 2011;27(12):1107–12.
16. Schofield S, Schutz J, Babl FE. Procedural sedation and analgesia for reduction of distal forearm fractures in the paediatric emergency department: a clinical survey. Emerg Med Australas. 2013;25(3):241–7.
17. Seith R, Theophilos T, Babl FE. Intranasal fentanyl and high concentration inhaled nitrous oxide for procedural sedation: a prospective observational pilot study of adverse events and depth of sedation. Acad Emerg Med. 2012;19(1):31–6.
18. American Academy of Pediatrics Committee on Drugs. Section on Anesthesiology. Guidelines for the elective use of conscious sedation, deep sedation, and general anesthesia in pediatric patients. Pediatrics. 1985;76:317–21.
19. American Academy of Pediatrics Committee on Drugs. Guidelines for monitoring and management of pediatric patients during and after sedation for diagnostic and therapeutic procedures: addendum. Pediatrics. 2002;110(4):836–8.
20. American Society of Anesthesiologists. Practice guidelines for sedation and analgesia by non-anesthesiologists: a report by the American Society of Anesthesiologists Task Force on Sedation and Analgesia by Non-Anesthesiologists. Anesthesiology. 1996;84:459–71.
21. American College of Emergency Physicians. Clinical policy for procedural sedation and analgesia in the emergency department. Ann Emerg Med. 1998;31(5):663–77.
22. Babl FE, Munro J, Kainey G, et al. Scope for improvement: hospital wide sedation practice at a Children's Hospital. Arch Dis Child. 2006;91:716–7.
23. Schechter NL, Blankson V, Pachter LM, Sullivan CM, Costa L. The ouchless place: no pain, children's gain. Pediatrics. 1997;99(6):890–4.
24. Schechter NL. From the ouchless place to comfort central: the evolution of a concept. Pediatrics. 2008;122 Suppl 3:S154–60.
25. Priestley S, Babl F, Krieser D, et al. Evaluation of the impact of a paediatric procedural sedation program on quality of care. Emerg Med Australas. 2006;18:498–504.
26. Babl FE, Krieser D, Belousoff J, Theophilos T. Evaluation of a paediatric procedural sedation training and credentialing program: sustainability of change. Emerg Med J. 2010;27:577–81.
27. Kelly A-M, Pannifex J, Cetiner E. Design and rollout of standardised approach to paediatric sedation in Victorian emergency departments. Emerg Med Australas. 2013;25:S1–14 (abstract).
28. Royal Children's Hospital Clinical Practice Guidelines. Procedural pain management guideline. Available at: http://www.rch.org.au/rchcpg/hospital_clinical_guideline_index/Procedural_Pain_Management/. Accessed 1 June 2013.
29. Ullman A, Long D, Horn D, Woosley J, Coulthard MG. The KIDS SAFE checklist for pediatric intensive care units. Am J Crit Care. 2013;22(1):61–9.

30. Anand KJ, Sippell WG, Aynsley-Green A. Randomised trial of fentanyl anaesthesia in preterm babies undergoing surgery: effects on the stress response. Lancet. 1987;1(8527):243–8.
31. Franck LS, Harris SK, Soetenga DJ, Amling JK, Curley MAQ. The Withdrawal Assessment Tool-1 (WAT-1): an assessment instrument for monitoring opioid and benzodiazepine withdrawal symptoms in pediatric patients. Pediatr Crit Care Med. 2008;9(6):573–80.
32. Royal Children's Hospital Clinical Practice Guidelines. Procedural sedation guideline. Available at: http://www.rch.org.au/rchcpg/hospital_clinical_guideline_index/Sedation_Procedural_Sedation_Guideline_Ward_and_Ambulatory_Areas/. Accessed 1 June 2013.
33. Agthe A, Kim G, Mathias K, Hendrix C, Chavez-Valdez R, Jansson L, Lewis T, Yaster M, Gauda E. Clonidine as an adjunct therapy to opioids for neonatal abstinence syndrome: a randomized, controlled trial. Pediatr Anesth. 2011;21:716–21.
34. American Academy of Pediatrics. Prevention and management of pain in the neonate: an update. Pediatrics. 2006;118(5):2231–41. Reaffirmed May 2010.
35. Duncan PG, Kobrinsky N. Prilocaine-induced methemoglobinemia in a newborn infant. Anesthesiology. 1983;59(1):75–6.
36. Taddio A, Ohlsson A, Einarson T, Stevens B, Koren G. A systematic review of lidocaine-prilocaine cream (EMLA) in the treatment of acute pain in neonates. Pediatrics. 1998;101(2):E1.
37. Harrison D. Australian College of Neonatal Nurses. Management of pain in sick hospitalised infants. Neonatal. Paediatr Child Health Nurs. 2006;9:27–9.
38. Harrison D, Beggs S, Stevens B. Sucrose for procedural pain management in infants. Pediatrics. 2012;130(5):918–25.
39. Slater R, Cornelissen L, Fabrizi L, Patten D, Yoxen J, Worley A, Boyd S, Meek J, Fitzgerald M. Oral sucrose as an analgesic drug for procedural pain in newborn infants: a randomised controlled trial. Lancet. 2010;376(9748):1225–32.
40. Frawley G, Bayley G, Chondros P. Laparotomy for necrotizing enterocolitis: intensive care nursery compared with operating theatre. J Paediatr Child Health. 1999;35(3):291–5.
41. Allegaert K, Anderson BJ, Verbesselt R, Debeer A, de Hoon J, Devlieger H, Van Den Anker JN, Tibboel D. Tramadol disposition in the very young: an attempt to assess in vivo cytochrome P-450 2D6 activity. Br J Anaesth. 2005;95(2):231–9.
42. Anderson BJ, Palmer GM. Recent developments in the pharmacological management of pain in children. Curr Opin Anaesthesiol. 2006;19(3):285–92.
43. Hodgkinson K, Bear M, Thorn J, Blaricum SV. Measuring pain in neonates: evaluating an instrument and development a common language. Aust J Adv Nurs. 1994;12(1):17–22.
44. Everitt I, Younge P, Barnett P. Paediatric sedation in emergency department: what is our practice? Emerg Med (Fremantle). 2002;14(1):62–6.
45. Bhatt M, Kennedy RM, Osmond MH, et al. Consensus-based recommendations for standardizing terminology and reporting adverse events for emergency department procedural sedation and analgesia in children. Ann Emerg Med. 2009;53:426–35.e4.
46. Mason K, Green SM, Piacevoli Q and International Sedation Task Force. Adverse event reporting tool to standardize the reporting and tracking of adverse events during procedural sedation: a consensus document from the World SIVA International Sedation Task Force. Br J Anaesth. 2012;108:13–20.
47. Borland ML, Jacobs I, Geelhoed G. Intranasal fentanyl reduces acute pain in children in the emergency department: a safety and efficacy study. Emerg Med (Fremantle). 2002;14:275–80.
48. Borland ML, Clark LJ, Esson A. Comparative review of the clinical use of intranasal fentanyl versus morphine in a paediatric emergency department. Emerg Med Australas. 2008;20:515–20.
49. Johnston S, Wilkes G, Thompson J, et al. Inhaled methoxyflurane and intranasal fentanyl for prehospital management of visceral pain in an Australian ambulance service. Emerg Med J. 2010;28(1):57–63.
50. Hallonsten AL, Jensen B, Raadal M, et al. EAPD guidelines on sedation in paediatric dentistry. Available at: http://www.eapd.gr/dat/5CF03741/file.pdf. Accessed 1 June 2013.
51. Scottish Dental Clinical Effectiveness Programme. Conscious sedation in dentistry, 2nd ed. 2012. Available at: http://www.sdcep.org.uk/index.aspx?o=2331. Accessed 1 June 2013.
52. Hosey MT. UK national clinical guidelines in paediatric dentistry. Int J Paediatr Dent. 2002;12:359–72.
53. National Institute of Health and Clinical Excellence. Clinical guideline 112. Sedation for diagnostic and therapeutic procedures in children and young people. 2010. Available at: http://www.nice.org.uk/nicemedia/live/13296/52130/52130.pdf. Accessed 1 June 2013.
54. Day PF, Power AM, Hibbert SA, Paterson SA. Effectiveness of oral midazolam for paediatric dental care: a retrospective study in two specialist centres. Eur Arch Paediatr Dent. 2006;7(4):228–35.
55. Prabhu NT, Nunn JH, Evans DJ, Girdler NM. Development of a screening tool to assess the suitability of people with a disability for oral care under sedation or general anesthesia. Spec Care Dentist. 2008;28(4):145–58.
56. Royal Australian and New Zealand College of Radiologists. Recommendations for imaging in children in non-dedicated paediatric centres. RANZCR. 2012. www.ranzcr.edu.au/Fdocuments-download/Fdoc_download/F1675-paediatric-imaging-guidelines. Accessed 1 June 2013.
57. Herd DW, McAnulty KA, Keene NA, Sommerville DE. Conscious sedation reduces distress in children undergoing voiding cystourethrography and does not interfere with the diagnosis of vesicoureteric reflux: a randomized controlled study. Pediatr Radiol. 2006;187:1621–6.
58. Royal Australian and New Zealand College of Radiologists. Position statement on the use of sedation and anaesthesia in paediatric imaging. RANZCR. 2012. Available at: www.ranzcr.edu.au/Fcomponent/Fdocman/Fdoc_download/F1654-position-statement-paediatric-imaging. Accessed 1 June 2013.
59. Duke J, Wood F, Semmens J, Edgar DW, Spilsbury K, Hendrie D, Rea S. A study of burn hospitalizations for children younger than 5 years of age: 1983–2008. Pediatrics. 2011;127(4):e971–7.
60. Gabbe B, Picton N, Loh I, Watterson D. Registry annual report. 1st July 2011–30th June 2012. Bi-National Burns Registry Project. Department of Epidemiology and Preventive Medicine, Monash University, Melbourne Victoria, Australia. 2012. Available at http://www.med.monash.edu.au/epidemiology/traumaepi/binbr-annual-report-y3.pdf. Accessed 20 July 2014.
61. Agbenorku M, Agbenorku PK, Fiifi-Yankson PK. Pediatric burns mortality risk factors in a developing country's tertiary burns intensive care unit. Int J Burns Trauma. 2013;3(3):151–8.
62. Barnes C, Downie P, Chalkiadis G, Camilleri S, Monagle P, Waters K. Sedation practices for Australian and New Zealand paediatric oncology patients. J Paediatr Child Health. 2002;38:170–2.
63. McCarthy M, Glick R, Green J, Plummer K, Peters K, Johnsey L, DeLuca C. Comfort First: an evaluation of a procedural pain management programme for children with cancer. Psychooncology. 2013;22:775–82.
64. Blount RL, Corbin SM, Sturges JW, Wolfe VV, Prater JM, James LD. The relationship between adults behavior and child coping and distress during BMA/LP procedures: a sequential analysis. Behav Ther. 1989;20:585–601.
65. Blount RL, Cohen LL, Frank NC, Bachanas PJ, Smith AJ, Manimala MR, Pate JT. The Child-Adult Medical Procedure Interaction Scale-Revised: an assessment of validity. J Pediatr Psychol. 1997;22:73–88.
66. Blount RL, Bunke VL, Cohen LL, Forbes CJ. The Child-Adult Medical Procedure Interaction Scale-Short Form (CAMPIS-SF): vali-

dation of a rating scale for children's and adults' behaviors during painful medical procedures. J Pain Symptom Manage. 2001;22:591–9.
67. Royal Children's Hospital. RCH Comfort kids. About Comfort Kids. Available at: http://www.rch.org.au/comfortkids/. Accessed 1 June 2013.
68. Royal Children's Hospital. RCH Comfort kids. Infant positioning. Available at: http://www.rch.org.au/uploadedFiles/Main/Content/comfortkids/ComfortKidsPositioningPoster.pdf. Accessed 1 June 2013.
69. Royal Children's Hospital. RCH Comfort kids. Positioning for procedures. Available at http://www.rch.org.au/uploadedFiles/Main/Content/comfortkids/KidsPositioning.pdf. Accessed 1 June 2013.
70. Royal Children's Hospital. RCH Kids Health Info. Reduce children's discomfort during tests and procedures. Available at: http://www.rch.org.au/kidsinfo/fact_sheets/Reduce_childrens_discomfort_during_tests_and_procedures/. Accessed 1 June 2013.
71. Auckland District Health Board. Pain management pathway. Available at: http://www.adhb.govt.nz/starshipclinicalguidelines/Pain%20management%20Pathway.htm#Procedural_Pain_Management. Accessed 1 June 2013.

Pediatric Sedation in the Underdeveloped Third World: An African Perspective—Models, Protocols, and Challenges

25

James A. Roelofse and Graeme S. Wilson

Abstract

Pediatric sedation remains a controversial issue, especially when combinations of drugs are used. The choice of using anesthetists or non-anesthetic personnel as sedation providers is an issue that is deliberated worldwide. In Sub-Saharan Africa, however, there is an acute shortage of sedation providers and other health care providers, which makes the provision of sedation services extremely difficult. Reasons for this shortage are discussed. Structured sedation training to train sedation providers in the provision of sedation services is unfortunately available only in a few centers. In this chapter, the challenges facing Sub-Saharan Africa as far as the provision of sedation services is concerned are discussed. Sedation models are presented, as well as protocols for drug administration. Case reports of typical cases that present for sedation are also presented.

Keywords

Sub-Saharan Africa • Sedation providers • Protocols • Challenges • Training • Drugs • Ketamine • Mobile sedation • South African Society of Anaesthesiologists (SASA) • South African Society of Sedation Practitioners (SOSPOSA) • National Institute of Health in the United Kingdom (NICE) Guidelines • International Liaison Committee on Resuscitation (ILCOR)

Introduction

Pediatric sedation for diagnostic and surgical procedures outside the operating room remains a controversial issue worldwide. There remains disquiet about safety and quality standards in the provision of sedation, especially the use of combinations of drugs and who should be the sedation providers. Health care centers are, however, experiencing an increasing demand for safe sedation. We may have reached the situation where the number of children requiring sedation outside the operating room exceeds the number of children requiring general anesthesia. Pediatric sedation is one of the fastest growing areas in patient care as it, in appropriate situations, offers a safe and cost-effective alternative to the limited capacity of general anesthesia in operating rooms. One of the challenges is that children probably represent a population with the highest risk/lowest error tolerance.

Pediatric sedation services can be defined as the formal allocation of identifiable resources and providers with the aim of providing scheduled sedation for children at various locations outside the operating room [1]. A wide variety of specialties and subspecialties, including non-anesthesiologists, are involved in pediatric sedation, utilizing a variety of different drugs, often administered by different routes. There is little agreement as to who should provide sedation,

J.A. Roelofse, M.B.Ch.B., M.Med. (Anes.) (✉)
Department of Anesthesiology, Tygerberg Hospital, 15 Sluysken Street Welgemoed, Bellville, Cape Province 7530, South Africa
e-mail: jar@sun.ac.za; jaroelofse@uwc.ac.za

G.S. Wilson
Department of Anesthesia, University of Cape Town, Red Cross War Memorial Children's Hospital, Rondebosch, Western Cape, South Africa
e-mail: Graeme.wilson@uct.ac.za

K.P. Mason (ed.), *Pediatric Sedation Outside of the Operating Room: A Multispecialty International Collaboration*,
DOI 10.1007/978-1-4939-1390-9_25, © Springer Science+Business Media New York 2015

which drugs be administered, or the sedation techniques employed. Practice settings and the use of support staff involved in pediatric sedation also remain contentious. Unfortunately, only a few institutions have dedicated and structured pediatric sedation services despite recommendations from a variety of organizations in this regard. A survey of North American hospitals confirms that structured programs are not common [2].

Sub-Saharan Africa is a densely populated and resource poor subcontinent that provides unique challenges in patient care. These challenges include a lack of facilities and staff for the performance of operative as well as non-operative procedures.

In a survey on anesthesia services in developing countries, the authors used a questionnaire to delineate the difficulties in providing anesthesia services in Uganda [3]. This survey provides us with insight of the availability of anesthesia services in other developing countries in Africa. The survey results show that 23 % of anesthetists have the facilities to deliver safe anesthesia to adults but only 13 % have facilities to deliver safe anesthesia to children. The questionnaire identified shortages of personnel, drugs, equipment, and training as major factors influencing service delivery. These factors had neither been quantified nor accurately described before. Training was also highlighted as problematic, with few physician anesthetists amongst the anesthesia providers. Most of the non-physician anesthetists had previously attended a training course or were currently in training. Anesthesia for children according to the results of the survey appears to be largely ketamine-based, mainly due to a "lack of disposable airway equipment such as tracheal tubes, facemasks and breathing circuits."

Ketamine is available in the majority of countries in Sub-Saharan Africa. It is an extremely important agent as it can provide anesthesia, sedation, and analgesia. Ketamine's inherent safety profile allows it to be used safely for procedures outside the operating room, provided that standard safety requirements are adhered to. Ketamine, used intramuscularly and intravenously, is regarded by many as the standard of care for the sedation of children in many developing countries, furthermore it is used by both anesthesiologists as well as "untrained personnel" for induction and maintenance of anesthesia. The authors in this chapter quantify and describe the problems and challenges faced by health care professionals in developing countries [3]. Their proposals could be used as guidance by health care professionals to improve, manage, and plan anesthesia and sedation services in developing countries.

Sedation can be considered a reasonable alternative to general anesthesia for certain surgical procedures in the Third World. Bearing in mind the common surgical conditions of childhood in developing countries in Africa, it becomes clear that there is a large potential market for sedation services [4]. Common surgical conditions encountered are fractures, burns, congenital abnormalities, infections, and dental problems, whereas hernia repairs form the bulk of the emergency surgical work. Widespread provision of safe sedation services would result in increased efficiency, reduced costs and personnel requirements, and a reduction in the pressure on the provision of general anesthesia.

Africa has a critical shortage of health care workers [5]. This remains one of the biggest challenges to Third World health facilities. The reasons for a lack of qualified personnel are multifactorial. The inability to train enough health care providers, training requirements, internal mal-distribution, and emigration of trained and skilled health care providers due to unacceptable working conditions contribute to the shortage of health care provision. Despite this, demand for sedation services for procedures outside the operating room exists and it will continue to increase, especially in rural areas. The ability to deliver pediatric sedation services will play an important role in providing sustainable, affordable health care in these settings. Training in pediatric sedation services remains a major obstacle and very few centers in Africa provide structured pediatric sedation training, let alone structures for the retention of competencies at all levels. A system is needed that can accredit individual sedation practitioners and furthermore training must be expanded to include other health care professionals in order to meet the growing demand for sedation services. The shortage of resources and the vast traveling distances in order to receive training and to maintain their clinical competence makes this no simple process.

The shortage of health care professionals to provide sedation services outside the operating room needs to be addressed. It is clear that there are simply not enough trained health care professionals available to meet these demands and, with an ever-growing population and the attending economic realities, this is unlikely to change in the near future. A lack of knowledge on sedation techniques and a lack of understanding that pediatric sedation can be a safe alternative to general anesthesia for certain procedures hampers the development of structured sedation services in many countries around the world. Dissemination of information on the value of sedation to help inform health care personnel on a safe alternative to general anesthesia is needed. In addition, more training opportunities for sedation practitioners must be created. This will only be possible by enthusiastic collaboration between the discipline of anesthesiology and other relevant health care disciplines or sub-disciplines, especially in undeveloped rural Africa with its unique problems. More research is necessary to assess the use of drugs and drug combinations that can be used for safe pediatric sedation outside the operating room in these circumstances.

The demand for sedation for procedures on children outside the operating room already seems to exceed the capacity for offering anesthetic services in the operating room. This is a serious problem that needs to be addressed to ensure that sufficient sedation providers are available to provide sedation services, and sufficient anesthesiologists to provide anesthetic services, especially in resource-poor settings. The shortage of providers and lack of training is probably the most common barrier to the development of universal pediatric sedation services. In an effort to address the problem, this author has spent the last decade and more in developing training programs for sedation practitioners and in developing protocols for safe sedation services. The results of these endeavors are outlined as follows.

Sedation Training

Certification of sedation training is a new concept in Africa. Structured sedation training in Africa was non-existent before the year 2000. Subsequently a postgraduate diploma in Sedation and Pain Control in the principles and techniques of both pediatric and adult sedation has been offered in South Africa to both anesthesiologists and non-anesthesiologists, first at Stellenbosch University and later at the University of the Western Cape. Both qualified anesthesiologists and dentists are tutors in this part-time modular program, presented over 2 years. The first year of training consists of three contact sessions lasting 3 days and incorporates both theoretical and practical training; this module includes both medical and dental clinical scenarios for sedation. Certification of appropriate airway skills—i.e., an Advanced Adult Life Support and Advanced Pediatric Life Support—is a prerequisite for all sedation students and certification must be updated regularly.

During their second year, students must write a 5,000 word referenced dissertation on a topic related to sedation and pain control. Students are encouraged to visit the University of the Western Cape at regular intervals for practical training and to develop their skills in sedation and pain control. After qualifying, students in possession of the diploma in sedation and pain control may then proceed to a master's degree. As few structured sedation-training programs are available elsewhere, the diploma and master's programs attract students from the whole of Africa and beyond. The majority of the students are non-anesthesiologists—usually medical practitioners with a special interest in sedation practice. Subsequently, other similar sedation programs have been developed in other areas of Africa. The author has since initiated sedation training at universities in Nairobi, Kenya, and at institutions in other African states. Health care providers across Africa are now recognizing that sedation for a variety of diverse procedures offers an acceptable viable alternative to general anesthesia.

To support the training of dental practitioners as operator/sedation practitioners, the Dental College of South Africa has approved an application for a diploma in Sedation and Pain Control (Dip Dent) through the College of Dentistry of South Africa. This will provide dentists with an opportunity to be involved as sedation providers in areas of need.

The South African Society of Sedation Practitioners (SOSPOSA), a special interest group of the South African Society of Anesthesiologists (SASA), is committed to uplifting sedation training in Africa. Annual sedation workshops are held to provide theoretical and practical training. SOSPOSA presents sedation symposia and workshops at the annual congress of the South African Society of Anesthesiologists (SASA). Further progress is being made in sedation training in southern Africa. A pediatric sedation training workshop, with national and international speakers, was presented as part of the Pediatric Anesthesia Congress of South Africa (PACSA) in 2012 and it is hoped that this too will become a permanent fixture.

As interest in the creation of formal sedation training programs grows, centers in developed countries are initiating sedation-training programs. A collaboration with University College London in the United Kingdom has been established, directed and taught by Dr. James Roelofse, the founder of the South African Postgraduate Diploma in Sedation. A postgraduate Certificate in Sedation and Pain Control is now offered in London. Lecturers from the University of Oslo, Norway have also become involved in sedation training at University of the Western Cape since 2011.

The chronic shortage of anesthesiologists in Africa results in a situation where supply of anesthesiologists cannot meet the demand for sedation providers. This begs an important and sometimes controversial question: Are non-anesthesiologists in the developing nations with limited resources capable of providing safe sedation to children? A review on sedation of children by non-anesthesiologists suggests that non-anesthesiologists can safely sedate pediatric patients, provided that they are given appropriate training [6]. Health care practitioners from all disciplines would need to be trained as pediatric sedation providers to meet the growing need [2]. Consequently, non-anesthesiologists are accepted into the aforementioned training programs, as they can play a vital role in providing sedation services, particularly in rural areas. Almost all the non-specialist anesthesiologists in our course have a diploma in anesthesia from the College of Medicine of South Africa. All candidates are required to have had some training in anesthesia. Non-anesthesiologists and anesthesiologists receive the same training for the diploma program. The diploma program provides didactic teaching on matters related to safe sedation practice. Emphasis is placed on patient safety and only American Society of Anesthesiologists (ASA) I and II patients qualify for sedation care outside of the operating room. The collaboration of anesthesiologists to train and educate non-anesthesia caregivers to safely sedate a clearly identified pediatric population (ASA I and II) is an important first step in Africa. By being involved in the training of non-anesthesiologists, the specialty of anesthesia will retain its influence on the quality and direction of patient care and sedation practice.

All health care professionals involved in sedation must be trained in specific sedation techniques and must follow accepted guidelines and protocols. This view was endorsed in 2007 by the Royal College of Anesthetists and the Faculty of Dental Surgery of the Royal College of Surgeons of England: The Standing Dental Committee in the United Kingdom published their guidelines on the "Standards for Conscious Sedation in Dentistry: Alternative Techniques" [7]. The guidelines state that it is essential that there is "evidence of training (even for anesthesiologists) in specific advanced sedation techniques, in an appropriate environment." Children under 12 years of age are specifically mentioned as a group for whom sedation providers must receive formal training. The American Society of Anesthesiologists (ASA) has published guidelines for sedation services provided by non-anesthesiologists [8], and the guidelines have been endorsed by the American Academy of Pediatrics (AAP) and the Joint Commission [9–11].

In 2010, the National Institute of Health in the United Kingdom (NICE) guidelines on "Sedation in children and young people" were published in the United Kingdom [12, 13]. This guideline also suggests that health care professionals involved in pediatric sedation must undergo theoretical and supervised clinical training. Keeping a logbook and airway certification are essential requirements for safe sedation practice.

Sedation Models

To find an acceptable pediatric sedation model that suits all patients, sedation practitioners, and locations is virtually impossible. Children undergoing diagnostic or therapeutic procedures are often frightened and uncooperative. Anxiety and fear is exacerbated by many different factors; in particular, previous unpleasant experiences. The need to provide analgesia together with sedation for painful procedures has resulted in the proliferation of multidrug sedation techniques. Subsequently, use of these techniques, with a higher incidence of adverse events and complications, has become commonplace. Provision of sedation services outside the operating room has also grown in demand in facilities that meet all the requirements for safe sedation practice [2]. Various pediatric sedation models that have been established throughout Africa will be reviewed as follows.

The Sedation Unit Model Within the Hospital

This model allocates a designated area of the hospital as a sedation room and a recovery area, which together represent an area for sedation, the procedure, and recovery. Training in a designated sedation unit creates awareness and makes students appreciative of the ideal environment for safe sedation practice. Designated sedation areas provide ideal conditions for sedation practitioners as they are not responsible for the supply of drugs and equipment. It however, remains the responsibility of the hospital to ensure that everything needed for safe sedation practice is provided.

This designated area should be adjacent to an operating room should failed sedation or surgical complication result in the need to progress to general anesthesia. Children usually receive oral or transmucosal sedation in the recovery area and are then transported to the procedure room, and back to the recovery area after the procedure. This area should also have a nitrous oxide/oxygen unit, with a sevoflurane vaporizer. Low concentrations of sevoflurane (0.3 %) can be added for very anxious children, delivered by the anesthesiologists or trained sedation practitioner. Parents or escorts are allowed to accompany the child into the sedation room until the child is comfortable, but should leave once the procedure has commenced.

We have primarily embraced the pediatric dental model for training purposes—this is a unique model as the airway is shared by both the sedation practitioner and the surgeon. This creates an ideal scenario for training safe sedation techniques. Pediatric dental care provides a challenging problem in developing countries as extensively damaged teeth often need multiple extractions. Many of these procedures are performed under intravenous sedation and require extensive dental surgery. Long periods of intravenous sedation using a variety of different agents are necessary to complete the work. In our sedation daycare unit, we provide intravenous sedation for more than 900 procedures a year. Only procedures on ASA I and II patients are performed outside the operating room. The sedation unit is staffed on a part-time basis by both anesthesiologists and non-anesthesiologists. Funding for the sedation service is provided by the South African government and the University of the Western Cape.

The University of the Western Cape has the biggest dental faculty in Sub-Saharan Africa. To improve capacity, the University of the Western Cape approved a pediatric emergency sedation dental clinic for minor dental procedures, such as extractions. Pre-school children under 6 years of age form the bulk of the clinic's patient load. These children are usually anxious, and to provide some form of anxiolysis we have recently been studying the use of intranasal midazolam.

Two doses of intranasal midazolam 0.3 and 0.5 mg/kg are being compared [14]. The drugs are administered intranasally 15 min before the procedure with a Mucosal Atomization Device (MAD®, LMA North America, San Diego, CA). Before local anesthesia is administered, a topical anesthetic is applied to the mucosa in the mouth. The study has shown some interesting preliminary results.

More than 90 % of children are calm with controlled behavior after the local anesthetic injection following intranasal administration of midazolam. All the children had oxygen saturation levels of above 95 %. More than 95 % of the children were discharged within 15 min after the procedure, meeting the requirements for safe discharge. The behavior of children leaving the emergency clinic was remarkably different than those who had no intranasal midazolam. No nausea, vomiting, and aspiration were reported in more than 150 cases. This single-drug technique is administered by an operator sedation practitioner and complies with the requirements of a simple or basic sedation technique as set out in the guidelines of the South African Society of Anesthesiologists [15].

The Mobile Sedation Model Within the Hospital

This model requires that sedation providers render a sedation service at a distant site within the hospital. This site is usually close to the inpatient hospital wards. Portable sedation equipment and appropriate drugs for sedating children are used in various locations in the hospital, e.g., bone marrow biopsies in an oncology ward [16]. Children are sedated and recovered at the site of the procedure by the sedation provider and support staff. This approach avoids the need for transporting the sedated child between the ward and procedure area and is very popular.

A Combined Sedation Model Within the Hospital

A combination of the aforementioned two models allows that some children are sedated in the unit and transported to fixed facilities, i.e., magnetic resonance imaging (MRI). The sedation unit is reserved for those procedures that may be performed onsite.

The Mobile Sedationist Model Outside the Hospital

A model that is growing in popularity in South Africa is administration of sedation in the office or other ambulatory center by a "mobile or traveling sedation practitioner." Mobile sedation practitioners are especially popular for pediatric dental procedures as well as minor plastic and dermatological procedures. They provide the practitioner the opportunity of performing procedures in their own environment, equipped with their own equipment. This is a cost-effective approach as it avoids the add-on costs generated when such procedures are performed in hospital operating rooms. This approach could potentially have substantial economic benefits for patients and their health insurance companies. As hospital-associated costs escalate, the demand for mobile sedation practitioners by different specialists, such as dermatologists and plastic surgeons, is increasing.

The increased demand for pediatric sedation services makes structured training in specific pediatric sedation techniques even more crucial. One concern is at what age can one safely sedate a child in a remote setting, especially if the sedation providers are not trained? In South Africa, the mobile sedation practitioner model is reserved and supported only for ASA I and II children and delivered by health care professionals appropriately trained in all areas of safe pediatric sedation practice.

The Operator-Sedationist Model

This model does not conform to guidelines and policies of some specialty societies outside Africa. However, it tends to be used for simple procedures with single drug administration. In this model, the sedation provider also performs the procedure. This model is practiced by dentists and other health care professionals, usually administering nitrous oxide/oxygen inhalation sedation, titrated doses of intravenous midazolam or oral sedatives for dental procedures or other minor procedures (i.e., suturing of lacerations, application of burn dressings, and cannulation of veins). According to the guidelines of the South African Society of Anesthesiologists [15], the activities of operator sedation practitioners should be confined to the use of single drugs, reserving combination drug therapy to the dedicated sedation provider model. The usual techniques for pediatric sedation by operator sedation practitioners include standard or simple sedation techniques with nitrous oxide and oxygen, oral/transmucosal benzodiazepines or titrated doses of intravenous midazolam but not a combination of the drugs. Intravenous routes of sedation delivery are not generally used by operator sedation practitioners for pediatric sedation. This model clearly has its restrictions and tends to offer sedation for a small group of children undergoing a limited type of procedure.

The Dedicated Sedationist Model

More advanced techniques of sedation delivery, which include continuous infusion of drugs, target-controlled infusions, and multidrug therapy, should only be used by dedicated sedation practitioners according to recognized guidelines. Ideally members of a pediatric sedation team using such advanced techniques must include at least two suitably qualified and experienced people. These techniques are especially valuable for sedation for painful and more complicated procedures, where single agent sedation is unsuitable.

Guidelines for Safe Pediatric Sedation in the Third World

Provision of safe pediatric sedation requires that established guidelines be rigorously followed. Sedation practitioners are encouraged to follow the guidelines of the Standing Dental Advisory Committee, Royal College of Anesthetists, American Academy of Pediatrics (AAP), the American Society of Anesthesiologists (ASA), the Joint Commission [7–11, 15] or the pediatric sedation guidelines from the South African Society of Anesthesiologists (SASA) [15]. (Refer to Chap. 2.)

These guidelines recognize that deep sedation is part of the spectrum of general anesthesia, and should only be administered by trained sedation personnel with formal anesthetic training. Hoffman et al. [17] have shown that adherence to formal guidelines (ASA and AAP guidelines) by non-anesthesiologists can reduce the risk of pediatric procedural sedation. They showed that adequate pre-sedation assessment achieves a reduction in complications of deep sedation. They furthermore showed that repeated assessment of sedation score reduces the risk of inadvertent deep sedation and attendant complications.

Sedation providers should be adequately qualified or trained. Education should include core training in both simple and advanced sedation techniques. Core competencies should include knowledge of anatomy, physiology, and pharmacology, whilst clinical competency in monitoring, airway examination, and ability to rescue the oversedated child are essential [15]. The concept of a sedation team is important. The team must include either the operator sedation practitioner (for basic sedation techniques) or a dedicated sedation practitioner, and support staff. Preferably two qualified and trained people should be available to assist with monitoring of the patient and must be able to render active support if the need for rescue should arise.

Practically, the safe practice of pediatric sedation can be broken down to three components:

1. Selection, assessment, and preparation of patients
2. Provision of sedation—here attention should be focused on safe practice, premises, equipment, and documentation
3. Recovery and discharge

Selection, Assessment, and Preparation of Patients

Correct pre-sedation selection and assessment of patients is critical to identify high-risk patients or situations where sedation is contraindicated or should not be performed outside the operating theater. Pre-sedation evaluation and assessment is mandatory as the history, clinical examination, and airway evaluation will direct triage decisions. Only ASA I and ASA II patients should be sedated outside the operating room and fasting guidelines must be adhered to (Table 25.1). Most guidelines emphasize that sedation for children less than 5 years of age should only to be performed by practitioners with extensive experience. Patients with potentially difficult airways (Table 25.2) should only be sedated in hospital by experienced personnel.

Written informed consent must be obtained and verbal and written instructions for, before and after the sedation procedure must be conveyed to a responsible person.

Provision of Sedation

Facilities must comply with the standards required for safe pediatric sedation outside the operating room. Attention should be focused on the procedure room where the appropriate staff, drugs, and equipment must be available to monitor and rescue a child.

Equipment for pediatric sedation should be appropriate for the intended procedure as well as the targeted depth of sedation. Monitoring equipment for all but the simple single agent (oral or inhalation) technique should include electrocardiogram (ECG), blood pressure, and pulse oximetry. If available, an end-tidal carbon dioxide monitor should be used. The precordial stethoscope remains an inexpensive and practical monitor, especially in under-resourced rural settings. The availability of a defibrillator is desirable wherever pediatric sedation performed, especially when combined drug techniques are employed [15]. (Refer to Chap. 3.)

Documentation and protocols must comply with contemporary guidance [7, 9, 16]. This includes documentation before, during, and after sedation. All parameters that are monitored during sedation must be documented and any adverse events entered on a sedation chart.

Recovery and Discharge

Recovery facilities must meet all the requirements for safe recovery of the child after sedation. No child should be sedated without an escort being available to accompany the child home. A protocol for back-up emergency services must be available for all cases done outside the operating room and ready access to ambulance services is advised wherever pediatric sedation is performed.

Table 25.1 Prudent limits of targeted depth of emergency department (ED) procedural sedation

STANDARD RISK				
ORAL INTAKE IN THE PRIOR 3 HOURS	**Urgency of the Procedure**			
	Emergent	***Urgent***	***Semi-Urgent***	***Non-Urgent***
Nothing	All levels of sedation	All levels of sedation	All levels of sedation	All levels of sedation
Clear liquids only	All levels of sedation	All levels of sedation	Up to and including brief deep sedation	Up to and including extended moderate sedation
Light snack	All levels of sedation	Up to and including brief deep sedation	Up to and including dissociative sedation; non-extended moderate sedation	Minimal sedation only
Heavy snack or meal	All levels of sedation	Up to and including extended moderate sedation	Minimal sedation only	Minimal sedation only
HIGHER RISK				
ORAL INTAKE IN THE PRIOR 3 HOURS	**Procedural Urgency**			
	Emergent Procedure	***Urgent Procedure***	***Semi-Urgent Procedure***	***Non-Urgent Procedure***
Nothing	All levels of sedation	All levels of sedation	All levels of sedation	All levels of sedation
Clear liquids only	All levels of sedation	Up to and including brief deep sedation	Up to and including extended moderate sedation	Minimal sedation only
Light snack	All levels of sedation	Up to and including dissociative sedation; non-extended moderate sedation	Minimal sedation only	Minimal sedation only
Heavy snack or meal	All levels of sedation	Up to and including dissociative sedation; non-extended moderate sedation	Minimal sedation only	Minimal sedation only

	Procedural Sedation and Analgesia Targeted Depth and Duration
↓ Increasing Potential Aspiration Risk ↓	Minimal sedation only
	Dissociative sedation; brief or intermediate-length moderate sedation
	Extended moderate sedation
	Brief deep sedation
	Intermediate or extended-length deep sedation

Brief: <10 min
Intermediate: 10–20 min
Extended: >20 min
Adapted from Green SM, Roback MG, Miner JR, Burton JH, Krauss B. Fasting and Emergency Department Procedural Sedation and Analgesia: A Consensus-Based Clinical Practice Advisory. Ann Emerg Med. 2007; 49(4): 454–461

Table 25.2 Patients with potentially difficult airways

Obstructive sleep apnea (OSA)
Large tonsils approaching the midline, or associated with loud snoring
Children who cannot lie flat because of airway obstruction
Stridor
Retropharyngeal masses
Neck masses
Tracheal deviation
Mallampati class 3 or 4
Neck mobility: decreased range of movement, including hydrocephalus with a large head
Syndromic features (e.g., Pierre-Robin, Treacher-Collins):
• Enlarged tongue
• Micrognathia
• Abnormal ears
Hemangiomas
Beware of children with malignancies: multiple level airway obstruction is possible

Reprinted with permission from Reed A, Thomas J, Roelofse JA, Gray R, de Kock M, Piercy J. Paediatric Procedural Sedation and Analgesia (PSA) Guidelines; South African Society of Anaesthesiologists. 2011

Guidelines for Mobile Sedation Practitioners

Safe practice of mobile sedation requires that the sedation practitioner takes responsibility for all the requirements of safe sedation practice. These include the suitability of the premises, the pre-sedation assessment, intraoperative care, documentation, and postoperative discharge of the child. A not unreasonable assumption is that the premises will provide only suction and light. The sedation practitioner must provide all the drugs, disposables, equipment (including resuscitation equipment) that may be needed. The sedation practitioner is also responsible for ensuring that suitably qualified health care professionals are available to assist with monitoring and rescue, if needed.

Routine equipment requirements should include: a stethoscope (preferably also a precordial stethoscope), blood pressure monitor, glucometer, and pulse oximeter. Mobile sedation practitioners are encouraged to use an ECG monitor and capnography, particularly when pediatric advanced sedation techniques are performed, or when deep sedation is intended. They are advised to carry a spare pulse oximeter. A thermometer is also advisable, especially as children often present with a runny nose and other respiratory symptoms for which an infectious process must be ruled out. It is also advisable to carry a glucometer. The mobile kit should also include items that improve patient comfort and safety, i.e., a blanket to keep the child warm, a cushion to put behind the shoulders to extend the neck, butterfly sponges to protect the airway from water in pediatric dental cases, and a radio with earphones to play music for the older child.

The kit should also contain emergency equipment such as oxygen, nasal cannulae, a self-inflating resuscitator, airways (nasal and oral), pediatric laryngoscope and blades, a suction catheter, endotracheal tubes, laryngeal mask airways, Magill's forceps, resuscitation drugs, and a defibrillator [15]. Mobile sedation practitioners usually operate in the private health care environment where the patients are responsible for the expenses and most carry medical insurance.

A mobile sedation practitioner must also have access to appropriate office infrastructure. This includes secretarial services to take care of appointments, the preparation of paperwork that should be sent to the parents ahead of time in respect of preoperative and postoperative instructions, and to gather information regarding the health status of the child. A patient follow-up system should be in place to allow the guardian to give postoperative feedback. The questionnaire allows for feedback on patient satisfaction and possible side effects, such as postoperative nausea and vomiting, pain during the procedure, double vision, and emotional disturbances. The form should also invite comment as to whether the parent and child would prefer sedation again; or rather opt for general anesthesia.

Behavioral Management of the Child

The single most important aspect of any successful sedation is to gain the child's trust. Earning a child's trust is not always easy, particularly if there have been past traumatic experiences with general anesthesia or sedation. All sedation techniques must include planning behavioral management strategies, empathy, understanding, and a patient approach. (Refer to Chap. 34.) The protocol for successful behavior management must incorporate two strategies: how to "read the mind" of the child [18] and how to use the specific practical guidelines. When trying to "read the mind" of the child, it is vital to try and establish a good personal relationship in order to gain their trust. This means placing yourself in the child's shoes and establishing rapport. Five important points to remember when interacting with a child are: (1) imagine you are the same age as the child you are dealing with, (2) use words that a child can understand, (3) do not lie to the child (this does not mean that one needs to disclose all details), (4) offer encouragement by telling him/her that he/she is good and brave to ensure that the child feels proud, and (4) use the information you get from the child to play mind games [18]. Always speak to children slowly and gently and talk to them about pleasant things, i.e., the smell of their favorite food, the ocean, paintings, etc. A child who does not want to make eye contact is not interested in what you are saying and will ignore attempts to establish rapport. Such children are difficult to sedate and may need a different approach and deeper levels of sedation.

The following practical hints may be useful for sedation practitioners and the team to establish a rapport with a child:

- The office/surgery, where procedures are to be performed, is a threatening environment for most children. Communication should not take place in the operating room but in a friendlier environment where the child can be made comfortable. He/she should be encouraged to ask questions and his/her consent should be obtained for the proposed sedation where possible.
- Wear casual, non-operating room clothing—appearing too formal may create anxiety in children, especially if they had previous negative experiences during general anesthesia.
- What you say is less important than how you say it. The attitude of the sedation practitioner is an important determinant of success. It is essential that the sedation practitioner shows confidence in what he or she is doing. The child and parent must be confident that the sedation provider knows exactly what is to be done, has the necessary experience, and can deliver safely on the promises. One should never afford the child or parent the opportunity to doubt one's professional ability. Always have a positive attitude that, at times, may be quite difficult. Show the child that you are enthusiastic about what you do and that you are excited to be in a position to be able to help. Confidence in one's own success as a sedation practitioner may convince the child that, even though his anxiety is valid, together the two of you can be successful. Never direct your conversation at the parent or escort; always involve the child irrespective of age. Always establish and maintain eye contact with the child—this simple gesture shows the child that you really care.
- Try to find an "ice-breaker" (a means of eliciting the child's trust and allaying his anxiety and fear) when first meeting the child by making a friendly non-threatening statement to start the conversation—this may be all that is needed to settle the child down. It is always good to find out about the interests of the child.
- Never look down at the child—if the child is seated or lying down, sit down beside him. It may even be advisable to sit on your haunches in front of the child. That way, your eyes are at the same level and it makes it much easier for the child to relate to the sedation practitioner.
- It is crucial that children never to be crowded—they need their personal space to feel respected.
- It is always wise to tell the child that you need his or her help and that sedation means a team effort.

Children are very susceptible to suggestion. Something like, "I cannot do this without your help" will go a long way toward making the child comfortable. In case of an intravenous cannulation, tell the child that a butterfly will come and sit on his/her hand. You are allowed to choose the color of the butterfly.

A final question: Do cultural factors play a role in the outcome, success rate, and/or achievability of multidrug sedation in children over the age of 5 years? A study of 354 children from eight different cultural groups showed that cultural factors do not influence the outcome, success, or achievability of multidrug sedation in children. The study, however, validated the importance of preoperative selection and assessment and the use of behavior management techniques [19].

Common Sedation Strategies in the Developing Nations

Oral Route: Single Agent

It is not routine practice to administer oral sedatives for surgical procedures. Children's behavior patterns vary and it is essential to do a behavioral assessment prior to the procedure. It is good practice to discuss this with the parent or guardian before sedation, as they usually can give the sedation practitioner guidance as to whether the child needs an oral sedative before surgery. Some children are, however, just too frightened due to previous traumatic experiences, and may thus need a sedative. An oral sedative must never be given to the child at home but in the facility where the procedure will be done.

Chloral hydrate is a sedative hypnotic still being used in some hospitals for sedation for children under the age of 3 years, especially for painless imaging [20]. The drug has no analgesic activities and the usual dose is 20–75 mg/kg, given orally.

Midazolam is a short-acting, water-soluble benzodiazepine with no analgesic properties. It is the most commonly used benzodiazepine for pediatric sedation and can be administered via various routes. The oral dose is 0.35 mg/kg, 20–30 min before surgery [21]. To make it easier to remember, we advise sedation providers to administer 7.5 mg orally to those children above 8 years of age, and 5 mg to those less than 8 years of age. The child must be constantly supervised and monitored after administration of the oral sedative. Midazolam is not available in a syrup formulation in Africa, so instead the tablet is crushed and diluted with paracetamol syrup. Alternatively, the aqueous formulation for intravenous midazolam is administered orally. Midazolam is a useful sedative in combination with other oral drugs.

Oral ketamine provides excellent sedation, analgesia, and amnesia and can also be used for painful procedures. In the developing world, it is usually combined with midazolam. Oral ketamine is useful for burn debridement in children at a dose of 10 mg/kg because of its excellent safety profile [22]. Acceptable sedation for dental procedures was achieved in children, 2–7 years of age, by the use of 12.5 mg/kg oral ketamine. The incidence of hallucinations was 16.6 % [23].

Ketamine administered orally is used extensively for analgesia and sedation during dressing changes in children suffering from burn injuries at the Red Cross War Memorial Children's hospital in South Africa [24]. A recent study from this institution in children between 1 and 8 years of age suggests that oral ketamine 5–10 mg/kg via a nasogastric tube with intravenous supplementation of 0.5–1 mg/kg provides reasonable sedation and analgesia for short dressing changes. Furthermore, oral ketamine administration results in high norketamine concentrations due to first-pass metabolism in turn contributing to good long-lasting post-procedural analgesia. Oral ketamine may serve as a valuable premedicant, sedative, and analgesic for children suffering from burn injuries.

Table 25.3 Dosing schedule for midazolam

Route	Dose (mg/kg)	Maximum dose	Time to peak effect (min)	Duration of action (min)
Oral	0.35	7.5 mg	10–30	60
Nasal	0.3–0.5	0.5 mg/kg	10–20	60
Rectal	0.5–1	1 mg/kg	10–15	60–90
Intravenous	0.025–0.1	1 mg	3–5	20–60

Reprinted with permission from Reed A, Thomas J, Roelofse JA, Gray R, de Kock M, Piercy J. Paediatric Procedural Sedation and Analgesia (PSA) Guidelines; South African Society of Anaesthesiologists. 2011

Nasal Route: Single Agent

Intranasal *midazolam* may be uncomfortable for children as it may cause a burning sensation. It is, however, useful in children who refuse to take medication by mouth, are vomiting, or are developmentally delayed. Although a tuberculin syringe can be used to administer 0.2 mg/kg midazolam intranasally, a Mucosal Atomization Device (MAD®, LMA North America, San Diego, CA) is available and makes nasal administration easier and more acceptable.

Rectal Route: Single Agent

Rectal administration of *midazolam* is useful for providing sedation for younger children (Table 25.3). Acceptance is high, particularly in small children. In some of the countries in Sub-Saharan Africa some parents prefer the rectal route for administration of sedative drugs. The administration of midazolam by this route may be indicated where children refuse to take oral drugs, are nauseous, vomiting, or very anxious. It can be used on its own for painless procedures or in combination with other drugs when analgesia is required. In a study, rectal midazolam administered at 1 mg/kg to children 30 min before dental surgery achieved satisfactory sedation and recovery whilst maintaining hemodynamic stability.

Rectal *diazepam* is a useful and cost-effective alternative sedative for midazolam, especially in rural areas, where the latter drug is often not available. Rectal diazepam, at a dose of 0.70 mg/kg, provides acceptable levels of sedation, and patient acceptance, when administered 30 min before a procedure [25]. Rectal *ketamine* at a dose of 5 mg/kg has also successfully been used in dental surgery and may be a useful alternative for pediatric sedation [26].

Intravenous Route: Single Agent

Any sedation administered by the intravenous route, using bolus or infusion techniques should be considered an advanced sedation technique [15], and should be administered by suitably trained and equipped personnel. Intravenous agents can be used as small boluses titrated to effect or as a continuous infusion. Unadjusted continuous infusion techniques may result in gradually rising plasma concentrations of sedative and necessitate constant intensive monitoring and airway vigilance.

Propofol is a short-acting phenol derivative. Its use as a sedative hypnotic agent outside the operating room remains contentious. Propofol has a narrow therapeutic index and the sedation practitioner should anticipate that deep sedation, airway obstruction, and apnea may occur rapidly and unpredictably. Although it is an effective sedative, it should be used only for brief procedures, as repeated doses or infusions are more likely to be associated with adverse events. The usual sedative dose in children is 0.3–0.5 mg/kg titrated to effect with a titration interval of at least 1 min. Target Controlled Infusion (TCI) of propofol may overcome some of the limitations of continuous infusions [27, 28]. TCI is an infusion controlled by a real-time pharmacokinetic model that employs algorithms to construct a variable rate infusion. (Refer to Chap. 31.) Two algorithms are available in South Africa: the Kataria and Paedfusor models. The Kataria model caters to children over the age of 3, whereas the Paedfusor model may be used in children over a year of age [29, 30]. As the effect site equilibration constant is not known in children, both models only allow use as plasma targeting. Usual plasma targets for sedation are between 0.5 and 2 mcg/mL, but like bolus dosing should be titrated to effect.

Table 25.4 Dosing schedule for ketamine

Route	Dose	Onset (min)	Time to peak effect (min)	Duration of action
Oral	2–5 mg/kg	5–10	20	4 h
Nasal	2–5 mg/kg	5–10	20	4 h
Rectal	2–5 mg/kg	5–10	20	4–6 h
Intravenous bolus	0.25–1 mg/kg	<1	3–5	10–15 min
Intravenous infusion	0.5–1 mg/kg/h	<1	3–5	10–15 min

Reprinted with permission from Reed A, Thomas J, Roelofse JA, Gray R, de Kock M, Piercy J. Paediatric Procedural Sedation and Analgesia (PSA) Guidelines; South African Society of Anaesthesiologists. 2011

Ketamine is probably the most widely used single intravenous sedative in the developing world. Ketamine induces a state of cortical dissociation with profound analgesia, sedation, and amnesia. At typical sedative doses, there is relative preservation of airway reflexes and tone. Emergence delirium is less common in children, and of a much smaller magnitude than adults and it correlates significantly with the degree of pre-procedural agitation. See Table 25.4 for dosing recommendations.

Midazolam is a short-acting benzodiazepine with potent amnestic, sedative, and anxiolytic properties. Paradoxical agitation may occur in up to 1.4 % of children and may necessitate treatment with flumazenil and use of an alternative agent. When given intravenously, most children should require no more than 1 mg [15]. See Table 25.3 for dosing recommendations.

Dexmedetomidine is an alpha 2-receptor agonist that has the ability to provide sedation without causing respiratory depression. A biphasic dose–response effect on hemodynamics has been described, characterized by decreases in arterial blood pressure and heart rate at low plasma concentrations and an increase in arterial blood pressure with further reductions in heart rate at higher plasma concentrations [31]. To minimize the hemodynamic effects of dexmedetomidine, the loading dose of 1 mcg/kg should be given as a slow intravenous injection over at least 10 min. This can be followed by a constant infusion of 0.2–0.7 mcg/kg/h.

Oral Route: Sedative and Analgesic Combination

No single drug is available that meets all the requirements of an ideal sedative. Drug combinations may therefore be necessary, particularly in the management of uncooperative children. Drug combinations do, however, increase the risk of complications and the sedation practitioner involved should be trained in advanced sedation techniques, and preferably have experience in general anesthesia. A combination of midazolam and ketamine is useful for sedation in short, painful procedures. Oral midazolam (0.35 mg/kg) combined with oral ketamine (5 mg/kg), in children has been shown to provide safe, effective, and practical sedation for minor oral surgical procedures under local anesthesia [32]. When oral ketamine and midazolam are used, in conjunction with an intravenous technique, the dose of oral ketamine should be reduced to 2 mg/kg. This dose of ketamine is also suitable for children under the age of 2 years [33] but they need to be monitored carefully for over sedation.

The safe and effective management of children for painful procedures outside the operating room remains a challenge. Dental procedures are common pediatric day-cases and are one of the commonly used research models used for studying the efficacy of minor analgesic agents [34]. Severity of postoperative pain is related to the number of teeth extracted, and an effective clinical research model has been established by studying children who have undergone six or more extractions [35]. This study gives valuable information regarding pain after pediatric dental procedures. Children aged 4–7 years, undergoing six or more dental extractions, received tramadol (1.5 mg/kg) or placebo 30 min before surgery. Both groups furthermore received oral midazolam (0.5 mg/kg) up to a maximum of 7.5 mg 30 min before surgery. Postoperative rescue analgesia was required by 19.4 % of the tramadol group, compared with 82.8 % of the placebo group [35]. This showed that the use of effective analgesic drugs, before sedation, minimized postoperative pain in children. Other studies have confirmed tramadol's analgesic efficacy, lack of significant respiratory depression and preservation of time to recovery when used in combination with other sedative agents [36, 37]. The combination of oral tramadol 1.5–3 mg/kg with midazolam is a useful combination for sedation and analgesia for children undergoing painful procedures outside the operating room. Another useful oral combination is trimeprazine (6 mg/mL) and methadone linctus (0.4 mg/mL) in a syrup base [23, 32]. The usual oral dose is 0.5 mL/kg of the mixture up to a maximum of 10 mL. This can be used as sedation for small, painful surgical procedures where local anesthesia is to be used. It is also a useful sedative combination for painless procedures as profound sedation is achieved. Unfortunately methadone, an opioid and trimeprazine a phenothiazine derivative have long elimination half-lives resulting in prolonged recovery. However, despite these limitations, the low cost of this combination makes it useful for oral pediatric sedation in the developing world. Deeper levels of sedation can be obtained by adding droperidol (0.1 mg/kg) to the mixture.

Nasal Route: Drug Combinations

Intranasal drug combinations have also been studied and show great promise, particularly in preschool children with separation anxiety in unfamiliar surroundings. Intranasal sufentanil (1.5–3 mg/kg) has been shown to facilitate separation of children from parents and provide effective postoperative analgesia [38].

Another intranasal drug combination study compared the combination of sufentanil (1 mcg/kg) and midazolam (0.3 mg/kg) with the combination of ketamine (5 mg/kg) and midazolam (0.3 mg/kg) in children undergoing six or more dental extractions [39]. Rapid onset of effective sedation and satisfactory postoperative pain control was demonstrated in both groups, however the sufentanil group required less rescue analgesia when compared to the ketamine group (72 % vs. 52 %).

Multimodal Routes: Drug Combinations

Due to a chronic lack of staff and resources it is not unusual to find advanced, neglected pathology in underdeveloped areas of the Third World. Multiple extractions and fillings are commonplace in dentistry and this compounds the problem of long waiting lists for general anesthesia. The need for alternative treatment options encourages the development of multidrug sedative plans and this often necessitates the use of intravenous drug combinations.

Multimodal Analgesia with Opioids

Multimodal therapy usually begins with a benzodiazepine, e.g., midazolam for anxiolysis. Midazolam may be administered by oral, nasal, intravenous, or rectal routes and sedation may be augmented by the use of one of the ultra-short-acting opioids [40, 41]. Phenylpiperidines are generally the drugs of choice, and, depending on the type of procedure, alfentanil or sufentanil are commonly used either by bolus administration or as part of an infusion technique. A study to establish the safe bolus dosages and infusion rates of alfentanil when combined with propofol, ketamine, and alfentanil was performed on 270 children under 8 years of age [42]. It is concluded that in children with stable vital signs and no respiratory depression, a titrated intravenous bolus dose of 1–2 mcg/kg alfentanil is a safe and effective technique. The bolus dose of alfentanil should be given 2 min before the expected painful stimulus and an intravenous infusion of 10–12 mcg/kg/h alfentanil is recommended (Table 25.5).

Table 25.5 Dosing schedule for alfentanil

Bolus	Titration interval	Infusion	Duration of action
0.5–1 μ(mu)g/kg	5 min	10–12 μ(mu)g/kg/h	<10 min

Reprinted with permission from Reed A, Thomas J, Roelofse JA, Gray R, de Kock M, Piercy J. Paediatric Procedural Sedation and Analgesia (PSA) Guidelines; South African Society of Anaesthesiologists. 2011

The safety and efficacy of combinations of sedative and analgesic drugs were studied in 254 children aged 5–9 years undergoing moderate sedation for dental procedures. All children received 0.5–1 mg of midazolam and alfentanil 1 mcg/kg slowly intravenously. This was followed by titrated doses of ketamine not exceeding 0.3 mg/kg/h and propofol 0.3 mg/kg to achieve the desired sedation level. In 83 % of the children, a workable environment was created for the dentist who was able to perform all dentistry as planned and showed that bolus administration of drugs is safe and efficacious in children. This study shows that combinations of drugs can be used safely for pediatric sedation and analgesia when administered by sedation practitioners trained in specific sedation techniques [43]. With a bolus technique sophisticated infusion pumps are not necessary and this could be a viable option in rural and other under resourced areas.

Remifentanil was studied for procedural sedation and analgesia as a 0.05 mcg/kg/min infusion in 154 children, aged 3–10 years, for dental procedures within the hospital setting. In a separate 20 mL syringe, 200 mg of propofol was mixed with 20 mg of ketamine and titrated to effect. A drop in oxygen saturation levels of <92 % occurred in 9 % of children. In children under the age of 5 years, desaturation occurred in 17 %, coincident with flexion of the head, depression of the chin by the dentist, or excessive oral irrigation. In children >8 years of age, there were no incidences of desaturation <92 % [44]. Remifentanil has also been used for analgesia for dermatology cases and laser treatments of the face, situations that do not permit injection of local anesthetic. Guidelines from the South African Society of Anesthesiologists on procedural sedation and analgesia do not support the use of remifentanil for procedures outside of the operating room [15].

Intravenous ketamine (0.1–0.5 mg/kg titrated) remains a valuable component of multidrug sedation regimes due to its unique sedative, analgesic, and amnestic properties. Ketofol, which consists of 50 mg ketamine mixed with 90 mg propofol in a 10-mL syringe, is a useful combination for sedation in shorter procedures [15]. The desired intravenous sedative dose is then titrated as necessary up to a maximum of 0.3 mg/kg of ketamine, which gives a maximum dose of 0.5 mg/kg of

Table 25.6 Dosing schedule for "Ketofol"

Route	Dose	Onset	Duration of action	Repeat dose	Titration interval
IV	0.05 mL/kg[a]	30–90 s	5–10 min	0.05 mL/kg	1–5 min

Ketofol: 5 mg/mL Ketamine, 9 mg/mL Propofol
Reprinted with permission from Reed A, Thomas J, Roelofse JA, Gray R, de Kock M, Piercy J. Paediatric Procedural Sedation and Analgesia (PSA) Guidelines; South African Society of Anaesthesiologists. 2011
[a]0.25 mg/kg ketamine and 0.045 mg/kg propofol

propofol (Table 25.6). This combination is especially valuable and often used for short medical and dental procedures.

We now have a better understanding of the pharmacokinetics and pharmacodynamics of sufentanil in pediatric practice [45]. Sufentanil can be used as part of a multidrug infusion technique and is particularly useful in children undergoing dental procedures lasting longer than 30 min. Propofol (100 mg), ketamine (25 mg), and sufentanil (2.5 μ[mu]g) are mixed in the same syringe and infused at a rate of 1–4 mg/kg/h (dose calculated according to the propofol concentration) titrated to response. In a study looking at 202 children who received this combination, no significant adverse events were seen; 78.5 % of children were able to maintain their airway without any support from the sedation practitioner, 16 % of children needed support to keep the airway patent whilst the dentist depressed the lower jaw, 4 % of children needed occasional airway support, and 1.5 % of children needed airway support most of the time. Loss of airway patency was seen particularly at deeper levels of sedation, and in patients with tonsillar hypertrophy [46]. None of the children needed supplemental oxygen and vital signs remained stable throughout the procedure.

Multimodal Analgesia Without Opioids

The use of non-opioid analgesic combinations helps to relieve and attenuate discomfort following painful procedures. Non-steroidal anti-inflammatory drugs, alpha 2-agonists, paracetamol, and ketamine can all provide beneficial analgesic effects when administered as part of a multimodal sedation regimen. For painful procedures, an intravenous infusion of 15 mg/kg paracetamol over 20 min is initiated 30 min before the procedure. Immediately before the procedure, ketorolac can be administered at a bolus dose of 0.5 mg/kg intravenously. For longer procedures, ketorolac can be administered as an infusion of 0.17 mg/kg/h and supplemented with 0.5 mg/kg ketamine as needed [47]. Propofol is another option, administered as bolus or infusion.

Conclusion

In conclusion, the ideal approach to pediatric sedation in underdeveloped countries should be based on the concept of multimodal pain management [48]. This is unfortunately not always possible. For painful procedures performed under sedation outside the operating room, an aggressive perioperative analgesic and sedative approach that provides safe effective analgesia, patient comfort, and sedation while causing minimal side effects is needed. In addition, postoperative analgesia is crucial and can be achieved with a multimodal approach, which may incorporate the use of opioids. Opioids, used with discretion, play a crucial role in polypharmacy for painful procedures. It is anticipated that non-opioid analgesic drugs will assume a future key role as synergists for painful procedures outside the operating room.

Most importantly, as Africa and developing countries move forward in their evolution of sedation delivery, the training of sedation providers must come to the forefront. With a scarcity of physicians and skilled sedation providers, Africa and the developing nations must prioritize the importance of training non-physician providers. It has been established that in developing countries, poor outcomes are a consequence of inadequate assessment, monitoring, treatment and resuscitation skills [49, 50]. The International Liaison Committee on Resuscitation (ILCOR) performs regular reviews in order to present, validate, and support international guidelines [51]. In 2010, the ILCOR specifically reviewed the outcomes of developing countries with respect to resuscitation training and outcomes [52]. The findings revealed that although training (including human/manikins) and education in resuscitation skills (pediatric and adult) were deemed to be important and of value by the health care providers, their utility in terms of improving patient outcome has not been validated or demonstrated. Furthermore, the educational methodology and approach was inconsistent between facilities. Future efforts must be made to determine the best approach to educate and train sedation providers not only in sedation delivery, but also in resuscitation skills. By establishing this best approach, Africa and developing nations will be better equipped to demonstrate that these skills can directly translate into improved patient outcomes.

Case Studies

The following case studies are examples of didactic and practical material, which is part of problem-based learning for the Postgraduate Diploma in Sedation Diploma Course and Pain Control.

Case 1

A 6-month-old child presented for vesiculocystourethrogram and an intravenous pyelogram for recurrent cystitis. This child had a failed sedation on a previous attempt. Reflux and congenital renal defects are suspected. The child weighs 10 kg and has a chronic runny nose.

Proposed procedure:

- Procedural sedation to be done in the radiology suite with no anesthetic facilities or trained assistance available.
- Sedation practitioner needs to provide all drugs and materials needed for the sedation.
- The infant needs to have an intravenous line inserted.
- Urethral catheterization for administration of contrast via an infusion into the bladder is necessary.
- The patient needs to lie still enough over a half-hour period with repeated X-rays being taken.
- Then the catheter is then removed and the infant needs to void the bladder via a spontaneous spinal reflex and be X-rayed in the process.

Problems facing the sedation practitioner:

- Working in an unfamiliar environment with colleagues and staff who are unfamiliar with the sedation procedure and not trained in resuscitation techniques.
- The need to have all regular and emergency equipment available at the premises.
- The challenge of balancing a sufficient level of sedation with drugs to overcome the pain of the procedure, while guarding against too deep a level of sedation.
- The need to place and protect monitoring equipment and intravenous lines on a moving surface while X-rays are being taken.
- Prevention of hypothermia in a hospital maintained air-conditioned unit, while exposing the perineum and legs, and infusing cold liquids.
- To maintain an adequate airway while the infant is some distance away from the sedation practitioner and placed under an X-ray unit.
- Possible anaphylaxis to contrast.

Procedural Sedation and Analgesia

The infant is assessed the day before the operation. Special attention is paid to airway evaluation.

A lidocaine/prilocaine eutectic mixture (EMLA®, AstraZeneca, NSW, Australia) is placed over a vein on the hand or foot for cannulation. The child is kept NPO, as advised in the guidelines of the South African Society of Anesthesiologists. A yellow 24-gauge cannula is placed in a vein on the hand. Glycopyrrolate 0.005 mg/kg is administered intravenously. Glycopyrrolate is an anti-cholinergic drug and can interfere with bladder voiding. Sedation by titration with ketamine 0.5 mg/kg intravenously is started. This is followed by propofol, which is slowly titrated via a diluted propofol bolus of 0.3 mg/kg. Induction time varies and so does response, so unhurried small doses are best given over 5 min, until achieving the desired effect. The infant is wrapped in a warm blanket and nasal drops are instilled to clear the nasal pathway; a portable suction is useful to clear the nose of secretions. The head and neck is slightly extended on a little pillow to keep the airway patent. Titrated ketamine doses of 0.25 mg/kg are repeated at 10-min intervals as required for any painful stimulus. A low-dose propofol infusion is administered via an infusion pump at 2–4 mg/kg/h.

Pulse oximetry and an ECG for monitoring are essential; capnography is helpful and use should be encouraged. It is often necessary to transfer the child from the radiology suite to another room for the intravenous pyelogram. A transfer of all equipment thus also needs to be done. The child should be monitored closely to detect any respiratory depression. Recovery may be longer in infants and the sedation practitioner must remain at the child's side until discharge criteria are met.

Case 2

A 5-year-old child weighing 20 kg with a diagnosis of attention-deficit hyperactivity disorder (ADHD) presented to the dentist for dental treatment.

This is a question that sedation practitioners often face; can one sedate a child with ADHD as they are usually extremely difficult to handle? This is a controversial issue. Maybe a qualified yes if:

- The child's pediatrician is happy that the child is on optimum treatment for his disability.
- Instructions can be followed that no chronic medication be stopped or altered before the sedation.
- Parents receive documentation provided by the sedation practitioner; regarding time of sedation, time to be nil per mouth, time and instructions for the Emla® (AstraZeneca, NSW, Australia) patch, time to be at the surgery, information on sedation, and contact number of the sedation practitioner.
- The child is booked early in the morning as the first appointment.

Problems facing the sedation practitioner:

- It is going to be a challenge as no child has the same degree of ADHD. One can never predict the outcome.

(continued)

(continued)

- Children are usually very anxious trying to cope with a threatening environment that they possibly do not know well, and need to be treated with sympathetic care and understanding. Be prepared and do not be unrealistic.
- Always have a plan B in case plan A fails.
- Take into consideration the circumstances of the family and support system: physical, emotional, and intellectual.
- Be especially careful as some of the children may suffer from epilepsy. Stay away from drugs that may trigger epilepsy and use drugs that are safe to use.
- Know the pharmacokinetics and pharmacodynamics of the common drugs used for ADHD and possible drug interactions with the sedatives you plan to use.
- If possible, postpone the operation for the following morning.
- If this is really an emergency, a general anesthetic should be considered as an alternative operation.

Day of Treatment

The sedation practitioner must arrive at the surgery early and prepare for any possible need; including checking the equipment of the dentist, i.e., suction that is in working order and possible excess water from the drill. The parents and child must arrive 30 min before the procedure. Plan to do the child first in the morning when there are no other people in the waiting room. Recommendations on How to Proceed

Step 1: Always try to do a child with ADHD as the first scheduled appointment of the morning. An unfamiliar environment and a crowded space can upset a child with ADHD severely. Let him bring his toys and his own blanket with him.

Never let him undress or take him away from the person he is most comfortable with, i.e., the mother, father, caretaker or the person with whom he spends the most time. Check the position of the Emla® patch to ensure painless cannulation.

Step 2: Try to administer midazolam 5 mg orally as a sedative. A 7.5 mg midazolam tablet crushes easily between two teaspoons. Cover it with sugar in the spoon. A trick that works well is to take your finger and dip it in the sugar mix, taste it and ask the patient to do the same. Then he/she will not be too reluctant to swallow the whole spoon of "sugar." It is advisable to administer a sedative as it gives a baseline sedation effect from where one can build on with the intravenous sedation drugs. Always let the child go to the bathroom before you continue with the procedure.

Spend time to communicate with the family and the child. Check the name, weight, medical history (especially snoring), medication, adverse reactions to medication, previous anesthetics, consent, and aftercare. It is most important to make the family comfortable about the proposed sedation. Convince them that you will take care of their child with a caring and sympathetic attitude. Remember these parents have been through a lot of trauma with this child already. Many practitioners are just so busy that they do not take time with the patient and family, but when you do this you will be rewarded with a more relaxed patient. It must be remembered, this is sedation and not a general anesthetic.

Inform the parents to expect a sleepy child for a few hours at home after the procedure, how to treat bleeding and pain, and what to eat or drink.

Step 3: Entering the procedure room. This can be very difficult. This child takes methylphenidate (Ritalin®) LA 20 mg daily and sodium valproate (Epilim®) 300 mg daily. He refused to sit in the dental chair, only on his father's lap in the corner of the room. Though he is 5 years old, he has the mental age of a child aged 3 years.

The only way forward is to get intravenous access. A small dose of ketamine 0.25 mg/kg is administered. Ketamine plus midazolam usually make children drowsy. The next step is to make the child comfortable. A hand towel is rolled and put under the shoulders to extend the neck. The child is covered with a blanket as the air conditioning in the room is usually set to suit the dentist's needs. An ECG and a pulse oximeter are used to monitor the heart rate and oxygen saturation. A dose of 1 mg of midazolam and 0.2 mg of glycopyrrolate is administered intravenously. A mixture of 120 mg propofol, 20 mg ketamine, and 0.5 mg alfentanil is administered as a continuous solution and titrated at a rate of 2–4 mg/kg/h.

The dentist was able to do a dental examination and inform the parents what to expect. Eight teeth had to be removed.

Local anesthesia was administered and the dentist asked to reduce the water flowing from the drill. High volume suction was constantly used to prevent the child from having excess water in the mouth and pharynx.

The child was kept sedated with the propofol infusion at a flow rate between 2 and 4 mg/kg/h. He had an uneventful recovery after the procedure.

Case 3

A 3-year-old boy weighing 16 kg presented for an outpatient abdominal MRI scan for a suspected Wilm's tumor (nephroblastoma). There is no MRI-compatible anesthetic machine at the facility and a previous attempt to sedate the child with chloral hydrate has failed.

This is not an uncommon scenario in the developing world. Due to high outlay costs, the acquisition of an

(continued)

(continued)
MRI scanner without the purchase of a MRI-compatible anesthetic machine is commonplace. A typical MRI examination consists of two to six imaging sequences, each lasting up to 15 min. The whole procedure may take anywhere from 20 min to 2 h to be completed. Chloral hydrate is the drug most commonly used in South Africa for non-painful imaging, but has a small but significant failure rate particularly during the longer scans. The long duration of MRI scans provides a significant challenge to the sedationist, and often requires the use of innovative techniques to provide safe and effective sedation.

Proposed procedure—Respiratory gated MRI of the abdomen:

- Whilst in the MRI scanner, the child will need to lie completely still for up to an hour and a half.
- Intravenous gadolinium will need to be given as a contrast agent.
- Respiratory gating of the MRI scanner improves image quality, but requires reasonable chest excursion to trigger the phase encoding.

Problems facing the sedation practitioner:

- Previously failed sedation with no option of inducing general anesthesia.
- The MRI environment precludes the use of equipment containing ferromagnetic metals. The sedationist needs to be aware of the limitations and dangers of working in an MRI environment. The sedationist must be aware of local protocols for resuscitation and emergency evacuation of the patient from the scanner, should the need arise.
- MRI facilities generally do not have sedation rooms, and auxiliary professional nurses are generally not trained in sedation and airway management.
- The child may have raised intra-abdominal pressure due to the abdominal mass, which may put him at risk of regurgitation—airway reflexes should preferably be maintained.
- Prolonged sedation without respiratory depression is required.
- Rapid recovery would expedite discharge and is particularly important for outpatient procedures.

Procedural Sedation

- The child is seen on admission and a eutectic mixture of lidocaine and prilocaine (Emla®) is applied over a vein on the hand or foot and an occlusive dressing applied. The dressing is left on for at least 60 min to achieve adequate dermal analgesia. A 22- or 24-gauge intravenous cannula is inserted. Ideally, intravenous cannulation should take place in the admissions or holding area where adequate lighting and assistance are more likely to be available prior to transfer to the radiology suite.
- The child is transferred to the MRI suite. In the holding area, patency of the intravenous cannula is ascertained with a bolus of 0.9 % saline. An oximeter probe is placed on the child in the waiting area. Dexmedetomidine 1 mcg/kg is manually infused over a period of 10 min whist the child is sitting on his parent's lap. The child's sedation level is monitored and when the child appears relaxed and calm the oximeter is removed and he is transferred into the MRI scanner.
- A fiber-optic oximeter and protective earphones are placed on the child. A three-way stopcock and extension line for administration of gadolinium is attached to the intravenous cannula.
- Intravenous dexmedetomidine 0.5 mcg/kg/h is infused by an Alaris Asena syringe driver placed and kept outside the 10 Gauss line (approximately 3 m from the magnet in a 1.5 T machine), and attached to extension tubing of suitable length.
- The child is monitored by the sedationist who remains in the MRI room for the duration of the scan. The infusion of dexmedetomidine may be stopped at the start of the last MRI sequence and it is imperative that the sedationist personally attends the recovery of the child until he is fit for discharge.

Case 4

A 4-year-old boy weighing 18 kg presents for a burns dressing change and removal of surgical clips. He was involved in a house fire and sustained 23 % full thickness burns, which required excision and grafting. He has had a protracted hospital stay and is traumatized and anxious. The placement of a peripheral intravenous catheter is documented as being extremely difficult.

In South Africa, an estimated US$ 26 million is spent annually for care of burns from kerosene (paraffin) cooking stove incidents. This directly impacts the availability of health care resources, and resource requirements for burn victims often outstrip availability. Whereas burns dressing changes in the developed world usually take place under general anesthesia in theater, patients in the developing countries are often not afforded that luxury.

Proposed procedure—Burns dressing change and removal of clips:

- Procedural sedation to be performed in the ward with no anesthetic facilities.

(continued)

(continued)

- Dressing changes are painful and require intense procedural analgesia as well as good post-procedural analgesia.

Problems facing the sedation practitioner:

- Pediatric burns patients are often uncooperative as they frequently have protracted hospital stays and are invariably severely traumatized and anxious.
- Intravenous access is often challenging.
- Tolerance to analgesic and hypnotics is common.

Procedural Sedation and Analgesia

- The child is kept nil per mouth as per SASA guidelines [15]. (Refer to Chap. 2.)
- The child is seen preoperatively, oral midazolam 7.5 mg and oral ketamine 180 mg (10 mg/kg) are prescribed to be given 1 h preoperatively. Oral atropine 0.15 mg is prescribed as an anti-sialagogue. Oral paracetamol 360 mg (20 mg/kg) is also given to facilitate postoperative analgesia. A eutectic mixture of lidocaine and prilocaine is applied over a vein on an unburned hand or foot and an occlusive dressing applied. The dressing is left on for at least 60 min to achieve adequate dermal analgesia.
- Resuscitation drugs and equipment are prepared in the ward. Pulse oximetry and an ECG for monitoring are essential; capnography is helpful and its use should be encouraged.
- Intravenous access with a 22- or 24-gauge cannula is attempted. If venous cannulation is possible sedation may be supplemented with small intravenous aliquots of ketamine (0.5 mg/kg) as needed. If intravenous cannulation is impossible then sedation can be supplemented with either 50 % nitrous oxide in 50 % oxygen (Entonox) or additional ketamine intramuscularly (2–4 mg/kg).
- The sedation practitioner monitors the child closely throughout the procedure, paying special attention to the airway and respiratory adequacy whilst the head, neck and thorax are being dressed.
- Monitoring of the airway, respiratory rate and pattern, heart rate, oxygen saturation, and level of consciousness should continue in the recovery area. The sedation practitioner should assume overall responsibility for the patient in the recovery area, and should not leave the premises until the discharge criteria are met.

References

1. Lowrie L, Weiss AH, Lacombe C. The pediatric sedation unit: a mechanism for pediatric sedation. Pediatrics. 1998;102:9. http://www.pediatrics.org/cgi/content/full/102/3/e30.
2. Lalwani K, Michel M. Pediatric sedation in North American children's hospitals: a survey of anesthesia providers. Paediatr Anaesth. 2005;15:209–13.
3. Hodges SC, et al. Anaesthesia services in developing countries: defining the problems. Anaesthesia. 2007;62:4–11.
4. Hodges SC, et al. Paediatric anaesthesia in developing countries. Anaesthesia. 2007;62:26–31.
5. Kumar P. Providing the providers—remedying Africa's shortage of health care workers. N Engl J Med. 2007;356:2564–7.
6. Smallman B. Pediatric sedation: can it be safely performed by non-anesthesiologists. Curr Opin Anaesthesiol. 2002;15:455–9.
7. Standards for conscious sedation in dentistry: alternative techniques. A report from the standing dental advisory committee. http://www.rcseng.ac.uk/fds/docs/SCSDAT%202007.pdf. August 2007.
8. American Society of Anesthesiologists. Practice guidelines for sedation and analgesia by non-anesthesiologists: a report of the American Society of Anesthesiologist's Task Force on sedation and analgesia by non-anesthesiologists. Anesthesiology. 2002;96:1004–17.
9. American Academy of Pediatrics Committee on Drugs. Guidelines for maintaining and management of pediatric patients during and after sedation for diagnostic and therapeutic procedures: an update. Pediatrics. 2006;118:2587–602.
10. Joint Commission on Accreditation of Healthcare Organizations. Comprehensive accreditation manual for hospitals. Oakbrook: JCAHO; 2005.
11. Statement on granting privileges for deep sedation to non-anesthesiologist sedation practitioners. (Approved by the ASA House of Delegates on October 20, 2010). http://www.asahq.org/publicationsandservices/sgstoc.htm
12. Sedation in children and young people NICE Guidance. http://www.guidance.nice.org.uk
13. Koh JL, Black DD, Leatherman IK, Harrison RD, Schmitz ML. Experience with an anaesthesiologist interventional model for endoscopy in a pediatric hospital. J Pediatr Gastroenterol Nutr. 2001;33(3):314–8.
14. Hardmeier M, Zimmermann R, Ruegg S, et al. Intranasal midazolam: pharmacokinetics and pharmacodynamics assessed by quantitative EEG in healthy volunteers. Clin Pharmacol Ther. 2012;91(5):856–62.
15. Reed A, Thomas J, Roelofse JA, Gray R, de Kock M, Piercy J. Paediatric procedural sedation and analgesia (PSA) guidelines. South African Society of Anaesthesiologists; 2011.
16. Von Heijne M, Bredlov B, Soderhall S, Olsson GL. Propofol-alfentanil anaesthesia for painful procedures in the pediatric oncology ward. Paediatr Anaesth. 2004;14:670–5.
17. Hoffman GM, et al. Risk reduction in pediatric procedural sedation by application of an American Academy of Pediatrics/American Society of Anesthesiologists process model. Pediatrics. 2002;109:236–43.
18. Engelbrecht DJS. Recommendations for the management of the anxious and phobic patient in dental conscious sedation. (Master's thesis). London: University of Stellenbosch; 2005.
19. De Vos WH. The influence of cultural factors on the success rate of conscious sedation in children in the United Kingdom. (Master's thesis). London, University of the Western Cape; 2008.
20. Sury MRJ, Harker H, Begent WK, Chong WK. The management of infants and children for painless imaging. Clin Radiol. 2005; 60:731–41.
21. Roelofse JA, Joubert JJ, Roelofse PG. A double-blind randomized comparison of midazolam alone and midazolam combined with ketamine for sedation of pediatric dental patients. J Oral Maxillofac Surg. 1996;54:838–44.
22. Green SM, Krauss B. Clinical practice guideline for emergency department ketamine dissociative sedation in children. Ann Emerg Med. 2004;44:460–71.
23. Roelofse JA, Joubert JJ, Swart LC, Stander I, Roelofse PG. An evaluation of the effect of oral ketamine and standard oral

premedication in the sedation of paediatric dental patients. J Dent Assoc S Afr. 1996;51:197–201.
24. Brunette KEJ, Anderson BJ, Thomas J, et al. Exploring the pharmacokinetics of oral ketamine in children undergoing burns procedures. Paediatr Anaesth. 2011;21(6):653–62.
25. Roelofse JA, Van der Bijl P. Comparison of rectal midazolam and diazepam for premedication in pediatric dental patients. J Oral Maxillofac Surg. 1993;51:525–9.
26. van der Bijl P, Roelofse JA, Stander I. Rectal ketamine and midazolam for premedication in pediatric dentistry. J Oral Maxillofac Surg. 1991;49:1050–4.
27. Wilson G. Target controlled infusion anaesthesia in children. S Afr J Anaesthesiol Analg. 2010;16(1):124–6.
28. Alexopoulos E, Hope A, Clark SL, McHugh S, Hosey MT. A report on dental anxiety levels in children undergoing nitrous oxide inhalation sedation and propofol target controlled infusion intravenous sedation. Eur Arch Paediatr Dent. 2007;8(2):82–6.
29. Absalom A, Amutike D, Lal A, White M, Kenny GNC. Accuracy of the Paedfusor' in children undergoing cardiac surgery or catheterization. Br J Anaesth. 2003;91(4):507–13.
30. Sepúlveda P, Cortínez LI, Sáez C, Penna A, Solari S, Guerra I, Absalom AR. Performance evaluation of paediatric propofol pharmacokinetic models in healthy young children. Br J Anaesth. 2011;107(4):593–600.
31. Mason KP. Incidence and predictors of hypertension during high-dose dexmedetomidine sedation for pediatric MRI. Paediatr Anaesth. 2010;20(6):516–23.
32. Roelofse JA, Louw LR, Roelofse PGR. A double-blind randomized comparison of oral trimeprazine- methadone and ketamine-midazolam for sedation for pediatric dental patients for oral surgical procedures. Anesth Prog. 1998;45:3–11.
33. Roelofse JA, Roelofse PGR. Oxygen desaturation in a child receiving a combination of ketamine and midazolam for dental extractions. Anesth Prog. 1997;44:68–70.
34. Littlejohn IH, Tarling MM, Flynn AJ, Ordman AJ, Aiken A. Postoperative pain relief in children following extraction of carious deciduous teeth under general anaesthesia: a comparison of nalbuphine and diclofenac. Eur J Anaesthesiol. 1996;13:359–63.
35. Roelofse JA, Payne KA. Oral tramadol: analgesic efficacy in children following multiple dental extractions. Eur J Anaesthesiol. 1999;16:441–7.
36. Payne KA, Roelofse JA, Shipton EA. Pharmacokinetics of oral tramadol drops for postoperative pain relief in children aged four to seven years—a pilot study. Anesth Prog. 2002;49:109–12.
37. Payne KA, Roelofse JA. Tramadol drops in children: analgesic efficacy, lack of respiratory effects, and normal recovery times. Anesth Prog. 1999;46:91–6.
38. Henderson JM, Brodsky DA, Fisher DM, et al. Pre-induction of anesthesia in pediatric patients with nasally administered sufentanil. Anesthesiology. 1988;68:671–5.
39. Roelofse JA, Shipton EA, de la Harpe CJ, Blignaut RJ. Intranasal sufentanil/midazolam versus ketamine/midazolam in the pediatric population prior to undergoing multiple dental extractions under general anesthesia: a prospective, double-blind, randomized comparison. Anesth Prog. 2004;51:114–21.
40. Scholz J, Steinfath M, Schulz M. Clinical pharmacokinetics of alfentanil, fentanyl and sufentanil—an update. Clin Pharmacokinet. 1996;31(4):275–92.
41. Egan TD, Kern SE, Muir KT, White J. Remifentanil by bolus injection: a safety, pharmacokinetic, pharma-codynamic, and age effect investigation in human volunteers. Br J Anaesth. 2004; 92(3):335–43.
42. Bester EJ. Multidrug sedation in children for dental procedures under the age of 8 years. (Master's thesis). Cape Town: University of the Western Cape; 2005.
43. Van Vuuren N Janse. Multidrug intravenous sedation in children aged 5–9 years for dental procedures. (Master's thesis). London: University of the Western Cape; 2009.
44. Roelofse J. Paediatric sedation. Br Dent J. 2009;206:55.
45. Lundeberg S, Roelofse JA. Aspects of pharmacokinetics and pharmacodynamics of sufentanil in pediatric practice. Paediatr Anaesth. 2011;21:274–9.
46. Swart E. The efficay and safety of intravenous sedation in children under the age of 10 years. (Masters thesis). Cape Town: University of the Western Cape; 2013.
47. Prins SA, Van Dijk M, Van Leeuwen P, Searke S, Andreson BJ, Tibboel D, et al. Pharmacokinetic and analgesic effects of intravenous propacetamol vs rectal paracetamol in children after major craniofacial surgery. Paediatr Anaesth. 2008;18: 582–92.
48. White PF. Editorial review: multimodal pain management—the future is now! Curr Opin Investig Drugs. 2007;8(7):517–8.
49. Nolan T, Angos P, Cunha AJ, et al. Quality of hospital care for seriously ill children in less-developed countries. Lancet. 2001;357: 106–10.
50. English M, Esamai F, Wasunna A, et al. Assessment of inpatient paediatric care in first referral level hospitals in 13 districts in Kenya. Lancet. 2004;363:1948–53.
51. Chamberlain DA, Cummins RO. Advisory statements of the International Liaison Committee on Resuscitation ('ILCOR'). Resuscitation. 1997;34:99–100.
52. Meaney PA, Topjian AA, Chandler HK, et al. Resuscitation training in developing countries: a systematic review. Resuscitation. 2010; 81(11):1462–72.

Part III

Safety in Sedation

Pediatric Sedatives and the Food and Drug Administration (FDA): Challenges, Limitations, and Drugs in Development

26

Lisa L. Mathis and Lynne P. Yao

Abstract

Imaging, invasive diagnostics, and minor surgical procedures on pediatric patients outside the operating room setting have increased, and there is a need for sedatives that have been properly assessed in the pediatric population for this indication. This chapter will review the process of obtaining Food and Drug Administration (FDA) approval of a drug or biologic for use in pediatric patients with a focus on sedation. The FDA approves products based on an independent review of evidence obtained from chemistry and manufacturing data, toxicology and pharmacology studies, and clinical trials. During the review of the marking application, the FDA must assess whether the drug is safe and effective in its proposed use(s), and whether the benefits of the drug outweigh the risks.

Keywords

Pediatric sedatives • Food and Drug Administration (FDA) • Pharmacokinetics (PK) • "Off-label" use • Food and Drug Modernization Act of 1997 (FDAMA) • Pediatric exclusivity • Best Pharmaceuticals for Children Act (BPCA) • Pediatric Research Equity Act (PREA) • Pharmacokinetics • Pharmacodynamics • Food • Food, Drug, and Cosmetic (FD&C) Act • Investigational New Drug (IND) Application • New Drug Application (NDA)

Introduction

In order for new medications to be marketed in the United States, they must be approved under the Food, Drug, and Cosmetic (FD&C) Act. The Food and Drug Administration (FDA) approves products based on an independent review of evidence obtained from chemistry and manufacturing data, toxicology and pharmacology studies, and clinical trials. Sponsors submit data for approval of a drug to the FDA in a marketing application.[1] Under the FD&C Act, drug manufacturers must demonstrate effectiveness of their products through the conduct of adequate and well-controlled studies to obtain marketing approval [1]. During the review of the marketing application, the FDA must assess whether the drug is safe and effective in its proposed use(s), and whether the benefits of the drug outweigh the risks. The FDA must also determine whether the methods used in manufacturing the drug and the controls used to maintain the drug's quality are adequate to preserve the drug's identity, strength, quality, and purity. Finally, the FDA must determine whether the drug's proposed labeling is appropriate and what it should contain.

Imaging, invasive diagnostics, and minor surgical procedures on pediatric patients outside the operating room setting have increased, and there is a need for sedatives that have

L.L. Mathis, M.D. (✉)
Department of Global Regulatory Affairs and Safety, Maternal and Pediatric Safety and Regulatory, Amgen Inc., Thousand Oaks, CA, USA
e-mail: lmathis@amgen.com

L.P. Yao, M.D.
Office of New Drugs, Center for Drug Evaluation and Research, US FDA, Silver Spring, MD, USA
e-mail: lynne.yao@fda.hhs.gov

[1] For the purposes of this chapter, future references to the term "drug" will include both drug and biologic products.

K.P. Mason (ed.), *Pediatric Sedation Outside of the Operating Room: A Multispecialty International Collaboration*, DOI 10.1007/978-1-4939-1390-9_26, © Springer Science+Business Media New York 2015

been properly assessed in the pediatric population for this indication. This chapter will review the process of obtaining the FDA approval of a drug or biologic for use in pediatric patients with a focus on sedation.

General Drug Development

Under current US regulations, any use of a drug or biologic not previously approved for marketing requires submission of an Investigational New Drug (IND) Application to the FDA. The data gathered during the IND phase (chemical analyses, animal studies, and human clinical trials) become part of the marketing application. The development of a medication for sedation is a stepwise process involving an evaluation of chemistry, nonclinical (i.e., animal), and clinical information (i.e., dosing, efficacy, and safety). While pediatric studies may begin during the IND phase for some products, for many products, including those used for sedation, it is likely that most of the clinical trials would begin after adult efficacy and safety have been established (Fig. 26.1).

Initial studies in humans (Phase 1 trials) are the first stage of testing in human subjects. Often, during this phase of development, a small number (e.g., 20–50 people) of healthy adult volunteers will be tested in trials designed to assess the first time use in humans for safety, tolerability, proof of concept for efficacy, and pharmacokinetics.

Pharmacokinetic (PK) parameters are often assessed in Phase 2 studies. PK studies provide information on the systemic exposure of a drug after administration. Important PK measurements include area under the curve (AUC) and maximum concentration (C_{max}), clearance (C), half-life ($T_{1/2}$), and volume of distribution (V_d). These parameters are all used to characterize a drug's absorption (A), distribution (D), metabolism (M), and elimination (E). The overall process (ADME) ultimately controls the systemic exposure to a drug and its metabolites after administration. Pharmacokinetic parameters must be considered when establishing the appropriate dose of a drug.

Once the first human exposure has been completed, and some PK parameters assessed, additional studies (Phase 2 studies) are performed on a larger number of participants (e.g., 20–300 patients) to assess the treatment effect size, provide safety assessments, and test the response to different doses in a larger group of volunteers and patients. The information obtained from Phase 2 studies is critical in designing the definitive Phase 3 studies.

The Phase 3 studies should leverage the data from all other nonclinical and clinical trials to determine an appropriate dose(s), and to estimate the number of patients required to demonstrate efficacy based on the expected treatment effect size. The clinical trials must also include sufficient numbers of patients with sufficient length of exposure to adequately assess the safety of the product for its intended use. Phase 3 studies are intended to provide substantial evidence of safety and effectiveness of the product and should therefore be designed as adequate and well-controlled studies [2].

A marketing application, or New Drug Application (NDA),[2] is submitted to the FDA once all required studies have been completed to support a new drug for marketing. A supplemental NDA (sNDA) may be submitted if the industry seeks to change the indication or population for a pharmaceutical product that has already been approved. The application must contain all information necessary to market the product including:

- A technical description of methods used in manufacturing (good manufacturing practice, GMP) and data on the drug's quality (supporting the drug's identity, strength, stability, and purity)

[2]Biologics Licensing Application (BLA) and supplement Biologics Licensing Application (sBLA) are submitted for biological products.

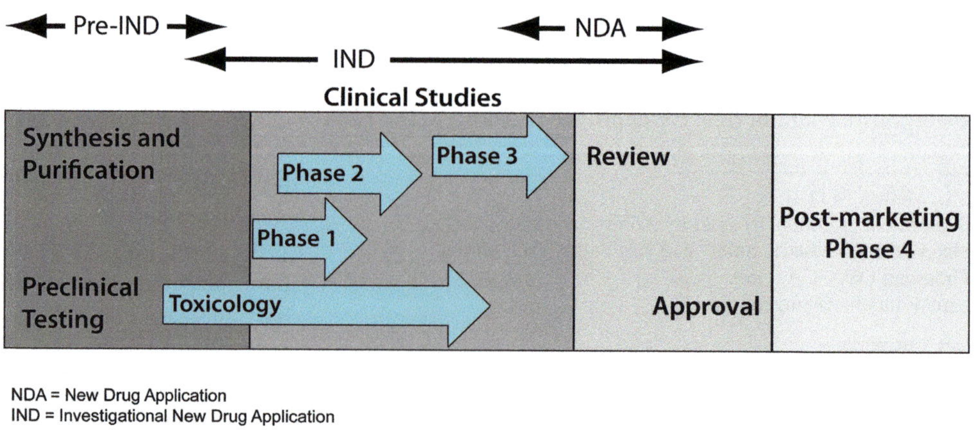

Fig. 26.1 Phases of drug development. *NDA* New Drug Application, *IND* Investigational New Drug Application

- Complete data from preclinical and clinical studies to support the safety and effectiveness of the drug in its proposed use(s)
- The drug's proposed labeling (package insert)

The product labeling describes the conditions of study, to include the patient population(s) studied, the dose(s) used, and the end point(s) assessed. Use(s) of the product under the specific conditions described in the product labeling is known as "on-label use." Uses of the product outside of these parameters, including any conditions or diseases, populations, or dosages not found in labeling, are known as "off-label" use.

Pediatric Legislation

Historically, many drugs, including those used in sedation, were not studied in pediatrics, and thus, the majority of drugs used in pediatric practice were "off label." Approximately 75 % of medicines used in children did not include specific pediatric prescribing information prior to implementation of legislation encouraging and requiring the study of medication in the pediatric population [3]. While the number of drugs with specific pediatric labeling information has improved under this process, the majority of commonly used sedatives continue to lack specific pediatric labeling or robust efficacy and safety data in children (Table 26.1).

Prior to the passage of important pediatric legislation, many pharmaceutical manufacturers were reluctant to study drugs in children due to ethical and financial constraints or trial design challenges [4]. However, the pediatric population accounts for 25 % of the US population and, therefore, represents a population that must be addressed during product development [5].

Because of the historic lack of data from adequate and well-controlled clinical trials, medications were often administered to children empirically, assuming that they were "little adults." This simplistic and often erroneous assumption resulted in pediatric dosing recommendations derived solely as fractions of adult dosing rather than on intrinsic factors based on known differences in growth and development (e.g., volume of distribution and maturation of metabolic pathways). Safety and efficacy were also simply assumed to be the same in the pediatric and the adult populations and did not take into account both known and potential safety and efficacy differences that may be present in a growing and developing pediatric patient.

The Food and Drug Modernization Act of 1997 (FDAMA) created an incentive program known as pediatric exclusivity. This provision allowed the FDA to issue a formal request, known as a Written Request, outlining the studies needed on a specific drug for one or more conditions or indications. The Written Request includes details of study design, number of patients needed, and important safety and efficacy endpoints to be measured. The Written Request also includes a due date for submission of the study data to the FDA. The FDA can grant 6 months of marketing exclusivity to sponsors who complete the voluntary pediatric studies using good scientific principles, blocking the approval of generics for the entire product line and all indications already approved, resulting in financial return for the sponsor who performed the studies [6]. Although FDAMA was to sunset on January 1, 2002, the incentive was reauthorized by the Best Pharmaceuticals for Children Act (BPCA) of 2002, 2007, and again in 2012. The most recent reauthorization of BPCA was permanent and does not sunset. Additionally, the ability to obtain pediatric exclusivity was extended to biologic products under the Patient Protection and Affordable Care Act of 2010.

After a patent expires for a drug, additional pediatric exclusivity provides no incentive for drug manufacturers to study the drug. Additionally, situations arise in which the FDA has issued a Written Request for a drug with existing patent protection but the sponsor declines the Written Request. In order to obtain important pediatric dosing, efficacy, and safety information in these drugs, an important section of BPCA was included to address these situations. This section of BPCA allows for the FDA to issue a Written Request first to the application holder(s), and then, if declined, forward it on to the National Institutes of Health (NIH), National Institute of Child Health and Human Development (NICHD).

Under these programs, almost one-third of the products studied had new, pediatric-specific safety information included in labeling. Among those safety findings were rare cases of seizures reported in pediatric patients in association with sevoflurane use for induction/maintenance of general anesthesia. Most cases were in children and young adults, most of whom had no medical history of seizures [7].

The Pediatric Research Equity Act (PREA), first enacted in 2003, requires pediatric assessments of new drugs for all new active ingredients, indications, dosage forms, dosing regimens, and routes of administration. The pediatric assessment must include data adequate to assess the dosing, safety, and effectiveness of the product for the claimed indications in all relevant pediatric subpopulations. PREA works in conjunction with BPCA, but unlike BPCA, PREA applies only to those drugs developed for diseases and/or conditions that occur in both the adult and pediatric populations. Drugs that have been granted Orphan Designation (i.e., intended to treat rare diseases) are exempt from PREA. PREA, like BPCA, was also permanently reauthorized under the Food and Drug Administration Safety and Innovation Act of 2012.

Implementation of BPCA and PREA has led to the addition of specific pediatric information in more than 500 product labels (1997–2013). Pediatric studies resulted in an

Table 26.1 Common sedatives and their use for children

Agent	Approved indication(s)[a]	Pediatric information
Chloral hydrate[b]	Manufacturing of chloral hydrate oral solution discontinued in 2012	Drug not approved by the FDA
Dexmedetomidine	• Sedation of initially intubated and mechanically ventilated patients during treatment in an intensive care setting • Sedation of nonintubated patients prior to and/or during surgical and other procedures	The efficacy, safety, and pharmacokinetics in patients less than 18 years of age have not been established. Therefore, this product should not be used in this population
Diazepam, injectable	• Adjunct for relief of skeletal muscle spasm due to reflex spasm to local pathology (such as inflammation of the muscles or joints, or secondary to trauma) • Spasticity caused by upper motor neuron disorders (such as cerebral palsy and paraplegia), athetosis, stiff-man syndrome, and tetanus • Adjunct in status epilepticus and severe recurrent convulsive seizures • Premedication (intramuscular) for relief of anxiety and tension in patients who are to undergo surgical procedures. Intravenously prior to cardioversion for the relief of anxiety and tension and to diminish the patient's recall of the procedure	• Although anxiolytic indication appears in labeling for adults, pediatric approval and dosing information are limited to use in tetanus and status epilepticus and recurrent convulsive seizures • Not approved below 30 days of life
Etomidate	Induction of general anesthesia	There are inadequate data to make dosage recommendations for induction of anesthesia in patients below the age of 10 years; therefore, such use is not recommended
Fentanyl citrate, injectable	• For analgesic action of short duration during the anesthetic periods, premedication, induction and maintenance, and in the immediate postoperative period (recovery room) as the need arises • For use as a narcotic analgesic supplement in general or regional anesthesia • For administration with a neuroleptic as an anesthetic premedication, for the induction of anesthesia, and as an adjunct in the maintenance of general and regional anesthesia • For use as an anesthetic agent with oxygen in selected high-risk patients, such as those undergoing open heart surgery or certain complicated neurological or orthopedic procedures	• The safety and efficacy of fentanyl citrate in children under 2 years of age have not been established • Rare cases of unexplained clinically significant methemoglobinemia have been reported in premature neonates undergoing emergency anesthesia and surgery, which included the combined use of fentanyl, pancuronium, and atropine. A direct cause-and-effect relationship between the combined use of these drugs and the reported cases of methemoglobinemia has not been established
Fospropofol	• A sedative–hypnotic agent indicated for the monitored anesthesia care (MAC) sedation in adult patients undergoing diagnostic or therapeutic procedures	Safety and effectiveness in pediatric patients have not been established because fospropofol has not been studied in patients <18 years of age. Fospropofol is not recommended for use in this population
Ketamine	• Sole anesthetic agent for diagnostic and surgical procedures that do not require skeletal muscle relaxation • Induction of anesthesia prior to the administration of other general anesthetic agents • To supplement low-potency agents, such as nitrous oxide	Safety and effectiveness in pediatric patients below the age of 16 have not been established
Lorazepam	• Treatment of status epilepticus • In adult patients for preanesthetic medication, producing sedation (sleepiness or drowsiness), relief of anxiety, and a decreased ability to recall events related to the day of surgery	• Pediatric pharmacokinetic data included in labeling • No pediatric dosing included in labeling • There are insufficient data to support the efficacy of injectable lorazepam as a preanesthetic agent in patients less than 18 years of age • Information in labeling about the "gasping syndrome" associated with benzyl alcohol, polyethylene glycol, and propylene glycol, components of lorazepam injection

Methohexital	In adults as follows: • IV induction of anesthesia prior to the use of other general anesthetic agents • IV induction of anesthesia and as an adjunct to subpotent inhalational anesthetic agents for short surgical procedures • Along with other parental agents, usually narcotic analgesics, to supplement subpotent anesthetic agents for longer surgical procedures • IV anesthesia for short surgical, diagnostic, or therapeutic procedures associated with painful stimuli • As an agent for inducing a hypnotic state	Methohexital can be used in pediatric patients older than 1 month as follows: • For rectal or IM induction of anesthesia prior to the use of other general anesthetic agents • For rectal or IM induction of anesthesia and as an adjunct to subpotent inhalational anesthetic agents for short surgical procedures • The safety and effectiveness of methohexital in pediatric patients below the age of 1 month have not been established. Studies of methohexital intravenously in pediatric patients have been reported in the published literature. The literature is not adequate to establish the safety and effectiveness in pediatric patients • Pediatric dosing information is included in labeling
Midazolam	• IM or IV for preoperative sedation/anxiolysis/amnesia • IV as an agent for sedation/anxiolysis/amnesia prior to or during diagnostic, therapeutic, or endoscopic procedures, such as bronchoscopy, gastroscopy, cystoscopy, coronary angiography, cardiac catheterization, oncology procedures, radiologic procedures, suture of lacerations, and other procedures either alone or in combination with other CNS depressants • IV for induction of general anesthesia, before administration of other anesthetic agents. IV midazolam can also be used as a component of intravenous supplementation of nitrous oxide and oxygen (balanced anesthesia) • Continuous intravenous infusion for sedation of intubated and mechanically ventilated patients as a component of anesthesia or during treatment in a critical care setting	• The safety and efficacy of midazolam for sedation/anxiolysis/amnesia following single-dose intramuscular administration, intravenously by intermittent injections, and continuous infusion have been established in pediatric and neonatal patients • Midazolam should not be administered by rapid injection in the neonatal population. Severe hypotension and seizures have been reported following rapid IV administration, particularly with concomitant use of fentanyl
Nitrous oxide[b]	This drug has not been found by the FDA to be safe and effective, and this labeling has not been approved by the FDA Safety and efficacy not established in children	Drug not approved by the FDA
Pentobarbital, injectable	• Sedatives • Hypnotics, for the short-term treatment of insomnia, since they appear to lose their effectiveness for sleep induction and sleep maintenance after 2 weeks • Preanesthetics • Anticonvulsant, in anesthetic doses, in the emergency control of certain acute convulsive episodes, e.g., those associated with status epilepticus, cholera, eclampsia, meningitis, tetanus, and toxic reactions to strychnine or local anesthetics	• No adequate well-controlled studies have been conducted in pediatric patients; however, safety and effectiveness of pentobarbital in pediatric patients are supported by numerous studies and case reports cited in the literature • The recommended pediatric dosage ranges from 2 to 6 mg/kg as a single IM injection not to exceed 100 mg
Propofol	• IV sedative–hypnotic agent that can be used for both induction and/or maintenance anesthesia as part of a balanced anesthetic technique for inpatient and outpatient surgery	• Approved for induction down to 3 years of age and maintenance of anesthesia down to 2 months of age • Not recommended for induction of anesthesia below the age of 3 years or for maintenance of anesthesia below the age of 2 months because its safety and effectiveness have not been established in those populations • Not indicated for use in pediatric ICU sedation since the safety of this regimen has not been established
Thiopental	Manufacturing of thiopental discontinued in 2011	No pediatric use or dosage information

[a]Based on most recent labeling as of September 2013

[b]Unapproved drugs: the Food, Drug, and Cosmetic Act generally requires that drugs marketed in the United States be shown to be both safe and effective prior to marketing and widespread use in the general population. The FDA's evidence-based system of drug approval and the OTC monograph system play essential roles in ensuring that drugs are both safe and effective. For a variety of historical reasons, some drugs, mostly older products, continue to be marketed illegally in the United States without required the FDA approval

approved pediatric sedation indication for midazolam, and an induction and/or maintenance of anesthesia indication for propofol. A Written Request for lorazepam has been issued, and studies are pending.

Dexmedetomidine was initially approved in the adult population for intubated and mechanically ventilated patients during treatment in an intensive care setting, and for sedation of nonintubated patients prior to and/or during surgical and other procedures. Subsequent to the studies performed under the pediatric legislation, dexmedetomidine labeling states that safety and efficacy have not been established for procedural or ICU sedation in pediatric patients based on one assessor-blinded trial in pediatric patients and two open-label studies in neonates. These studies did not meet their primary efficacy endpoints.

Both lorazepam and ketamine have been placed on a priority list by NIH to be studied under BPCA, and pediatric studies using lorazepam are currently underway. A randomized, double-blind, dose-controlled clinical trial of fospropofol disodium injection in adolescent patients (12–18 years old) undergoing upper endoscopy and randomized, double-blind, dose-controlled clinical trial in infants and very young children (ages 1 month up to 3 years old) undergoing sedation for procedures such as lumbar puncture and/or magnetic resonance imaging (MRI) are still pending as a PREA study requirement. The studies of the youngest patients will not be conducted until nonclinical studies in animals delineating risks of apoptosis are complete.

Drug Development for Pediatrics

Rational drug development depends on a thorough evaluation of all available data, including both nonclinical and clinical studies, prior to initiation of pediatric studies. Evaluation of these data should be used to inform a study design in pediatric patients that will best support the dosing, safety, and efficacy of the drug.

The timeframe for consideration of trials in the pediatric population depends on what is known about the compound and the circumstances surrounding clinical use of the product. Planning for pediatric studies should begin early and as soon as there is evidence that the product may provide benefit to the pediatric population. Drug development for the pediatric population requires a unique focus, and a full review must be performed of the chemistry, manufacturing, nonclinical, and clinical data to assess the potential for effects unique to the pediatric population. Under the Food and Drug Administration Safety and Innovation Act signed into law in 2012, drug manufacturers are required to submit their plans for pediatric drug development earlier in development. The goal of this law is to encourage drug developers to evaluate products for use in pediatric populations sooner when feasible, ultimately leading to faster incorporation of pediatric-specific use information in drug labeling.

Chemistry, Manufacturing, and Controls

While most chemistry, manufacturing, and control (CMC) issues are resolved once a product has been developed for adults, there are unique CMC aspects for pediatrics that must be addressed. Many medications that are administered by mouth are marketed initially as tablets or capsules. Not all children are capable of swallowing tablets or capsules, particularly young children or those with physical or cognitive impairment. Most children 6 years of age and older can swallow tablets or capsules, but even up to 10 % of patients aged 6–12 years cannot swallow this dosage form. PREA requires the development of an age-appropriate formulation unless the sponsor can show reasonable attempts to produce a formulation have failed. Examples of age-appropriate formulations include, but are not limited to, oral suspensions and solutions; sprinkles; dissolvable strips, tablets, and capsules; and intravenous/intramuscular solutions. Stratification for a study of an oral agent may involve dividing patients into two groups: those capable of swallowing the tablet or capsule (e.g., patients >6 years of age) and those who cannot.

In addition to the need for development of specific formulations for a given age group, the route of administration may also affect stratification due to dosing issues as well as safety concerns. For example, absorption of oral medications in infants may be unpredictable due to erratic and delayed gastric emptying, alkaline gastric pH, and diminished intestinal and biliary secretion [8]. Thus, drugs administered by mouth may require enrichment of patient enrollment in younger age groups.

Not only is appropriate formulation development important for pediatrics, so is the availability of a flexible dosage form. Unlike adults, most pediatric patients are dosed on a milligram per kilogram basis; thus, dosage forms must be flexible to allow for this. Additionally, formulations that appear ready to use in all populations (intravenous or oral solution) may contain excipients that may be harmful to specific pediatric populations. For example, benzyl alcohol, a preservative used in some products for intravenous administration, can cause gasping syndrome in preterm infants and thus render the product unsafe for use in this population [9].

Nonclinical Studies

Nonclinical studies are required for the approval of all drugs and biologics; however, additional toxicology testing may be needed before proceeding into the pediatric population.

The nonclinical safety evaluation of drugs intended for use in pediatrics should primarily focus on potential effects on growth and development that have not been studied or identified in previous nonclinical and/or clinical studies. Juvenile animal testing may be useful in assessing potential developmental age-specific toxicities and differences in sensitivity between adult and juvenile animals.

The known pharmacological and toxicological properties of the drug relative to the proposed patient population should be considered. Juvenile animal studies are especially relevant when known target organ toxicity occurs in adults in tissues that undergo significant postnatal development, such as the nervous system. This is particularly relevant for the sedative class because the mechanism of action results from effects on the central nervous system.

Both rodent and primate studies have demonstrated a potential risk of apoptosis in the developing brain when anesthetics such as ketamine are administered [10–12]. Drugs that act as *N*-methyl-D-aspartate (NMDA) receptor antagonists and those that act in an agonistic manner at the aminobutyric acid (GABA) receptor (aka GABA-mimetics) induce neuronal injury and death in the brains of juvenile rodents [13]. Drugs that exert their effects at one or both of these receptors include benzodiazepines, inhaled anesthetics, chloral hydrate, etomidate, propofol, ketamine, and nitrous oxide. While evidence of neuronal susceptibility to neurotoxic insult has come from recent studies, these data also demonstrate variability in susceptibility to toxicity based on development, dose, and duration of exposure. While these findings have led to a recommendation to delay surgeries requiring sedation if possible, no specific changes in clinical practice guidelines have been recommended at this time [14]. The methodologies for assessing this type of toxicity in humans have not been developed, and while concerning, the clinical relevance of these findings in humans remains unknown. It is even more difficult to determine how these data translate into the risk for pediatric patients requiring sedation for a necessary procedure outside of the operating room (e.g., lumbar puncture, bone marrow aspirate, orthopedic intervention, suturing, dental work, etc.).

During drug development, there is not only a need for the toxicological assessments to focus primarily on the active chemical ingredient, but testing the inactive ingredients in the clinical formulation can also be important, particularly when a drug's ADME profile is altered by the inactive ingredients or when uncharacterized excipients are present.

Clinical Trials

Ultimately, in order to establish substantial evidence of effectiveness and safety of a product in a pediatric population, clinical trials must be performed. Both the appropriate timing of such studies and the types of studies to be conducted depend on the treatment and condition being studied. There are many important factors that must be considered in designing a successful pediatric clinical trial, including protection of pediatric study participants, determination of the correct dose(s) and study endpoints, extrapolation of efficacy, recruitment and retention of an adequate number of patients, and choice of controls.

Ethics

Studies in pediatric patients have specific ethical considerations that must be followed. These principals are described fully in 21CFR part 50, subpart D, "Additional Protections for Children Involved as Subjects in Research." Children may be involved in biomedical research only after there is some evidence that the product may provide benefit to the pediatric population, and this should be established in the adult population, if possible. The regulation also requires that for any treatment or procedure performed in pediatric investigations that constitutes more than a minor increase over minimal risk, there must be the potential for the enrolled child to benefit from the treatment. Furthermore, a minor child cannot legally consent to participate in a study, and this, coupled with the fact that the child must have the potential for direct benefit, means that generally, only children with the condition of interest can be enrolled in the clinical trials. This principle holds for pharmacokinetic and pharmacodynamic studies as well as studies assessing safety and efficacy. Therefore, studies that can be performed in healthy adults, such as bioavailability studies, cannot be performed in healthy children.

Pharmacokinetics and Pharmacodynamics

Pediatric pharmacokinetics can differ from adult pharmacokinetics due to intrinsic factors, such as organ development, body weight, and body surface area. Growth and development can also lead to changes in pharmacokinetic parameters. In children, growth and development are rapid; therefore, adjustment in dose within a single patient over the treatment period may be important to maintain a stable systemic exposure for both appropriate safety and efficacy evaluations.

The pediatric population includes a broad range of ages, from newborns to teenagers—groups that are different in many ways. Generally, age groupings for pediatric studies are outlined as in Table 26.2, but may differ based on characteristics of the underlying condition, of the drug, or of the patient population.

While traditional PK studies in the adult population may require intensive blood sampling, there are times when an

Table 26.2 Age groups for pediatric studies

Age groups
≥1 to <6 months
6 months to <2 years
2 to <6 years
6 to <12 years
12–18 years

alternate approach in pediatrics is required because of their limited blood volume. One strategy for obtaining adequate PK information in pediatric populations is to perform a population PK study rather than a traditional PK study. This approach relies on infrequent (sparse) sampling of blood from a larger population than would be used in a standard pharmacokinetic study. Samples can be collected at various times of day and/or repeatedly over time in a given patient. Estimates of both population and individual means, as well as estimates of intra- and intersubject variability, can be obtained if the population PK study is properly designed. A large number of patients are generally needed, which can be a challenge in some pediatric diseases and conditions. Additionally, as mentioned previously, adult PK studies can often be performed in healthy volunteers, but this is not the case in pediatrics. Under most circumstances, only children with the condition of interest can be enrolled in the clinical trials because of special protections afforded to special populations under 21CFR part 50, subpart D.

Pharmacokinetic studies should be designed to identify a lowest *effective dose* for the drug (i.e., the lowest dose that demonstrates a clinically meaningful treatment effect) and a range of doses that can be used in the Phase 3 trials. Multiple doses should be evaluated for each age group; for example, the Written Request for rocuronium (for use during anesthesia) required three doses to be studied. The selection of the doses to be used in a pharmacokinetic study can be informed by literature, current medical practice, and/or dosing in adults.

The term pharmacodynamics (PD), or the response component of the exposure–response measurement, refers to measurement of both the desired and the undesired effects of the drug. Pharmacodynamic endpoints should also be measured when collecting blood and/or urine samples to provide some understanding of concentration–response relationships for both efficacy and safety. When possible, both PK and PD data in pediatric trials should be collected and analyzed to determine how the two are linked, i.e., the PK/PD (or exposure–response) relationship. For studies evaluating drugs for pediatric sedation, age-appropriate sedation scale(s) must be used for Phase 2 and Phase 3 studies. Since the studies will likely be multicenter, the same age-appropriate instruments must be used at each study site.

Although additional validation is needed, several scales may be considered for use in nonverbal children, particularly the COMFORT/COMFORT-behavioral scale and the University of Michigan Sedation Scale (UMSS). The studies supported by the NIH/NICHD in response to a Written Request issued by the FDA for the use of lorazepam for sedation used the COMFORT scale to measure sedation. In an objective measure derived from electroencephalogram (EEG) recordings, the bispectral index (BIS) may also be useful for monitoring the depth of sedation. Additionally, capnography, along with pulse oximetry, should be used to monitor for hypoventilation.

The data from the Phase 2 studies should be carefully reviewed to inform the appropriate study design and statistical analysis plan for Phase 3 studies. In addition, data collected from Phase 2 studies can be used as additional support for extrapolation of efficacy from adequate and well-controlled adult trials (see following section).

Extrapolation

Extrapolation from adult efficacy data to the pediatric population describes the reliance on adequate and well-controlled efficacy studies in adults to support a finding of efficacy in the pediatric population. When extrapolation is used, it is generally supplemented by additional studies in the pediatric population, usually pharmacokinetic and safety studies. Extrapolation is based on a prior conclusion that the course of the disease or condition and the effects of the drug are sufficiently similar in adults and pediatric patients to allow extrapolation. Additionally, extrapolation from one pediatric age group to another (e.g., older to younger or vice versa) may preclude the necessity for separate studies in each pediatric age group. However, the safety profile of any drug may be different in adults when compared to children, and thus, safety cannot be extrapolated.

In general, efficacy of sedative medications cannot be extrapolated from adults or older pediatric patients to younger pediatric patients. However, there may be times when Phase 2 studies can serve as proof of concept that the product has the dose–response relationship that is similar to adults and thus can serve as a basis for utilizing extrapolation. In this case, the Phase 2 study may provide both dosing information and support for efficacy, leaving safety to be assessed. While safety studies can be difficult and large, the overall study burden is reduced with the introduction of extrapolation.

Phase 3 Safety and Efficacy Studies

For approval of a new drug in adult and adolescent patients (aged 12 years and older), at least two adequate and well-controlled Phase 3 clinical trials are generally required to support either an indication for sedation in the intensive care unit or for procedural sedation.

Phase 3 trials in the intensive care population are expected to be conducted in the same population that will use the medication if it is approved. Thus, studies should be designed to enroll a representative range of patient demographics and disease likely to be encountered in clinical practice. Clinical trials evaluating procedural sedation should enroll patients for a specific procedure and include a representative range of pediatric patients. For example, studies of a product for suturing and fracture reduction would generally only include pediatric patients who are ambulatory, not chronically ill, hospitalized patients. Studies for lumbar puncture or imaging should include pediatric patients down to the newborn period, not just patients 12 years of age and older.

For drugs used for sedation, many efficacy-related outcome measures in children are the same as for adults, including time to sedation, time to reemergence and/or discharge, and the success of procedure (performance conditions). Assessing the depth of sedation in children is critical as an unintended level of deep sedation places children at higher risk for respiratory depression and other complications [15]. On the other hand, too little sedation may increase the incidence of intraoperative awareness or prevent the procedure from being completed successfully [16]. Consensus regarding a "gold standard" for assessing sedation in young children has not been reached [17].

Enrollment of an adequate number of patients to detect a statistically significant, clinically meaningful treatment effect is a common challenge in pediatric drug development. Multiple centers must be utilized to recruit a sufficient number of patients. Some strategies to improve enrollment include conducting multinational trials (other international regulatory authorities such as the European Medicines Agency also require development of products for children), opening enrollment at centers where procedural sedation is common (a large children's hospital with a busy emergency department, a high-acuity neonatal intensive care unit, a large hematology/oncology service), and/or utilizing expert networks.

The choice of a control group can also be a challenge for pediatric sedation trials. It would be difficult to justify the use of a placebo for sedation, as difficult to find parents and guardians willing to enroll their children into a placebo-controlled trial. The use of an active comparator is also a challenge as most of the drugs commonly used for sedation in pediatrics, with the exception of midazolam, are not studied or approved by the FDA for this indication. It is difficult to assess the difference in treatment effect between the active control and drug under study if a treatment effect for the active control has not been clearly established. Concerns can be founded about use of an unlabeled product in the study even if that same product is the standard of care.

Important safety considerations for study protocols include monitoring of vital signs, in particular, airway, ventilation, oxygenation, and hemodynamic variables. Monitoring must be assessed by personnel who are able to safely rescue patients from oversedation. Laboratory assessments such as blood chemistries, liver function testing, and complete blood count are needed. Special pediatric subpopulations such as preterm infants need to be carefully monitored for the development of comorbidities of prematurity, such as intraventricular hemorrhage, necrotizing enterocolitis, sepsis, and persistent ductus arteriosus, and an adjudication of the relationship of any adverse event to the use of the study drug must be made. All patients participating in studies must be monitored in a postanesthetic care setting or equivalent by appropriately trained health-care providers until discharge criteria have been met.

Patient assessment and management of residual effects of study drugs after criteria for discharge must be incorporated into clinical protocols. For example, protocols must assess when the patient may again safely operate a motor vehicle (adolescents only) or perform cognitively intensive tasks. Some patients may require multiple procedures that require sedation. Pharmacokinetic and other laboratory data may be required to determine the interval when repeat sedation may be performed safely. Study protocols must indicate how adverse events will be appropriately categorized, adjudicated, and followed until resolution. Additionally, whenever normal limits of safety laboratory studies have been exceeded or when reversal agents or other interventions are needed to prevent an adverse event or to sustain clinical vitality, these should be appropriately documented as adverse events.

Assessing the depth of sedation in pediatric patients is critical. Pediatric patients younger than 6 years of age and those who are developmentally delayed may require deep levels of sedation to achieve appropriate procedural sedation. In addition, this age group is especially vulnerable to the effects of the sedative medication on respiratory drive, airway patency, and protective reflexes [15]. Since a child's ability to cooperate with a procedure is dependent on the child's chronological and developmental age, it is important to develop and validate assessment metrics that are appropriate for the patient's age and state of development, to include verbal and nonverbal measures. As such, different metrics for younger pediatric subpopulations may be needed for comprehensive study of the entire age range of pediatric patients likely to be exposed to the drug in medical practice. The appropriateness of sedation scales or scores to be used in young patients or nonverbal patients must be assessed and validated.

Although extrapolation of efficacy may be appropriate, safety cannot be extrapolated from older to younger patients. Since developing systems may respond differently from mature adult organs, some drug interactions and adverse events that occur in pediatric patients may not be identified in adults or older pediatric patients. However, in general, the nature of the acute safety monitoring of clinical trials is expected to be similar to that required in adults. Evaluation of safety must account for physiologic variations related to maturation and development. Pediatric patients may experience novel adverse events or toxicities of higher severity compared with adults. Extended follow-up may be required to assess developmental progress in patients receiving sedation during periods of neuronal expansion and interconnection. Evidence of behavioral abnormalities may be a clinical finding resulting from accelerated neuronal apoptosis. Therefore, follow-up for such clinical findings may be required after administration of medication in suspected drug classes.

Conclusion

With the passage of historic pediatric legislation, and increasing experience in conducting studies in the pediatric population, significant advances have been made in obtaining adequate and well-controlled studies of drugs in infants and children [18]. In addition, there have been advances in assessing both the short- and long-term safety of the sedatives in the developing child [19]. Despite this progress, most products used for pediatric sedation have not been approved for this use by the FDA. Thus, future clinical development programs should be focused on narrowing the knowledge gap between what is known about the use of these products in adults and children.

Disclaimer The views expressed herein represent those of the authors and do not necessarily represent the views or practices of the authors' employers or any other party. No official support or endorsements by the US FDA is provided or should be inferred. No commercial interest or other conflict of interest exists between L. Yao and the pharmaceutical companies. L. Mathis is employed by Amgen, Inc.

References

1. US Food and Drug Administration. Code of Federal Regulations Title 21 Subpart D: Drugs for Human Use, Part 314.126. Washington, DC: US Government Printing Office; 2012.
2. US FDA. Guidance for Industry. Providing clinical evidence of effectiveness for human drug and biological products. 1998. Available at: http://www.fda.gov/downloads/Drugs/GuidanceComplianceRegulatoryInformation/Guidances/ucm078749.pdf. Accessed 4 Nov 2013.
3. Wilson JT. An update on the therapeutic orphan. Pediatrics. 1999;104(3):585–90.
4. Roberts R, Rodriguez W, Murphy D, et al. Pediatric drug labeling: improving the safety and efficacy of pediatric therapies. JAMA. 2003;290:905–11.
5. U.S. Census Bureau. Current population reports. http://www.childstats.gov/americaschildren. Accessed 2 Nov 2010.
6. Li J, Eisenstein E, Grabowski H, et al. Economic return of clinical trials performed under the pediatric exclusivity program. JAMA. 2007;297(5):480–8.
7. Benjamin D, Smith B, Sun J, et al. Pediatric drug trials: safety and transparency. Arch Pediatr Adolesc Med. 2009;163(12):1080–6.
8. Anand K. Analgesia and anesthesia for neonates: study design and ethical issues. Clin Ther. 2005;27(6):814–43.
9. Gershanik J, Boecler B, Ensley H, McCloskey S, George W. The gasping syndrome and benzyl alcohol poisoning. N Engl J Med. 1982;307(22):1384–8.
10. Young C, Jevtovic-Todorovic V, Qin YQ, et al. Potential of ketamine and midazolam, individually or in combination, to induce apoptotic neurodegeneration in the infant mouse brain. Br J Pharmacol. 2005;146:189–97.
11. Rudin M, Ben-Abraham R, Gazit V, et al. Single-dose ketamine administration induces apoptosis in neonatal mouse brain. J Basic Clin Physiol Pharmacol. 2005;16:231–43.
12. Slikker W, Zou X, Hotchkiss CE, et al. Ketamine-induced neuronal cell death in the perinatal rhesus monkey. Toxicol Sci. 2007; 98:145–58.
13. Mellon RD, Simone AF, Rappaport BA. Use of anesthetic agents in neonates and young children. Anesth Analg. 2007;104:509–20.
14. McGowan FX, Davis PJ. Anesthetic-related neurotoxicity in the developing infant: of mice, rats, monkeys and, possibly, humans, editorial. Anesth Analg. 2008;106(6):1599–602.
15. Cote C, on Wilson S and the Work Group Sedation. Guidelines for monitoring and management of pediatric patients during and after sedation for diagnostic and therapeutic procedures: an update. Pediatrics 2006;118(6):2587–98.
16. Johansen J. Update on bispectral index monitoring. Best Pract Res Clin Anaesthesiol. 2006;20(1):81–99.
17. Litalien C, Jouvet P. Validation of a sedation scale for young mechanically ventilated children: a painful challenge? Pediatr Crit Care Med. 2006;7(2):183–4.
18. Rappaport B, Mellon RD, Simone A, Woodcock J. Defining safe use of anesthesia in children. N Engl J Med. 2011;364(15): 1387–90.
19. Ramsay JG, Rappaport BA. SmartTots: a multidisciplinary effort to determine anesthetic safety in young children. Anesth Analg. 2011;113(5):963–4.

Is There Evidence for Long-Term Neurocognitive Effects of Sedatives?

27

Sulpicio G. Soriano and Laszlo Vutskits

Abstract

The potential neurotoxic effects of drugs used for anesthesia and sedation have captured the attention of pediatric care providers. As early as in 1953, personality changes have been documented in children receiving anesthetic and sedative drugs. Despite this early observation, the utilization of anesthetics and sedatives to facilitate painful and distressing procedures on infants and children has become the standard of care. However, the irrefutable laboratory reports documenting the neurotoxic effect of anesthetic and sedative drugs on the developing brain have sparked public awareness to this potential side effect. Given the public health implications of this phenomenon, this chapter will discuss relevance of these issues in the context of the management of sedation in pediatric patients undergoing diagnostic and painful procedures.

Keywords

Neurotoxic • Pediatric • Anesthesia • Sedation • Neuroapoptosis • Anesthetic-induced developmental neurotoxicity (AIDN)

Introduction

The potential neurotoxic effects of drugs used for anesthesia and sedation have captured the attention of pediatric care providers [1, 2]. As early as in 1953, personality changes have been documented in children receiving anesthetic and sedative drugs [3]. Despite this early observation, the utilization of anesthetics and sedatives to facilitate painful and distressing procedures on infants and children has become the standard of care. However, the irrefutable laboratory reports documenting the neurotoxic effect of anesthetic and sedative drugs on the developing brain have sparked public awareness to this potential side effect. Two extensive reviews of the neurotoxic potential of sedation in neonatal and pediatric intensive care settings have been published [4, 5]. However, the relevance of neurotoxicity of the different classes of sedative drugs for procedural sedation has not been fully reviewed. Given the public health implications of this phenomenon, we will discuss relevance of these issues in the context of the management of sedation in pediatric patients undergoing diagnostic and painful procedures.

Sedative-Induced Developmental Neurotoxicity

Sedative drugs are potent modulators of the central nervous system but reversibly making patients unresponsive and insensate to diagnostic and therapeutic procedures [6]. Exposure to anesthetic and sedative drugs during the perinatal period leads to neuroapoptosis (cell death) and subsequent

S.G. Soriano, M.D. (✉)
Department of Anesthesiology, Perioperative and Pain Medicine, Boston Children's Hospital, 300 Longwood Avenue, Boston, MA 02115, USA
e-mail: sulpicio.soriano@childrens.harvard.edu

L. Vutskits, M.D., Ph.D.
Department of Anesthesiology, Pharmacology and Intensive Care, University Hospital of Geneva, 4, Rue Gabrielle-Perret-Gentil, Geneva 1205, Switzerland
e-mail: laszlo.vutskits@unige.ch

K.P. Mason (ed.), *Pediatric Sedation Outside of the Operating Room: A Multispecialty International Collaboration*,
DOI 10.1007/978-1-4939-1390-9_27, © Springer Science+Business Media New York 2015

Table 27.1 Known neurotoxicity of common sedatives

Drug	Neurotoxicity/ altered plasticity	Reference
Propofol	Yes	[10, 11, 19, 26, 40, 42]
Midazolam	Yes	[11, 18]
Pentobarbital	Yes	[26]
Chloral hydrate	Yes	[29, 54]
Ketamine	Yes	[8, 11, 27, 33, 38, 39]
Dexmedetomidine	No	[14]

neurocognitive deficits in laboratory rodent and monkey models [7, 8]. It should be noted that high dose of the sedative drug and prolonged duration of the exposure (4–6 h) mediate anesthetic-induced developmental neurotoxicity (AIDN) in laboratory models. Given the low doses administered and brief exposure to the drugs, the relevance of AIDN in the setting of sedation may be superfluous. Susceptibility to AIDN is not limited to the postnatal period, but to the fetus as well. Perinatal exposure to anesthetic and sedative drugs leads to neuroapoptosis and stunted dendritic growth [9, 10]. While administration of anesthetics to juvenile rats led to enhanced dendritic formation and synaptic density, the clinical significance for this finding is unknown [11, 12]. Similar dendritic morphology has been observed in psychiatric and neurological disorders [13].

Sedative drugs are primarily *N*-methyl-D-aspartate (NMDA) antagonists (ketamine) and γ(gamma)-aminobutyric acid (GABA) agonists (midazolam, propofol, pentobarbital, and chloral hydrate). Currently, dexmedetomidine has been the only drug that does not induce neuroapoptosis and have been also shown to attenuate isoflurane-induced neuroapoptosis (Table 27.1) [14]. It should be noted that most preclinical studies on AIDN utilized high doses and long exposure times. Furthermore, these experimental paradigms were conducted in the absence of concurrent noxious stimulation, which does not account for the interaction of sedation and stressful/painful procedures. Recent reports of neonatal rats receiving ketamine during the application of noxious stimuli resulted in less neuronal cell death [15, 16]. These experimental paradigms do not reflect clinical conditions associated with procedural sedation in pediatric patients [17]. Subanesthetic doses of midazolam or propofol induces neuroapoptosis in neonatal mice [18, 19]. Multiple short (1 h) anesthetics with sevoflurane (an inhaled GABA agonist) resulted in increased neuroapoptosis in neonatal rats, while a single exposure did not [20]. An enhanced environment mitigated the degree of neuroapoptosis in this rodent model [21]. Taken together, these preclinical observations demonstrate causality between anesthetic exposure during a vulnerable developmental period with synaptic modeling and plasticity.

Mechanisms of Aberrant Neuronal Development from Sedative Drugs

Normal development of the immature brain undergoes physiologic pruning mediated by neuronal apoptosis [22]. The developing central nervous system is exquisitely sensitive in its internal milieu. Peak synaptogenesis occurs between the third and seventh postnatal weeks in rats [23]. This is equivalent to the period between 25 gestational week and 1 year of age in humans. However, neurogenesis and context-dependent modulation of neural plasticity continues throughout life from the perinatal period to adulthood. In fact, the rate of neurogenesis peaks in different brain regions in an age-dependent fashion, with a majority of this process occurring primarily during the perinatal period and less during adulthood. It appears that newly born neurons are most vulnerable to the neuroapoptotic effect of anesthetic and sedative drugs [24, 25]. Therefore, nonphysiologic exposure to various drugs and stressors (painful stimuli, maternal deprivation, hypoglycemia, hypoxia, and ischemia) during this critical window may induce neurodegeneration. These findings beg the question of whether other confounding variables are involved in this process. The potential contribution of coexisting medical conditions and undiagnosed genetic syndromes to neurodevelopment has to be considered in light of the potential neurotoxic effects of drugs used for sedation.

The molecular mechanisms that produce immobility, analgesia, and amnesia are still unknown. This fundamental gap hinders the ability of investigators to identify the specific mechanisms that impact the developing central nervous system. Although the anesthetic mechanisms of NMDA antagonists and GABA agonists are divergent, both clearly induce neurodegenerative and neurocognitive changes in animal models [26]. Transient pharmacological blockade of the NMDA receptor with the noncompetitive pharmacological antagonist MK801, phencyclidine, or ketamine induced developmental stage-dependent widespread apoptosis in the developing brain [27]. The initial response from the scientific community was that anesthetic and anticonvulsant drugs and ethanol accelerate this normal "pruning" or apoptotic process. However, this notion was dismissed by a report that commonly used anesthetics (midazolam, isoflurane, and nitrous oxide) induced neuroapoptosis and subsequent derangements in long-term potentiation (an electrophysiological correlate of learning) and neurobehavioral performance [28]. A large number of experimental data from several research groups have confirmed these results [7]. Of note, the proapoptotic effect depends on the developmental stage: being most pronounced at postnatal day 7 and inexistent in 15-day-old rodents. Chloral hydrate has been shown to induce neuroapoptosis in neonatal rats, and lithium protects against this neurotoxic reaction [29]. These preclinical reports clearly demonstrate that drugs that are routinely utilized to sedate pediatric patients have neurotoxic properties.

Several lines of investigation have implicated other neuronal cell death mechanisms such as excitotoxicity, mitochondrial dysfunction, aberrant cell cycle reentry, trophic factor dysregulation, and disruption of cytoskeletal assembly [30–36]. A combination of these and other parallel neurodegenerative pathways likely mediate the neurotoxic effects of anesthetic drugs.

On the surface, the notion that sedative drugs can be excitotoxic can be a contradiction. However, GABA agonists stimulate immature neurons due to a developmental variation of the chloride channels [37]. Subsequent reports on the mechanism of GABAergic-induced seizures in newborn rats revealed that the NKCC1 chloride channel blocker, bumetanide, attenuated the both neuroapoptosis and epileptiform activity [31]. Prolonged exposure to a NMDA antagonist such as ketamine leads to an upregulation of the NMDA receptor, leading to an increased accumulation of excitotoxic intracellular calcium [30]. Excitotoxic insults are also linked to mitochondrial dysfunction in neurons, and prolonged exposure to anesthetic drugs incites a comparable response [32].

Sedative drugs induce neuronal apoptosis in fetal and neonatal rhesus monkeys in a dose- and duration-dependent fashion [38–40]. A 3-h-long exposure to ketamine did not seem to affect cell death, while a 5-h-long exposure has been shown to induce apoptosis both in the fetal and early postnatal brains. This experimental paradigm resulted in persistent cognitive deficits assessed by an operant test battery [8]. Monkeys receiving a 24-h-long ketamine anesthesia at postnatal day 5 showed impaired motivation and learning but no problems with short-term memory when tested up to 3.5 years post-exposure. Propofol anesthesia for 5 h resulted in apoptosis of neurons and oligodendrocytes in fetal and neonatal nonhuman primates [40].

Exposure to sedative drugs during brain development not only induces neuronal cell death but can also impair neurogenesis and synaptogenesis in an age-dependent manner. Postnatal rat pups had decreased neuronal progenitor proliferation and persistent deficits of hippocampal function, while older rats increased progenitor proliferation and neuronal differentiation, and this was correlated with improved memory function [41]. Propofol impairs the survival and maturation of adult-born hippocampal neurons in a developmental stage-dependent manner by inducing a significant decrease in dendritic maturation and survival of newly born neurons that were 17 days old but not at 11 days [25]. The developmental stage-dependent effects of anesthesia exposure during brain maturation are also true in the context of synaptogenesis. Exposure of 7-day-old pups to different kinds of anesthetics and sedatives consistently lead to a rapid and permanent decrease in the number of synapses in the hippocampus and the cerebral cortex. In contrast, when these drugs were administered at later stages of the brain growth spurt, neuronal viability is preserved with a significant increase in synaptic density [11, 42].

Taken together, three factors appear to induce AIDN in laboratory models:

1. Developmental susceptibility during synaptogenesis
2. High dose of the anesthetic
3. Prolonged duration of exposure

Clinical Evidence for Sedative-Induced Neurological Sequelae

Most of the clinical reports that examine the effect of anesthetic exposure on neurocognitive development are based on retrospective observations of pediatric patients undergoing surgery and presumably general anesthesia. These reports do not specifically identify the classes of anesthetic and sedative drugs administered. Furthermore, these reports do not consider the direct effects of surgery and underlying comorbidities. Although most of the studies have attempted to control for obvious confounders, the retrospective nature of these investigations make it impossible to control for all the known and unknown confounders. Of note, there is no consensus from the published retrospective analyses of the behavioral sequelae after anesthesia and surgery during infancy and children.

Several retrospective reports demonstrate an association between surgery/anesthesia and learning and behavioral disorders. In a series of retrospective reports, the Mayo Clinic group examined a cohort born from 1976 to 1982 for learning disabilities. The patients who were exposed to surgery and anesthesia before the age of four had increased incidence of learning disabilities at age 19 years [43]. Risk factors included more than one anesthetic exposure and general anesthesia lasting longer than 2 h. A similar study, using matched cohorts, revealed that children under the age of 2 who had more than one anesthetic were almost twice as likely to have speech and language disabilities than those who had a single or no anesthetic exposure [44]. In contrast, a cohort study from a birth registry from Australia reported that even a single exposure to general anesthesia before age 3 years was related to decrease performance on receptive and expressive language and cognitive testing done at 10 years [45]. A similar retrospective report derived from Iowa revealed a negative correlation between the duration of surgery/anesthesia and scores on academic achievement tests [46]. Data analysis from the Medicaid database indicates that, even after adjustment for potential confounding factors, children who underwent hernia repair before the age of 3 years were twice as likely as children in the comparison group to be subsequently diagnosed with a developmental or behavioral disorder [47]. When this group was controlled for gender and birth weight, there was still a nearly twofold increase in these issues. A follow-up study that matched patients with non-anesthetic-exposed siblings found that the former had a 60 % greater association between exposure to anesthesia and later neurologic and developmental problems [48].

Meanwhile other investigators report no evidence of an association between exposure to general anesthesia at a young age and later school problems. An analysis of a twin–twin registry from the Netherlands comparing the educational achievements of identical twin pairs revealed that twin pairs exposed to general anesthesia had lower educational achievements than unexposed twin pairs [49]. However, when one twin was exposed and the other was not, there were no differences in educational achievements. These findings imply that exposure to general anesthesia was not associated with impaired educational performance. A Danish birth cohort compared average test scores at ninth grade in infants who had inguinal hernia study and reported no statistically significant differences from the naïve cohorts after adjusting for known confounders [50]. A similar analysis of infants undergoing pyloromyotomies revealed no difference in their educational performance to a surgery-naïve cohort [51]. Since these retrospective reports are based on patients undergoing surgery and presumably general anesthesia, they may not have been relevant in the setting of procedural sedation.

Several reports have been published on the effect of sedation on neurocognitive parameters in intensive care patients. In a review of premature neonates receiving sedation for mechanical ventilation, prolonged sedation was not associated with a poor neurological outcome [52]. A similar report examining the impact of perioperative administration of sedatives in pediatric cardiac surgery found no association between the dose and duration of these drugs and adverse neurodevelopmental outcome at 18–24 months [53]. A reevaluation of these children at kindergarten age demonstrated that the number of days on chloral hydrate was associated with lower-performance intelligence quotient, and the cumulative dose of benzodiazepines was associated with lower visual motor integration (VMI) scores [54]. The Beery-Buktenica VMI scores reflect the ability to integrate visual and motor abilities and screen for possible learning, neuropsychological, and behavioral problems [55]. These sedation studies in the intensive care unit may reveal a mild association between GABA agonists and neurodevelopmental deficits. However, the overwhelming impact of severe illness [56] and prolonged administration of the sedative drugs cannot be discounted. Dexmedetomidine is the only sedative that does not have overt neurotoxic properties in preclinical settings. Its use as a primary sedative for preterm and term neonates has been shown to be effective without major side effects [57]. A direct comparison between dexmedetomidine and lorazepam on septic adults revealed a significant reduction in brain dysfunction with the former [58]. Dexmedetomidine maintains cognitive function in adult intensive care patients requiring cooperative sedation [59]. The effect of dexmedetomidine on both short- and long-term cognitive domains in pediatric patients remains to be investigated.

Conclusions from Preclinical and Clinical Investigations

Extrapolation of these preclinical and clinical studies to procedural sedation in pediatric patients is problematic. Since millions of young children undergo sedation every year worldwide, the public health impact of developmental anesthesia neurotoxicity, if it exists, could be a major issue in humans. These individual studies were conducted on relatively homogenous populations in terms of ethnic and socioeconomic distribution and may not be applicable to the diverse group of pediatric patients undergoing sedation. Furthermore, the retrospective nature of these reports may have unaccounted confounders that may instigate neurological deficits. Furthermore, these studies cannot separate the effects of anesthesia from coexisting condition, surgery, or stress of hospitalization. Clearly, rigorous clinical research is needed to resolve this issue.

These concerns have led to a risk assessment by the Food and Drug Administration's Life Support Advisory Committee in March of 2007, stating that the "existing and well-understood risks of anesthesia (hemodynamic and respiratory) continue to be the overwhelming considerations in designing an anesthetic (sedation), and the understood risks of delaying surgery (procedure) are the primary reasons to determine the timing" [60]. Although the risk is exceedingly low, respiratory and cardiac morbidities associated with the administration of sedatives should be seriously considered in the context of the "potential neurotoxicity" in these drugs [61]. Recently, the SmartTots initiative issued a statement acknowledging these preclinical findings: "Discuss with parents and other caretakers the risks and benefits of procedures requiring anesthetics or sedatives, as well as the known health risks of not treating certain conditions" [62, 63]. A recent international seminar confirmed that evidence from laboratory investigations definitively demonstrate that anesthetic and sedative drugs lead to neuroapoptosis and subsequent neurocognitive deficits at the extremes of age [64]. Furthermore, evidence from retrospective clinical reports in pediatric surgical populations is still inconclusive. Since the use of sedative drugs is standard practice and unavoidable in pediatric patients, the clinician should be aware of the evolving investigations and be up to date on best clinical practices.

References

1. Loepke AW, Soriano SG. An assessment of the effects of general anesthetics on developing brain structure and neurocognitive function. Anesth Analg. 2008;106(6):1681–707.
2. Rappaport B, Mellon RD, Simone A, Woodcock J. Defining safe use of anesthesia in children. N Engl J Med. 2011;364(15): 1387–90.
3. Eckenhoff JE. Relationship of anesthesia to postoperative personality changes in children. AMA Am J Dis Child. 1953;86(5):587–91.
4. Durrmeyer X, Vutskits L, Anand KJS, Rimensberger PC. Use of analgesic and sedative drugs in the nicu: Integrating clinical trials and laboratory data. Pediatr Res. 2010;67(2):117–27.
5. Loepke AW. Developmental neurotoxicity of sedatives and anesthetics: a concern for neonatal and pediatric critical care medicine? Pediatr Crit Care Med. 2010;11(2):217–26.
6. Rudolph U, Antkowiak B. Molecular and neuronal substrates for general anaesthetics. Nat Rev Neurosci. 2004;5(9):709–20.
7. Stratmann G. Review article: Neurotoxicity of anesthetic drugs in the developing brain. Anesth Analg. 2011;113(5):1170–9.
8. Paule MG, Li M, Allen RR, Liu F, Zou X, Hotchkiss C, et al. Ketamine anesthesia during the first week of life can cause long-lasting cognitive deficits in rhesus monkeys. Neurotoxicol Teratol. 2011;33(2):220–30.
9. Li Y, Liang G, Wang S, Meng Q, Wang Q, Wei H. Effects of fetal exposure to isoflurane on postnatal memory and learning in rats. Neuropharmacology. 2007;53(8):942–50.
10. Vutskits L, Gascon E, Tassonyi E, Kiss JZ. Clinically relevant concentrations of propofol but not midazolam alter in vitro dendritic development of isolated gamma-aminobutyric acid-positive interneurons. Anesthesiology. 2005;102(5):970–6.
11. De Roo M, Klauser P, Briner A, Nikonenko I, Mendez P, Dayer A, et al. Anesthetics rapidly promote synaptogenesis during a critical period of brain development. PLoS One. 2009;4(9):e7043.
12. Briner A, De Roo M, Dayer A, Muller D, Habre W, Vutskits L. Volatile anesthetics rapidly increase dendritic spine density in the rat medial prefrontal cortex during synaptogenesis. Anesthesiology. 2010;112(3):546–56.
13. Penzes P, Cahill ME, Jones KA, Vanleeuwen J-E, Woolfrey KM. Dendritic spine pathology in neuropsychiatric disorders. Nat Neurosci. 2011;14(3):285–93.
14. Sanders RD, Xu J, Shu Y, Januszewski A, Halder S, Fidalgo A, et al. Dexmedetomidine attenuates isoflurane-induced neurocognitive impairment in neonatal rats. Anesthesiology. 2009;110(5):1077–85.
15. Anand KJ, Garg S, Rovnaghi CR, Narsinghani U, Bhutta AT, Hall RW. Ketamine reduces the cell death following inflammatory pain in newborn rat brain. Pediatr Res. 2007;62(3):283–90.
16. Liu JR, Liu Q, Li J, Baek C, Han XH, Athiraman U, et al. Noxious stimulation attenuates ketamine-induced neuroapoptosis in the developing rat brain. Anesthesiology. 2012;117(1):64–71.
17. Anand KJ, Soriano SG. Anesthetic agents and the immature brain: Are these toxic or therapeutic? Anesthesiology. 2004;101(2):527–30.
18. Young C, Jevtovic-Todorovic V, Qin YQ, Tenkova T, Wang H, Labruyere J, et al. Potential of ketamine and midazolam, individually or in combination, to induce apoptotic neurodegeneration in the infant mouse brain. Br J Pharmacol. 2005;146(2):189–97.
19. Cattano D, Young C, Straiko MM, Olney JW. Subanesthetic doses of propofol induce neuroapoptosis in the infant mouse brain. Anesth Analg. 2008;106(6):1712–4.
20. Shih J, May LD, Gonzalez HE, Lee EW, Alvi RS, Sall JW, et al. Delayed environmental enrichment reverses sevoflurane-induced memory impairment in rats. Anesthesiology. 2012;116(3):586–602 [Research Support, Non-U.S. Gov't].
21. Shen X, Dong Y, Xu Z, Wang H, Miao C, Soriano SG, et al. Selective anesthesia-induced neuroinflammation in developing mouse brain and cognitive impairment. Anesthesiology. 2013;118(3):502–15.
22. Buss RR, Sun W, Oppenheim RW. Adaptive roles of programmed cell death during nervous system development. Annu Rev Neurosci. 2006;29:1–35.
23. Dobbing J, Sands J. Comparative aspects of the brain growth spurt. Early Hum Dev. 1979;3(1):79–83.
24. Hofacer RD, Deng M, Ward CG, Joseph B, Hughes EA, Jiang C, et al. Cell-age specific vulnerability of neurons to anesthetic toxicity. Ann Neurol. 2013;73(6):695–704.
25. Krzisch M, Sultan S, Sandell J, Demeter K, Vutskits L, Toni N. Propofol anesthesia impairs the maturation and survival of adult-born hippocampal neurons. Anesthesiology. 2013;118(3):602–10.
26. Fredriksson A, Ponten E, Gordh T, Eriksson P. Neonatal exposure to a combination of n-methyl-d-aspartate and gamma-aminobutyric acid type a receptor anesthetic agents potentiates apoptotic neurodegeneration and persistent behavioral deficits. Anesthesiology. 2007;107(3):427–36 [Research Support, Non-U.S. Gov't].
27. Ikonomidou C, Bosch F, Miksa M, Bittigau P, Vockler J, Dikranian K, et al. Blockade of nmda receptors and apoptotic neurodegeneration in the developing brain. Science. 1999;283(5398):70–4 [Research Support, Non-U.S. Gov't Research Support, U.S. Gov't, P.H.S.].
28. Jevtovic-Todorovic V, Hartman RE, Izumi Y, Benshoff ND, Dikranian K, Zorumski CF, et al. Early exposure to common anesthetic agents causes widespread neurodegeneration in the developing rat brain and persistent learning deficits. J Neurosci. 2003; 23(3):876–82.
29. Cattano D, Straiko MM, Olney JW. Chloral hydrate induces and lithium prevents neuroapoptosis in the infant mouse brain. Anesthesiology. 2008;109:A315.
30. Slikker Jr W, Paule MG, Wright LK, Patterson TA, Wang C. Systems biology approaches for toxicology. J Appl Toxicol. 2007;27(3):201–17 [Review].
31. Edwards DA, Shah HP, Cao W, Gravenstein N, Seubert CN, Martynyuk AE. Bumetanide alleviates epileptogenic and neurotoxic effects of sevoflurane in neonatal rat brain. Anesthesiology. 2010;112(3):567–75.
32. Sanchez V, Feinstein SD, Lunardi N, Joksovic PM, Boscolo A, Todorovic SM, et al. General anesthesia causes long-term impairment of mitochondrial morphogenesis and synaptic transmission in developing rat brain. Anesthesiology. 2011;115(5):992–1002.
33. Soriano SG, Liu Q, Li J, Liu J-R, Han XH, Kanter JL, et al. Ketamine activates cell cycle signaling and apoptosis in the neonatal rat brain. Anesthesiology. 2010;112(5):1155–63.
34. Liu JR, Baek C, Han XH, Shoureshi P, Soriano SG. Role of glycogen synthase kinase-3beta in ketamine-induced developmental neuroapoptosis in rats. Br J Anaesth. 2013;110 Suppl 1:i3–9.
35. Lu LX, Yon J-H, Carter LB, Jevtovic-Todorovic V. General anesthesia activates bdnf-dependent neuroapoptosis in the developing rat brain. Apoptosis. 2006;11(9):1603–15.
36. Lemkuil BP, Head BP, Pearn ML, Patel HH, Drummond JC, Patel PM. Isoflurane neurotoxicity is mediated by p75ntr-rhoa activation and actin depolymerization. Anesthesiology. 2011;114(1):49–57.
37. Ben-Ari Y. Excitatory actions of gaba during development: The nature of the nurture. Nat Rev Neurosci. 2002;3(9):728–39 [Review].
38. Slikker W, Zou X, Hotchkiss CE, Divine RL, Sadovova N, Twaddle NC, et al. Ketamine-induced neuronal cell death in the perinatal rhesus monkey. Toxicol Sci. 2007;98(1):145–58.
39. Brambrink AM, Evers AS, Avidan MS, Farber NB, Smith DJ, Martin LD, et al. Ketamine-induced neuroapoptosis in the fetal and neonatal rhesus macaque brain. Anesthesiology. 2012;116(2):372–84.
40. Creeley C, Dikranian K, Dissen G, Martin L, Olney J, Brambrink A. Propofol-induced apoptosis of neurones and oligodendrocytes in fetal and neonatal rhesus macaque brain. Br J Anaesth. 2013;110 Suppl 1:i29–38.
41. Stratmann G, Sall JW, May LD, Bell JS, Magnusson KR, Rau V, et al. Isoflurane differentially affects neurogenesis and long-term

neurocognitive function in 60-day-old and 7-day-old rats. Anesthesiology. 2009;110(4):834–48 [Research Support, Non-U.S. Gov't].
42. Briner A, Nikonenko I, De Roo M, Dayer A, Muller D, Vutskits L. Developmental stage-dependent persistent impact of propofol anesthesia on dendritic spines in the rat medial prefrontal cortex. Anesthesiology. 2011;115(2):282–93.
43. Wilder RT, Flick RP, Sprung J, Katusic SK, Barbaresi WJ, Mickelson C, et al. Early exposure to anesthesia and learning disabilities in a population-based birth cohort. Anesthesiology. 2009;110(4):796–804 [Multicenter Study Research Support, N.I.H., Extramural Research Support, Non-U.S. Gov't].
44. Flick RP, Katusic SK, Colligan RC, Wilder RT, Voigt RG, Olson MD, et al. Cognitive and behavioral outcomes after early exposure to anesthesia and surgery. Pediatrics. 2011;128(5):e1053–1061.
45. Ing C, DiMaggio C, Whitehouse A, Hegarty MK, Brady J, von Ungern-Sternberg BS, et al. Long-term differences in language and cognitive function after childhood exposure to anesthesia. Pediatrics. 2012;130(3):e476–485.
46. Block RI, Thomas JJ, Bayman EO, Choi JY, Kimble KK, Todd MM. Are anesthesia and surgery during infancy associated with altered academic performance during childhood? Anesthesiology. 2012;117(3):494–503.
47. DiMaggio C, Sun LS, Kakavouli A, Byrne MW, Li G. A retrospective cohort study of the association of anesthesia and hernia repair surgery with behavioral and developmental disorders in young children. J Neurosurg Anesthesiol. 2009;21:286–91.
48. Dimaggio C, Sun L, Li G. Early childhood exposure to anesthesia and risk of developmental and behavioral disorders in a sibling birth cohort. Anesth Analg. 2011;113:1143–51.
49. Bartels M, Althoff RR, Boomsma DI. Anesthesia and cognitive performance in children: No evidence for a causal relationship. Twin Res Hum Genet. 2009;12(3):246–53.
50. Hansen TG, Pedersen JK, Henneberg SW, Pedersen DA, Murray JC, Morton NS, et al. Academic performance in adolescence after inguinal hernia repair in infancy: A nationwide cohort study. Anesthesiology. 2011;114:1076–85.
51. Hansen TG, Pedersen JK, Henneberg SW, Morton NS, Christensen K. Educational outcome in adolescence following pyloric stenosis repair before 3 months of age: A nationwide cohort study. Paediatr Anaesth. 2013;23(10):883–90.
52. Roze JC, Denizot S, Carbajal R, Ancel PY, Kaminski M, Arnaud C, et al. Prolonged sedation and/or analgesia and 5-year neurodevelopment outcome in very preterm infants: Results from the epipage cohort. Arch Pediatr Adolesc Med. 2008;162(8):728–33.
53. Guerra GG, Robertson CM, Alton GY, Joffe AR, Cave DA, Dinu IA, et al. Neurodevelopmental outcome following exposure to sedative and analgesic drugs for complex cardiac surgery in infancy. Paediatr Anaesth. 2011;21(9):932–41.
54. Guerra GG, Robertson CM, Alton GY, Joffe AR, Cave DA, Dinu IA, et al. Neurotoxicity of sedative and analgesia drugs in young infants with congenital heart disease: 4-year follow-up. Paediatr Anaesth. 2014;24(3):257–65.
55. Beery KE, Buktenica NA. Beery-buktenica developmental test of visual motor inegration. 5th ed. Minneapolis: NCS Pearson Inc.; 2004.
56. Moser JJ, Veale PM, McAllister DL, Archer DP. A systematic review and quantitative analysis of neurocognitive outcomes in children with four chronic illnesses. Paediatr Anaesth. 2013; 23(11):1084–96.
57. Chrysostomou C, Schulman SR, Herrera Castellanos M, Cofer BE, Mitra S, da Rocha MG, et al. A phase II/III, multicenter, safety, efficacy, and pharmacokinetic study of dexmedetomidine in preterm and term neonates. J Pediatr. 2013;164(2):276–82.e1-3.
58. Pandharipande PP, Sanders RD, Girard TD, McGrane S, Thompson JL, Shintani AK, et al. Effect of dexmedetomidine versus lorazepam on outcome in patients with sepsis: An a priori-designed analysis of the mends randomized controlled trial. Crit Care. 2010;14(2):R38.
59. Goodwin HE, Gill RS, Murakami PN, Thompson CB, Lewin 3rd JJ, Mirski MA. Dexmedetomidine preserves attention/calculation when used for cooperative and short-term intensive care unit sedation. J Crit Care. 2013;28(6):1113.e1117–0.
60. FDA. The neurotoxicity of anesthetic and sedative drugs in juvenile animals and the implications for pediatric patients undergoing surgical, medical or diagnostic procedures requiring exposure to these agents. 2007. http://www.fda.gov/ohrms/dockets/ac/07/transcripts/2007-4285t1.pdf
61. Cravero JP, Beach ML, Blike GT, Gallagher SM, Hertzog JH, Pediatric Sedation Research Consortium. The incidence and nature of adverse events during pediatric sedation/anesthesia with propofol for procedures outside the operating room: a report from the pediatric sedation research consortium. Anesth Analg. 2009; 108(3):795–804.
62. SmartTots. Consensus statement on the use of anesthetics and sedatives in children. 2012. http://www.smarttots.org/resources/consensus.html
63. Ramsay JG, Rappaport BA. SmartTots: a multidisciplinary effort to determine anesthetic safety in young children. Anesth Analg. 2011;113(5):963–4.
64. Jevtovic-Todorovic V, Absalom AR, Blomgren K, Brambrink A, Crosby G, Culley DJ, et al. Anaesthetic neurotoxicity and neuroplasticity: an expert group report and statement based on the bja salzburg seminar. Br J Anaesth. 2013;111(2):143–51.

28 Incidence and Stratification of Adverse Events Associated with Sedation: Is There a Benchmark?

Mark G. Roback

Abstract

A significant and growing number of children receive sedation for procedures performed outside of the operating room each year. While a large number of studies have reported on adverse events occurring in association with procedural sedation in many of these settings, benchmarks for sedation adverse event rates have not been formally established. The intent of this chapter is to add some clarity to the concept that, unlike adverse outcomes (e.g., death, permanent neurologic injury) that are largely preventable and should not occur, the occurrence of adverse events is unavoidable, and acceptable rates of adverse events should exist. Once acceptable rates of sedation adverse events are established, sedation providers and programs should be able to compare their individual outcomes to these national and international standards. This chapter will examine current sedation practice outside the operating room and associated adverse events. It will focus on important barriers that must be overcome before meaningful adverse event rates may be determined and best practice guidelines established.

Keywords

Sedation • Anesthesia • Adverse events • Benchmarks • Best practice guidelines • Closed Claims Project • Quebec Guidelines • Pediatric Sedation Research Consortium (PSRC) • World Society of Intravenous Anesthesia (World SIVA) • International Sedation Task Force (ISTF) • Objective Risk Assessment Tool for Sedation (ORATS)

Background

A significant and growing number of children receive sedation for procedures performed outside of the operating room each year [1–4]. For largely elective procedures, this increase has been estimated to be 10 % annually in a sedation research network of 38 centers [5]. The range of procedures performed and number of different providers of sedation have also expanded appreciably [6]. While a large number of studies have reported on adverse events occurring in association with procedural sedation in many of these settings [1–18], benchmarks for sedation adverse event rates have not been formally established.

The intent of this chapter is to add some clarity to the concept that, unlike adverse outcomes (e.g., death, permanent neurologic injury [19]) that are largely preventable and should not occur, the occurrence of adverse events is unavoidable, and acceptable rates of adverse events should exist. Once acceptable rates of sedation adverse events are established, sedation providers and programs should be able to compare their individual outcomes to these national and international standards. This chapter will examine current sedation practice outside the operating room and associated adverse events. It will focus on important barriers that must be overcome before meaningful adverse event rates may be determined and best practice guidelines established.

M.G. Roback, M.D. (✉)
Department of Pediatrics, University of Minnesota Children's Hospital, M653 East Building, 2450 Riverside Avenue, Minneapolis, MN 55454, USA
e-mail: mgroback@umn.edu

K.P. Mason (ed.), *Pediatric Sedation Outside of the Operating Room: A Multispecialty International Collaboration*, DOI 10.1007/978-1-4939-1390-9_28, © Springer Science+Business Media New York 2015

Introduction

Procedural sedation and analgesia, commonly referred to as "sedation," is the use of anxiolytic, sedative, analgesic, or dissociative drugs to attenuate pain, anxiety, and motion to facilitate the performance of a necessary diagnostic or therapeutic procedure, provide an appropriate degree of amnesia or decreased awareness, and ensure patient safety [20]. The American College of Emergency Physicians defines procedural sedation and analgesia as "a technique of administering sedatives or dissociative agents with or without analgesics to induce a state that allows the patient to tolerate unpleasant procedures while maintaining cardiorespiratory function" [21]. Comprehensively, we wish to successfully complete necessary procedures for children by providing them sedation, analgesia, and amnesia while maintaining safety.

The depth of sedation experienced by patients is a continuum, dependent on multiple factors including type of drug and dose administered, route and rate of administration, and characteristics of the child receiving the sedation [22, 23]. Children can easily move from one level of sedation to a deeper level [24, 25]. Regardless of the depth of sedation that is targeted, a subset of children will become more sedated than intended, and some will become unresponsive and experience loss of airway-protective reflexes (general anesthesia) for at least a brief period of time during sedation. Stratification of risk for sedation-related adverse events, based on the depth of sedation continuum, is imperfect due to the subjective nature of the tools used to determine depth of sedation. A recent editorial acknowledges the limitations of using responsiveness to verbal and/or tactile stimuli to determine depth of sedation and proposes the development of objective mechanisms to predict the ongoing risk of serious adverse events [26].

Regardless of the mechanism for determining depth of sedation, the uncertainty of achieving targeted levels of sedation is one of the reasons for which we believe that children represent a subgroup of patients at highest risk and with the lowest error tolerance [19, 27]. Importantly, serious adverse events associated with the sedation of children such as cardiopulmonary arrest, apnea, laryngospasm, and pulmonary aspiration, although uncommon, have been reported by many providers, using an array of sedation drugs, in a variety of settings [12–15, 28, 29]. It is incumbent on sedation providers to recognize adverse events and make appropriate interventions—perform rescue—to prevent adverse outcomes from occurring [19].

Sedation services are provided for children by a range of providers in various settings including sedation units, emergency departments, dental and gastroenterology offices, radiology/imaging suites, hospital wards, and in outpatient settings [1–4, 30, 31]. We should expect that sedation provided by anesthesiologists, pediatric intensivists, hospital medicine physicians, dentists, gastroenterologists, pediatricians, emergency and pediatric emergency physicians, certified registered nurse anesthetists, advanced practice nurses, pediatric nurse practitioners, registered nurses, physicians' assistants, pediatricians, and radiologists may have inherent differences [1–4, 32–39]. Sedation providers will differ in the types of patients for whom they provide sedation as well as the variety of procedures for which these patients receive sedation [1, 2]. The drugs administered and routes of administration used will also differ based on the depth of sedation targeted. Similarly, the procedures for which sedation is provided may also influence adverse event profiles. Sedation provided by a pediatric emergency physician in the emergency department for a painful procedure will differ from sedation provided by the same individual in radiology for a magnetic resonance imaging (MRI) scan, which is not painful but requires children to be motionless.

When we propose rates of "acceptable" adverse events, we must consider not only the characteristics of the patient and provider but also the nature and setting of the procedure performed (i.e., elective, emergent, painful, motionless), as well as the choice of sedative, dose, and route of administration. Considerable controversy exists over whether the risk of sedation-related adverse events is related to the training of the provider [40]. However, in a study of more than 130,000 pediatric procedural sedation cases performed in a large sedation consortium by a variety of pediatric specialists (14 % anesthesiologists), the rates of major complications were not found to differ by provider [5].

As we present the existing current sedation literature in this chapter, we will examine specific characteristics of the sedation event that may be expected to influence adverse event rates. We must also recognize that different providers will define and report adverse events differently based on their training and experience. Regardless of the variables involved in determining acceptable rates of adverse events, the end result of sedation services for children must always be the same: safe, effective sedation provided to facilitate the successful provision of necessary, oftentimes painful, procedures [22, 23].

Setting the Standards for Safety

Determining acceptable rates of adverse events associated with sedation is important due to the potential impact of adverse events on overall patient safety. Most of our knowledge regarding safety of sedation provided to children outside of the operating room comes from small, single-center studies, which comment on adverse events but are underpowered to draw definitive conclusions about safety or particular risk factors for adverse events [41]. As a result, current sedation practice guidelines are not evidence-based, but rather are largely derived from incomplete data sets or are the products of consensus opinion [21, 42–51]. Additionally, specific specialty-based practice guidelines exist, which may provide divergent recommendations regarding similar sedation practice [22, 36, 39, 44, 52].

Perhaps the most significant improvements in patient safety have been achieved for patients who receive general anesthesia. Anesthesia-related mortality in patients undergoing general anesthesia in operating rooms has been reduced from 1 in 20,000 in the 1950s to a current rate of approximately 1 in 200,000 [53]. The Closed Claims Project was established in 1984 by the American Society of Anesthesiologists (ASA) to identify anesthetic-related complications and their mechanism of occurrence with the goal of improving patient safety [54]. This dramatic improvement in the safety of general anesthesia was found to be largely due to improvements in how patients were monitored [55]. A recent study of monitored anesthesia care found that appropriate use of monitoring, vigilance, and early resuscitation could have prevented many of the adverse events seen [56]. However, to make further improvement in the safety of anesthesia, to definitely address the many issues pertaining to anesthesia risk, and to further develop best practice guidelines, prospective multicenter studies designed to examine large numbers of patients must be conducted [57].

Anesthesiologists have developed strategies to improve the safety of general anesthesia by examining critical events. In 2000, Coté and his colleagues published a critical incident analysis of adverse events associated with sedation provided to children outside the operating room identified through retrospective evaluation of national reporting systems over 27 years [19, 27]. This critical incident analysis attempted to identify factors that contribute to adverse sedation events associated with sedation provided to children undergoing procedures. Factors identified to be associated with adverse outcomes (i.e., permanent neurologic injury and death) include sedation that occurred in a nonhospital-based facility, sedation performed with inadequate or inconsistent physiologic monitoring, sedation administered without adequate presedation medical evaluation, sedation performed in the absence of an independent observer with inadequate recovery procedures, and sedation performed with the occurrence of medication errors. Drug overdoses and drug interactions, particularly when three or more drugs were used, were commonly associated with adverse sedation events [27]. Importantly, all routes of administration and all classes of drugs used for sedation were associated with serious adverse events.

The authors of this critical incident analysis of sedation outside the OR concluded that adverse outcomes associated with sedation were most likely related to the *failure of healthcare providers to rescue patients* from sedation-related adverse events like apnea and oxygen desaturations. They further postulate that individual patient characteristics were less important than failure to rescue patients from the progression of less serious adverse events to serious adverse outcomes.

This important work reinforces the belief that improvements in patient safety related to sedation may be made and acceptable rates of adverse events determined. However, the Closed Claims Project critical incident analysis identified characteristics of complications only. No information about the hundreds of thousands of cases that occurred without complication was gathered for comparison. Although the safety of general anesthesia and sedation outside the operating room has improved with strict adherence to monitoring guidelines and timely intervention or rescue from adverse events, most would agree that more work is needed for further progress to be made. Additional data describing the circumstances and conditions surrounding sedation events with and without complications is required to make critical comparisons. From these data, acceptable rates of adverse events may be determined, and the goal of developing best practice guidelines designed to eliminate poor outcomes will be realized. Ideally, by identifying the rates of adverse events and their predictors, it may be possible to design strategies to reduce the risks. Green and Mason proposed an Objective Risk Assessment Tool for Sedation (ORATS). (Refer to Chap. 38, Table 38.1.) The ORATS would suggest specific variables, physiologic parameters, and thresholds that predict the risk of serious adverse events at escalating depths of sedation.

Disparities in Adverse Event Rate Reporting

A wide range of rates of adverse events (2–26 %) associated with emergency department sedation has been reported in recent studies of children [4, 12–15]. The three largest prospective studies of emergency department sedation in children receiving a variety of sedation/analgesia drugs for the breadth of emergency procedures provide a good example of the variability in reported adverse event rates. Despite being conducted in three similar, large, urban children's hospital emergency departments, these studies report distinctly different rates of common adverse events such as oxygen desaturations (8.6 % versus 13.9 % versus 0.8 %) and vomiting (7.2 % versus 1.1 % versus 0.3 %) as well as total adverse event rates (17.0 % versus 17.8 % versus 2.3 %) [4, 12, 13]. Closer scrutiny of these studies provides some insight into the disparity in adverse event rate reporting. Centers differed with respect to drugs administered, routes of administration employed, use of supplemental oxygen, and the definitions used for oxygen desaturations. Any or all of these factors may be postulated to affect reported adverse event rates. Additionally, the largest of these studies investigated only 2,500 children [4]. Much larger studies are needed to develop adverse event rates of less common potential complications of sedation such as apnea, laryngospasm, pulmonary aspiration, and cardiopulmonary arrest.

In another example, comparisons between like single-center studies, significant disparities in adverse event reporting remain despite having similar settings (emergency departments), types of procedure performed (painful), and sedation drug (ketamine) administered. Only the route of administration differed (intravenous versus intramuscular) in these studies—yet reported adverse event rates such as vomiting still varied considerably from 3.8 to 18.7 % [4, 12, 14, 58–63].

Adverse event rates reported with sedation provided with propofol are a further example of disparities in adverse event reporting despite use of a common agent. With the administration of propofol, the variability of reported adverse event rates such as oxygen desaturation (0–30 %) and apnea necessitating the use of positive pressure ventilation (0–2.5 %) may be due to differences in providers (pediatric intensivists versus emergency physicians), setting (sedation unit versus emergency department versus radiology), type of procedure (painful versus not painful, emergent versus elective), and presence of co-administered analgesic such as fentanyl [3, 7, 64–72]. In emergency department studies of sedation provided using propofol-based regimens, rates of adverse events varied from low 3.5 % [73] to highs of 31 % [62] and 33 % [5]. One study of sedation using propofol with fentanyl reported complications in an extremely high rate (84 %) of patients [74]. Given the high degree of variability of adverse event rates observed when current studies are compared, it is impossible to draw conclusions about the effectiveness of sedation and safety.

Clinically apparent pulmonary aspiration is an important, although infrequently reported, complication of sedation outside the operating room [1–3, 29, 30, 75]. As part of the assessment of patients about to receive sedation or anesthesia, careful history addressing recent oral intake is undertaken with the goal of minimizing the risk of pulmonary aspiration by adhering to preprocedural fasting recommendations [76]. Clinically apparent pulmonary aspiration events have been reported to have occurred in association with sedation in settings where ASA preprocedural fasting guidelines are routinely followed such as dedicated sedation units [1–3] and for radiological procedures and bronchoscopy [30, 31]. However, in emergency departments, where adherence to preprocedural fasting guidelines has not been shown to be rigorously applied [9–11], aspiration has never been reported to have occurred in a child [49, 77, 78].

Examples of the range of rates of adverse events are presented in this section to emphasize that multiple factors contribute to the incidence of adverse events in any given setting. In order to begin to understand these interactions, we must ensure that comparisons are made that control for as many of these factors as possible. Reasons for differences in adverse event reporting may be obvious such as the rate of respiratory depression associated with propofol administered intravenously as opposed to that observed with oral chloral hydrate. Further reasons for disparities in adverse event reporting may be as basic as how we define and report adverse events of interest.

Definition of Adverse Events and Reporting Recommendations

In addition to the clinical parameters described in the previous section, some of the variability of reported rates of adverse events associated with sedation provided outside the operating room may be attributed to existing widespread differences in definitions of adverse events and reporting practices. The rate of total adverse events is dependent on how these events are defined and which events individual providers and sedation services choose to report as significant. For example, an anesthesiologist may consider sonorous breathing resulting in a pulse oximeter reading of 87 % (relieved by a simple jaw thrust) as inherent to sedation with propofol and not report its occurrence as an adverse event. By contrast, a pediatric emergency physician may respond exactly the same way to an identical event with similar results yet report it as partial airway obstruction and oxygen desaturation. In another example, if oxygen desaturation is defined as an oximeter reading less than 90 % in room air for greater than 30 s, a child who experiences oxygen desaturation from 100 % at the beginning of sedation to 90 % during the procedure and who responds positively to an airway maneuver and the administration of oxygen would not be reported as having experienced an adverse event.

Efforts to develop evidence-based practice guidelines designed to prevent the occurrence of adverse events have been limited by an inability to aggregate adverse event results from existing studies. As described previously, sedation practice varies widely, and the rate of adverse events is reported inconsistently. An important reason for this variability is that investigators do not have a standardized set of definitions and reporting guidelines to follow [9, 12, 13, 70, 79]. In order to facilitate comparisons between studies and the aggregation of data from multiple studies, definitions to describe sedation practices, interventions, and adverse events must be developed and routinely used. Only after clear definitions for adverse events and recommendations for reporting exist, and are consistently followed in studies of large numbers of patients receiving sedation, will meaningful adverse event rates be established. Once standard adverse event rates are established, sedation providers and programs may accurately and critically assess their work.

To address the wide disparities that exist in the reporting of adverse events, the Quebec Guidelines for sedation provided

Table 28.1 Intervention-based definitions for sedation-associated adverse events

Adverse events	Interventions performed in response
1. Oxygen desaturation	• Vigorous tactile stimulation • Airway repositioning • Suctioning • Oral or nasal airway placement
2. Apnea: central versus obstructive (partial versus complete)	• Administration of reversal agents • Supplementing/increasing oxygen • Application of positive pressure ± ventilation with bag mask • Tracheal Intubation
3. Clinically apparent pulmonary aspiration	• Extended observation or admission to hospital
4. Retching/vomiting	• Administration of antiemetic
5. Cardiovascular events Bradycardia Hypotension	• Chest compressions • Administration of medications • IV fluid administration
6. Excitatory movements	• Procedure was delayed, interrupted, or not completed
7. Paradoxical response to sedation	• Administration of reversal agents
Unpleasant recovery reactions	• Administration of sedation drugs • Allocation of additional personnel to care for the patient • Delay in discharge or disposition
8. Permanent complications (neurologic injury or death)	

to children in the emergency setting were devised by consensus of an expert panel of pediatric emergency physicians and pediatric anesthesiologists [20]. Intervention-based definitions for adverse events were chosen because the panel believed that this framework would yield the greatest possibility of uniform data collection for clinically important events. Definitions using this approach require specific clinical criteria to be present (e.g., decrease in oxygen saturation) *and* for one or more interventions (e.g., tactile stimulation and administration of blow-by oxygen) to be performed with the intention of treating or managing the event [20]. Table 28.1 provides a list of adverse events that should be documented and reported as recommended by the Quebec Guidelines, as well as examples of interventions that may be performed in response to these events. The Appendix provides complete Quebec Guidelines recommendations for definitions of adverse events within a template that may be used for data collection and documentation.

The Quebec Guidelines were intended to provide researchers with a template on which adverse events may be consistently documented and reported with the purpose of consistently collecting data that will allow uniform data sets and meaningful comparisons of sedation studies. Although the guidelines were developed for use in children receiving sedation in the emergency department, an accompanying editorial states that the Quebec Guidelines are broadly applicable to all forms of sedation research or adverse event monitoring [80]. More directly, despite the pediatric intent, each definition and recommendation applies readily to adults. This approach and the principles put forth also extrapolate to any setting in which sedation is performed with appropriate personnel and monitoring [22, 23, 80].

Once data is generated from multicenter studies of large populations of patients using standardized definitions and reporting schemes, meaningful adverse event rates may be established and definitive clinical care guidelines may be devised that will improve our ability to ensure the safety of sedation provided to children outside of the operating room.

Multicenter Investigations

Until just recently no studies of sufficiently large numbers of children who received sedation outside the operating room existed to allow for evaluation of acceptable rates of adverse events. The Pediatric Sedation Research Consortium (PSRC) has published an observational study of more than 30,000 children who received sedation at 26 institutions for mostly elective procedures (8 % emergency), performed by different providers (pediatric intensivists 28.4 %, emergency physicians 27.9 %, and anesthesiologists 19.2 %) using mostly the following drugs singly or in combination: propofol (50.1 %), midazolam (27.1 %), ketamine (13.6 %), or chloral hydrate (11.7 %) [1]. In this large cohort of children, they observed zero deaths, 1 cardiac arrest, 1 case of pulmonary aspiration, 13 episodes of laryngospasm, and 73 patients experienced unexpected apnea. All patients were successfully rescued from potentially adverse outcomes, and 1 in 1,500 sedation events resulted in unexpected admission to the hospital.

A subsequent study examined propofol administration under circumstances similar to their first study in almost 50,000 children [2]. Again, no deaths were observed; however, apnea or airway obstruction was common (5.75 %) and cardiac arrest ($n=2$), pulmonary aspiration ($n=4$), and laryngospasm ($n=96$) occurred. The authors emphasized that safety depends on the providers' ability to identify potentially serious adverse events, usually respiratory in nature, and provide appropriate rescue. Further data is needed to identify specific patients who may be at an increased risk for adverse events and to establish rates of adverse events in the emergency setting and in those receiving sedation drugs other than propofol.

In 2011, the PSRC published a comparison of major complication rates by provider for 131,751 pediatric procedural sedation cases [5]. Aspiration, death, cardiac arrest, unplanned admission to the hospital, increase in patient's level of care, and requirement for emergency anesthesia consultation were considered major complications and occurred between 7.6 and 12.4 per 10,000 for anesthesiologists, emergency physicians, intensivists, pediatricians, and other pediatric providers. Given the large sample size, these complication rates may be considered benchmarks for large, elective sedation services staffed by highly trained sedation providers primarily administering propofol.

Ketamine has become the most commonly administered drug for the sedation of children in the emergency department [22, 23, 45, 46, 48, 81–83]. A recent individual patient data meta-analysis of more than 8,000 ketamine administrations to children in 32 emergency departments sheds some light on adverse event rates and risk factors for emergency sedation with ketamine. Green et al. reported an overall incidence of airway and respiratory adverse events of 3.9 % [81]. Clinically apparent pulmonary aspiration did not occur in any of these patients. From this fact we can infer that the rate of aspiration associated with emergency department administered ketamine is very low, but we must consider what the risk actually may be. As illustrated in a *JAMA* article "If nothing goes wrong is everything alright?," we need to be cautious about reporting rates of rare adverse events and consider the maximum risk of occurrence [84]. Although this study represents the largest sample of children receiving emergency department ketamine sedation to date and provides important information, larger studies are required to definitively determine the maximal risk for rare adverse events such as aspiration.

Prospective studies of large cohorts of children, using standardized definitions and reporting structures for adverse events are required to generate the data needed to examine carefully the multitude of factors that contribute to adverse events before meaningful "acceptable" adverse event rates may be established.

Future Directions

As described previously, the work of the Pediatric Sedation Research Consortium and the ketamine individual patient data meta-analysis are important first steps toward generating the data required to carefully assess sedation practice in children outside the OR [1, 2, 81]. Recently, the World Society of Intravenous Anesthesia (World SIVA) established an International Sedation Task Force (ISTF) represented by 25 members from multispecialties, both adult and pediatric, from 11 countries. In a recently published manuscript, the ISTF has proposed an Adverse Event Reporting Tool designed to standardize the collection of sedation outcome data worldwide (Table 28.2) [85]. This tool will be an open-access web-based tool, available to providers globally.[1] The data collected will be available to individual and institutional users and will, in addition, populate the global ISTF sedation database. The collection of large data from multi-specialists globally will be an important first step to identify and carefully evaluate the range of variables that affect sedation-related adverse event rates. Such studies must be broad reaching in scope yet flexible enough to consider new developments in sedation techniques and monitoring as well as the use of the ever-emerging new sedation drugs that become available.

Only through rigorous adherence to the use of standardized adverse events definitions and reporting structures, such as described in the Quebec Guidelines and by the ISTF, will standardized data sets be compiled. This will allow for the aggregation of data and meaningful comparisons of sedation studies. National and international multispecialty collaborations will be required to develop databases with sufficient patient numbers and the clinical data required to develop and evaluate sedation practice based on patient populations and providers, procedures performed, and drugs administered. The feasibility of such a collaborative endeavor requires not only cooperation of multiple specialties using cutting-edge data collection technology but also a level of funding that to date has not been realized.

Conclusion

From the discussion presented here we can conclude that adverse event rates will vary depending on individual patient characteristics, procedures performed, sedation drugs and doses employed, and the setting in which patients receive care. In addition, the definitions used to identify adverse events and existing reporting structures will also impact on rates of adverse events observed.

A large sedation research consortium has provided us with initial data regarding expected rates of major complications of elective sedation performed by specialized sedation services [5]. As further studies of large numbers of children are performed using standardized definitions and reporting of adverse events, we will gain a clearer picture of what may be expected and acceptable adverse event rates for sedation performed outside the OR. Further multicenter, prospective research of international populations of children who receive sedation to identify risk factors for adverse events is needed so that true evidence-based sedation best practice guidelines may be established.

Standards of adverse event rates will vary based on the characteristics of the sedation experience as described previously. However, patient safety will ultimately be ensured by the careful assessment of risks and benefits of sedation that is performed in carefully monitored and controlled settings by skilled providers prepared to provide cardiorespiratory rescue when needed.

[1] www.AESedationReporting.com or www.InternationalSedationTaskForce.com

Table 28.2 International Sedation Task Force Adverse Event Sedation Reporting Tool (www.AESedationReporting.com)

World SIVA adverse sedation event recording tool configured for a web page or paper form				
Step 1: Was there one or more adverse events associated with this sedation encounter?				
• No, this form is now complete		• Yes, fill out remainder of form below		
Step 2: Please DESCRIBE the adverse event(s). Check all that apply				
Minimal risk descriptors	*Minor risk descriptors*	*Sentinel risk descriptors*		
• Vomiting/retching	• Oxygen desaturation (75–90 %) for <60 s	• Oxygen desaturation, severe	• Other specify below	
• Subclinical respiratory depression[a]	• Apnea, not prolonged	(<75 % at any time) or prolonged		
• Muscle rigidity, myoclonus	• Airway obstruction	(<90 % for >60 s)		
• Hypersalivation	• Failed sedation[e]	• Apnea, prolonged (>60 s)		
• Paradoxical response[b]	• Allergic reaction without anaphylaxis	• Cardiovascular collapse/shock[g]		
• Recovery agitation[c]	• Bradycardia[f]	• Cardiac arrest/absent pulse		
• Prolonged recovery[d]	• Tachycardia[f]			
	• Hypotension [f]			
	• Hypertension[f]			
	• Seizure			
Step 3: Please note the INTERVENTIONS performed to treat the adverse events(s). Check all that apply				
Minimal risk	*Minor risk*	*Moderate risk*	*Sentinel intervention*	
• No intervention performed	• Airway repositioning	• Bag valve mask-assisted ventilation	• Chest compressions	• Other, specify below
Administration of:	• Tectile stimulation or the administration of:	• Laryngeal mask airway	• Tracheal intubation or the administration of:	
• Additional sedative (s)	• Supplemental oxygen, new or increased	• Oral/nasal airway	• Neuromuscular blockade	
• Antiemetic	• Antisialagogue	• CPAP or the administration of:	• Pressor/epinephrine	
• Antihistamine		• Reversal agents	• Atropine to treat bradycardia	
		• Rapid IV fluids		
		• Anti convulsant IV		
Step 4: Please note the OUTCOME of the adverse event(s). Check all that apply				
Minimal risk outcome	*Moderate risk outcome*	*Sentinel outcome*	• Other specify below	
• No adverse outcome	• Unplanned hospitalization or escalation of care[h]	• Death		
		• Permanent neurological deficit		
		• Pulmonary aspiration syndrome[i]		
Step 5: Assign a SEVERITY rating to the adverse event(s) associated with this sedation encounter				
• It there are any options checked in the Sentinel columns above, then this is a *Sentinel*[j] adverse event				
• If the most serious option(s) checked above are Moderate risk, then this is a *Moderate*[k] risk adverse event				
• If the most serious option(s) checked above are Minor risk, then this is a *Minor*[l] risk adverse event				
• If the most serious option(s) checked above are Minimal risk, then this is a *Minimal*[m] risk adverse event				

Additional details (including "other" entries):

[a]"Subclinical respiratory depression" is defined as capnographic abnormalities suggesting respiratory depression that do not manifest clinically

[b]"Paradoxical response" is defined as unanticipated restlessness or agitation in response to sedatives

[c] "Recovery agitation" is defined as abnormal patient affect or behaviors during the recovery phase that can include crying, agitation, delirium, dysphoria, hallucinations, or nightmares

[d]"Prolonged recovery" is defined as failure to return to baseline clinical status within 2 h

[e]"Failed sedation" is defined as inability to attain suitable conditions to humanely perform the procedure

[f]Alteration in vital signs (bradycardia, tachycardia, hypotension, hypertension) is defined as a change of >25 % from baseline

[g]"Cardiovascular collapse/shock" is defined as clinical evidence of inadequate perfusion

[h]Examples of "Escalation of care" include transfer from ward to intensive care and prolonged hospitalization

[i]"Pulmonary aspiration syndrome" is defined as known or suspected inhalation of foreign material such as gastric contents into the respiratory tract associated with new or worsening respiratory signs

[j]"Sentinel" adverse events are those critical enough to represent real or serious imminent risk of serious and major patient injury. Once recognized, they warrant immediate and aggressive rescue interventions. Once clinically concluded, they warrant immediate reporting within sedation care systems and the highest level of peer scrutiny for continuous quality improvement

[k]"Moderate" adverse events are those that, while not sentinel, are serious enough to quickly endanger the patient if not promptly managed. Once clinically concluded, they warrant timely reporting within sedation care systems and periodic peer scrutiny for continuous quality improvement

[l]"Minor" adverse events are those encountered periodically in most sedation settings and those pose little threat given appropriate seditionist skills and monitoring

[m]"Minimal" adverse events are those that alone present no danger of permanent harm to the patient

Appendix: Recommended Documentation for Sedation Research

A. SEDATION DOCUMENTATION
1. Pre-Sedation Behavioral State

Definition: The patient's behavioral state immediately prior to sedation.

1. Indicate the state that best describes the child's behavior immediately prior to the administration of the sedation drugs:
□ Calm (eg, not crying)
□ Agitated but responds to comforting (eg, briefly stops crying)
□ Agitated and does not respond to comforting (eg, continuous ciying)

2. Efficacy of Sedation

Definition: A successful sedation creates conditions necessary to safely facilitate completion of a procedure through attenuation of pain, anxiety and movement with amnesia or decreased awareness. Patient must fulfill all criteria for a sedation to be considered successful.

1. Sedation was efficacious □YES □ NO
If YES, indicate which of the following criteria were met during the sedation
□ The patient does not have unpleasant recall of the procedure
□ The patient did not experience a sedation-related adverse event, resulting in the abandonment of the procedure
□ The patient did not experience a permanent complication
□ The patient did not have an unplanned admission to hospital or prolonged ED observation
□ The patient did not actively resist or require physical restraint for completion of the procedure

B. ADVERSE OUTCOME DOCUMENTATION
1. Oxygenation
1.1 Oxygen Desaturation □YES □ NO

Definition: Oxygen desaturation AND one or more intervention(s) are performed with the intention of improving the saturation

1. Baseline oxygen saturation on room air prior to PSA ______%
2. Oxygen delivered at start of Sedation phase □ NO □ YES
If YES, Method of oxygen delivery: □ nasal canula □ blow-by □ face mask □ face mask + non-rebreather
Flow rate delivered: ______ litres/minute
3. Indicate the interventions performed in response to the oxygen desaturation *(indicate ALL that apply)*
□ Vigorous tactile stimulation
□ Airway repositioning
□ Suctioning
□ Supplementing/increasing oxygen
□ Oral or nasal airway placement
□ Application of positive pressure +/ventilation with bag mask
□ Tracheal Intubation
□ Other ______________________
4. Lowest reliable oxygen saturation measured during the sedation ________%

2. Ventilation
2.1Apnea: central □ YES □ NO

Definition: Cessation or pause of ventilatory effort AND one or more intervention(s) are performed with the intention of stimulating or assisting ventilation.

1. Indicate the criteria used for recognition *(indicate ALL that apply)*
□ Visual confirmation of cessation/pause of ventilation
□ Cyanosis
□ Oxygen desaturation
□ Loss of $C0_2$ waveform
□ Other________________
2. Indicate the interventions performed in response to the apnea *(indicate ALL that apply)*

□ Vigorous tactile stimulation □ Application of bag mask with assisted ventilation
□ Administration of reversal agents □ Tracheal intubation
□ Other

2.2 Apnea: Obstructive
2.2.1 Partial Upper Airway Obstruction □YES □ NO

Definition: Manifested by stridor, snoring OR chest wall and suprasternal retractions AND one or more intervention(s) are performed with the intention of relieving the partial airway obstruction.

1. Indicate the criteria used for recognition (indicate ALL that apply)
   □ Stridor □ Oxygen desaturation
   □ Snoring □ Other_______________
   □ Chest wall or suprasternal retractions

Source: Bhatt M, Kennedy RM, Osmond MH, Krauss B, McAllister JD, Ansermino JM, Evered LM, Roback MG; Consensus Panel on Sedation Research of Pediatric Emergency Research Canada (PERC) and the Pediatric Emergency Care Applied Research Network (PECARN). Consensus-based recommendations for standardizing terminology and reporting adverse events for emergency department procedural sedation and analgesia in children. *Ann Emerg Med.* 2009;53(4):426-435.e4. Reprinted with permission from the American College of Emergency Physicians

References

1. Cravero JP, Blike GT, Beach ML, et al. Incidence and nature of adverse events during pediatric sedation/anesthesia for procedures outside the operating room: report from the Pediatric Sedation Research Consortium. Pediatrics. 2006;118(3):1087–96.
2. Cravero JP, Beach ML, Blike GT, et al. The incidence and nature of adverse events during pediatric sedation/anesthesia with propofol for procedures outside the operating room: a report from the Pediatric Sedation Research Consortium. Anesth Analg. 2009;108(3):795–805.
3. Vespasiano M, Finkelstein M, Kurachek S. Propofol sedation: intensivists' experience with 7304 cases in a children's hospital. Pediatrics. 2007;120:e1411–7.
4. Roback MG, Wathen JE, Bajaj L, Bothner JP. Adverse events associated with procedural sedation and analgesia in a pediatric emergency department: a comparison of common parenteral drugs. Acad Emerg Med. 2005;12:508–13.
5. Couloures KG, Beach M, Cravero JP, et al. Impact of provider specialty on pediatric procedural sedation complication rates. Pediatrics. 2011;127:e1154–60.
6. Havidich JE, Cravero JP. The current status of procedural sedation for pediatric patients in out-of-operating room locations. Curr Opin Anaesthesiol. 2012;25:453–60.
7. Mallory MD, Baxter AL, Yanosky DJ, Cravero JP. Emergency physician administered propofol sedation: a report on 25 433 sedations from the pediatric sedation research consortium. Ann Emerg Med. 2011;57:462–468.e1.
8. Srinivasan M, Turmelle M, Depalma LM, et al. Procedural sedation for diagnostic imaging in children by pediatric hospitalists using propofol: analysis of the nature, frequency, and predictors of adverse events and interventions. J Pediatr. 2012;160:801–806.e1.
9. Roback MG, Bajaj L, Wathen J, Bothner J. Preprocedural fasting and adverse Events in procedural sedation and analgesia in a pediatric emergency department – are they related? Ann Emerg Med. 2004;44:454–9.
10. Agrawal D, Manzi SF, Gupta R, et al. Preprocedural fasting state and adverse events in children undergoing procedural sedation and analgesia in a pediatric emergency department. Ann Emerg Med. 2003;42:636–46.
11. Babl FE, Puspitadewi A, Barnett P, et al. Preprocedural fasting state and adverse events in children receiving nitrous oxide for procedural sedation and analgesia. Pediatr Emerg Care. 2005;21:736–43.
12. Pitetti RD, Singh S, Pierce MC. Safe and efficacious use of procedural sedation and analgesia by nonanesthesiologists in a pediatric emergency department. Arch Pediatr Adolesc Med. 2003;157:1090.1096.
13. Pena BMG, Krauss B. Adverse events of procedural sedation and analgesia in a pediatric emergency department. Ann Emerg Med. 1999;34:483–91.

14. Green SM, Rothrock SG, Lynch EL. Intramuscular ketamine for pediatric sedation in the emergency department: safety profile in 1,022 cases. Ann Emerg Med. 1998;31:688–97.
15. Newman DH, Azer MM, Pitetti RD, et al. When is a patient safe for discharge after procedural sedation? The timing of adverse effect events in 1,367 pediatric procedural sedations. Ann Emerg Med. 2003;42:627–35.
16. Malviya S, Voepel-Lewis T, Eldevik OP, et al. Sedation and general anaesthesia in children undergoing MRI and CT: adverse events and outcomes. Br J Anaesth. 2000;84:743–8.
17. Malviya S, Voepel-Lewis T, Prochaska G, Tait AR. Prolonged recovery and delayed side effects of sedation for diagnostic imaging studies in children. Pediatrics. 2000;105:e42.
18. Malviya S, Voepel-Lewis T, Tait AR. Adverse events and risk factors associated with the sedation of children by nonanesthesiologtists. Anesth Analg. 1997;85:1207–13.
19. Coté CJ, Notterman DA, Karl HW, et al. Adverse sedation events in pediatrics: a critical incident analysis of contributing factors. Pediatrics. 2000;106:633–44.
20. Bhatt M, Kennedy R, Osmond MH, et al. Consensus-based recommendations for standardizing terminology and reporting adverse events for emergency department procedural sedation and analgesia in children. Ann Emerg Med. 2009;53:426–435.e4. Epub 2008 Nov 19.
21. American College of Emergency Physicians. Clinical policy for procedural sedation and analgesia in the emergency department. Ann Emerg Med. 1998;31:663–77.
22. Krauss B, Green SM. Sedation and analgesia for procedures in children. N Engl J Med. 2000;342:938–45.
23. Krauss B, Green SM. Procedural sedation and analgesia in children. Lancet. 2006;367:766–80.
24. The Joint Commission on Accreditation of Healthcare Organizations (JCAHO), Accreditation Manual for Hospitals, 2006:253.
25. Ramaiah R, Bhananker S. Pediatric procedural sedation and analgesia outside the operating room: anticipating, avoiding and managing complications. Expert Rev Neurother. 2011;11:755–63.
26. Green SM, Mason KP. Stratification of sedation risk: a challenge to the sedation continuum. Paediatr Anaesth. 2011;21:924–31.
27. Coté CJ, Karl HW, Notterman DA, et al. Adverse sedation events in pediatrics: analysis of medications used for sedation. Pediatrics. 2000;105:805–14.
28. Parker RI, Mahan RA, Biugliano D, Parker MM. Efficacy and safety of intravenous midazolam and ketamine as sedation for therapeutic and diagnostic procedures in children. Pediatrics. 1997;99:427–31.
29. Brown ET, Corbett SW, Green SM. Iatrogenic cardiopulmonary arrest during pediatric sedation with meperidine, promethazine, and chlorpromazine. Pediatr Emerg Care. 2001;17:351–3.
30. Hoffman GM, et al. Risk reduction in pediatric procedural sedation by application of an AAP/ASA process model. Pediatrics. 2002; 109:236–43.
31. Sanborn PA, Michna E, Zurakowski D, et al. Adverse cardiovascular and respiratory events during sedation of pediatric patients for imaging examinations. Radiology. 2005;237:288–94.
32. Sweeney H, Marai S, Kim C, et al. Creating a sedation service for pediatric urodynamics: our experience. Urol Nurs. 2008;28(4): 273–8.
33. Farrell MK, Drake GJ, Rucker D, et al. Creation of a registered nurse-administered nitrous oxide sedation program for radiology and beyond. Pediatr Nurs. 2008;34(1):29–35.
34. Woodthorpe C, Trigg A, Alison G, et al. Nurse led sedation for paediatric MRI: progress and issues. Paediatr Nurs. 2007;19(2):14–8.
35. Wood C, Hurley C, Wettlaufer J, et al. Retrospective comparison of emergency department length of stay for procedural sedation and analgesia by nurse practitioners and physicians. Pediatr Emerg Care. 2007;23(10):709–12.
36. Pershad J, Gilmore B. Successful implementation of a radiology sedation service staffed exclusively by pediatric emergency physicians. Pediatrics. 2006;117(3):e413–22.
37. King WK, Stockwell JA, DeGuzman MA, et al. Evaluation of a pediatric-sedation service for common diagnostic procedures. Acad Emerg Med. 2006;13(6):673–6. Epub 2006 May 2.
38. Yamamoto LG. Initiating a hospital-wide pediatric sedation service provided by emergency physicians. Clin Pediatr. 2008;47(1): 37–48.
39. Shankar VR. Sedating children for radiological procedures: an intensivist's perspective. Pediatr Radiol. 2008;38 Suppl 2:S213–7.
40. Webb ST, Hunter DN. Is sedation by non-anaesthetists really safe? Br J Anaesth. 2013;111(2):136–8.
41. Miner JR, Krauss B. Procedural sedation and analgesia research: state of the art. Acad Emerg Med. 2007;14:170–8.
42. American Academy of Pediatrics Committee on Drugs. Guidelines for monitoring and management of pediatric patients during and after sedation for diagnostic and therapeutic procedures. Pediatrics. 1992;89(pt 1):1110–5.
43. American Society of Anesthesiologists Task Force on Sedation and Analgesia by Non-Anesthesiologists. Practice guidelines for sedation and analgesia by non-anesthesiologists. *Anesthesiology* 2002;96:1004-17.
44. American Academy of Pediatrics. Guidelines for monitoring and management of pediatric patients during and after sedation for diagnostic and therapeutic procedures: Addendum. Committee on Drugs. Pediatrics. 2002;110:836–8.
45. American College of Emergency Physicians. Clinical policy: evidence-based approach to pharmacologic agents used in pediatric sedation and analgesia in the emergency department. Ann Emerg Med. 2004;44:342–77.
46. American College of Emergency Physicians. Clinical policy: procedural sedation and analgesia in the emergency department. Ann Emerg Med. 2005;45:177–96.
47. Miner JR, Burton JH. Clinical practice advisory: emergency department procedural sedation with propofol. Ann Emerg Med. 2007;50:182–7.
48. Green SM, Roback MG, Kennedy R, et al. Clinical practice guideline for emergency department ketamine dissociative sedation: 2011 update. Ann Emerg Med. 2011;57:449–61.
49. Cote CJ, Wilson S. Guidelines for monitoring and management of pediatric patients during and after sedation for diagnostic and therapeutic procedures: an update. Pediatrics. 2006;118:2587–602.
50. Green SM, Roback MG, Miner JR, et al. Fasting and emergency department procedural sedation and analgesia: a consensus-based clinical practice advisory. Ann Emerg Med. 2007;49:454–61.
51. American Academy of Pediatric Dentistry. Guidelines for the elective use of pharmacologic conscious sedation and deep sedation in pediatric dental patients. Pediatr Dent. 1993;15:297–9.
52. O'Connor RE, Sama A, Burton JH, et al. Procedural sedation and analgesia in the emergency department: recommendations for physician credentialing, privileging, and practice. Ann Emerg Med. 2011;58(4):365–70.
53. Cote CH. Strategies for preventing sedation accidents. Pediatr Ann. 2005;34:625–33.
54. Lee LA, Bomino KB. The closed claims project has it influenced anesthetic practice and outcome? Anesthesiol Clin North America. 2002;20:485–501.
55. Tinker JH, Dull DL, Caplan RA, et al. Role of monitoring devices in prevention of anesthetic mishaps: a closed claims analysis. Anesthesiology. 1989;71:541–6.
56. Bhananker SM, Posner KL, Cheney FW, et al. Injury and liability associated with monitored anesthesia care. A closed claims analysis. Anesthesiology. 2006;104:228–34.
57. Petty WE, Kremer M, Biddle C. A synthesis of the Australian patient safety foundation anesthesia incident monitoring study, the

American society of anesthesiologists closed claims project, and the American association of nurse anesthetists closed claims study. AANA J. 2002;70:193–202.
58. Roback MG, Wathen JE, Mackenzie T, Bajaj L. A Randomized, Controlled Trial of IV versus IM Ketamine for Sedation of Pediatric Patients Receiving Emergency Department Orthopedic Procedures. Ann Emerg Med. 2006;48:605–12.
59. Dachs RJ, Innes GM. Intravenous ketamine sedation of pediatric patients in the emergency department. Ann Emerg Med. 1997; 29:146–50.
60. McCarty EC, Mencio GA, Anderson Walker L, et al. Ketamine sedation for the reduction of children's fractures in the emergency department. J Bone Joint Surg Am. 2000;82:912–8.
61. Green SM, Rothrock SG, Harris T, et al. Intravenous ketamine for pediatric sedation in the emergency department: safety profile with 156 cases. Acad Emerg Med. 1998;5(10):971–6.
62. Heinz P, Geelhoed GC, Wee C, et al. Is atropine needed with ketamine sedation? A prospective, randomized, double blind study. Emerg Med J. 2006;23:206–9.
63. McGlone RG, Fleet T, Durham S, et al. A comparison of intramuscular ketamine with high dose intramuscular midazolam with and without intranasal flumazenil in children before suturing. Emerg Med J. 2001;18:34–8.
64. Godambe SA, Elliot V, Matheny D, et al. Comparison of propofol/fentanyl versus ketamine/midazolam for brief orthopedic procedural sedation in a pediatric emergency department. Pediatrics. 2003;112:116–23.
65. Guenther-Skokan E, Pribble C, Bassett KE, et al. Use of propofol sedation in a pediatric emergency department: a prospective study. Clin Pediatr. 2001;40:663–71.
66. Bassett KE, Anderson JL, Pribble CG, et al. Propofol for procedural sedation in children in the emergency department. Ann Emerg Med. 2003;42:773–82.
67. Shah A, Mosdossy G, McLeod S, et al. A blinded, randomized controlled trial to evaluate ketamine-propofol versus ketamine alone for procedural sedation in children. Ann Emerg Med. 2011; 57:425–33.
68. Hertzog JH, Dalton HJ, Anderson BD, et al. Prospective evaluation of propofol anesthesia in the pediatric intensive care unit for elective oncology procedures in ambulatory and hospitalized children. Pediatrics. 2000;106:742–7.
69. Andolfatto G, Abu-Laban RB, Zed PJ, et al. Ketamine-propofol combination (ketofol) versus propofol alone. for emergency department procedural sedation and analgesia: a randomized double-blind trial. Ann Emerg Med. 2012;59(6):504–12.e1-2.
70. Barbi E, Gerarduzzi T, Marchetti F, et al. Deep sedation with propofol by nonanesthesiologists : a prospective pediatric experience. Arch Pediatr Adolesc Med. 2003;157:1097–103.
71. Hasan RA, Shayevitz JR, Patel V. Deep sedation with propofol for children undergoing ambulatory magnetic resonance imaging of the brain: experience from a pediatric intensive care unit. Pediatr Crit Care Med. 2003;4:454–8.
72. Pershad J, Godambe SA. Propofol for procedural sedation in the pediatric emergency department. J Emerg Med. 2004;27:11–4.
73. Willman EV, Andolfatto G. A prospective evaluation of "ketofol" (ketamine/propofol combination) for procedural sedation and analgesia in the emergency department. Ann Emerg Med. 2007;49:23–30.
74. Messenger DW, Murray HE, Dungey PE, et al. Subdissociative dose ketamine versus fentanyl for analgesia during propofol procedural sedation: a randomized controlled trial. Acad Emerg Med. 2008;15:877–86.
75. Cheung KW, Watson M-L, Field SG, et al. Aspiration pneumonitis requiring intubation after procedural sedation and analgesia: a case report. Ann Emerg Med. 2007;49(4):462–4. Epub 2006 Nov 3.
76. American Society of Anesthesiologists. Practice guidelines for preoperative fasting and the use of pharmacologic agents to reduce the risk of pulmonary aspiration: application to healthy patients undergoing elective procedures. Anesthesiology. 1999;90:896–905.
77. Green SM. Fasting is a consideration—not a necessity—for emergency department procedural sedation and analgesia. Ann Emerg Med. 2003;42:647–50.
78. Green SM, Krauss B. Pulmonary aspiration risk during ED procedural sedation: an examination of the role of fasting and sedation depth. Acad Emerg Med. 2002;9:35–42.
79. Sacchetti A, Stander E, Ferguson N, et al. Pediatric procedural sedation in the community emergency department: results from the ProSCED registry. Pediatr Emerg Care. 2007;23:218–22.
80. Green SM, Yealy DM. Procedural sedation goes Utstein: the Quebec guidelines. Ann Emerg Med. 2009;53(4):436–8. Epub 2008 Dec 21.
81. Green SM, Roback MG, Krauss B, et al. Predictors of airway and respiratory adverse events of ketamine sedation in the emergency department: an individual-patient data meta-analysis of 8,282 children. Ann Emerg Med. 2009;54(2):158–68.e1-4.
82. Bhargava R, Young KD. Procedural pain management patterns in academic pediatric emergency departments. Acad Emerg Med. 2007;14:479–82.
83. Haley-Andrews S. Ketamine—the sedative of choice in a busy pediatric emergency department. J Emerg Nurs. 2006;32:186–8.
84. Hanley JA, Loppman-Hand A. If nothing goes wrong is everything all right? Interpreting zero numerators. JAMA. 1983;249(13):1743–5.
85. Mason KP, Green SM. Piacevoli Q and the International Sedation Task Force. Adverse event reporting tool to standardize the reporting and tracking of adverse events during procedural sedation: a consensus document from the World SIVA International Sedation Task Force. Br J Anaesth. 2012;108(1):13–20.

29 Medicolegal Risks and Outcomes of Sedation

Steven M. Selbst and Stewart L. Cohen

Abstract

Most children who receive sedation outside the operating room have good outcomes and benefit from efforts to reduce pain and anxiety during a procedure. However, administration of sedative and analgesic agents to children in the outpatient setting always carries some risk to the patient. If a child has an adverse outcome after sedation, and there is evidence of substandard care then there is the potential for a professional liability ("malpractice") claim against the providers and/or the facility. It is difficult to track with any reliability the actual results of all such claims throughout the USA, in part because there is no uniform national system to report jury verdicts and judgments in state courts that are not appealed. Further, if a malpractice case is settled prior to a jury verdict, the details of those settlements are often kept confidential by the agreement of parties, typically at the request of the medical providers or their insurance carriers. A review of publicly available reports has identified several pediatric sedation claims of alleged negligence. In each of these malpractice cases, the allegations were that the care provided by the professionals (and/or institution) was below an established standard of care, that there was a breach of that standard and that the breach caused injury to the patient. Standard of care is defined as that care which a reasonable physician in a particular specialty would have given to a similar patient, under similar circumstances. Because most clinicians have similar access to information and knowledge, they are usually held to a national standard of care regardless of how remotely the individual may practice.

Keywords

Medicolegal risks • Sedation • Malpractice • Litigation • Negligence • Standard of care • Breach • Jury verdict • Indemnity • Informed consent • Civil action • Complaint • Defense • Certificate of merit • Defendant • Plaintiff • Prosecution • Civil lawsuit • Homicide • Involuntary manslaughter • Criminal negligence

Introduction and Background

Most children who receive sedation outside the operating room have good outcomes and benefit from efforts to reduce pain and anxiety during a procedure [1–3]. However, administration of sedative and analgesic agents to children in the outpatient setting always carries some risk to the patient [1–5]. It is reported that 4 % of children who received ketamine in the emergency department have airway and respiratory adverse events and that up to 17 % of pediatric procedural

S.M. Selbst, M.D. (✉)
Department of Pediatrics, Nemours/Alfred I. duPont Hospital for Children and Sidney Kimmel Medical College at Thomas Jefferson University, 1600 Rockland Road, Wilmington, DE 19803, USA
e-mail: sselbst@nemours.org

S.L. Cohen, Esq.
Cohen, Placitella & Roth, P.C., Two Commerce Square, Suite 2900, 2001 Market St., Philadelphia, PA 19103, USA
e-mail: scohen@cprlaw.com

K.P. Mason (ed.), *Pediatric Sedation Outside of the Operating Room: A Multispecialty International Collaboration*, DOI 10.1007/978-1-4939-1390-9_29, © Springer Science+Business Media New York 2015

sedations result in some type of complication [3, 4]. Most adverse events are respiratory in nature and 1 in every 200 requires interventions to maintain a patent airway and ventilate the patient. One in every 1,500 sedations results in an event that requires unanticipated admission to the hospital [3]. If a child has an adverse outcome after sedation, and there is evidence of substandard care then there is the potential for a professional liability ("malpractice"[1]) claim against the providers and/or the facility. It is difficult to track with any reliability the actual results of all such claims throughout the USA, in part because there is no uniform national system to report *jury verdicts*[2] and judgments in state courts that are not appealed.[3] Further, if a malpractice case is settled prior to a jury verdict, the details of those settlements are often kept confidential by the agreement of parties, typically at the request of the medical providers or their insurance carriers [6]. (Refer to Chap. 30, section "Closed Claims Settlements for Cases Outside the Operating Room.") A review of publicly available reports has identified several pediatric sedation claims of alleged *negligence*[4]. In each of these malpractice cases, the allegations were that the care provided by the professionals (and/or institution) was below an established *standard of care*[5], that there was a *breach*[6] of that standard and that the breach caused injury to the patient (see Case Studies 1–6 at end of chapter). Standard of care is defined as that care which a reasonable physician in a particular specialty would have given to a similar patient, under similar circumstances. Because most clinicians have similar access to information and knowledge, they are usually held to a national standard of care regardless of how remotely the individual may practice [7].

Most malpractice lawsuits are resolved prior to trial. Less than 10 % reach a *jury verdict* [8, 9]. Still, these legal actions can be quite burdensome, expensive, and emotionally draining for both professionals, patients, and their families. On average, a medical malpractice claim costs a minimum of $23,000 to defend. Claims that go to trial are generally more costly [8]. The mean *indemnity payout*[7] (money paid to the plaintiff) is about $275,000, a figure that almost doubles for pediatricians [10].

Adverse outcomes can occur in the absence of substandard care. When litigation ensues, the hospital/facility along with the physicians and nurses may all be named in the lawsuit. Many states require that, prior to filing any professional negligence claim, the lawyer for the injured party file some type of *certificate of merit*[8] to substantiate that a licensed professional has reviewed the claim and agrees that there is merit to the allegations of substandard care and causation [11]. Claims against medical facilities can be founded on the employer/employee relationship [12] or the institution's direct negligence [13] and/or failure to establish adequate written policies and procedures as required under federal law and/or state licensing requirements [14]. A hospital or an outpatient facility may be sued for the conduct of an anesthesiologist practicing at the facility even though the physician is not a direct employee: because the anesthesiologist provides care at the facility, it is implied that he is an employee [15].

Preventing Litigation

Professional negligence lawsuits are a risk of medical practice. A legitimate lawsuit is based on the breach of a recognized standard of care. Malpractice claims can be minimized, or at least reduced, if the medical staff and institution are committed to practicing "good" medicine, communicating well with family members and other hospital staff, and documenting the "good" care that is delivered [7]. Compliance with the standard of care and the establishment and strict compliance with established policies and procedures are the "best practices."

[1]Please refer to section "Glossary" at the end of chapter.

[2]Please refer to section "Glossary" at the end of chapter.

[3]Federal law requires all insurance companies to report the details of every medical malpractice payment to the Federal Government 42 U.S.C. § 11131. This information however is not available to the public. Specifically the law requires the following:

§11131 Requiring reports on medical malpractice payments.

(a) In general. Each entity (including an insurance company) which makes payment under a policy of insurance, self-insurance, or otherwise in settlement (or partial settlement) of, or in satisfaction of a judgment in, a medical malpractice action or claim shall report, in accordance with section 424 [42 USCS § 11134], information respecting the payment and circumstances thereof.

(b) Information to be reported. The information to be reported under subsection (a) includes:

(1) The name of any physician or licensed health care practitioner for whose benefit the payment is made.

(2) The amount of the payment.

(3) The name (if known) of any hospital with which the physician or practitioner is affiliated or associated.

(4) A description of the acts or omissions and injuries or illnesses upon which the action or claim was based.

(5) Such other information as the Secretary determines is required for appropriate interpretation of information reported under this section.

(c) Sanctions for failure to report. Any entity that fails to report information on a payment required to be reported under this section shall be subject to a civil money penalty of not more than $ 10,000 for each such payment involved. Such penalty shall be imposed and collected in the same manner as civil money penalties under subsection (a) of section 1128A of the Social Security Act [42 USCS § 1320a-7a] are imposed and collected under that section.

[4]Please refer to section "Glossary" at the end of chapter.

[5]Please refer to section "Glossary" at the end of chapter.

[6]Please refer to section "Glossary" at the end of chapter.

[7]Please refer to section "Glossary" at the end of chapter.

[8]Please refer to section "Glossary" at the end of chapter.

Practice "Good" Medicine

Malpractice claims arise from adverse outcomes. If there is no injury, there is no basis to bring a claim. Accordingly, the most effective way to prevent a malpractice lawsuit is to prevent an adverse outcome (see Table 29.1).

Sedation providers must be qualified, credentialed, and experienced [5, 16]. Qualifications and credentials may be verified with background checks. Experience, however, is more ephemeral. For example, consider the situation of a nurse, caring for a child in sedation recovery, who is educated and qualified to perform pediatric resuscitation but has no experience in actually resuscitating a baby. Should a child under her care suffer a catastrophic injury as a result of substandard care, one basis of a claim may be that this inexperienced nurse was left solely responsible and that her employers failed to establish, implement, and enforce policies and procedures to prevent this occurrence.

Hospitals and medical facilities are required to develop written policies and procedures to hire, train, and retain experienced, qualified, and credentialed sedation providers. This responsibility is mandated under federal regulations and Joint Commission accreditation standards [17]. A hospital may even be liable for services it renders at a "free-standing" facility, which it does not own, if it retains overall responsibility and authority to provide these services[9] [18]. There is no universal rule on what the credentialing process must entail. For example, some facilities require the clinician to be certified in Pediatric Advanced Life Support (PALS), Basic Life Support (BLS), and possibly take a course or complete an online sedation module. Other facilities recommend simulation-based training of non-anesthesiologists to improve patient safety during pediatric sedation [19]. Although there are no international or national standards for credentialing, training, policies, and procedures, there are "assumed" competencies:

1. While training may vary at different institutions, the clinician must be thoroughly knowledgeable about the sedative agents, their use, and potential complications.
2. The clinician must realize that along the sedation continuum, a deeper depth of sedation may occur.

Table 29.1 Preventing adverse outcomes

Provider must be qualified and credentialed
Provider must have skills to rescue patient
Provider must have knowledge of medications and potential complications
Provider must prepare for a deeper level of sedation than anticipated
Perform a pre-sedation evaluation
Consult anesthesia for high-risk cases
Check medications and dosages prior to administration
Observe patients until back to baseline
Develop and follow hospital policies and procedures

3. The clinician and staff must have appropriate skills to rescue a sedation-related complication.
4. The institutions are responsible for ensuring that policies, procedures, and staff are in place to support such a rescue.

Clinicians who work in a free-standing facility (such as a dental office or a gastroenterology suite) must operate with caution and be prepared to activate emergency medical services (EMS) when needed. They must have proper equipment available and the necessary skill to use this equipment appropriately while awaiting help [20]. In the event of an adverse outcome, sedation providers at an office setting remote from a hospital may be held to the same standards as those who operate in a hospital.

The practice of prescribing sedatives as a pre-anxiolytic to be taken at home, administered by a parent prior to arrival, should be avoided. This practice is associated with an increased risk for airway obstruction at home or during transport [21]. Furthermore, the clinician must choose appropriate sedatives and dosing to achieve the intended depth of sedation [22]. For example, if a sedative achieves deep sedation in a case intended for anxiolysis, this may lead to litigation based on a breach of the standard of care [23].

The Sedation Process

The sedation of a child begins even before the child arrives. It involves a process that begins with the pre-screening of the patient, continues through the child's arrival for sedation, and then follows the child through the sedation and through discharge from the recovery room and follow-up with the family at 24 h post-discharge. This section will review the medicolegal implications and provide advice for the sedation provider at each step of the sedation process.

Pre-sedation Evaluation/Decisions

The sedation provider is responsible for the final evaluation of the child prior to administration of sedation. Inadequate

[9]Under federal regulations that apply whenever a Hospital accepts Medicare and Medicaid funds, the governing body of a hospital must assure, where emergency services are provided outside the hospital, that the medical staff has written policies and procedures for appraisal of emergencies, initial treatment and referral when appropriate. 42 C.F.R. § 482.12 (f)(2) Under the Joint Commission of Accredited Healthcare Organization standards, the hospital is required to ensure that services provided by contractual arrangements are provided safely and effectively. Pursuant to those standards, the hospital "retains overall responsibility and authority for services furnished under a contract." Standard LD.3.50 (2007).

evaluation prior to the sedation has been found to be a factor in many adverse events [21]. A pre-sedation health evaluation should at a minimum include the patient's age, weight, allergies, medications, vital signs, relevant family history, and past medical history (including physical abnormalities, history of snoring, and neurologic impairment that may increase potential for airway obstruction). A focused physical examination and assessment of the airway is crucial; large tonsils or anatomic airway abnormalities should be noted as they may increase the risk for airway obstruction [20, 22].

The non-anesthesia sedation provider should consult anesthesia for high-risk patients. In general, high-risk patients are those with snoring, stridor, craniofacial abnormalities, chronic lung disease, abnormal airway, vomiting, gastroesophageal reflux, bowel obstruction, asthma exacerbation, active respiratory disease (pneumonia), complex medical problems (mediastinal mass, prematurity, cardiac disease), hypovolemia, or neuromuscular disorder. An anesthesia consult is also suggested for children younger than 1 year of age or those with an American Society of Anesthesiologists (ASA) classification of three or greater [20, 24].

Medication dosages should be double-checked before administration and all resuscitation equipment and medications should be available. The SOAPME—Suction, Oxygen, Airway (appropriate-sized equipment), Pharmacy (drugs needed), Monitors, Equipment (perhaps a defibrillator)—checklist is a helpful and easy to remember pneumonic for sedation preparation [20, 22]. A "time out" must be performed before any medication is given in order to verify the correct patient, site, and medications [25]. It is important to anticipate and be prepared for complications, such as laryngospasm [26]. The Joint Commission and American Academy of Pediatrics (AAP) emphasize the concept of "sedation rescue," which is essential to safe sedation [20, 25].

Medication Errors

Every time a sedative or analgesic is administered there is always a chance for error. Each year, 1.5 million preventable adverse drug events occur. As many as 7,000 people die as a result of avoidable medication errors. Although hospitals and pharmacies have adopted computerized prescriptions and bar-coding equipment to decrease the chance of a medication error, errors still occur [27]. One study found that there are 3.99 errors for every 1,000 medications ordered for inhospital patients. Many are potentially serious [28]. This is due in part to look-alike and sound-alike drugs. Hospitals and clinicians must be careful to keep these look-alike and sound-alike medications separated and clearly labeled.

Many medication errors are due to incorrect computation. Some of these errors may be preventable by computer-based order sets, which have prescribing limits that restrict drug doses. Serious medication errors with a misplaced decimal point can result in a tenfold error. It is thus recommended that a zero be placed before a decimal point to express any number less than one (e.g., 0.5 mL). Alternatively, one should never use a terminal zero (e.g., 5.0), since failure to note this decimal point may result in a tenfold overdose. Avoid abbreviations (cc, μ, mL, MSO_4, N_2O) because these are not universally understood and may be misinterpreted. Preventable errors occur when the health care provider fails to either obtain an adequate history of food or medication allergies, or to read the medical history that documents an allergy [29]. Furthermore, proper supervision of sedation trainees is important. Trainees often prescribe and administer sedation to children. Lack of trainee supervision is a common factor in medical errors and resulting malpractice lawsuits [30].

Post-sedation/Discharge

Observation of the patient for an appropriate period of time following sedation and in the recovery period is critical. While it is important to establish written criteria for discharge, it is also important as a matter of administration and policy to identify who will decide when discharge criteria have been met. For example, does a nurse make the discharge decision based solely on established written criteria? Should a physician perform a final examination before discharge? Every child who receives sedation must be discharged following criteria proposed by the AAP [5, 20]. Whether the criteria has been met, and how those protocols and procedures are implemented and enforced are left to the discretion of the practitioner and the facility. The proper exercise of this discretion can raise questions of Standard of Care. A minimum return to baseline medical and cognitive status is usually expected: Cardiovascular function, an intact gag reflex, a patent airway, adequate hydration, and baseline respiratory status are critical. The child should be easily aroused and as responsive to verbal and tactile stimuli as he was prior to sedation. Younger children or those with neurologic dysfunction should return to their pre-sedation level of function before discharge. Consider a prolonged recovery stay if the accompanying and responsible guardian is alone (driving the car) or if the child has a significant underlying medical problem (neurologic impairment, respiratory disease, history of sedation-related complications) [20]. Failure to give adequate instructions and advice concerning limitation of activity and appropriate dietary precautions and a premature discharge can have disastrous consequences. Each child should be provided with a 24-h phone number that parents can call with any questions about their child's sedation or behavior [24].

Policies and Protocols

Hospitals are required under federal law and Joint Commission standards to develop, publish, teach, enforce, and drill sedation policies and procedures. Written policies are defined in the Joint Commission standards as "the formal, approved description of how a governance, management or clinical process is defined, organized and carried out." Simply stated, policies are mandatory and should be distinguished from advisory guidelines. Failure to have written policies in place is not only a violation of law but also a violation of the federal funding requirements under Medicare. This failure could lead to a claim of a violation of standard of care against a facility, institution, and responsible administration. Although sedation providers at non-Joint Commission facilities may not be required to have such written policies and procedures, absence of or non-adherence to these policies/procedures can be evidence of a deviation from the standard of care. Hospital protocols and policies should be reasonable, so that clinicians understand and are able to adhere to them. For instance, capnography is "encouraged" for sedated children in AAP and ASA guidelines [20, 31]. However, if the hospital does not routinely use or provide end-tidal CO_2 monitoring for sedated patients, capnography should not be a requirement in the policy and procedure manual of the hospital.

The Joint Commission mandates that each institution develop its own specific protocols for any patient at risk of losing his protective airway reflex during sedation [25]. The standard of care must be consistent throughout the hospital, regardless of the location at which the sedation is administered (emergency department, clinic, radiology suite, etc.) [25]. The institution must standardize the documentation process in terms of history, physical exam, and events during the procedure and recovery period. Guidelines for *informed consent*[10] for procedures must be consistent throughout the institution (see section "Informed Consent"). Monitoring guidelines and requisite skills of the sedation providers must be uniform within the institution [25]. Standards for how long a child must take nothing by mouth (NPO) prior to sedation must be consistent. Although NPO guidelines have been recently challenged due to lack of published validation pertaining to outcome, hospitals must establish, maintain, and update these policies. Even in the emergency department, the administration of sedatives must be preceded by a thorough evaluation of food and fluid intake. The hospital policy may provide for modification of NPO guidelines in an emergency situation after careful consideration and documentation of the risk versus benefits of proceeding. This hospital policy should reflect that in an emergency, when proper fasting cannot be ensured, the increased risk of sedation must be weighed against its benefits [5]. In general, the minimum needed depth of sedation should be targeted in these emergency situations [20].

Hospital policy should define which clinicians can prescribe or administer specific sedative medications. For example, many hospitals permit non-anesthesiologists to administer agents such as propofol or ketamine after specific training. Others prohibit this. Such decisions are generally left to the discretion of the individual hospital, as the standard of care allows non-anesthesiologists to use such medications within appropriate guidelines [16]. The package insert information is important, but does not necessarily dictate clinical practice. Particularly for children in the USA, many medications are not approved by the Food and Drug Administration (FDA) and are administered "off label." Accordingly, off-label use of some sedatives (propofol, for example) has been incorporated into specialty guidelines (American College of Emergency Physicians (ACEP) and American College of Gastroenterology). (Refer to Chaps. 2, 18, and 19.) In the event of a malpractice lawsuit involving sedative agents, evidence-based research and clinical usage protocols are considered. If such evidence demonstrates safe and effective outcomes for the agents utilized, the clinician may offer that as evidence to defend the use and administration of agents, such as propofol.

Hospital policies should specify which medications can or cannot be administered by nursing staff. In many states, nurses are not permitted to administer certain sedative agents. Nurses must follow the state, local, and hospital regulations. In the event of an unintended adverse outcome with sedation, deviation from these rules will be closely scrutinized.

Finally, hospital policies should address the issue of photographs and video recording of patients during sedation. In general, images of a patient during his medical care become part of the patient's permanent medical record. They are subject to the same legal scrutiny as other parts of the medical record and may be used as evidence in the event of a malpractice lawsuit. An exception may be for images acquired by a treating physician for purposes other than medical care (such as for use in publications, lectures, or a clinical trial).

Clinical Guidelines

Several specialty organizations have published sedation guidelines to guide health care professionals. The AAP published guidelines for sedation in 2006 [20], as did the ACEP in 2008 [32]. (Refer to Chap. 2.) The Joint Commission defines practice guidelines as "tools that describe processes found by clinical trials or by consensus opinion of experts to be the most effective in evaluation and/or treating a patient who has a specific symptom, condition, or diagnosis, or

[10] Please refer to section "Glossary" at the end of chapter.

describe a specific procedure. Synonyms include practice parameter, protocol, preferred practice pattern and guidelines." All who administer sedation should be familiar with published clinical care guidelines. This is especially true of the guidelines accepted by a specialty. It is important that a specialist adhere to his own specialty guidelines or document his rational for deviation. Failure to follow them may well be the basis of the claim that there was a deviation from the standard of care [33]. Guidelines from major organizations such as the AAP have great impact in court. In general, a guideline supports a standard of care. It may well be viewed by the courts and juries as establishing the "rules of the road." Surprisingly, a recent study showed that monitoring guidelines suggested by ACEP, AAP, and ASA for non-anesthesiologists were followed in only about half the pediatric cases analyzed [34]. The failure to adhere may be the basis of a claim for a liability against the sedation provider.

Guidelines for fasting (NPO) prior to sedation are consensus based rather than evidence based and thus they are debatable. Regardless, one should not disregard the fasting status of the patient [20, 22, 32, 35–37]. Documentation of the last oral intake is good practice and a Joint Commission requirement [25]. When NPO status is not adhering to guidelines and sedation proceeds regardless, documentation is critical. Consider and document the risk-to-benefit ratio, weighing NPO status against the urgency of the procedure. This will help prevent an adverse event and will help defend the care provided.

Communicate Well

It is very important for those involved with sedation to communicate effectively with families and show compassion [38]. Clinicians should listen well and speak clearly. Advise the family on what to anticipate and keep them informed as the procedure and sedation evolves. Develop a sense of trust with the family. The clinician's dress, posture, and manners can impact the ability to develop a sense of trust.

Failure to communicate is often a factor in malpractice lawsuits. As many as 70 % of lawsuits can involve patient and/or family concerns about a clinician's communication style or attitude [39]. Patients who sued reported that the physicians inadequately explained the diagnosis or treatment to the family, failed to communicate effectively, failed to understand their perspective, and often discounted or devalued their views. In many cases the family felt rushed. In this study, 13 % reported the doctor would not listen, 32 % reported the doctor did not talk openly, 48 % indicated the doctor attempted to mislead them, and 70 % said the doctor did not warn them about their baby's outcome [40].

Informed Consent

Informed consent is more than just obtaining a parent's signature on a piece of paper. The family of a child who receives sedation is entitled to receive and understand pertinent information about the procedure and the medications to be used. Parents have the right to know about the risks and benefits of the treatment, and any available alternatives. Their consent normally must be obtained prior to administration of any sedatives. A general consent form signed upon arrival at an outpatient facility does not usually imply consent for sedation. Separate consent for sedation is strongly advised. Whether consent should be in written or verbal form depends on local, state, and institutional requirements. In many states, verbal consent is adequate for most emergency procedures. However, the best evidence of consent in the event of a subsequent lawsuit is a signed consent form. Written consent forms educate the guardian with respect to the procedure and provide some protection to the caregiver by documenting the steps taken to inform the family. However, signing a form does not necessarily equate to an informed consent [41, 42]. The guardian may still claim that the risks and benefits were not adequately explained. In the event that a specific consent form was not used, the record should clearly document what the parents were told and their verbal agreement and understanding. In a true emergency, informed consent is not needed; it is implied and assumed that a reasonable parent would want immediate necessary care [42].

For example, Pennsylvania law defines informed consent as providing the consenting person with a description of the procedure and the risks and alternatives such that a "reasonably prudent person" would be able to make an informed decision about whether to undergo the procedure. This patient-focused concept of informed consent is followed by most states. If they are not told of the risk of and alternative to the treatment, the parents could conceivably bring a lawsuit against a physician for failing to obtain informed consent. If the child suffers harm from the sedation, the parents would have to prove that reasonable people, properly advised, and fully informed would not have consented to the procedure [7].

Parents should be informed consumers. Information given should include objectives and alternatives to the medical procedure itself, as well as of the sedation and anticipated changes in behavior during and after the sedation. Parents should be informed of alternatives such as the use of local anesthesia, regional anesthesia, general anesthesia, and alternate routes of administration. One study identified that parents most often wanted information regarding induction, adverse events, emergence reactions, and pain relief [43].

Information should be given in a clear straightforward manner. The care provider should be sure that the guardian understands the information given. It may be useful to ask the parent to paraphrase what they have been told. If a serious

Table 29.2 Important items of informed consent

Provide a clear explanation
Describe risks and benefits of sedation
Review medication effects, anticipated change in behavior, possible emergence reactions, pain relief
List all potential serious complications
List potential common, minor complications
Discuss alternative treatments—local or general anesthesia
Make sure the family understands the information

complication could result from treatment, then the caregiver should inform the family of all but the most remote risks. On the contrary, if the potential injury is minor, the family need only be informed of the risks that are common [20, 22, 44, 45]. In general, no parent should be forced to make a specific treatment decision for a child. Most parents desire the opinion and advice of the experienced provider in order to make a reasonable determination of what is best for the child. Table 29.2 summarizes important features of the informed consent process.

Communicate Well with Colleagues

Good communication among all staff members involved with sedation is essential. Do not demean other staff members in front of parents. Instead, it is best to "manage up" and praise other staff in front of families. Avoid joking or stray comments as families may believe (misinterpret) that the staff is not concentrating on their child. Communication among colleagues with respect and support is as important as communication to ensure adequate transfer of pertinent patient information. Numerous medical malpractice errors relate to the poor transfer of medical information between the responsible staff. Change of shift can be particularly dangerous, as pertinent medical information is not always communicated during handoffs [46–48].

Document Carefully

Careful documentation of the use of sedatives and analgesics is extremely important. In any medical negligence case, the child's medical record will be reviewed by an attorney and consulting expert physicians in order to determine whether an injury was the result of negligence. The standard of care and statutes in the various states establish that the medical record must contain a minimum amount of sufficient and accurate information. This information should identify the patient, support the diagnosis, justify the treatment, document the medical course and outcome, and promote continuity of care among health care providers. The medical record could either be your best defense or the plaintiff's best evidence. If the medical care relied upon to defend the case is not described in the medical record, the patient/guardian, or their experts, may testify that "it didn't happen." Although a complete and thorough medical record may not always prevent a lawsuit, it may help the health care provider to defend a claim. Often, there is an extended length of time between the patient encounter and a subsequent malpractice suit. A complete, well-prepared record may be helpful when memory of the event has faded. The chart should reflect a neat, professional appearance and it should be maintained as if it were a public document [7, 41].

Adequate documentation is important. If an inpatient or outpatient chart already exists, there is no need to repeat the information previously documented. However, a brief note to indicate that the chart was reviewed before administration of sedative agents is recommended. Indicate the child's presedation status. Note that the patient's condition has not changed since arrival or since the last exam in the record [20].

Documented history should include the child's age and abnormalities of the airway (snoring, sleep apnea) or other relevant diseases. A review of systems, previous hospital admissions, and relevant family history is noteworthy. The record should indicate any history of allergies or adverse drug reactions, medications used prior to sedation, and the patient's last oral intake [20, 24].

Document a careful physical exam with a focus on the patient's airway and cardiovascular system. Record the patient's correct weight, *in kg only*. Of course, it is important to record vital signs and oxygen saturation at specific intervals [20, 24].

A well-designed, time-based record will make it easier to find and record essential information. The patient's weight and allergies should be placed in an obvious location in the record so they can be easily noticed when medications are ordered. Checklists in the record may serve to remind the caregiver to ask specific questions or perform a specific part of the physical examination [24]. A time-based record should include details of drug administration and the patient's name (route, site, military time of dosing, dosage, and effect). Any adverse effects should be recorded as well as necessary vital signs at regular intervals. Document the child's level of consciousness during the procedure (how he/she responds to verbal commands or tactile stimulation) [20, 24].

Careful documentation is important not only prior to and during the sedation process, but also during the recovery phase. Prior to the patient's discharge from the sedation unit, document the child's level of consciousness and oral intake. Discharge instructions may be preprinted and must be reviewed with the child's guardian before the patient is allowed to go home. The discharge instructions should remind the parents that the child should not be involved in play that requires coordination such as bike riding or skateboarding for 24 h. Recommend adult supervision at home.

Unsupervised bathing, use of electrical devices, or other dangerous items should not be permitted for at least 8 h. The family should be told who and when to call if there are questions or concerns. Provide and encourage that the parents use a 24-h telephone number to call with questions. Discuss safe transport home with the provided guardian [20, 24].

Never Alter Medical Records

It is never wise to alter a patient's medical record or to make a late entry after an adverse event has occurred. Altered, missing, or "misplaced" records create the appearance of a "cover-up" and can result in sanctions. It is the responsibility of all providers involved in a child's care to maintain and secure the medical record.

With electronic medical records (EMR) all subsequent and non-sequential entries are obvious and apparent. Even handwritten notes can be analyzed by a forensic expert in order to uncover late entries. The authors advise that in order to correct a handwritten note, draw a single line through the error and initial and date it. Do not attempt to cover up the mistake by blacking out words or phrases. Should litigation ensue, it will be easier to explain missing facts or a poor record than it will be to defend a record that has been altered [49].

Managing Medical Errors in the Event of an Adverse Event

When a sedation-related complication occurs, a full investigation is needed. In the event of hospital-related events, the hospital's risk management office should be contacted immediately. This office is the division of the hospital that manages adverse outcomes and aims to prevent them by careful monitoring of hospital "systems." Risk managers will generally guide and support the hospital staff through documentation of the event and recommend any further action if applicable. Subsequent treatment rendered to the patient should be documented in the medical record. Some recommend that lengthy details of any possible medical errors not be discussed in the record, but rather should be documented in an incident report. The incident report should be written as soon after the adverse event as possible, and the hospital risk management office should receive the only copy. The incident report should contain a description of the incident: full names of all those who were involved, date, time of the event, clinical impact of the problem, and actions taken. Remember that incident reports may be discoverable. Never include a written apology or conclusion assigning blame to an individual. It is not advisable to make self-serving or defensive statements in the medical record [50].

When an error has occurred, full disclosure to the family is recommended. Offering a sincere apology to the family may diffuse anger and prevent a malpractice lawsuit. Studies have shown families are more likely to sue if they believe the doctor concealed the truth. Disclosure can preserve a good doctor–patient relationship and thus reduces litigation risk. Families often retain an attorney in order to gain information and a better understanding of what happened to their child. Open communication following an error may prevent the need to retain an attorney [51, 52].

When to Contact an Attorney

Following an untoward event or outcome (even if no substandard care is involved), it is advisable to alert the hospital risk management office. In some cases, even when the physician is not expecting a lawsuit, he or she may receive written notification of legal action, known as a "Civil Action" or a "Complaint." This should be taken seriously, even if you disagree with everything in the Complaint (charges may be exaggerated). Never ignore a Civil Action or Complaint. The Complaint may list statements that are demoralizing or insulting; remember that they are unchallenged allegations. The complaint may misstate or ignore facts.

As soon as the complaint is received, those named in the complaint should notify their hospital risk manager and the malpractice insurance company to confirm that a *defense*[11] attorney will be assigned. The attorney, once assigned to the case, will discuss the matter with his assigned "client" and respond with an "Answer" to the Complaint (generally denying the allegations) within a certain timeframe [7, 53]. The clinician has a right to hire a "private" attorney to represent him or her, but this is usually at the clinician's expense. Some situations may warrant a private attorney: for example, when the insurance company wishes to either settle or continue to defend the case, when the clinician disagrees with the malpractice carrier, or when the same defense lawyer represents multiple parties. A single attorney representing multiple providers may raise concern of Conflicts of Interest for the defense lawyer and when there may be insufficient insurance funds to cover any potential payout claim. There have been claims made by physicians against lawyers assigned by their malpractice insurance carrier to defend them. It is prudent for a physician to seek a second opinion from personal counsel if they do not agree with or are unsure of the course of action (such as a no settlement position) recommended by the insurance company's attorney [53].

Being named in a malpractice lawsuit does not mean that the physician is a "bad" clinician, or that the doctor even did anything wrong. Make some recommendations to your

[11] Please refer to section "Glossary" at the end of chapter.

attorney for a possible expert witness for your defense. Do not discuss the facts of the case with colleagues. Do not call the patient's family to discuss the matter [7, 53]. Tell your attorney all you know about the incident in order to help him/her develop the case. In many instances, early in the litigation the medical negligence (or lack of such) has been acknowledged and cases are easily resolved. This early resolution is only possible if the clinicians involved are able and willing to accept and acknowledge their own responsibility.

Quality Improvement

The Joint Commission requires each facility to perform quality improvement reviews of sedation practices. Each facility should track adverse events, which should include the need for airway intervention, apnea, oxygen desaturation, and prolonged or unsatisfactory sedation. These events should be examined to detect system flaws, and to reduce risk in the future [5, 20, 24].

Family Member Presence for Procedures

No studies have been done to evaluate how the presence of family members affects litigation. However, studies do show that most family members who witness a procedure report favorable opinions of the process. This favorable opinion by families holds true for cardiopulmonary resuscitation, even in cases of patient death. In one study, 71 % of surveyed family members believed their presence at the resuscitation comforted their child, 67 % believed they adjusted better to the loss of the child by witnessing the resuscitation, and 63 % would recommend being present during cardiopulmonary resuscitation [54]. To date, there is no literature to support that family member presence during sedation and procedures will increase legal risks for a clinician. Rather, a satisfied parent may decrease the likelihood of a lawsuit, as satisfied family members are generally less likely to file a lawsuit [54, 55].

Case Studies

Case 1

A young man presents to an Illinois emergency department for treatment after he was hit in the head with a baseball bat during an altercation [56]. The patient had a markedly elevated blood alcohol level, was intoxicated and combative. The emergency physicians were concerned about an intracranial injury and ordered a computerized tomography (CT) scan of his head. He was given midazolam for sedation for the CT scan. Two hours following the midazolam, he suffered a cardiorespiratory arrest. The emergency medical staff attempted to resuscitate him. His trachea was intubated, mechanically ventilated, then disconnected from the ventilator when declared irreversibly brain dead.

The family sued the hospital and contended that the cause of death was the respiratory depression from midazolam in combination with alcohol intoxication. They claimed that midazolam was contraindicated in an intoxicated patient, an excessive dose of midazolam administered, and that the hospital failed to properly monitor the patient. The physicians argued that midazolam is short acting and was not the cause of his respiratory arrest. They maintained that it was a reasonable choice of sedative for a combative patient who required a CT scan to rule out an intracranial bleed.

The verdict was in favor of the physicians and the hospital.

Teaching Point

This case reminds us that physicians who order sedatives must understand their effects and side effects. They must be familiar with drug interactions when the patient has another medication (or substance such as alcohol) in his system. Midazolam should not be administered to patients with acute alcohol intoxication with depressed vital signs. Concomitant use of midazolam with alcohol may increase the risk of hypoventilation or apnea and may contribute to profound or prolonged drug effect. Clearly, all patients who receive sedation for a CT scan must be appropriately monitored.

Case 2

A 12-year-old patient with Crohn's disease presents to a Minnesota clinic for an endoscopy [57]. The gastroenterologist and a nurse administered fentanyl and midazolam for sedation. After the very brief procedure, after the gastroenterologist had left the room and the nurse was finishing up her paperwork in the procedure room, the patient's pulse oximeter alarm went off, the oxygen saturation was noted to be very low (90 %), and a nasal cannula was placed. The physician was summoned. Over the next several minutes, pharmacological reversal agents for midazolam and fentanyl were administered, but assisted breathing (ventilation) was not initiated. About 7–8 min into the event, the patient suffered a cardiac arrest. Chest compressions

(continued)

were begun and a defibrillator established a viable cardiac rhythm. An oral pharyngeal airway was eventually placed and breathing was assisted with a bag-valve mask device. The patient suffered an anoxic brain injury and allegedly will require assisted living in an institution for the rest of his life.

The patient and family sued the clinic and the physician for negligence. The clinic denied liability. A $3.1 million settlement was reached during mediation.

Teaching Point

This clinic was not prepared for the rare, but serious complications of sedation. Although there were physiologic monitors and pulse oximetry was being followed, it appears that the oxygen desaturation was identified after a delay. The most significant fault is the failure to have a rescue plan in place. All personnel must know how to react in the event of an adverse event. The clinic and personnel should be trained and prepared to identify and manage an emergency. Simulations and/or mock drills can assist in the acquisition of competence and familiarization of sedation and emergency protocols.

Case 3

A healthy 2-year-old child with no prior medical history presented to an Illinois emergency department (ED) after he suffered a generalized seizure at home [57]. The seizure lasted at least 20 min, until it was stopped with anticonvulsant medications. The child's trachea was intubated, while he was stabilized in the emergency department. A decision was made to obtain a CT scan of the head before transferring the child to another hospital for additional monitoring and treatment. By emergency department protocol, the intubated child would have been transferred sedated to and from the CT scanner with physiological monitors and manual hand ventilation. There was no specific entry in the medical records, however, to confirm that such monitors were used. Two nurses, a respiratory therapist, and a medical student accompanied the child to and from the CT scan. During the subsequent litigation, none of these individuals had a clear memory of monitors being used, alarms being set, or any vital signs being taken during the 24-min transport. Upon return to the ED after the CT scan, he was discovered to be in cardiopulmonary arrest. After almost an hour of unsuccessful resuscitation efforts, he was pronounced dead.

The family sued the ED and claimed that the endotracheal tube became dislodged during the transport to the CT scan. They also claimed that because the child was not properly monitored, no one noticed that he was not breathing when he was removed from the CT scanner. They argued that he was in unrecognized cardiac arrest for more than 5 min, making resuscitation impossible. The *defendants* (health care providers) claimed that the death was due to the onset of a sudden cardiac arrest upon his return to the ED and that this was a complication of status epilepticus. One of the nurses testified that when she returned with the child to the ED, she switched the EKG leads from the portable monitor to the permanent monitor, "got nothing" and thought there was a malfunction with the electrocardiogram leads. When she replaced the leads, the monitor showed ventricular fibrillation, which then quickly changed to asystole.

A jury ruled in favor of the family and awarded them $3,662,221.

Teaching Point

A sedated child must be carefully monitored by qualified personnel who are trained and prepared to identify adverse events and initiate resuscitation. This case also reminds us of the importance of careful documentation. It is difficult to believe that an intubated patient went to the CT scanner without a physiologic monitor. However, there was no documentation of the presence of a cardiac monitor and none of the caretakers could remember him being on a monitor. Although it is not known if his death was preventable, clearly, there should have been better observation and documentation.

Case 4

A 3-year-old child went to a dental office with his mother to have a tooth filled. Prior to the appointment, the mother was given a bottle of chloral hydrate by the dentist's office to administer to her son prior to arrival in order to sedate him. After the dentist completed the procedure, the child began choking and vomiting. The child then stopped breathing and smelling salts were administered with no discernible effect. The dentist attempted to clear the child's airway and used an ambu bag with a face mask to ventilate the patient. Paramedics were called. When the paramedics arrived the child was apneic and asystolic. The paramedics then intubated the child's trachea and made unsuccessful attempts to resuscitate. The child died a short time thereafter. An

(continued)

autopsy was performed and it was determined that the child died of acute trichloroethanol (a metabolite of chloral hydrate) intoxication.

The mother of the deceased child filed a wrongful death suit against the dentist claiming that the defendant:

1. Negligently prescribed an excessive dose of chloral hydrate
2. Negligently instructed the mother to administer the medication at home, rather than having him monitored continuously from the time the medication was first given to him
3. Negligently failed to properly monitor the child while he was in the office
4. Negligently failed to possess the necessary equipment to properly monitor and resuscitate
5. Negligently failed to timely initiate appropriate resuscitation on the child

The case was settled after a mediation session for $350,000.

Teaching Point

Clinicians who work in a free-standing facility must be particularly cautious and they must have a well-delineated plan to activate EMS in the event of an adverse event. They must have proper equipment available and the necessary skill to use this equipment appropriately while awaiting help. It is dangerous and unadvisable to have parents administer sedative medications at home. When administering and prescribing sedatives, the pharmacokinetics, pharmacodynamics, and dosing limits must be carefully followed. It is preferable to have a health care professional administer the sedative before the procedure.

Case 5

A child underwent an elective upper endoscopy to determine if she was suffering from a blockage of gallstones or stenosis. The procedure was performed by a gastroenterologist who administered sedation for the procedure. During the procedure the patient began moving while the gastroenterologist inserted a papillotome to open the ampulla in order to enable drainage of bile from the common bile duct. To minimize patient movement the gastroenterologist administered more sedation but was unsuccessful in stopping the movement. As a result of these movements, the papillotome lacerated the bile duct. A subsequent surgery was required to repair the laceration.

As a result of the laceration, the patient sued the gastroenterologist on a theory that the doctor was negligent in not adequately sedating the patient. A jury returned a verdict in favor of the patient in the amount of $305,000.

Teaching Point

This case illustrates the importance of achieving the proper level of sedation in order to avoid adverse outcomes. Inadequate sedation led to the patient's movement during the procedure. Care must be taken to sufficiently sedate the patient for successful completion of the intended procedure while at the same time avoiding oversedation.

Case 6

A 4-year-old boy presented to a Michigan hospital for a magnetic resonance imaging (MRI) study to evaluate a leg mass. He was given midazolam, fentanyl, and pentobarbital sedation for the MRI. The patient suffered a cardiopulmonary arrest during the MRI. He was left with permanent central nervous system damage, resulting in cerebral palsy and mental retardation. The family sued and alleged that inappropriate amounts of medication were utilized and that the hospital staff failed to not only monitor the patient but also to ensure appropriate oxygen delivery. They believed that the permanent and severe brain injuries were a result of the incident. The hospital contended that the child was appropriately monitored but was unusually sensitive to the medications. The case was settled for $2,950,000 [58].

Teaching Point

While details are unavailable, one has to question whether the patient in this case was appropriately monitored. One should also question the use of a multimodal sedative regimen that included fentanyl for a painless MRI procedure. Sedation may have been desirable, but a narcotic analgesic seems unnecessary and perhaps dangerous in this case. The clinician should have a clear understanding of the goals of sedation and then choose and dose the drugs wisely [22].

Case 7

An otherwise healthy 2-year-old boy was brought to a Texas emergency department (ED) for treatment of a tongue laceration. The boy was given midazolam and

(continued)

morphine sedation to repair the laceration. Naloxone was administered following the procedure to reverse the somnolence and hasten discharge. The patient was discharged from the ED 8 h after the procedure, apparently still asleep. He never woke up at home, and was later pronounced dead. The parents sued the hospital and the treating physician, claiming that the medication was given inappropriately and the child was not properly monitored. The hospital settled the case for $975,000 [59].

Teaching Point

Premature discharge of a sedated patient from the ED can have disastrous consequences. Before discharge, this child should have returned to baseline neurologic state, had normal cardiovascular function, an intact gag reflex, and a patent airway. He should meet established criteria and guidelines for discharge. The child should have been able to sit and talk at discharge. Younger children or those with neurologic dysfunction should be close to their pre-sedation level of function before discharge [20].

Case 8

A 17-year-old boy arrived at a Minnesota hospital for his scheduled iron infusion. He required premedication to avoid a rash and hives from the iron transfusion. He was given 50 mg of diphenhydramine intravenously, 100 mg of steroids, and 2 mg of lorazepam. Despite premedication, he developed a reaction when iron was infused and subsequently received an additional 50 mg of diphenhydramine and 2 mg of lorazepam intravenously. The patient was soon discharged, without a responsible adult to pick him up. Fifteen minutes after leaving the hospital, the car that the patient was driving rolled over at high speed in a single vehicle crash. He suffered catastrophic head injuries and died. The state trooper who investigated the crash concluded that the patient fell asleep while driving.

The family sued the hospital that administered the sedatives after it was revealed that the nurses who gave the medications were not familiar with the drugs nor their actions. The family believed the nurses were negligent for failing to make certain the patient was discharged to a responsible adult. The case was settled before trial for $2.35 million [60].

Teaching Point

Medical personnel caring for the sedated patient must be familiar with the drugs that are given and their actions. The patient must be carefully monitored until he or she meets established discharge criteria. A pediatric patient (teenager) should not be permitted to drive home alone after receiving sedation for a procedure. Since it is difficult for a parent to care for her child while driving, one should consider prolonged observation at the medical center if the only adult present has to drive the car [20].

Case 9

A 15-year-old boy with obstructive sleep apnea and a home apnea monitor underwent sedation for a dental procedure (wisdom tooth extraction) at a hospital in Utah. He was administered 5 mg of intravenous morphine during the procedure and an additional 50 mg of intravenous meperidine was administered while he was in the Recovery Room. The patient was still somnolent after 2 h in recovery but was discharged home in the care of his parents soon before the evening closure of the recovery room. The parents helped the patient to get dressed and he was awake long enough to get into their car. At home he fell asleep on the couch and later he was found with no pulse or respiration. Paramedics were called to the scene and the patient was transported by ambulance to a hospital where he was declared dead.

The family sued and claimed that the patient should not have been discharged, as he had been too somnolent to meet discharge criteria. They also claimed that with his history of sleep apnea and home apnea monitor, he should have remained in the hospital overnight for observation and apnea monitoring. The coroner suggested that the postmortem level of meperidine in the patient's blood suggested that he had taken more of this medication after discharge from the hospital. The parents denied this and claimed that the boy had refused an additional dose of the medication offered by a nurse before leaving the hospital. The family argued that the coroner failed to take into account postmortem redistribution of drug levels.

A confidential settlement was reached [61].

Teaching Point

This was a preventable death, and the case would have been difficult to defend in court. Despite the dosage of narcotics received, the hospital had a clearly defined overnight policy, requiring hospital admission for any patient on a home apnea monitor. The same day discharge violated the hospital's own policy. Even should

(continued)

this patient not have had a history of sleep apnea and home monitoring, the closing of a Day Surgery Recovery Room (implied but not confirmed in this case) does not justify early discharge of a patient who is recovering from sedation or anesthesia [61].

Conclusion

The majority of children who receive sedation and analgesia outside the operating room have a good outcome, and benefit from efforts to reduce pain and anxiety during a procedure. Occasionally, there is a preventable complication that is the result of substandard care. Those providing care to sedated children must vigilantly assess, formulate a plan, and monitor the child in order to minimize potential adverse outcomes. Develop and follow written policies and procedures to guide care. Act reasonably. Provide high quality care and be prepared to rescue a patient if there is an adverse event. Communicate well with patients, families, and staff. Finally, careful documentation of the good care delivered will be important to defend any litigation (Table 29.3).

Table 29.3 Preventing malpractice lawsuits related to sedation

Practice "good medicine"
• Take precautions to prevent adverse outcomes
• Ask for help when needed
Communicate well
• Listen to family members and keep them informed
• Speak in terms the family can understand
• Develop a sense of trust with the family
• Communicate carefully with other staff members
• Be cautious during patient handoffs
Document carefully
• Use a well-designed, time-based record
• Keep the medical record neat and professional in appearance
• Indicate that information previously obtained was reviewed
• Never alter the medical record after discharge of the patient
• Correct errors appropriately
• Provide written discharge instructions:
– Document that these were reviewed verbally
Manage errors appropriately
• Follow hospital policies
• Contact Risk Management Office
• Do not attempt to cover up
• Investigate errors thoroughly
• Disclose errors to families
• Apologize when appropriate

Glossary

The following are general lay definitions of terms common to the practice of criminal and civil law. Some of the precise definitions vary from state to state according to that state's laws and practice.

Breach The violation of an obligation, engagement, or duty.

Certificate of merit A certificate filed in a medical malpractice action. Under court rules, it is filed by the plaintiff's attorney with the complaint (the document that begins the lawsuit and contains the plaintiff's allegations). In a certificate of merit, the plaintiff's attorney certifies that he/she has reviewed the facts of the case, and has consulted with a medical expert and concluded that the plaintiff's action has merits.

Civil lawsuit A legal case brought on behalf of an individual (plaintiff) against another individual or entity (defendant) who acted negligently (below some standard of care) and thereby caused them harm. This case is brought for a monetary recovery for damages sustained by the plaintiff. The plaintiff's burden of proof in a civil lawsuit is typically by a preponderance of the evidence, a lesser burden of proof than in a criminal *prosecution*[12]. A successful civil lawsuit usually results in the payment of money for the losses sustained by the plaintiff.

Criminal Negligence Acting in a grossly negligent manner. Typically this involves the conscious disregard of a known risk of death or serious injury.

Defense Those responsible for representing a defendant in a criminal case or a *civil lawsuit*[13]. The defense does not have the burden of proving innocence or lack of fault.

Homicide The unlawful taking of another's life. Homicide ranges from first degree murder, the taking of a life with specific intent to kill and with malice, to *involuntary manslaughter*[14], an accidental killing where the defendant acts unintentionally and without malice but with *criminal negligence*[15].

Indemnity A contractual insurance agreement whereby the insurer agrees to pay for the insured's loss or claims arising from some contemplated act, such as professional negligence.

Informed consent The consent given by a patient to a doctor that allows the doctor to perform a certain procedure or render particular treatment. The consent is "informed" because the doctor has explained the specifics of the procedure or treatment to the patient, including the risks and

[12] Please refer to section "Glossary."

[13] Please refer to section "Glossary."

[14] Please refer to section "Glossary."

[15] Please refer to section "Glossary."

alternatives, who has then made a knowing, informed decision about whether they want to proceed.

Involuntary manslaughter The unlawful taking of another's life without intent to kill or to harm and without malice, but the act is committed with criminal negligence.

Jury verdict The definitive answer(s) given by the Jury to the court concerning the issues or questions of fact committed to the jury for their deliberation and determination. Depending on the jurisdiction, verdicts in civil lawsuits may not require unanimity.

Malpractice Professional negligence. This is an act of negligence committed by a professional such as a doctor, a lawyer, an engineer, etc., while acting within their profession. The negligent conduct is measured by the standard of care in that profession and in that specialty in which the professional practices. A doctor who commits malpractice is said to have breached the standard of care in their area of specialty.

Negligence Failing to act in a reasonably prudent manner.

Prosecution Charging an individual (defendant) with a violation of criminal law, marshaling the evidence against that individual, presenting the evidence to a court or jury and, if a conviction is obtained, proceeding to sentencing against the individual. The prosecutor represents the people of the state where the crime occurred and technically not the victim of the crime, although the prosecutor often speaks on behalf of the victim. The prosecutor bears the burden of proving guilt beyond a reasonable doubt. If a conviction is obtained, the defendant faces incarceration.

Standard of care The standard according to which negligence in a particular situation is determined. The care that an ordinary prudent person would exercise under similar circumstances.

References

1. King WK, Stockwell JA, Deguzman MA, et al. Evaluation of a pediatric sedation service for common diagnostic procedures. Acad Emerg Med. 2006;13:673–6.
2. Pena BM, Krauss B. Adverse events of procedural sedation and analgesia in a pediatric emergency department. Ann Emerg Med. 1999;34:483–91.
3. Cravero JP, Bilke GT, Beach M, et al. Incidence and nature of adverse events during pediatric sedation/anesthesia for procedures outside the operating room: Report from the pediatric sedation research consortium. Pediatrics. 2006;118:1087–96.
4. Green SM, Roback MG, Krauss B, et al. Predictors of airway and respiratory adverse events with ketamine sedation in the emergency department: An individual patient data meta-analysis of 8282 children. Ann Emerg Med. 2009;54:158–68.
5. Fein JA, Zempsky WT, Cravero JP, American Academy of Pediatrics Committee on Pediatric Emergency Medicine and Section on Anesthesiology and Pain Medicine. Relief of pain and anxiety in pediatric patients in emergency medicine systems. Pediatrics. 2012;130:e1391–405.
6. Furrow BR. The patient injury epidemic: medical malpractice litigation as a curative tool. Drexel L Rev. 2011;4:41–76.
7. Selbst SM, Korin JB. Preventing malpractice lawsuits in pediatric emergency medicine. Dallas: American College of Emergency Physicians; 1997. p. 1–196.
8. Carroll AE, Parikh PD, Buddenbaum JL. The impact of defense expenses in medical malpractice claims. J Law Med Ethics. 2012;40(1):135–42.
9. Selbst SM, Friedman MJ, Singh SB. Epidemiology and etiology of malpractice lawsuits involving children in US emergency departments and urgent care centers. Pediatr Emerg Care. 2005;21:165–9.
10. Jena AB, Seabury S, Lakdawalla DL, et al. Malpractice risk according to physician specialty. N Engl J Med. 2011;365:629–38.
11. Pa. R.C.P. 1042.3; 18 Del. C. § 6853; 735 ILCS 5/2-622; N.J. Stat. § 2A:53A-27; and Ohio Civ. R. 10(D)(2).
12. *Bing v. Thunig*, 143 N.E.2d 3, 9, (N.Y. 1957); *Weldon v. Seminole Municipal Hospital*, 709 P.2d 1058, 1059 (Okla. 1985).
13. *Barkes v. River Park Hosp*., Inc., 328 S.W.3d 829 (Tenn. 2010).
14. *Thompson v. Nason Hosp*., 527 Pa. 330 (Pa. 1991); *Welsh v. Bulger*, 548 Pa. 504 (Pa. 1997).
15. *Seneris v. Haas*, 45 Cal. 2d 811 (Cal. 1955).
16. American College of Emergency Medicine. Policy statement-sedation in the emergency department. Ann Emerg Med. 2011; 57(5):469.
17. *See* 42 C.F.R. § 482.52; Joint Commission Standards 13.20-13.40. (2007); States sometimes also have similar regulations. *See e.g.*28 Pa. Code § 555.31 et seq.
18. Joint Commission Standards 42 C.F.R. § 482.12 (f)(2) Standard LD.3.50 (2007).
19. Shavit I, Keidan I, Hoffman Y, et al. Enhancing patient safety during pediatric sedation-The impact of simulation -based training of non-anesthesiologists. Arch Pediatr Adolesc Med. 2007;161(8):740–3.
20. American Academy of Pediatrics, American Academy of Pediatric Dentistry, Cote CJ, Wilson S, Work Group on Sedation. Guidelines for monitoring and management of pediatric patients during and after sedation for diagnostic and therapeutic procedures: an update. Pediatrics. 2006;118(6):2587–602.
21. Cote CJ, Karl HW, Notterman DA, et al. Adverse sedation events in pediatrics: a critical incident analysis of contributing factors. Pediatrics. 2000;106:633–44.
22. Mandt MJ, Roback MG. Assessment and monitoring of pediatric procedural sedation. Clin Pediatr Emerg Med. 2007;8:223.
23. Rutman MS. Sedation for emergent diagnostic imaging studies in pediatric patients. Curr Opin Pediatr. 2009;21:306–12.
24. Pershad J, Kost S. Emergency department based sedation services. Clin Pediatr Emerg Med. 2007;8:253–61.
25. Joint Commission on Accreditation of Healthcare Organizations. Comprehensive accreditation manual for hospitals: the official handbook by the JCAHO. Oakbrook Terrace: Joint Commission on Accreditation of Healthcare Organizations; 2005.
26. Green SM, Roback MG, Krauss B. Laryngospasm during emergency department ketamine sedation. A case-control study. Pediatr Emerg Care. 2010;26(11):798–802.
27. Wright AA, Katz IT. Bar Coding for Patient Safety, 353 *New Eng.* J Med. 2005;329(330).
28. Lesar TS, Briceland L, Stein DS. Factors related to errors in medication prescribing. JAMA. 1997;277:312–7.
29. Levine SR, Cohen MR, Blanchard NR, et al. Guidelines for preventing medication errors in pediatrics. J Pediatr Pharmacol Ther. 2001;6:426–42.
30. Singh H, Thomas EJ, Petersen LA, et al. Medical errors involving trainees. A study of closed malpractice claims from 5 insurers. Arch Intern Med. 2007;167:2030–6.
31. American Society of Anesthesiologists Committee of Origin: Standards and Practice Parameters. Standards for Basic Anesthetic Monitoring. Last amended on October 20, 2010. http://www.asahq.

org/~/media/For%20Members/documents/Standards%20 Guidelines%20Stmts/Basic%20Anesthetic%20Monitoring%20 2011.ashx
32. Mace SE, Brown LA, Francis L, et al. Clinical policy: Critical issues in sedation of pediatric patients in the ED. Ann Emerg Med. 2008;51:378.
33. Noah L. Medicine's epistemology: mapping the haphazard diffusion of knowledge in the biomedical community. Ariz L Rev. 2002;373:462–3.
34. Langhan ML, Mallory M, Hertzog J, et al. Physiologic monitoring practices during pediatric procedural sedation. Arch Pediatr Adolesc Med. 2012;166(11):990–8.
35. Green SM, Roback MG, Milner JR, et al. Fasting and emergency department procedural sedation and analgesia: a consensus- based clinical practice advisory. Ann Emerg Med. 2007;49:454–61.
36. Roback MG, Bajaj L, Wathen JE, et al. Pre-procedural fasting and adverse events in procedural sedation and analgesia in a pediatric emergency department: are they related? Ann Emerg Med. 2004;44:454–9.
37. American Society of Anesthesiologists Committee on Standards and Practice Parameters. Practice guidelines for preoperative fasting and the use of pharmacologic agents to reduce the risk of pulmonary aspiration: Application to healthy patients undergoing elective procedures. Anaesthesioliogy. 2011;114:495–511.
38. Cronan K. Patient complaints in a pediatric emergency department: averting lawsuits. Clin Ped Emerg Med. 2003;4(4):235–42.
39. Beckman HB, Markalis KM, Suchman AL, et al. The doctor-patient relationship and malpractice. Lessons learned from plaintiff depositions. Arch Intern Med. 1994;154:1365.
40. Hickson GB, Clayton EW, Githens PH, et al. Factors that prompted families to file malpractice claims following perinatal injuries. JAMA. 1992;267:1359–63.
41. Selbst SM. Risk management and medico-legal aspects of procedural sedation. In: Krauss B, Brustowicz RM, editors. Pediatric procedural sedation and Analgesia. Philadelphia: Lippincott Williams and Wilkins; 1999. p. 115–23.
42. American Academy of Pediatrics, Committee on Pediatric Emergency Medicine and Committee on Biothetics. Consent for emergency medical services for children and adolescents. Policy Statement. Pediatrics. 2011;128(2):427–33.
43. Wisselo TL, Stuart C, Muris P. Providing parents with information before anesthesia; what do they really want to know? Pediatr Anaesth. 2004;14:299–307.
44. Kasuto Z, Vaught W. Informed decision making and refusal of treatment. Clin Pediatr Emerg Med. 2003;4:285–91.
45. Applebaum PS, Grisso T. Assessing patients' capacities to consent to treatment. N Engl J Med. 1988;319:1635–8.
46. Kachalia A, Gandhi TK, Puopolo AL, et al. Missed and delayed diagnoses in the emergency department: a study of closed malpractice claims from 4 liability insurers. Ann Emerg Med. 2007;49: 196–205.
47. Dhingra KR, Elms A, Hobgood C. Reducing error in the emergency department: A call for standardization of the sign-out process. Ann Emerg Med. 2010;56(6):637–42.
48. Yu KT, Green RA. Critical aspects of emergency department documentation and communication. *Emerg Clin NA* 2009; 27(4): 641-54, ix.
49. Barratt K, Schwid B, Schwid M. Don't doctor your records. Wis Med J. 1996;95:385–7.
50. Selbst SM. The difficult duty of disclosing medical errors. Contemp Pediatr. 2003;20:51–63.
51. O'Connor E, Coates HM, Yardley IE, et al. Disclosure of patient safety incidents: a comprehensive review. Int J Qual Health Care. 2010;22(5):371–9.
52. Mitka M. Disclosing medical errors does not mean greater liability costs. JAMA. 2010;304(13):1656–7.
53. Westgate A. You've been served-now what? *Physicians Practice* 2012;115–20.
54. Tinsley C. Experience of families during cardiopulmonary resuscitation in a pediatric intensive care unit. Pediatrics. 2008; 122(4):e799–804.
55. Dingeman RS, Mitchell EA, Meyer EC, et al. Parent presence during complex invasive procedures and cardiopulmonary resuscitation: A systematic review of the literature. Pediatrics. 2007;120:842–54.
56. Selbst SM. Pediatric emergency medicine: legal briefs. Pediatr Emerg Care. 1998;14(6):430.
57. Selbst SM. Pediatric emergency medicine: legal briefs. Pediatr Emerg Care. 2011;27(10):992–4.
58. Selbst SM. Pediatric emergency medicine: legal briefs. Pediatr Emerg Care. 2003;19:46.
59. Selbst SM. Pediatric emergency medicine: legal briefs. Pediatr Emerg Care. 1996;12:309.
60. Selbst SM. Pediatric emergency medicine: legal briefs. Pediatr Emerg Care. 2005;21:353–4.
61. Selbst SM, Osterhoudt K. Pediatric emergency medicine: legal briefs. Pediatr Emerg Care. 2008;24:700–4.

Additional Reading

Coombs v. Curnow, 219 P.3d 453, 462 (Idaho 2009)

Government Accountability Office. Medical malpractice: implications of rising premiums on access to health care. Washington DC: GAO; Aug. 29, 2003.

Institute of Medicine. To err is human: building a safer health care system. Washington, DC: IOM, National Academies Press; 1999.

Martinez v. Driscoll Found. Children's Hosp., 1997 Tex. App. LEXIS 4602 (Tex. App. Corpus Christi Aug. 28, 1997).

NAIC. Countrywide summary of medical malpractice insurance calendar years 1991–2008. Washington, DC: National Association of Insurance Commissioners; 2009.

Scheinfeld N. Photographic images, digital imaging, dermatology and the law. Arch Dermatol. 2004;140:473–6.

Selbst SM. Pediatric emergency medicine: legal briefs. Pediatr Emerg Care. 2000;16:459.

Improving the Safety of Pediatric Sedation: Human Error, Technology, and Clinical Microsystems

30

Craig S. Webster, Brian J. Anderson, Michael J. Stabile, and Alan F. Merry

Abstract

Recent years have seen significant improvements in the safety of a number of areas of health care. However, evidence would suggest that the practice of pediatric sedation outside of the operating room is an area where unaddressed complexities and risks in care remain. In addition, the number of children receiving sedation outside of the operating room is on the increase, emphasizing the need to realize opportunities to improve safety. We outline the risks inherent in sedating children in the context of both the human factors and system factors perspectives. We incorporate examples from other high-technology industries such as aviation and nuclear power generation to allow a better understanding of why things go wrong during sedation. The value of prior risk assessment, communication, checklists, and formalized recovery pathways are discussed, and new directions for the development of safety initiatives are identified. Finally a number of practical steps based on existing successful safety approaches are given, with an emphasis on the demonstration of efficacy and the sharing of successful safety solutions.

Keywords

Safety • Pediatric sedation • Human error • Systems • Risk • Technology • World Society for Intravenous Anesthesia (World SIVA) • International Sedation Task Force (ISTF) • Root cause analysis • Nuclear power

C.S. Webster, B.Sc., M.Sc., Ph.D. (✉)
Centre for Medical and Health Sciences Education, University of Auckland, Private Bag 92-019, Auckland 1142, New Zealand
e-mail: c.webster@auckland.ac.nz

B.J. Anderson, Ph.D., F.A.N.Z.C.A., F.J.F.I.C.M.
Department of Anaesthesiology, University of Auckland School of Medicine, Auckland, New Zealand
e-mail: briana@adhb.govt.nz

M.J. Stabile, M.D., M.B.A.
Department of Anesthesia, Centennial Medical Center, Nashville, TN, USA

St. Louis University School of Medicine, St. Louis, MO, USA
e-mail: alfa45@aol.com

A.F. Merry, F.A.N.Z.C.A, F.P.M.A.N.Z.C.A.
Department of Anaesthesiology, University of Auckland and Auckland City Hospital, Auckland, New Zealand
e-mail: a.merry@auckland.ac.nz

Introduction

Children undergoing health-care procedures have specific needs different to those of adults. Alleviating the pain and anxiety that comes with frightening or painful procedures is one important example. While parental presence, reassurance, and other strategies are important, pharmacologic sedation is often required, and this comes with attendant risks. Furthermore, the number of children undergoing procedures with sedation alone is increasing, particularly in locations outside the operating room. This is attributable in large part to the increasing variety of available imaging and diagnostic technologies [1, 2].

Initiatives to improve the safety of health care have gained momentum since the publication of the Institute of Medicine report in 2000, which called for a 50 % reduction in adverse

K.P. Mason (ed.), *Pediatric Sedation Outside of the Operating Room: A Multispecialty International Collaboration*,
DOI 10.1007/978-1-4939-1390-9_30, © Springer Science+Business Media New York 2015

Table 30.1 Summaries of contemporary large-scale studies estimating the rates of adverse events during hospitalized care

Study	Sample	When sampled	AE rate	Percentage preventable
Harvard Medical Practice Study [4, 5]	30,121 records 51 hospitals	1984	3.7 %	Majority
Quality in Australian Health Care Study [6]	14,179 records 28 hospitals	1992	16.6 %	48 %
Utah and Colorado Study [7]	15,000 records 13 hospitals	1992	2.9 %	–
London Study [8]	500 records 2 hospitals	1998	10.8 %	48 %
New Zealand Study [9]	15,000 records 13 hospitals	1998	12.9 %	35 %

events across all health-care domains [3]. However, much of what we know about the rates of adverse events in health care comes from retrospective record reviews of hospitalized general-patient populations—five large-scale landmark studies of this type, employing comparable methods, are summarized in Table 30.1 [4–9]. An adverse event (AE) in these studies was defined as an injury caused by medical management (rather than the underlying disease) and that prolonged hospitalization or produced a disability at the time of discharge, or both [4, 5]. Rates of reported AEs varied from 3.7 to 16.6 %. Findings from these studies relating to the adult population were widely reported, but analyzes on pediatric populations were not conducted [10]. Less is therefore known about the frequency with which things can go wrong during procedures on children, particularly under sedation in various locations. However, in a recent large-scale multinational study involving 26 institutions, the incidence of complications during sedation in pediatric patients conducted outside of the operating room was examined in 30,037 cases [1]. Participating clinicians were asked to submit data for each case, prospectively, using a structured Web-based tool. The most common type of procedure for which sedation was required was radiologic (62 %), and 98 % of these were magnetic resonance imaging (MRI) or computed tomography (CT) scans that were not painful, but potentially distressing. Overall, 5.3 % (n=1,601) of children in the study were involved in some kind of undesirable event or complication. The most common event was a reduction in arterial oxygen saturation (SpO_2) to below 90 % (n=470, 29 %). More concerning complications included cardiac arrest (n=1), aspiration (n=1), laryngospasm (n=13), allergic reaction (n=17), prolonged sedation (n=41), prolonged recovery (n=67), vomiting (n=142), the requirement for bag-mask ventilation (n=192), and inability to complete the procedure because of inadequate sedation (n=267). These data are not directly comparable with data from populations of hospitalized, adult general patients, in part because the latter patients would typically be undergoing more invasive procedures than those requiring only sedation (Table 30.1). Nevertheless, it is worrying that children undergoing minor or noninvasive procedures under sedation should experience complication rates higher than those seen in two previous estimates of the rate of adverse events in hospitalized adult patients—and this remains true even if events involving oxygen desaturation below 90 % are excluded. In adult patients in general hospitals, at least 35 % of adverse events have been judged to be preventable (Table 30.1). A recent review of notes for 11,247 discharged hospital patients suggests that a higher proportion of adverse events are preventable in infants and adolescents than in adult patients (78 % and 79 % versus 41 %, respectively). In the same study children were found to be 1.35 times more likely than adults to experience preventable adverse events during diagnostic procedures (which are the commonest indication for sedating children outside the operating room [10]). These findings suggest risk factors and complexities to the care of pediatric patients that are currently not being adequately addressed. Children have a low tolerance for errors. Furthermore, there are many challenges to providing sedation outside the operating room (Table 30.2). Even when following appropriate guidelines, difficulties are common. A study of 1,140 children undergoing sedation in a unit in which the American Academy of Pediatrics guidelines were in use found that 13 % received inadequate sedation while 5.3 % experienced a respiratory event associated with oversedation [11].

The Need for a Paradigm Shift

The Institute of Medicine in the United States claimed in 2000 that "health care is a decade or more behind other high-risk industries in its attention to ensuring basic safety" and called for a paradigm shift in the quality of patient care [3]. Responding to this call, the *100,000 Lives Campaign*, introduced by the Institute of Healthcare Improvement, reported in 2006 the saving of 122,300 lives over a period of 18 months in American hospitals through the implementation of six evidence-based practices [12, 13]. Although this campaign

Table 30.2 Factors that may increase risk in children undergoing sedation, especially outside the operating room

• Weight-based and off-label use of drugs[a]
• Changing physiology and dose and drug effect with age[a]
• Sedation monitoring systems and scores that vary and change with age[a]
• Limited reserves to tolerate dose inaccuracies[a]
• Difficulty in maintaining homeostasis because of small size and immature physiology[a]
• Congenital conditions and comorbidities[a]
• The increasing number and complexity of sedation cases conducted in children[a]
• Sedation performed under urgency
• Sedation performed in a variety of different locations with no standardized backup or safety equipment
• Sedation performed by a variety of staff, including anesthesiologists, emergency ward staff, cardiologists, nurses, and house officers
• Variability in target depth of sedation and in sedation training

[a]Those particularly applicable to pediatric patients

is highly commendable in terms of engaging health-care providers and has led to the further *5 Million Lives Campaign* [14], it has also been criticized for being unable to demonstrate what aspects of the intervention were actually effective in achieving the result, or that much of the observed reduction in mortality was not due to other influences [12, 15]. While systematic approaches to improving safety have recently been shown to produce benefits in some areas [16–19], the improvement of safety in health care has been uneven, and in many areas little or no improvement has occurred. We suggest that the sedation of children is one such area and that preventable adverse events still occur too often in this context. Medication errors are a leading source of adverse events in pediatric patients [1, 20–23]. Among other things, these contribute to both inadequate sedation and excessive sedation with consequent airway complications, cardiovascular instability, and prolonged recovery. In many settings the management of many of these complications may be almost routine, rendering the complications inconsequential (e.g., by the provision of supplemental oxygen and jaw thrust) [24]. However, this rapid and easy management highlights the importance of many of the system, monitoring, training, and perioperative communication issues that are critical for the safe sedation of children.

Efforts to improve pediatric sedation have focused on many of the issues in Table 30.2, and proxy markers are often used as measures of safety or risk for this purpose. Proxy markers are indicators that are associated with, but occur more frequently than, rare outcomes of interest. They tend to focus on structures and processes rather than outcomes and so tend to be easier to measure [25]. Examples of markers of safety in sedation include the documentation of fasting for solids and liquids, the recording of weight, allergies, consent, risk assessment, and appropriate vital signs including depth of sedation, the presence of appropriate staff, written drug orders, and provision of a discharge handout [26].

Medication Errors

Medication errors (in any age group) may occur through commission or omission [27, 28]. The former involves the wrong drug, the right drug inadvertently repeated (so-called insertion errors), the wrong dose, the wrong route, or the wrong time. In addition, failure to correctly record administered medications may also be considered an error because of the critical importance of an accurate record in planning ongoing patient care [22, 29]. In errors of commission, harm may occur through unintended effects of incorrect actions (e.g., sedation from dexmedetomidine instead of dexamethasone for nausea). In errors of omission, harm may occur through the absence of intended effects (e.g., awareness or unwanted movement during inadequate sedation). The "six rights" of medication administration have been promulgated in response to these known failure modes, namely, the right patient, dose, medication, time, route, and record of the administration [22].

Experience from pediatric anesthesia suggests unintentional additional medication doses are the most prevalent drug error, but wrong drug, wrong dose, and wrong route errors are also common; errors with analgesics and antibiotics are particularly common [30, 31]. In intensive care or high dependency units, errors are frequent in both the administration and the prescribing of drugs [32]. In addition, adverse respiratory events arising from sedatives and analgesics often reflect poor choices of drugs and inadequate understanding and application of pharmacology, particularly when using combinations of drugs [33]. For example, respiratory adverse events are more common with fentanyl/ketamine combinations than with ketamine alone [34].

Dosage errors are also particularly common in children [5, 31, 35]. The patient's growth, maturation, and size are critical determinants of dose. Clearance, the pharmacokinetic parameter dictating maintenance dose, is immature at birth and matures over the first few years of life. Bupivacaine toxicity has occurred in infants receiving continuous regional neuronal blockade through failure to appreciate immature clearance [36]. Clearance has a nonlinear relationship to weight [37]: when clearance is expressed using a linear function (e.g., $L\ h^{-1}\ kg^{-1}$), it is highest in the 1- to 2-year-old age band and decreases throughout childhood until adult rates are achieved in late adolescence. Drug doses scaled directly from an adult dose (in $mg\ kg^{-1}$) will typically be inadequate. Consequently, propofol when used as an infusion for sedation in children requires a proportionately higher dose rate to achieve the same target concentration as in adults [38].

Similarly, the use of remifentanil parameters derived from adult studies for infusions in children results in lower concentrations than anticipated because clearance expressed per kilogram is higher in children [39].

There is substantial between-subject variability of response to any given dose. Pharmacodynamics has been inadequately studied in children and especially in infants. It follows that reliance on dose is not enough to judge effect reliably, and sedation must be monitored. This is difficult in young children, partially because of a lack of objective measures of effect in this group (e.g., processed EEG); instead it is necessary to rely on observation and on measurement tools (such as sedation scores) based on observation. However, observation may be difficult when children are undergoing certain radiological procedures, such as MRIs, for example. This difficulty in assessing sedation increases in children who have preexisting cerebral pathology [40] or behavior disorders [41] or who are very young [42].

The paucity of integrated pharmacokinetic-pharmacodynamic (PK-PD) studies of intravenous sedation in children, particularly sedation involving multiple drugs, predisposes to inadequate or excessive dose. Drug interactions may occur with mixtures used for sedation, but they may also be consequent to longer-term therapy with other drugs. For example, phenobarbital, used for seizure control, induces CYP3A4, an enzyme responsible for ketamine clearance. Thus, the sedative effect of ketamine, which is metabolized by CYP3A4, is reduced in children on long-term phenobarbital therapy [43, 44].

Infants are unable to swallow pills, but pediatric oral formulations are not available for the majority of commercially available medications. When no liquid oral formulation is available, intravenous preparations are often administered orally (e.g., of midazolam or ketamine) without adequate information about their absorption characteristics, hepatic extraction ratio, or the effect of any diluent used to improve palatability; this may lead to inappropriate dosing [45].

Children generally require smaller doses than adults. Because medications are packaged for adult use, dilution is commonly required in pediatric anesthesia. This further predisposes to dosage errors [5, 35], often in the form of tenfold overdoses because mistakes with the decimal place are easy to make [46]. Technique is particularly important in the administration of medications to small children and babies. Some of the intended dose of a medication may easily be retained in the dead space of any part of an intravenous administration set, or in a syringe, with the result that the desired effect may not be obtained. Subsequently, an unintended dose of this medication may be given inadvertently, flushed from the dead space by the later injection of another medication. The effect then may be excessive, untimely and potentially lethal [47]. Apnea, bradycardia, hypotension, and hypotonia have been reported in a premature neonate weighing 1.6 kg after an overdose of morphine, arising from medication unintentionally retained in a syringe [48].

Although medications are usually prescribed on a weight basis (e.g., in mg kg^{-1}), children are often not weighed. A survey of 100 children's notes in a busy emergency department revealed that only 2 % were weighed prior to the prescribing of medication [49]. Twenty-nine percent of physicians' estimates, 40 % of nurses' estimates, and 16 % of parents' estimates differed from actual weight by more than 15 % [50]. The accuracy of methods used to estimate weight also varies [51, 52].

Given the many factors that predispose to medication error in small children (Table 30.2), the importance of monitoring (particularly the degree of sedation) is obvious. Stress should also be placed on protocols (e.g., for measuring weight) and training (e.g., in the differences of PK-PD pharmacology between children and adults). Finally, guidelines, technology, and equipment need to be suitable for children rather than simply adapted from adult applications.

The Clinical Microsystem as a Unit of Analysis

A clinical microsystem is a group of "clinicians and staff working together with a shared clinical purpose to provide care for a population of patients" [53]. Understanding the operation of the clinical microsystem that delivers pediatric sedation is the key to identifying aspects for improvement. The elements of this microsystem include the patients, the clinicians, support staff, information technology, supplies, equipment, and care processes—and elements may be spread over various locations within the organization or beyond into the community. Certain roles, such as the person administering sedatives, may be held by individuals from different professional groups from instance to instance. The training of these individuals, and the approaches and standards used by them, may differ. In addition, sedation occurs in a variety of locations, which contributes to the variation in the staff available to perform the sedation, the equipment used, and the available safety and backup systems. This variation in location creates risks that do not apply to a team that performs in a fixed location, such as an operating room. In an operating room, the team typically has a designated number of defined roles filled from specified professional groups (such as nurses, anesthesiologists, and surgeons). Equipment tends to be reasonably standardized, and the way in which the members of the team perform their duties and interact with each other is relatively formalized.

To understand the operation of a clinical microsystem, the first step is to identify the personnel and other components that comprise the microsystem and then map the functional relationships of each to the others. Such a map can then be used as a guide to collect information on the operation of the microsystem and to identify gaps between how the microsystem is intended to operate and how it actually does operate. Strengths should be identified as well as weaknesses. The concept of "positive deviance" is that in any domain a few individuals facing risk will follow "uncommon, beneficial practices" and therefore experience better outcomes than their counterparts [54]. Once identified, these positively deviant strengths can be formalized, shared, and promoted more widely. The ultimate goal is to find ways to improve the connections between the elements of the microsystem, enhance its performance, and promote better outcomes [55–57].

Although the clinical microsystem seems likely to be a useful unit of analysis for the purposes of improving clinical safety during pediatric sedation, it is also necessary to consider the nature of its constituent parts, namely, humans and technology, and the way these interact. The complexity of technology used in health care today and the psychological determinants of human error remain important and underappreciated factors in the genesis of poor clinical outcomes.

People Versus Systems

Traditionally, safety in medicine has largely depended on the resolve and vigilance of individual clinicians to anticipate and avoid dangerous outcomes. Such an approach to safety has been called the person-centered approach, because all responsibility for safety rests on the shoulders of the individuals in the workplace [58, 59]. For the majority of the time, the person-centered approach works reasonably well in most organizations. Even in error-prone environments, skilled personnel can often perform adequately or even very well, finding inventive and creative ways to keep operational activities within desired limits despite deficiencies in technical and organizational aspects of their environment [60]. People should not be expected to perform like machines, which execute the same tasks repeatedly without deviation. Indeed, recovery from an unexpected event or other departure from the routine is one of the strengths of human intelligence (and a weakness of machines) and is a key feature of the avoidance of adverse events in complex endeavors. However, personal resolve to avoid bad outcomes is not sufficient: simply deciding to avoid error is, on its own, doomed to failure. In work environments where perfect performance is required every time and where error may lead to devastating consequences, the person-centered approach is insufficient to guarantee the requisite levels of safety and performance in the long term.

An important consequence of the person-centered approach is that the search for the reasons that things go wrong is typically not expanded further than those individuals immediately involved in the accident. All clinicians, no matter how resolved, will sooner or later make errors—simply because they are human and error is a statistically inevitable concomitant of being human [58, 59, 61]. Under the person-centered approach, when clinicians make mistakes, as they inevitably will, they are typically blamed for their carelessness and told to try harder to avoid error. Typically, little or no effort is made to identify the features of the system that predisposed or contributed to the error. This leaves such features active in the environment to precipitate similar errors in the future. Reason has called these features "passive errors" [58] or "latent factors" [62]. In the ultimate person-centered response, eliminating (e.g., through dismissal) the person who made the error simply sets up the replacement person for the same error to happen again. All medical systems contain many features that can only be described as accidents waiting to happen, and the relentless increase in the complexity of medical technology and treatment means that resolve and vigilance alone are increasingly inadequate to ensure the safety of patients [63–66].

Making Sense of Uncommon Adverse Events

Repeat even a safe activity often enough and eventually an accident will result—this phenomenon has been called the law of large numbers [67, 68]. The simple realization that the probability of an accident or failure can never be absolutely zero is one of the central ideas to come from the study of high-technology systems, including aviation, nuclear power, and space exploration [66, 69, 70]. Health care is a highly developed technological system, and the number and complexity of patients continues to increase year on year. It follows that the number of patients harmed by their procedures must also increase (given a constant, or even slowly decreasing underlying risk of harm). Thus, even though health care is almost certainly safer today than it has ever been in terms of relative risk (at least in high-income countries), it is causing harm to a record number of patients. However, relative risk estimates or Bayesian inference do not come intuitively to many people when they are required to interpret the occurrence of such adverse events [71]. Humans tend to focus on the total number of bad outcomes, regardless of the associated number of trouble-free outcomes [72–75]—on the numerator alone, rather than the ratio of numerator to denominator. We tend to have a fixed idea of how many plane crashes or medical mishaps are tolerable each year, regardless of the total number of planes in the sky, or patients treated. The current alarm about the safety of health care suggests that the number of patients harmed each year may be approaching the fixed level over which many people will cease to view health care as safe (Fig. 30.1). A further consequence of the law of large numbers is the fact that an adverse

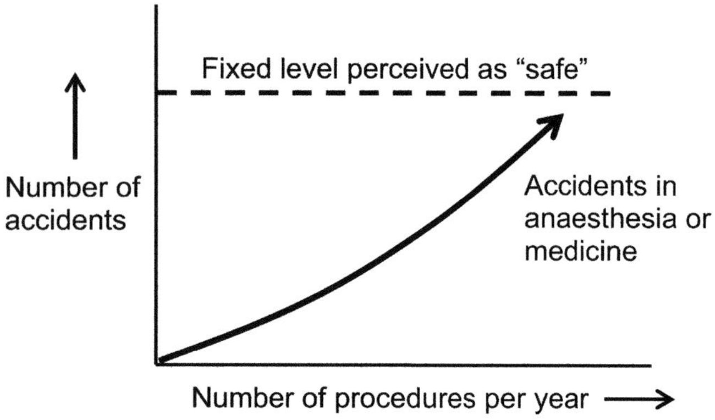

Fig. 30.1 What is considered safe is generally perceived as a fixed level of accidents for any particular technology (reproduced from Webster CS. Why anesthetizing a patient is more prone to failure than flying a plane. Anaesthesia. 2002;57:819–820, with permission from John Wiley and Sons)

event of any particular type will not be seen often, or at all, by any particular clinician—thus, clinical impressions can be considerably biased in relation to the true rate and importance of the adverse event [76]. Such bias can lead either to an underestimate (if the adverse event has never been encountered—the clinician perhaps believing that this is because his or her practice is better than average) or to an overestimate (if the clinician has been unfortunate enough to have had perhaps two or three bad experiences with the adverse event). Quantifying the true rate of any infrequent adverse event requires a systematic approach. It is trivial to estimate statistically the sample size needed to gain a reasonable estimate of any particular low incidence phenomenon: such studies often require data collection from thousands of patients, which can be prohibitive. Both these consequences of the law of large numbers, that is, not considering the denominator and the bias present in clinical impressions, impede the development of effective algorithms for dealing with uncommon adverse events and present a significant challenge for evidence-based health care. To continue to be viewed as safe, all technologies must become progressively safer with increasingly widespread use. Many aspects of medical technology have so far failed to achieve this.

One of the most promising approaches to the improvement of safety in health care involves the adoption of what has been called the systems approach [64, 77–79]. This differs from the human-centered approach in that it widens the focus of safety initiatives from the individual to include the "system" in which individuals work and emphasizes the elimination of unsafe aspects of equipment, procedures, work environments, and organizations. There are good examples of changes to particular aspects of systems that have dramatically improved safety, such as the inclusion of anti-hypoxic devices in modern anesthetic machines to prevent the omission of oxygen [80]. However, many of the straightforward opportunities for simple improvements through engineering innovations have been taken, and further implementation of the systems approach in health care will increasingly depend on a deeper understanding of the nature of human error, the factors that engage humans in changing behavior, and the way specific health-care systems fail. Critically, this better understanding will need to be followed through to the redesign of specific unsafe features within health-care systems.

The Nature of Human Error

Human errors are not random events. Their nature in any particular circumstance, and even the frequency with which they occur, can be predicted to a large degree through an understanding of the underlying mechanisms of human psychology [58, 81–86]. The capacities of our cognitive faculties are finite and imperfect. We can absorb, store, and process only a small portion of the information or stimuli in the world at any given time. We often act on "autopilot" without being consciously aware of many of the details of our actions, yet remain distractible. In addition, our memories are selective and dynamic. We remember certain events better than others on the basis of their significance to us as individuals, our recent similar experience, or the task we were engaged in at the time. Even once committed to memory, information in our heads changes over time, and recall can be partial and slow. Most of these limitations, far from being shortcomings, are in fact coping mechanisms honed by millions of years of human evolution [85, 87, 88]. Likewise, being able to carry out sequences of behavior in an automatic manner, without being consciously aware of the individual actions that make each up, allows us to perform more than one action at a time and frees up limited cognitive resource to monitor life-threatening or otherwise important events in the environment. For example, while engrossed in reading a book, we remain able to react appropriately to developing circumstances around us, for example, by noticing that the house is on fire. The upside of the nature of our cognitive faculties is that we perform quickly, often creatively, and typically very well for the vast majority of the time [89]. The downside is that under certain circumstances, we can be predisposed to make particular types of error [58, 83].

Error Types[1]

Psychologist James Reason, drawing on the work of Jens Rasmussen in particular, has defined a theoretical framework

[1]Some of the material in the section *Error Types* is drawn from the first author's PhD thesis: Webster CS. *Implementation and Assessment of a New Integrated Drug Administration System (IDAS) as an Example of a Safety Intervention in a Complex Socio-technological Workplace.* Auckland: University of Auckland, 2004.

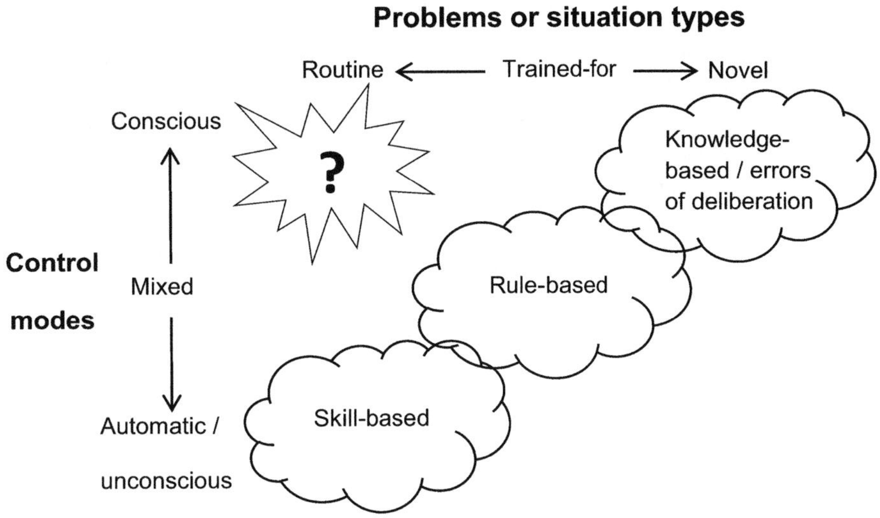

Fig. 30.2 The three modes of human performance (in clouds) and their relationship to the control modes and situations in which they are employed (adapted from Reason [58, 62]). Many attempts to improve safety in health care simply call for clinicians to pay more attention to their work, but fully conscious control of routine work is a mode of performance that is not sustainable in human nature (this imaginary zone in human performance is indicated by the question mark). We must look elsewhere for better and more effective methods of safety improvement

called the generic error-modeling system (GEMS) by which human behavior and errors can be classified [58, 62, 90, 91]. In the GEMS, human behavior is seen as being controlled by either conscious or automatic processes or a mixture of these two control modes (Fig. 30.2). Such control modes lead to three relatively distinct forms of human behavior. The three forms of human behavior also lead to three general classes of human error.

Knowledge-Based Errors (or Errors of Deliberation)

At the highest level of conscious awareness, the conscious control mode is slow, prone to error, requires effort, and operates sequentially (i.e., it deals with one thing at a time) [58, 62]. However, it can deal with completely novel and complex problems and is a primary source of human knowledge. The increased cognitive effort required when learning a new task appears to be directly reflected in the physiological activity of the brain. Novelty requires a "full-brain" conscious response, resulting in a large increase in brain activity [92]. In contrast, a familiar situation where an existing skill or rule can be applied results in little increased brain activity yet leads to smoother behavioral performance. Typically, we resort to the conscious control mode only when our stock of existing rules has become exhausted. This is not because we are mentally lazy, but because in most circumstances reasoning from first principles, using the conscious control mode, would take much too long. In addition, the operation of the conscious control mode (or the process of deliberation [85]) is probably the most error-prone human control mode. Furthermore, this process is often based on an incomplete or inaccurate "knowledge base"; some of this knowledge may reside in our minds and be amenable to training, but much of it is in the world, including in other people's minds. Thus, faulty decisions often reflect mental models that are subtly out of line with reality. This is the source of the term "knowledge-based errors," but in fact this phenomenon can promote rule-based errors as well. In addition, human deliberation suffers from a number of known biases, including confirmation bias (arriving at a conclusion and then adapting the facts to fit it), frequency bias (using the first information to mind), and similarity bias (attempting to solve two superficially similar, but different, problems in the same way) [58, 85]. Attempts to remove or mitigate such biases have been made, most recently through a process called cognitive debiasing, which proposes a suite of educational and mentally reflective initiatives aimed at "recalibrating" the mind in order to improve clinical tasks such as diagnoses [93, 94]. All such initiatives, however, start with gaining a better understanding of human psychology.

Rule-Based Errors

Rule-based behavior is the next level down in terms of the degree of conscious awareness required for the execution of a behavior—using the intermediary or mixed control mode (Fig. 30.2) [58, 62]. Acting in a rule-based way typically involves the conscious recognition of a familiar set of circumstances and the application of a learned rule. Applying an existing rule is much faster and less effortful than deliberation, and the majority of decisions in health care involve the application of rules in this way. Appropriately, the bulk of education in health care focuses on the acquisition of a very large rule base. Rule-based errors typically involve either the misinterpretation of a set of circumstances and hence the application of a good rule in the wrong situation or the application of a bad or inadequate rule that is thought to suffice. As an individual's repertoire of rules increases, with ongoing education and experience, he or she becomes more expert and is able to apply an appropriate rule in a much larger number of circumstances. Thus, an expert is likely to be equipped with a much greater, and typically more reliable, resource of rules than a novice [85] and will need to resort to deliberation (i.e., actively reasoning from first principles) less often.

Skill-Based Errors

The unconscious control mode is fast (often reflex-like), efficient, but rigid. It is the control system that allows "automatic" or skill-based behavior and comprises a collection of highly learned, frequently used routines or skills. Skill-based behavior tends to be so well learned that once started a sequence will often run through to completion without much further involvement from conscious awareness, for example, tying shoelaces or signing your name. In addition, the recognition of subtle cues and patterns by experts is often done at the unconscious level, leading to masterly and rapid performance that the individual often has difficulty explaining after the fact other than in terms of intuition, often stating simply that "they just knew" [84].

Experts have a large repertoire of skill-based behaviors, which allow them to perform at higher levels of efficiency than novices. Skill-based performance allows multitasking while requiring the least cognitive effort of any form of human performance. A novice will often labor over a single task that an expert can perform in seconds, and simultaneously with other tasks, simply because the novice has yet to acquire the ability to perform the task at the skilled-based level [58, 62].

Without skilled-based behavior, few of us would be able to perform even the simplest of everyday tasks, yet ironically skill-based expertise can also predispose us to make certain errors [95]. The ability to drive to work by an accustomed route while mentally planning the morning's activities is usually advantageous. However, if your workplace has recently changed, it is possible to find yourself halfway to the old, familiar address before realizing that you are traveling in entirely the wrong direction. Errors like these do not usually matter, because under normal conditions there is time to compensate for them—recovering from error is one of the greatest strengths of human intelligence [89, 96]. However, in certain error-intolerant environments, such as health care, typical everyday errors can lead to disaster so quickly that there is no time to prevent the consequences. The ability of a clinician to administer a drug while simultaneously calling further treatment instructions to an assistant in an emergency is a situation where the advantages of skill-based behavior may make the difference between life and death. However, such circumstances may also predispose a clinician to administer the wrong drug if drugs are poorly labeled and are used in an environment with inadequate safeguards. Novices are less likely to make such drug errors, simply because they do not possess the skill base with which to perform many of the actions involved at the unconscious level. However, a novice is likely to respond too slowly to provide effective patient care in a life-and-death emergency.

Two of the commonest categories of skill-based error are slips, in which an expert correctly performs a well-learned skill in incorrect circumstances (e.g., injection of the wrong drug), and lapses, in which an expert misses a step in a well-learned and otherwise correctly executed skill sequence because of momentary interruption from the environment or concurrent tasks (e.g., a busy clinician failing to record the administration of a drug) [29, 95, 97]. Both kinds of errors occur because the expert is able to perform skill-based behaviors largely unconsciously. Therefore, unlike performance of the rule-based type, greater expertise does not reduce the chance of error in skill-based performance. It is little appreciated that experts, in fact, can be expected to commit more slips and lapses than novices simply because they have a larger skill base at their disposal [58].

Technical Errors

A further kind of skill-based error common in health care has been described by Runciman and colleagues as the technical error [98]. A technical error can occur when the correct rule is employed, when no slip or lapse occurs, but where the desired outcome is not achieved because of a mismatch between the required technical skill and the applied technical skill. In the placement of an epidural catheter, for example, the tip may be inserted too far, resulting in the complication of dural tap, or it may not enter the epidural space at all, resulting in no anesthetic effect. The primary factor contributing to such technical errors is variability of patients and of physicians. During the insertion of an epidural catheter, the physiology of some patients may make insertion more difficult than others and some physicians are more skilled than others. Physicians also have good and bad days. If the difficulty of a particular patient is beyond the skill of a particular physician on the particular day, a dural tap or failed insertion may occur. Whether this is an error or not is a normative matter. If the epidural was one that a reasonable practitioner could usually have achieved, then, arguably it was a technical error. However, some tasks in medicine, including some epidural insertions, are technically impossible for the vast majority of practitioners with contemporary equipment and techniques. It seems unreasonable to refer to failure in these circumstances as error. Error should not be judged primarily by the outcome but by the process involved in its commission. Many anesthesiologists will know the feeling, in realizing that they have performed a dural tap (in this example), that they somehow just got it wrong—that they made a technical error. Golf provides a good illustration of this idea. No golfer living today would classify failing to get a hole in one from a distance of 150 m as a technical error, but many would readily relate to the idea that an uncharacteristic slice into the rough of a drive from the tee was a technical error.

The challenge of patient variability should not be underestimated. Unlike many high-technology endeavors where a great deal of standardization is possible, health care clearly must contend with the subtle physical variations and abnormal anatomies that exist in individuals—differences that are often unknown and unknowable before the procedure has begun. This is quite a different situation than with a manufactured artifact, such as an aircraft, where its exact structure and function can be known and where these details are documented. As Atul Gawande has put it, "a study of forty-one thousand trauma patients in the state of Pennsylvania—just trauma patients—found that they had 1,224 different injury-related diagnoses in 32,261 unique combinations. That's like having 32,261 kinds of airplane to land" [99]. Furthermore, unlike aircraft, none of these 32,261 unique trauma cases came with a manual.

Exhortation and Protocols

Despite these complexities, typically little training or education on the psychology of error or the nature of human behavior is provided during a health-care career. Efforts aimed at reducing error in health care often involve exhortation to be more careful at worst or the creation of new safety procedures and protocols at best [59, 100, 101]. Both these approaches to error reduction focus on the individual clinician and so are consistent with the human-centered approach. This view holds that all error is due to forgetfulness, inattention, poor motivation, carelessness, negligence, and recklessness [102]—paying more attention or following often lengthy safety protocols is therefore expected to stop error. Exhortation alone to be more careful, particularly with respect to skill-based performance, is equivalent to asking clinicians to perform all their duties with the conscious control mode. However, fully conscious control of routine behavior is a human performance mode that is not sustainable for anything more than *very* short periods, especially when individuals are required to possess a skill base related to the tasks they are being asked to perform. In Fig. 30.2 this imaginary zone in human performance is indicated with a question mark.

The Effects of Fatigue

Physical and mental fatigue increase with sleep deprivation, and increased fatigue leads to increased likelihood of the occurrence of the error types previously mentioned [103, 104]. Humans also experience a normal circadian cycle in sleepiness through the 24-h day, increasing in late afternoon (from 2 PM to 6 PM) and early morning (from 2 AM to 6 AM) where performance can be impaired [105, 106]. For example, the circadian nadir of human performance has been implicated in a number of notorious industrial accidents such as the Bhopal chemical plant accident in 1984 that killed 3,787 people; the Chernobyl nuclear reactor accident in 1986, which it has been estimated may eventually kill 27,000 people internationally through cancer; and the Three Mile Island nuclear reactor accident in 1979 (discussed in more detail later) [70].

Much of the research into the effects of fatigue involves test tasks, notably the psychomotor vigilance task (PVT), administered over short periods in a quiet room with no distractions—conditions that have little in common with the work of an anesthesiologist. Furthermore, increased mental effort and the effects of adrenaline may counter the effects of fatigue, at least temporarily, and so some doubt remains over whether the risk of error during anesthesia is necessarily increased by moderate degrees of sleep deprivation [104, 107, 108]. Evidence that fatigue impairs surgical performance is also less than clear [109]. On the other hand, some participants in a simulation-based study of anesthesia residents fell asleep for brief periods [110], and 48.8 % of respondents to a survey of Certified Registered Nurse Anesthetists had witnessed a colleague asleep during a case [111]—events that seem hard to defend. Other studies in health care have demonstrated increased risk of significant medical errors, adverse events, and attentional failures associated with fatigue [108, 112–114]. For example, on the basis of 5,888 h of direct observation, interns working traditional schedules involving multiple extended-duration shifts ($\geq$24 h) per month have been found to make 20.8 % more serious medication errors and 5.6 times more serious diagnostic errors than when working without extended-duration shifts [115]. It is also relevant that Dawson has shown that shifts of 16 h or more are associated with reductions in performance equivalent to the effects of alcohol intoxication as legally defined [116]. However, the causes of human fatigue are not confined to the work place, and it is also unclear that all recommended fatigue countermeasures are effective in improving patient care. For example, reducing the work hours of residents has resulted in more handovers of care, and these in themselves are a known source of patient risk due to communication failure [117, 118]. Attempts to reduce working hours for clinicians have been made in various countries, but, in many, current hours worked remain higher than in other safety-critical industries such as the aviation industry [114, 119]. Furthermore, limitations to residents' hours of work are more common than limitations to the hours that senior doctors may from time to time be asked to work [120]. In general, though, some reasonable limits on work hours are appropriate. Strategic napping may also be effective in bringing relief from fatigue [106, 119], and facilities should be provided to allow this.

Human Factors and the Culture of Safety

In recent years there has been growing interest in the adoption of the "safety culture" of the aviation industry in anesthesia, and the analogy of the anesthetist as the "pilot" of his or her patient has become well known [121, 122]. The aviation industry in the United States began adopting systematic approaches to improving safety in the 1920s when the first laws were passed to require that aircraft be examined, pilots licensed, and accidents properly investigated. The first safety rules and navigation aids were then introduced. The first aviation checklist was introduced following the crash of the Boeing Model 299 in 1935, killing two of the five flight crew, including the pilot, Major Ployer Hill [99, 123]. The Model 299 was a new, more complex aircraft than previous models, and during the more involved process of flight preparation, Major Hill omitted a critical step—he forgot to release a catch, which on the ground locked the aircraft's control flaps. Once in the air this mistake rendered the aircraft uncontrollable. The crash investigators realized that there was probably no one better qualified to fly the aircraft than Major Hill and that despite this the fatal error was still made. Some initially believed that the new aircraft was too complicated to be flyable. Given the circumstances of the accident, the investigators realized that further training would not be an effective response to prevent such an event from occurring again. Thus, the idea of a checklist emerged: a simple reminder list of critical steps that had to occur before the aircraft could leave the ground. With this checklist in use, the Model 299 (and later versions of it) remained in safe operation for many years.

A teamwork improvement system called Crew Resource Management (CRM), primarily focused on nontechnical skills such as communication in the cockpit, followed checklists in aviation in the early 1980s [75, 123]. Aviation checklists have subsequently been applied to many other routine and emergency aspects of aircraft operation and are today organized hierarchically in a binder such that in an uneventful flight only the topmost checklist is required. However, if operating conditions deviate for the routine, the checklist hierarchy forms a decision tree through which additional relevant checklists are brought to bear on each abnormal set of conditions, for example, managing an engine fire [99, 124]. In this way checklists coordinate the actions of those in the cockpit with each other and with members of the wider microsystem of aircraft operation, including members of the cabin crew, aircraft traffic control personnel, and through traffic control, other aircraft. It should be emphasized, however, that checklists do not substitute for training and expertise; they are simply a form of aide-memoire to assist in making training and expertise more effective. The ongoing training of pilots is itself a model for safety improvement that health care is only now beginning to adopt.

Today, much technical and nontechnical flight training occurs in sophisticated immersive flight simulators. The result of this on-going program of training in human factors relevant to flying is an enviable safety record for the aviation industry. Commercial air travel is now by far the safest form of transportation by distance—resulting in only 0.05 deaths per billion kilometers traveled, compared with 3.1 and 108 deaths per billion kilometers traveled by car and motorcycle transportation, respectively [123]. It is worth noting that even the latter risks are much lower than that of anesthesia. This can be seen if the risk of death attributable to anesthesia is assumed to be 1 in 200,000 cases (and we believe this to be an optimistic estimate) [125, 126], and both this and the rates for road transportation are converted to a time basis. People are generally much more likely to die in a road accident than during an anesthetic, but that is because of the relative exposures to these risks, rather than to the rates of risk themselves.

Simulation and Safety

Modern manikin-based simulators were first introduced in health care in the 1960s and have since been used primarily for technical skills training such as airway management and life support. In the 1980s, more immersive simulation environments incorporating such manikins were developed and training began to include crisis management during rare events and the safety of care [127]. A version of CRM for anesthesia was first promoted in the early 1990s, but nontechnical skills training for complete clinical teams, including surgical staff, is (surprisingly) a recent innovation [128, 129]. The slower uptake of simulation in health care probably reflects the greater technical challenge of simulating the human body and its various responses to health-care interventions. Considerable realism can be achieved today [130, 131], but a key deficit in anesthesia simulation lies in the fact that the simulators require an operator. Although some of the physiologic models are impressive on their own, there is a long way to go before a simulator will automatically respond to the interventions of anesthesia in the way a healthy patient does, let alone the way patients with various pathologies might do. Again, this reflects the fact that anesthesia, involving human patients, is much more complex than aviation, in which pilots expect to work with standardized and fully functional aircraft. Certainly weather varies, but if safety is in doubt, flights are deferred. With many acute patients, the avoidance of risky conditions is not possible. Furthermore, although there is emerging evidence of the transfer of learning in clinical simulators to the real world, much work needs to be done to assess the validity of many aspects of health-care simulation [131, 132]. While flight simulators have for many years been sufficiently immersive and realistic that a pilot trained entirely in the simulator can step into a real aircraft and fly it without further training, it will be many years before simulation in health care reaches this level of sophistication.

Teamwork and Communication

An additional challenge for modern health care is that its multi-professional nature hinders the changing of work culture and increases the risk of poor teamwork and communication failure [133–135]. Communication strategies used by hospital personnel have not kept pace with the increasing complexity of care and have changed little, if any, in decades. A clinical team is often comprised of a disparate set of individuals from different schools of training with different skill sets and world views who must somehow work together to bring about a successful outcome for a unique patient with a unique presentation—and this is likely to be particularly the case during sedation outside the operating room. As a consequence, observational research in health care demonstrates that failures in teamwork and communication are relatively common, particularly when handing over patient care from one health-care team to another and when a patient is receiving multidisciplinary care involving a number of professional groups simultaneously [133, 136, 137]. Furthermore, the communication that does occur during multidisciplinary care often happens in silos, that is, within a professional group rather than between groups. Professional silos manifest an unwillingness to speak up to challenge others, a lack of engagement in team decision making, and poor agreement on shared goals [133, 138]. Poor communication of this sort has been associated with compromised patient safety, increased rates of procedural errors, patient harm, significant additional costs, and work place dissatisfaction [56, 139]. However, team processes can be improved. A recent systematic review of 28 qualifying papers reports on team processes such as communication, coordination, leadership, and non-technical skills; from 66 comparisons of a team process variable with a performance variable, 40 (61 %) were found to be significantly related [140]. Of the 11 studies reporting team process interventions, 7 (66 %) showed significant improvements after the intervention.

Salas et al. [141] have proposed a model for teamwork based on empirical evidence from teams across diverse organizations that is informative in efforts to improve teamwork in pediatric sedation. Five dimensions of effective teamwork are described: team orientation, team leadership, mutual performance monitoring, backup behavior, and adaptability. These dimensions are underpinned by three coordinating factors: mutual trust, closed loop communication, and shared mental models within the team.

Team orientation is probably the most important factor. Mutual trust and shared mental models are unlikely to occur if the people providing sedation for diverse procedures in children, and the different proceduralists with whom they are working, do not even identify as a team. Lack of team orientation is a substantial barrier to improvement, and there would be great value in the simple step of getting all relevant practitioners together and obtaining agreement that the care for pediatric patients undergoing sedation actually warrants the formation of an explicit team that works together to standardize and improve their equipment and processes [142, 143].

Leadership is interesting in this context. In the clinical setting, leadership will need to be dynamic depending on the issue in question and the training and experience of the practitioners involved. If present, an anesthesiologist would be expected to lead the management of a crisis that developed during a procedure, for example, but decisions about aspects of the procedure itself are more likely to be initiated by the proceduralist. An agreed approach is required to ensure that the best decisions are made and this requires discussion and consensus building away from the demands of managing patients. This raises the important question of the overall leadership of the team. There is obviously a need for regular meetings of the team members to discuss approaches, set expectations, agree on needed equipment, and adopt guidelines, among many other important aspects of practice. There is no particular reason for such a leader to be an anesthesiologist, a surgeon, or a member of any other particular group—the role here is really one of coordination and consensus building.

An effective way to build teamwork is to provide training for the whole team in communication and other nontechnical skills. As previously discussed, simulation provides a powerful tool for doing this. Briefing sessions of the whole team at the beginning of every clinical session are very helpful to plan the day and to ensure that mental models are indeed shared in respect of anticipated problems and the plans for dealing with them. Not only do such sessions improve safety, they also greatly improve the flow and efficiency of the day. Debriefing at the end of each session is also valuable. This can be very brief and should focus on what went well and what opportunities for improvement were noticed.

If patients are regularly transferred at the end of procedures to postanesthetic care rooms, high dependency rooms, or even wards, attention should be paid to standardization of the process of handover or handoff. The work of de Leval and his group has resulted in important gains in safety and efficiency when taking patients from the operating room to the intensive care unit [144]. Similar gains are likely in the context of pediatric sedation.

Some team process improvements may be enhanced by the adoption of process tools. The World Health Organization (WHO) Safe Surgery Checklist was specifically designed to promote better communication and enhance teamwork. Some of the benefits that have been demonstrated with its use were found in categories not specifically targeted by checklist items [17]. The authors of the checklist have speculated that these additional benefits may be due to the more global effects of better team communication engendered by the act of carrying out the steps of the checklist itself, including individual team members introducing themselves by name [99]. This has two advantages. It promotes directed communication in which people are addressed by name. It also activates people; once a person has spoken, he or she is more likely to speak again. This increases the likelihood of speaking up if an error is noticed.

The Nature of System Failures

The complexity and design of systems is also a significant contributor to human error. Complexity theory asserts that some systems behave in ways that are inexplicable on the basis of only a knowledge of the systems' individual components—that is, the behavior of the whole depends on more than a knowledge of its parts [57, 145]. Typical examples of such complex systems are living organisms, stock markets, and the weather. Socio-technological systems contain human operators or workers as vital components in their everyday function and are thus distinguished from purely technological systems that are capable of essentially automatic operation [3, 83, 146, 147]. Specific work environments, clinical microsystems, or large-scale technological systems can be understood as complex socio-technological systems in this sense. Despite this, health care remains one of the last industries to adopt the kind of systematic approach to safety that has proved successful in many other high technologies [66, 69, 121, 148–150].

Characteristics of Safe and Unsafe Systems

In Charles Perrow's *Normal Accidents Theory*, a "normal accident" is one that occurs in a complex system through the unanticipated interaction of multiple failures. The complexity of the system both predisposes to the occurrence of simultaneous multiple failures and masks the many potential ways in which such individual failures may interact in a dangerous way [66]. Perrow also suggests that the function of any system can be classified along two dimensions: interaction and coupling. A task or process can be said to have *complex* interaction between parts if there are many alternative subtasks at any point in its completion or *linear* if it is comprised of a set of fixed steps carried out in rigid sequence. The coupling dimension describes the extent to which an action in the task or process is related to its consequences. A system is *tightly* coupled if consequences occur immediately after an action. Hence, tightly coupled systems result in more accidents because minor mistakes, slips, or lapses can become serious accidents before they can be corrected. A *loosely* coupled system is more forgiving of error and allows greater opportunity for an error to be corrected in time to avoid serious consequences [151]. These two dimensions form Perrow's interaction/coupling space with which human activities can be classified [66].

For example, baggage handling by airlines is a relatively safe organizational activity because it is both loosely coupled and has linear interaction between parts (bottom left quadrant of Fig. 30.3). That is, a bag tends to progress through a fixed number of independent steps on the way to being delivered to its owner, and there are many opportunities to correct mistakes in the process. Furthermore, the consequences of failure are typically irritating and correctable rather than catastrophic. At the opposite side of the interaction/coupling space, a nuclear power plant by comparison is potentially dangerous because it has both complex interaction and tight coupling between parts or subsystems (top right quadrant in Fig. 30.3). Errors in the operation of a nuclear power plant may very quickly lead to dangerous outcomes. In addition, complex interaction makes the system inherently more difficult to control because such complexity increases the chance that unanticipated system interactions may cause the system to spontaneously depart from the desired path of operation. While it is widely understood that nuclear power plants are complex and tightly coupled, it is less well appreciated that health-care systems also fall into the most dangerous quadrant of the interaction/coupling space (the upper right-hand quadrant) and have similar characteristics [152, 153]. In fact, health care is probably more challenging than nuclear power plants, because it combines tightly coupled elements with loosely coupled elements and varies from simple through complicated to complex and indeed chaotic (or dynamical) [99]. On the other hand, the potential for truly catastrophic consequences on a grand scale is larger with nuclear power plants. Human beings are complex (physiological and psychological) systems and so appear on the extreme high end of the complexity dimension. A normal awake patient would fall on the loose side of the midline of the coupling dimension because of the homeostatic and self-regulating subsystems of the body. However, a human being undergoing anesthesia or sedation is a decidedly more tightly coupled system than a fully awake individual, necessitating close monitoring and an array of techniques to maintain the patient's safety. Consequently a sedated patient migrates to a location within the interaction/coupling space significantly closer to the most potentially dangerous top corner (Fig. 30.3)—a zone in closer proximity to a nuclear plant than an aircraft.

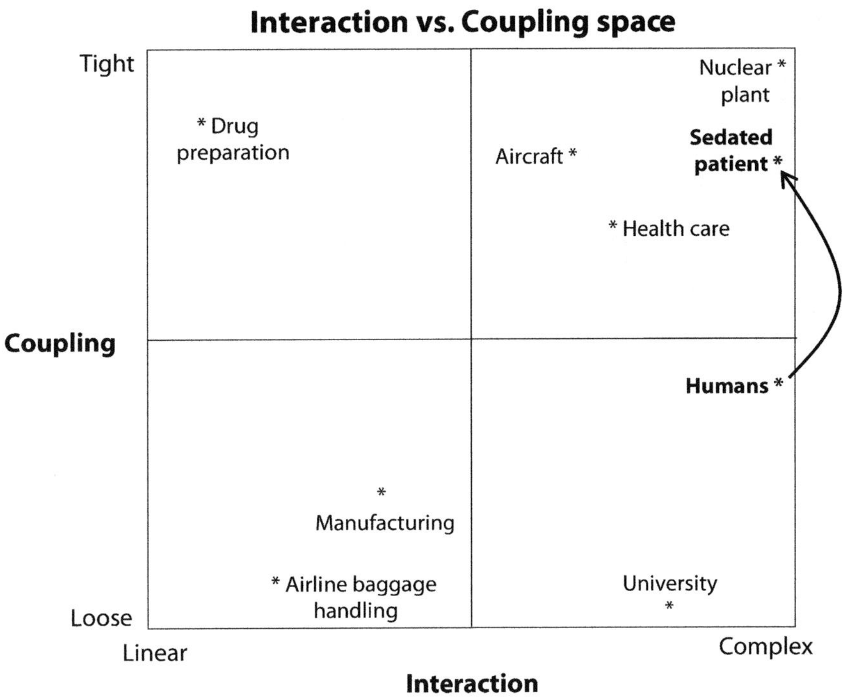

Fig. 30.3 The interaction/coupling space (adapted from Perrow [66]) with which human activities and organizations can be classified. Note that health care falls in the most potentially dangerous, upper right-hand quadrant, in which organizations and activities are both tightly coupled and have complex interactions. Human beings as complex (physiological) systems and the migration within the space of humans when they become sedated patients is shown

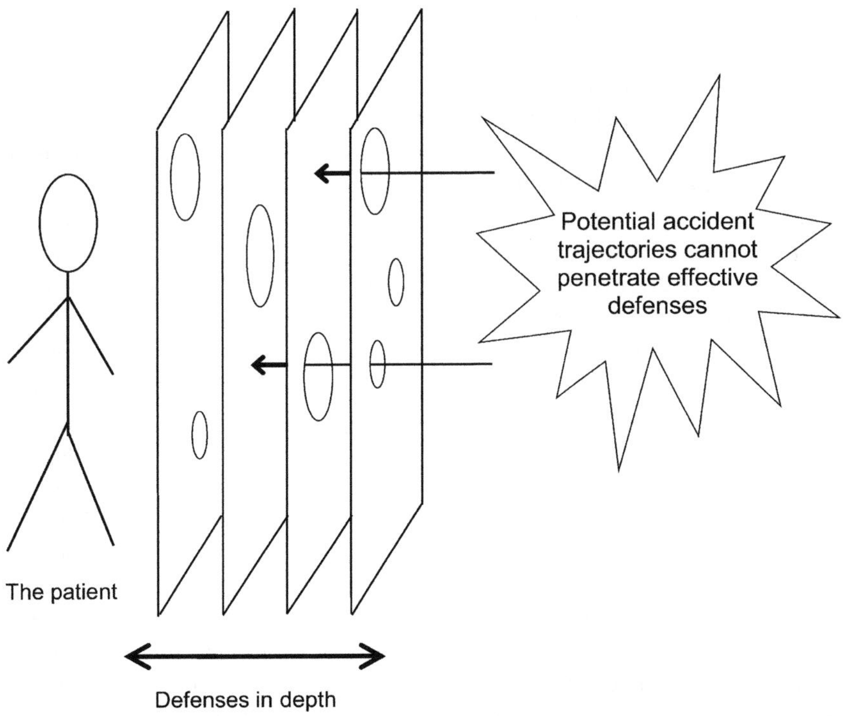

Fig. 30.4 The role of multiple defenses in preventing system failure. Despite inevitable defects, multiple layers of system defenses effectively shield the patient (adapted from Reason's "Swiss cheese" model [58, 62])

Barriers to System Failure

Even in tightly coupled complex systems, barriers exist to stop mistakes or faults leading to disaster, and most of the time these work successfully. Factors such as good design, effective safety devices, tolerance limits, and recommended operating procedures can all be seen as a system's defenses against an accident or system failure. When represented schematically these defenses form overlapping layers that protect the system from accident (Fig. 30.4). Inevitably, such defenses are imperfect. Defects in design, unexpected changes in supplies, violations such as not following correct procedures, a lack of agreement on the best approach in any particular circumstance, a lack of proper maintenance,

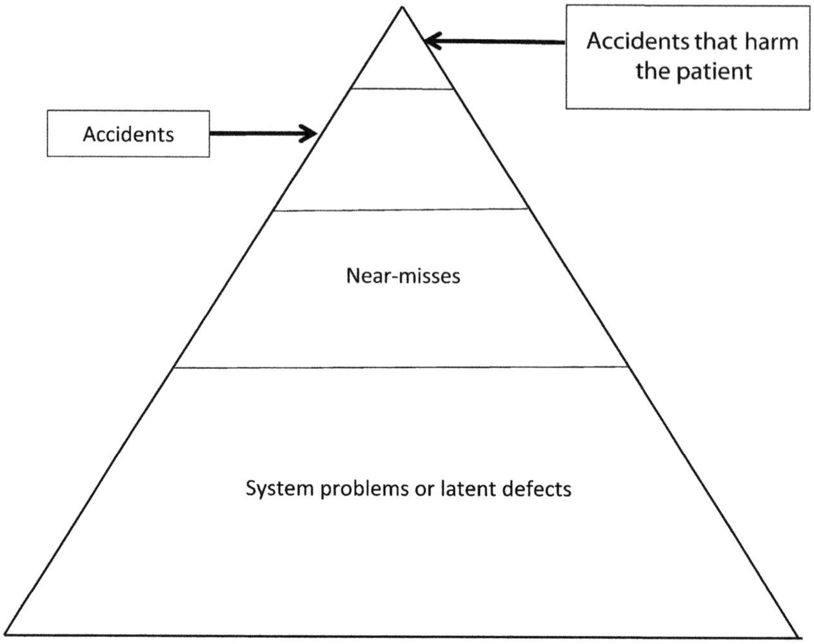

Fig. 30.5 The incident pyramid. The largest portion of the pyramid is made up of system problems or latent factors. The apex or "sharp end" of the pyramid comprises accidents that harm the patient and is the most visible part, not least because this is typically where the operator or clinician acts as the final trigger for the occurrence of an active failure

poor team communication, or simple human error may be represented as holes in the layers of defenses. The size of these holes (or latent factors) depends on the severity of the design problem or risk-taking behavior of the practitioner. Such factors lie dormant or are latent because they exist within the organization, usually undetected, until a series of events occurs in which they are discovered through their mutual contribution to an accident. A defect in the system's defenses in one layer is usually compensated for by an intact barrier at another. However, when a set of defects coincide, an accident trajectory is created through all layers of the system's defenses, and a system failure or accident will occur [58, 62, 98]. Having fewer layers of system defenses increases the chance of an accident occurring as it means it is more likely that latent factors will coincide. Conversely, increasing the number of layers of defense decreases the chance that a combination of latent factors will coincide, presuming that every layer is independent. The systems approach recognizes that no defense or safety mechanism is perfect under all circumstances (including the human in the system). However, given enough layers of defense, good system protection can be achieved even in the presence of imperfections (Fig. 30.4). The systems approach does not remove the need for the human operator to monitor the safety of proceedings as the final system defense, but it does remove some of the burden of this task and facilitates his or her ability to monitor effectively and function safely.

In the industrial setting, systematic approaches to the prevention of industrial accidents have a relatively long history compared with efforts to prevent injury and harm in health care. In the fourth edition of his book entitled *Industrial Accident Prevention*, published in 1959, Heinrich states that "industrial accident prevention has come of age" and that "safety begins with safe tools, safe machines, safe processes and safe environment" [154]. In health care, however, there is a lingering belief that all a doctor really needs to prevent mistakes is appropriate resolve and vigilance—the realization that this is not the case has been slow [98, 155]. No one would claim that the prevention of iatrogenic harm in health care has come of age.

As accidents are less common than near misses, and not all accidents cause injury, the proportional makeup of these events is often represented diagrammatically as a pyramid [78, 154]. Heinrich has described this pyramid in the industrial setting with his 300-29-1 ratio, which states that for every major injury there will be, on average, 29 minor injuries and 300 no-injury accidents [154]. A similar hierarchical arrangement seems certain to exist in health care, although the proportions are likely to be different and to vary from example to example. For example, it has been estimated that incidents are 3,300 times more likely than accidents in health care and that only about 1 % of drug administration errors cause injury to patients [148, 156]. Latent system problems or defects can be added to the hierarchy at the lowest level below near misses as the system features, which predispose the events above them in the pyramid [101] (Fig. 30.5).

The apex of the pyramid represents the sharp end of the system and is the most visible part in any organization because it is where accidents and patient harm occur and typically where the human operator or clinician is found as the last failed barrier against system failure. However, the single largest part of the pyramid is its base, which contains the unsafe aspects of equipment, procedures, and organizations. These factors contribute to the vast majority of accidents but generally remain unknown until they precipitate an accident. The largest and most sustainable safety gains are to be had by addressing the base of the pyramid with safety strategies designed to remove latent system defects [81]. Such an approach will have a substantial knock-on effect through the higher layers of the pyramid and will be more effective and long lasting than exhorting individuals at the sharp end to be more careful [65, 148, 157].

Traversing the Incident Pyramid

Root Cause Analysis

Root cause analysis (RCA) is a formal analytical method developed in other high-reliability organizations that works backwards from an accident or adverse event in order to determine the event's underlying causes and predisposing factors, such that these can be removed or redesigned to prevent the accident from reoccurring in the future. An RCA may be initiated after any accident, but many organizations have a policy to initiate an RCA after the occurrence of any of a predetermined set of events of interest or so-called sentinel events. The Joint Commission defines a sentinel event as any unanticipated event in a health-care setting resulting in death or serious physical or psychological injury to a patient or patients, not related to the natural course of the patient's illness [158]. The effectiveness of the RCA method in health care is suggested by a recent study of 139 Veterans Affairs medical centers over 3 years. This study demonstrated that centers that conducted an average of 4.8 RCAs per year had lower postoperative complication rates than centers that completed fewer than 4.0 RCAs per year [159].

The advantages of RCA include that the method is a system-based approach and so widens the scope of accident investigation from the human at the accident site to the wider system in which personnel work—thus allowing the identification of more sustainable and effective corrective actions. However, despite its usefulness, RCA remains a reactive method—an accident or sentinel event needs to occur before an RCA can be undertaken. In this sense, RCAs work from the apex of the incident pyramid to the base, meaning that only a subset of underlying causal factors may be discovered during the investigation.

Failure Mode and Effect Analysis

Failure mode and effect analysis (FMEA) was first used to understand military systems in the 1950s. It is a standardized approach that first identifies elements in an organization that carry risk of causing harm, then prioritizes the identified elements and remediates the most dangerous [160, 161]. The advantages of this method are that it is a proactive and system-based approach—in safety-critical systems, it can be carried out before an accident or serious incident occurs, thus helping to ensure the continued accident-free operation of the organization. While FMEA may allow the possibility of system improvement in health care before the occurrence of harm to the patient, one disadvantage is that the method is relatively costly in terms of time and resources. However, the cost of any safety initiative needs to be weighed against the very large human and financial cost of continuing to harm and kill patients during their care [61]. As FMEA starts with the elements of an organization that predispose accidents (often called accident precursors), this method can be seen to work from the bottom of the incident pyramid to the top. A recent FMEA conducted in the pediatric department of a 213-bed university hospital found that none of the steps in the drug administration process were free from potential failures modes. The highest-risk failure mode in all pediatric units was found to be the calculation of medication doses, especially for infusion administration [160].

Lessons from the Development of Safety in the Nuclear Power Industry

The US nuclear power industry has spent more time and money on safety than the health-care industry, including making early use of incident reporting, simulation training, and system redesign [70, 162–164]. In addition, given the close proximity of a sedated patient and a nuclear plant in the Perrow space (Fig. 30.3), it is instructive to consider the safety response from the nuclear industry in the face of one of the most significant nuclear power plant accidents in US history.

The Three Mile Island Nuclear Power Plant Accident

As in health care, a nuclear power plant constitutes a complex socio-technical work environment where an everyday human error or minor system fault can lead to a cascading sequence of events that ends in disaster or serious accident. Charles Perrow's influential *Normal Accidents Theory*, discussed above and which has been widely applied to the understanding of accidents in health care, has its origins in the analysis of the Three Mile Island Number 2 (TMI-2) nuclear power plant accident in 1979. The accident sequence began during routine maintenance at just after 4 AM on March 28, during which a minor deviation from normal conditions triggered a series of events that led to the malfunction of a pilot-operated relief valve (PORV). At about 2 min into the accident sequence the PORV failed to close, this resulted in the loss of much needed coolant from the reactor core for approximately the next 3 h [66, 69, 70]. Operators were scrambling to understand and control the rapidly evolving crisis but were unaware that the PORV remained open—this information being lost in the confusion of alarm signals. The particular sequence of failures caused the reactor to behave in a way outside anything in the operators' previous experience and the reactor's standard operating procedures. Despite confusion over the state of the reactor, the operators followed what they believed to be standard procedure in the circumstances. However, with the PORV still open, these actions actually exacerbated the crisis, and the reactor core began to melt. About 2 h later "fresh eyes" entered the room in the form of reactor operator Brian Mehler, who, reasoning from first principles, closed a manual valve to the PORV, suspecting it may still be open. This regained control of the reactor, but by then it had been damaged beyond repair. Subsequent analysis suggested that the reactor may have been as little as half an hour away from a complete meltdown, resulting in a likely breach of the reactor vessel, and possible widespread release of radioactive material [66].

It seems likely that fatigue compromised the abilities of the plant operators to diagnose the correct state of the reactor and to take appropriate and timely action. They were also more likely to suffer confirmation bias in their interpretation of the plant's instruments: this group of experts believed the PORV was closed, despite some control panels indicating the opposite. They therefore proceeded to take action consistent with their existing incorrect diagnosis—actions that actually made matters worse. Mehler was less likely to be suffering from confirmation bias when he brought a fresh pair of eyes into the room, as he had not been present from the start of the accident sequence and had no fixed diagnosis of the reactor in mind.

From reports of clinical disasters, we know that clinicians, not surprisingly, can suffer from the same kind of confirmation bias as the TMI-2 operators did and that their expert understanding of clinical crises is often incomplete. As a consequence, a fresh pair of eyes can be immediately beneficial in resolving a clinical crisis [85, 153, 165]. In addition, rules can run out during clinical care, and clinicians can fail to assimilate vital information about rapidly evolving complex situations despite its apparently obvious presentation [166]. The combination of uncommon events, poor team communication, and conflicting or incomplete information from patient monitors can significantly increase the risk of an adverse event for patients. For example, although it has been available in operating rooms for many years, capnography monitoring is often not used during patient sedation elsewhere. This can delay the detection of hypoventilation and desaturation, even while monitoring patients with pulse oximetry. In such circumstances the routine use of supplemental oxygen may mask declining oxygen saturation levels until they have fallen precipitously—a dangerous situation that may take several minutes to detect [2]. The sedating clinician therefore may not be aware of the state of the patient or have an opportunity to act to correct the desaturation before sequelae occur, with the consequence that once detected more aggressive forms of corrective action must be taken.

A State-Space Approach to Failure in Complex Systems

An approach that allows system failure and the value of incident reporting to be visualized is the state-space approach [153]. In any complex system, the set of all possible system states is very large and much larger than the subset of known states (Fig. 30.6). Desired states (e.g., where a patient is safely sedated) are a subset within the set of known system states. Some *known* states lead to disaster—and only this relatively small subset of states or "credible accidents" can be specifically guarded against with the use of safety systems and procedures (the hatched area in Fig. 30.6). However, a probably larger subset of *unknown* system states can also lead to disaster—these pathways are much more difficult to guard against because the causal mechanisms involved are simply unknown, and this represents a blind spot in system safety.

For example, applying the state-space approach to the TMI-2 accident, we can see that although the nightshift operators were aware that the reactor was off-normal, they believed its state remained within the boundaries of known states—that is, they believed the reactor's state had migrated from A to B in Fig. 30.6. Their attempts to move back to a desired state therefore made use of standard procedures. In fact, the reactor's state had migrated all the way to point C and was possibly within 30 min of attaining state D (meltdown). In any complex system, migration to D from either A or B is difficult by design (e.g., because of an attentive care team and the use of effective monitoring during sedation, or due to a nuclear plant's safety subsystems). Migration from C to D, however, is via the system safety blind spot, which bypasses known safety systems. Moving the system back to a desired state from anywhere within the set of unknown states requires at least some degree of knowledge-based or deliberative reasoning because there can be no specific rules for dealing with unknown states. Thinking from first principles can be particularly difficult when one is fatigued, or during the pressures of a crisis.

The Role of Incident Reporting

The state-space approach also demonstrates the value of incident reporting. Incident reports increase the set of known

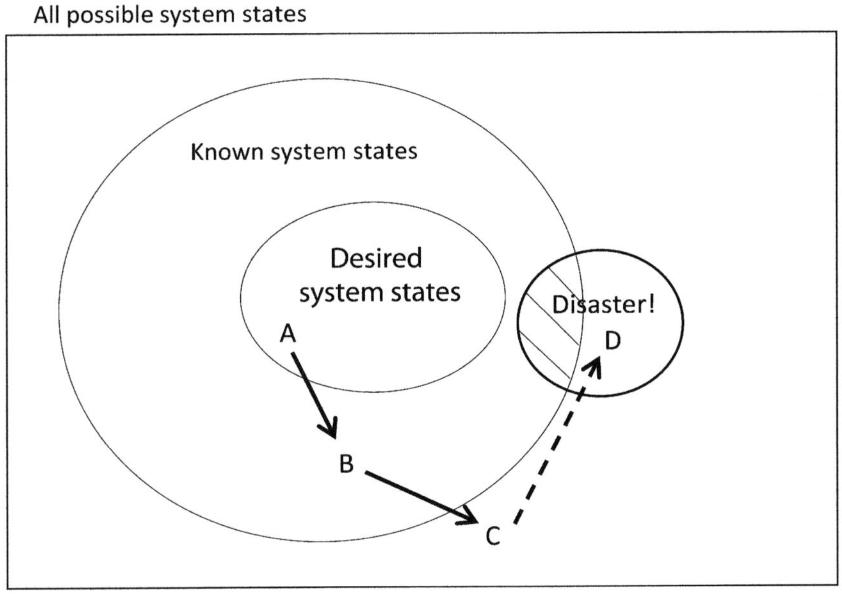

Fig. 30.6 State-space diagram for an accident in a generic complex system. Known system states are a subset of the larger set of all possible system states. Some known states lead to disaster, and only these can be specifically guarded against with safety systems and procedures (the hatched area). However, a probably larger set of unknown system states also leads to disaster, but these cannot be guarded against specifically because the causal mechanisms involved are unknown (Reproduced from Webster CS. The nuclear power industry as an alternative analogy for safety in anaesthesia and a novel approach for the conceptualisation of safety goals. Anaesthesia. 2005;60:1115–1122, with permission from John Wiley and Sons)

system states at the cost of unknown states, thus expanding the known-state circle (shown as the new solid line in Fig. 30.7). This allows better and more inclusive procedures to be developed for previously unexpected system behavior—thus, effortful, error-prone knowledge-based or deliberative reasoning will be required less often. The safety initiatives undertaken in response to the TMI-2 accident are listed in Table 30.3, all of which increased the set of known states [69, 70]. It is worth noting that these go far beyond that typically undertaken in health care when disaster occurs—this is despite the fact that the number of patient deaths due to preventable adverse events in health care greatly outnumber deaths due to nuclear accidents of any variety [70]. The less robust safety response in health care almost certainly reflects the persistent person-centered approach, a less systematic approach to the analysis of failures, and the fact that disaster in health care, although no less tragic, generally has a lower profile, killing patients one at a time.

The Value of Incident-Based Recovery Pathways

Figure 30.7 shows the execution of a successful recovery path in a generic complex system. Incident reporting has allowed the set of known states to be expanded. The accident pathway from A to C is identical to that in Fig. 30.6, but now, point C is included in the set of known states for which a standard, rule-based procedure has been developed. Timely implementation of the new procedure allows a recovery pathway to be executed (C to A) to restore the system to a desired state before disaster or harm occurs. Recovery pathways are critically important in the complex socio-technical systems such as health care. In his landmark paper, Cooper found that 93 % of more than 1,089 reported critical incidents during anesthesia could be recovered from without harm to the patient, underscoring the effective use of recovery pathways in the operating room [165]. By contrast, anesthesia and sedation conducted in more remote locations such as emergency departments and nonhospital-based facilities demonstrate poorer outcomes for patients [167–169], suggesting that the facilities or skilled personnel needed to conduct effective recoveries are not available in these locations to the same extent.

Closed Claims Settlements for Cases Outside the Operating Room

Closed claims cases collected by the American Society of Anesthesiologists (ASA) represent adverse patient outcomes where a lawsuit was subsequently taken against the clinicians or organization involved. These data provide insights into events at the tip of the incident pyramid where some

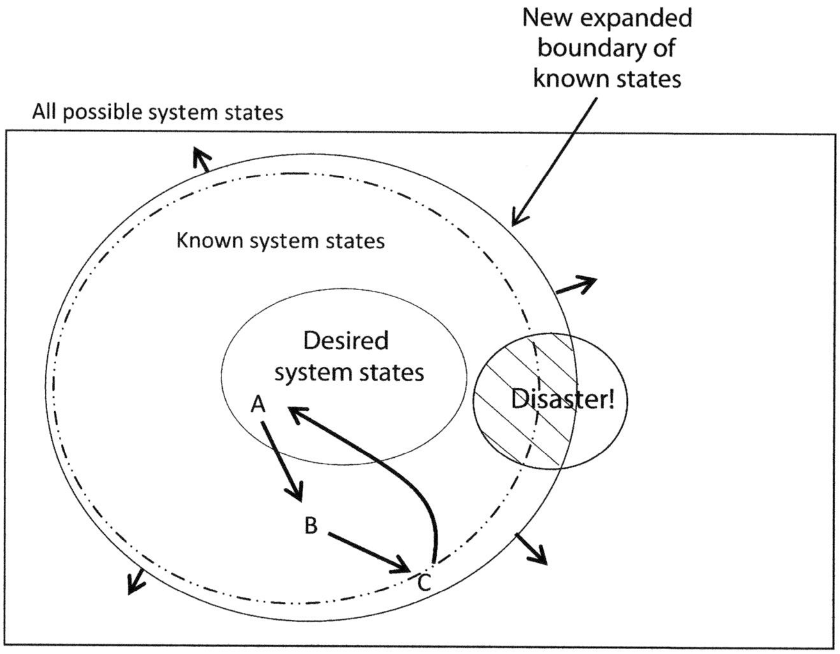

Fig. 30.7 State-space diagram for the successful implementation of a recovery path (C to A) in a generic complex system. Incident reporting has allowed the number of known system states to be increased. This has allowed better procedures to be developed, thus guarding against a larger set of known disaster states—this is reflected in an increased hatched area (compare Fig. 30.6) (Reproduced from Webster CS. The nuclear power industry as an alternative analogy for safety in anaesthesia and a novel approach for the conceptualisation of safety goals. Anaesthesia. 2005;60:1115–1122, with permission from John Wiley and Sons)

Table 30.3 The safety response of the US nuclear industry to the 1979 Three Mile Island accident

1. Extensive revisions of standard procedures taking into account new known failure modes such as open-PORV events
2. An expanded training program for TMI-1 personnel, much of it taking place in an $18 million, full-scale simulator of the plant control room[a]
3. Establishment of a more active incident reporting scheme with a lower threshold for the reporting of incidents, most of which will be precursors to accidents
4. More than 100 safety modifications to twin TMI-1 reactor, costing $95 million[a]
5. Inherently safer reactor designs developed for future construction

[a]US$ amounts not adjusted for inflation

kind of patient harm has typically occurred (Fig. 30.5) [167]. Table 30.4 shows all cases in the database relating to the use of MRI or sedation outside of the operating room in the 10 years from 1995. While these data are unlikely to be representative of the depth or breadth of harm caused during pediatric sedation or the system problems related to it, it is of note that 5 out of 6 of the cases in Table 30.4 involve a ventilation problem, or sequelae thereof, as the damaging event. Many of the known risk factors for sedation in children are also present in these reports, including young age, congenital conditions, comorbidities, and off-label drug use. Case 6 in Table 30.4 involved a severely agitated patient who produced copious secretions but was not suctioned in a timely way, because this task had fallen to the MRI technician—thus reflecting poorly defined roles of responsibility and a lack of effective communication in the sedation team. Case 3 suggests poor saturation monitoring where the last SpO_2 reading was taken several minutes before bradycardia occurred. These reports suggest that better assessment of risk before the procedure begins could prevent sedated patients incurring harm. Furthermore, better monitoring throughout could allow early detection of potential problems and rapid application of recovery pathways before patient harm occurs (Fig. 30.7) [170, 171].

The Value of Best Practice Guidelines in Procedural Sedation

The aforementioned observations based on closed claims cases are supported by a number of empirical findings. An analysis of 118 notifiable adverse drug events relating to pediatric sedation concludes that adverse patient outcome is not determined by the characteristics of the patient but rather a failure to rescue the patient from developing adverse events [168]. A study by Hoffman and colleagues of the value of best practice guidelines during pediatric procedural sedation reaches similar conclusions [170]. The authors developed a program of procedural sedation for nonanesthesiologists modeled on guidelines of the American Academy of Pediatrics (AAP) and the American Society of Anesthesiologists (ASA), including monitoring standards, a guided pre-sedation risk assessment, nil by mouth guidelines, a sedation scoring system, time-based recordings of sedation status, monitored recovery until awake, and assessment of fitness for discharge. Data were collected prospectively from 960 patient records for 3 months, yielding an overall complication rate of 4.2 %. Performance of the pre-sedation risk assessment

Table 30.4 Closed claims cases in the 10 years from 1995 involving MRI or sedation outside the operating room

Case no.	Age	ASA	Procedure	Anesthetic care	Appropriateness of anesthetic care	Contributing factors	Damaging event	Settlement payment (US$)[a]	Severity of injury[b]
1	21 months	2	Upper endoscopy	SpO_2, BP, EKG, 0_2 via nasal cannula, sedation with 60–80 mg propofol	Less than appropriate	Immunoglobulin deficit, congenital heart disease; child became cyanotic after the removal of monitors; code was called; ET tube may have been mispositioned	Inadequate oxygenation/ ventilation	$275,620 against anesthesiologist	9
2	19 months	3–5	MRI	Sedation with propofol TIVA	Appropriate	Tetralogy of Fallot/pulmonary atresia, significant comorbidities, multiple interventional cardiac catheters resulting in seizure post-completion before MRI, off-label propofol use, respiratory obstruction, multiorgan failure	Inadequate oxygenation/ ventilation	$3,119,480	9
3	8 years	2	Esophagogastro-duodendoscopy	SpO_2, sedation with fentanyl, midazolam, propofol	Impossible to judge	Fragile X disease, mental retardation, likely missed respiratory arrest, last SpO_2 reading several minutes before bradycardia, unresponsive to glycopyrrolate/atropine	Cardiac arrest	$7,798,710 ($1,250,000 against anesthesia team)	8
4	13 months	3	MRI	GA with nitrous oxide, sevoflurane and propofol	Less than appropriate	History of sickle cell anemia, laryngospasm and desaturation leading to cardiac arrest, delayed intubation	Airway obstruction	$328,170	9
5	9 months	2–3	MRI	GA	Appropriate	Born 6 weeks premature, seizure disorder, respiratory distress after MRI completed, possible aspiration pneumonia	Poor patient condition	$18,619	4
6	6 months	3	MRI	Sedation with propofol	Less than appropriate	Cardiac murmur, suffered seizures due to meningitis, patient agitation and copious secretions, delayed suction by MRI tech	Respiratory event	$18,633	4

[a]Payment amounts are reported in 2012 inflation adjusted US dollars

[b]Severity of injury: 9 = patient death; 8 = grave permanent injury (severe brain damage, quadriplegia, lifelong care, or fatal prognosis); 4 = major temporary injury (brain damage, nerve damage, unable to work, prolonged hospitalization)

reduced the complication rate by 50 % overall ($p=0.041$), and this reduction was most pronounced in the patients who underwent targeted deep sedation where the complication rate was reduced by 90 % ($p<0.018$).

The Future of Safety in Pediatric Sedation

There are several practical things that any institution should be doing now to improve the safety of pediatric sedation [142, 143] (Table 30.5). Other opportunities to identify points at which the safety of the clinical microsystem of procedural sedation can be improved are likely to involve the adaptation of successful safety initiatives from other areas of health care. It is perhaps surprising that it has taken more than 70 years since their use in aviation for checklists to become popularized in health care [99]. However, the value of checklists to ensure that error-prone or often-forgotten critical steps in clinical procedures are carried out has demonstrated a number of dramatic improvements in health-care processes. Pronovost and colleagues have demonstrated a 66 % reduction in bloodstream infections associated with the use of central venous catheters in a study of 375,757 catheter days—estimating that in the state of Michigan alone such a reduction could save approximately 2,000 lives and US$ 200 million a year in avoided postinfection costs [16, 172]. Haynes and colleagues have shown a 36 % reduction in a host of postoperative complications in a multinational study of 3,733 patients undergoing a wide range of procedures with the use of the WHO Surgical Safety Checklist [17, 173].

Checklists such as these are a kind of cognitive safety net, ensuring that errors or omissions are avoided during the exigencies of clinical care. Adoption of the WHO checklist has been uneven. The routine use of this checklist during sedation of children would be one of the most effective single measures available today at low cost to enhance the safety of these patients. In addition to providing checks, the pre-sedation risk assessment in Hoffman's study of procedural guidelines is essentially a checklist to ensure that risks are not overlooked before medication is given, and it seems likely that such checklist techniques could be applied more widely during pediatric sedation [170]. Their implementation may also involve aspects of system redesign. For example, in Pronovost's work it was found that the best way to ensure compliance with the checklist for central venous catheter insertion was to have a designated trolley for this purpose on which all the materials needed were always available [172]. In the same way, greater standardization of equipment and drugs, and of the way in which these are presented, would enhance safety during the sedation of pediatric patients.

Table 30.5 Some practical suggestions for improvement in the safety of sedation for procedures in children

1. Teamwork: create identified teams and build consensus over approaches to care
2. Standardization: standardize the equipment and medications used within each institution
3. Guidelines: adopt existing best practice guidelines for procedural sedation and develop institution-specific guidelines where gaps exist
4. Training: establish regular simulation-based training sessions for the whole team with a focus on nontechnical skills, particularly communication
5. Checklists: adopt the WHO Surgical Safety Checklist and engage in its effective use
6. Medications: adopt the APSF New Paradigm for medication administration [142]
7. Briefings and debriefings: begin every session with a team briefing to ensure that the day is planned, and the mental models for patient care are shared. End each session with a short debriefing to identify what has gone well and what can be improved

More extensive system redesign has been used in a safety initiative in our own research group where a multimodal approach was taken to reduce drug administration error during anesthesia. This approach involved color coding, bar coding, improved layout, voice prompts, and prefilled syringes. Compared with conventional methods, the use of the redesigned system was associated with a 35 % reduction in drug administration error in an incident monitoring study of 74,478 anesthetic cases and a 21 % reduction in drug recording and administration error in an observational study of 1,075 cases [18, 174]. Other areas where safety research is likely to have relevance to pediatric sedation would include computerized provider (or physician) order entry (CPOE) systems, and during patient handover. CPOE systems involve two primary safety strategies: forcing functions, which typically involve choosing the drugs the patient will receive from predetermined electronic lists, thus eliminating entry errors, and automatic alerts for known contraindications such as allergies and drug interactions. The use of such systems has shown reductions in drug prescription errors of around 50 % in various studies, including in pediatric patient populations [175, 176]. The handover or handoff for a child undergoing or having undergone sedation can be a critical point for the occurrence of error or information loss as this is where the clinical team administering the sedation interfaces with other parts of the wider clinical microsystem in other locations [117]. Clinical microsystem mapping may be particularly useful here to determine whether handoffs are proceeding as they should and the points at which problems are arising [53]. One study at a children's hospital identified four transition points on the patient pathway to and from the operating room and MRI suite and developed formal handover checklists for each transition [177]. In the 12 months after introduction, no errors had occurred on either the surgical or MRI pathways, with each checklist taking less than 10 s to execute on each occasion. The use of simulation is also likely to play an increasingly important role in teaching and assessment of communication skills, in determining compliance with sedation guidelines and safety procedures, and in assessing the potential usefulness of new approaches [178, 179].

New Approaches to Incident Reporting and Safety Monitoring

Although incident reporting is widely used in anesthesia, the threshold for the reporting of events remains at least a magnitude higher than in the nuclear power industry, and at least historically, has been primarily in response to accidents [153, 163]. A high reporting threshold means that accidents and incidents that are reported in anesthesia tend to be from the top of the incident pyramid and therefore offer less information about how to remove predisposing factors to error inherent in the wider system. This difference in reporting thresholds represents one of the obstacles in transitioning health care from a very safe to an ultrasafe industry [180]. It also suggests that considerable scope exists for improvement in the quantity and quality of data on the performance of health-care systems—shortcoming that is of particular concern in higher-risk areas such as pediatric sedation [162, 181]. An additional barrier to the improvement of safety in health care is the relatively poor sharing of information on hazards and their remedies. By contrast, any identified critical system fault in an aircraft or nuclear power plant is shared throughout these industries, so that the fault can be rapidly removed or that procedures to deal with it can be uniformly applied by pilots and operators [70].

Recently, systems that allow the lowering of the reporting threshold have been introduced in anesthesia. A Web-based system that allows the reporting of accidents and accident precursors became available in Australia and New Zealand in October 2010 and has collected almost 2,000 reports to date from 55 participating hospitals [182]. A similar Web-based system was introduced in the United States in 2011 by the Anesthesia Quality Institute [183]. Specializing in procedural sedation, a Web-based adverse event reporting tool developed by the World Society for Intravenous Anesthesia (World SIVA) and the International Sedation Task Force is also now available for the reporting of sedation-related adverse events and accident precursors [184]. (Refer to Chap. 28; Table 28.2.) Importantly the World SIVA tool is based on a standardized set of definitions developed as part of a consensus document drawing on definitions from the Institute of Medicine, World Health Organization, the European Medicines Agency, and the US Food and Drug Administration [185, 186]. Such reporting tools benefit anesthesia in a similar way as reporting systems in other high-technology industries by allowing comparable data to be collected internationally, thus informing policy, clinical guidelines, and safety initiatives. Once hazards have been identified by these systems, warnings can be given to all participants. Thus, such systems can potentially address both the information underreporting and information sharing problems in health care.

Incident reporting provides insights into many risks, and over time, changes in patterns can provide evidence of progress [18, 187]. However, when an effective remedy for a known risk has been developed, there are other more powerful methods for quantifying changes in the safety levels achieved with its use. For example, the strategy of so-called "care bundles" has been introduced by the Institute for Health Improvement [188]. A bundle is a collection of 3–5 relatively independent care interventions with strong clinical agreement (elements of which may include checklists) and used within a defined population of patients. Compliance with the bundle is measured in an all-or-none way and reported regularly, using combined process and outcome indicators. The aim of monitoring safety levels using combined indicators is to remain focused on the goal of improving outcomes while simultaneously tracking key processes that are involved in achieving the outcome. Such an approach reduces the possibility of gaming. Data collection on safety levels achieved with use of the bundle therefore become an embedded part of clinical practice. Areas where care bundles have already shown benefits include central venous line use, hand hygiene, and the prevention of ventilator-associated pneumonia [189–191], but similar effective strategies could be adopted for the improvement and maintenance of safety in pediatric sedation in specific populations of patients or locations.

Conclusion

We may be at the beginning of a new era in evidence-based patient safety. For the first time in decades, relatively simple interventions have been shown to have surprisingly dramatic effects in terms of the reduction of treatment-caused harm in health care. We are beginning to understand how to change the operation of health-care organizations for the better—reducing injury, death, and costs. Given the magnitude of the reductions in harm achieved in specific areas, the Institute of Medicine's goal of a 50 % reduction in error across the board no longer seems excessively ambitious. However, much work remains to be done. We need to better understand why errors happen, both in terms of the psychology of those who make them and the system factors that predispose to them. We need to widen the focus of accident investigation from the individual clinician at the sharp end to include the wider system in which clinical microsystems of many clinicians operate. Combining such a systems perspective with a lowered threshold for the reporting of incidents, so that precursors to accidents are also reported, will allow a better understanding of why things go wrong and will identify points in the care process where risk is raised, and interventions to manage such risk can be adopted. It is also important to ask the how and why questions in this process in order to better understand how to generalize safety initiatives from one health-care domain to another and to avoid wasting resource on approaches that do not work. Many effective approaches to bringing about safety improvements are available, based on similar endeavors in other complex industries, and many of these are already being applied in health care. Successes and failures in the use of these safety initiatives should be shared, so that others can spread the successes and avoid the failures. Risk management needs to involve screening for risk preemptively and adjusting care appropriately, while also anticipating recovery pathways that may be needed and ensuring all resources are available for their use. Finally, approaches that do work need to be institutionalized, as does the data collection needed to monitor their ongoing use. Clinicians take great pride and satisfaction from improving the lives of their patients, and rightly so. What is needed is at least a similar degree of interest in improving the systems that will ensure the safety of the patient who undergoes such care.

Acknowledgements We would like to thank Dr. Karen Domino, Dr. Karen Posner, and the American Society of Anesthesiologists Closed Claims Project for supplying the data in Table 30.4.

Authors Craig S. Webster, Michael Stabile, and Alan F. Merry own shares in Safer Sleep Limited, a company that aims to improve safety in medicine and which manufactures the new system mentioned in references [18] and [174]. Alan F. Merry founded and is a Director of Safer Sleep Limited.

Alan F. Merry chairs the Board of the Health Quality and Safety Commission in New Zealand. He is Head of the School of Medicine in Auckland, which includes the Simulation Centre for Patient Safety (in which some of the research referenced in this chapter was conducted). He was the anesthesia lead for the development of the WHO Surgical Safety Checklist.

The remaining author has no competing interests to declare.

References

1. Cravero JP, Blike GT, Gallagher SM, Hertzog JH, Havidich JE, Gelman B. Incidence and nature of adverse events during pediatric sedation/anesthesia for procedures outside the operating room: report from the pediatric sedation research consortium. Pediatrics. 2006;118:1087–96.
2. Langhan ML, Mallory M, Hertzog JH, Lowrie L, Cravero JP. The Pediatric Sedation Research Consortium. Physiologic monitoring practices during pediatric procedural sedation. Arch Pediatr Adolesc Med. 2012;166:990–8.
3. Institute of Medicine. To err is human—building a safer health system. Washington: National Academy; 2000.
4. Brennan TA, Leape LL, Laird NM, Hebert L, Localio AR, Lawthers AG, et al. Incidence of adverse events and negligence in hospitalized patients. Results of the Harvard Medical Practice Study I. N Engl J Med. 1991;324:370–6.
5. Leape LL, Brennan TA, Laird N, Lawthers AG, Localio AR, Barnes BA, et al. The nature of adverse events in hospitalized patients. Results of the harvard medical practice study II. N Engl J Med. 1991;324(6):377–84.
6. Wilson RM, Runciman WB, Gibberd RW, Harrison BT, Newby L, Hamilton J. The quality in Australian health care study. Med J Aust. 1995;163:458–71.
7. Thomas EJ, Studdert DM, Burstin HR, Orav EJ, Zeena T, Williams EJ, et al. Incidence and types of adverse events and negligent care in Utah and Colorado. Med Care. 2000;38:261–71.
8. Vincent C, Neale G, Woloshynowych M. Adverse events in British hospitals—preliminary retrospective record review. BMJ. 2001;322:517–9.
9. Davis P, Lay-Yee R, Schug S, Briant R, Scott A, Johnson S, et al. Adverse events in New Zealand public hospitals—principal findings from a national survey. Occasional paper 3. Wellington: Ministry of Health; December 2001.
10. Woods D, Thomas E, Holl J, Altman S, Brennan T. Adverse events and preventable adverse events in children. Pediatrics. 2005; 115:155–60.
11. Malviya S, Voepel-Lewis T, Tait AR. Adverse events and risk factors associated with the sedation of children by nonanesthesiologists. Anesth Analg. 1997;85:1207–13.
12. Berwick DM, Hackbarth AD, McCannon CJ. IHI replies to "the 100,000 lives campaign: a scientific and policy review". Jt Comm J Qual Patient Saf. 2006;32:628–33.
13. McCannon CJ, Schall MW, Calkins DR, Nazem AG. Quality improvement—saving 100,000 lives in US hospitals. BMJ. 2006;332:1328–30.
14. McCannon CJ, Hackbarth AD, Griffin FA. Miles to go: an introduction to the 5 million lives campaign. Jt Comm J Qual Patient Saf. 2007;33:477–84.
15. Wachter RM, Pronovost PJ. The 100,000 lives campaign: a scientific and policy review. Jt Comm J Qual Patient Saf. 2006;32: 621–7.
16. Pronovost P, Needham D, Berenholtz S, et al. An intervention to decrease catheter-related bloodstream infections in the ICU. N Engl J Med. 2006;355:2725–32 [erratum appears in N Engl J Med. 2007 Jun 21;356:2660].
17. Haynes AB, Weiser TG, Berry WR, Lipsitz SR, Breizat AS, Dellinger EP, et al. A surgical safety checklist to reduce morbidity and mortality in a global population. N Engl J Med. 2009; 360:491–9.
18. Webster CS, Larsson L, Frampton CM, Weller J, McKenzie A, Cumin D, et al. Clinical assessment of a new anaesthetic drug administration system: a prospective, controlled, longitudinal incident monitoring study. Anaesthesia. 2010;65:490–9.
19. Webster CS. Overcoming complexity and improving the safety of medical systems. Prometheus. 2012;30:320–6.
20. Cook TM, Woodall N, Frerk C. Major complications of airway management in the UK: results of the Fourth National Audit Project of the Royal College of Anaesthetists and the Difficult Airway Society. Part 1: anaesthesia. Br J Anaesth. 2011;106:617–31.
21. Cook TM, Woodall N, Harper J, Benger J. Major complications of airway management in the UK: results of the Fourth National Audit Project of the Royal College of Anaesthetists and the Difficult Airway Society. Part 2: intensive care and emergency departments. Br J Anaesth. 2011;106:632–42.
22. Merry AF, Anderson BJ. Medication errors—new approaches to prevention. Paediatr Anaesth. 2011;21:743–53.
23. Cudny ME, Wang NE, Bardas SL, Nguyen CN. Adverse events associated with procedural sedation in pediatric patients in the emergency department. Hosp Pharm. 2013;48:134–42.
24. Roback MG, Wathen JE, Bajaj L, Bothner JP. Adverse events associated with procedural sedation and analgesia in a pediatric emergency department: a comparison of common parenteral drugs. Acad Emerg Med. 2005;12(6):508–13.
25. Donabedian A. An introduction to quality assurance in health care. New York: Oxford University Press; 2003.

26. Babl FE, Krieser D, Belousouff J, Theophilos T. Evaluation of a paediatric procedural sedation training and credentialing programme: sustainability of change. Emerg Med J. 2010;27:577–81.
27. Linsky A, Simon SR. Medication discrepancies in integrated electronic health records. BMJ Qual Saf. 2013;22(2):103–9.
28. Zhang Y, Dong YJ, Webster CS, Ding XD, Liu XY, Chen WM, et al. The frequency and nature of drug administration error during anaesthesia in a Chinese hospital. Acta Anaesthesiol Scand. 2013;57:158–64.
29. Merry AF, Webster CS, Mathew DJ. A new, safety-oriented, integrated drug administration and automated anesthesia record system. Anesth Analg. 2001;93:385–90.
30. Maclennan AI, Smith AF. An analysis of critical incidents relevant to pediatric anesthesia reported to the UK National Reporting and Learning System, 2006–2008. Paediatr Anaesth. 2011;21(8): 841–7.
31. Llewellyn RL, Gordon PC, Wheatcroft D, Lines D, Reed A, Butt AD, et al. Drug administration error—a prospective survey from three South African teaching hospitals. Anaesth Intensive Care. 2009;37:93–8.
32. Thomas AN, Panchagnula U. Medication-related patient safety incidents in critical care: a review of reports to the UK national patient safety agency. Anaesthesia. 2008;63(7):726–33.
33. Pitetti R, Davis PJ, Redlinger R, White J, Wiener E, Calhoun KH. Effect on hospital-wide sedation practices after implementation of the 2001 JCAHO procedural sedation and analgesia guidelines. Arch Pediatr Adolesc Med. 2006;160(2):211–6.
34. Green SM, Roback MG, Krauss B, Brown L, McGlone RG, Agrawal D, et al. Predictors of airway and respiratory adverse events with ketamine sedation in the emergency department: an individual-patient data meta-analysis of 8,282 children. Ann Emerg Med. 2009;54(2):158–68. e151–4.
35. Barker KN, Allan EL. Research on drug-use-system errors. Am J Health Syst Pharm. 1995;52(4):400–3.
36. Berde C. Convulsions associated with pediatric regional anesthesia. Anesth Analg. 1992;75:164–6.
37. Anderson BJ, Meakin GH. Scaling for size: some implications for paediatric anaesthesia dosing. Paediatr Anaesth. 2002;12(3): 205–19.
38. McFarlan CS, Anderson BJ, Short TG. The use of propofol infusions in paediatric anaesthesia: a practical guide. Paediatr Anaesth. 1999;9:209–16.
39. Rigby-Jones AE, Priston MJ, Sneyd JR, McCabe AP, Davis GI, Tooley MA, et al. Remifentanil-midazolam sedation for paediatric patients receiving mechanical ventilation after cardiac surgery. Br J Anaesth. 2007;99(2):252–61.
40. Kannikeswaran N, Mahajan PV, Sethuraman U, Groebe A, Chen X. Sedation medication received and adverse events related to sedation for brain mri in children with and without developmental disabilities. Paediatr Anaesth. 2009;19(3):250–6.
41. Isik B, Baygin O, Kapci EG, Bodur H. The effects of temperament and behaviour problems on sedation failure in anxious children after midazolam premedication. Eur J Anaesthesiol. 2010;27(4):336–40.
42. Litman RS, Soin K, Salam A. Chloral hydrate sedation in term and preterm infants: an analysis of efficacy and complications. Anesth Analg. 2010;110(3):739–46.
43. Sumpter A, Anderson BJ. Phenobarbital and some anesthesia implications. Paediatr Anaesth. 2011;21(10):995–7.
44. Eker HE, Yalcin Cok O, Aribogan A, Arslan G. Children on phenobarbital monotherapy requires more sedatives during MRI. Paediatr Anaesth. 2011;21:998–1002.
45. Larsson P, Nordlinder A, Bergendahl HT, Lonnqvist PA, Eksborg S, Almenrader N, et al. Oral bioavailability of clonidine in children. Paediatr Anaesth. 2011;21(3):335–40.
46. Koren G, Barzilay Z, Greenwald M. Tenfold errors in administration of drug doses: a neglected iatrogenic disease in pediatrics. Pediatrics. 1986;77(6):848–9.
47. Ma H, Lovich MA, Peterfreund RA. Quantitative analysis of continuous intravenous infusions in pediatric anesthesia: safety implications of dead volume, flow rates, and fluid delivery. Paediatr Anaesth. 2011;21(1):78–86.
48. Zenk KE. Intravenous drug delivery in infants with limited i.v. access and fluid restriction. Am J Hosp Pharm. 1987;44(11):2542–5.
49. Greig A, Ryan J, Glucksman E. How good are doctors at estimating children's weight? J Accid Emerg Med. 1997;14(2):101–3.
50. Harris M, Patterson J, Morse J. Doctors, nurses, and parents are equally poor at estimating pediatric weights. Pediatr Emerg Care. 1999;15(1):17–8.
51. Black K, Barnett P, Wolfe R, Young S. Are methods used to estimate weight in children accurate? Emerg Med (Fremantle). 2002;14(2):160–5.
52. Luscombe MD, Owens BD, Burke D. Weight estimation in paediatrics: a comparison of the APLS formula and the formula 'weight=3(age)+7'. Emerg Med J. 2011;28:590–3.
53. Barach P, Johnson JK. Understanding the complexity of redesigning care around the clinical microsystem. Qual Saf Health Care. 2006;15:i10–6.
54. Marsh DR, Schroeder DG, Dearden KA, Sternin J, Sternin M. The power of positive deviance. BMJ. 2004;329:1177–9.
55. Lingard L, Espin S, Evans C, Hawryluck L. The rules of the game: interprofessional collaboration on the intensive care unit team. Crit Care. 2004;8:R403–8.
56. Lingard L, Regehr G, Orser B, et al. Evaluation of a perioperative checklist and team debriefing among surgeons, nurses, and anesthesiologists to reduce failures in communication. Arch Surg. 2008;143:12–8.
57. Zibrowski EM, Singh SI, Goldszmidt MA, Watling CJ, Kenyon C, Schultz V, et al. The sum of the parts detracts from the intended whole: competencies and in-training assessments. Med Educ. 2009;43:741–8.
58. Reason J. Human error. New York: Cambridge University Press; 1990.
59. Webster CS. Human psychology applies to doctors too. Anaesthesia. 2000;55:929–30.
60. Reason J. The human contribution—unsafe acts, accidents and heroic recoveries. Surrey: Ashgate; 2008.
61. Webster CS. The iatrogenic-harm cost equation and new technology [editorial]. Anaesthesia. 2005;60:843–6.
62. Reason J. Managing the risks of organisational accidents. Aldershot: Ashgate; 1997.
63. Webster CS, Merry AF. British syringe label "standards" are an accident waiting to happen. Anaesthesia. 2000;55:618.
64. Webster CS. Doctors must implement new safety systems, not whinge about them. Anaesthesia. 2002;57:1231–2.
65. Nolan TW. System changes to improve patient safety. BMJ. 2000;320:771–3.
66. Perrow C. Normal accidents—living with high risk technologies. New York: Basic Books; 1984.
67. Seife C. Fingers crossed—NASA's space station plans reveal a remarkable faith in rocket reliability. New Scientist. 1998;158 (2133):4–5.
68. Seife C. ISS titanic. New Scientist. 1998;160(2160):38–41.
69. Chiles JR. Inviting disaster—lessons from the edge of technology. New York: Harper Collins; 2001.
70. Schlager N, editor. When technology fails—significant technological disasters, accidents, and failures of the twentieth century. Detroit: Gale Research; 1994.
71. Anonymous. Bayesian inference. http://en.wikipedia.org/wiki/Bayesian_inference. Accessed 5 June 2013.

72. Ross JF. The polar bear strategy—reflections on risk in modern life. Reading: Perseus Books; 1999.
73. Lomax GP. From breeder reactors to butterflies—risk, culture and biotechnology. Risk Anal. 2000;20:747–53.
74. Starr C. Hypothetical fears and quantitative risk analysis. Risk Anal. 2001;21:803–6.
75. Maurino DE, Reason J, Johnston N, Lee RB. Beyond aviation human factors—safety in high technology systems. Aldershot: Ashgate; 1995.
76. Altman DG, Bland JM. Absence of evidence is not evidence of absence. BMJ. 1995;311:485.
77. Webster CS. Why anaesthetising a patient is more prone to failure than flying a plane. Anaesthesia. 2002;57:819–20.
78. Department of Health. An organisation with a memory—report of an expert group on learning from adverse events in the NHS. London: Stationery Office; 2000.
79. Spath PL, editor. Error reduction in health care—a systems approach to improving patient care. San Francisco: Jossey-Bass; 2000.
80. Saunders DI, Meek T. Almost 30% of anaesthetic machines in UK do not have anti-hypoxia device. BMJ. 2001;323:629.
81. Reason J. The contribution of latent human failures to the breakdown of complex systems. Philos Trans R Soc Lond B Biol Sci. 1990;327:475–84.
82. Reason J, Lucas D. Absent-mindedness in shops—its incidence, correlates and consequences. Br J Clin Psychol. 1984;23:121–31.
83. Dorner D. The logic of failure—recognizing and avoiding error in complex situations. Reading: Addison-Wesley; 1997.
84. Klein G. Sources of power—how people make decisions. Cambridge, MA: MIT; 1999.
85. Merry AF, McCall SA. Errors, medicine and the law. Cambridge: Cambridge University Press; 2001.
86. Runciman B, Merry A, Walton M. Safety and ethics in healthcare—a guide to getting it right. Aldershot: Ashgate; 2007.
87. Dennett DC. Consciousness explained. London: Penguin; 1991.
88. Marshall J. Unforgettable. New Scientist. 2008;197(2643):30–3.
89. Norman D. Things that make us smart—defending human attributes in the age of the machine. Reading: Perseus; 1993.
90. Rasmussen J. Human errors: a taxonomy for describing human malfunction in industrial installations. J Occup Acc. 1982;4: 311–33.
91. Rasmussen J. Skills, rules, and knowledge: signals, signs, and symbols, and other distinctions in human performance models. IEEE Trans Syst Man Cybernet. 1983;13(3):257–66.
92. McCrone J. States of mind. New Scientist. 1999;161(2178):30–3.
93. Croskerry P, Singhal G, Mamede S. Cognitive debiasing 1: origins of bias and theory of debiasing. BMJ Qual Saf. 2013;22 Suppl 2:ii58–64. doi:10.1136/bmjqs-2012-001712.
94. Croskerry P, Singhal G, Mamede S. Cognitive debiasing 2: impediments to and strategies for change. BMJ Qual Saf. 2013;22 Suppl 2:ii65–72. doi:10.1136/bmjqs-2012-001713.
95. Merry AF, Webster CS. Labelling and drug administration error. Anaesthesia. 1996;51:987–8.
96. Salas E, editor. Human-technology interaction in complex systems. Stamford: JAI; 1999.
97. Keers RN, Williams SD, Cooke J, Ashcroft DM. Causes of medication administration errors in hospitals: a systematic review of quantitative and qualitative evidence. Drug Saf. 2013;36:1045–67. doi:10.1007/s40264-40013-40090-40262.
98. Runciman WB, Sellen A, Webb RK, Williamson JA, Currie M, Morgan C, et al. Errors, incidents and accidents in anaesthetic practice. Anaesth Intensive Care. 1993;21:506–19.
99. Gawande A. The checklist manifesto—how to get things right. New York: Metropolitan Books; 2009.
100. Webster CS, Anderson DJ. A practical guide to the implementation of an effective incident reporting scheme to reduce medication error on the hospital ward. Int J Nurs Pract. 2002;8:176–83.
101. Anderson DJ, Webster CS. A systems approach to the reduction of medication error on the hospital ward. J Adv Nurs. 2001;35:34–41.
102. Reason J. Human error—models and management. BMJ. 2000;320:768–70.
103. Krueger GP. Sustained work, fatigue, sleep loss and performance: a review of the issues. Work and Stress. 1989;3:129–41.
104. Samkoff JS, Jacques CHM. A review of studies concerning effects of sleep deprivation and fatigue on residents' performance. Acad Med. 1991;66:687–93.
105. Roth T, Roehrs TA, Carskadon MA, Dement WC. Daytime sleepiness and alertness. In: Kryger MH, Roth T, Dement WC, editors. Principles and practice of sleep medicine. 2nd ed. Philadelphia: WB Saunders; 1994. p. 40–9.
106. Broughton RJ. Chronobiological aspects and models of sleep and napping. In: Dinges DF, Broughton RJ, editors. Sleep and alertness—chronobiological, behavioural and medical aspects of napping. New York: Raven; 1989. p. 71–98.
107. Cheeseman JF, Webster CS, Pawley MDM, Francis MA, Warman GR, Merry AF. Use of a new task-relevant test to assess the effects of shift work and drug labelling formats on anesthesia trainees' drug recognition and confirmation. Can J Anaesth. 2011;58:38–47.
108. Gander PH, Millar M, Webster CS, Merry AF. Sleep loss and performance of anaesthesia trainees and specialists. Chronobiol Int. 2008;25:1077–91.
109. Sturm L, Dawson D, Vaughan R, Hewett P, Hill AG, Graham JC, et al. Effects of fatigue on surgeon performance and surgical outcomes: a systematic review. ANZ J Surg. 2011;81(7–8):502–9 [Research Support, Non-U.S. Gov't Review].
110. Howard SK, Gaba DM, Smith BE, Weinger MB, Herndon C, Keshavacharya S, et al. Simulation study of rested versus sleep-deprived anesthesiologists. Anesthesiology. 2003;98(6):1345–55. discussion 1345A.
111. Biddle C, Aker J. The national study of sleep-related behaviors of nurse anesthetists: personal and professional implications. AANA J. 2011;79(4):324–31.
112. Barger LK, Ayas NT, Cade BE, Cronin JW, Rosner B, Speizer FE, et al. Impact of extended-duration shifts on medical errors, adverse events, and attentional failures. PLoS Med. 2006;3:e487.
113. Howard SK, Rosekind MR, Katz JD, Berry AJ. Fatigue in anesthesia—implications and strategies for patient and provider safety. Anesthesiology. 2002;97:1281–94.
114. Gaba DM, Howard SK. Fatigue among clinicians and the safety of patients. N Engl J Med. 2002;347:1249–55.
115. Landrigan CP, Rothschild JM, Cronin JW, Kaushal R, Burdick E, Katz JT, et al. Effect of reducing interns' work hours on serious medical errors in intensive care units. N Engl J Med. 2004;351:1838–48.
116. Dawson D, Reid K. Fatigue, alcohol and performance impairment. Nature. 1997;388:235.
117. Manser T, Foster S, Flin R, Patey R. Team communication during patient handover from the operating room: more than facts and figures. Hum Factors. 2013;55:138–56.
118. Hannaford N, Mandel C, Crock C, Buckley K, Magrabi F, Ong M, et al. Learning from incident reports in the Australian medical imaging setting: handover and communication errors. Br J Radiol. 2013;86: DOI: 10.1259/bjr.20120336.
119. Veasey S, Rosen R, Barzansky B, Rosen I, Owens J. Sleep loss and fatigue in residency training—a reappraisal. J Am Med Assoc. 2002;288:1116–24.
120. Gander PH, Merry AF, Millar MM, Weller J. Hours of work and fatigue-related error: a survey of New Zealand anaesthetists. Anaesth Intensive Care. 2000;28(2):178–83.
121. Helmreich RL, Merritt AC. Culture at work in aviation and medicine. Aldershot: Ashgate; 2001.
122. de Leval MR. Human factors and surgical outcomes—a cartesian dream. Lancet. 1997;349:723–5.

123. Anonymous. Aviation safety. http://en.wikipedia.org/wiki/Aviation_safety. Accessed 6 June 2013.
124. Hunt P. Safety in aviation. Perfusion. 1988;3:83–96.
125. Gibbs N, (editor). Safety of anaesthesia—a review of anaesthesia-related mortality reporting in Australia and New Zealand 2003–2005. Australian and New Zealand College of Anaesthetists; 2009.
126. Merry AF, Webster CS. Has anesthesia care become safer and is anesthesia-related mortality decreasing? F1000 Med Rep. 2009;1:69. doi:10.3410/M3411-3469.
127. Gaba DM, DeAnda A. A comprehensive anesthesia simulation environment: re-creating the operating room for research and training. Anesthesiology. 1988;69:387–94.
128. Gaba DM, Howard SK, Fish KJ, Smith BE, Sowb YA. Simulation-based training in anesthesia crisis resource management (ACRM): a decade of experience. Simul Gaming. 2001;32:175–93.
129. Cumin D, Boyd MJ, Webster CS, Weller JM. A systematic review of simulation for multidisciplinary team training in operating rooms. Sim Healthcare. 2013;8:171–9.
130. Weller J, Henderson R, Webster CS, Shulruf B, Torrie J, Davies E, et al. Building the evidence on simulation validity: comparison of anesthesiologists' communication patterns in real and simulated cases. Anesthesiology. 2014;120:142–8. doi:10.1097/ALN.1090b1013e3182a1044bc1095.
131. Weller JM, Frengley R, Torrie J, Webster CS, Tomlinson S, Henderson K. Change in attitudes and performance of critical care teams after a multi-disciplinary simulation-based intervention. Int J Med Educ. 2012;3:124–31.
132. Gaba DM. The future vision of simulation in health care. Qual Saf Health Care. 2004;13 Suppl 1:i2–10.
133. Lingard L, Espin S, Whyte S, Regehr G, Baker GR, Reznick R, et al. Communication failures in the operating room: an observational classification of recurrent types and effects. Qual Saf Health Care. 2004;13:330–4.
134. Small SD, Barach P. Patient safety and health policy: a history and review. Hematol Oncol Clin North Am. 2002;16:1463–82.
135. Stratman RC, Wall MH. Implementation of a comprehensive drug safety program in the perioperative setting. Int Anesthesiol Clin. 2013;51:13–30.
136. Roth EM, Christian CK, Gustafson M, Sheridan TB, Dwyer K, Gandhi TK, et al. Using field observations as a tool for discovery: analysing cognitive and collaborative demands in the operating room. Cogn Tech Work. 2004;6:148–57.
137. Christian CK, Gustafson ML, Roth EM, Sheridan TB, Gandhi TK, Dwyer K, et al. A prospective study of patient safety in the operating room. Surgery. 2006;139:159–73.
138. Manser T. Teamwork and patient safety in dynamic domains of healthcare: a review of the literature. Acta Anaesthesiol Scand. 2009;53:143–51.
139. Mishra A, Catchpole K, McCulloch P. The Oxford NOTECHS System: reliability and validity of a tool for measuring teamwork behaviour in the operating theatre. Qual Saf Health Care. 2009;18:104–8.
140. Schmutz J, Manser T. Do team processes really have an effect on clinical performance? A systematic literature review. Br J Anaesth. 2013;110:529–44.
141. Salas E, Sims DE, Burke CS. Is there a "big five" in teamwork? Small Gr Res. 2005;36:555–99.
142. Eichhorn JH. Apsf hosts medication safety conference—consensus group defines challenges and opportunities for improved practice. APSF Newsletter. 2010;25(1):2–8.
143. Australian and New Zealand College of Anaesthetists. Guidelines on sedation and/or analgesia for diagnostic and interventional medical, dental or surgical procedures (PS9). Melbourne: The College; 2010.
144. Catchpole KR, de Leval MR, McEwan A, Pigott N, Elliott MJ, McQuillan A, et al. Patient handover from surgery to intensive care: using formula 1 pit-stop and aviation models to improve safety and quality. Paediatr Anaesth. 2007;17:470–8.
145. Plsek PE, Greenhalgh T. The challenge of complexity in health care. BMJ. 2001;323:625–8.
146. Tenner E. Why things bite back—technology and the revenge of unintended consequences. New York: Vintage Books; 1997.
147. Wiener LR. Digital woes—why we should not depend on software. New York: Addison-Wesley; 1993.
148. Barach P, Small SD. Reporting and preventing medical mishaps—lessons from non-medical near miss reporting systems. BMJ. 2000;320:759–63.
149. Sagan SD. The limits of safety—organizations, accidents, and nuclear weapons. Princeton: Princeton University Press; 1993.
150. Morone JG, Woodhouse EJ. Averting catastrophe—strategies for regulating risky technologies. Los Angeles: University of California Press; 1986.
151. Weick KE. Educational organizations as loosely coupled systems. Admin Sci Quart. 1976;21:1–19.
152. Cook R, Rasmussen J. "Going solid": a model of system dynamics and consequences for patient safety. Qual Saf Health Care. 2005; 14:130–4.
153. Webster CS. The nuclear power industry as an alternative analogy for safety in anaesthesia and a novel approach for the conceptualisation of safety goals. Anaesthesia. 2005;60:1115–22.
154. Heinrich HW. Industrial accident prevention—a scientific approach. 4th ed. New York: McGraw-Hill; 1959.
155. Runciman WB, Webb RK, Lee R, Holland R. System failure—an analysis of 2000 incident reports. Anaesth Intensive Care. 1993;21:684–95.
156. Bates DW. Medication errors—how common are they and what can be done to prevent them. Drug Saf. 1996;15:303–10.
157. Berwick DM. Not again! Preventing errors lies in redesign—not exhortation. BMJ. 2001;322:247–8.
158. Anonymous. The joint commission—sentinel event policy and procedures. http://www.jointcommission.org/Sentinel_Event_Policy_and_Procedures/. Accessed 5 June 2013.
159. Percarpio KB, Watts BV. A cross-sectional study on the relationship between utilization of root cause analysis and patient safety at 139 department of veterans affairs medical centers. Jt Comm J Qual Patient Saf. 2013;39:32–7.
160. Lago P, Bizzarri G, Scalzotto F, Parpaiola A, Amigoni A, Putoto G, et al. Use of FMEA analysis to reduce risk or errors in prescribing and administering drugs in paediatric wards—a quality improvement report. BMJ Open. 2012;2:e001249.
161. Kuo F-Y, Huang W-C, Chiou K-R, Mar G-Y, Cheng C-C, Chung C-C, et al. The effect of failure mode and effect analysis on reducing percutaneous coronary intervention hospital door-to-balloon time and mortality in st segment elevation myocardial infarction. BMJ Qual Saf. 2013;22:626–38.
162. Webster CS, Merry AF, Larsson L, McGrath KA, Weller J. The frequency and nature of drug administration error during anaesthesia. Anaesth Intensive Care. 2001;29:494–500.
163. Belles RJ, Cletcher JW, Copinger DA, Dolan BW, Minarick JW, O'Reilly PD. 1994 accident sequence precursor program results. Nucl Saf. 1996;37:73–83.
164. Perin C. Operating as experimenting—synthesizing engineering and scientific values in nuclear power production. Sci Technol Hum Val. 1998;23:98–128.
165. Cooper JB, Newbower RS, Kitz RJ. An analysis of major errors and equipment failures in anesthesia management—considerations for prevention and detection. Anesthesiology. 1984;60:34–42.
166. Cooper JO, Cullen BF. Observer reliability in detecting surreptitious random occlusions of the monaural esophageal stethoscope. J Clin Monit. 1990;6:271–5.
167. Metzner J, Posner KL, Domino KB. The risk and safety of anesthesia at remote locations: the US closed claims analysis. Curr Opin Anaesthesiol. 2009;22:502–8.

168. Cote CJ, Notterman DA, Karl HW, Weinberg JA, McCloskey C. Adverse sedation events in pediatrics—a critical incident analysis of contributing factors. Pediatrics. 2000;105:805–14.
169. Lee HH, Milgrom P, Starks H, Burke W. Trends in death associated with pediatric dental sedation and general anesthesia. Paediatr Anaesth. 2013;23:741–6.
170. Hoffman GM, Nowakowski R, Troshynski TJ, Berens RJ, Weisman SJ. Risk reduction in pediatric procedural sedation by application of an American Academy of Pediatrics/American Society of Anesthesiologists process model. Pediatrics. 2002; 109:236–43.
171. von Ungern-Sternberg B, Krisztina B, Chambers NA, Rebmann C, Johnson C, Sly PD, et al. Risk assessment for respiratory complications in paediatric anaesthesia: a prospective cohort study. Lancet. 2010;376:773–83.
172. Pronovost P, Vohr E. Safe patients, smart hospitals. London: Hudson Street Press; 2010.
173. Anonymous. World alliance for patient safety. WHO guidelines for safe surgery. Geneva: World Health Organisation; 2008. http://www.who.int/patientsafety/safesurgery.
174. Merry AF, Webster CS, Hannam J, Mitchell SJ, Edwards K, Jardim A, et al. Multimodal system designed to reduce errors in recording and administration of drugs in anaesthesia: a prospective randomised clinical evaluation. BMJ. 2011;343:d5543. doi:10.1136/bmj.d5543.
175. Radley DC, Wasserman MR, Olsho LEW, Shoemaker SJ, Spranca MD, Bradshaw B. Reduction in medication errors in hospitals due to adoption of computerized provider order entry systems. J Am Med Inform Assoc. 2013;20:470–6.
176. Sard BE, Walsh KE, Doros G, Hannon M, Moschetti W, Bauchner H. Retrospective evaluation of a computerized physician order entry adaptation to prevent prescribing errors in a pediatric emergency department. Pediatrics. 2008;122:782–7.
177. Low DK, Reed MA, Geiduschek JM, Martin LD. Striving for a zero-error patient surgical journey through adoption of aviation-style challenge and response flow checklists: a quality improvement project. Paediatr Anaesth. 2013;23:571–8.
178. Tobin CD, Clark CA, McEvoy MD, Reves JG, Schaefer JJ, Wolf BJ, et al. An approach to moderate sedation simulation training. Simul Healthc. 2013;8(2):114–23.
179. Arriaga AF, Bader AM, Wong JM, Lipsitz SR, Berry WR, Ziewacz JE, et al. Simulation-based trial of surgical-crisis checklists. N Engl J Med. 2013;368:246–53.
180. Amalberti R, Auroy Y, Berwick D, Barach P. Five system barriers to achieving ultra safe health care. Ann Intern Med. 2005;142:756–64.
181. Runciman B, Merry A, McCall Smith A. Improving patients' safety by gathering information—anonymous reporting has an important role. BMJ. 2001;323:298.
182. Anonymous. Webairs, anaesthetic incident reporting system, Australasian and New Zealand College of Anaesthetists (ANZCA). http://www.anztadc.net/Demo/IncidentTabbed.aspx. Accessed 7 June 2013.
183. Anonymous. The anesthesia incident reporting system (airs), anesthesia quality institute. http://www.aqihq.org. Accessed 27 Nov 2013.
184. Mason KP, Green SM, Piacevoli Q. Adverse event reporting tool to standardize the reporting and tracking of adverse events during procedural sedation: a consensus document from the World SIVA International Sedation Task Force. Br J Anaesth. 2012;108:13–20.
185. Cravero JP, Havidich JE. Pediatric sedation—evolution and revolution. Paediatr Anaesth. 2011;21:800–9.
186. World Health Organization. WHO draft guidelines for adverse event reporting and learning systems. Geneva: WHO; 2005.
187. Webb RK, Currie M, Morgan CA, Williamson JA, Mackay P, Russell WJ, et al. The Australian incident monitoring study—an analysis of 2000 incident reports. Anaesth Intensive Care. 1993; 21:520–8.
188. Griffin RR, Haraden C, Nolan TW. Using care bundles to improve health care quality. Cambridge, MA: Institute for Healthcare Improvement; 2012. http://www.ihi.org.
189. Anonymous. Health quality and safety commission New Zealand. http://www.hqsc.govt.nz/. Accessed 10 Sep 2013.
190. Robb E, Jarman B, Suntharalingam G, Higgens C, Tennant R, Elcock K. Using care bundles to reduce in-hospital mortality: quantitative survey. BMJ. 2010;340:c1234.
191. Resar R, Pronovost P, Haraden C, Simmonds T, Rainey T, Nolan T. Using a bundle approach to improve ventilator care processes and reduce ventilator-associated pneumonia. Jt Comm J Qual Patient Saf. 2005;31:243–8.

Part IV

Sedation into the Twenty-Second Century

31 Intravenous Infusions for Sedation: Rationale, State of the Art, and Future Trends

Anthony R. Absalom

Abstract

When sedation outside of the operating room is required, possible routes of administration of sedative agents include the inhalational, oral, intranasal, intramuscular, and intravenous routes.

Although administration of low doses of volatile anesthetic agents by inhalation can provide adequate sedation (and analgesia if nitrous oxide is also used), this mode of sedative administration is often not feasible outside the operating room. With oral or enteral, transnasal, rectal, or intramuscular administration, the administered drug forms a depot that is absorbed slowly. Agents administered by the oral or enteral route are then subjected to significant first-pass metabolism. This problem is avoided with intramuscular injection, but this route is seldom used because it is painful. For all these routes, the rate at which the drug reaches the systemic circulation is highly variable, since it also depends on factors such as gastric emptying, peristalsis, local pH, other contents of the gut, cardiac output, and mucosal or muscular blood flow.

The problems of variable absorption and first pass effects are avoided by intravenous administration as the entire administered dose reaches the systemic circulation. There remains considerable inter- and intra-individual variability in the relationship between administered dose and the blood concentration profile achieved (i.e., pharmacokinetics), but this variability is far less than with other routes of administration.

Keywords

Intravenous infusion • Sedation • Pharmacokinetic • Pharmacodynamic • Steady state • Blood concentration • Effect-site concentration • Ketamine • Etomidate • Propofol • Dexmedetomidine • Total intravenous anesthesia (TIVA) • Context-sensitive half-time (CSHT) • Patient-maintained sedation (PMS) • Closed loop • Target controlled infusion (TCI) • Effect site • Sedasys • NONMEM

Introduction

Benefits of the Intravenous Route of Administration

When sedation outside of the operating room is required, possible routes of administration of sedative agents include the inhalational, oral, intranasal, intramuscular, and intravenous routes.

A.R. Absalom, M.B.Ch.B., F.R.C.A., F.H.E.A., M.D. (✉)
Department of Anesthesiology, University Medical Center Groningen, PO Box 30.001, 9700 RB, Groningen, The Netherlands
e-mail: a.r.absalom@umcg.nl

K.P. Mason (ed.), *Pediatric Sedation Outside of the Operating Room: A Multispecialty International Collaboration*, DOI 10.1007/978-1-4939-1390-9_31, © Springer Science+Business Media New York 2015

Although administration of low doses of volatile anesthetic agents by inhalation can provide adequate sedation (and analgesia if nitrous oxide is also used), this mode of sedative administration is often not feasible outside the operating room. The bulky apparatus required to administer the agent, oxygen, and nitrous oxide, and to scavenge waste gases, is a significant limitation. Furthermore, distressed children are unlikely to cooperate sufficiently to tolerate a face mask or a "physiological" mouthpiece, as well as the odor and taste of the agent, throughout the period of administration.

With oral or enteral, transnasal, rectal, or intramuscular administration, the administered drug forms a depot that is absorbed slowly. Agents administered by the oral or enteral route are then subjected to significant first-pass metabolism. This problem is avoided with intramuscular injection, but this route is seldom used because it is painful. For all these routes, the rate at which the drug reaches the systemic circulation is highly variable, since it also depends on factors such as gastric emptying, peristalsis, local pH, other contents of the gut, cardiac output, and mucosal or muscular blood flow. This results in considerable inter- and intra-individual variability in bioavailability when these routes are used. In patients who are in pain, distressed, or unwell, absorption and systemic penetration of orally administered agents may be minimal. Thus, administration of standard doses of sedatives by these routes results in very variable blood concentrations and clinical effects, making it very difficult to judge in advance the required dose.

The problems of variable absorption and first pass effects are avoided by intravenous administration as the entire administered dose reaches the systemic circulation. There remains considerable inter- and intra-individual variability in the relationship between administered dose and the blood concentration profile achieved (i.e., pharmacokinetics), but this variability is far less than with other routes of administration.

For any sedative agent, the blood and effect-site concentrations that will provide adequate sedation will depend on the sensitivity of the patient to the drug (pharmacodynamics), which can change with time and can be profoundly and unpredictably altered by co-administration of analgesics and other drugs. The required concentrations will also depend on the nature and severity of any noxious stimuli. Since the stimuli involved with any intervention change over time, as can the patient's susceptibility to the agent, so too will the effect-site concentration required for optimal sedation.

The inhalational route offers the ability to titrate the dose against the clinical effect, but suffers from the practical disadvantages previously discussed. Of the remaining available routes of administration, only the intravenous route enables fine control of the blood concentration and clinical effects, particularly with newer agents that have "fast" kinetics, such as propofol. When administered as a single bolus, propofol has both a rapid onset and offset of action—the rapid onset is because the drug crosses the blood–brain barrier rapidly, and the rapid offset is because extensive redistribution to well-perfused tissues causes a rapid fall in blood concentrations and thus a decline in effect-site concentrations. With repeated boluses or an infusion, there is extensive redistribution of the drug into different tissues, but overall the drug does not "accumulate" significantly, in the sense that when administration ceases, blood concentrations fall fairly rapidly because hepatic metabolism is rapid compared with the rate of return of drug from the peripheral tissues.

If sedation with propofol is inadequate, then blood and effect-site concentrations can be rapidly increased by the administration of one or more boluses, or an infusion. If on the other hand sedation is excessive, then cessation of further drug administration should result in a rapid decline in blood concentrations and clinical effect. The ability to make rapid and fine adjustments to the depth of sedation is probably the major advantage of intravenous administration.

With almost all intravenously administered anesthetic drugs fixed-rate infusions result in blood concentrations that increase significantly over time. One exception is remifentanil, which reaches steady-state blood concentrations after about 15 min of infusion at a fixed rate. The problem of increasing blood concentrations at constant infusion rates can be a trap for the unwary, since the relationship between infusion rate and clinical effect will change over time. A patient that is initially safe and adequately sedated, may later become excessively sedated, with potentially life-threatening compromise of the airway and respiratory drive, despite there being no increase in the infusion rate. Steady-state blood concentration profiles are made possible by target-controlled infusion (TCI) systems, which facilitate titration of the blood concentration to the clinical effect, and will be discussed in detail later in this chapter.

Naturally, a disadvantage of intravenous administration is that intravenous access is required. Many children find this distressing, particularly if venous access is difficult because of obesity or obliteration of the veins caused by prior administration of irritant drugs. The pain and discomfort of intravenous cannulation can be limited by prior application of a topical local anesthetic formulation, by distraction by a parent or play therapist, by the use of small gauge cannulae, and of course by rapid completion of the procedure by an experienced and skilled physician.

Choice of Agents

Pharmacokinetic and pharmacodynamic factors influence our choice of agents. Pharmacokinetics describe the relationship between drug dose and blood concentration, whereas pharmacodynamics is the study of the clinical effects themselves and of the relationship between blood concentration and clinical effect.

Ideally, a drug used for sedation should have a rapid onset of action and also a rapid offset of action. This requires an agent with a combination of favorable pharmacokinetic properties and pharmacodynamic properties, such as rapidly reached steady-state blood concentrations during infusion, a rapid rate of blood–effect-site equilibration, lack of accumulation, a rapid decline in blood concentrations on stopping the infusion [and ideally a context-insensitive half-time (CSHT)]. By definition then, agents that are able to provide rapid, titratable and controllable sedation must usually be administered by continuous infusion. Fentanyl is a good illustrative example. After a single dose, or a short duration infusion, fentanyl has rapid kinetics. Once repeated doses or an infusion lasting more than an hour have been given, the kinetics become slower and the CSHT increases significantly, making it unsuitable for use by infusion outside of the operating room (OR) or intensive care unit (ICU). Other intravenous agents that accumulate significantly and are not suitable for use by infusion or multiple bolus administration outside of the ICU are morphine, midazolam, and thiopentone. Perhaps the most promising drug, particularly with regard to pharmacokinetics and dynamics, is remimazolam, which is metabolized by nonspecific tissue esterases, and has a fast onset and offset of effect [1, 2]. This drug is currently undergoing further phase II and III evaluation.

Of the currently available drugs, those with suitable pharmacokinetics for use by infusion include ketamine, etomidate, propofol, and dexmedetomidine. Unfortunately, although ketamine has many suitable characteristics, such as maintained cardiorespiratory stability, bronchodilation, and potent analgesia, it can cause problematic psychiatric phenomena. In subsedative doses in adults it has been shown to cause several of the negative symptoms of schizophrenia [3, 4].

At sedative and anesthetic doses, troublesome emergence phenomena are common, particularly when ketamine is used as the sole agent. These phenomena are less severe in children and can be attenuated by concomitant benzodiazepine administration. Etomidate commonly causes pain on injection and nausea and vomiting, and when used by infusion it is associated with significant adrenal suppression [5]. Indeed, in unwell adults, even single doses were shown to interfere with adrenal function for 24 h [6].

Another suitable agent is methohexitone, but unfortunately it is no longer widely available. Thus, the only remaining agents that are suitable for use by infusion are propofol and dexmedetomidine.

Pharmacodynamics of Propofol and Dexmedetomidine

Propofol

The introduction into clinical practice of the intravenous hypnotic agent propofol has led to a significant increase in the popularity of the technique of total intravenous anesthesia (TIVA) in most of the world. TIVA is the exclusive use of the intravenous route for induction and maintenance of anesthesia. Strictly speaking, a technique involving intravenous infusions supplemented by nitrous oxide, for example, is not a TIVA technique. Exclusive use of the intravenous route for sedation is a natural extension of TIVA, since propofol and most other intravenous hypnotic agents produce anxiolysis and sedation at lower doses.

Part of the reason for the popularity of propofol is the favorable pharmacokinetic profile (see above and later discussion) and the availability of infusion equipment to simplify and facilitate accurate and precise administration such as "calculator" infusion pumps and TCI systems. "Calculator" infusion pumps are simpler systems that can be programmed with the patient's weight so that the user can input a dose in mass-based units such as a bolus dose size in μ(mu)g/kg or an infusion rate in μ(mu)g/kg/min. Another reason for the increase in popularity of TIVA is propofol's beneficial pharmacodynamic profile. At subsedative doses, propofol induces anxiolysis and amnesia [7, 8].

For procedures and environments that are frightening to children, these effects are highly desirable. In addition to anxiolysis it produces a sense of well-being and is associated with a very low incidence of nausea and vomiting [9, 10]. In fact, propofol has been shown to possess direct antiemetic properties at subhypnotic doses [11]. This is particularly beneficial in painful procedures requiring supplementary use of opioid analgesics that are likely to induce nausea and vomiting. With increasing doses, propofol produces dose-dependent sedation, with a gradual, stepwise loss of higher cognitive functions. For example, although functional imaging studies suggest that neurophysiological responses associated with processing of complex sentences are lost at very light levels of sedation [8], basic auditory perception of words continues for some time after loss of responses to command [12]. Propofol does, of course, possess some undesirable pharmacodynamic effects. These include pain on initial intravenous injection and dose-related cardiorespiratory depression. Pain on injection can be attenuated by many methods and virtually eliminated by using a new propofol formulation containing medium chain triglycerides with added lidocaine [13].

The problems of respiratory and cardiovascular depression are dose dependent, but can be somewhat unpredictable, particularly in unwell patients. Propofol causes modest reductions in myocardial contractility and more marked effects on systemic vascular resistance. At lower doses there is a reduction in respiratory rate and tidal volume, obtunded airway reflexes, and obtunded responses to hypercarbia and hypoxemia. An anesthetic induction dose commonly causes a brief period of apnea. Moreover, when other agents are co-administered marked synergism can occur, particularly with the opioids. Modest doses of propofol and remifentanil have been shown to increase the apnea threshold and markedly obtund the ventilatory response to hypercarbia [14]. These adverse cardiorespiratory effects of propofol are part of the reason why, in some quarters, it is felt that sedation with propofol should only be administered by anesthesiologists [15, 16].

The ASA guidelines on safe sedation practices are not quite as proscriptive in the use of propofol by nonanesthesiologists, and rather only state that "practitioners administering propofol should be qualified to rescue patients from any level of sedation, including general anesthesia" [17].

Dexmedetomidine

Dexmedetomidine is an effective sedative agent, producing a state of sedation that is unique among intravenous agents because the patient remains rousable even from relatively deep sedation. This difference is probably related to the fact that most other intravenous sedatives exert their clinical effects via a different mechanism (an agonist effect on $GABA_A$ receptors on inhibitory neurons in the thalamus and other areas), whereas dexmedetomidine acts as a highly selective α(alpha)2 adrenergic agonist (i.e., having minimal effects on the α[alpha]1 receptor subtype), which results in enhanced activity in non-Rapid Eye Movement (NREM) sleep-promoting pathways [18].

An agonist effect on α(alpha)2 receptors results in inhibition of the locus coeruleus, which is thought to disinhibit the ventrolateral preoptic (VLPO) nucleus, causing increased GABA release from VLPO neurons resulting in decreased activity in the tubo-mamillary nucleus (TMN). Natural NREM sleep is also associated with increased firing of VLPO neurons. Since the TBM is the only neuronal source of histamine, which causes arousal, this action on the TBM results in reduced histamine release and sleep or sedation.

In addition to the benefit of rousability, the promotion of natural sleep may bring other benefits such as the restorative functions of sleep. Disturbances of natural sleep are known to cause cognitive and mood changes, and to have adverse effects on immunity. In addition, recent work suggests that dexmedetomidine may modulate the inflammatory response in critically ill patients and in septic animals [19, 20].

Finally dexmedetomidine (and other α[alpha]2 adrenergic receptor agonists) have several other beneficial effects. These include analgesia and an opioid sparing effect when used during painful procedures, and slowing of the heart rate and protection against myocardial ischemia (shown in adults). In high doses dexmedetomidine can cause vasoconstriction, but in lower doses it causes mild vasodilation and only minor effects on the blood pressure. Respiratory drive is well maintained. In adult intensive care patients, sedation with dexmedetomidine is associated with less delirium than other agents [21].

These pharmacodynamic benefits, coupled with a pharmacokinetic profile that makes it suitable for use by infusion, have led to increased use of dexmedetomidine for sedation. When used as the sole agent for sedation for computed tomography (CT) and magnetic resonance imaging (MRI) studies, dexmedetomidine has been shown to produce reliable and effective sedation with acceptable hemodynamic stability and no adverse effects on respiratory parameters [22–25].

Basic Principles of Pharmacokinetics

What is a Pharmacokinetic Model and How is it Derived?

A pharmacokinetic model is a mathematical model that can be used to predict the blood concentration profile of a drug after a bolus dose or an infusion of varying duration. Some types of models, such as recirculatory models, approximate human physiology by estimating blood volume, cardiac output, and blood flow to different organs or groups of organs [26–30].

The most commonly used models are the so-called mamillary, compartmental models, as illustrated in Fig. 31.1. In order to understand these models, some understanding of the mathematics of exponential processes is necessary (see below). It is important to remember that compartmental models are mathematical constructs. They are typically derived by measuring the arterial or venous plasma concentration of a drug after a bolus or infusion in a group of patients or volunteers, and then estimating the pharmacokinetic parameters of the drug under investigation by performing nonlinear mixed effects modeling with software such as NONMEM® (Globomax LLC, Hanover, MD, USA). During this process, the investigators typically begin with a simple model and then make stepwise increases in the complexity of the model. Increases in complexity that do not significantly improve the ability of the model to predict measured blood concentrations are rejected in favor of the simpler model.

Important Mathematical Concepts for Understanding of Pharmacokinetic Models

Many physiological processes depend on concentration gradients and so display first-order kinetics (Fig. 31.1). For most anesthetic agents, the enzymes involved in metabolism are not saturable at clinical concentrations, and thus the amount of drug metabolized during any unit of time depends on the plasma drug concentration at that time.

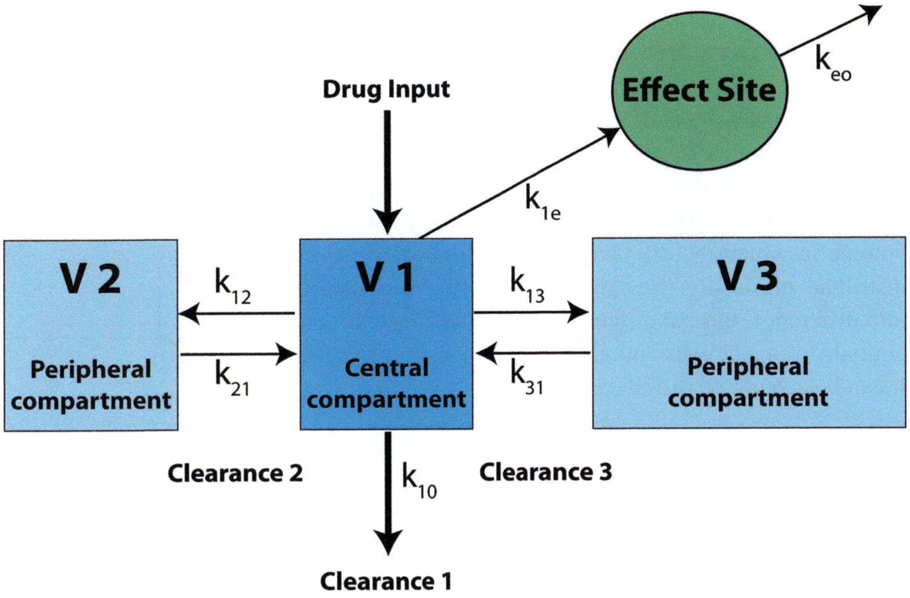

Fig. 31.1 The three-compartment pharmacokinetic model enlarged with an effect compartment. (Adapted from [94])

Similarly, redistribution of most anesthetic drugs is a passive process in which the rate and direction of redistribution depend on the concentration gradient between the blood and other tissues.

For any first-order process, the variable of interest changes in an exponential manner. Depending on the process, the variable may either increase or decrease exponentially. When the variable of interest is an amount (e.g., the mass of drug or the number of millimoles of drug) then the changes in this variable over time can be described mathematically in the following general way (the formula applies equally well to other exponential process such as population growth or the arterial blood pressure changes during diastole):

$$A(t) = A(0) \times e^{k.t}$$

where $A(0)$ is the amount at time zero, t is the time since the start of the process, $A(t)$ is the amount at time t, k is the rate constant (with units of the inverse of time—typically $\min^{-1}$), and e is an irrational constant approximately equal to 2.7182. The rate constant k describes the proportional change over a unit of time. If $k = 1$, then $A(t)$ increases by a multiple of e^1 in each unit of time, i.e., $A(t)$ increases by 271.8 % in each unit of time. On the other hand if $k = -1$, then $A(t)$ changes by a factor of e^{-1} ($= 1/e = 0.367$) in each unit of time, which means that $A(t)$ decreases by 63.3 % in each unit of time.

The rate of change of $A(t)$ at time t can be calculated mathematically as the first differential of $A(t)$ as follows:

$$\frac{dA(t)}{dt} = k \times A(0) \times e^{k.t} = k \times A(t)$$

Thus although the proportional change is constant, the absolute change over a unit of time changes according to the amount, $A(t)$, present during that unit of time.

In pharmacology we are often more interested in concentrations than amounts, and we are commonly dealing with situations where gradients decline over time. For these situations the following general equation will apply:

$$C(t) = C(0) \times e^{-k.t}$$

where $C(0)$ is the concentration at time zero, t is the time since the start of the process (e.g., the time since drug administration), $C(t)$ is the concentration at time t, and k is the rate constant.

Half-Life, Time Constant, and Rate Constant

The time constant, τ(tau), is another rate descriptor, but with units of time. Mathematically it is the inverse of the rate constant (i.e., $1/k$) and represents the time taken for a change by a factor of e (i.e., an increase of 271 % or a decrease of 63 %).

Rate and time constants are not intuitively easy to understand, and thus the pharmacology literature often uses half-lives to describe the time course of exponential processes. Simply put, the half-life describes the time it takes for a change by a factor of 2, i.e., for the amount to change to double or half the initial value. By definition the half-life is shorter than the time constant. Mathematically the half-life can be calculated as follows:

$$t\frac{1}{2} = \tau(\text{tau}) \times \ln 2 = \tau(\text{tau}) \times 0.693 = \frac{1}{k} \times 0.693$$

Volume of Distribution

If serial measurements of the concentration of a drug can be performed, then it is possible, with knowledge of the time course of drug administration, and appropriate mathematical techniques, to calculate a volume of distribution (an apparent volume in which the drug has been distributed). Few drugs distribute uniformly throughout the body. Most distribute into different tissues at different rates. In these situations, an "initial volume of distribution" (V1 or Vc) is often described. It can be calculated as follows:

$$\mathrm{Vd} = \frac{\mathrm{Dose}}{C(0)}$$

Since drugs do not mix instantaneously on injection, $C(0)$ is calculated by extrapolating the time–concentration curve back to time zero. If the volume of distribution, Vd, is larger than the circulating blood volume, then the drug is likely to have rapidly mixed in the blood and extracellular fluids.

The volume of distribution at steady state, Vdss, is the apparent volume of distribution once adequate time has been allowed for complete equilibration of the drug across all tissues. In multicompartmental models, Vdss is the mathematical sum of the volumes of all compartments in the model. For drugs with extensive protein binding and/or high lipid solubility, the peripheral tissues will have a large capacity to absorb the drug, resulting in a Vdss greater than the volume of the entire body.

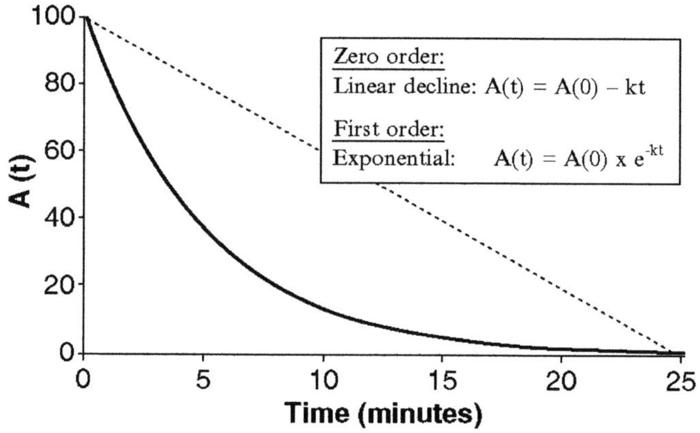

Fig. 31.2 Exponential versus linear decay. The (*dotted*) *straight line* represents linear decay, in which the amount of drug at time t is a linear function of the initial amount. The curve (*solid*) illustrates exponential decay in which the amount of drug at time t is an exponential function of the initial amount

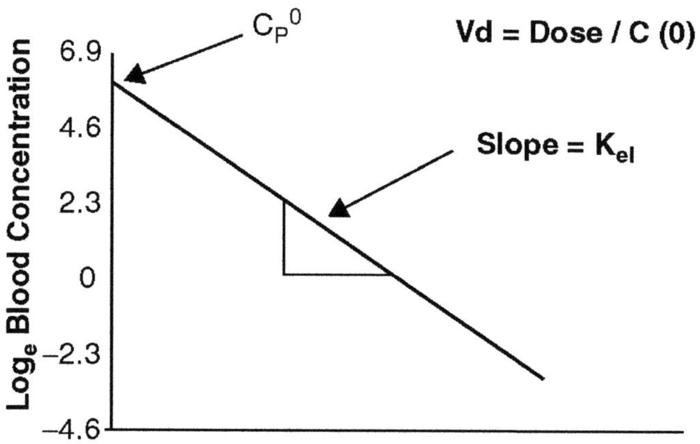

Fig. 31.3 The relationship between log e drug concentration and time after a bolus of a drug with single compartment kinetics. The slope of the elimination curve is constant

Single Compartment Pharmacokinetic Models

The behavior of a drug that does not undergo redistribution can be described by a single compartment mathematical model. On injection, the drug distributes uniformly throughout a single volume, V, and the drug concentration in this compartment is the same as the plasma concentration. After a single bolus or an infusion, the drug concentration will decline because of metabolism or elimination, as described by the following equation:

$$C_{\mathrm{p}}(t) = C_{\mathrm{p}}(0) \times \mathrm{e}^{-kel.t}$$

where $C_{\mathrm{p}}(t)$ is the plasma concentration at time t, $C_{\mathrm{p}}(0)$ is the initial plasma concentration, k_{el} is the elimination rate constant, and $t = 0$ is the time of the bolus or the time at which the infusion ceased. Clearance (mL/h) can be calculated from k_{el} as follows:

$$\text{Clearance, Cl} = k_{\mathrm{el}} \times \mathrm{V},$$

If the relationship between drug concentration and time is plotted on linear axes then the exponential decline results in a curved graph (Fig. 31.2). If however, a semilogarithmic graph is used (i.e., the logarithm of the concentration is plotted) a straight line will result. Figure 31.3 shows the relationship between $\log_e C_{\mathrm{p}}(t)$ and time.

As shown the elimination rate constant can be calculated from the slope of the line in Fig. 31.3. If the natural logarithm ($\log_e$ or "ln") of the drug concentration is plotted against time, then the slope is simply equal to k_{el}. As there is only one rate constant influencing the rate of decline in drug concentration, the decline in plasma concentrations has a constant $t_{1/2}$ that can be calculated from k_{el} as shown previously.

Three Compartment Models

The pharmacokinetics of most anesthetic drugs are best described by three compartment models. Each model describes the number of compartments, and their volumes, the rate of drug metabolism or elimination, and the rate of transfer of drug between the different compartments. The concept is summarized in Fig. 31.1.

By convention, the compartment into which the drug is injected is called the central compartment (V1 or Vc), which may be thought of as including the blood volume, although it can be larger than the blood volume. It is sometimes referred to as the initial volume of distribution. Elimination of active drug by metabolism usually occurs from within this compartment (as in the case of hepatic or renal metabolism). The rate of elimination is described interchangeably by a rate constant (k_{10}) or a clearance (Clearance $= k_{10} \times \text{V1}$). The second compartment, V2, is referred to as the "rapid redistribution" compartment since drug concentrations in V2 equilibrate rapidly with those in the central compartment. The rate constants k_{12} and k_{21} are used to describe the rate of drug transfer from V1 to V2 and from V2 to V1, respectively. Fast redistribution clearance, "Clearance 2," can be calculated as:

$$\text{Clearance 2} = k_{12} \times \text{V1} = k_{21} \times \text{V2}$$

The third compartment, V3, is often referred to as the "slow" compartment (because there is rather slower drug distribution between V1 and V3). Here the rate constants k_{13} and k_{31} are used to describe the rate of drug transfer from V1 to V3 and from V3 to V1, respectively. Slow redistribution clearance, "Clearance 3," can be calculated as:

$$\text{Clearance 3} = k_{12} \times \text{V1} = k_{21} \times \text{V2}$$

The second and third compartments are sometimes referred to as the "vessel rich" and "vessel poor" compartments, respectively, but these terms are best avoided since they encourage the false impression that these compartments represent distinct anatomical or physiological entities. The sum of V1, V2, and V3 gives the "volume of distribution at steady state," Vd_{ss}.

The site of action of the anesthetic agents is, of course, not in the vascular system, but in the brain at a vaguely defined "effect site." Thus, many models now also include the effect site as a fourth compartment, with the rate constant k_{eo} being used to describe the rate of equilibration between the central and effect-site compartments.

For a drug showing three compartment kinetics (such as propofol), the change in concentrations after a bolus or infusion cannot be described by a single rate constant or half-life. The decline in plasma concentration is more complex because it is influenced by several simultaneous exponential processes, each with a different rate constant, so that the time required for the concentration to fall by 50 % (or any other proportion) changes over time. Figure 31.4 shows a typical curve of the relationship between blood concentration and time after a single bolus dose of an anesthetic drug. The time course of changes in plasma concentration shown

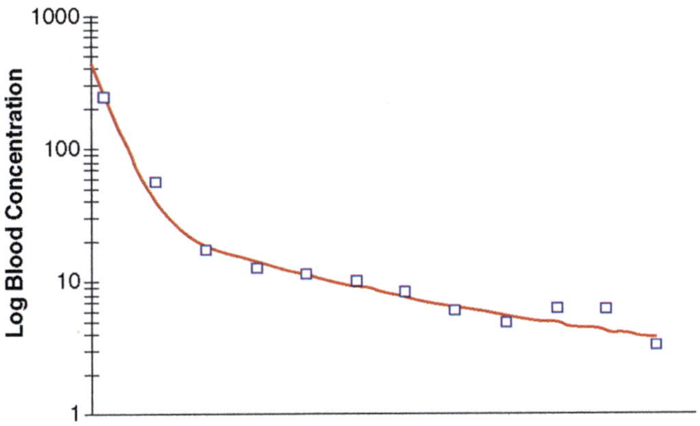

Fig. 31.4 Relationship between plasma concentration (after a bolus dose) and time for a typical anesthetic agent, displaying tricompartment kinetics. The *squares* represent typical measured concentrations and the *red line* represents a curve generated the sum of three exponentials

in Fig. 31.4 can be described mathematically as the sum of three exponential processes as follows:

$$C_p(t) = A.e^{-\alpha(\text{alpha})t} + B.e^{-\beta(\text{beta})t} + C.e^{-\gamma(\text{gamma})t}$$

where A, B, C, α(alpha), β(beta), and γ(gamma) are constants. As can be seen in Fig. 31.4, in the early phase after a bolus dose, the plasma concentration falls rapidly, being mostly influenced by rapid redistribution (described by a rate constant α[alpha]). Later on the rate of decline in plasma concentrations is influenced mostly by redistribution to less well-perfused tissues (described by a rate constant β[1]). Eventually the predominant factor is elimination (rate constant γ[gamma]). From these parameters the time-honored redistribution and elimination half-lives can be calculated.

During and after administration of repeated bolus doses or infusions, the changes in drug concentrations vary in a complex matter since they are influenced by several simultaneous exponential processes, and the relative contributions of the different processes change for most anesthetic drugs as the duration of infusion increases. These factors make it difficult to predict drug concentrations without the assistance of computer programs.

Context-Sensitive Half-Time

The concept of "context-sensitive half-time" (CSHT) has been introduced as a simple metric that provides a summary of the interplay of time and the different half-lives after an infusion [31].

It describes the time taken for blood concentration of a drug to fall by 50 % after the end of an infusion of a specified duration—the context is thus the duration of infusion. The influence of duration of infusion on CSHT indicates the degree of drug accumulation and the balance between redistribution and metabolism/elimination. This metric only describes the time taken for the first decline of 50 %—the time taken for subsequent 50 % falls will be different. Also, it does not necessarily describe when clinical effects will cease, since these depend on the initial concentration, and pharmacodynamic factors such as the sensitivity of the patient to the drug. Nonetheless, it gives the physician a useful indicator of the rate at which drug concentrations will decline after an infusion and an indication of the influence of duration of infusion.

Pharmacokinetic Models for Propofol

During the early 1990s a study of the predictive accuracy of the "Marsh" adult propofol model in 20 children showed that it significantly overestimated the blood concentrations (i.e., measured blood concentrations were less than expected) [32]. This was consistent with other work showing that the pharmacokinetics of propofol differ between children and adults [33, 34].

The Marsh model was then revised to produce a model specific to children (the size of the central compartment volume was increased, but remained a linear function of body weight), and when prospectively tested, the predictive performance was improved compared with the adult model [32].

Since then several other models specific to children have been produced. Schüttler published a complex model in 2000 based on a combined analysis of data from several other studies [35]. This model, which contains multiple covariates, and adjusts for mode of drug administration (bolus versus infusion) and sampling site (arterial versus venous), was designed for use in a wide range of patients including children. The Short model, on the other hand, was designed specifically for the pediatric population [36], but like the Schüttler model it is seldom used in clinical practice.

The Kataria and Paedfusor models (Table 31.1) are the most commonly used models at present and are available in commercially available TCI systems available in most countries of the world (but not the USA). Despite the fact that the models were developed in different ways, and that weight is incorporated in a different way in each model, the overall model parameters are fairly similar. Figure 31.5 shows a comparison of the cumulative propofol dose for children weighing 14 and 20 kg when the Kataria and Paedfusor

Table 31.1 Kataria and Paedfusor pediatric propofol models

	Paedfusor [38, 93]		Kataria [37] Weight proportional		Kataria [38] Weight proportional, age adjusted	
	Model	20 kg patient	Model	20 kg patient	Model	5 years, 20 kg patient
V1	0.458 L/kg	9.2 L	0.52 L/kg	10.4 L	0.41 L/kg	8.2 L
V2	1.34 L/kg	26.8 L	1.0 L/kg	20 L	0.78 L/kg + (3.1 × age)–16	15.1 L
V3	8.20 L/kg	163.9 L	8.2 L/kg	164 L	6.9 L/kg	138 L
K_{10} (min^{-1})	70 × Weight$^{-0.3}$/458.4	0.062	0.066	0.066	0.0854	0.0854
K_{12} (min^{-1})	0.12	0.12	0.113	0.113	0.1878	0.1878
K_{13} (min^{-1})	0.034	0.034	0.051	0.051	0.0634	0.0634
K_{21} (min^{-1})	0.041	0.041	0.059	0.059	0.077 × weight/V2	0.1020
K_{31} (min^{-1})	0.0019	0.0019	0.0032	0.0032	0.0038	0.0038

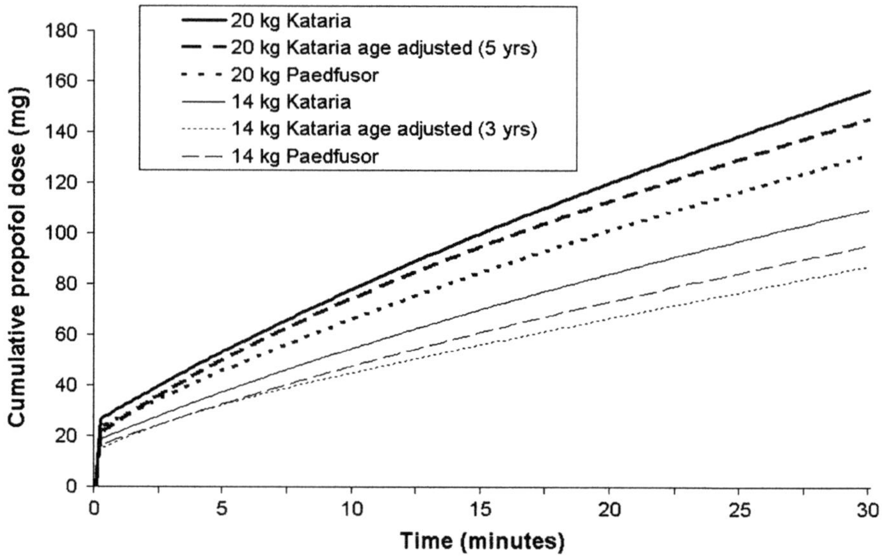

Fig. 31.5 Cumulative propofol doses administered to children weighing either 12 or 20 kg, by TCI systems programmed with the Kataria or Paedfusor pharmacokinetic models for propofol (target concentration 2.5 μ[mu]g/mL)

models are used to administer a target blood concentration of 2.5 μ(mu)g/mL.

Kataria et al. used three different pharmacokinetic modeling techniques in an extended group of children between 3 and 11 years and found that the pharmacokinetics of propofol could be described by a three compartment model [37]. They found that a weight-proportional model performed significantly better than a model with fixed volumes and rate constants. Adjusting V2 (and hence k_{12} and k_{21}) according to age produced a further (modest) improvement. Although Kataria recommended that the weight proportional model be used, some investigators have used the weight proportional model with age adjustment. The equation used to adjust V2 for age is likely to yield an anomalous (negative) V2 for children younger than 3 years, and thus the age-adjusted, weight-proportional model should not be used in children younger than 3 years.

The Paedfusor model [38] was adapted from one of the preliminary models developed by Schüttler prior to the publication of his final model [35] and was incorporated in a pediatric TCI pump developed and used in Glasgow. In the Paedfusor model the central compartment volume and clearance have a nonlinear correlation with weight, whereas in the final Schüttler model all variables have a nonlinear correlation with age and weight.

A recent study investigated the predictive performance of eight existing pediatric propofol models in children between 3 and 26 months of age [39]. Most models performed acceptably, but interestingly the Short model was found to perform best.

With increasing size, pharmacokinetic parameters change in a complex nonlinear way, and the scaling techniques used in the models described earlier do not deal optimally with size-related changes in very young and small children. It is increasingly being recognized that allometric scaling best describes the relationships between clearances and size [40]. Recent work in Groningen, using allometric scaling for size, and a maturation function (to deal with changes in organ and enzyme function in the early months after month), has produced a single pharmacokinetic model for propofol that appears to accurately predict propofol concentrations from 6 months through to old age [41].

Pediatric Propofol Infusion Regimens

Disadvantages of Repeated Bolus Dose Administration

Although it is possible to maintain sedation or anesthesia with repeated boluses of an intravenous sedative agent, this is far from ideal. Firstly, stable levels of sedation are not possible since the blood and effect-site concentrations will be constantly either rising or falling. If the bolus size is too big, the patient state will oscillate from excessive sedation/anesthesia, with the attendant risks, to inadequate sedation. Secondly, it is difficult to judge the dose required to produce adequate, but not excessive blood concentrations. Finally, it is also difficult to judge the required interval between doses. Figure 31.6 shows the estimated blood concentrations arising from repeated 40 mg boluses of propofol administered to a 20 kg child. In these simulations, a bolus was administered each time the estimated concentration fell to 2 μ(mu)g/mL. As can be seen, as drug accumulates in peripheral tissues, the rate of decline in blood concentration after successive doses gradually decreases, resulting in an increase in the interval between doses.

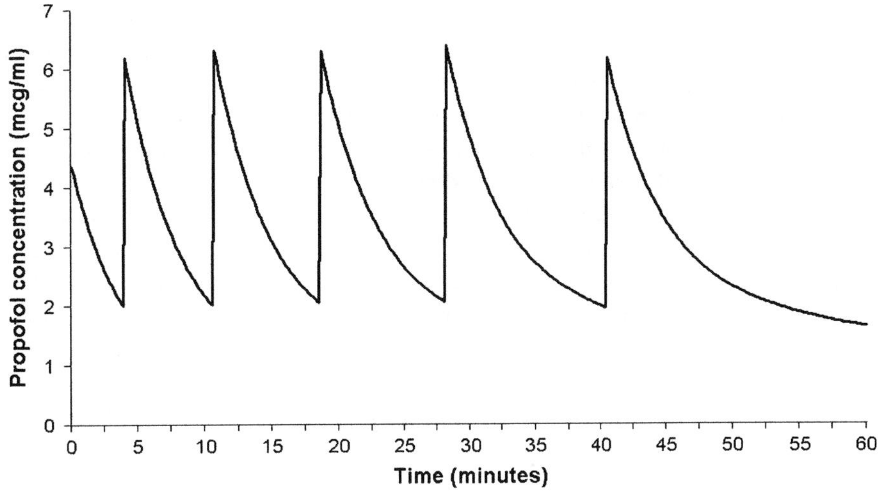

Fig. 31.6 Estimated blood propofol concentrations resulting from repeated 40 mg boluses of propofol in a 20 kg child. In this simulation, a repeat bolus was administered each time the estimated concentration fell to 2 μ(mu)g/mL. Note how the rate of decline in concentration after successive doses gradually decreases; resulting in an increase in the interval between doses

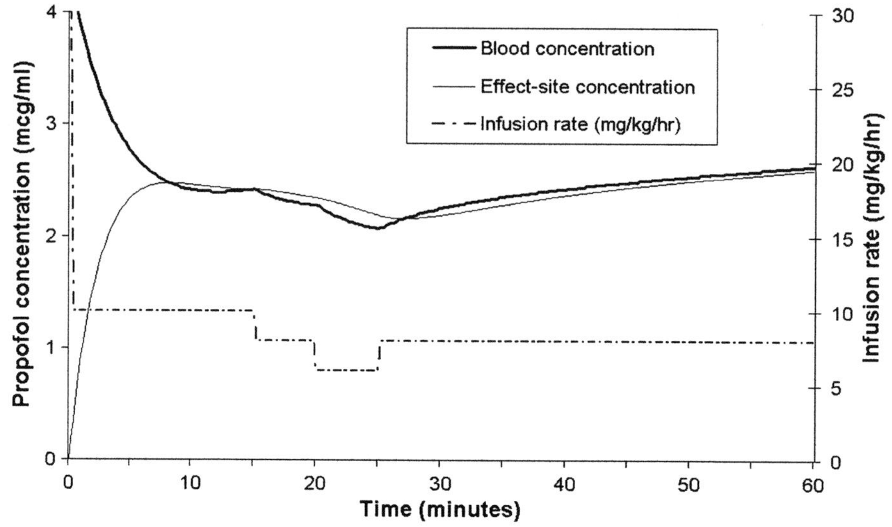

Fig. 31.7 Blood and effect-site concentrations (*heavy* and *light continuous lines*, respectively, as estimated by the Paedfusor model with a k_{eo} of 0.91 min^{-1}), arising from an initial bolus of 2 mg/kg, followed by an infusion initially at 10 mg/kg/h. Note the slow blood and effect-site concentration changes after step changes in infusion rate at 15, 20, and 25 min. Also, note that the concentrations continue to rise when the infusion rate is kept constant

Commonly Used Regimens

Typically, blood concentrations of the order of 2–3 μ(mu)g/mL are required for sedation in children. Naturally the concentration required is influenced by multiple other factors such as co-administered drugs. Thus, it is not surprising that after cardiac surgery, Murray et al. found that the mean measured propofol concentration at recovery of consciousness was only 0.97 μ(mu)g/mL [42], whereas Rigouzzo et al. found that the EC50 (of measured blood propofol concentration at steady state) associated with loss of consciousness in healthy children was 4.0 μg/mL [43].

A commonly used deep sedation regimen for is an initial bolus of 2 mg/kg followed by an infusion at 10 mg/kg/h (in children <1 year of age, higher doses may be required, e.g., an initial bolus of 3 mg/kg and higher initial infusion rates). Figure 31.7 shows a simulation of the regimen, with the concentrations estimated by the Paedfusor model. At about 10 min after the initial bolus the blood concentrations reach a nadir of ~2.5 μ(mu)g/mL. If the infusion rate is kept constant at 10 mg/kg/h, the blood and effect-site concentrations, and clinical effect will gradually increase (reaching ~5 μ[mu]g/mL after several hours), which is why downward titration of the infusion rate is commonly required.

In a recent study, Koroglu and colleagues administered a 3 mg/kg bolus followed by infusions of 10–15 μ(mu)g/kg/min (i.e., 6–9 mg/kg/h) of propofol to 30 children between 1 and 7 years of age for sedation during MRI scans [22]. With this propofol regimen, sedation was adequate in 27 of the 30 children, cardiorespiratory stability was reasonable, and mean recovery and discharge times were 18 and 27 min, respectively.

PK Models for Dexmedetomidine

Pharmacokinetic models for dexmedetomidine in children have recently been produced from studies involving single bolus administration [44], after short infusions [45], and after longer infusions [46] for postoperative sedation. Further studies are needed to compare the predictive accuracy of these models to determine which perform optimally in clinically relevant situations.

Infusion Regimens for Dexmedetomidine

Despite the low α(alpha)1 affinity of dexmedetomidine, rapidly administered boluses cause bradycardia and hypertension. Typical infusion regimens thus usually comprise an initial bolus over 10 min, followed by a continuous infusion. Mason used an initial bolus of 2 μ(mu)g/kg over 10 min (repeated if Ramsay sedation score [47] of 4 not reached) followed by an infusion at 1 μ(mu)g/kg/min, in 62 patients with mean age 2.8 years and mean weight 15 kg, undergoing CT imaging [23]. Of these patients, 10 % were able to undergo their scan during the initial loading dose, 16 % required a second loading dose, and 90 % required the maintenance infusion. Two patients became agitated during the loading dose and were given alternative agents for sedation.

Subsequently, Mason reported the results of a study of the use of higher doses of dexmedetomidine in >700 patients undergoing MRI scanning, which is more stimulating, and in which movement causes significant image degradation [24]. With time their regimen evolved from an initial bolus of 2–3 μ(mu)g/kg and from an initial infusion rate of 1 μ(mu)g/kg/h to 1.5 and 2 μ(mu)g/kg/h. The highest doses were associated with successful sedation and image acquisition in 97.6 % of patients, but with reasonable cardiorespiratory safety.

Koroglu and colleagues used smaller doses for sedation during MRI scanning in 30 children with a mean age of 4 and mean weight of 14 kg; the bolus dose was 1.0 μ(mu)g/kg over 10 min, and this was followed by an infusion at 0.5 μ(mu)g/kg/h initially, but increased to 0.7 μ(mu)g/kg/h if a Ramsay score of 5 was not reached within 25 min [22, 24]. With this regimen, additional midazolam was required in 16 % of patients to facilitate successful scan completion.

Target Controlled Infusions

Definition

A TCI is an infusion of a drug administered by an infusion pump controlled by a computer or microprocessor that is programmed to calculate and implement the drug infusion rates required to achieve in a patient the blood or effect-site concentrations required by the user. Simply put, with these systems, the user inputs a desired "target" concentration, and the system uses the parameters of a pharmacokinetic model for that drug and the patient parameters included as covariates in the pharmacokinetic model to calculate the infusion rates estimated to be necessary to achieve that concentration.

Rationale for TCI

As previously explained, bolus doses of intravenous drugs for sedation are generally only suitable for short procedures. Although infusions do provide more stable conditions, they still do not provide stable blood concentrations. Even for propofol, a drug with rapid kinetics, blood concentrations continue rising for several hours when fixed rate infusions are used (see Fig. 31.7). There is thus a poor correlation between infusion rate and clinical effect. During the course of any procedure, the effect-site concentration required for adequate sedation will vary widely according to several other factors such as the influence of co-administered drugs (especially opioid analgesics), the onset of natural sleep, changes in the environment, and the severity of any noxious stimuli. The changing relationship between infusion rate and effect-site concentration, and the delay in blood–effect-site concentration equilibration, makes rational, precise, and rapid titration of the infusion very difficult. As can be seen in Fig. 31.7, stepwise changes in the infusion rate of 2 mg/kg/h result in very slow changes in blood and effect-site concentrations, so that it is difficult to assess the response to an infusion rate adjustment. These difficulties form an important part of the rationale for TCIs, where a computer or microprocessor is used to implement the infusion rates required to maintain steady-state blood concentrations. Since steady-state blood concentrations arise quite quickly, TCI systems allow the user to judge the clinical effect of a blood concentration and to then adjust the target blood concentration accordingly, rather than adjusting the infusion rate accordingly. An analogy is to compare the control a car driver has over the speed of his car, when he has a speedometer and cruise control system versus the control he would have with only a gas pedal and no cruise control system or speedometer.

When k_{eo} values for children have been validated and effect-site targeting is sufficiently developed for use in children, then a further refinement will be added since users will then be able to titrate the effect-site concentration titrate according to observed patient responses.

With blood and effect-site concentration targeting, absolute accuracy of the pharmacokinetic model is not important, since steady-state concentrations arise very quickly, and there remains wide variability in pharmacodynamic sensitivity among different patients to given blood and effect-site concentrations. Thus, even with the most accurate models and systems, titration according to pharmacodynamic responses will be required.

Principles of TCI

With TCI the user is able to set and alter a desired "target" drug concentration. The target is usually a blood concentration (although algorithms do exist for effect-site targeting [48] and have been implemented for propofol, remifentanil, and sufentanil use in adults). TCI systems use compartmental pharmacokinetic models with complex mathematical algorithms to calculate and implement the infusion rates required to achieve the target concentration. The system software calculates the drug amount in each of the compartments every 10 s, taking into account the amount of drug infused over the previous 10 s, the movement of drug into and out of the central compartment by redistribution, and the rate of removal of active drug from the central compartment by metabolism or elimination. It then calculates and implements the infusion rate required to maintain the target concentration over the subsequent 10 s.

The theoretical foundations for a system designed to maintain and achieve steady-state blood concentrations were laid by Kruger-Thiemer in 1968 [49] and later developed and refined by Vaughan and Tucker [50, 51] and Schwilden [52] (who developed the first clinical application of this theory: the "computer-assisted total intravenous anesthesia system"). The schemes developed by these pioneers for drugs conforming to two-compartment models became known as BET (**B**olus, **E**limination, **T**ransfer) schemes, so-called because they comprised an initial bolus to fill the central compartment (size in mg = target concentration × V1), followed by two superimposed infusions: one to replace drug lost by elimination and one to replace drug lost by redistribution. Modern TCI systems continue to use methods based on this approach, except that most modern models comprise of three compartments. After the initial bolus, three superimposed infusions are computed. When the target concentration is constant, drug lost by elimination is replaced by a constant rate infusion, since a fixed proportion of the total

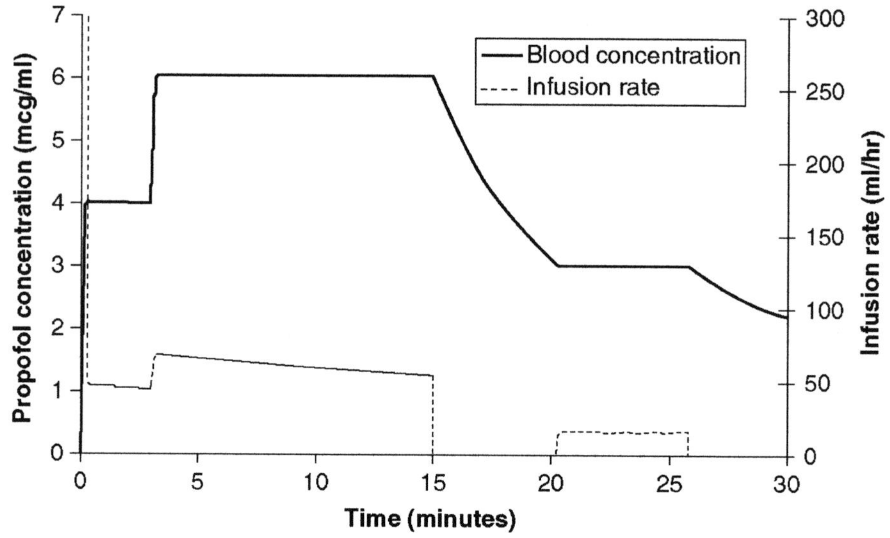

Fig. 31.8 Blood concentration targeted TCI, showing the infusion rates required by the Paedfusor model for a child weighing 20 kg. At time zero the target is set at 4 μ(mu)/mL, at 3 min it is increased to 6 μ(mu)g/mL, and at 15 min the target is reduced to 3 μ(mu)g/mL

amount of drug in the central compartment is eliminated in each unit of time. In contrast, the amount of drug distributed to peripheral tissues declines exponentially as the gradient between the central compartment and the peripheral compartments decreases. Thus, two infusions at exponentially declining rates are required to replace drug "lost" from the central compartment by fast and slow redistribution. The sum of these three infusions is an infusion at a decreasing rate.

When the user decreases the target concentration, the infusion system stops infusing drug until it calculates that the blood concentration has decreased to the target concentration, whereupon the infusion restarts (see Fig. 31.8).

The first commercially available TCI systems contained the Diprifusor®, a microprocessor that was embedded in intravenous infusion pumps sold by several manufacturers from 1996 onwards (in numerous countries around the world, but not in the USA). The development of the Diprifusor® has been described in detail [53, 54]. TCI pumps controlled by it could only administer TCIs of propofol, and only if the microprocessor was able to detect the presence of single-use prefilled glass syringes of 1 % or 2 % propofol purchased from AstraZeneca. These syringes contain a programmable metallic strip in the flange that is detected by a sophisticated process called programmed magnetic resonance.

In the years since the release of the first generation of TCI systems, the patent for propofol has expired and significantly cheaper generic forms of propofol are now available. This has led to the development and launch of second-generation TCI systems, the so-called Open TCI systems. In addition to the use of generic propofol, these systems also can be used for TCI of a variety of drugs, from a variety of syringe types and sizes. Two commonly used commercially available systems are the Alaris Asena PK® (Alaris Medical Systems, Basingstoke, UK) and the Base Primea (Fresenius, Brezins, France).

Choice of Propofol Target Concentration

In general, blood concentrations between 2 and 3 μ(mu)g/mL are required for sedation in children. However, there are no hard and fast rules, and it is important to remember that use of a TCI system does not remove the requirement for titration of the target concentration according to the clinical response, since there is very broad intra- and inter-individual pharmacodynamic variability. Unfortunately there is very little data at present on the target concentrations required during sedation. There have been some studies of the concentrations required for loss of consciousness and so, for safe sedation, it is worth bearing these in mind. Hammer and colleagues investigated the TCI propofol requirements for preventing a movement or hemodynamic response to esophagogastroduodenoscopy in 12 children between 3 and 11 years of age [55]. The EC50 (i.e., the propofol concentration estimated by the age-adjusted Kataria model at which 50 % of patients did not respond) in this group was 3.55 μ(mu)g/mL when calculated using Dixon's up–down method [55] and 3.7 μ(mu)g/mL when recalculated using logistic regression [56]. In 45 children between 6 and 13 years of age, Rigouzzo found that the mean target propofol concentration (Kataria age-adjusted model) associated with a BIS (Bispectral Index) of 50 (i.e., surgical anesthesia) was 3.0 μ(mu)g/mL, and the mean measured propofol concentration associated with BIS 50 was 4.3 μ(mu)g/mL [43].

Predictive Performance of PK Models During TCI

Most studies of the validity and accuracy of models used for TCI have used the parameters recommended by Varvel for assessing the predictive performance of a model during

TCI: bias, imprecision, wobble, and divergence [57]. Generally, bias <20 % and imprecision <40 % are considered acceptable [58, 59]. Although not yet common in clinical practice, there is a growing body of experience of TCI administration of propofol in children. Some studies have studied predictive performance of TCI systems during anesthesia in children. Absalom and colleagues assessed the predictive performance of the Paedfusor model in 29 children aged between 1 and 15 years who were undergoing cardiac surgery or cardiac catheterization [38]. Predictive performance was well within the acceptable range. Bias was 4.1 % indicating that on average the measured blood concentrations were 4 % higher than predicted; while the imprecision was 9.7 %, indicating that 50 % of measured blood concentration samples were in the range from 90.3 to 109.7 % of the target concentration [38]. Engelhardt and colleagues used a simple manual infusion regimen designed to manually target three different propofol concentrations in children, and then assessed the ability of the Kataria model to predict the measured concentrations [60]. In this study the bias was 6.98 % and the imprecision 17.3 %. Rigouzzo and colleagues used the age-adjusted Kataria model for TCI administration of propofol at target concentrations varying between 2 and 6 μ(mu)g/mL [43]. They did not perform a formal analysis of predictive performance, but reported that the Kataria model generally underestimated measured concentrations; mean measured concentrations at target concentrations of 2, 3, and 6 μ(mu)g/mL were 2.4, 4.7, and 12.2 μ(mu)g/mL, respectively [43].

There are, as yet, no studies of the predictive performance of PK models for dexmedetomidine in children and no studies specifically investigating the predictive performance of pharmacokinetic models for propofol in children undergoing sedation.

Future Directions

Model Development and the Open TCI Initiative[1]

TCI systems are in common use for propofol sedation and anesthesia in adult patients in more than 100 countries. A factor that is limiting the use of this technology in the pediatric population is the paucity of published data verifying the validity and accuracy of the current pediatric models in different settings and patient groups. One of the goals of the recently established "Open TCI Initiative" is to set up multicenter collaborations to investigate model performance at the extremes of age. It is hoped that more extensive validation, and possibly the availability of a "universal" model [41], will lead to increased use of TCI technology for sedation and anesthesia in children.

[1] http://www.opentci.org/doku.php. Accessed 6 Dec 2008.

Drug Interactions

Studies in adults over the past 20 years have made advances in our understanding of interactions between different classes of anesthetic agents. These interactions include pharmacokinetic interactions, in which the presence of one drug causes measured concentrations of another drug to be different from those expected, and pharmacodynamic interactions, in which the presence of one drug alters the clinical effects of another drug. It is clear that in adults, pharmacokinetic interactions are common among anesthetic agents, and usually result in higher than expected concentrations, and that pharmacodynamic interactions between hypnotics and opioids result in potent synergism for the sedative, anesthetic, respiratory, and cardiovascular effects of the hypnotic agents [8–16, 61–66]. Newer monitors, which incorporate real-time information about the strength of pharmacodynamic interactions in adults, have been developed [67, 68].

Drover studied the pharmacodynamic interaction of propofol and modest doses of remifentanil in children undergoing endoscopy and found that remifentanil reduced the target propofol concentration (Kataria age-adjusted model) required for tolerance of endoscopy from 3.7 to 2.8 μ(mu)g/mL [56].

At present there is very little other published data concerning the magnitude and significance of anesthetic drug interactions in children. An understanding of this subject is important since it enables anesthesiologists to practice more safely, and sometimes to use these interactions for the benefit of patients. It is thus likely that much more work will be done on this subject, and that infusion and monitoring systems for children will display advisory messages based on real-time estimates of the interactions between co-administered agents.

Effect-Site Targeted TCI Systems

So far we have focused on blood-targeted TCI systems, which attempt to achieve the target blood concentration set by the user, while the effect-site concentration follows passively with a time delay determined by the rate of blood–effect-site equilibration. When a suitable k_{eo} exists for a given drug, pharmacokinetic model, and population group, then it can be used in conjunction with the pharmacokinetic parameters to "target" the effect site instead of the blood concentration. Because the anesthetic drugs have their mechanism of action in the brain rather than the blood, effect-site targeting is intuitively more appealing than blood concentration targeting and offers the potential for more rapid and precise control of the depth of sedation or anesthesia.

TCI systems operating in effect-site targeting mode manipulate the blood concentration to bring about the target (effect-site) concentration as rapidly as possible, by implementing an overshoot in blood concentration when the user increases the target effect-site concentration, and a blood concentration undershoot when the user decreases the target effect-site concentration. For effect-site targeting, the choice of k_{eo} value is critical, since it will determine the degree of overshoot or undershoot required. If the k_{eo} is too small for the patient and model, then excessively large under- and over-shoots will occur, and these may compromise patient safety. Effect-site targeting has been implemented in commercially available TCI systems programmed with pharmacokinetic models suitable for use with propofol and remifentanil in adults. Unfortunately, there are differences in the way that effect-site targeting is implemented in the different pumps, resulting in significantly different infusion profiles for the same model in some patient groups [69].

It is hoped that the Open TCI initiative will be able to also resolve this controversy.

Although the commercially available TCI devices generally are also programmed with one or more pediatric propofol models, effect-site targeting has not been implemented for children. This is largely because there is currently no validated and generally accepted k_{eo} value for use with the pediatric propofol models. Munoz and colleagues recently used the time to peak effect methodology recommended by Minto [70] to calculate k_{eo} values for use with the Paedfusor and Kataria models. Further studies are likely to be necessary to demonstrate the safety and benefit of effect-site targeting in children before this technique is widely used in pediatric practice.

Patient-Maintained Sedation

A patient-maintained sedation (PMS) system is a TCI system in which the patient is able to alter (increase) the target (blood or effect-site) concentration by pressing a button on a handset. Safety is enhanced by having a preset lockout period during which further target increases are not allowed, and by having automatic decreases in target concentration if the handset is not operated within preset time limits [70–75]. These systems thus combine the benefits of TCIs (stable blood and effect-site concentrations) with the psychological and safety benefits of patient control.

The Food and Drug Administration (FDA) in the United States has recently approved the Sedasys sedation system (Johnson & Johnson, Ethicon, NJ, USA) for adults over age 18 years. Approved in May 2013, the system monitors pulse oximetry, noninvasive blood pressure, electrocardiogram, capnography, and patient responses. It analyzes and integrates the data in order to regulate the delivery of intravenous propofol via a TCI-like infusion (i.e., aiming for stable concentrations). The system has a safety algorithm that uses patient responses and physiological data to regulate the delivery of propofol (it stops propofol delivery if the data indicates impending respiratory depression). This unique and novel approach thus merges the benefits of TCI technology with traditional monitoring principles. In comparing the safety of Sedasys to that of the manual administration of propofol, the Sedasys was found to be superior in its ability to maintain oxygen saturation, achieve and maintain minimal to moderate sedation, decrease recovery time, decrease the incidence of adverse events, and provide sedation with higher patient and clinician satisfaction [76].

Although not intended to be utilized on high-risk patients [77], the Sedasys shows promise and has even prompted some to wonder whether "robotic" delivery of anesthesia may someday replace human controlled delivery [78]. These systems have shown great promise in adult groups, but have not yet been investigated in children. It is highly likely that PMS systems suitable for use by children will be developed once issues regarding PK model validity have been addressed and safety of PMS has been demonstrated.

Closed Loop Control

Automated control systems are almost omnipresent in modern life and are accepted without question. They control household appliances, fly airplanes, and control the flow of road and train traffic. Computer systems capable of automatic control of anesthesia and sedation have been developed and tested in adults [79–86].

More recently, Liu and colleagues have developed a system capable of dual control of propofol and remifentanil infusions and tested its performance in many hundreds of patients [87, 88]. Their system has been shown to improve the stability and control of anesthesia and to reduce anesthesiologist workload [89]. In a study in sedated adult intensive care patients, the system achieved more accurate control of sedation, while reducing propofol requirements by half and decreasing vasopressor requirements [90]. In another study among adults undergoing rigid bronchoscopy, system performance was equivalent (but not superior) to manually controlled TCI infusions [91].

Since the problems of dose titration for sedation and anesthesia apply to children as well as to adults, it is likely that this technology will one day be used to improve the accuracy of drug administration for sedation in children. Indeed, preliminary work on closed loop systems for children is already underway [92].

References

1. Antonik LJ, Goldwater DR, Kilpatrick GJ, Tilbrook GS, Borkett KM. A placebo- and midazolam-controlled phase I single ascending-dose study evaluating the safety, pharmacokinetics, and pharmacodynamics of remimazolam (CNS 7056): part I. Safety, efficacy, and basic pharmacokinetics. Anesth Analg. 2012; 115(2):274–83.
2. Wiltshire HR, Kilpatrick GJ, Tilbrook GS, Borkett KM. A placebo- and midazolam-controlled phase I single ascending-dose study evaluating the safety, pharmacokinetics, and pharmacodynamics of remimazolam (CNS 7056): part II. Population pharmacokinetic and pharmacodynamic modeling and simulation. Anesth Analg. 2012;115(2):284–96.
3. Morgan HL, Turner DC, Corlett PR, Absalom AR, Adapa R, Arana FS, Pigott J, Gardner J, Everitt J, Haggard P, Fletcher PC. Exploring the impact of ketamine on the experience of illusory body ownership. Biol Psychiatry. 2011;69(1):35–41.
4. Corlett PR, Cambridge V, Gardner JM, Piggot JS, Turner DC, Everitt JC, Arana FS, Morgan HL, Milton AL, Lee JL, Aitken MR, Dickinson A, Everitt BJ, Absalom AR, Adapa R, Subramanian N, Taylor JR, Krystal JH, Fletcher PC. Ketamine effects on memory reconsolidation favor a learning model of delusions. PLoS One. 2013;8(6):e65088.
5. Ledingham IM, Watt I. Influence of sedation on mortality in critically ill multiple trauma patients. Lancet. 1983;1(8336):1270.
6. Absalom A, Pledger D, Kong A. Adrenocortical function in critically ill patients 24 h after a single dose of etomidate. Anaesthesia. 1999;54(9):861–7.
7. Leslie K, Sessler DI, Schroeder M, Walters K. Propofol blood concentration and the bispectral index predict suppression of learning during propofol/epidural anesthesia in volunteers. Anesth Analg. 1995;81(6):1269–74.
8. Davis MH, Coleman MR, Absalom AR, Rodd JM, Johnsrude IS, Matta BF, Owen AM, Menon DK. Dissociating speech perception and comprehension at reduced levels of awareness. Proc Natl Acad Sci U S A. 2007;104(41):16032–7.
9. Tang J, Chen L, White PF, Watcha MF, Wender RH, Naruse R, Kariger R, Sloninsky A. Recovery profile, costs, and patient satisfaction with propofol and sevoflurane for fast-track office-based anesthesia. Anesthesiology. 1999;91(1):253–61.
10. Raeder J, Gupta A, Pedersen FM. Recovery characteristics of sevoflurane- or propofol-based anaesthesia for day-care surgery. Acta Anaesthesiol Scand. 1997;41(8):988–94.
11. Borgeat A, Wilder-Smith OH, Saiah M, Rifat K. Subhypnotic doses of propofol possess direct antiemetic properties. Anesth Analg. 1992;74(4):539–41.
12. Heinke W, Fiebach CJ, Schwarzbauer C, Meyer M, Olthoff D, Alter K. Sequential effects of propofol on functional brain activation induced by auditory language processing: an event-related functional magnetic resonance imaging study. Br J Anaesth. 2004; 92(5):641–50.
13. Rochette A, Hocquet AF, Dadure C, Boufroukh D, Raux O, Lubrano JF, Bringuier S, Capdevila X. Avoiding propofol injection pain in children: a prospective, randomized, double-blinded, placebo-controlled study. Br J Anaesth. 2008;101(3):390–4.
14. Nieuwenhuijs DJ, Olofsen E, Romberg RR, Sarton E, Ward D, Engbers F, Vuyk J, Mooren R, Teppema LJ, Dahan A. Response surface modeling of remifentanil-propofol interaction on cardiorespiratory control and bispectral index. Anesthesiology. 2003; 98(2):312–22.
15. Perel A. Non-anaesthesiologists should not be allowed to administer propofol for procedural sedation: a Consensus Statement of 21 European National Societies of Anaesthesia. Eur J Anaesthesiol. 2011;28(8):580–4.
16. Network SIGN. Safe sedation of children undergoing diagnostic and therapeutic procedures. Edinburgh: SIGN; 2006.
17. American Society of Anesthesiologists Task Force on Sedation and Analgesia by Non-Anesthesiologists. Practice guidelines for sedation and analgesia by non-anesthesiologists. Anesthesiology. 2002;96(4):1004–17.
18. Nelson LE, Lu J, Guo T, Saper CB, Franks NP, Maze M. The alpha2-adrenoceptor agonist dexmedetomidine converges on an endogenous sleep-promoting pathway to exert its sedative effects. Anesthesiology. 2003;98(2):428–36.
19. Memis D, Hekimoglu S, Vatan I, Yandim T, Yuksel M, Sut N. Effects of midazolam and dexmedetomidine on inflammatory responses and gastric intramucosal pH to sepsis, in critically ill patients. Br J Anaesth. 2007;98(4):550–2.
20. Taniguchi T, Kurita A, Kobayashi K, Yamamoto K, Inaba H. Dose- and time-related effects of dexmedetomidine on mortality and inflammatory responses to endotoxin-induced shock in rats. J Anesth. 2008;22(3):221–8.
21. Riker RR, Shehabi Y, Bokesch PM, Ceraso D, Wisemandle W, Koura F, Whitten P, Margolis BD, Byrne DW, Ely EW, Rocha MG. Dexmedetomidine vs midazolam for sedation of critically ill patients: a randomized trial. JAMA. 2009;301(5):489–99.
22. Koroglu A, Teksan H, Sagir O, Yucel A, Toprak HI, Ersoy OM. A comparison of the sedative, hemodynamic, and respiratory effects of dexmedetomidine and propofol in children undergoing magnetic resonance imaging. Anesth Analg. 2006;103(1):63–7.
23. Mason KP, Zgleszewski SE, Dearden JL, Dumont RS, Pirich MA, Stark CD, D'Angelo P, Macpherson S, Fontaine PJ, Connor L, Zurakowski D. Dexmedetomidine for pediatric sedation for computed tomography imaging studies. Anesth Analg. 2006;103(1):57–62.
24. Mason KP, Zurakowski D, Zgleszewski SE, Robson CD, Carrier M, Hickey PR, Dinardo JA. High dose dexmedetomidine as the sole sedative for pediatric MRI. Paediatr Anaesth. 2008;18(5):403–11.
25. Mason KP, Zgleszewski SE, Prescilla R, Fontaine PJ, Zurakowski D. Hemodynamic effects of dexmedetomidine sedation for CT imaging studies. Paediatr Anaesth. 2008;18(5):393–402.
26. Upton RN, Ludbrook G. A physiologically based, recirculatory model of the kinetics and dynamics of propofol in man. Anesthesiology. 2005;103(2):344–52.
27. Upton RN. The two-compartment recirculatory pharmacokinetic model—an introduction to recirculatory pharmacokinetic concepts. Br J Anaesth. 2004;92(4):475–84.
28. Weiss M, Krejcie TC, Avram MJ. A minimal physiological model of thiopental distribution kinetics based on a multiple indicator approach. Drug Metab Dispos. 2007;35(9):1525–32.
29. Avram MJ, Krejcie TC. Using front-end kinetics to optimize target-controlled drug infusions. Anesthesiology. 2003;99(5):1078–86.
30. Krejcie TC, Avram MJ. What determines anesthetic induction dose? It's the front-end kinetics, doctor! Anesth Analg. 1999; 89(3):541–4.
31. Hughes MA, Glass PS, Jacobs JR. Context-sensitive half-time in multicompartment pharmacokinetic models for intravenous anesthetic drugs. Anesthesiology. 1992;76(3):334–41.
32. Marsh B, White M, Morton N, Kenny GN. Pharmacokinetic model driven infusion of propofol in children. Br J Anaesth. 1991; 67:41–8.
33. Saint-Maurice C, Cockshott ID, Douglas EJ, Richard MO, Harmey JL. Pharmacokinetics of propofol in young children after a single dose. Br J Anaesth. 1989;63(6):667–70.
34. Murat I, Billard V, Vernois J, Zaouter M, Marsol P, Souron R, Farinotti R. Pharmacokinetics of propofol after a single dose in children aged 1–3 years with minor burns. Comparison of three data analysis approaches. Anesthesiology. 1996;84(3):526–32.

35. Schuttler J, Ihmsen H. Population pharmacokinetics of propofol: a multicenter study. Anesthesiology. 2000;92(3):727–38.
36. Short TG, Aun CS, Tan P, Wong J, Tam YH, Oh TE. A prospective evaluation of pharmacokinetic model controlled infusion of propofol in paediatric patients. Br J Anaesth. 1994;72(3):302–6.
37. Kataria BK, Ved SA, Nicodemus HF, Hoy GR, Lea D, Dubois MY, Mandema JW, Shafer SL. The pharmacokinetics of propofol in children using three different data analysis approaches. Anesthesiology. 1994;80(1):104–22.
38. Absalom A, Amutike D, Lal A, White M, Kenny GN. Accuracy of the 'Paedfusor' in children undergoing cardiac surgery or catheterization. Br J Anaesth. 2003;91(4):507–13.
39. Sepulveda P, Cortinez LI, Saez C, Penna A, Solari S, Guerra I, Absalom AR. Performance evaluation of paediatric propofol pharmacokinetic models in healthy young children. Br J Anaesth. 2011;107(4):593–600.
40. Anderson BJ, Holford NH. Mechanistic basis of using body size and maturation to predict clearance in humans. Drug Metab Pharmacokinet. 2009;24(1):25–36.
41. Eleveld DJ, Proost JH, Cortinez LI, Absalom AR, Struys MM. A general purpose pharmacokinetic model for propofol. Anesth Analg. 2014;118:1221–37.
42. Murray DM, Thorne GC, Rigby-Jones AE, Tonucci D, Grimes S, Tooley MA, Wolf AR. Electroencephalograph variables, drug concentrations and sedation scores in children emerging from propofol infusion anaesthesia. Paediatr Anaesth. 2004;14(2):143–51.
43. Rigouzzo A, Girault L, Louvet N, Servin F, De-Smet T, Piat V, Seeman R, Murat I, Constant I. The relationship between bispectral index and propofol during target-controlled infusion anesthesia: a comparative study between children and young adults. Anesth Analg. 2008;106(4):1109–16.
44. Potts AL, Warman GR, Anderson BJ. Dexmedetomidine disposition in children: a population analysis. Paediatr Anaesth. 2008; 18(8):722–30.
45. Petroz GC, Sikich N, James M, van Dyk H, Shafer SL, Schily M, Lerman J. A phase I, two-center study of the pharmacokinetics and pharmacodynamics of dexmedetomidine in children. Anesthesiology. 2006;105(6):1098–110.
46. Diaz SM, Rodarte A, Foley J, Capparelli EV. Pharmacokinetics of dexmedetomidine in postsurgical pediatric intensive care unit patients: preliminary study. Pediatr Crit Care Med. 2007;8(5):419–24.
47. Ramsay MA, Savege TM, Simpson BR, Goodwin R. Controlled sedation with alphaxalone-alphadolone. Br Med J. 1974;2(920): 656–9.
48. Shafer SL, Gregg KM. Algorithms to rapidly achieve and maintain stable drug concentrations at the site of drug effect with a computer-controlled infusion pump. J Pharmacokinet Biopharm. 1992;20(2): 147–69.
49. Kruger-Thiemer E. Continuous intravenous infusion and multicompartment accumulation. Eur J Pharmacol. 1968;4(3):317–24.
50. Vaughan DP, Tucker GT. General theory for rapidly establishing steady state drug concentrations using two consecutive constant rate intravenous infusions. Eur J Clin Pharmacol. 1975;9(2–3):235–8.
51. Vaughan DP, Tucker GT. General derivation of the ideal intravenous drug input required to achieve and maintain a constant plasma drug concentration. Theoretical application to lignocaine therapy. Eur J Clin Pharmacol. 1976;10(6):433–40.
52. Schwilden H. A general method for calculating the dosage scheme in linear pharmacokinetics. Eur J Clin Pharmacol. 1981;20(5): 379–86.
53. Glen JB. The development of 'Diprifusor': a TCI system for propofol. Anaesthesia. 1998;53 Suppl 1:13–21.
54. Gray JM, Kenny GN. Development of the technology for 'Diprifusor' TCI systems. Anaesthesia. 1998;53 Suppl 1:22–7.
55. Hammer GB, Litalien C, Wellis V, Drover DR. Determination of the median effective concentration (EC50) of propofol during oesophagogastroduodenoscopy in children. Paediatr Anaesth. 2001;11(5):549–53.
56. Drover DR, Litalien C, Wellis V, Shafer SL, Hammer GB. Determination of the pharmacodynamic interaction of propofol and remifentanil during esophagogastroduodenoscopy in children. Anesthesiology. 2004;100(6):1382–6.
57. Varvel JR, Donoho DL, Shafer SL. Measuring the predictive performance of computer-controlled infusion pumps. J Pharmacokinet Biopharm. 1992;20(1):63–94.
58. Swinhoe CF, Peacock JE, Glen JB, Reilly CS. Evaluation of the predictive performance of a 'Diprifusor' TCI system. Anaesthesia. 1998;53 Suppl 1:61–7.
59. Schuttler J, Kloos S, Schwilden H, Stoeckel H. Total intravenous anaesthesia with propofol and alfentanil by computer-assisted infusion. Anaesthesia. 1988;43(Suppl):2–7.
60. Engelhardt T, McCheyne AJ, Morton N, Karsli C, Luginbuehl I, Adeli K, Walsh W, Bissonnette B. Clinical adaptation of a pharmacokinetic model of Propofol plasma concentrations in children. Paediatr Anaesth. 2008;18(3):235–9.
61. Vuyk J, Lim T, Engbers FH, Burm AG, Vletter AA, Bovill JG. The pharmacodynamic interaction of propofol and alfentanil during lower abdominal surgery in women. Anesthesiology. 1995; 83(1):8–22.
62. Vuyk J, Mertens MJ, Olofsen E, Burm AG, Bovill JG. Propofol anesthesia and rational opioid selection: determination of optimal EC50-EC95 propofol-opioid concentrations that assure adequate anesthesia and a rapid return of consciousness. Anesthesiology. 1997;87(6):1549–62.
63. Bouillon T, Bruhn J, Radu-Radulescu L, Bertaccini E, Park S, Shafer S. Non-steady state analysis of the pharmacokinetic interaction between propofol and remifentanil. Anesthesiology. 2002; 97(6):1350–62.
64. Bouillon TW, Bruhn J, Radulescu L, Andresen C, Shafer TJ, Cohane C, Shafer SL. Pharmacodynamic interaction between propofol and remifentanil regarding hypnosis, tolerance of laryngoscopy, bispectral index, and electroencephalographic approximate entropy. Anesthesiology. 2004;100(6):1353–72.
65. Bruhn J, Bouillon TW, Radulescu L, Hoeft A, Bertaccini E, Shafer SL. Correlation of approximate entropy, bispectral index, and spectral edge frequency 95 (SEF95) with clinical signs of "anesthetic depth" during coadministration of propofol and remifentanil. Anesthesiology. 2003;98(3):621–7.
66. Luginbuhl M, Schumacher PM, Vuilleumier P, Vereecke H, Heyse B, Bouillon TW, Struys MM. Noxious stimulation response index: a novel anesthetic state index based on hypnotic-opioid interaction. Anesthesiology. 2010;112(4):872–80.
67. Kennedy RR. Seeing the future of anesthesia drug dosing: moving the art of anesthesia from impressionism to realism. Anesth Analg. 2010;111(2):252–5.
68. Gin T. Clinical pharmacology on display. Anesth Analg. 2010; 111(2):256–8.
69. Schnider T, Minto C. Pharmacokinetic models of propofol for TCI. Anaesthesia. 2008;63(2):206.
70. Minto CF, Schnider TW, Gregg KM, Henthorn TK, Shafer SL. Using the time of maximum effect site concentration to combine pharmacokinetics and pharmacodynamics. Anesthesiology. 2003;99(2):324–33.
71. Irwin MG, Thompson N, Kenny GN. Patient-maintained propofol sedation. Assessment of a target-controlled infusion system. Anaesthesia. 1997;52(6):525–30.
72. Henderson F, Absalom AR, Kenny GN. Patient-maintained propofol sedation: a follow up safety study using a modified system in volunteers. Anaesthesia. 2002;57(4):387–90.
73. Stonell CA, Leslie K, Absalom AR. Effect-site targeted patient-controlled sedation with propofol: comparison with anaesthetist administration for colonoscopy. Anaesthesia. 2006;61(3):240–7.

74. Leitch JA, Anderson K, Gambhir S, Millar K, Robb ND, McHugh S, Kenny GN. A partially blinded randomised controlled trial of patient-maintained propofol sedation and operator controlled midazolam sedation in third molar extractions. Anaesthesia. 2004; 59(9):853–60.
75. Anderson KJ, Leitch JA, Green JS, Kenny GN. Effect-site controlled patient maintained propofol sedation: a volunteer safety study. Anaesthesia. 2005;60(3):235–8.
76. Pambianco DJ, Vargo JJ, Pruitt RE, Hardi R, Martin JF. Computer-assisted personalized sedation for upper endoscopy and colonoscopy: a comparative, multicenter randomized study. Gastrointest Endosc. 2011;73(4):765–72.
77. Martin JF, Bridenbaugh P, Gustafson M. The SEDASYS System is not intended for the sedation of high-risk patients. Gastrointest Endosc. 2011;74(3):723.
78. Hemmerling TM, Terrasini N. Robotic anesthesia: not the realm of science fiction any more. Curr Opin Anaesthesiol. 2012;25(6): 736–42.
79. Kenny GN, Mantzaridis H. Closed-loop control of propofol anaesthesia. Br J Anaesth. 1999;83(2):223–8.
80. Mortier E, Struys M, De Smet T, Versichelen L, Rolly G. Closed-loop controlled administration of propofol using bispectral analysis. Anaesthesia. 1998;53(8):749–54.
81. Struys MM, De Smet T, Versichelen LF, Van DV, Van den BR, Mortier EP. Comparison of closed-loop controlled administration of propofol using bispectral index as the controlled variable versus "standard practice" controlled administration. Anesthesiology. 2001;95(1):6–17.
82. Leslie K, Absalom A, Kenny GN. Closed loop control of sedation for colonoscopy using the bispectral index. Anaesthesia. 2002; 57(7):693–7.
83. Absalom AR, Sutcliffe N, Kenny GN. Closed-loop control of anesthesia using bispectral index: performance assessment in patients undergoing major orthopedic surgery under combined general and regional anesthesia. Anesthesiology. 2002;96(1):67–73.
84. Absalom AR, Kenny GN. Closed-loop control of propofol anaesthesia using bispectral index: performance assessment in patients receiving computer-controlled propofol and manually controlled remifentanil infusions for minor surgery. Br J Anaesth. 2003; 90(6):737–41.
85. Struys MM, De Smet T, Greenwald S, Absalom AR, Binge S, Mortier EP. Performance evaluation of two published closed-loop control systems using bispectral index monitoring: a simulation study. Anesthesiology. 2004;100(3):640–7.
86. De Smet T, Struys MM, Neckebroek MM, Van den Hauwe K, Bonte S, Mortier EP. The accuracy and clinical feasibility of a new bayesian-based closed-loop control system for propofol administration using the bispectral index as a controlled variable. Anesth Analg. 2008;107(4):1200–10.
87. Liu N, Chazot T, Hamada S, Landais S, Boichut N, Dussaussoy C, Trillat B, Beydon L, Samain E, Sessler DI, Fischler M. Closed-loop co-administration of propofol and remifentanil guided by the bispectral index. A randomized multicenter study. Anesth Analg. 2011;112(3):546–57.
88. Liu N, Le Guen M, Benabbes-Lambert F, Chazot T, Trillat B, Sessler DI, Fischler M. Feasibility of closed-loop titration of propofol and remifentanil guided by the spectral M-entropy monitor. Anesthesiology. 2012;116(2):286–95.
89. Dussaussoy C, Peres M, Jaoul V, Liu N, Chazot T, Picquet J, Fischler M, Beydon L. Automated titration of propofol and remifentanil decreases the anesthesiologist's workload during vascular or thoracic surgery: a randomized prospective study. J Clin Monit Comput. 2014;28(1):35–40.
90. Le Guen M, Liu N, Bourgeois E, Chazot T, Sessler DI, Rouby JJ, Fischler M. Automated sedation outperforms manual administration of propofol and remifentanil in critically ill patients with deep sedation: a randomized phase II trial. Intensive Care Med. 2013; 39(3):454–62.
91. Liu N, Pruszkowski O, Leroy JE, Chazot T, Trillat B, Colchen A, Gonin F, Fischler M. Automatic administration of propofol and remifentanil guided by the bispectral index during rigid bronchoscopic procedures: a randomized trial. Can J Anaesth. 2013;60(9):881–7.
92. van Heusden K, Ansermino JM, Soltesz K, Khosravi S, West N, Dumont GA. Quantification of the variability in response to propofol administration in children. IEEE Trans Biomed Eng. 2013; 60(9):2521–9.
93. Absalom A, Kenny G. 'Paedfusor' pharmacokinetic data set. Br J Anaesth. 2005;95(1):110.
94. Absalom A, Struys MMRF. An overview of TCI and TIVA. Ghent: Academia; 2005. p. 13.

Usage of Complementary and Alternative Medicine in Pediatric Sedation

32

Yuan-Chi Lin

Abstract

Complementary and alternative medicine includes those acceptable health care approaches outside of our conventional medicine. The National Center for Complementary and Alternative Medicine classified these therapies from a complete medical system of premise and practice; biological-based practices; mind-body medicine; manipulative and energy medicine.

Music therapy, hypnotherapy, guided imagery, and acupuncture-related techniques have been applied for pediatric sedation. These therapies can easily work in conjunction with available conventional medical treatments for pediatric sedation.

Keywords

Complementary and alternative medicine • Pediatric sedation • Music therapy • Hypnosis • Guided imagery • Acupuncture • Acupressure

Introduction

Complementary and alternative medicine (CAM) describes any health care approach outside the area of conventional medicine. It is a group of diverse medical and health systems, practices, and products, and is commonly used in conjunction with conventional medicine.

The National Center for Complementary and Alternative Medicine groups these therapies into several domains (Table 32.1). It can come from a complete medical system of premise and practice, including homeopathic medicine, naturopathic medicine, traditional Chinese medicine, ayurveda, and Tibetan medicine.

Commonly utilized forms of CAM include biologically based practice, mind-body medicine, manipulative and body-based practice, and energy medicine. Biologically based practices of CAM employ the use of the substances from nature, including herbs, nutrition, vitamins, and dietary supplements. Mind-body medicine involves a variety of techniques designed to enhance the mind's capacity to affect bodily functions and symptoms. Some examples of mind-body medicine include meditation, biofeedback, relaxation, guided imagery, prayer, and music therapy. (Refer to Chap. 34: *Non-pharmacological Distraction Techniques as Sedation Adjunct.*) Manipulative practices are based on manipulation and movement of the body. These include massage, chiropractic or osteopathic manipulation. Energy medicine employs the usage of energy fields. Some examples include acupuncture, qigong, reiki, and therapeutic touch.

Use of CAM in the pediatric population is increasing in popularity. In the United States, approximately 38 % of adults and 12 % of children currently use some form of complementary medicine [1]. The surgical environment is one in which CAM has become particularly popular with pediatric patients, families, and health care professionals. Pediatric patients require sedation more often than adults for medical procedures. They are at higher risk for respiratory depression and life-threatening hypoxia, and peri-procedure anxiety is directly related to fear, unfamiliar environments, and a loss of control. CAM can be used as a noninvasive modality for decreasing patients' anxiety and assisting with sedation.

Y.-C. Lin, M.D., M.P.H. (✉)
Department of Anesthesiology, Perioperative and Pain Medicine, Boston Children's Hospital, Harvard Medical School, 300 Longwood Avenue, Boston, MA 02115, USA
e-mail: Yuan-Chi.Lin@childrens.harvard.edu

K.P. Mason (ed.), *Pediatric Sedation Outside of the Operating Room: A Multispecialty International Collaboration*, DOI 10.1007/978-1-4939-1390-9_32, © Springer Science+Business Media New York 2015

Table 32.1 Major types of complementary and alternative medicine (adapted from NCCAM, National Institutes of Health, Bethesda, Maryland)

Whole medical systems
• Homeopathic medicine
• Naturopathic medicine
• Traditional Chinese medicine
• Ayurveda
• Tibetan medicine
Biologically based practices
• Herbal products
• Nutritional supplements
• Vitamins
• Dietary supplements
Mind-body medicine
• Meditation
• Biofeedback
• Relaxation
• Guided imagery
• Prayer
• Music therapy
• Tai Chi Chuan
Manipulative practices
• Chiropractic manipulation
• Massage
• Osteopathic manipulation
Energy medicine
• Acupuncture
• Qigong
• Reiki
• Therapeutic touch

Music

Music has been widely used for healing purposes through the ages. It is recognized as a safe, inexpensive, and effective anxiolytic adjunct to medical procedures. Music therapy employs the use of experiencing or making music for therapeutic purposes. It can serve as an adjuvant therapy in critically ill patients. In a randomized controlled trial, ten critically ill patients were allocated to a music or a no-music group. The music group received a special selection of slow movements from Mozart's piano sonatas, which had been analyzed for compositional elements for relaxation. The music was delivered for 1 h via headphones, where the control subjects wore headphones without music. Music application was shown to significantly reduce the amount of sedative medication needed to achieve a comparable degree of sedation. In those receiving the music intervention, plasma concentrations of growth hormone increased, whereas those of interleukin-6 and epinephrine decreased. The reduction in systemic stress hormone levels was associated with a significantly lower blood pressure and heart rate. Music may exert its sedative effects by a neurohumoral pathway involving interactions between the hypothalamo-pituitary axes with the adrenal medulla via mediators of the unspecific immune system [2]. A multicenter randomized controlled trial utilized music therapy to help reduce anxiety and sedation among 373 patients receiving mechanical ventilation for acute respiratory failure. The music intervention group (126 patients) could select their preferred pieces of music to listen to as they wanted. The patient-directed music listening group had relative decreases of about 36 % in anxiety, sedation intensity, and sedation frequency as compared with usual care [3].

The use of intraoperative music in awake patients decreases patient-controlled sedative and analgesic requirements. A randomized controlled study of 35 adults undergoing urologic procedures with spinal anesthesia and patient-controlled intravenous propofol sedation randomly assigned patients to intraoperative music via headset or to no intraoperative music. The patients in the music group required significantly less propofol for sedation than patients in the control group [4]. A randomized controlled study of 43 adults undergoing lithotripsy treatment of renal or ureteral calculi and receiving patient-controlled intravenous opioid analgesia also randomly assigned patients to either a music or no-music group. The patients who listened to music had a significant reduction in alfentanil requirements [4]. By using self-report validated behavioral and physiological measures of anxiety, 93 adult patients were evaluated before, during, and after surgery. Patients who listened to music of their choice during the preoperative period reported less anxiety [5].

A randomized controlled trial of 70 children undergoing surgical procedures indicated that children are less anxious and show increased compliance during induction when exposed to a single care-provider in a dimmed, quiet operating room with background music [6]. In another study, 123 children were randomly assigned into one of three groups: interactive music therapy, oral midazolam, and a control group. The children who received midazolam were significantly less anxious during the induction of anesthesia than the children in the music therapy and control groups. There was no difference in anxiety during the induction of anesthesia between children in the music therapy group and children in the control group. Music therapy may be helpful on separation and entrance to the operating room, depending on the therapist; however, it does not appear to relieve anxiety during the induction of anesthesia [7].

Sixty pediatric patients receiving either chloral hydrate or music therapy for electroencephalography testing revealed that music therapy may be a cost-effective, risk-free alternative to pharmacological sedation [8]. There has been report of a high success rate of utilizing music for pediatric patients undergoing computerized tomography scans, echocardiograms, initiation of intravenous lines, and electroencephalograms (EEGs). Music therapy is a cost-effective intervention for most pediatric facilities [9]. It can be used as an adjuvant therapeutic measure in pediatric sedation.

Hypnotherapy

Hypnotherapy is the induction of a trance-like state to facilitate relaxation of the conscious mind. The hypnotic trance is neither a sleep state nor a state of unconsciousness. It is a state of altered consciousness in which attention can be focused on some things to the exclusion of others. Relaxation, immobilization, and altering or abolishing painful stimuli are frequently seen with hypnosis. A study of 49 embolization procedures on 30 patients utilizing medical hypnosis revealed that 45 of the procedures were successfully performed using hypnosis [10].

Faymonville et al. did a study of positron emission tomography in 11 healthy volunteers to identify the brain areas in which hypnosis modulates cerebral responses to a noxious stimulus. Hypnosis decreased both pain sensation and the unpleasantness of noxious stimuli. Noxious stimulation caused an increase in regional cerebral blood flow in the thalamic nuclei and anterior cingulate and insular cortices. The hypnotic state induced a significant activation of a right-sided extrastriate area and the anterior cingulate cortex. The interaction analysis showed that how the activity in the anterior cingulate cortex was related to pain perception and unpleasantness was different from the hypnotic state than in control situations. Both intensity and unpleasantness of the noxious stimuli were reduced during the hypnotic state [11].

Lang and colleagues did a randomized study of 236 women referred for large core needle breast biopsy to receive standard care, structured empathic attention, or self-hypnotic relaxation during their procedures. The study demonstrated that hypnosis can be successfully integrated to core needle biopsy for the diagnosis of breast cancer. The adjunctive use of hypnosis by trained members of the procedure team resulted in substantially less anxiety and a reduction in pain, compared to two other randomized conditions: routine care and sympathetic assistance. After more than an hour, the hypnotic analgesia was clearly superior to that obtained in standard care or the nonspecific empathy conditions [12].

A study explored the use of hypnosis for pain and anxiety management in six colonoscopy patients who received a hypnotic induction and instruction in self-hypnosis on the day of their colonoscopy, compared to ten consecutive patients who received standard care. Hypnosis appeared to be a feasible method of managing anxiety and pain associated with colonoscopy, reduced the need for sedation, and may have other benefits, such as reduced vasovagal events and recovery time [13].

Ghoneim et al. did a randomized controlled trial of 60 patients to evaluate the usefulness of tape-recorded hypnosis instruction on perioperative outcome in surgical patients. The hypnosis group received an audio tape to listen to daily for the immediate preoperative week. The controlled group did not receive a tape. Anxiety was reduced before surgery by means of the audio tape containing hypnotic instructions, however, for no discernible reason, and there was an increase in the incidence of vomiting [14]. Balini et al. studied 46 patients undergoing percutaneous transluminal coronary angioplasty of the left anterior descending coronary artery. They were randomized to receive medication or hypnotic sedation during the procedure. The increase in cardiac sympathetic activity associated with balloon inflation and myocardial ischemia during percutaneous transluminal coronary angioplasty of the left anterior descending coronary artery was selectively eliminated by hypnosis but not by drug sedation [15].

A meta-analysis performed on 18 controlled trials suggested that the addition of hypnosis substantially enhanced treatment outcome. The average client receiving cognitive-behavioral hypnotherapy showed greater improvement than at least 70 % of clients receiving non-hypnotic treatment. Hypnotherapy enhances the effects of cognitive-behavioral psychotherapy, including anxiety, insomnia, pain, and obesity [16].

Hypnotherapy is one of the oldest forms of psychotherapy. It encourages the patient to use his or her imagination to improve health and health behaviors. While most of the current research is on its use in the adult population, hypnotherapy may be integrated into pediatric sedation in the future.

Guided Imagery

Patients who undergo sedation usually experience some fear and apprehension about their procedures. Guided imagery is a simple, low-cost therapeutic tool that can help counteract these feelings. A randomized controlled trial of 130 patients underwent elective colorectal surgical procedures. They were assigned to receive either routine perioperative care or listen to guided imagery tapes for 3 days before their procedures, during the peri-procedure period, and for 6 days after the intervention. The patients in the guided imagery group experienced considerably less preoperative and postoperative anxiety and pain, and required nearly 50 % less narcotic medications than patients in the control group [17].

Guided imagery was successfully utilized in 56 patients undergoing radiology interventional procedures. They were enrolled in a standardized protocol with script guided imagery to produce a state of self-hypnotic relaxation. Each of the patients developed an imagery scenario. Although there were common trends in the chosen imagery, such as nature, travel, family, home, and personal skills, the chosen topics were highly individual. This variable made prerecorded tapes or provider-directed imagery unlikely to be equally successful [18].

Anodyne imagery technique consists of conditioned relaxation, induction of a trance state, and guided processing of the patient's internal imagery. A study involved 100 patients undergoing interventional radiologic procedures. Anodyne imagery eased patients' anxiety and fears and reduced the amount of midazolam and fentanyl used during interventional radiologic procedures, possibly improving procedural safety and augmenting the speed of recovery [19].

Guided imagery technique can produce analgesia and anxiolysis. Though the technique is highly individualized, it has a potential to be integrated into pediatric sedation in the future.

Acupuncture and Related Techniques

Used for more than two millennia, acupuncture is one of the oldest medicinal practices in the world. It is part of traditional Chinese medicine. Since its reintroduction in the United States in the early 1970s, acupuncture has become a widely used complementary medical therapy, used to maintain and restore health through the stimulation of acupuncture points by the insertion of hair-thin needles through the skin. In traditional Chinese Medicine and acupuncture, illness is caused by imbalance of a person's energy called *qi*. Qi is created between heaven and earth. Qi flows through the entire body of living creatures. Acupuncture promotes the flow of "qi," which is equivalent to energy. Endogenous opioid peptides in the central nervous system play a major role in mediating the effect of acupuncture [20]. Several acupuncture-related techniques, including electro-acupuncture, moxibustion, cupping, acupressure, and auricular therapy, are commonly applied. Complications from acupuncture treatment are rare.

Acupuncture can be used to assist upper endoscopic and colonoscopy procedures. In a study of 106 patients, those receiving midazolam rated the procedure as slightly less troublesome than those receiving acupuncture. Oxygen saturation, blood pressure, and heart rate were significantly lower in patients receiving midazolam [21]. In a randomized controlled trial of 55 patients who received colonoscopy examination with either electro-acupuncture analgesia or meperidine analgesia, the analgesic effect of both groups was the same. The electro-acupuncture group has fewer side effects, particularly in regard to dizziness. Serum concentration of beta-endorphin in both groups showed similar trends of change during colonoscopy. Changes in serum concentration of epinephrine, norepinephrine, dopamine, cortisol, and beta-endorphin were also similar between these two groups [22]. Another study of 30 patients undergoing colonoscopy was randomized to receive acupuncture, sham, or no acupuncture. Midazolam was used for sedation for all three groups. The acupuncture group experienced less pain and required less midazolam than the other two groups. The demand for sedative drugs during colonoscopy was decreased through the use of acupuncture by reducing the discomfort and anxiety of the patients [23].

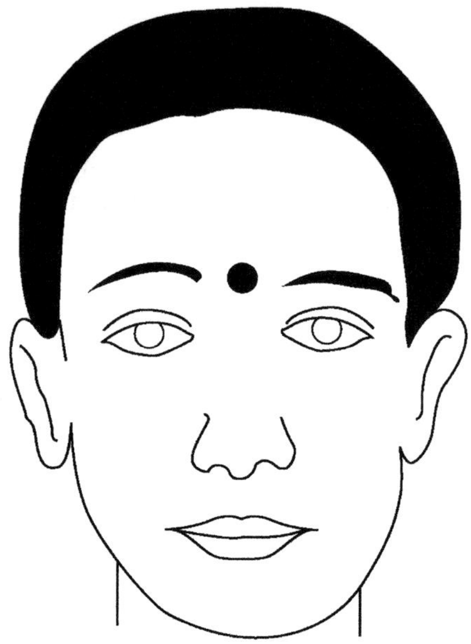

Fig. 32.1 Extra-one, EX-HN3, (Yin-Tang) acupuncture point locates on the forehead, at the midpoint between the eyebrows

In a study of 56 patients undergoing lithotripsy procedures, patients were enrolled into either an acupuncture or sham group. Using a combination of auricular and body acupuncture, patients had less pre-procedural anxiety and required less intra-procedural analgesia [24]. Another study involving 35 patient undergoing lithotripsy procedures showed that electro-acupuncture was an effective method for inducing sedation with analgesia without any demonstrable side effects [25].

Acupuncture or acupressure on the extra-one, EX-HN3, (Yin-Tang) acupuncture point is effective in producing sedation. The extra-one, EX-HN3, (Yin-Tang) acupuncture point is located on the forehead, at the midpoint between the eyebrows (Fig. 32.1).

A prospective, randomized, single-blind, controlled study assigned 52 patients either to acupuncture on Yin-Tang or to a sham acupuncture group. The bispectral index (BIS) values in the acupuncture group were significantly lower than in the sham group [26].

A study of 50 patients was randomly assigned to acupuncture of the Yin-Tang point or control point. Acupuncture application significantly decreased the BIS value compared to the control group [27].

Acupressure over this point produces analgesic and sedative effects. A study of 52 children undergoing endoscopic procedures was randomized to receive acupressure bead intervention either at the extra-one (Yin-Tang) acupuncture point or at a sham point. Anesthetic techniques were standardized and maintained with intravenous propofol infusion.

Children receiving the acupressure on the extra-one (Yin-Tang) point experienced reduced anxiety. There were no significant changes in BIS values between the groups, and the total intra-procedural propofol requirements did not differ between them. Acupressure bead intervention at the extra-one (Yin-Tang) acupuncture point reduced pre-procedural anxiety in children undergoing endoscopic procedures, however [28]. A study involving 22 healthy female volunteers was randomized to receive acupressure on either the extra-one (Yin-Tang) point or a sham point. Acupressure at the extra-one (Yin-Tang) point significantly reduced needle insertion pain compared to acupressure at the sham point. Acupressure at the extra-one (Yin-Tang) acupuncture point significantly reduced the low frequency/high frequency ratio of heart rate variability responding to needle insertion. This implies a reduction in sympathetic nervous system activity [29].

A crossover study of volunteers indicated that acupressure on the extra-one (Yin-Tang) acupuncture point can significantly reduce BIS values and verbal stress scores [30, 31]. In a randomized controlled trial of 48 volunteers, 5 min of acupressure on the extra-one (Yin-Tang) acupuncture point significantly reduced the EEG spectral entropy values [29]. A randomized trial of 61 parents indicated that acupressure at the extra-one (Yin-Tang) acupuncture point can have anxiolytic and sedative effects on parents in the preoperative holding area before their children's surgery [32].

Ear acupuncture (Fig. 32.2), also known as auricular therapy, is based on the principles of traditional Chinese medicine. It is practiced as a sole treatment or in conjunction with body acupuncture therapy, and is an effective treatment for acute anxiety. Ear acupuncture can decrease preoperative anxiety in adults undergoing outpatient surgery [33]. A study of 67 patients undergoing dental extraction compared the efficacy of auricular acupuncture, intranasal midazolam, placebo acupuncture, and no treatment for reducing dental anxiety. Patients having dental extractions were randomized to one of four groups: auricular acupuncture, placebo acupuncture, intranasal midazolam, and a no-treatment group. Anxiety was assessed before the interventions, after 30 min, and after the dental extraction. The auricular acupuncture group and the midazolam group were significantly less anxious at 30 min compared to patients in the placebo acupuncture group. Patient compliance assessed by the dentist was significantly improved if auricular acupuncture or application of intranasal midazolam had been performed [34].

Auricular acupuncture points may be stimulated for a longer period of time by using ear seeds or ear tacks. Ear seeds can be small seeds from the dry Vaccaria plant or can be made from stainless steel. These seeds are held in place on the ear with a small piece of adhesive tape (Fig. 32.3). Auricular acupressure is an effective treatment for anxiety during ambulance transport. In a study of 36 patients who required ambulance transport to medical facilities, patients were randomized to receive auricular acupressure at the relaxation point or at a sham point. Patients in the auricular acupressure group reported significantly less anxiety than

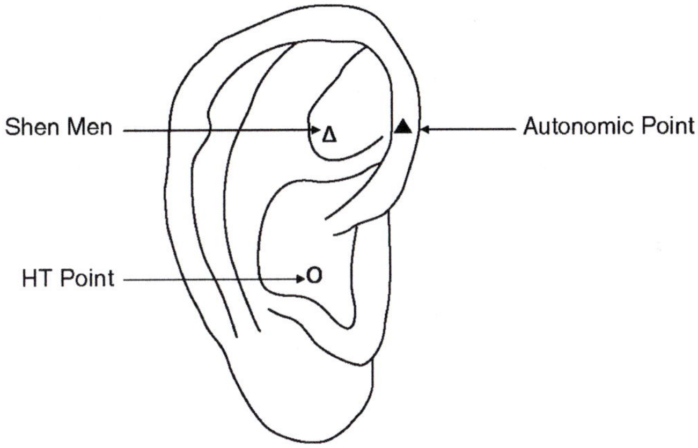

Fig. 32.2 Location of auricular acupuncture points

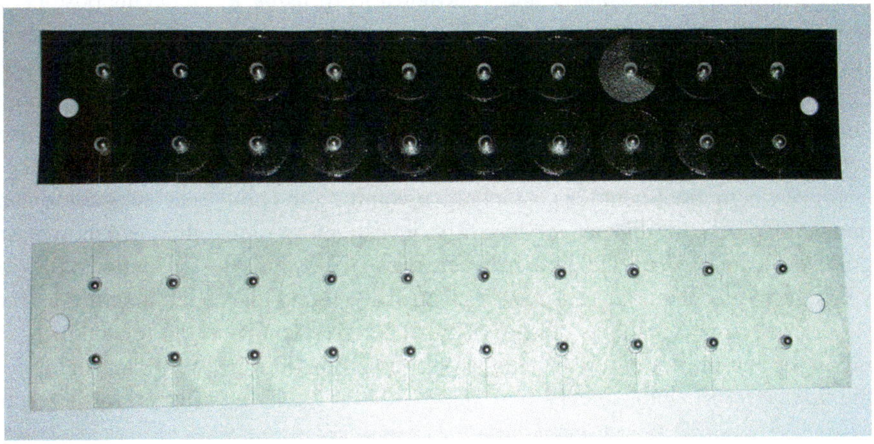

Fig. 32.3 Auricular acupressure press pellets; 1.2 mm diameter stimulating press pellets are made from stainless steel

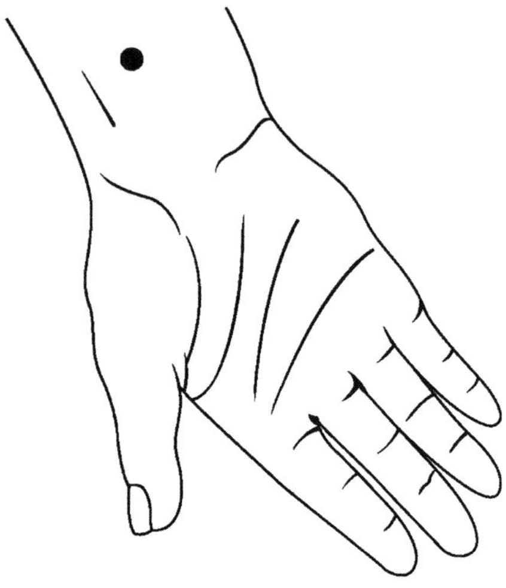

Fig. 32.4 PC 6 acupuncture point locates on the anterior forearm, three finger breadths proximal to the transverse wrist crease, between the tendons of palmaris longus and flexor carpi radialis muscles

patients in the sham group on arrival at the hospital [35]. Another randomized controlled trial of 38 patients with acute hip fractures received either bilateral auricular acupressure or the sham control during ambulance transport. Patients in the true intervention groups had less pain and anxiety and lower heart rates on arrival at the hospital [36].

Acupressure is the application of pressure to the acupuncture points with the finger, which can achieve significant clinical effects. In a double-blinded design study of 60 minor trauma patients, patients were randomly assigned into one of three groups: true acupressure, sham acupressure, and no acupressure. The group of patients who received true acupressure experienced significantly less pain, anxiety, and had a lower heart rate, and reported greater satisfaction than the other two groups [37].

Post-sedation nausea and vomiting is a significant problem that occurs frequently in the post-sedation recovery care unit. It can cause electrolyte imbalance, delay discharge, and other complications. Schlager and colleagues [38], using a low level of laser stimulation of the PC 6 acupuncture point (Fig. 32.4) in children undergoing strabismus surgery, found that the intervention significantly decreased postoperative vomiting. Chu and colleagues [39] applied acupressure with acu-plaster to BL-10, BL-11, and GB-34 acupuncture points as prophylactic treatment for postoperative vomiting in children undergoing strabismus surgery. The investigators randomized a total of 65 children between ages of 3 and 14 years into a placebo or an acu-plaster group. They found that significantly fewer patients developed postoperative vomiting in the acu-plaster group than in the placebo group during the first 24 h following surgery.

Schlager and colleagues [40] applied acupressure to acupuncture points in the hand 30 min before induction and kept the acupressure in place for 24 h in a group of children undergoing strabismus surgery. They found children in the acupressure group had a significantly lower incidence of vomiting as compared to the placebo group. Somri and colleagues [41] compared the antiemetic effect of P6 acupuncture with ondansetron and a placebo in a group of children receiving dental surgery. They found a significant decrease in the number of patients who vomited and also in the total number of vomiting episodes in two treatment groups as compared with the placebo group. There was no difference between the acupuncture and ondansetron groups.

Rusy and colleagues [42] used electrical stimulation of acupuncture point P6 as a prophylactic postoperative nausea and vomiting treatment for children undergoing tonsillectomy with or without adenoidectomy. The investigators also found that children who received true electrical stimulation at acupuncture points PC6 had significantly less postoperative nausea and vomiting. Butkovic et al. [43] compared the use of laser acupuncture and metoclopramide in preventing the development of postoperative nausea and vomiting. The investigators found that bilateral laser acupuncture PC6 stimulations are as effective as metoclopramide in preventing the development of postoperative nausea and vomiting in children. Yeh et al. did a crossover randomized auricular acupuncture points study of children with cancer who had a history of chemotherapy-induced nausea and vomiting. They used auricular acupuncture points stimulation utilizing the application of small seeds and adhesive tape over the ear acupuncture points to prevent the incidence of nausea and vomiting [44].

Kabalak and colleague [45] found that transcutaneous electrical acupuncture point stimulation, utilizing skin surface electrodes applied 20 Hz and 10 mA for 5 min to the P6 acupuncture points, was as effective as ondansetron in preventing postoperative vomiting following pediatric tonsillectomy. A meta-analysis of the acupuncture point's stimulation effect on postoperative nausea and vomiting in children indicates that acupressure and acupuncture are as effective as medication in reducing postoperative vomiting in children [46].

Most of the available studies involve the adult population, rather than pediatric patients. Evidence-based medical research has indicated that acupuncture and related techniques can be used for analgesic, anxiolytic, and sedative effects. It is very effective in prevention and treatment of peri-procedure nausea and vomiting [47]. It is estimated that there are more than 20,000 licensed acupuncture providers in the United States, among them 3,000 physicians who perform acupuncture as part of their medical practice. Acupuncture and related techniques can be used in conjunction with conventional therapy for sedation and prevention and can ease discomfort after the procedure.

Sucrose Sucking in Infants

Sweetening agents have been recommended in position statements and consensus documents for procedural pain management in neonates. In a randomized study, 113 healthy term newborns, whose heels were pricked for the Guthrie test to detect phenylketonuria, were randomized into four groups: the first receiving 2 mL of 30 % sucrose, the second 10 % glucose, the third 30 % glucose, and the fourth distilled water. The study showed that 30 % sucrose was superior to 10 and 30 % glucose solutions in relieving pain [48].

Johnston et al. studied 85 preterm infants (between 25 and 34 weeks post-conceptual age) randomly assigned to oral sucrose and or simulated rocking 15 min before a routine heel stick procedure. Utilizing 0.05 mL of 24 % sucrose placed on the anterior surface of the tongue just prior to the lancing of the heel diminished pain from minor procedures in preterm infants [49]. A single-blind randomized crossover study of 90 preterm neonates undergoing heel-lancing procedures indicated the sensorial stimulations from skin-to-skin contact that include tactile, olfactory sensations from the mother are sufficient to decrease pain response in premature neonates. Other stimulations such as rocking, sucking, and music were also efficacious for neonatal sedation [50]. There is strong evidence to support sucrose for minor invasive procedures, and combinations of medications for tracheal intubation in neonates [51].

Conclusion

Sedation for pediatric procedures can be distressing for children and their families. Studies related to using CAM, non-pharmacological methods for reducing anxiety and improving cooperation, show that these methods may avoid the adverse effects of sedation. (Refer to Chap. 34: *Non-pharmacological Distraction Techniques as Sedation Adjunct*.) A Cochrane review assessed 17 trials of the effects of CAM non-pharmacological interventions in assisting induction of anesthesia in children by reducing their anxiety or distress or by increasing their cooperation. Eight trials assessed parental presence; none showed significant differences in anxiety or cooperation of children during induction, except for one in which parental presence was significantly less effective than midazolam in reducing children's anxiety at induction. In children undergoing hypnosis, there was a nonsignificant trend toward reduced anxiety during induction compared with midazolam. Children of parents having acupuncture compared with parental sham-acupuncture were less anxious during induction and more children were cooperative. The presence of parents during induction of general anesthesia does not reduce their child's anxiety. There are promising CAM non-pharmacological interventions, such as parental acupuncture, clown doctor, hypnotherapy, low sensory stimulation, and handheld video games [52]. A recent publication has indicated that acupuncture sedation can be an adjunct therapy for gastroscopy, extracorporeal shock wave therapy, and dental anxiety [53].

Most medical procedures increase pediatric patients' and their family's fears and anxiety, which are commonly addressed by sedatives. Insufficient treatment of pain and anxiety can cause cardiovascular strain and restlessness, possibly jeopardizing the success of the procedure. Pharmacologic oversedation can provoke respiratory and cardiovascular depression, thereby increasing the procedural risks and delaying the patient's recovery. Pediatric sedation should be individually tailored to each child for personal situation. CAM interventions can be integrated as part of pediatric sedation procedures. It may not be the sole therapy, but CAM can be used in conjunction with conventional medical therapies to assist with sedation and decrease patients' pain and anxiety.

Case Studies

Case 1

Margie is an 8-year-old patient with severe burns. Her life is challenged with daily dressing changes. Her mom is concerned that morphine has made her very tired and sleepy. Other opioids also made her to have itchy skin. This would complicate her skin care.

Are there any other therapies that can be utilized for her daily dressing changes?

Suggestions

Hypnosis, guided imagery, music therapy, meditation, or acupuncture can be used on post-procedure pain in the pediatric population. Hypnosis and guided imagery have been proposed as particularly appropriate intervention for children since children are generally more susceptible to hypnosis and guided imagery than adults. Children are more willing to absorb in fantasy than adults. Creative arts, including music therapy, art therapy, and movement therapy, can be used for the pediatric population. Older children can learn self-meditation to ease various painful and traumatic procedures. Acupuncture is effective in easing procedure-related pain and rarely has any serious adverse effect.

(continued)

Case 2

John is a pediatric registered nurse and a member of an emergency transport team. Anxiety is a common problem during transport. He inquires if there is anything he can do to ease patient anxiety during transport?

Suggestions

John applied auricular acupressure for his patient to ease anxiety and pain prior to the patient's transport to the Emergency Room. Auricular acupuncture points may be stimulated for a longer period of time by using ear seeds or ear tacks. Ear seeds can be small seeds from the dry Vaccaria plant or can be made from stainless steel. These seeds are held in place on the ear with a small piece of adhesive tape. Auricular acupressure is an effective treatment for anxiety during ambulance transport. In a study of 36 patients who required ambulance transport to medical facilities, patients were randomized to receive auricular acupressure at the relaxation point or at a sham point. Patients in the auricular acupressure group reported significantly less anxiety than patients in the sham group on arrival to the hospital. Another randomized controlled trial of 38 patients with acute hip fractures received either bilateral auricular acupressure or the sham control during ambulance transport. Patients in the true intervention groups had less pain and anxiety and lower heart rates on arrival at the hospital.

Case 3

Sean is an 11-year-old, 38 kg, boy with acute lymphocytic leukemia. He has ongoing chemotherapy including intrathecal medication. The peri-procedure lumbar puncture sedatives included intravenous midazolam 4 mg and fentanyl 200 μg. In the post-procedure recovery room, he complained about severe nausea and vomiting. In spite of intravenous fluid, zofran, reglan, and scopolamine patch, he continued suffering from intractable nausea and vomiting. What is next?

Suggestions

Post-sedation nausea and vomiting is a significant problem that occurs frequently in the post-sedation recovery care unit. It can cause electrolyte imbalance, delay discharge, and other complications. Sean received acupuncture treatment in the post-procedure recovery room. He felt better and was able to go home afterward. The American Society of Anesthesiologists (ASA) Consensus Guidelines for the Management of Postoperative Nausea and Vomiting [54], acupuncture, acupressure, and acupoint stimulation had antiemetic efficacy rates comparable with that of pharmacologic therapy. Acupuncture treatment can be utilized for the prevention of, as well as treatment for, nausea and vomiting.

References

1. Sawni-Sikand A, Schubiner H, Thomas RL. Use of complementary/alternative therapies among children in primary care pediatrics. Ambul Pediatr. 2002;2(2):99–103.
2. Conrad C, Niess H, Jauch KW, Bruns CJ, Hartl W, Welker L. Overture for growth hormone: requiem for interleukin-6? Crit Care Med. 2007;35(12):2709–13.
3. Chlan LL, Weinert CR, Heiderscheit A, Tracy MF, Skaar DJ, Guttormson JL, et al. Effects of patient-directed music intervention on anxiety and sedative exposure in critically ill patients receiving mechanical ventilatory support: a randomized clinical trial. JAMA. 2013;309(22):2335–44.
4. Koch ME, Kain ZN, Ayoub C, Rosenbaum SH. The sedative and analgesic sparing effect of music. Anesthesiology. 1998;89(2):300–6.
5. Wang SM, Kulkarni L, Dolev J, Kain ZN. Music and preoperative anxiety: a randomized, controlled study. Anesth Analg. 2002;94(6):1489–94, table of contents.
6. Kain ZN, Wang SM, Mayes LC, Krivutza DM, Teague BA. Sensory stimuli and anxiety in children undergoing surgery: a randomized, controlled trial. Anesth Analg. 2001;92(4):897–903.
7. Kain ZN, Caldwell-Andrews AA, Krivutza DM, Weinberg ME, Gaal D, Wang SM, et al. Interactive music therapy as a treatment for preoperative anxiety in children: a randomized controlled trial. Anesth Analg. 2004;98(5):1260–6, table of contents.
8. Loewy J, Hallan C, Friedman E, Martinez C. Sleep/sedation in children undergoing eeg testing: a comparison of chloral hydrate and music therapy. Am J Electroneurodiag Technol. 2006;46(4):343–55.
9. DeLoach Walworth D. Procedural-support music therapy in the healthcare setting: a cost-effectiveness analysis. J Pediatr Nurs. 2005;20(4):276–84.
10. Bank WO, Kerber CW. Medical hypnosis during therapeutic embolizations of the carotid and vertebral arteries. Neuroradiology. 1979;17(5):249–52.
11. Faymonville ME, Laureys S, Degueldre C, DelFiore G, Luxen A, Franck G, et al. Neural mechanisms of antinociceptive effects of hypnosis. Anesthesiology. 2000;92(5):1257–67.
12. Lang EV, Berbaum KS, Faintuch S, Hatsiopoulou O, Halsey N, Li X, et al. Adjunctive self-hypnotic relaxation for outpatient medical procedures: a prospective randomized trial with women undergoing large core breast biopsy. Pain. 2006;126(1–3):155–64.
13. Elkins G, White J, Patel P, Marcus J, Perfect MM, Montgomery GH. Hypnosis to manage anxiety and pain associated with colonoscopy for colorectal cancer screening: case studies and possible benefits. Int J Clin Exp Hypn. 2006;54(4):416–31.
14. Ghoneim MM, Block RI, Sarasin DS, Davis CS, Marchman JN. Tape-recorded hypnosis instructions as adjuvant in the care of patients scheduled for third molar surgery. Anesth Analg. 2000; 90(1):64–8.

15. Baglini R, Sesana M, Capuano C, Gnecchi-Ruscone T, Ugo L, Danzi GB. Effect of hypnotic sedation during percutaneous transluminal coronary angioplasty on myocardial ischemia and cardiac sympathetic drive. Am J Cardiol. 2004;93(8):1035–8.
16. Gearan P, Schoenberger NE, Kirsch I. Modifying hypnotizability: a new component analysis. Int J Clin Exp Hypn. 1995;43(1):70–89.
17. Tusek DL, Church JM, Strong SA, Grass JA, Fazio VW. Guided imagery: a significant advance in the care of patients undergoing elective colorectal surgery. Dis Colon Rectum. 1997;40(2):172–8.
18. Fick LJ, Lang EV, Logan HL, Lutgendorf S, Benotsch EG. Imagery content during nonpharmacologic analgesia in the procedure suite: where your patients would rather be. Acad Radiol. 1999; 6(8):457–63.
19. Hatta T, Koike M, Langman P. Laterality of mental imagery generation and operation: tests with brain-damaged patients and normal adults. J Clin Exp Neuropsychol. 1994;16(4):577–88.
20. Han JS. Acupuncture and endorphins. Neurosci Lett. 2004; 361(1–3):258–61.
21. Melchart D, Steger HG, Linde K, Makarian K, Hatahet Z, Brenke R, et al. Integrating patient preferences in clinical trials: a pilot study of acupuncture versus midazolam for gastroscopy. J Altern Complement Med. 2002;8(3):265–74.
22. Wang HH, Chang YH, Liu DM, Ho YJ. A clinical study on physiological response in electroacupuncture analgesia and meperidine analgesia for colonoscopy. Am J Chin Med. 1997;25(1):13–20.
23. Fanti L, Gemma M, Passaretti S, Guslandi M, Testoni PA, Casati A, et al. Electroacupuncture analgesia for colonoscopy. A prospective, randomized, placebo-controlled study. Am J Gastroenterol. 2003;98(2):312–6.
24. Wang SM, Punjala M, Weiss D, Anderson K, Kain ZN. Acupuncture as an adjunct for sedation during lithotripsy. J Altern Complement Med. 2007;13(2):241–6.
25. Resim S, Gumusalan Y, Ekerbicer HC, Sahin MA, Sahinkanat T. Effectiveness of electro-acupuncture compared to sedo-analgesics in relieving pain during shockwave lithotripsy. Urol Res. 2005;33(4):285–90.
26. Acar HV, Cuvas O, Ceyhan A, Dikmen B. Acupuncture on Yintang point decreases preoperative anxiety. J Altern Complement Med. 2013;19(5):420–4.
27. Paraskeva A, Melemeni A, Petropoulos G, Siafaka I, Fassoulaki A. Needling of the extra 1 point decreases bis values and preoperative anxiety. Am J Chin Med. 2004;32(5):789–94.
28. Wang SM, Escalera S, Lin EC, Maranets I, Kain ZN. Extra-1 acupressure for children undergoing anesthesia. Anesth Analg. 2008;107(3):811–6.
29. Arai YC, Ushida T, Osuga T, Matsubara T, Oshima K, Kawaguchi K, et al. The effect of acupressure at the extra 1 point on subjective and autonomic responses to needle insertion. Anesth Analg. 2008;107(2):661–4.
30. Fassoulaki A, Paraskeva A, Patris K, Pourgiezi T, Kostopanagiotou G. Pressure applied on the extra 1 acupuncture point reduces bispectral index values and stress in volunteers. Anesth Analg. 2003;96(3):885–90, table of contents.
31. Fassoulaki A, Paraskeva A, Kostopanagiotou G, Tsakalozou E, Markantonis S. Acupressure on the extra 1 acupoint: the effect on bispectral index, serum melatonin, plasma beta-endorphin, and stress. Anesth Analg. 2007;104(2):312–7.
32. Wang SM, Gaal D, Maranets I, Caldwell-Andrews A, Kain ZN. Acupressure and preoperative parental anxiety: a pilot study. Anesth Analg. 2005;101(3):666–9, table of contents.
33. Wang SM, Peloquin C, Kain ZN. The use of auricular acupuncture to reduce preoperative anxiety. Anesth Analg. 2001;93(5):1178–80, table of contents.
34. Karst M, Winterhalter M, Munte S, Francki B, Hondronikos A, Eckardt A, et al. Auricular acupuncture for dental anxiety: a randomized controlled trial. Anesth Analg. 2007;104(2):295–300.
35. Kober A, Scheck T, Schubert B, Strasser H, Gustorff B, Bertalanffy P, et al. Auricular acupressure as a treatment for anxiety in prehospital transport settings. Anesthesiology. 2003;98(6):1328–32.
36. Barker R, Kober A, Hoerauf K, Latzke D, Adel S, Kain ZN, et al. Out-of-hospital auricular acupressure in elder patients with hip fracture: a randomized double-blinded trial. Acad Emerg Med. 2006;13(1):19–23.
37. Kober A, Scheck T, Greher M, Lieba F, Fleischhackl R, Fleischhackl S, et al. Prehospital analgesia with acupressure in victims of minor trauma: a prospective, randomized, double-blinded trial. Anesth Analg. 2002;95(3):723–7, table of contents.
38. Schlager A, Offer T, Baldissera I. Laser stimulation of acupuncture point p6 reduces postoperative vomiting in children undergoing strabismus surgery. Br J Anaesth. 1998;81(4):529–32.
39. Chu YC, Lin SM, Hsieh YC, Peng GC, Lin YH, Tsai SK, et al. Effect of bl-10 (tianzhu), bl-11 (dazhu) and gb-34 (yanglinquan) acuplaster for prevention of vomiting after strabismus surgery in children. Acta Anaesthesiol Sin. 1998;36(1):11–6.
40. Schlager A, Boehler M, Puhringer F. Korean hand acupressure reduces postoperative vomiting in children after strabismus surgery. Br J Anaesth. 2000;85(2):267–70.
41. Somri M, Vaida SJ, Sabo E, Yassain G, Gankin I, Gaitini LA. Acupuncture versus ondansetron in the prevention of postoperative vomiting. A study of children undergoing dental surgery. Anaesthesia. 2001;56(10):927–32.
42. Rusy LM, Hoffman GM, Weisman SJ. Electroacupuncture prophylaxis of postoperative nausea and vomiting following pediatric tonsillectomy with or without adenoidectomy. Anesthesiology. 2002; 96(2):300–5.
43. Butkovic D, Toljan S, Matolic M, Kralik S, Radesic L. Comparison of laser acupuncture and metoclopramide in PONV prevention in children. Paediatr Anaesth. 2005;15(1):37–40.
44. Yeh CH, Chien LC, Chiang YC, Lin SW, Huang CK, Ren D. Reduction in nausea and vomiting in children undergoing cancer chemotherapy by either appropriate or sham auricular acupuncture points with standard care. J Altern Complement Med. 2012;18(4):334–40.
45. Kabalak AA, Akcay M, Akcay F, Gogus N. Transcutaneous electrical acupoint stimulation versus ondansetron in the prevention of postoperative vomiting following pediatric tonsillectomy. J Altern Complement Med. 2005;11(3):407–13.
46. Dune L. Integrating tuina acupressure and traditional Chinese medicine concepts into a holistic nursing practice. Explore. 2006;2(6):543–6.
47. Gan TJ, Meyer TA, Apfel CC, Chung F, Davis PJ, Habib AS, et al. Society for ambulatory anesthesia guidelines for the management of postoperative nausea and vomiting. Anesth Analg. 2007;105(6):1615–28, table of contents.
48. Atilla H, Isikay CT, Kansu T. Isolated sixth nerve palsy from pontine infarct. Acta Neurol Belg. 2000;100(4):246–7.
49. Johnston CC, Stremler RL, Stevens BJ, Horton LJ. Effectiveness of oral sucrose and simulated rocking on pain response in preterm neonates. Pain. 1997;72(1–2):193–9.
50. Johnston CC, Filion F, Campbell-Yeo M, Goulet C, Bell L, McNaughton K, et al. Enhanced kangaroo mother care for heel lance in preterm neonates: a crossover trial. J Perinatol. 2009; 29(1):51–6.
51. Lago P, Garetti E, Merazzi D, Pieragostini L, Ancora G, Pirelli A, et al. Guidelines for procedural pain in the newborn. Acta Paediatr. 2009;98(6):932–9.
52. Yip P, Middleton P, Cyna AM, Carlyle AV. Non-pharmacological interventions for assisting the induction of anaesthesia in children. Cochrane Database Syst Rev. 2009;(3):CD006447.
53. Lin JG, Chen K, Lee YC. Sedation. In: Lin YC, Hsu E, editors. Acupuncture for pain management. New York: Springer; 2014.
54. Gan TJ, Diemunsch P, Habib AS, et al. Consensus guidelines for the management of postoperative nausea and vomiting. Anesth Analg. 2014;118(1):85–113.

Pediatric Research: Designing, Implementing, and Interpreting Strong Trials

33

Andrew Davidson

Abstract

Clinical research is vital to generate the evidence to guide clinical practice. Clinical research may be qualitative or quantitative, and observational or interventional. A trial is an important form of interventional research designed to assess the effectiveness of a therapy. Trials may be efficacy trials focused on assessing efficacy in ideal circumstances or effectiveness trials conducted in wider real-life populations.

The most important aspect of good research is the research question. A good question is relevant and clearly defined. To be useful, a research study must be well designed and conducted well. Qualified statistical input is needed for nearly all high-quality research projects—particularly trials.

Research in children is challenging for many reasons including ethics, heterogeneity, and a paucity of validated outcome measures and basic pharmacological knowledge.

Keywords

Clinical research • Pediatrics • Clinical trial • Study design • Statistics • Translation • Statistical significance • Qualitative research • Quantitative research • Good clinical practice (GCP)

Introduction

Research is the systematic collection and analysis of information to create knowledge. Knowledge is information that can be used beyond the context of its collection to better understand and predict the natural world. In medicine, knowledge is used to better understand the cause and natural course of disease to develop new therapies or diagnostic tests, to improve medical practice, or to change the environment or human behavior. The ultimate goal is to improve health outcomes. In clinical care, research forms the backbone of evidence to guide best practice.

Researchers are driven by many motives: the desire to improve the health and care of their own patients, to create knowledge to benefit the wider population, curiosity and the thrill of discovery, or they just simply enjoy the intellectual challenge. Hospitals promote and support research to directly improve care of their patients, to increase the academic standing of the institution and hence to attract better clinical staff, and to create an academic enquiring culture that will foster the uptake of evidence-based practice and hence improve patient care. Not all clinicians should be expected to actively lead research; however, participating in and understanding the basic principles of research helps all clinicians to critically appraise any new evidence applicable to their practice.

This chapter briefly outlines the principles of clinical research. It is not intended to provide an exhaustive account of research design or biostatistics. For those wishing more detail, several texts are listed at the end of this chapter.

A. Davidson, M.B.B.S., M.D., F.A.N.Z.C.A. (✉)
Department of Anaesthesia and Pain Management,
The Royal Children's Hospital Melbourne, Murdoch Children's Research Institute, Melbourne, VIC, Australia
e-mail: andrew.davidson@rch.org.au

K.P. Mason (ed.), *Pediatric Sedation Outside of the Operating Room: A Multispecialty International Collaboration*,
DOI 10.1007/978-1-4939-1390-9_33, © Springer Science+Business Media New York 2015

Challenges Doing Pediatric Clinical Research

Children are often referred to as therapeutic orphans due to the paucity of data about even common therapies. Many drugs are "off label" in children. One reason for this is the lack of basic pharmacokinetic, pharmacodynamic, efficacy, and safety data in children. Recent government incentives in both the USA and Europe have increased the amount of drug research in children; however, there is still a long way to go. In March, 2014 the American Academy of Pediatrics and its Committee on Drugs published a policy statement on off-label drugs in children. The policy concluded that "evidence, not label indication, remains the gold standard from which practitioners should draw when making therapeutic decisions for their patients." The statement made recommendations for off-label drug administration and the advocating of off-label drug research and publication [1]. (Refer to Chap. 26.)

There are several reasons why clinical research falls behind in children:

1. Children are a heterogeneous group. They range from the premature neonate to the large adolescent. This range of weight and organ development means that studies may have to be done in multiple age strata. This increases the cost and complexity of research.
2. Children are not altruistic and children cannot volunteer for early phase clinical studies. Research ethical standards may be more rigorous in children as they are regarded as a vulnerable population. This may lengthen the approval process and may limit any invasive interventions or tests.
3. The market for therapies in children may not be as large as in adults. A sizable proportion of the total pediatric illness burden is made up of many separate rare diseases. There is less financial incentive for pharmaceutical industries to develop drugs for children.
4. Pediatric clinical studies require environments suited specifically to children. This limits the number of sites that can do pediatric research.

Apart from the above there are other aspects of pediatric studies that differ from adult studies. When designing a pediatric clinical study the following points must be considered before the study is developed:

1. Is the mechanism underlying the premise understood? If the pathology or physiology is not understood, it is very difficult to interpret clinical studies. For example, without knowing why awareness occurs in children it is difficult to design any clinical study to prevent awareness and difficult to know how to generalize the results from the study population of children to another population.
2. Is the outcome measure relevant and validated in children? Is it appropriate for the ages to be studied? Many measures are valid in adults but have never been properly validated in children. For example, adult measures of coagulation are often not relevant to children and indeed normal reference ranges for children have only recently been developed. Similarly, adult measures of consciousness cannot be applied to young children and quality of recovery scores are not well developed in children.
3. Are the outcome measures valid across the ages to be studied? For example, some form of pain scores may be valid in one age group but not ideal in another.
4. If the study is a drug study, are the doses appropriate for children? Have the basic pharmacokinetic and pharmacodynamic studies been performed to determine optimal dose and blood level? For example, we have little idea what is the optimal plasma level for propofol in young children.
5. Are the outcomes developmentally relevant? For example, neurobehavioral outcomes before the age of 2 are of limited value as many children will catch up with their peers regardless of the intervention.

Organizationally pediatric research also requires staff, equipment, and general environments that are suited for children.

Observational Research

Broadly speaking, clinical research may be divided into observational or interventional research. In observational research, data are collected without controlling or introducing new therapies. In interventional research, an intervention or therapy is applied according to a study protocol rather than the usual clinical decision-making practice.

Qualitative Research

Observational research may be qualitative or quantitative. Quantitative research deals with data based on some form of numerical scale. Qualitative research describes the nature of a phenomenon or experience. Qualitative data may need to be collected with open-ended questions or interviews. Analyzing the data consists of identifying common themes or dimensions of experience. Qualitative research is frequently useful before quantitative research. For example, before researching postoperative outcomes after total intravenous anesthesia (TIVA) the researcher needs to know what outcomes are important. Discovering important outcomes for the patient and family requires interviewing, open-ended questions, and exploring all types of families and patient experiences. Once common themes are identified, important outcomes can be defined and the researcher can then go on to quantitative research and count how often the relevant outcomes occur. Unfortunately, there is often a temptation to launch into quantitative research without sufficient preceding qualitative research. Qualitative research is particularly important in pediatric research where outcome measures have often been poorly developed.

Quantitative Research: Data Types

When counting or measuring outcomes it is vital to consider what type the data are. The type of data will dictate how you present, summarize, and analyze the data. Data may be described as categorical, ordinal, discrete, and continuous.

Categorical data are groups with no particular order amongst groups; for example, gender, operation type, ethnicity. Categorical data are usually summarized with counts, percentages, rates, or proportions.

Ordinal data is when there is a natural order or rank between groups without a direct mathematical relationship; for example, American Society of Anesthesiologists (ASA) status or grade of tumor. Ordinal data are usually summarized with counts, percentages, rates, or proportions, but also can be summarized with medians and ranges.

Numerical data is when the data is on a scale that has a constant mathematical relationship. *Discrete data* is numerical data when the numbers are whole integers; for example, numbers of vomits. *Continuous data* is when the data are on a continuous scale; for example, weight or drug concentration. Numeric data is presented with a measure of central tendency such as mean or median and a measure of spread such as standard deviation or interquartile range. When it comes to analysis, some tests (parametric tests) assume that data are numerical and normally distributed.

Sometimes it is unclear if data should be regarded as ordinal or numerical. For example, some verbal rating pain scores or the outputs of anesthesia depth monitors such as bispectral index (BIS).

Quantitative Research: Study Designs

Observational research may be retrospective, cross sectional, or prospective. Retrospective studies look at data already collected. Cross-sectional studies look at data at a particular time point, and prospective data collects data in a planned way moving forward in time from the present.

Case reports report single patient events or characteristics. A *case series* may report several similar patients or events.

A case control study starts with an outcome of interest and then looks backward to examine possible causes. The case is matched with similar subjects to see if exposures of interest are more common in cases compared to the controls. Case control studies are useful for rare outcomes.

Cohort studies are the most common observational studies. A cohort study starts with a group and follows the group forward in time and then compares characteristics of those in the cohort that develop a relevant outcome to those that did not determine possible cause of the outcome. A cohort study may be retrospective where the group is selected retrospectively.

Once qualitative research determines the outcomes of interest, observation studies may be simply descriptive—determining the prevalence or frequency of an event or outcome. Observational data may also be used to determine associations in analytic studies. Causation may then be further established prospectively in intervention studies.

Bias and Confounding

Bias and confounding can limit the validity of observational studies. Bias is a lack of accuracy where the variable does not represent what it is intended to measure due to systematic error. There are a number of causes of bias. *Selection bias* occurs when group allocation is uneven for some reason and this leads to an alteration in outcome of interest. *Detection bias* may occur if observation is poorer in quality in one group compared to the other. *Observer bias* occurs where there is a conscious or subconscious distortion of reporting or measuring by the observer; for example, by using leading questions in an interview. *Instrument bias* may occur if an instrument is poorly calibrated. *Reporting bias* is when the subject distorts their self-report of an outcome either consciously or subconsciously.

There is also a *response bias* if only a particular subsection of a population consents to a study. This reduces the generalizability or external validity of the study. Lastly, *publication bias* is where studies that find strong evidence for a difference in outcome are more likely to be published than those that find no evidence for a difference in outcome.

The Hawthorne effect is a particular type of bias where involvement in the study itself can influence the result beyond the effect of the intervention or exposure of interest; for example, if the process of consent or measurement influences outcome.

Confounding occurs when a factor influences both the likelihood of exposure (or baseline characteristics) and outcome, leading to the false assumption that the exposure or intervention causes the outcome. For example, premature babies are both at risk of poor neurobehavioral outcome and also at risk of having a hernia. This could lead to the false assumption that hernia repairs cause poor neurobehavioral outcome. Confounding is one of the most troublesome problems in observational studies. It may be reduced with matching or with adjustment for likely confounding factors in regression analysis, but such adjustments are never perfect and it is always possible that unknown factors are causing confounding. Increasing sample size in observational studies does not reduce confounding as the degree of confounding simply grows with the size of the study. Reducing confounding is the strongest argument for randomized trials.

Causality and Association

Observational studies can demonstrate associations between exposures (or interventions) and outcomes but because of confounding they have a limited capacity to demonstrate causation. In a classic publication, Sir Bradford Hills described nine factors that can assist with determining causation from mere association [2]:

1. Strength of association: there is a large effect size and the precision or evidence is strong and the methodology is rigorous
2. Consistency: the same effect is seen in multiple similar studies
3. Specificity: the effect or outcome is clearly defined and circumscribed
4. Temporality: the outcome clearly follows the exposure or intervention
5. Biological gradient: the effect size is greater with greater dose or duration of exposure
6. Plausibility: there is a mechanistic explanation based on preclinical work
7. Coherence: the outcome is similar in different populations
8. Experiment: the effect can be modified by modifying the exposure or intervention
9. Analogy: similar exposures or interventions have similar effects

Trials

A trial is a systematic study to determine the effect of an intervention. It usually refers to those studies where the intervention is determined by a protocol. A randomized controlled trial is where treatment allocation is randomized. If treatment is randomized, there cannot be a systematic relationship between an external factor and treatment allocation, thus confounding is minimized. Randomized trials are always prospective.

Trials may be blinded where the subject, observer, and researchers may be unaware of treatment allocation until analysis is complete. Blinding is important as it reduces the possibility bias. In a randomized controlled trial there may be one or more different treatment groups and a control group. The control group may get "usual" treatment or no active treatment (placebo). Results are easiest to interpret where there are simply two groups: new treatment and established treatment. Trials may be unblinded or "open label" where researchers and subjects know which treatment is being given. Open label studies may be performed where blinding is impossible or impractical; for example, comparing a spinal versus general anesthesia.

Other trial designs include a *crossover trial* where the same subject receives both treatments one after the other. They may or may not be given in random order. This design reduces patient variability as the same subject gets both treatments; however, other bias may be introduced if the first treatment has a carryover effect into the next treatment period.

An *n of one trial* is where a treatment or series of different treatments is tried on just one patient.

Cluster trials are when groups are randomized rather than individuals. This is done where it is impractical to randomize within departments or clinics. For example, when assessing an educational program, a whole class at school may receive an educational program rather than trying to give each individual subject a different program. Cluster trials are weaker due to cluster bias. When subjects are randomized by group, this reduces the inter-subject variability, which may make differences look more certain than they really are. This bias can be partly adjusted for.

Phase of Trials

Drug trials are often described as occurring in different phases.

- Phase I: Studies to determine pharmacokinetics and safety, usually conducted in healthy volunteers, or unresponsive patients
- Phase II: Studies to determine dose–response curves and benefits in small populations
- Phase III: Trials to determine the benefits in larger, more heterogeneous, and clinically relevant populations
- Phase IV: Post-marketing surveillance studies for additional safety data

It is very unusual to have "first-in-man" studies in children. Drugs are usually first tested in healthy volunteer adults or adults with refractory disease.

Efficacy and Effectiveness

Clinical trials may be further defined as efficacy and effectiveness studies. Efficacy trials are designed to determine if a therapy works in ideal circumstances; usually with narrow inclusion criteria. Effectiveness studies are designed to see if therapies work in real-life circumstances, usually with larger samples and broader inclusion criteria. Efficacy is usually established before effectiveness. Both are needed to guide clinical decisions. If only efficacy studies are performed, it may be doubted if therapies work in real clinical situations.

Heath Service Delivery Research

Health service delivery research is research into how the health system works. For example, this may include systematically investigating how to increase throughput in a hospital or the operating room. It could also be more community based; for example, determining how best to provide a service and meet patient needs across the state or country. Health service research is closely linked to Quality (see later). To be effective, health services research requires reliable and valid measures of health outcomes or quality of life or recovery; in children there are very few such measures that are proven to be reliable and valid [3]. As the cost of health steadily increases, governments, hospitals, and insurers are increasingly interested in promoting health service delivery research.

Implementation Science

Enormous amounts of knowledge are generated by medical research. This is largely wasted if it does not result in clinicians changing practice. Implementation science (also known as knowledge transfer) is the study of clinician behavior, educational modalities, and health care systems to determine how knowledge can most effectively and efficiently lead to change in practice and hence improved health outcomes. Like health service delivery research, implementation science is being seen as increasingly important to provide a cost-efficient health system. Implementation science and health services delivery research may involve a variety of research designs including trials.

Translation

Research translation has become a buzz word in medical research. The translational pathway is the concept that knowledge generated in one modality of research can be passed down the pathway from basic science to clinical research to change in practice and improved outcomes (Fig. 33.1). Research translation is the process of passing that knowledge along and translational research is any research that has potential to be passed along [4].

The focus on translation is due to the ever-increasing research budgets in the face of stubbornly stable global or national health indices. Research that has no potential for translation may be regarded as having less potential value. It is harder for basic science researchers to follow areas of interest or curiosity with no clear idea of how the outcomes of the research might eventually make a difference to health outcomes.

Traditionally the pathway has gone from basic science to clinical to community; discovery to innovation to application. However, the pathway can and should go both ways. For greater efficiency, public health imperatives should drive the questions that drive the basic science research.

There are two well-described blocks in translation. The first is often known as T1 and is the bottleneck between basic science discovery in the lab and early phase clinical studies. Many promising therapies never make it over the "valley of death" into clinical trials [5]. For every successful drug in clinical trials, dozens are tested in the lab. This greatly increases the cost of developing new drugs. The second block, known as T2, is between successful trials and change in practice and improved outcomes [6]. Implementation science addresses this block.

An important concept is research *into* translation. Funding bodies and pharmaceutical companies are looking for ways to improve the process of translation to make the whole medical research system more efficient using such technologies as advanced modeling and bioinformatics [7].

Quality Improvement

Quality improvement (QI) involves formal analysis of performance followed by the use of systematic efforts to improve it. The Institute of Medicine in the USA defines quality along six dimensions: safety, effectiveness, patient-centered, timeliness, efficiency, and equity [8].

Strictly speaking, outcomes reported in quality improvement programs are institution specific. Thus they are not generalizable knowledge and the results themselves are not publishable [9]. However, this distinction may be blurred. QI

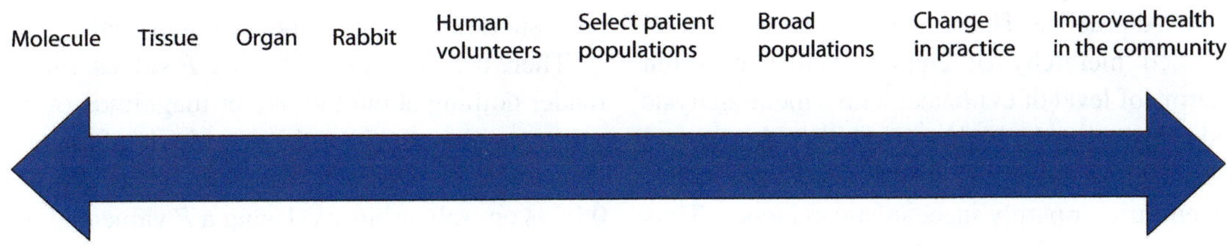

Fig. 33.1 The translational pathway

activity may reveal novel associations or insights into therapy that are indeed new, generalizable, and publishable; thus, while the QI data was not primarily collected for research, research may be performed on the data. As more and more data are accumulated by QI projects, more research studies are performed "mining" this data. There are, however, significant limitations inherent in this data mining (see later).

QI may also be publishable as a report of the system itself rather than the results. Such QI reports are an integral part of health service delivery research.

Audit is a term often used to mean the systematic collection of new or examination of existing clinical data. To avoid confusion, it is preferable to try and avoid the term if possible. If the study is a cohort study, then it is best to call it a cohort study rather than an audit. If the audit is part of a QI project, then indicate it is part of a QI project.

The Theory of Research

To fully understand the limitations of research requires an understanding of the theory and philosophy underlying research.

Mechanistic and Empiric Research

In ancient Greece, medical practitioners were either empiricist or dogmatists. An empiricist made no attempt to describe or understand the mechanism underlying disease but could predict an outcome from having seen the outcome after a large number of similar observations. A dogmatist relied on underlying truths or universal laws to explain mechanisms and hence predict the outcome. The two were merged by Galen who thought that treatment was best based on both reason and experience. In some ways, modern medicine is still a mix of empiricist and dogmatist. The dogmatist philosophy is that the molecular or even genomic mechanisms underlying disease and therapy can help clinicians understand what is going on with their patient and hence how best to treat them. On the other hand, the empiricist approach is to guide therapy based on large well-conducted observational studies. Sir Bradford Hills echoed Galen when he stated that causation was best proven with both strength of association and biologic plausibility. Clinicians seek to follow evidence-based practice. That evidence is based on both the well-described hierarchy of empiric evidence (often expressed in terms of level of evidence, with a meta-analysis of randomized trials being the highest level of evidence) and on an understanding of the mechanisms. Clinicians rarely rely on purely empiric or purely mechanistic evidence. Thus research can be either mechanistic or empiric and both are equally needed to guide practice. When designing studies, it sometimes helps to think if you are seeking empiric or mechanistic evidence. For example, is your study seeking to determine the pharmacokinetics of propofol in children, or is it seeking to see if propofol TIVA improves recovery? Mechanistic studies seek tightly controlled experimental conditions to reduce natural variability.

Hypotheses

Research is often centered on hypotheses. It is important to understand the limitations of hypothesis-driven research. Inductive reasoning is the generation of a "law" or "truth" based on a number of observations. In contrast, deductive reasoning is applying general laws to predict a particular outcome. The validity of inductive reasoning is inherently limited as the number of observations is always limited. For example, a man may see many white swans without ever seeing a black swan and incorrectly deduce that all swans are white.

In the early twentieth century, the hypothetico-deductive method was introduced to address the limitations of inductive reasoning. This involves a hypothesis being generated and then tested with an experiment or observation. If the hypothesis does not fit with the observation, it is rejected. To test a hypothesis, the null hypothesis is first generated; a statement that the intervention has no effect on the outcome of interest. The complementary alternative hypothesis is that the intervention does have some effect. In clinical research, a sample is tested and an inference made on the population from which the sample is drawn. In particular, the null hypothesis is that there is no effect seen in the population from which the sample was drawn. The P value is the probability that the result seen in the sample could have occurred randomly or by chance. If the P value is less than an arbitrary set point (often 0.05), then the null hypothesis is rejected and it is thus assumed that the intervention has some effect. A type I error is if the null hypothesis is incorrectly rejected while a type II error is if the null hypothesis is incorrectly accepted.

Most trials are superiority trials where the null hypothesis is that there is no effect. A trial may also be designed as an equivalence trial where the null hypothesis is that the effect is greater than some set level (a point predetermined as being clinically significant). Equivalence and superiority trials have subtle differences in design and analysis.

There are limitations in using P values. Firstly, it tells the reader nothing about the size or magnitude of the effect. A P value may be <0.05 but the magnitude of the effect or difference might be clinically irrelevant. Secondly, the set point of 0.05 is entirely arbitrary. Using a P value and the underlying hyothetico-deductive method forces clinical research into a dichotomous outcome; either something has an effect or not.

This is not well suited to clinical research where we may be more interested in the size or magnitude of an effect. Both the *P* value and hypotheses are likely to be gradually phased out of clinical research.

Instead of testing hypotheses and generating *P* values, a superior method is to consider a trial as a way to estimate the size of effect along with an indication of the precision around the estimate of that effect. This is expressed as reporting the actual effect (often a difference in means, risk ratio, odds ratio, or something similar) and the 95 % confidence intervals around the effect. This gives the reader an idea of the magnitude of the effect and the precision around the estimate.

The word "statistical significance" is often used to indicate a result with a *P* value <0.05. In contrast, "clinical significance" is used to indicate that the magnitude of the effect is enough to be clinically important. Using the word "significant" alone is ambiguous and thus meaningless. As mentioned before, "statistically significant" is entirely arbitrary and should perhaps be avoided. Similarly "clinically significant" can also be problematic; as what is clinically important may vary between populations and clinicians. If the words "clinically significant" are to be used, then it is optimal to justify why that size of effect is indeed important.

Problems also arise differentiating "no difference" from "equivalence." These problems are more acute if *P* values are used. No difference usually means the *P* value is greater than 0.05. However, this does not mean equivalence. Firstly, strictly speaking, equivalence can only be determined if the trial was designed and analyzed as an equivalence trial. Secondly, equivalence can only be assumed if the 95 % confidence interval around the observed difference does not cross what would be regarded as a clinically significant difference.

Lastly, as previously mentioned, even if the *P* value is >0.05, the breadth of the 95 % confidence interval still needs to be considered in terms of what might be clinically relevant. If the 95 % confidence interval is entirely beneath what would be regarded as clinically relevant, then the result shows a "statistically significant" difference that is "clinically insignificant." If the *P* value is >0.05 and the 95 % interval partly lies below what may be regarded as clinically relevant. The result is "statistically significant" and possibly "clinically significant."

In summary, it is best to avoid *P* values and better to report 95 % confidence intervals. Authors should only claim there is a difference, no difference, or equivalence if the magnitude and precision of the result clearly fit these criteria. If there is any doubt, then report the findings and let the reader decide if the precision and magnitude of effect warrant a conclusion that the result is a clinically relevant difference, no difference, or equivalence.

Doing a Clinical Research Project

For research to be useful and not misleading, it must be of high quality. Doing high-quality research is not a simple task. The study must be well designed and carefully conducted. Researchers now rarely work in isolation. The simple questions have been answered and the remaining more challenging questions require efficient and effective research teams maximizing collaboration and sharing skills and resources; the wise saying of "publish or perish" has been replaced by "collaborate or collapse."

The Research Question

The most important element in any research study is the research question. Without a clear prospective research question, there is no research project. If you have ever read a research paper and had no idea what the paper was about, then the researchers either had no coherent questions or they were unable to clearly articulate their question. The question drives all stages of the project: from protocol, to conduct, to analysis, and publication.

A good research question is relevant, original, feasible, plausible, and defined.

Relevant: There is no point in answering a question when nobody cares what the answer might be. The question must have the capacity for translation. When considering relevance, ask if the appropriate qualitative research has been done. Do you know what the relevant outcome actually is? Is it relevant to all stakeholders: patient, family, community, health dollar provider, and clinician? It is easy to know what is relevant for clinicians, but more important to find out what is relevant to *all* the stakeholders. Engaging stakeholders when formulating the research question will increase the chance that the research will be translated and change practice.

Original: There is less interest in answering a question that is already answered. A thorough literature search will show that most of your ideas have been thought of before. However, replication is also important. Going back to Sir Bradford Hills, consistency increases the veracity of results and the likelihood that causation is real. Increasingly, journals are realizing that replication studies are important if the question is important.

Feasible: There is no point trying to answer an unanswerable question. For example, we cannot know if TIVA reduces nausea in neonates as we have no way of measuring nausea in a neonate. Feasibility may also be limited by available subjects, resources, funds, and ethics. Pilot studies may be necessary to determine if a protocol is feasible, i.e., will people actually follow it and can the data be successfully collected. For example, a pilot study might be needed to see if clinicians can actually follow a protocol that requires aiming for a very low or high blood concentration of anesthetic.

Plausible: A clinical study should be based on some biologic plausibility. There should be some mechanistic rationale for the study; for example, determining if the color of the premedication influences emergence delirium incidence is probably a bad research question. A purist following hypothetico-deductive theory, however, would argue that all research should have no preconceived idea of likely outcome. In reality, we are Bayesian and we tend to do research with some idea of what we expect. This leads to more efficient use of resources, but does increase the risk of propagating incorrect dogma.

Defined: a research question is usually defined in terms of PICOT for interventional studies and PECOT for observational studies:

- Population
- Intervention or Exposure
- Comparator
- Outcome
- Time frame

Defining the question and indicating how it is relevant, original, and plausible will form the background of the protocol and the introduction of the paper.

One of the challenges in clinical research is finding original ideas and good research questions. Good questions are driven by clinical need and/or innovation or discovery further up the translational pathway; for example, new drugs or new technologies. Good questions often arise in academic departments where researchers and clinicians work together. Research questions may arise from quality improvement activities, or when knowledge holes are identified when attempting to write clinical practice guidelines.

Developing the Protocol

Once a good research question has been defined, the next step is to write the protocol. It is very wise to use a protocol template recognized by your IRB or ethics committee. A full protocol is essential for every research project—even a simple retrospective cohort study reviewing patient notes. Note that by defining the question with PICOT or PECOT the inclusion criteria and outcome measures have already been prepared.

The collection of baseline data should be described and the intervention also should be described in great detail. Similarly the protocol should explain exactly how the subjects will be recruited, randomized, and provide details of all blinding procedures.

A particularly important aspect of the protocol is defining the outcome measures. There should be one primary outcome measure and this measure should be that which is most closely linked to the research question. There may be multiple secondary outcomes. These are usually related in some way to the primary outcome. All outcomes and measures should be defined in the protocol.

The protocol should include a justification for the number of subjects enrolled. Enrolling too few may result in a study with inadequate power leading to inadequate precision. Enrolling an excess may be unethical and waste resources. To determine the number of subjects, the researchers need to first define the primary outcome of interest. Then there needs to be an estimate of the variability or standard deviation in that outcome if it is numerical data or the frequency of the event of interest if it is categorical or ordinal. The researchers should also decide what level of precision they would accept.

Protocols should have version numbers and dates of drafting. If the study is at multiple sites, the same protocol should be used at each site. Any significant modification of the approved protocol requires ethical and other regulatory review.

Some trials will require an independent safety and data monitoring committee and/or a formal trial steering committee. If an interim analysis is planned, criteria for this must be carefully determined before the trial starts.

Pilot Studies

Pilot studies are frequently needed prior to a trial. The pilot study answers a question that will help answer the larger question in the definitive study. A pilot study may be required to identify the frequency of outcome if it is a dichotomous event or variability in a numerical outcome. Pilot studies may also involve qualitative research to better refine or justify the outcome of interest.

Sometimes pilot studies test the feasibility of the protocol. Can researchers actually enrol subjects, follow the protocol, and obtain the outcome data in real-life clinical situations? This is important for complex protocols and for large studies.

Ethical Approval

All human research requires some form of ethical review and oversight. Trials are often regarded as higher risk than observational studies as the researcher is essentially experimenting on a human being.

Research ethics is based on a number of core principles:

- *Beneficence*: Where possible every effort should be made to benefit the subject and not cause unnecessary harm, burden, or risk.
- *Respect for persons*: The rights of the individual should be respected. Obtaining informed and free consent is a crucial aspect of respect. Respecting privacy is also important.
- *Justice*: Research should not unduly benefit or harm a subsection of the population for the benefit of the broad population. Vulnerable subjects should be protected. Research should also not ignore a subsection of the population.
- *Merit and integrity*: Ethical research must be well designed, well conducted, and useful to the community. Research that is irrelevant, poorly designed, underpowered, or sloppily conducted produces results that are either useless or misleading. That is unethical.

To maximize beneficence, trials should strive for equipoise. Equipoise is when the risks and benefits in each arm of the study are judged to be equal. The need for equipoise can make using a placebo difficult as this would only be ethical if it were fairly certain that the therapy did not have any effect. In reality there is often some plausible reason to expect that one treatment arm is more likely to be effective. This may be ethical if the individual is informed of risks and likely benefits and then consents.

There are added dimensions to ethical research in children. Children are often too young to understand and thus cannot consent. They are also vulnerable to coercion, making free consent more difficult. They may also be too young to be regarded as acting altruistically. Thus there is closer scrutiny of trials in children; risk and burden must be minimal and the equipoise should be more certain. It is, however, recognized that it would be unethical to make it harder to conduct research in children, thus there is a tension between principles. Lastly, research in children is unethical if it is not conducted in an environment suited to children and with methods applicable to children.

Regulatory Issues

As well as ethical approval, research studies require a variety of governance and regulatory standards. Researchers should be trained in GCP (Good Clinical Practice). GCP is an internationally recognized code of conduct that ensures high-quality data collection. It focuses on research ethics, ensuring the data are collected appropriately and verifiable, adequate documentation, ensuring the research team functions and communicates well, that researchers have appropriate qualifications, and there is appropriate supervision with defined reporting lines. It also covers how adverse events should be defined, detected, and reported.

Trials must also be registered before commencement on a public trials registration website (such as http://clinicaltrials.gov). Registration is mandatory for most high impact journals. Registration provides an indicator of how many trials are performed but not published. This is to help reduce publication bias—the risk that trials that report finding a difference are more likely to be published than those that do not. It also allows readers and editors to check that the trial was performed the way it was intended to be performed. This is important for the validity of the trial and reduces the risk that post hoc analyses are published without declaring they are post hoc (see later).

Before starting a trial, the case record form should be thoroughly reviewed. Data must be collected in an unambiguous manner. Numerical and categorical data are far easier to enter into a database and analyze than free text. Also researchers should avoid collecting excessive amounts of data as this will increase the burden for data collectors and increase the risk that data will be incorrect or incomplete.

Every research project should also have a delegation log clearly indicating who can perform all the various functions in the study team, along with documentation supporting qualifications needed to perform these tasks. If the trial is run at multiple sites, there must be formal written agreements between sites outlining responsibilities.

Analysis Plan

An analysis plan is essential. It should be written in detail before any data are seen or analyzed. Ideally, it would be written before the data are collected. If the study involves a retrospective analysis of existing data, the analysis plan must be written before looking at any of the data in any form.

A prospectively written analysis plan helps avoid data- or outcome-driven research. With the increased amount of data now collected electronically, data-driven research is becoming a major problem for biomedical research (data mining). Data-driven research occurs when the researchers have seen the data in some form and thus have an idea of possible outcome before they decide exactly how to analyze the data. The danger in the form of analysis will be chosen to maximize the chance of identifying the effect or association that the researcher suspects or wants—even subconsciously. Inevitably there are many subtle variations in how data can be analyzed. All choices in the analysis should be made prospectively on carefully considered clinical or biological grounds.

Problems can also arise if multiple analyses are performed on the same data set, particularly if multiple unrelated hypotheses are tested. If $P<0.05$ is taken as "significant," then it is inevitable that the more hypotheses there are, the more likely some will be deemed significant purely by chance. Traditionally this can be partly accounted for by accepting only lower P values as "significant." However, this is unsatisfactory for all the reasons already mentioned and an alternative approach is to consider such analyses as "hypothesis generating" rather than "hypothesis testing" and report no P values at all.

Need for Statistical Help

There are many statistical challenges in the design and reporting of trials. From a statistical perspective there is no such thing as a simple trial. Therefore, all trials should have strong statistical input. For a large and complex trial, this should be from a statistician with experience in large complex trials. Statistical input is needed throughout the trial from defining the research question to preparing the final paper.

Running the Project

Principles of GCP should be followed during the study. Protocol violations and adverse events must be identified, recorded, and reported appropriately. Nobody should be allowed to analyze the outcome data before the trial is closed except within the criteria of any predetermined interim analysis. Running a large trial is like running a small business; it requires careful budgeting, good team management and planning, and managing external relationships. To maintain momentum, all stakeholders and relevant staff should be informed about trial progress, ideally through regular presentations or newsletters.

During the trial, the data should be queried as needed and entered into a database. The database should meet the basic requirements for recording trial data, including proper security, specific log in codes, and means to identify when and by whom any entries are altered.

When recruitment is complete, data is cleaned and final queries answered before the database is closed, and a single primary analysis is performed following the predetermined analysis plan. If secondary analyses are performed, it must be clearly noted in any presentation or publication that the analysis was secondary (post hoc). Secondary analyses run the risk of being outcome driven as previously mentioned and hence have less validity than the primary analysis.

Reporting Results

Once the analysis is finished, all stakeholders should be informed of the results. Results should be published quickly while there is still momentum [10]. For trials, results should be reported using the CONSORT format [11]. Authorship should follow standard authorship guidelines and ideally decided well before the study is completed. At this stage the researchers should follow their plan for translation; informing important stakeholders and policy makers, and, if need be, incorporating the results into new clinical practice guidelines.

Big Trials

Large trials have greater power and can recruit faster, answering important questions sooner. Large trials also reduce the risk of random imbalance between groups confounding the trial results. Multicenter trials have the added advantage of having a more heterogeneous population increasing the generalizability of the results. A diverse population may also enable hypothesis-generating post hoc sub-analyses in particular subpopulations.

Large multisite trials are more difficult to perform as there needs to be close coordination between sites and agreement over protocol, intellectual property, and authorship. Data management can also be challenging. Particular attention is needed to keep the group cohesive and momentum going. Successful collaborations inevitably lead to networks that spawn bigger and better trials.

Funding

After a decade of having steadily risen, funding for clinical research has now plateaued in many countries. Funding bodies are increasingly looking for more "bang for their buck." It is thus even more important that research questions are relevant. Funding agencies have also recognized the importance of collaboration and, being more risk averse, are particularly interested in proven feasibility and a track record of quality research.

Traditionally pediatrics has been relatively underfunded compared to adult medicine; however, recent US and European Union government incentives have begun to result in an increase in pediatric clinical research.

Conclusion

Future Challenges and Possibilities in Pediatric Research

Genomics and other "omics" will potentially greatly increase our mechanistic understanding of disease and guide new therapies. (Refer to Chap. 11.) It can be argued that in all trials, DNA should be taken for future analysis as we understand more about how genetics may influence pharmacology and disease.

Another future challenge is the huge increase in the amount of population and clinical data now available; particularly with electronic medical records and better data linkage. The ease of collecting data may fundamentally change how we do observational studies. Such research, however, is only as good as the data entered.

References

1. American Academy of Pediatrics Committee on Drugs. Policy statement: off-label use of drugs in children. Pediatrics. 2014;133(3):563–7.
2. Hill AB. The environment and disease: association or causation? Proc R Soc Med. 1965;58:295–300.
3. McCormick MC, Flores G, Freed GL, Homer CJ, Johnson KB, DeFriese GH. Challenge to child health services research: report from the Committee on Pediatric Health and Health Care Quality Measures. Acad Pediatr. 2011;11(4):257–9.
4. Davidson A. Translational research: what does it mean? Anesthesiology. 2011;115(5):909–11.
5. Butler D. Translational research: crossing the valley of death. Nature. 2008;453(7197):840–2.
6. Woolf SH. The meaning of translational research and why it matters. JAMA. 2008;299(2):211–3.
7. Collins FS. Reengineering translational science: the time is right. Sci Transl Med. 2011;3(90):90cm17.
8. Varughese AM, Hagerman NS, Kurth CD. Quality in pediatric anesthesia. Paediatr Anaesth. 2010;20(8):684–96.
9. Shafer SL. Anesthesia & Analgesia policy on institutional review board approval and informed consent for research. Anesth Analg. 2011;112(3):494–5.
10. Davidson AJ, Carlin JB. What a reviewer wants. Paediatr Anaesth. 2008;18(12):1149–56.
11. Rennie D. How to report randomized controlled trials. The CONSORT statement. JAMA. 1996;276(8):649.

Recommended Reading

Myles PS, Gin T. Statistical methods for anaesthesia and intensive care. Oxford: Butterworth Heinemann; 2000.

Hulley SB, Cummings SR, Browner WS, Grady DG, Newman TB. Designing clinical research. Philadelphia: Lippincott Williams & Wilkins; 2013.

Non-pharmacological Distraction Techniques as Sedation Adjunct

34

Daniela Hearst

Abstract

While great progress has been made in the last 35 years to make hospitals and hospital procedures more user friendly and child oriented, being in a hospital, even as a day case, can be a bewildering and frightening experience for many children and young people who have to cope with many unfamiliar sights, sounds, smells, and the hustle and bustle of adults in unfamiliar clothing. This chapter seeks to place procedural anxiety within a developmental framework and describes evidence-based preparation and interventions that can work alongside pharmacological agents to minimize distress for invasive and noninvasive medical procedures. General principles for good practice are proposed and different techniques described. The limitations of the research base are discussed and suggestions for managing the uncooperative child are made. Case studies are given in conclusion.

Keywords

Augmentative and alternative communication (AAC) • Non-pharmacological • Distraction • Uncooperative child • Anxiety • Fear • Distress • Stress • Behavioral intervention • Guided imagery • Relaxation • Breathing • Rehearsal • Reinforcement • Hypnosis • Developmental stage • Special needs • Child life specialist • Clinical psychologist • Autistic spectrum disorder (ASD) • Children's Hospital of Eastern Ontario Pain Scale (CHEOPS) • Face, Legs, Activity, Cry, and Consolability Scale (FLACC) • Procedural Behavior Rating Scale (PBRS) • Pediatric Behavior Checklist (PBCL) • Child-Adult Medical Procedures Interaction Scale (CAMPIS) • Modified Yale Perioperative Anxiety Scale (m-YPAS) • Induction Compliance Checklist (ICC) • Emotionality, Activity and Sociability Scale (EAS) • Post-hospital Behavioral Questionnaire (PBHQ) • Non-communicating Children's Pain Checklist (NCCPC) • Revised FLACC Scale (FLACC-R)

Introduction

I work in a specialist children's hospital as a clinical psychologist with expertise in pediatrics. My role is to facilitate the child's and family's adaptation to illness or medical condition and treatment, reduce psychological distress, promote optimal development, and help improve their sense of well-being and health outcomes. When I walk through the reception and outpatient areas, I see children with nasogastric tubes, metal frames on legs and faces, and children who look different in a variety of ways as a result of congenital anomalies or treatment. A combination of tedium and anxiety pervades the waiting areas for investigations. This is my work environment and I choose to be there. Our patients and their parents usually do not. While great progress has been made in the last 35 years to make hospitals and hospital procedures more user friendly and child oriented, being in a

D. Hearst, B.Sc. (Hons)., M.Phil. (✉)
Department of Paediatric Psychology, Psychosocial and Family Services, Great Ormond Street Hospital for Children NHS Foundation Trust, London, UK
e-mail: Daniela.Hearst@gosh.nhs.uk

K.P. Mason (ed.), *Pediatric Sedation Outside of the Operating Room: A Multispecialty International Collaboration*,
DOI 10.1007/978-1-4939-1390-9_34, © Springer Science+Business Media New York 2015

hospital, even as a day case, can be a bewildering and frightening experience for many children and young people who have to cope with many unfamiliar sights, sounds, smells, and the hustle and bustle of adults in unfamiliar clothing.

This chapter seeks to place procedural anxiety within a developmental framework and describes evidence-based preparation and interventions that can work alongside pharmacological agents to minimize distress for invasive and noninvasive medical procedures. General principles for good practice are proposed and different techniques described. The limitations of the research base are discussed and suggestions for managing the uncooperative child are made. Case studies are given in conclusion.

It has long been recognized that children find hospitals and hospital procedures stressful. In 1941, Pearson reported the adverse emotional reactions young children displayed undergoing anesthesia for surgery [1]. Children show their distress in a variety of ways: ceasing to talk or play, becoming agitated, restless, appearing frightened, trembling, crying, sudden urination, increased muscle tone, or even attempting to run away from medical staff [2, 3]. Hospital procedures including injections, venipunctures, lumbar punctures, bone marrow aspirations, insertion of lines and drains, and dressing changes are all potential stressors. Children are afraid of (1) separation from parents; (2) physical pain, death, or mutilation; (3) strange environment and procedures; (4) humiliation through loss of control and competence; and (5) uncertainty about what is acceptable behavior [4]. Even "minor" nonpainful procedures such as X-ray, computerized tomography (CT) and magnetic resonance imaging (MRI) scans, swallowing pills, a dental examination, or having a plaster cast fitted or removed can be experienced as malign, distressing, and stressful. For parents there is the additional underlying fear of investigations delivering bad news.

Stress can be conceptualized as an interaction between a person and their environment that is perceived as taxing and a threat to personal well-being. Stress causes physiological, cognitive, emotional, behavioral, and interpersonal changes. Physiological changes include raised heart, respiration rates, rise in blood pressure, and elevated skin temperature. Cognitive information processing can become overly pessimistic and hopeless. Emotional responses include anger, fear, and depression. Behavioral changes include avoidance, self-soothing (e.g., thumb sucking or nail biting), and inability to concentrate. Interpersonal responses include impaired communication with and perceptions of others. Thus hospital-induced stress can create a feeling of threat. This threat—the perception of danger by physical injury or psychological damage to self—causes both fear and anxiety, and it is useful to distinguish between the two. Anxiety, implying potential rather than immediate threat, is characterized by wariness, watchfulness, apprehension, and inhibition [5] and can be present in children as early as 6–9 months old [6]. Fear—physiological, emotional, cognitive, and behavioral—is the reaction to threatening and harmful stimulus and the response to immediately dangerous situations, leading to a flight or fright response. In young children, this produces urgent seeking for physical proximity to the parent or primary attachment figure. In older children flight might be literal as they bolt from the procedure room. In fear and anxiety states, a child's attention becomes narrow and concentrated on the source of threat. Fear and anxiety can become debilitating and cause transient or long-term behavioral disturbance, particularly when the threat is repeated or prolonged. However, it is not uncommon for medical professionals to see a child's anxiety as out of proportion to the procedure; the child is then labeled as having procedural phobia and is referred for psychological therapy. A phobia is an inappropriately exaggerated and prolonged response to a harmless or benign stimulus and medical procedures are rarely perceived by children as a benign experience. It is more useful to speak about anticipatory anxiety or distress.

Why is it important to try to reduce procedural anxiety? It prevents later problems and is cost effective. Despite their resilience, children experience the anticipatory anxiety associated with a procedure as the most distressing aspect of healthcare [7]. Procedures involving needles are particularly aversive for children; a recent survey found that approximately two-thirds of children are frightened of needles [8]. When procedures have to be repeated (for example, a child with leukemia may have 8–15 invasive procedures in the first month of induction therapy) [9], children may become sensitized to the procedures such that these become not only distressing but also traumatic, with negative effects on behavior and well-being. Children remember their experiences and, while a child's age is predictive of distress, children do not simply "grow out of it." It has been estimated that around one-quarter of adults are afraid of needles [10] and for approximately 10 % the fear is such that they neglect their routine dental care and vaccinations [11, 12]. A distressed child produces a distressed parent, who may feel helpless to alleviate their child's suffering. Anger directed at their parents for allowing "nasty people to hurt me" may adversely affect family relationships and parental confidence in supporting their child's care at subsequent hospital visits. It is not just parental confidence that can be undermined; it is equally difficult for medical staff when their patients become very distressed and resistant. There are also cost benefits both to hospital and the family in reducing procedural distress: reduced time for procedures, fewer cancelled or rescheduled appointments, and higher parental satisfaction with the service.

There is a wide variation in pain and distress responses in children, related to individual characteristics of the child and their parents as well as environmental/contextual factors.

The Child

Children aged 1–5 years show the most behavioral distress and pain responses compared to older children [13]. Shy children with poorer social skills and lower adaptability to change tend to be more anxious. Lower adaptability, low mood, and high emotionality have been shown to be associated with higher levels of distress [14]. Children who are sensitive to change and new situations and those with developmental delay are more likely to be anxious in an unfamiliar hospital setting. The outer calm or apparent disdain of adolescents may belie a fear of waking up during a sedated procedure or not waking up at all.

The Parents

Parental physiological responses—heart rate, salivary amylase levels [15, 16]—correlate with their child's behavior during procedures. Children of highly anxious parents are themselves more anxious, as are children of divorced or separated parents. Mothers tend to be more anxious compared to fathers. When a child's condition is chronic, requiring regular hospital visits and in-patient episodes, parental anxiety is increased; it is also related to the child's temperament [17].

The Context of Treatment

The behavior of medical staff can affect anxiety levels in the child if they inadvertently give verbal and nonverbal cues that convey irritation or impatience. Machinery, vials with blood, and instruments can all be anxiety provoking. Even the application of a local topical anesthetic can induce fear [18]. Children who unexpectedly attend emergency departments for isolated, acute conditions may have little previous experience or acquired knowledge of hospitals and medical procedures compared to those children whose chronic conditions require frequent hospital attendance. A routine and identical procedure can cause greater distress in children who are unfamiliar with hospital staff and procedures [19].

Assessing Anxiety

Clinicians who are used to working with children will often accurately judge a child's mood or state within a few minutes in their presence. Indeed, pediatric anesthetists can often predict children's anxiety better than their mothers [20]. However, subjective assessment can be unreliable and more formal assessment may be helpful, particularly in situations where a child is receiving sequential procedures over an extended time period. There are many measures of assessing pain and distress using self-report, report by others, observational measures, and physiological measures, but there is no agreed gold standard. Each measure has its strength and limitations with varying suitability for different situations. While self-report by children may be considered the ideal of measurement, there are recognized limitations and issues for reliability that become evident in a clinical setting: Very young children cannot complete measures; highly anxious and distressed children may over- or underreport their pain and distress and tend to use the extreme ends of scales—ignoring middle values; and children with cognitive impairments and global developmental delay may have major difficulties in using self-report [21].

Measures are most useful when used well in advance of a procedure so that specific and targeted interventions can be delivered, as necessary. For an overview of pediatric pain measures, see Cunnington [22] and Chorney and McMurtry [23]. In selecting an appropriate scale for use in clinical practice, there are a number of issues to consider:

1. That the behaviors measured may not exclusively relate to pain but can also describe other negative reactions provoked by an acute and invasive procedure. For example, crying or shouting can indicate a child's fear, anger, or distress as well as pain. It should not automatically be assumed that the behaviors before a procedure signal distress while behaviors during and after a procedure purely reflect pain. Such behaviors are not discrete and independent of each other; there are clear similarities and overlap. This is important in terms of the different interventions that might be offered. Further research is necessary to fine tune the differentiation and measurement of a range of emotions that are expressed in externally identical behaviors [24].
2. That the majority of measures have been developed and validated in Western cultures on English-speaking populations. The limited literature on cultural differences in pain behavior suggests that there are localized and individual differences [25] and generalizations about universal applicability of pain measures may be inappropriate.
3. That scales may have evolved for use in different clinical situations from those used in the original validation, e.g., Children's Hospital of East Ontario Pain Scale (CHEOPS) was conceived as a measure of postoperative pain [26] but is now also used to measure procedural pain (see Table 34.1).
4. That some measures (e.g., those requiring training, additional personnel, video recording, coding of data) may be more appropriate to research and less suitable for a clinical setting. A clinical situation can change rapidly and measures may not be sufficiently flexible to detect sudden changes.

The following are some illustrative examples of measures that can be used in various clinical situations.

Table 34.1 Children's Hospital of Eastern Ontario Pain Scale (CHEOPS)

Item	Behavioral		Definition	Score
Cry	No cry	1	Child is not crying	
	Moaning	2	Child is moaning or quietly vocalizing silent cry	
	Crying	2	Child is crying, but the cry is gentle or whimpering	
	Scream	3	Child is in a full-lunged cry; sobbing; may be scored with complaint or without complaint	
Facial	Composed	1	Neutral facial expression	
	Grimace	2	Score only if definite negative facial expression	
	Smiling	0	Score only if definite positive facial expression	
Child verbal	None	1	Child not talking	
	Other complaints	1	Child complains, but not about pain, e.g., "I want to see mommy" or "I am thirsty"	
	Pain complaints	2	Child complains about pain	
	Both complaints	2	Child complains about pain and about other things, e.g., "It hurts. I want my mommy"	
	Positive	0	Child makes any positive statement or talks about other things without complaint	
Torso	Neutral	1	Body (not limbs) is at rest; torso is inactive	
	Shifting	2	Body is in motion in a shifting or serpentine fashion	
	Tense	2	Body is arched or rigid	
	Shivering	2	Body is shuddering or shaking involuntarily	
	Upright	2	Child is in a vertical or upright position	
	Restrained	2	Body is restrained	
Touching	Not touching	1	Child is not touching or grabbing at wound	
	Reach	2	Child is reaching for but not touching wound	
	Touch	2	Child is gently touching wound or wound area	
	Grab	2	Child is grabbing vigorously at wound	
	Restrained	2	Child's arms are restrained	
Legs	Neutral	1	Legs may be in any position but are relaxed; includes gentle swimming or separate-like movements	
	Squirm/kicking	2	Definitive uneasy or restless movements in the legs and/or striking out with foot or feet	
	Drawn up/tensed	2	Legs tensed and/or pulled up tightly to body and kept there	
	Standing	2	Standing, crouching, or kneeling	
	Restrained	2	Child's legs are being held down	

To assess procedural and brief episodes of pain:

1. Children's Hospital of Eastern Ontario Pain Scale (CHEOPS)
   Originally developed as a measure of postoperative pain, this is now an established measure of behaviors during brief episodes of pain in infants and children up to 18 years, and can be used to measure the outcomes of interventions to alleviate pain. The measure comprises six items of behavior—cry, facial, child verbal, torso, touch, and legs—each item being given a score of 1–3 from which a total pain score can be derived (see Table 34.1). The CHEOPS has been used extensively in many countries and contexts for venipunctures, immunizations, and surgery. However, some consider it to be complicated to score and less practical compared to other observational scales.
2. Face, Legs, Activity, Cry, and Consolability Scale (FLACC) [27]
   This scale measures both procedural and postoperative pain, originally designed for children up to 7 years but subsequently modified for use up to late adulthood, with five indicators—face, legs, activity, cry, and consolability—each rated on a three-point scale (0–2) (see Table 34.2). This scale is used for a large variety of procedures, including venipuncture, catheterization, laceration repair, and chest drain removal. It is a low burden scale, translated for use in many countries.

To assess procedural distress and interactions:

1. Procedure (or Procedural) Behavioral Rating Scale (PBRS) [28]
   This scale for children from 8 months to 18 years records the presence or absence of 11 distress-related behaviors for three phases of the procedure—pre-procedure, procedure, and recovery—producing summated scores for each phase of the procedure and across the three phases (see Table 34.3). The measure can be scored relatively quickly to obtain a gross overall score for each phase and has been used to record distress during venipunctures, lumbar punctures, immunizations, and treatments for burns.
2. Pediatric Behavior Checklist (PBCL) [29]
   This measure, originally designed for children and young people undergoing bone marrow aspiration, has been

Table 34.2 Face, Legs, Activity, Cry, and Consolability Scale (FLACC) [27]

	Scoring		
Category	0	1	2
Face	No particular expression or smile	Occasional grimace or frown Withdrawn Disinterested	Frequent to constant quivering chin Clenched jaw
Legs	Normal position or relaxed	Uneasy Restless Tense	Kicking or legs drawn up
Activity	Lying quietly Normal position Moves easily	Squirming Shifting back and forth Tense	Arched, rigid, or jerking
Cry	No cry (awake or asleep)	Moans or whimpers Occasional complaint	Crying steadily Screams or sobs Frequent complaints
Consolability	Content Relaxed	Reassured by occasional touching, hugging, or being talked to Distractable	Difficult to console

Table 34.3 Procedural Behavior Rating Scale [28]

Behavioral Item	Operational Definition
Cry	Tears in eyes or running down face
Cling	Physically holds on to parent, significant other, or nurse
Fear verbal	Says "I'm scared," "I'm afraid," etc.
Pain verbal	Says "Ow," "Ouch," "It hurts," "You're hurting me," etc.
Scream	No tears, raises voice, verbal or nonverbal
Stall	Verbal expression of delay ("Wait a minute," "I'm not ready yet," etc.) or behavioral delay (ignores nurse's instructions)
Carry	Has to be physically carried into or out of room or placed on table, not because of physical inability to do so on his or her own
Flail	Random gross movements of arms or legs, but no intention to make aggressive contact
Refusal position	Does not follow instructions with regard to body placement on treatment table
Restrain	Has to be held down due to lack of cooperation
Muscular rigidity	Any of following behaviors: clenched fists, white knuckles, gritted teeth, clenched jaw, wrinkled brow, eyes clenched shut, contracted limbs, body stiffness
Emotional support	Verbal or nonverbal solicitation of hugs, physical comfort, or expression of empathy from parent, significant other, or nurse
Requests termination	Verbally asks/pleads that procedure be stopped
The following items were subsequently eliminated from the original list:	
Groan	Nonverbal, vocal expression of pain or discomfort
Laugh	Smiling with a chuckling sound
Stoic silence	Child does not respond to questions or remarks of others. May appear "trancelike"
Nausea verbal	Says "I'm sick," "I feel nauseous," "My stomach feels like I'm going to throw up"
Vomit	Includes retching, dry heaves
Urinate/defecate	Soils or wets self
Kick	Intentional aggressive movement of leg(s) to make physical contact
Hit	Intentional aggressive movement of arm(s) or hand(s) to make physical contact
Bite	Intentional aggressive closing of jaw to make physical contact
Verbal hostility	Says "I hate you," "You're mean," etc.
Curse	Utters profanity
Questions	Nondelay, information-seeking verbal behavior ("What are you doing now?" "Is it over yet?" etc.)

Table 34.4 Pediatric Behavior Checklist [29]

Behavioral item	Operational definition
Muscle tension	Displays any of the following behaviors: eyes tightly shut, clenched jaw, stiff body, clenched fists, gritted teeth (contraction of any observable body part)
Screaming	Raises voice or yells (can be with or without words)
Crying	Tears or sobs
Restraint	Has to be held down
Pain verbalized	Says "Ow," "Ouch," or "You're hurting me," etc.
Anxiety verbalized	Says "I'm scared" or "I'm afraid"
Verbal stalling	Expresses verbal delay such as "Stop," "I'm not ready," or "I want to tell you something"
Physical resistance	Moves around, will not stay in position, or tries to climb off table

modified to rate ten behaviors on a 1–5 scale, before, during, and after the procedure, akin to the PBRS described previously (see Table 34.4). It can be used for a variety of medical procedures and has been recommended as an outcome measure of procedural distress in pediatric pain clinical trials [30].

3. Child-Adult Medical Procedure Interaction Scale-short form (CAMPIS-SF) [31]
   This scale measures categories of behavior—child distress, child coping, adult distress promoting, and adult coping promoting—with scoring on a five-point scale (see Table 34.5). The scale requires a training period of 1–2 days, but videos can then be coded in real time. It can be used for venipunctures, bone marrow aspirations, immunizations, and voiding cystourethrograms.

Table 34.5 CAMPIS-SF codes and descriptive statistics

	Mean	Standard deviations	Minimum range	Maximum range
CAMPIS-SF codes				
Child coping	6.0	2.7	3	13
Child distress	6.8	3.3	3	14
Parent coping promoting	6.4	2.9	3	14
Parent distress promoting	4.3	1.5	3	8
Nurse coping promoting	5.3	1.8	3	10
Nurse distress promoting	4.2	1.1	5	8
Proportions of CAMPIS-R codes				
Child coping	0.42	0.28	0	1.00
Child distress	0.49	0.31	0	1.00
Parent coping promoting	0.26	0.14	0	0.58
Parent distress promoting	0.15	0.13	0	0.46
Nurse coping promoting	0.25	0.13	0.03	0.52
Nurse distress promoting	0.12	0.07	0.02	0.33
Validity measures				
OSBD distress	13.2	17.3	0	76.8
BAADS approach/avoidance	15.6	3.3	6	22
BAADS distress	10.2	7.7	5	60
Parent fear	41.3	27.8	0	100
Parent pain	52.7	27.4	2	100
Nurse distress	20.3	29.3	0	100
Nurse cooperation	81.1	31.7	0	100
Child fear	2.4	1.7	1	5
Child pain	3.4	1.6	1	5

Reprinted with permission from Blount RL, Bunke V, Cohen LL, Forbes C. The Child-Adult Medical Procedures Interaction Scale-Short Form (CAMPIS-SF): validation of a rating scale for children's and adults' behaviors during painful medical procedures. J Pain Symptom Manage 2001;22:591–599

To assess perioperative behavior and distress:

1. Modified Yale Preoperative Anxiety Scale (m-YPAS) [32]
   This 27-item scale measures anxiety across five domains of behavior (activity, emotional expressivity, arousal state, vocalization, and dependence on parents) in children over 2 years of age, prior to induction of anesthesia (see Table 34.6). It is quick to administer and can track rapidly changing states in the child.
2. The Induction Compliance Checklist (ICC) [33]
   This is an 11-point scale developed for use as an observational measure to quantify the level of compliance in a children aged 0–17 years undergoing induction of anesthesia by inhalation (see Table 34.7). Scores range from 0 to 10, where 0 is considered to be the ideal induction without anxiety or behavioral disturbance in the child, with a cut-off score of 6 for poor compliance with induction.
3. Emotionality, Activity and Sociability Scale (EAS) [34]
   This is a measure of child temperament containing 20 items, each item being rated by parents on a five-point scale, with a score obtained for each of the three temperaments (see Table 34.8). It is a useful measure to obtain preoperatively to predict a child's distress at the time of anesthesia.
4. Post-hospital Behavioral Questionnaire (PHBQ) [35]
   This questionnaire, completed by parents at home following discharge from hospital, assesses behavioral changes in the child. It consists of 27 items to assess general anxiety, separation anxiety, sleep disorders, eating difficulties, aggression, and apathy (see Table 34.9). The parent is asked to compare typical behavior in their child compared to behavior shown during the first week after hospitalization, using a five-point scale.

To assess pain in children with intellectual impairment:

1. Non-communicating Children's Pain Checklist (NCCPC) [36]
   This is the most widely validated measure for assessing pain in children with cognitive impairments and is designed to be used by parents and caregivers (see Table 34.10). The checklist comprises 30 items rated 0–3 on seven subscales (vocal behavior, social, facial expression, active, body and limbs, physical signs, and

Table 34.6 Modified Yale Preoperative Anxiety Scale [32]

Activities
1. The child looks around, is curious, plays with toys, reads (or other behavior that is appropriate for the age group); moves around the pre-anesthetic/treatment room to get toys or seeks family members; might move toward the equipment in the surgery room
2. The child does not explore or play, may look down, plays with own hands, or sucks own thumb (blanket); may stay close to family while playing, or exhibits a manic quality while playing
3. The child moves without concentration from toy to family members, movements are not connected to the activity; movements or play are frantic/agitated; twisting, moving on the table; may push the mask or grab family members
4. Child tries to escape, pushes with arms and feet, may move entire body; in the waiting room, the child runs around without purpose, does not look at toys, does not want to be separated from family, clings on desperately
Vocalization
1. Reads (vocalization not adequate for the activity), asks questions, makes comments, stutters, laughs, answers questions promptly, but generally may be quiet; child is too young to speak in social situations or too absorbed in play to answer
2. Answers adults, but whispers; uses "baby talk"; only responds with shaking or nodding of head
3. Quiet, no sound or does not answer adults
4. Weeping, moaning, grunting, silent crying
5. Child cries, may scream "No"
6. Crying—high pitched and sustained
Expressing emotions
1. Happy, smiling, concentrating on playing
2. Neutral, no discernible facial expression
3. From worried (sad) to frightened, sad, worried, or teary eyes
4. Distressed, crying, extreme upset, eyes may be wide open
State of arousal
1. Alert, looks around occasionally, notices or watches the anesthesiologist's actions (could be relaxed)
2. Withdrawn, calm and silent, may suck thumb, or face turned into adult
3. Attentive, quickly looks around, may be startled by sounds, eyes wide, body tense
4. Panicked whining, may cry, may shun others, turns body away
Interaction with family members
1. Child concentrates on playing, sits idle, or shows age-appropriate behavior, does not need family members; may interact with parent if the parent initiates the interaction
2. Seeks family members (moves close and speaks to otherwise silent parent), seeks and accepts comfort, may lean against family member
3. Looks silently to family members, apparently observes their actions, does not seek contact or comfort, but will accept it if offered; or clings to parent
4. Keeps family members at a distance or leaves area when family members appear, might push away parent or else desperately cling to parent and not let them go away

eating/sleeping). A version of the NCCPC (NCCP-PO) is available to use postoperatively.

2. Face, Legs, Activity, Cry, and Consolability Scale-Revised (FLACC-R)

Table 34.7 Induction Compliance Checklist [33]

Check off all applicable behavior:	Score
Perfect induction (does not exhibit negative behavior, fear, or anxiety)	Score 0
Crying, tears in eyes	
Turns head away from mask	
Verbal refusal, says "no"	
Verbalizes fear or worry, such as "Where's Mommy?" or "Will it hurt?"	
Pushes mask away with hands, pushes away nurse/anesthetist with hands or feet	
Covers mouth/nose with hands/arms or buries face	
Hysterical crying, may scream	
Kicks, flails legs/arms, arches back, or general struggling	
Requires physical restraint	
Completely passive, either rigid or limp	
Total Score (number of items ticked)	

Table 34.8 Emotionality, Activity and Sociability Scale example [34]

EAS Scales	Rating
Shyness	
Tends to be shy	
Makes friends easily	
Is very sociable	
Takes a long time to warm up to strangers	
Is very friendly with strangers	
Sociability	
Likes to be with people	
Prefers playing with others rather than alone	
Finds people more stimulating than anything else	
Is somewhat of a loner	
Activity	
Is always on the go	
When he moves about, he usually moves slowly	
Is off and running as soon as he wakes up in the morning	
Is very energetic	
Prefers quiet, inactive games to more active ones	
Emotionality	
Cries easily	
Tends to be somewhat emotional	
Often fusses and cries	
Gets upset easily	
Reacts intensely when upset	
When alone, he feels isolated	

This is a revised version of the FLACC described previously for use with children with cognitive impairment (see Table 34.11).

Summary features of the tests are given in Table 34.12.

We now turn to preparation for procedures. This needs to take a systemic family focus as children and their parents are interdependent and psychologically "joined at the hip."

Table 34.9 Post-hospital Behavioral Questionnaire example [35]

Questions:
1. Do you have frequent headaches?
2. Do you have lack of appetite?
3. Do you have trouble sleeping?
4. Do you get scared easily?
5. Do you feel your hands shaking?
6. Do you feel nervous, tense, or worried?
7. Do you have digestion problems?
8. Do you have trouble thinking clearly?
9. Have you felt sad lately?
10. Have you cried more than usual?
11. Have you experienced difficulty in carrying out your daily activities with satisfaction?
12. Do you find it difficult to make decisions?
13. Do you have difficulties with your work?
14. Are you unable to play a useful role in your life?
15. Have you lost interest in things?
16. Do you feel useless, not diligent?
17. Have you thought about killing yourself?
18. Do you feel tired all the time?
19. Have you had unpleasant feelings in your stomach?
20. Do you get tired easily?

Table 34.10 Non-communicating Children's Pain Checklist revised

Vocal subscale
• Moaning, whining, or whimpering (fairly soft)
• Crying (moderately loud)
• Screaming or yelling (extremely loud)
• A sound or word expressing pain
Eating/sleeping subscale
• Eating less, disinterested in food
• Increased sleep
• Decreased sleep
Social subscale
• Uncooperative, cranky, irritable, unhappy
• Reduced social interaction, withdrawn
• Seeking comfort or physical closeness
• Difficult to distract, cannot be satisfied or pacified
Facial subscale
• Furrowed brow
• A change in eyes, including squinting, eyes wide, eyes frowning
• Mouth turned down into a frown, unsmiling
• Lips puckered up, drawn tight, pouting, or quivering
• Clenching or grinding teeth, chewing or thrusting out tongue
Activity subscale
• Unmoving, reduced activity, quiet
• Jumps around, agitated, fidgety
Body/limb subscale
• Floppy body
• Stiff, spastic, tense, rigid body
• Points out or touches part of body that hurts
• Protects, favors, or guards part of the body that hurts
• Flinches or moves away body part, being sensitive to touch
• Moving the body in specific way to show pain (e.g., head thrown back, arms down, body curled up)
Physiological signs subscale
• Shivering
• Change in skin color, pallor
• Sweating, perspiring
• Tears
• Sharp intake of breath, gasping
• Breath holding

Modified from [36]

Helping Parents Help Their Children

Anxious children instinctively turn to their parents for protection and support, and most children will want their parents to be present during a frightening procedure. In turn, parents want to protect their child from threat and most parents would choose to be with their children during all procedures and for as long as possible when the procedure involves anesthesia for surgery [37].

Interestingly, the research evidence (based on studies of induction of anesthesia in an operating theater) for the effectiveness of parental presence alone in reducing a child's anxiety and distress is not strong [38]. Multiple randomized controlled trials indicate that the presence of parents at their child's anesthetic induction does not of itself reliably reduce a child's anxiety [39]. It is how parents behave that makes the difference. Parents whose own anxiety is overwhelming and who instruct, criticize, or even reassure excessively can increase anxiety and distress in their child [40, 41].

A series of studies has shown that anxious children with calm parents present during anesthetic induction were significantly less anxious than anxious children whose parents were not present at induction. Calm children with highly anxious parents present were significantly more anxious than calm children whose parents were not present at induction [42].

Parents can be taught psychological interventions including distraction and supported to act as coaches to help their child prepare for anesthetic induction and increase the effectiveness of hospital preparation programs in reducing anxiety in the child, pre- and post-surgery [43], reducing postoperative delirium and analgesia required, and allowing quicker discharge from hospital [44].

The advantages of parental presence therefore are:

1. Calm, positive, proactive, and focused parental support can help reduce both parental and child anxiety and distress [45].
2. Parents can acquire new skills to enhance both their own and their child's coping mechanisms, which is particularly useful for any future procedures a child might have to undergo.
3. Surgery represents a major life event for the whole family and potentially challenges parents' perceptions of their

Table 34.11 Revised FLACC Scale

	Scoring		
Category	0	1	2
Face	No particular expression or smile	Occasional grimace or frown Withdrawn Disinterested **Sad, appears worried**	Frequent to constant quivering chin Clenched jaw **Distressed looking face** **Expression of fright/panic**
Legs	Normal position or relaxed **Usual tone and motion to limbs**	Uneasy Restless Tense **Occasional tremors**	Kicking or legs drawn up **Marked increase in spasticity** **Constant tremors** **Jerking**
Activity	Lying quietly Normal position Moves easily **Regular rhythmic respirations**	Squirming Shifting back and forth Tense **Tense/guarded movements** **Mildly agitated** **Shallow/splinting respirations** **Intermittent sighs**	Arched, rigid, or jerking **Severe agitation** **Head banging** **Shivering** **Breath holding** **Gasping** **Severe splinting**
Cry	No cry (awake or asleep)	Moans or whimpers Occasional complaint **Occasional verbal outbursts** **Constant grunting**	Crying steadily Screams or sobs Frequent complaints **Repeated outbursts** **Constant grunting**
Consolability	Content Relaxed	Reassured by occasional touching, hugging, or being talked to Distractable	Difficult to console **Pushing caregiver away** **Resisting care or comfort measures**

Revisions in *bold*

Table 34.12 Summary features of assessment tests

Scale	Age range	Rater	Behaviors assessed	Test characteristics	Clinical application	Comments
1. To assess procedural pain						
CHEOPS	4 months to 18 years	Health professional Researcher	Cry Facial Child verbal Torso Touch Legs	Six items Rating scales: 0–2 1–3 1–2	Perioperative Venipuncture Intramuscular injections Immunizations Dental procedures Bone marrow aspirations Severe pain	May be more suitable for research contexts
FLACC	15 days to 80+ years	Health professional Researcher	Face Legs Activity Cry Consolability	Five items Rating scale: 0–2	Wide range: as above plus Minimally conscious patients Urethral catheterization Nasogastric tube insertion Chest drain removal Fracture reduction	Used in a variety of countries
2. To assess procedural distress and interactions						
PBRS	8 months to 18 years	Health professional Researcher	Distress behaviors	11 items Scored over three phases of procedure	Wide range: Perioperative Venipuncture Lumbar puncture Chemotherapy Burns	

(continued)

Table 34.12 (continued)

Scale	Age range	Rater	Behaviors assessed	Test characteristics	Clinical application	Comments
PBCL	1 month to 19 years	Health professional	Muscle tension	Eight items	Wide range: as above plus	Useful outcome measure for clinical trials
		Researcher	Screaming	Rated 1–5	Nasendoscopy	
			Crying		Pediatric assessments	
			Restraint used			
			Pain verbalized			
CAMPIS-SF	2–18 years	Researcher	Adult coping promoting	Four items/subscales	Wide range: as above	
			Adult distress promoting	Scored over three phases of procedure		
			Child coping			
			Child distress			
3. To assess perioperative behavior and distress and postoperative distress						
m-YPAS	>2 years	Health professional	Five domains of behavior activity	27 items	Assesses perioperative anxiety	Rapid to complete
			Vocalization			Can be used in rapidly changing clinical situations
			Emotional expression			
			Arousal			
			Parental dependence			
ICC	0–17 years	Health professional	Observation of behaviors	11 items	Assess compliance at anesthetic induction by inhalation	
EAS		Parents	Rating scale	20 items	Assesses child temperament	
			Three domains emotionality	Five-point scale		
			Activity			
			Sociability			
PHBQ	6 months to 16 years	Parents	Assesses	27 items	Child's behavior at home following surgery	Possibility of parental bias
			General anxiety			
			Separation anxiety			
			Sleep disorders			
			Eating problems			
			Aggression			
			Apathy			
4. To assess pain in children with intellectual impairment						
NCCPC		Parents	Vocal behavior	30 items		Version NCCP-PO available
		Caregivers	Social	Rated 1–3		For postoperative assessment
			Facial expression			
			Active			
			Body and limbs			
			Physical signs			
			Eating/sleeping			
FLACC-R		Health professional				Modified version of FLACC
		Researcher				

own control and effectiveness. Health professionals can enhance their relationships with families by including them as active partners in the preparatory stages of their child's surgery as well as at anesthetic induction.

4. Parents report higher satisfaction with the hospital service when their child is less anxious [46]. This is important as measures of parent- and patient-reported experience are increasingly used as indicators of quality and process of healthcare delivery.

Preparation

This should not be considered as an optional "frill" in medical care but fundamental to enhancing a child's sense of control, mastery, and self-esteem as well as reducing distress by facilitating the successful completion of a procedure [47]. Children and their parents should receive information that is specific, accurate, and developmentally appropriate [48]. Anxious parents may not hear (or even be able to listen to) information given verbally. Leaflets, DVDs, websites, interactive books, etc. giving clear detailed explanations enable parents to absorb information at their own pace and convey this to their children. Children also need to understand the sensory elements of a procedure, i.e., what they are likely to see, hear, taste, smell, and feel. Many resources are available through hospital websites—e.g., Great Ormond Street Hospital for Children's "Children's Zone" [49], Contact a Family [50]—or organizations such as Action for Sick Children, a charity in the UK that publishes family-friendly medical information and campaigns to improve services and attitudes to the way in which sick children and young people are treated [51]. Advance consideration of the clinic environment is necessary and how psychological coping mechanisms are going to affect any pharmacological agents that will be used, e.g., topical anesthetics. If a child or young person has had a previously adverse experience or has difficult access to veins, then an experienced clinician should perform the procedure. Children soon identify who the good "needle sticker" is in a team.

The following general principles underlie good practice for procedures:

1. First and foremost, take the time to establish a rapport with the child and their family using developmentally appropriate language. It is useful to attend to one's own nonverbal cues as well as to the child's, e.g., crossing one's arms can unwittingly convey impatience and irritation. A positive working relationship is key to helping a child through procedures and treatment. This does not have to take up undue time. Ask what the child likes doing or observe what the child has with them or is playing with. A few minutes of coloring in can pay dividends with later cooperation. Humor is useful, but care needs to be taken that the child does not perceive that the clinician is making fun of them.
2. Enhance parental preparation and participation so parents can become coaches for their children. It is important to check out what the parents have (or have not) told their child about the procedure. Some parents tell their children little or nothing, believing it is kinder to the child not to worry them in advance; however, their child may arrive for the procedure suspicious and highly vigilant knowing something "is up" but unsure what. It is helpful to formulate a plan with parents, who are the experts of their child and to elicit the best way to support their child with interactive coping strategies, i.e., the skill set of thoughts and actions a child can use in an anxiety-provoking situation.
3. Build on a child's resilience and existing skills for coping. Ask the child about any previous experience and what if anything they might find hard to manage. Correct any misconceptions about a procedure, e.g., a needle for a venipuncture will not go right through the arm and out the other side. Ask what has been helpful in the past, including the use of topical anesthetic agents. Develop a coping strategy together giving the child limited choices where possible. Some children choose to be involved with the procedure, some prefer to be distracted. Young people require appropriate privacy and might want to be seen without their parents.
4. Give developmentally appropriate information about the procedure and its duration in terms of an activity already familiar to the child, e.g., the time it takes to sing a familiar nursery rhyme or song. When explaining what the child is likely to experience, frame the sensation in a positive way, e.g., the lubricating gel for an ultrasound can be described as "jelly on the belly." The loud noises on the machine or equipment can be likened to a motorbike or helicopter or indeed anything the child might find positive and interesting.
5. Create a plan together with the child and their parents. This may include the opportunity to become familiar with the medical equipment, e.g., mask. Decide with the child where and how they will sit or lie for the procedure, if appropriate. Give limited choices where possible.
6. Consider the room and environment where the procedure will be performed. It is better to use a specific treatment room and avoid "safe areas" like the child's bed or playroom so the child knows there are places where nothing painful or aversive will happen to them. Have medical equipment and machinery out of direct view, if possible, to reduce the anxiety this might otherwise provoke. Remove unnecessary equipment and have child-friendly decoration and toys. A token mobile is not sufficient. Have the minimum number of personnel needed in the room and try to restrict unnecessary comings and goings. The atmosphere should be as calm and soothing as possible, irrespective of the child's age.
7. A child held in a comfortable position during a procedure (e.g., on a parent's lap) enhances feelings of security and this can significantly reduce distress [52, 53]. Infants and toddlers can be held in a face-to-face embrace with their parents leaving an arm free. This is an example of therapeutic holding (see later section). During the procedure, only one person should talk to the child at any given time. The reality is that everyone is under time pressure but it is helpful to try and go at the child's pace. Again, give the child limited choices to enable the child to feel a sense of control. It is important to tell the child what they can do rather than what they cannot. It is better to say "hold your arm as still as you can" rather than "don't move." Allow the child to make a loud noise, e.g., an animal roar or sing a loud note that can be heard down the corridor. A bellow or shout can be a surprising and distracting behavior for a child who would be normally expected to have to show polite and restrained behavior. This is not always popular

with clinicians but is effective for some children. Encourage the child and praise effort (e.g., "you are doing really well to hold your arm still") but clinicians and parents should not apologize. Other examples of helpful and unhelpful language are given by Cohen [54].

8. Whether the procedure has gone well or badly, it is important to talk to the child and parents afterwards about aspects that did go well and what might be more helpful next time. This is particularly necessary for procedures that have to be repeated regularly. The clinician can praise the child for trying irrespective of outcome. A plan can be made to enhance further preparation and consolidate coping strategies. If this step is omitted, there is a risk that the child thinks they have managed on this one occasion purely by chance but would not be able to cope again with future procedures.

Psychological Interventions

Painful stimuli reach awareness through the attention-control mechanism. Effective psychological interventions for pain and concomitant distress focus attention away from the sensation causing pain and toward competing pleasurable stimuli [55]. There is empirical support for behavioral interventions, including distraction, guided imagery, relaxation, breathing, rehearsal, and reinforcement for appropriate behavior [56–58]. Such interventions are primarily based on cognitive behavioral therapy (CBT), which identifies negative beliefs relating to anxiety and replaces them with more positive thoughts to promote adaptive behavior:

1. Distraction
   This is not about creating a diversion but an active shifting and refocusing of attention from anxiety-provoking stimuli (e.g., the needle) toward a pleasing stimulus. Distraction stimuli and activities need to be varied and engaging using sensory, physical, and cognitive elements [59]. Above all, distraction should be easy and fun to perform. Distraction works best when it is interactive and a parent can act as a child's coach, as children rarely engage in active coping mechanisms without an adult initiating these [60]. Distraction has been found to be effective for infants up to young adults [61]. It is important that a distraction activity is used before, during, and after the procedure to hasten recovery. Distraction activities can include interactive electronic games, virtual reality goggles, music, storytelling, counting backwards in groups of numbers, or spotting an error in an adult reciting multiplication tables. Children can be involved in creating a distractor that is interesting and personal to them. Depending on age, this could be a favorite toy or character that acts as a superhero who can give a child a magic cloak or glove to wear that reduces the sensation of pain.

   Distraction provided by parents or medical staff is easy to use and is of low cost. It is only contraindicated if a child is known to cope best by focusing on the details of the procedure [62]. The effect of a particular distractor can wear off, so it is advisable to keep something novel for use for when the procedure occurs.
2. Relaxation with guided imagery
   Relaxation can be defined as "state of relative freedom from anxiety and skeletal muscle tension, a quietening or calming of mind and muscles" [63]. In a relaxed state, heart and respiratory rates are decreased, and skin resistance and muscle tone reduced. Physiological arousal can be reduced through slow breathing and the tensing and releasing of muscle. Techniques often aim to tense and relax different muscle groups around the body in a progressive manner. This can be particularly helpful when the insertion of a catheter is required. Relaxation is a skill that requires time and practice to learn, so it needs to be rehearsed well before the procedure is scheduled. There are commercial tapes or stories for children to use, but it is often more effective when children create these themselves. The child can be asked to invent a detailed story around a place they find highly pleasurable with great attention to the detail of what the child would do and what they would experience. Clinical experience shows that what is relaxing to an adult (lying on a beach or by a mountain lake) is not necessarily relaxing to a child. Many a child has chosen a theme park, with stomach-churning rides, as the most relaxing place to be.
3. Hypnosis
   This is a natural state of heightened awareness where attention can be diverted from peripheral stimuli and refocused with increased receptivity to new ideas. In this state of increased suggestibility in combination with deep relaxation, a person is receptive to suggestions made by the therapist for changes in thoughts, emotions, and behaviors as well as perception and experience. There is no universal operational definition of hypnosis; indeed there is some controversy over the theoretical underpinnings as to whether hypnosis represents an altered and trance state of consciousness that is distinct from ordinary, day-to-day attention [64] or whether hypnotic phenomena are not unique and can occur without a concomitant state of altered consciousness [65]. The different theoretical explanations are not mutually exclusive and no one theory explains all the phenomena associated with hypnosis. Interventions using hypnosis are particularly suitable for children as they are naturally curious and creative and have vivid imaginations with looser boundaries between reality and fantasy, compared to adults. Hypnosis has been found to be effective in reducing anxiety and pain in children undergoing invasive procedures such as venipunctures, lumbar punctures, bone marrow aspirations, and voiding cystograms [66]. Children can be taught how to

self-administer hypnotic techniques in anxiety-provoking medical procedures; however, the research evidence indicates that direct parental involvement is critical to maintaining a positive therapeutic effect [67].

Developmental Stages and Understanding of Illness

From Infant to Toddler: 0–2 Years

The baby is developing rapidly to coordinate their sensory and motor responses through acting on their environment, to distinguish self from others and to achieve control, to learn about cause and effect and achieve object permanence. Essential to a baby's sense of security is the relationship established by consistent caregiving, by parents or main caregivers. In the first weeks, babies, while able to discriminate between people, will accept care from unfamiliar adults. After 3 months they respond differently to familiar and unfamiliar people. Fear of separation triggers anxiety. At around 6–9 months of age with heightened attachment to parents, babies will begin to develop a fear of strangers. As language develops, babies understand more than they can express including their fears, which can increase their distress. Before 2 years of age, babies probably have little understanding of illness but will absorb their parents' anxiety and distress and can show fear in response to painful stimulation.

Interventions

Effective intervention is aimed at calming and soothing the infant with gentle, physical, and sensory stimulation. The parent can hold, cuddle, rock, and massage their baby in an environment that is quiet and low lit, before, during, and after the procedure [68]. Holding a baby against a parent's chest with skin-to-skin contact (kangaroo care) has been shown to be helpful in reducing pain behavior [69]. Swaddling a baby can also have a calming effect [70]. Sucrose water, given on a pacifier or by syringe, can also reduce pain behavior [71]. Infants can also be distracted by developmentally appropriate toys offered by parents or nurses [72]. It may be instinctive for a parent to reassure or even apologize to their baby, but this may actively increase an infant's distress [73].

Toddler to Preschool: 3–5 Years

The rapid acquisition of language and symbolic thinking underpins this period of increasing physical independence, assertion, and self-control. This is the age of "I do it." Unable to understand another's point of view, they may strongly resist being "done to" both verbally and physically. They have no clear boundaries between reality and fantasy and are very imaginative. Children of this age see health and illness as distinct and separate entities. Good health is linked with parents, while the child can feel responsible for their illness: "I'm ill because I was naughty." Treatment can feel like a punishment for being bad. They may feel guilty for causing family disruption as a result of illness and treatment. Effects of illness are not easily distinguished from side effects of treatment, so having to swallow medicine can be as aversive as the symptom it is designed to alleviate. Children of this age have little concept of future time, so reassurance that a procedure will not last long is meaningless and pain can feel overwhelming.

Interventions

Useful distraction activities for this age group include blowing bubbles with encouragement to watch the bubbles float away or pop, playing with toys that make a noise or light up when manipulated, or imagining making a feather dance on a hand. This helps produce regulated controlled breathing and a state of relaxation.

From Primary School to Early Adolescence: 6–10 Years

This stage is characterized by the child's increasing physical, academic, social skills, and achievements. Acceptance by peers is key: who is most popular, who is best at mathematics, who runs the fastest, etc. Illness that interferes with daily life and cherished skills highlights a child's difference from his peers, just when he needs to be like the others. If chronic illness causes long absences from school, self-esteem may suffer. Children accept that their thoughts and actions do not cause illness, but have a relatively unsophisticated understanding of the disease process; causation is external by germs as a universal contagion theory. While death is understood as a permanent state, it can become personalized as a monster stealing a child from his family.

Interventions

Children, with the support of their parents, can choose what they would find most helpful. Some will want to actively engage with activities such as playing electronic games, interactive word or number games, squeezing balls, or an enhanced blowing bubble game where the child chooses a color associated with anxious feelings and this sits on the bubble. As the bubble is blown away, the child imagines the color changing to one associated with one of calm, happy, and relaxed feelings. Other children may prefer more passive strategies including listening to music of their choice or being read to.

Adolescence: 11–15 Years

The young person has developmental tasks to achieve. These include:

- Gaining a stable self-concept through trying out different identities
- Achieving psychosexual development
- Preparing for emotional and economic interdependence with family
- Preparing for a future career and employment
- Learning to make decisions

The influence of and acceptance by peers is extremely important. There can be power struggles with parents and authority figures, including their doctors. At this age, young people understand that illness is about understanding malfunctioning body systems and can have multiple causes and is also exacerbated by stress and emotions. They also understand that illnesses have an end point and are not all or nothing events—you can be a little bit ill. Thinking is egocentric and can lead to the assumption that everyone sees things the adolescent's way. The young person wishes to avoid loss of face and can feel that it is unacceptable to show fear or distress. Body image is very important and medical interventions can be perceived as threatening the desired look.

Interventions

With a strong need to maintain dignity, composure and "save face," procedures should occur in a room where some degree of privacy is possible. Young people should choose who is present to support them and the type of distraction they would prefer. Again, games on electronic devices are helpful, as is conversation, use of guided imagery as a story, and active focus on controlled breathing.

Summary

The interventions described are not mutually exclusive and can be even more effective when used in combination. There are a number of protocols available to guide the clinician in which interventions to use, how and when. Examples of these include Gaskell [74], Royal College of Australasian guidelines [75], and Cunnington [22]. While these are extremely useful as a clinical tool, it should be remembered that children and young people have highly individual and often unpredictable reactions to a procedure, even one they have experienced before. When acutely ill, anxious children often regress to an earlier developmental level and prefer strategies a clinician might associate with a younger child. These strategies should be observed and honored. It is not helpful to label a child "babyish." The active planning and selection of a distracting intervention by a child, whatever form it takes can, in itself, promote mastery and coping.

It should also be noted that research evidence for effective psychological, non-pharmacological interventions specifically relates to studies of children undergoing anesthetic induction for surgery in an operating theater. Moreover, research studies often exclude children with chronic illness, syndromes, cognitive impairment, and previous episodes of surgery and hospitalization; these are the very children and young people clinicians will assess and treat on a daily basis and who can present particular challenges.

Special Needs

Children with special needs, whether physical, sensory, cognitive, or in combination, are likely to need additional support. These children have chronic neurological, developmental, and/or physical impairments. "Special needs" can include learning disability (IQ < 70), which affects approximately 2 % of the population in the UK [76]; language and communication disorders; sensory impairments and reduced mobility; and self-help and independent living skills. These impairments singly or in combination can produce compromised behavior in the hospital setting that is unfamiliar and perceived as threatening. Such children are particularly vulnerable to high anxiety and distress, which can result in a lack of cooperation or outright physical defiance to a medical procedure, as effective communication between child and clinician may be compromised. The child may not be able to effectively describe symptoms, understand the given instructions, or indeed the reason for a procedure. Distress, physical discomfort, or pain may be communicated by oppositional and physically disruptive behavior. The child may find the change in routine intolerable, e.g., a long wait in a busy waiting area or prolonged fasting.

Children diagnosed with autistic spectrum disorder (ASD) can present particular challenges. ASD is a lifelong developmental disorder characterized by three main areas of impairment:

- *Social Interaction*—difficulty with social relationships and understanding others' intentions and perspectives.
- *Social Communication*—difficulty in understanding verbal or nonverbal communication.
- *Social Imagination*—difficulty with understanding the intentions of others and how their own behavior affects other people. Children often have a very literal view of the world and cannot generalize information.

It is important to note that these children may be of below average intelligence, but equally can be of normal or high intelligence. Additionally the child with ASD might have repetitive behavioral patterns and be resistant to changes in routine. They can be hypo- or hypersensitive to sound, light, touch, and pain.

The optimal care for children with special needs, and ASD in particular, requires careful and coordinated preparation by the clinical team. Before the appointment or admission, the child's physical and psychological needs can be established by gaining information from parents/caregivers or community resources of the child's physical and developmental status, severity of condition, mobility, level of understanding, likes, dislikes and fears, and means of communication [77]. A plan can be drawn up to facilitate the smooth completion of the procedure. In general, children with ASD would benefit from:

1. Waiting in a quiet area, ideally in a separate room where stimulation is reduced.
2. Allowing more time for the procedure.
3. Having a familiar parent or caregiver present to "interpret" for the child and provide physical security and comfort.
4. Having a familiar toy or activity that calms the child and provides security and comfort.
5. Being first on the list to reduce waiting and fasting times.

Children with impaired verbal communication may use a type of augmentative and alternative communication (AAC) [78], which can include pictures, objects, sign language, gestures, facial expression, or computer software symbols.

It is helpful for the clinician to:

- Check out the level of the child's understanding
- Speak quietly and clearly
- Use simple clear language and gestures, avoiding jargon or metaphor
- Warn the child before making any physical contact
- Avoid surprising the child

It is generally unhelpful to:

- Raise the voice; shouting distorts the shape of the mouth, creating an angry expression, leading to misunderstanding by the child
- Use complex language with metaphor
- Hurry the child

The presence of parents and familiar caregivers can be essential to "interpret" the child's responses and ensure that the best coping strategies for that child are in place. Adaptation to standard practice may be required. For a child with a significant hearing impairment, a clinician needs to engage the child's full attention and maintain good eye contact to ensure that the child understands what is happening. Speech and gestures need to be clear with background noise minimized. Children with learning difficulties and/or who are on the spectrum of autistic disorders should be allowed extra time and preferably be first or last on the investigation list. Waiting for a procedure is particularly challenging for these children and if possible it should be kept to a minimum in a quiet area, with fewer stimuli. Waits of 10 min or longer have been shown to contribute to the need for preoperative sedation [79].

When a Problem Arises: If a Child Refuses or the Procedure Is Unsuccessful

Occasionally a child becomes too distressed and/or physically resistant and withdraws cooperation to the point where the procedure is halted. Where possible, it is preferable to abandon the procedure and arrange another time so that additional coping skills can be mobilized with the help of a child life specialist or, when necessary, a child clinical psychologist. Even when a procedure cannot go ahead, it is important to end on as positive a note as possible, praising the child for what they have been able to achieve and planning further interventions to aid the next attempt at the procedure. Children need to feel that the repeat of procedure is not their punishment for being "naughty."

Figure 34.1 shows a simple flow diagram for dealing with uncooperative or resistant children. Despite everyone's best best intentions, this noncompliance can cause irritation and frustration in clinicians and overt anger at their child by parents. Staff and parents need to keep as calm as possible and avoid verbal conflict. The child's best interests and safety must be at the heart of subsequent actions and these interests include the child's dignity and self-esteem as well as the maintenance of a good relationship between the child and their clinician. Children are often very ashamed of their "failure" in relation to their parents' and clinicians' expectations and may want a "second chance" (though often at some unspecified point in the future). If it is possible to take a short break, the child and parents should be allowed to leave the room to regain composure before returning for a second attempt.

It may be possible to negotiate therapeutic holding with the child to enable sedation or local anesthesia to be applied. *Therapeutic*, *supportive*, or *clinical holding* all describe the use of limited force applied with the child's assent to achieve the necessary immobilization for a procedure to be effectively performed. School-aged children and young people may well agree to being wrapped up in a sheet as an aid to keeping still. If a child's assent cannot be obtained, therapeutic holding ceases to be "therapeutic" as far as the child is concerned and can leave the child feeling out of control and even more anxious and distressed [80].

Circumstances will arrive when the medical team may consider it necessary to apply greater physical restraint to the child to achieve the required level of immobility or access. Physical restraint for procedures has been an accepted part of standard medical care in order to act in the child or young person's best interests [81]. The terms *restraint*, *forced immobilization*, and *restrictive physical interaction* all can be defined as the "positive application of force with the intention of overpowering the child" [82]. Restraint can be used to "administer medication or carry out a procedure to which a child objects or refuses" [83]. The child's assent

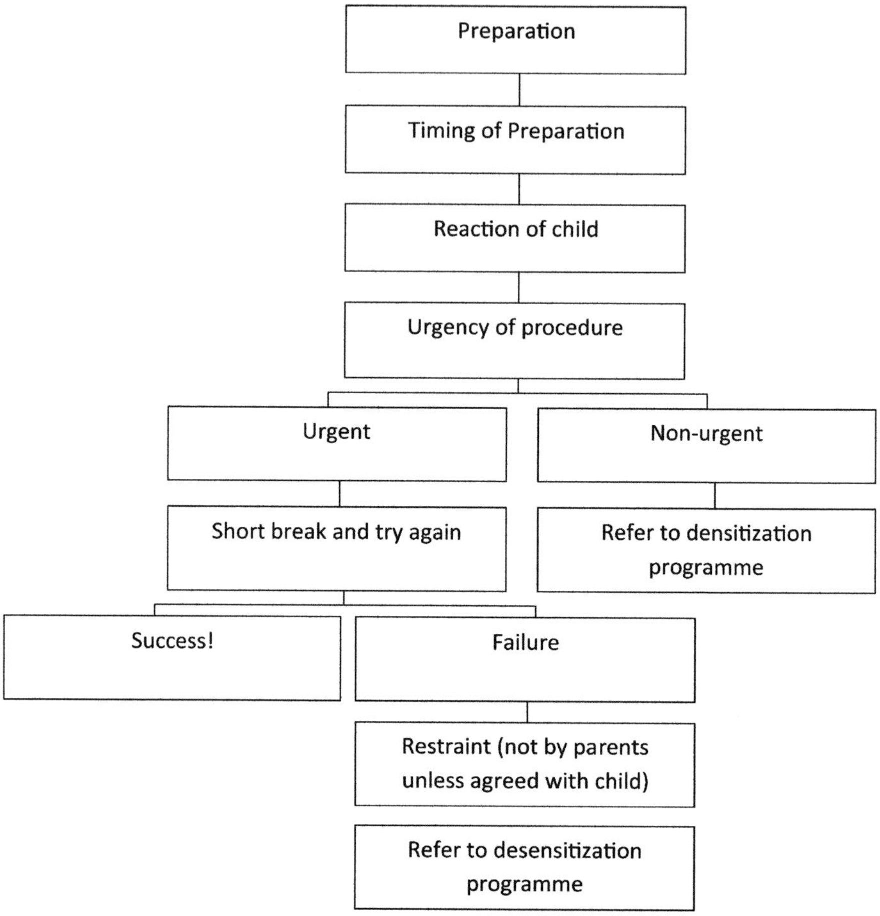

Fig. 34.1 A simple flow diagram for dealing with uncooperative or resistant children

may or may not have been sought or will not have obtained. Reasons for using restraint during a procedure include:

- Medical necessity and urgency
- The child risks harm to himself or herself through physical resistance
- Insufficient capacity by the child to understand the reason and necessity for the procedure

There is an equal obligation on clinical staff to cause no harm, to respect life, and to respect autonomy. By choosing to apply restraint and acting against a child's wishes, the team must evaluate whether the child's medical interests outweigh the potential negative consequences of physically overpowering the child: it is a balance between medical necessity and risk of psychological trauma, which can include fear and distrust of all medical care, lowered self-image, and even posttraumatic stress disorder [84]. Restraint should be used as a last resort technique and never as a convenience to the hospital schedule. It should be remembered that imposition of restraint may be more traumatic for the child than the treatment itself and make any future procedure all the more problematic [85, 86].

Staff considering the use of restraint must be aware of their institution's policies, local and national protocols or guidelines, and the appropriate legal frameworks [87, 88]. These will include when and how physical restraint should be used, time limits for attempting a procedure, and how incidents are reported.

Where possible, the child should be informed calmly and clearly in developmentally appropriate language what restraint will and will not involve. The minimum force necessary to achieve the procedure must be used, e.g., use of splints or wrapping. The family needs to be supported by a staff member not involved in the physical restraint. After the procedure has been carried out, if possible have a debriefing session with the child and parents to clarify, explain, and allow the child to express their opinions.

Restrictive physical intervention (restraint) should only be carried out by trained staff with the written consent of parents. Details of an intervention involving physical restraint need to be carefully documented in the child's medical record. Not all staff might agree with a decision to use restraint and will need an opportunity to discuss their concerns.

Parents may wish to be involved in holding down their child but this may not be the best option, as they are unlikely to have the necessary training and there might be a lasting adverse impact on the relationship between the child and parent, with loss of trust.

Protocols and guidelines are essential; however, there will be unavoidable situations where despite best intentions, therapeutic handling or restraint leaves the child, parents, and staff angry and distressed. In medical emergencies, there may not be time to prepare the parents and child sufficiently. With large and physically strong adolescents, where the patient has comorbidities, psychiatric problems, and/or learning difficulties, restraint may be extremely difficult. It is all the more important for everyone involved to have an opportunity to debrief so that lessons can be learned and preparations made for any future intervention.

Conclusion

There is broad agreement on a clinical and ethical obligation to reduce the anxiety, pain, and distress of children and young people undergoing invasive procedures outside of the operating theater. Pain and distress reduction is cost effective, yet in practice can be harder to achieve in healthcare systems that are too often inflexible, with restrictions placed on time and resources.

It is necessary to adopt a truly family-centered approach where the clinician can work collaboratively with children and their parents to achieve the best medical outcomes and psychological well-being [89, 90]. The child can be encouraged to be an active participant in his or her care rather than a passive recipient. The desired ethos is "patient before procedure."

Non-pharmacological interventions are effective in:

- Reducing anxiety, pain, and distress
- Developing and enhancing coping skills in children and their parents
- Minimizing the use of restraint
- Facilitating cooperation with future procedures
- Increasing family satisfaction with medical services

Child life specialists are essential members of the multidisciplinary team involved in pediatric healthcare. They are professionals who "promote effective coping through play, preparation, education and self-expression activities. They provide emotional support for families and encourage optimum development of children facing a broad range of challenging experiences, particularly those related to healthcare and hospitalisation, including painful procedures" [91]. In America, training to be a child life specialist requires a bachelor's degree in child life, child development, psychology, or associated field plus a child life internship leading to professional certification.

Child life specialists will work with inpatients and outpatients and their families to assess and offer interventions. Clinical psychologists specializing in pediatrics have an honors degree in psychology plus postgraduate clinical experience and professional training at a doctoral level. They offer assessment and therapy for those children with severe distress or major behavioral or emotional difficulties that interfere with the delivery of medical care. However, non-pharmacological techniques and interventions can and should be used by everyone in the team.

Clinical practice must be evidence based and underpinned by high quality research. Research to date has largely focused on psychological issues and interventions for children undergoing anesthesia in an operating theater. This research methodology has primarily used pediatric populations with isolated medical problems undergoing single event procedures. These children have been selected to fit in Class I (normally healthy patient) or Class II (a patient with mild systemic disease, i.e., mild asthma) in the American Society of Anesthesiologists (ASA) physical status classification. Useful as these studies are in guiding assessments and interventions, more research is required for children with permanent complex conditions and comorbidities being treated over many years, who need to have multiple and repeated procedures. A case studies approach may be beneficial for these populations to develop and implement individualized programs of preparation and intervention.

Case Studies

Case 1

Susie, aged 11 years, was a girl from Sweden who had undergone emergency neurosurgery at a specialist children's hospital in London. She had made a stormy recovery and required lumbar punctures on three successive days. She was extremely distressed and physically resistant to the procedure.

Behavioral Management

The psychologist was called to the treatment room where the lumbar puncture was being attended. She had not met Susie before, but was immediately able to comment on her excellent command of English. A few minutes conversation established that Susie was a keen and competent skier. The psychologist's own skiing ability was rudimentary but together with Susie she constructed a detailed story whereby Susie was skiing down her favorite piste and experiencing the exhilaration of speed and elegant style. A scenario that would have terrified the psychologist gave enormous pleasure to Susie. She was asked to shut her eyes and hold the small pillow she had used as a baby. She listened as the psychologist repeated the story using a lot

(continued)

of detail and delivered in a low-key tone. At the end of the story, Susie asked when the procedure was going to begin and was told it had been completed. The medical personnel present remarked how relaxed they also felt. Susie was very proud of her achievement but was worried she would not be able to tolerate the procedure if the psychologist was not present to tell the story. The next day the psychologist returned for the second lumbar puncture but stood silently by the bedside while Susie narrated the story to herself without speaking. The lumbar puncture was successfully completed and there was no indication from Susie's behavior that she experienced the procedure as painful. The next day the third lumbar puncture was successfully completed without the psychologist being present. Susie was very impressed with her new skills in coping with medical procedures.

Case 2

Richard, aged 7 years, has a recurrent tumor requiring repeated resections and biopsies under anesthetic. Additionally and unrelated, he has severe eczema, requiring frequent hospitalization for treatment. Initially cooperative and appearing to enjoy the hospital and the special attention afforded to him, he had become increasingly resistant to all investigations, invasive and noninvasive, such that it was very difficult to get him into the car to travel to outpatient appointments. He required a computerized tomography (CT) scan and a functional MRI with a contrast dye, requiring cannulation. This had always been difficult for Richard, despite the expertise of experienced nurses inserting the cannula. An acute eye infection necessitated a stay in a children's ward of a general adult hospital where he was frightened by the loud noises of machinery and bustle of an adult radiology service. He understood that scans do not hurt and that the reason he was having them was to confirm that he was tumor free but nevertheless he was very frightened and could not promise that he could go through with the scans back at the children's hospital.

Behavioral Management

He worked with the child life specialist, visited the scanning rooms, and practised games to rehearse lying still. His mother supported him by setting clear boundaries, not being overly apologetic and conveying the message that these tests needed to be done and reinforcing the coping strategies selected. Richard was not able to have the topical anesthetic cream because it inflamed

(continued)

his eczema, nor would he accept the cold spray, but though crying, was able to keep his hand still. He lay still throughout the scans and was delighted with his success. He said he still hated coming to hospital.

Key Points

Non-pharmacological techniques are not magic but can sometimes have a magical effect in a situation of acute distress. It is possible to build a rapport with a child and create a collaborative intervention in a short space of time that enables the procedure to proceed and the child to gain a sense of mastery and competence. The intervention for Susie (see Case 1) used distraction and guided imagery to focus attention away from the locus of pain.

Richard has undergone 2 years of hospital attendances, multiple surgeries, and invasive investigations, disrupting life at home and at school. It is not possible to promise him that the tumor will not recur or tell him with certainly how much more treatment he will need and when. His disfiguring skin condition distresses him as he feels ugly and a freak and that his peers stare at him and avoid him. His refusal to cooperate is a measure of his anger at being a victim of illness. In withholding his cooperation with hospital visits and investigations, Richard is exerting the only control he feels he has. Distraction techniques are helpful in managing specific investigations, but further work with the child and family is required to be undertaken by the child life specialist and clinical psychologist to address the wider issues imposed by Richard's illnesses.

References

1. Pearson G. Effect of operative procedures on the emotional life of a child. Am J Dis Child. 1941;62:716–29.
2. Vernon D, Foley J, Sipowicz R, Shulman J. The psychological responses of children to hospitalization and illness. Springfield, MA: Thomas Books; 1965. p. 1–5.
3. Burton L. Anxiety relating to illness and treatment. In: Verma V, editor. Anxiety in children. New York, NY: Mathuen Croom Helm; 1984. p. 151–72.
4. Vistainer MA, Wolfer JA. Psychological preparation for surgical pediatric patients: the effects on children's and parents' stress responses and adjustment. Pediatrics. 1975;56:187–202.
5. Schwarzer R, Schulz U. The role of stressful life events. In: Nezu AM, Nezu CM, Geller PA, editors. Handbook of psychology, Health psychology, vol. 9. New York, NY: Wiley; 2002. p. 27–49.
6. Kagen J, Snidman N. The long shadow of termperament. Boston, MA: Harvard University Press; 2004.
7. Schechter NL, Blankson V, Pachter LM, Sullivan CM, Costa L. Ouchless place. No pain, children's gain. Pediatrics. 1997;99: 890–4.

8. http://www.painfoundation.org/media/resources/pain-surveys.html. Accessed 14 Jan 2014.
9. Shockey DP, Menzies V, Glick DF, Taylor AG, Boitnott A, Rovnyak V. Preprocedural distress in children with cancer: an intervention using biofeedback and relaxation. J Pediatr Oncol Nurs. 2013;30(3):129–38.
10. Taddio A, Ipp M, Thivakaran S, et al. Survey of the prevalence of immunisation non-compliance due to needle fears in adults and children. Vaccine. 2012;30:4807–12.
11. Hamilton JG. Needle phobia: a neglected diagnosis. J Fam Pract. 1995;41:169–75.
12. Sokolowski CJ, Giovannati Jr JA, Boyes SG. Needle phobia: etiology, adverse consequences and patient management. Dent Clin North Am. 2010;54:731–44.
13. Kleiber C, Schutte D, McCarthy A, Floira-Santos M, Murray J, Hanharan K. Predictors of topical anesthesia effectiveness in children. J Pain. 2007;8:168–74.
14. Ranger M, Campbell-Yeo M. Temperament and pain response: a review of the literature. Pain Manag Nurs. 2008;9:2–9.
15. Arai YC, Kandatsu N, Ito H, et al. Induction and emergence behavior of children undergoing general anesthesia correlates with maternal salivary amylase activity before the anesthesia. Acta Anaesthesiol Scand. 2008;52(2):285–8.
16. Arai YC, Ueda W, Ushida T, Kandatsu N, Ito H, Komatsu T. Increased heart rate variability correlation between mother and child immediately pre operation. Acta Anaesthesiol Scand. 2009;53(5):607–10.
17. Kain ZN, Maclaren J, Mayes LC. Perioperative behavior stress in children. In: Cote CH, Lerman J, Todres ID, editors. A practice for anesthesia for infants and children. Philadelphia, PA: Saunders Elsevier; 2009. p. 26.
18. Duff AJA, Bliss AK. Reducing stress during venepuncture. In: David TJ, editor. Recent advances in paediatrics, vol. 22. London: Royal Society of Medicine; 2005. p. 149–57.
19. Bauchner H, Vinci R, May A. Teaching parents how to comfort their children during common medical procedures. Arch Dis Child. 1994;70:548–50.
20. McLaren JE, Thompson C, Weinberg M, et al. Prediction of preoperative anxiety in children: who is most accurate? Anesth Analg. 2009;108(6):1777–82.
21. Schaiavenato NL, Craig KD. Pain assessment a social transaction beyond the gold standard. Clin J Pain. 2010;26:667–76.
22. Cunnington PMD. Management of the uncooperative frightened child. In: Bingham R, Thomas AL, Sury M, editors. Hatch & Sumner's textbook of paediatric anesthesia. London: Hodder Arnold; 2007. p. 369–81.
23. Chorney JM, McMurtry CM. Behavioral measures of pain. In: McGrath PJ, Stevens BJ, Walker SM, et al., editors. Oxford textbook of paediatric pain. Oxford: Oxford University Press; 2013.
24. Bird L, McMurty CM. Fear in pediatric acute pain: role and measurement. Pain Manag. 2012;2:527–9.
25. Pedro H, Barros L, Moleiro C. Brief report: parents and nurses' behaviors associated with child distress during routine immunization in a Portuguese population. J Pediatr Psychol. 2010;35: 602–10.
26. McGrath PJ, Johnston G, Goodman JT, Dunn J, Chapman J. CHEOPS: a behavioral scale or rating postoperative pain in children. In: Fields HL, Dubner R, Cervero F, editors. Advances in pain research and therapy, vol. 9. New York: Raven; 1985. p. 395–402.
27. Merkel SI, Voepel-Lewis T, Shayevitz JR, Malviya S. The FLACC; a behavioral scale for scoring postoperative pain in young children. Pediatr Nurs. 1997;23:293–7.
28. Katz EG, Kellerman J, Ellenberg L. Hypnosis in the reduction of acute pain and distress in children with cancer. J Pediatr Psychol. 1987;12:379–94.
29. LeBaron S, Zeltzer L. Assessment of acute pain and anxiety in children and adolescents by self-reports, observer reports and a behavior checklist. J Consult Clin Psychol. 1984;52:729–38.
30. McGrath PJ, Walco GA, Turk DC, et al. Core outcome domains and measures for pediatric acute and chronic/recurrent pain clinical trials: PedIMMPACT recommendations. J Pain. 2008;9: 771–83.
31. Blount RL, Bunke V, Cohen LL, Forbes C. The Child-Adult Medical Procedures Interaction Scale-Short Form (CAMPIS-SF): validation of a rating scale for children's and adults' behaviors during painful medical procedures. J Pain Symptom Manage. 2001;22:591–9.
32. Kain ZN, Mayes LC, Cicchetti DV, et al. The Yale Preoperative Anxiety Scale: how does it compare with a 'gold standard'? Anesth Analg. 1997;85(4):783–8.
33. Kain ZN, Caramico LA, Mayes LC, et al. Preoperative preparation programs in children: a comparative examination. Anaesth Analg. 1998;87(6):1249–55.
34. Buss AH, Plomin R. Temperament: early developing personality traits. Hillsdale, NJ: Lawrence Erlbaum; 1984.
35. Vernon DT, Schulman JL, Foley JM. Changes in children's behavior after hospitalization. Some dimensions of response and their correlates. Am J Dis Child. 1966;111(6):581–93.
36. Breau LM, McGrath PJ, Camfield CS, Finley GA. Psychometric properties of the non-communicating children's pain checklist-revised. Pain. 2002;99:349–57.
37. Bauchner H, Vinci R, Waring C. Pediatric procedures: do parents want to watch? Pediatrics. 1989;84:907–9.
38. Piira T, Sugiura T, Champion GD, Donnelly N, Cole ASJ. The role of parental presence in the context of children's medical procedures; a systematic review. Child Care Health Dev. 2005;31: 233–43.
39. Kain ZF, Caldwell-Andrews AA, Mayes LC, et al. Family-centered preparation for surgery improves perioperative outcomes in children. Anesthesiology. 2007;106:65–74.
40. Liossi CL, White P, Franck L, Hatira P. Parental pain expectancy as a mediator between child expected and experienced procedure-related pain intensity during painful medical procedures. Clin J Pain. 2007;23(5):392–9.
41. Kain ZN, Maclaren J, Mayes LC. Perioperative behavior stress in children. In: Cote CH, Lerman J, Todres ID, editors. A practice for anesthesia for infants and children. Philadelphia, PA: Saunders Elsevier; 2009. p. 27.
42. Kain ZN, Mayes LC, Caldwell-Andrews AA, Karas DE, McClain BC. Preoperative anxiety, postoperative pain and behavioral recovery in young children undergoing surgery. Paediatrics. 2006;118:651–8.
43. Li HCW, Lopez V, Lee TLI. Psychoeducational preparation of children for surgery: the importance of parental involvement. Patient Educ Couns. 2007;65(1):34–41.
44. Kain ZW, Caldwell-Andrews AA, Mayes LC, et al. Family-centred preparation for surgery improves perioperative outcomes in children. Anaesthesiology. 2007;106(65):65–74.
45. Cohen LL, Blount RL, Panopoulos G. Nurse coaching and cartoon distraction: an effective and practical intervention to reduce child, parent, and nurse distress during immunizations. J Pediatr Psychol. 1997;22(3):355–70.
46. Lew VK, Lalwani K, Palermo TM. Factors affecting parental satisfaction following pediatric procedural sedation. J Clin Anesth. 2010;22:29–34.
47. Jaaniste T, Hayes B, von Bayer CL. Providing children with information about forthcoming medical procedure: a review and synthesis. Clin Psychol Sci Pract. 2007;14:124–43.
48. Department of Health. Getting the right start: National Service Framework for Children-Standard 7: services for children and young people in hospital. London: The Stationary Office; 2003.

49. http://www.gosh.nhs.uk/children/. Accessed 14 Jan 2014.
50. www.cafamily.org.uk. Accessed 14 Jan 2014.
51. http://www.actionforsickchildren.org/. Accessed 14 Jan 2014.
52. Sparks LA, Setlik J, Luhrman J. Parental holding and positioning to decrease IV distress in young children: a randomized controlled trial. J Pediatr Nurs. 2007;22:440–7.
53. Duff AJA, Gaskell SL, Jacobs K, Houghton JM. Management of distressing procedures in children and young people: time to adhere to the guidelines. Arch Dis Child. 2012;97(1):1–4.
54. Cohen LL. Behavioral approaches to anxiety and pain management for pediatric venous access. Pediatrics. 2008;122 Suppl 3:S134–9.
55. Blount RL, Zempsky WT, Janniste T. Management of pediatric pain and distress due to medical procedures. In: Roberts C, Steele R, editors. Handbook of pediatric psychology. 4th ed. New York: Guilford Press; 2010. p. 171–88.
56. Christie D, Wilson C. CBT in pediatric and adolescent health settings: a review of practice-based evidence. Paediatr Rehabil. 2004;8(4):241–7.
57. Uman LS, Chambers CT, McGrath PJ, Kisely S. A systematic review of randomised control trials examining psychological interventions for needle-related procedural pain and distress in children and adolescents: an abbreviated Cochrane review. J Paediatr Psychol. 2008;33:842–54.
58. Yip P, Middleton P, Cyna AM, Carlyle AV. Non-pharmacological interventions for assisting the induction of anesthesia in children. Cochrane Database Syst Rev. 2009;(3):CD006447. doi:10.1002/14651858.CD006447.pub2.
59. Dahlquist LM, Pendley JS, Landtrip DS, Jones CL, Steuber CP. Distraction interventions for pre-schoolers undergoing intramuscular injections and subcutaneous port access. Health Psychol. 2002;21:94–9.
60. Pringle B, Hilley L, Gelfand K, et al. Decreasing child distress during needle sticks and maintaining treatment gains over time. J Clin Psychol Med Settings. 2001;8(2):119–30.
61. Koller D, Goldman RD. Distration techniques for children undergoing procedures: a critical review of pediatric research. J Pediatr Nurs. 2011;27:652–81.
62. Christiano B, Russ SW. Matching preparatory intervention to coping style: the effect of children's distress in the dental setting. J Pediatr Psychol. 1998;23(1):17–27.
63. McCaffery M, Beebe A. Pain, clinical manual for nursing practice. London: Mosby; 1994.
64. Hilgard ER, Hilgard JR. Hypnosis in the relief of pain. New York: Brunner/Mazel; 1994.
65. Chaves JF. Hypnosis in pain management. In: Rhue JW, Lynn SJ, editors. Handbook of clinical hypnosis. Washington, DC: American Psychological Association; 1993. p. 511–32.
66. Liossi C, Kuttner L, Wood C, Zeltzer L. Hypnosis and relaxation. In: McGrath P, Stevens B, Walker S, Zempsky WT, editors. Oxford textbook of paediatric pain. Oxford: Oxford University Press; 2013. p. 560–8.
67. Liossi C, White P, Hatira P. A randomized clinical trial of a brief hypnosis intervention to control venepuncture-related pain of paediatric cancer patients. Pain. 2009;142:255–63.
68. Stevens B, Petryshen P, Hawkins J, Smith B, Taylor P. Developmental versus conventional care: a comparison of clinical outcomes for very low birth weight infants. Can J Nurs Res. 1996;28(4):97–113.
69. Johnston CC, Stevens B, Pinelli J, et al. Kangaroo care is effective in diminishing pain response in diminishing pain response in preterm neonates. Arch Pediatr Adolesc Med. 2003;157(11):1084–8.
70. Campos RG. Rocking and pacifiers: two comforting interventions for heal stick pain. Res Nurs Health. 1994;17(5):321–31.
71. Stevens B, Yamada J, Ohlsson A. Sucrose for analgesia in newborn infants undergoing painful procedures. Cochrane Database Syst Rev. 2004;(3):CD001069. doi:10.1002/14651858.CD001069.pub2.
72. Cohen LL, Bernard RS, NcClellan CB, MacLaren JE. Assessing medical room behavior during infants' painful medical procedures: the Measure of Adult and Infant Soothing and Distress (MAISD). Child Health Care. 2005;34:81–9.
73. Blount RL, Simons LE, Devine KA, et al. Evidence-based assessment of coping and stress in paediatric psychology. J Pediatr Psychol. 2008;33:1021–45.
74. Gaskell S. Evidence-based guidelines for the management of invasive and/or distressing procedures with children. Position paper. Leicester: British Psychological Society (BPS); 2010.
75. Royal Australasian College of Physicians. Management of procedure related pain n children and adolescents. Guideline statement: paediatric and health division. J Paediatr Child Health. 2006;42:51–529.
76. Emerson E, Hatton C, Robertson J, et al. People with learning disabilities in England 2010. Durham: Improving Health and Lives: Learning Disabilities Observatory; 2010.
77. Van der Walt JH, Moran C. An audit of the perioperative management of autistic children. Paediatr Anaesth. 2001;11:401–8.
78. Beukelman DR, Mirenda P. Augmentative and alternative communication: supporting children and adults with complex communication needs. 3rd ed. Baltimore: Brookes; 2005.
79. Kim JE, Jo BY, Choi HS, Lee Y. High anxiety, young age and long waits increase the need for preoperative sedatives in children. J Int Med Res. 2012;40:1381–9.
80. Lambrenos K, McArthur E. Introducing a clinical holding policy. Paediatr Nurs. 2003;15(4):30–3.
81. Folkes K. Is restraint a form of abuse? Paediatr Nurs. 2005; 17(6):41–4.
82. Department of Health. Guidance on permissible forms of control in children's residential care. London: The Stationary Office; 1993.
83. Jeffrey K. Therapeutic restraint of children: it must always be justified. Paediatr Nurs. 2002;14(9):20–2.
84. Brenner M. Child restraint in the acute setting of paediatric nursing: an extraordinarily stressful event. Issues Compr Pediatr Nurs. 2007;30(1–2):29–37.
85. Robinson S, Collier J. Holding children still for procedures. Paediatr Nurs. 1997;9(4):12–4.
86. McGrath P, Forrester K, Fox-Young S, Huff N. "Holding the child down" for treatment in paediatric haematology: the ethical, legal and practice implications. J Law Med. 2002;10(1):84–96.
87. Nunn J, Foster M, Master S et al. Consent and the use of physical intervention in the dental care of children. British Society of Paediatric Dentistry. 2008;18(Suppl.1):39–46.
88. Royal College of Nursing. Restrictive physical intervention and therapeutic holding for children and young people. London: Royal College of Nursing; 2010.
89. Chorney JM, Kain Z. Family-centered pediatric perioperative care. Anesthesiology. 2010;112(3):751–5.
90. Visitainer MA, Wolfer JA. Psychological preparation for surgical pediatric patients: the effect on children's and parent's stress responses and adjustment. Pediatrics. 1975;56:187–202.
91. Child Life Council. The child life profession. 2012. Available at: htto://www.childlife.org/The%20Child%20Life%20Profession/. Accessed July 2013.

The Role of Simulation in Safety and Training

35

James J. Fehr and Itai M. Pessach

Abstract

Simulation has advanced from the days of Resusci-Annie and basic cardiopulmonary resuscitation training. High-fidelity, computer-controlled mannequins allow early learners and advanced clinicians to explore various domains of sedation practice and prepare for unusual or life-threatening events. This modality has the advantage of permitting deliberative practice toward mastery without putting patients at risk. With increasing demands for patient safety and provider accountability, simulation is likely to play an increasing role in provider training.

Keywords

Simulation • Mannequin • Patient safety • Pediatrics • Sedation • Education • Crisis resource management (CRM) • Andragogy

History of Medical Simulation

The development of mannequins for teaching basic life support techniques signaled the entry of simulation into medical training. In the 1950s, Dr. Peter Safar introduced the principles of basic life support [1, 2]. With his collaborators Dr. James Elam and Dr. Bjørn Lind, these techniques were brought into medical training through the development of Resusci-Annie [3]. In 1969, a computer-controlled patient simulator was created by Denson, representing the progenitor of current computerized mannequins [4]. The greater processing power and increasingly compact nature of modern computer systems have expanded possible simulation applications. Contemporary computer-controlled mannequins can simulate a range of physiologic findings including reactive pupils, a range of auscultatory cardiac and respiratory sounds, palpable pulses, seizures, and more. These mannequins can be intubated, defibrillated, receive chest compressions, have an intraosseous needle placed, and undergo needle decompression of a pneumothorax or cardiac tamponade. Their physiologic modeling can demonstrate vital signs on a computer monitor that respond with high fidelity to pharmacologic interventions. Present day mannequins can simulate all aspects of the worst imaginable clinical day. They are used in the teaching and assessment of individuals and teams in training programs worldwide.

Pilots and physicians share many job characteristics as both have to deal with complex settings involving stress, multidisciplinary teams, interaction with advanced technology, and human lives. These similarities led to the adoption of many techniques and methods initially developed for aviation into the practice of medicine. Simulation-based training is one of the most important techniques that have been applied to medicine [5]. The "blue box" flight simulator designed by Edwin Link in the 1920s was built to teach new pilots how to fly by the instrument panel. This historic mechanical engineering device provided accurate instrument flight readings in response to the pilot's operation of the

J.J. Fehr, M.D. (✉)
Department of Anesthesiology and Pediatrics, St. Louis Children's Hospital, St. Louis, MI, USA
e-mail: fehrj@wustl.edu

I.M. Pessach, M.D., Ph.D.
Israel Center for Medical Simulation (MSR), Sheba Medical Center, Tel-Hashomer, Israel
e-mail: Itai.pessach@sheba.health.gov.il

K.P. Mason (ed.), *Pediatric Sedation Outside of the Operating Room: A Multispecialty International Collaboration*,
DOI 10.1007/978-1-4939-1390-9_35, © Springer Science+Business Media New York 2015

simulator controls and is considered to be the first mechanical flight simulator. Its purpose was twofold: To train pilots without exposing them to the risk of flying solo prior to any hands-on practice and to save expenses [6].

With the remarkable developments in computer science, robotics, virtual reality, and gaming technology as well as in education and adult learning theories, simulation-based training has evolved to become an integral and important part of flight crew training. In fact, no airline or agency will allow pilots to fly if they have not completed the necessary simulator-based certification or recertification. This standard has also been adopted by many other fields in which errors may have catastrophic consequences (military, nuclear power).

Aircraft accidents are rare events that can lead to significant casualties and place the public at risk. As research has previously shown that more than 70 % of aviation accidents involve human error, flight simulators are used to train not only for technical flying skills but also for teamwork training: to train teams to work together and to provide a safe learning environment that allows for the exploration of personal physiological and psychological limitations. (Refer to Chap. 30.) In recent years, the promotion of safety and the prevention of error in medicine are receiving an increasing focus, which further boosts the integration of simulation-based training into daily practice [7].

With the improvement in simulation tools, Gaba and Howard focused on improving team communication and dynamics in the medical sphere with the introduction of Crisis Resource Management (CRM) [8]. This was an adaptation of crew resource management that was developed for pilots in response to analyses of airline disasters. The goal of CRM is to help providers develop greater situational awareness so that during an emergency they effectively utilize all available clinical resources. Simulation-based training incorporates facilitated debriefing as a teaching tool. One approach to debriefing is advocacy-inquiry, which demands good judgment to support reflective practice [9].

There are numerous examples of simulation in the literature that describe its application to various aspects of sedation. Rosenberg and colleagues reported on the use of a mock magnetic resonance imagining (MRI) scanner to prepare children for an actual unsedated scan [10]. The simulated MRI experience resulted in a decreased heart rate and lessened self-reported distress. LaPierre and colleagues described the pharmacologic simulation of common propofol and propofol-remifentanil dosing regimens for upper endoscopy in adults [11]. This study involved human volunteers receiving target-controlled infusions (TCI) to various serum plasma drug concentrations, which simulated published recommended doses. A 42F bougie was passed 40 cm into the esophagus of the sedated volunteers to simulate placement of an endoscope. These approaches to simulation are focused on the delivery of sedation. The remainder of the chapter will concentrate on the role of simulation for sedation providers.

Medical simulation refers to any of a number of processes or techniques that present scenarios with clinically relevant content and encourage deliberative practice [12]. Refinement and increasing integration of simulation has led to a vast array of options: from task trainers to high-fidelity mannequins and from code reenactments to interview training with standardized patients. Simulation scenarios can present the novice with basic concepts, provide a forum to review important principles, and challenge experienced practitioners with complex clinical problems. Simulation enables individuals as well as teams from any medical domain to be trained, assessed, evaluated, and refined. Simulation is integral to enhancing patient safety without putting actual patients at risk: Initial training can be provided, baseline competency can be assessed, and preliminary steps toward mastery can be achieved.

Andragogy, the theory of adult education, describes the strategies that adults use to learn. Traditional learning employs the lecture-centric model of education. Adults, however, have an extensive repertoire of experiences and approach the acquisition of new information differently from younger students. Adult learners have been shown to benefit from educational experiences that allow them flexibility, opportunities for reflection, hands-on practice, and team learning. Education delivery guided by neurobiology would provide a milieu where active involvement, engagement, visualization, and repetition occur [13]. Simulation incorporates these educational strategies and strives to provide an engaging educational environment that can be adapted to the individual learning styles of adults.

In cognitive psychology there is a well-described decay in memory that occurs after learners are taught new information or infrequently used skills. Roediger has demonstrated this after undergraduates learn new words and Larsen has confirmed this in follow-up of pediatric residents confronted with new medical information [14, 15]. Simulation can be used to address this predictable memory decay through assessment, retraining, retesting, and the process of test-enhanced learning [16].

Simulation for Sedation Safety and Training

In *To Err is Human*, published in 2000, the Institute of Medicine identified medicine as a perilous undertaking. It estimated that 44,000–98,000 unnecessary deaths from adverse events occur annually in the United States during hospitalization [17]. A decade later, these estimates have been reaffirmed and expanded [18, 19]. In general, pediatric sedation is associated with a low incidence of significant adverse events when administered by well-trained sedation providers. The Pediatric Sedation Research Consortium demonstrated that during propofol sedation for children out of the operating room there were no deaths, a low rate of adverse events, and a low rate of hospital admission [20]. Regardless, severe adverse outcomes in healthy children undergoing sedation do occur. Especially when a patient's level of consciousness is altered, there is an increased potential risk of severe adverse events [21].

Traditional medical education has followed the "see one, do one, teach one" paradigm and the education of pediatric sedation providers tends to follow this approach. Medicine is traditionally approached as an apprenticeship. Efforts have been made to organize and standardize the training of sedation providers to be concordant with the recommendations of the American Academy of Pediatrics (AAP), the Society for Pediatric Anesthesiology (SPA), and the American Society of Anesthesiologists (ASA). However, with restriction of trainees' hours, demands for greater supervision, and increasing focus on patient safety, it is challenging to guarantee that present trainees have sufficient experience in sedation. The AAP guidelines encourage the use of patient simulators to train sedation providers in the management of rare events [22]. (Refer to Chap. 2.) The value of simulation is not limited to only physicians. Farnsworth and colleagues reported in 2000 on the use of an anesthesia simulator to teach and evaluate nurses involved in sedation [23]. They demonstrated an improvement in test scores and an overall satisfaction with the educational experience. In 2004, Babl developed a comprehensive sedation training program for an academic and a nonacademic hospital in Australia. The course was taught by nurse educators and included a standardized sedation checklist, educational materials, and a multiple choice test. Six months later, a follow-up query revealed that the participants believed that the training had significantly improved proxy markers of patient safety. This benefit, however, recedes over time. Retraining is critical. At a 3-year follow-up, the same study revealed deterioration in these proxy markers of patient safety at both sites [24]. More recently, in Canada, Schneeweiss and colleagues compared self-directed and educated sedation providers with those that received 4 h of formal simulation-based sedation training. The group that underwent sedation training outperformed the self-directed learners in knowing and understanding sedation guidelines and practices [25].

Tobin and colleagues have described a moderate sedation course that included an online didactic component, basic airway management training, and a simulation component [26]. They demonstrated the feasibility of using such a multimodal method of teaching moderate sedation but were not able to demonstrate a T3 level of translational research: improved clinical outcomes as measured by reduction of adverse events such as severe hypoxemia.

Simulation for Pediatric Sedation

Simulation has been incorporated into the training of sedation providers for both adults and children. This trend is an extension of current integration of simulation into medical school curricula, nursing education, and medical training of physician trainees.

Although to date there are no studies to support improved outcomes as a direct result of simulation, intellectually simulation has been embraced as of value to train and evaluate sedation providers [27]. Simulation has been applied to identify latent systems failures during pediatric procedural sedation [28].

Sedation of children occurs in varied locations: emergency rooms, intensive care units, operative suites, and free-standing ambulatory procedural centers. The training and background of individuals who sedate children is diverse. Multiple specialties interface in the sedation of children: nursing, pediatrics, anesthesiology, intensive care, dental medicine, gastrointestinal medicine, radiology, surgery, and others. Simulation is an attempt to standardize the basic skill set of novice sedation providers, to reinforce concepts previously encountered but not mastered, and to remediate individuals whose skills are not at the level of their peers. Teams may also be trained, refined, and enhanced using simulation.

Crisis management and team training is critical for simulation. Most sedation teams are limited to a sedation provider and a nurse. When adverse events occur, an emergency code team usually assists in the patient management. The sedation provider must be prepared to coordinate and/or lead crises so that this care is delivered effectively and expeditiously. Simulation will develop the management skill set. Simulation can enhance the provider's confidence, clarity, and communication effectiveness during such emergencies.

Schinasi and colleagues have reported a needs assessment of pediatric residents during procedural sedation [29]. These residents represented different stages of training and varying degrees of simulation experience. A performance evaluation checklist was created for a simulated adverse event of apnea and oxygen desaturation during the procedural sedation of a simulated child during a fracture reduction; 97 % of the participants recognized the desaturation event and delivered oxygen (95 %) within 60 s. Positive pressure ventilation was performed by 75 % within 97 s from the onset of hypoventilation. These data demonstrate the value of simulation to identify a learning and skill gap and then address it through performance assessment and debriefing. Although a post-test confidence self-assessment demonstrated improvement after increased years of training, it correlated poorly with actual performance in the actual simulation scenario.

Keidan and colleagues also reported the use of a patient simulator to evaluate pediatric trainee performance in recognizing

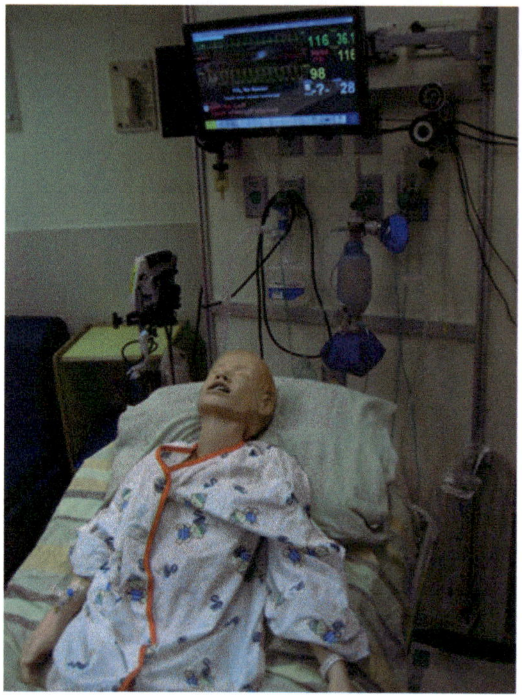

Fig. 35.1 Contemporary simulation mannequin

and responding to apnea and hypoventilation. In this study, pediatric residents were slower to respond if the simulated pediatric patient was receiving oxygen as compared to those who were not receiving oxygen [30]. This study is a good example of how simulation can identify clinical deficits of providers, and their potential risks to actual patients.

In the domain of sedation for pediatric dentistry, Tan applied simulation to present dental residents and dental assistants with crisis situations [31]. Participants managed four scenarios: anaphylaxis, laryngospasm, sedative overdose, and cardiac arrhythmia. Following the simulation, each participant completed a survey that queried their prior clinical experience; only 29 % reported having been involved with a similar real-life medical crisis. The survey and post-simulation debriefing revealed that a majority were unfamiliar with the equipment, and that the majority felt that simulation was a good tool for them to learn CRM.

Simulation is an important teaching tool for individuals and teams to participate in "real-life" scenarios on a high-fidelity mannequin (Fig. 35.1) in a close-to-real-life environment. The simulation process can also be performed "in situ," referring to the actual environment where sedation occurs such as the emergency department, the clinic treatment room, or the pediatric intensive care unit. This unique opportunity not only allows for the training and practice of extreme and rare events, but also highlights critical aspects in patient safety, such as the applicability of protocols, ergonomics (the setup of the space where sedation is to be administered), the location and availability of necessary equipment, and many other important details that only become evident during a critical event.

Principles of Simulation-Based Training for Pediatric Sedation

Initial Training

Approaches to the development of simulation-based training for pediatric sedation are not fundamentally different than training for other competencies. There are some obvious prerequisites. In most cases some experience in pediatric care is required as well as certification in Pediatric Advanced Life Support (PALS). Training is typically preceded by theoretical preparations using didactic presentations and self-learning of material, which includes important topics in pediatric sedation: patient evaluation and preparation, pharmacology, physiologic monitoring, protocols, policies, and regulations.

Simulation-based training is usually a tiered evolution of skill acquisition. This begins with the acquisition of task-specific skills relevant to pediatric sedation. This encompasses proficiency in essential rescue measures such as head positioning and suctioning, oxygen supplementation, bag-mask ventilation, and recovery positions. It can include the appropriate use of pharmacologic reversal agents and the proper use and interpretation of physiologic monitoring technologies including pulse oximetry and capnography. The skill training is best when individualized and will serve to achieve a common foundation of knowledge and language for trainees from various disciplines and backgrounds. Often these skills are taught by demonstration and practice on mannequins during short sessions with an instructor.

After acquiring basic sedation skills, the next "tier" of training progresses to "real-life" sedation scenarios that challenge multiple members of the team. These scenarios require the application, practice, and integration of the basic sedation concepts with effective communication, crisis management, and advanced life support skills. Each session is followed by a facilitated debriefing session that allows for reflective practice and learning enhancement. The use of videotaping during the simulation sessions provides an objective reference for participants and facilitators during the debriefing. Videotaping encourages a learner-centered approach of self-reflection and transparency, thus maximizing the learning opportunity.

In 2003, the Israeli ministry of health instituted mandatory training for medical providers of pediatric sedation. To meet the growing need for training, the Israeli Center for Medical Simulation (MSR) has developed a simulation-based training

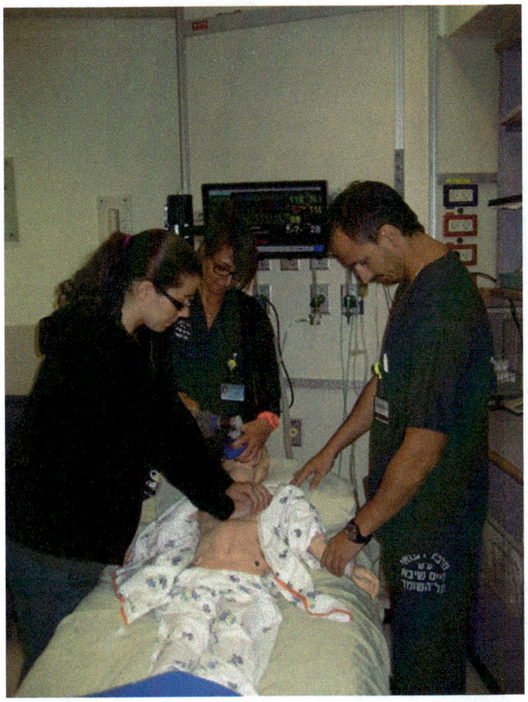

Fig. 35.2 Team training in the pediatric intensive care unit at Sheba Medical Center, Tel-Hashomer, Israel

Table 35.1 A curriculum of patient safety during pediatric sedation

Learning objectives
• To acquire proficiency in the use of medication regimens
• To understand decision making in the context of pediatric sedation medications and patient safety.
• To become competent in diagnosing and managing adverse sedation reactions
• To understand and use monitoring technologies including capnometry and capnography
• To acquire proficiency in essential rescue measures such as airway management, head and recovery positioning, suction, oxygen supplementation, bag-mask ventilation and use of reversal agents, position.
Course outline:
• Advanced E-learning theoretical presentation and pretest
• Introduction
• Simulation-based skill training for—monitoring technologies, positioning, airway management, and bag-mask ventilation
• Practice of pediatric sedation simulation-based scenarios:
– Oversedation leading to airway compromise
– Sedative overdose leading to apnea and bradycardia
Minimum requirements for successful completion of the course
Upon completion of the course, participants are required to pass a written multiple choice examination and a simulated safety-skills session, which includes an evaluation of the participant's ability to assess and manage airway complications

program for patient safety during pediatric sedation based on the aforementioned principles (Fig. 35.2). An example of a curriculum for simulation-based basic training in patient safety during pediatric sedation is shown in Table 35.1.

In the decade that followed, hundreds of providers, including pediatric residents, fellows, senior physicians, and pediatric nurses were trained using this platform. This type of simulation-based training has significantly improved patient safety and led to better adherence to pediatric sedation protocols by nonanesthesiologists that routinely perform procedural sedation outside the operating room [32]. It demonstrated that following completion of simulation-based training, unsupervised pediatric residents performed procedural sedation in a manner that was safe and comparable to that performed by certified pediatric emergency physicians [33].

Advanced Training

The use of simulation for training and maintaining competencies in pediatric sedation does not end with the completion of the basic initial training. The use of in situ simulation (performing in the clinical setting where procedures take place) is growing rapidly and many units and institutions have developed these capabilities in recent years. In situ simulation enables providers to engage in their own setting, with their own equipment. This can uncover unidentified challenges and variables that could not have been otherwise anticipated [34, 35]. In situ simulation can also serve to monitor and test the efficiency, effectiveness, and applicability of various safety measures and protocols that are used for pediatric sedation [36, 37].

Future Trends

Contemporary medicine is confronted with escalating medical care costs and expanding demands for patient safety. Health care systems must balance the need for safe and high-quality care with the costs of training and assessing the provider competency. As technological developments lead to an ever-expanding diagnostic toolbox and novel potential therapies, there are increasing demands for sedation of children. Pediatric sedation is substantially safer than it was a generation ago. As pediatric sedation becomes safer, the risk of the sedation provider experiencing unintended consequences decreases. Simulation provides an opportunity to experience these increasingly rare events. It is one mechanism by which trainees and providers can be challenged to think beyond their routines and to develop a greater awareness of the complexity and potential hazards of their practice.

Simulation provides flexibility for different levels of experience and adaptability to different clinical domains and social situations. The limitations of simulation are related to financial expense and the limited outcome data. The costs include the purchase and maintenance of the mannequins, the salaries of the simulation staff, and the storage of equipment. A separate simulation center is not required; mobile simulation carts can provide the same experience at a more modest cost [38]. A dedicated simulation center, if remote from areas of clinical service, may actually limit simulation experience by depriving participants of experiencing the actual locations in which sedation is delivered.

Sedation providers for children are required to be certified in basic and advanced life support techniques for children. Current Advanced Cardiac Life Support (ACLS) and PALS courses present computer-based simulation scenarios that must be satisfactorily completed prior to application on the mannequin. Students are becoming familiar with this method of training, and have come to anticipate the stresses and challenges of the simulation environment. They are able to repeat the simulation when their performance does not reach their goal and practice until satisfactory performance is achieved.

Pediatric Sedation Simulation Scenario

A pediatric sedation simulation can be created using the most expensive of computer-controlled mannequins or with more modest simulators. Designing and delivering a meaningful simulation experience requires consideration of the purpose of the exercise: Who are the intended participants? What resources are available? What are the curricular goals? The content of simulation scenarios can be adjusted to serve participants of differing experiential levels. For example, a scenario built around a 3-year-old child being sedated for an MRI might be adapted for the early learner to practice MRI safety and basic sedation techniques. It could also be used to introduce more challenging problems such as laryngospasm, anaphylaxis, or pneumothorax. Complicating factors may be built into the scenario to increase their difficulty and make them more appropriate for advanced practitioners. Such content could include communication challenges, medical errors, and delivering bad news to the family. Sedation scenarios are also described in the literature that can be used to guide simulation development. Chen and colleagues described a simulation scenario for airway rescue during pediatric sedation. This was a comprehensive scenario of a 2-year-old child with Acute Lymphoblastic Leukemia undergoing sedation for PICC line placement and provides a template to follow [39]. The journal *Simulation in Healthcare* is dedicated to simulation-based investigation and is a resource for obtaining scenarios for program development.

The equipment necessary to run a scenario does not have to be prohibitively expensive and does not require a de dicated onsite simulation suite. It begins with a simulation mannequin. Mannequins are available from numerous vendors with a broad range of prices, sizes, and capabilities. Most can be intubated, can receive chest compressions, and provide cardiac and respiratory sounds. They are usually computer controlled, and some of the most recently developed are controlled by smart pad computers, which have the advantages of ease of use and portability. The vital signs are presented on a computer screen and can be altered by the controller or change in response to the participant's actions during a scenario. Ultimately, equipment selection is guided by available resources and educational goals. For simulation scenarios, the mannequin does not have to be an expensive high-fidelity computer-controlled machine. Basic pediatric CPR trainers can be used, even without a computer monitor. In such cases, the vital signs and scenario development should be scripted and read to the participant as the scenario unfolds.

Simulation is being increasingly recognized by the Accreditation Council for Graduate Medical Education (ACGME) as a method to mark the achievement of milestones by residents and fellows. The methodology of simulation is familiar to medical students who, since 2004, have taken the United States Medical Licensing Examination (USMLE) Step 2 Clinical Skills. This exam involves interacting appropriately with simulated patients, taking a medical history, performing a clinical exam, and then writing a summary including a differential diagnosis. Simulation has also been integrated into recertification training for experienced practitioners. The American Board of Anesthesiology's Maintenance of Certification in Anesthesia (MOCA) program has incorporated simulation as a component of practice performance assessment and improvement for recertification. Participants typically spend a day working on recognition and response to crisis situations, crew resource management, and team training [40].

Simulation also can be incorporated more informally as a component workshop at national meetings. The logistics of securing meeting space can be challenging. Such simulations may involve a group of individuals participating in a scenario while the audience observes, or small groups rotating through simulation stations. The latter model has been used at the Pediatric Sedation Outside of the Operating Room conference[1] of Boston Children's Hospital and Harvard Medical School [41], which is presented in a hotel room (Fig. 35.3). In this model, participants in groups of four to eight rotate for 1 h through a scenario. Five or six scenarios run concurrently and are repeated throughout the day. A range of topics can be covered including crisis resources management, laryngospasm, anaphylaxis, oversedation, airway obstruction, airway foreign body, and the challenging parent. With

[1] www.PediatricSedationConference.com

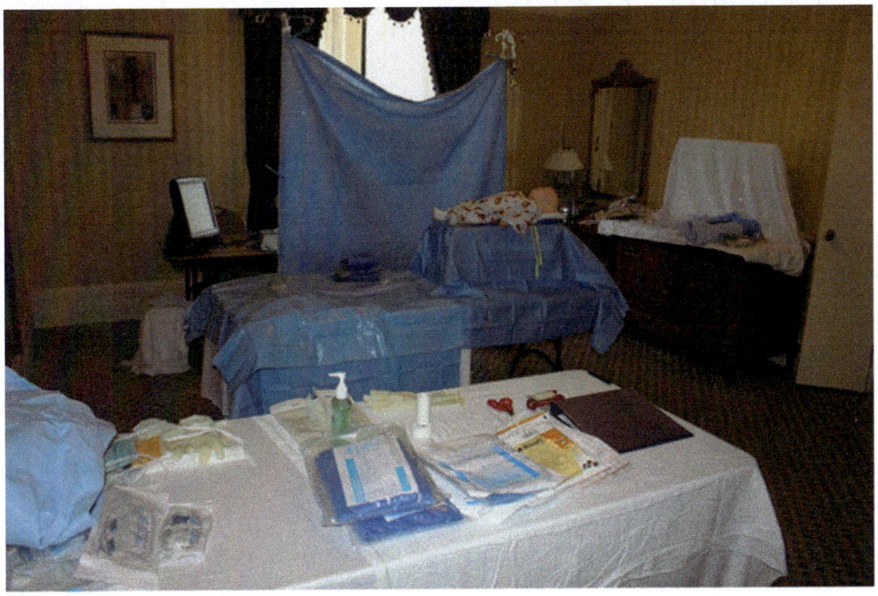

Fig. 35.3 Setup for onsite simulation in hotel room at the Pediatric Sedation Outside of the Operating Room conference in Boston (www.PediatricSedationConference.com)

Table 35.2 Suggested equipment for pediatric sedation simulations

Pediatric mannequin	Computer-controlled mannequin. (Could substitute with simple mannequin and scripted vital signs)
Airway	Laryngoscope, endotracheal tubes, stylet, oral airways, LMA
Breathing	CPAP bag, Ambu bag, oxygen source, capnometer
Circulation	IV tubing, IV catheters, intraosseous needle
Resuscitation equipment	Defibrillator, chest tubes
Radiographs	Chest X-ray
Simulated medications	Propofol, atropine, succinylcholine, epinephrine
Miscellaneous	Clean syringes, IV bag and tubing
Prop	Infusion pump

two to four faculty members participating, there is an extremely favorable student-to-faculty ratio and these sessions are generally positively reviewed.

In considering how one might use simulation in an educational or evaluative sense, it is helpful to explore a hypothetical scenario. The following pediatric simulation case provides a construct for thinking about how to design, develop, and utilize simulation to train individuals in pediatric sedation. It can be adapted to local situations and modified to prevailing needs. Presented in Table 35.2 is some basic equipment that might be utilized in such a simulation and a proposed scenario template is provided in Table 35.3. The following scenario includes suggestions for equipment to consider making available for the simulation, the simulation script, and a potential checklist of key actions that one might consider should be accomplished by the participant. These key actions are suggested, not validated, and do not represent an absolute gold standard of performance.

Sedation Scenario

Patient is a 5-year-old child undergoing a lumbar puncture for new onset seizures. The child was healthy until a recent episode of decreased responsiveness. Lumbar puncture is ordered under sedation.

Past Medical History: term birth, uncomplicated pregnancy
Medications: none
Allergies: none
Past Medical History: none
Past Surgical History: none
Family History: noncontributory
Review of Systems: normal development

Physical Examination
Weight: 20 kg
Vital Signs: HR 136, RR 32, BP 112/74, SpO_2 99 % (room air), afebrile
Airway: no loose teeth, Mallampati I
CV: regular rate and rhythm, no murmur
Resp: clear to auscultation
GI: non-tender, non-distended, soft
Neuro: grossly intact, fussy but consolable

Teaching Points

1. To review the guidelines for pediatric sedation from the AAP and ASA
2. To review basic airway management
3. To identify and manage hypoventilation and apnea during sedation
4. To consider how CRM can be utilized to improve management of children undergoing sedation

Table 35.3 Template for simulated scenario actions

Template for Scenario Actions (Hypoventilation during Lumbar Puncture)	
Initial State	
HR 136, RR 32, BP 112/74, SpO_2 99% fussy & consolable	Patient identified, time out confirmed, participant assumes care of the patient. Administers titrated doses of fentanyl (1 microgram/kg) and versed (0.1 mg/kg).
Sedation	
HR 116, RR 18, BP 82/54, SpO_2 98% (1.0 FiO_2) somnolent	Following the initial dose of fentanyl and versed, the child is still moving. The proceduralist is complaining that they cannot do the procedure. Additional doses of fentanyl (1 microgram/kg) and versed (0.1 mg/kg) are administered.
Desaturation	
Hypoventilation & Apnea HR 76, RR 0, SpO_2 74%	The child develops hypoventilation and becomes apneic.
Recovery	
HR 116, RR 18, BP 82/54, SpO_2 98% (1.0 FiO_2)	Following stabilization of the child the vital signs return to normal and the debriefing can begin.

Scenario Checklist: Hypoventilation During Lumbar Puncture
Participant Specialty: ______________________
Participant Level of Training: ______________________

Scenario:

5-year-old undergoing monitored sedation for an LP to evaluate new onset seizures.

Child desaturates following administration of second dose of fentanyl and versed.

Place a checkmark by the tasks the participant completes (Table 35.4).

Based on the expectations of a sedation provider to independently sedate pediatric patients, please evaluate this participant using the scale in Table 35.5.

Table 35.4 Sedation scenario completion checklist

1.	Recognizes desaturation
2.	Informs the person performing the LP that the patient is desaturating
3.	Asks the person performing the LP to stop
4.	Moves the patient to supine
5.	Repositions head with chin lift
6.	Administers oxygen
7.	Places an oral airway
8.	Inspects for chest rise
9.	Auscultates breath sounds
10.	Performs positive pressure ventilation
11.	Performs positive pressure ventilation in less than 60 s

Table 35.5 Sedation scenario participant assessment scale

The care provided was:								
Unsatisfactory			**Satisfactory**			**Superior**		
1	**2**	**3**	**4**	**5**	**6**	**7**	**8**	**9**

References

1. Safar P. Ventilatory efficacy of mouth-to-mouth artificial respiration. JAMA. 1958;167(3):335–41.
2. Safar P, Brown TC, Holtey WJ, Wilder RJ. Ventilation and circulation with closed-chest cardiac massage in man. JAMA. 1961; 176(7):92–4.
3. Tjomsland N, Laerdal T, Baskett P. Bjørn Lind—the ground-breaking nurturer. Resuscitation. 2005;65:133–8.
4. Denson JS, Abrahamson S. A computer-controlled patient simulator. JAMA. 1969;208:504–8.
5. d'Agincourt-Canning LG, Kissoon N, Singal M, Pitfield AF. Culture, communication and safety: lessons from the airline industry. Indian J Pediatr. 2011;78(6):703–8.
6. Rosen KR. The history of medical simulation. J Crit Care. 2008;23(2):157–66.
7. Beaubien JM, Baker DP. The use of simulation for training teamwork skills in health care: how low can you go? Qual Saf Health Care. 2004;13 Suppl 1:i51–6.
8. Howard SK, Gaba DM, Fish KJ, et al. Anesthesia crisis resource management training: teaching anesthesiologists to handle critical incidents. Aviat Space Environ Med. 1992;63(9):763–70.
9. Rudolph JW, Simon R, Rivard P, Dufresne RL, Raemer DB. Debriefing with good judgment: combining rigorous feedback with genuine inquiry. Anesthesiol Clin. 2007;25:361–76.
10. Rosenberg DR, Sweeney JA, Gillen JS, Kim J, et al. Magnetic resonance imaging of children without sedation: preparation with simulation. J Am Acad Child Adolesc Psychiatry. 1997; 36(6):853–9.
11. LaPierre CD, Johnson KB, Randall BR, Egan TD. A simulation study of common propofol and propofol-opioid dosing regimens for upper endoscopy. Anesthesiology. 2012;117:252–62.
12. Weinstock PH, Kappus LJ, Kleinman ME, Grenier B, Hickey P, Burns JP. Toward a new paradigm in hospital-based pediatric education: the development of an onsite simulator program. Pediatr Crit Care Med. 2005;6:635–41.
13. Friedlander MJ, Andrews L, Armstrong EG, Aschenbrenner C, Kass JS, et al. What can medical education learn from the neurobiology of learning? Acad Med. 2011;86:415–20.
14. Roediger HL, Karpicke J. Test-enhanced learning: taking memory tests improves long-term retention. Psychol Sci. 2006;17:249.
15. Larsen DP, Butler AC, Roediger HL. Repeated testing improves long-term retention relative to repeated study: a randomised controlled trial. Med Educ. 2009;43:1174–81.
16. Larsen DP. When I, say…test-enhanced learning. Med Educ. 2013;47:961.
17. Kohn L, Corrigan J, Donaldson M, editors. Errors in healthcare: a leading cause of death and injury: from *To Err is Human*. Washington, DC: National Academies Press; 2000. p. 26–48.
18. Landrigan CP, Parry GJ, et al. Temporal trends in rates of patient harm resulting from medical care. N Engl J Med. 2010; 363:2124–34.
19. James J. A new, evidence-based estimate of patient harms associated with hospital care. J Patient Saf. 2013;9(3):122–8.
20. Cravero JP, Beach ML, Blike GT, Gallagher SM, Hertzog JH. The incidence and nature of adverse events during pediatric sedation/anesthesia with propofol for procedures outside the operating room: a report from the pediatric sedation research consortium. Anesth Analg. 2009;108:795–804.
21. Metzner J, Domino KB. Risks of anesthesia or sedation outside the operating room: the role of the anesthesia care provider. Curr Opin Anaesthesiol. 2010;23:523–31.
22. Cote C, Wilson S. Guidelines for monitoring and management of pediatric patients during and after sedation for diagnostic and therapeutic procedures: an update. Pediatrics. 2006;118:2587.
23. Farnsworth ST, Egan TD, Johnson SE, Westenskow D. Teaching sedation and analgesia with simulation. J Clin Monit. 2000; 16:273–85.
24. Babl FE, Krieser D, Belousoff J, Theophilos T. Evaluation of a paediatric procedural sedation training and credentialing programme: sustainability of change. Emerg Med J. 2010;27:577–81.
25. Schneeweiss S, Ratnapalan S. Impact of a multifaceted pediatric sedation course: self-directed learning versus a formal continuing medical education course to improve knowledge of sedation guidelines. Can J Emerg Med. 2007;9(2):93–100.
26. Tobin CD, Clark CA, McEvoy MD, Reves JG, et al. An approach to moderate sedation simulation training. Simul Healthc. 2013; 8:114–23.
27. Cravero JP, Havidich JE. Pediatric sedation—evolution and revolution. Pediatr Anaesth. 2011;21:800–9.
28. Blike GT, Christoffersen K, Cravero JP, Andeweg SK, Jensen J. Method for measuring system safety and latent errors associated with pediatric procedural sedation. Anesth Analg. 2005;101: 48–58.
29. Schinasi DA, Nadel FM, Hales R, Boswinkel JP, Donoghue AJ. Assessing pediatric residents' clinical performance in procedural sedation. Pediatr Emerg Care. 2013;29(4):447–52.
30. Keidan I, Gravenstein D, Berkenstadt H, Ziv A, Shavit I, Sidi A. Supplemental oxygen compromises the use of pulse oximetry for detection of apnea and hypoventilation during sedation in simulated pediatric patients. Pediatrics. 2008;122:293–8.
31. Tan GM. A medical crisis management simulation activity for pediatric dental residents and assistants. J Dent Educ. 2011;5(6): 782–90.
32. Shavit I, Keidan I, Hoffmann Y, et al. Enhancing patient safety during pediatric sedation: the impact of simulation-based training of nonanesthesiologists. Arch Pediatr Adolesc Med. 2007;161(8): 740–3.
33. Shavit I, Steiner IP, Idelman S, Mosleh M, Hadash A, Biniamini L, Lezinger M, Kozer E. Comparison of adverse events during procedural sedation between specially trained pediatric residents and pediatric emergency physicians in Israel. Acad Emerg Med. 2008; 15:617–22.
34. Rosen MA, Hunt EA, Pronovost PJ, Federowicz MA, Weaver SJ. In situ simulation in continuing education for the health care professions:

a systematic review. J Contin Educ Health Prof. 2012;32(4):243–54.

35. Patterson MD, Geis GL, Lemaster T, Wears RL. Impact of multidisciplinary simulation-based training on patient safety in a paediatric emergency department. BMJ Qual Saf. 2013;22(5):383–93.
36. Kobayashi L, Dunbar-Viveiros JA, Devine J, Jones MS, Overly FL, Gosbee JW, Jay GD. Pilot-phase findings from high-fidelity in situ medical simulation investigation of emergency department procedural sedation. Simul Healthc. 2012;7(2):81–94.
37. Patterson MD, Geis GL, Falcone RA, Lemaster T, Wears RL. In situ simulation: detection of safety threats and teamwork training in a high risk emergency department. BMJ Qual Saf. 2013;22(6):468–77.
38. Weinstock PH, Kappus LJ, Garden A, Burns JP. Simulation at the point of care: reduced-cost, in situ training via a mobile cart. Pediatr Crit Care Med. 2009;10(2):176–81.
39. Chen MI, Edler A, Wald S, DuBois J, Huang YM. Scenario and checklist for airway rescue during pediatric sedation. Simul Healthc. 2006;2:194–8.
40. http://www.theaba.org/Home/anesthesiology_maintenance. Accessed 13 Dec 2013.
41. www.PediatricSedationConference.com. Accessed 13 Dec 2013.

Michael Jackson: Medical Ethics and What Went Wrong

36

Gail A. Van Norman and Joel S. Rosen

Abstract

In June of 2009, Michael Jackson died following a cardiac arrest. Jackson suffered from severe insomnia and anxiety, and Dr. Conrad Murray, a physician hired to look after Jackson's medical needs during preparations for a major world tour, had apparently undertaken to treat Jackson's insomnia in his home using a drug with known deadly potential: propofol. This is not a pediatric case, nor is it even typical in cases of medical negligence. But the Michael Jackson case illustrates many issues concerning legal standards with regard to negligence when it results in a patient death and practice standards with regard to sedation, professionalism, and the ethical obligations of physicians. In this chapter, we will undertake to discuss the Jackson case from both legal and professional perspectives, and then to compare elements of the Jackson case with that of another case of sedation that also ended in patient death, but not in criminal charges of homicide.

Keywords

Michael Jackson • Propofol • Medical ethics • Legal standards • Negligence • Involuntary manslaughter • Standard of care • Malpractice • Voluntary manslaughter • Professionalism • Criminal negligence • People v. Stanley Burroughs • Insomnia • Beneficence • Deontology • Nonmaleficence • Homicide • Prosecution • Civil lawsuit • Defense • Malpractice • Informed consent

Introduction

In June of 2009, Michael Jackson (see Fig. 36.1) died following a cardiac arrest. Mr. Jackson suffered from severe insomnia and anxiety, and Dr. Conrad Murray, a physician hired to look after Mr. Jackson's medical needs during preparations for a major world tour, had apparently undertaken to treat Mr. Jackson's insomnia in his home using a drug with known deadly potential: propofol.

This is not a pediatric case, nor is it even typical in cases of medical *negligence*.[1] But the Michael Jackson case illustrates many issues concerning legal standards with regard to negligence when it results in a patient death and practice standards with regard to sedation, professionalism, and the

[1]Please refer to glossary for definition.

G.A. Van Norman, M.D. (✉)
Department of Anesthesiology and Pain Medicine, University of Washington Medical Center, 1959 Pacific Street, Seattle, WA 98195, USA

Department of Biomedical Ethics, University of Washington Medical Center, 1959 Pacific Street, Seattle, WA 98195, USA
e-mail: gvn@uw.edu

J.S. Rosen, Esq.
Cohen, Placitella & Roth, P.C., Two Commerce Square, Suite 2900, 2001 Market Street, Philadelphia, PA 19103, USA
e-mail: jrosen@cprlaw.com

K.P. Mason (ed.), *Pediatric Sedation Outside of the Operating Room: A Multispecialty International Collaboration*, DOI 10.1007/978-1-4939-1390-9_36, © Springer Science+Business Media New York 2015

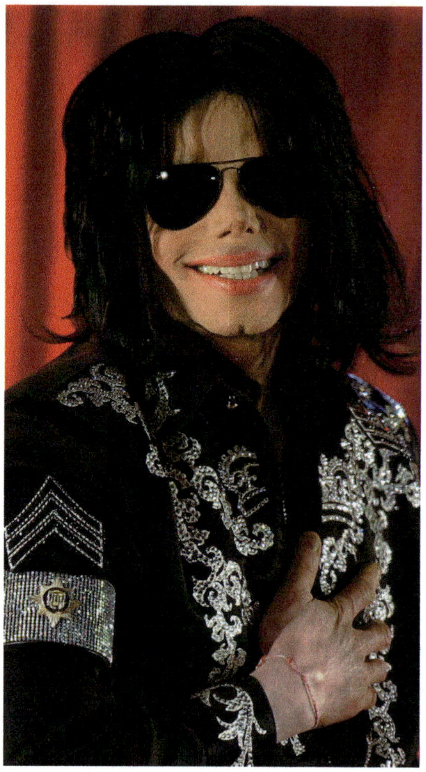

Fig. 36.1 Michael Jackson, the King of Pop (© Joel Ryan//AP/Corbis)

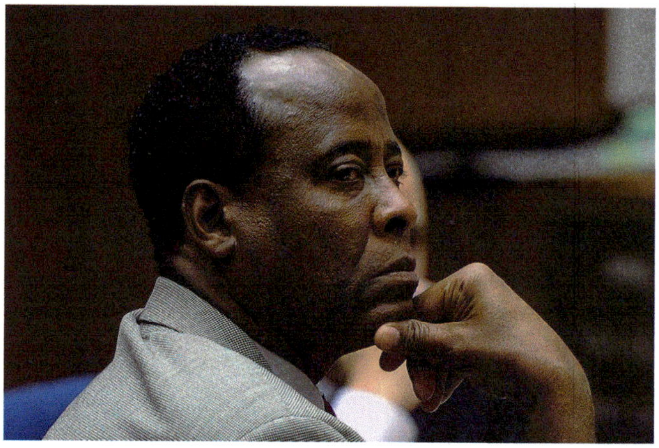

Fig. 36.2 Dr. Conrad Murray in the court room during the trial (© KEVORK DJANSEZIAN/Reuters/Corbis)

ethical obligations of physicians. In this chapter, we will undertake to discuss the Jackson case from both legal and professional perspectives, and then to compare elements of the Jackson case with that of another case of sedation that also ended in patient death, but not in criminal charges of *homicide*.[2]

Legal Versus Professional Standards and Ethics

When discussing ethics and professionalism in medicine, it is nearly impossible not to stray into discussion of legal issues. (Refer to Chap. 29.) Legal standards are not equivalent to professional or ethical standards in medicine, though they often parallel each other. Nevertheless, what is legal may not in fact be ethical, while what is considered ethical is not in all cases legal. Take, for example, the case of lethal injection. A physician's participation in lethal injection ordered by the courts is most certainly legal; but use of medical skills to perform a nonmedical task, such as carrying out executions for the state, is considered unethical by every major medical association in the Western world. On the other hand, performing an abortion in Northern Ireland, even to save the life of the mother, would be illegal, although most medical associations of the Western world would consider such an act not only ethical, but in some cases even a physician's professional duty.

It is rare in the medical world for actions related to medical care to violate criminal law. More commonly, questionable medical care is examined in the light of professional standards and medical competencies. Substandard medical care resulting in injury can lead to *civil lawsuits*[3] alleging *malpractice*.[4] Unprofessional conduct as well as substandard care may additionally lead to regulatory sanctions such as withdrawal of medical licensure, cancelation of hospital staff privileges, and expulsion from professional organizations. In the Michael Jackson case, it was found that egregious and willful acts of negligence that were later deemed to be the cause of the subsequent death of Mr. Jackson were actually criminal and deserved criminal penalties. In addition to violations of the criminal code, many ethical and professional standards were also breached.

The Death of Michael Jackson: A Legal Perspective

Dr. Conrad Murray was arrested and charged with *involuntary manslaughter*[5] in connection with the death of Michael Jackson (see Fig. 36.2). Dr. Murray was an interventional cardiologist whose main practice consisted of performing angioplasty procedures. He was not an anesthesiologist, nor was he board certified in anesthesiology. The following facts are taken from the transcript of the trial of Dr. Murray, mostly opening and closing arguments.

[2]Please refer to glossary for definition.

[3]Please refer to glossary for definition.

[4]Please refer to glossary for definition.

[5]Please refer to glossary for definition.

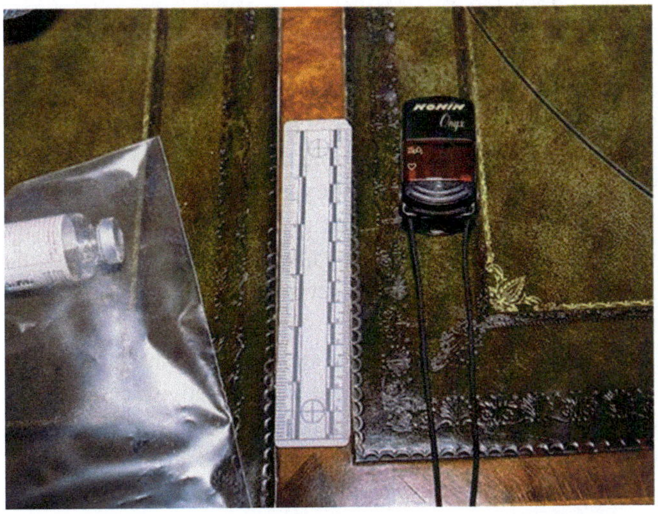

Fig. 36.3 This photo from the Los Angeles Police Department shows medication and medical equipment (a pulse oximeter) found at the home of Michael Jackson

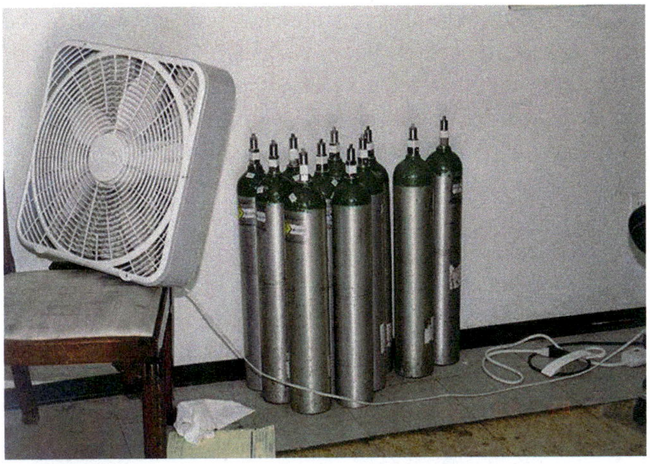

Fig. 36.4 This photo from the Los Angeles Police Department shows oxygen tanks that were in Michael Jackson's home

Dr. Murray met Michael Jackson in 2006 through a friend who was a security guard for Jackson. He had subsequently treated Jackson for some minor medical conditions. At the time of his death, Jackson was in the final rehearsal stages leading up to a world concert tour with full rehearsals and staging taking place at the Staples Center in Los Angeles. Jackson had contacted Dr. Murray in 2009 and requested that Murray accompany him on the tour to provide general medical care, emergency medical care, and reasonably requested services. A contract was drawn up for Dr. Murray whereby he was to be paid $150,000 per month for that care, which was signed by Dr. Murray, but never by anyone representing Jackson. Nevertheless, Dr. Murray cancelled his own practice and, by the time of rehearsals, was providing Jackson with medical care as anticipated by this contract.[6]

On June 25, 2009, Michael Jackson died in his home from what the coroner found was acute propofol intoxication with contributing benzodiazepine effect.[7] The facts surrounding his death are established largely through the evidence found at the scene (see Figs. 36.3, 36.4, 36.5, and 36.6) and a statement given by Dr. Murray to police in the presence of his attorney several days after the incident. What is undisputed is that Dr. Murray had provided medical services to Michael Jackson for more than 2 months. He was at Jackson's home every day for at least 6 days a week. Jackson was unable to sleep without the assistance of medication, and every night Dr. Murray would administer propofol to enable Jackson to get to sleep at home.[8]

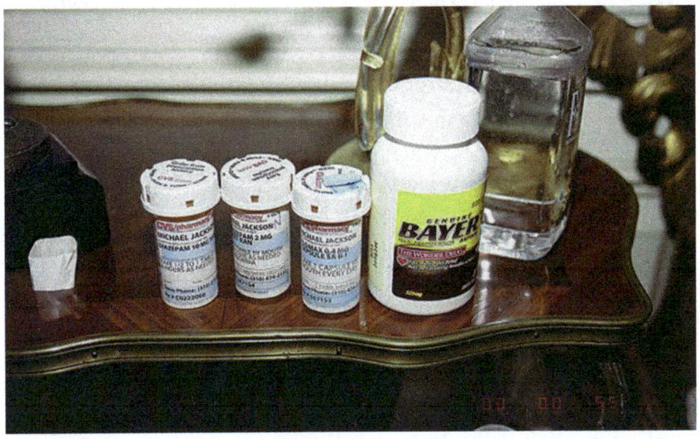

Fig. 36.5 This photo from the Los Angeles Police Department shows medications that were found at the Carolwood residence where Michael Jackson lived

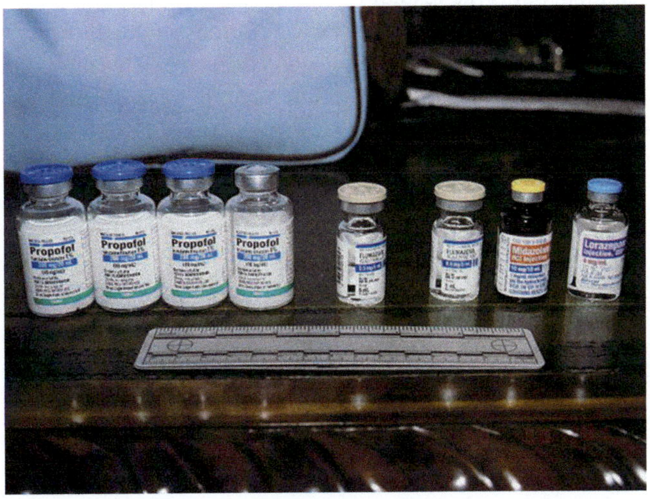

Fig. 36.6 This photo from the Los Angeles Police Department shows medication (propofol included) found in Michael Jackson's home

---

[6] *Opening statements of David Walgren and Ed Chernoff from trial.*
[7] *County of Los Angeles Autopsy Report 2009-04415.*
[8] *Opening statements of David Walgren and Ed Chernoff from trial.*

According to Dr. Murray's statement, on the night of the incident he started an IV line in Jackson's leg to hydrate him. Dr. Murray administered in succession lorazepam and valium for sleep, to no avail. According to Dr. Murray, Jackson requested the propofol and he gave Jackson 25 mg of propofol diluted with lidocaine after which Jackson went to sleep. He monitored him for a period of time, and then left Jackson alone in his bed to go to the bathroom for about 2 min. When he returned, he saw that Jackson was not breathing. He started to perform CPR and called for help. Eventually an ambulance was called, but Jackson was dead upon their arrival.[9]

Dr. Murray was charged with a single crime: Involuntary Manslaughter, Section, Section 192(b) of the California Penal Code. Involuntary manslaughter is defined under that code as follows:

> Manslaughter is the unlawful killing of a human being without malice. It is of three kinds: (b) Involuntary—in the commission of an unlawful act, not amounting to a felony; or in the commission of a lawful act which might produce death, in an unlawful manner, or without due caution and circumspection.

Involuntary manslaughter is distinguished from voluntary manslaughter, which in turn is different than murder. To get a full understanding of how involuntary manslaughter fits in with the other forms of homicide that can be charged in California, it is helpful to see how the statutes define those other forms. Manslaughter is distinguished from murder, which is an unlawful killing of a human being with malice aforethought.[10] Malice is a specific term of art in the law that is defined either as express malice, where there is an act manifesting a deliberate unlawful intention to take away a life, or implied malice, which is a killing without provocation or under circumstances that show an abandoned or malignant heart.[11] Manslaughter is an unlawful killing without malice. It is either voluntary—a killing that occurs from a sudden quarrel or heat of passion; or involuntary—a killing that is unintentional but is the result of *criminal negligence*.[12,13]

These definitions under the California statutes are very typical of how homicide is defined in different states throughout the country. A murder occurs when there is a homicide committed with malice.[14] If there is no malice, then an unlawful killing is manslaughter. There are two types of manslaughter, voluntary and involuntary. Typically, an unlawful killing committed in "the heat of passion" or in the "unreasonable belief of self-defense" is voluntary manslaughter because the actor is said to have committed the crime without the requisite mental state to prove that they had malice, but the killing itself is done pursuant to an intentional act. This is in contrast to an unlawful killing committed due to criminal negligence, which is involuntary manslaughter. There is no intent to kill or even necessarily to do harm to the victim. The death occurs from what is typically described as gross negligence, or conduct that demonstrates a reckless disregard for the value of human life.[15]

Because of the way state homicide statutes are written, the only homicide charge that would typically apply for negligent conduct of a doctor is involuntary manslaughter. The theory of a *prosecution*[16] would be that the conduct of the doctor is so outside the bounds of the accepted standard of care that it amounts to criminal negligence, or gross negligence. It is the concept of criminal negligence that usually distinguishes a potential criminal prosecution from a case where there may only be civil liability. But clearly, in the context of medical treatment, the facts would have to be extremely egregious to give rise to a potential criminal prosecution.

Under the California Penal Code, there are two types of acts that could constitute the crime of involuntary manslaughter in that state. One occurs when a person is committing an unlawful act that is not an "inherently dangerous" felony under the California Penal Code, and during the commission of that unlawful act there is a killing. The second occurs when a person is committing a perfectly lawful act, but is doing so with criminal negligence.

The case of *The People v. Stanley Burroughs* provides some insight into how the California Courts apply the homicide statute to the practice of medicine, although this case did not quite deal with the legitimate practice of medicine. The defendant in that case was a self-styled healer who

[9] *Transcript of Recorded Interview of Conrad Murray.*

[10] California Penal Code, Section 187(a).

[11] California Penal Code, Section 188.

[12] Please refer to glossary for definition.

[13] California Penal Code, Section 192.

[14] Pennsylvania—*Commonwealth v. Yuknovich, 295 A.2d 290 (1972)*; Virginia—*Moxley v. Commonwealth*, 77 S.E.2d 389, 393 (Va. 1953) (stating that "malice is the essence of murder"); Georgia Code Sec. 16 5 1, defining murder as a killing committed with malice aforethought.

[15] Pennsylvania—18Pa.C.S. Sec. 2504, requiring an act committed in a grossly negligent or reckless manner, *Commonwealth v. Agnew*, 398 A.2d 209 (Pa.Super.Ct. 1979), defining criminal negligence as a great departure from the standard of ordinary care evidencing disregard for human life; Texas Penal Sec. 19.04, defining manslaughter as occurring when the actor causes a death through reckless acts, with recklessness defined as being aware of but consciously disregarding a substantial risk that death will occur. Sec. 19.05, defining criminally negligent homicide as occurring when the actor causes a death through criminal negligence, further defined as occurring through an act that one ought to be aware creates a substantial risk death; Virginia—*Gallimore v. Commonwealth*, 436 S.E.2d 421, 445 (Va. 1993), stating that gross negligence, required for involuntary manslaughter, is a reckless or indifferent disregard of the rights of others, under circumstances reasonably calculated to produce injury; Georgia Code Sec. 16-5-3, defining involuntary manslaughter as causing the death of another in the commission of an unlawful act, other than a felony, or in the commission of a lawful act in an unlawful manner likely to cause death or great bodily harm; Illinois—720 ILCS 5/9-3, defining involuntary manslaughter as killing an individual by an act that is likely to cause death or serious bodily injury, when that act is performed recklessly.

[16] Please refer to glossary for definition.

"treated" a 24-year-old man who was diagnosed with leukemia.[17] After unsuccessful treatment from conventional doctors, the victim turned to the defendant, who claimed to have successfully cured a number of people suffering from cancer through the use of certain drinks, exposure to light, and massage therapy. The victim quickly became seriously ill and was experiencing severe pain in his abdomen. The defendant first convinced the young man to postpone a bone marrow test. He then treated the victim with deep abdominal massages on two successive days. This "treatment" resulted in convulsions and excruciating pain, followed by a massive hemorrhage of the mesentery in the abdomen, which led to the victim's death. Evidence at trial showed that the hemorrhage was caused by the massages performed by the defendant.

Clearly, the defendant did not intend to kill or even harm the victim. However, the defendant was tried and convicted of second-degree felony murder based upon the jury's determination that he was engaged in the unlicensed practice of medicine, which is a felony. The question for the California Supreme Court was whether that underlying felony was one that was "inherently dangerous to human life." If it was, then the defendant would be guilty of second-degree murder, also known as felony murder. If the underlying felony was not inherently dangerous to human life, then the defendant would only be guilty of involuntary manslaughter for committing an unlawful act that resulted in a death. The Supreme Court found that the act of practicing medicine without a license was not so inherently dangerous that, by its very nature, it could not be committed without creating a substantial risk that someone would be killed.[18] It did rule, however, that the defendant's acts constituted involuntary manslaughter because they were unlawful acts that led to the death of the victim.

Obviously, the facts of the *Burroughs* case can best be described as on the fringe of common experience. This was not legitimate medical treatment, nor was it treatment provided by a physician. But the facts surrounding the Conrad Murray prosecution could also be described as extreme, even though he was a licensed physician. In that case, a powerful sedating agent was administered repeatedly outside the confines of a hospital, treatment center, or even a doctor's office. It was administered by a physician who was not an anesthesiologist. It was administered far outside the scope of its normal use. And it was administered under circumstances that were very unusual.

In a footnote to the *Burroughs* decision, the Supreme Court also addressed the meaning of criminal negligence. The court defined it as:

> Such a departure from what would be the conduct of an ordinarily prudent or careful man under the same circumstances as to be incompatible with a proper regard for human life, or, in other words, a disregard of human life or indifference to consequences.[19]

This dual definition of involuntary manslaughter was applied to the prosecution of Dr. Murray. Although charged with only one count of involuntary manslaughter, the prosecution advanced two theories of guilt under that statute. First, it argued that Dr. Murray performed a lawful act, but did so with criminal negligence, and that act caused the death of Michael Jackson. As described later, the prosecution laid out a number of different acts committed by Dr. Murray in the course of his medical treatment of Michael Jackson that were acts that were done with criminal or gross negligence. Second, the prosecution argued that Dr. Murray had a legal duty to Michael Jackson that he failed to perform that legal duty, that this failure amounted again to criminal negligence, and that this failure to act caused the death of Michael Jackson. The legal duty claimed by the prosecution and recognized by the court was the legal duty of a physician to a patient. As stated by the trial judge to the jury at the trial, a physician who has assumed the responsibility to treat and care for a patient has a legal duty to treat and care for that patient.[20] This legal duty was given to the jury as a fact in the judge's charge on the law, so that it was for them to determine whether Dr. Murray failed to treat and care for his patient, and whether this failure amounted to criminal negligence.

Any experienced trial lawyer will be aware of the specific charge on the law that the judge will give to the jury at the end of the case, and tailor their arguments to the evidence and to the law that the jury has to follow. The Murray case was no exception. The opening argument of the prosecutor highlighted those themes from the beginning of his case. He told the jury that Dr. Murray acted with gross negligence (necessary to prove involuntary manslaughter), that Murray repeatedly denied appropriate care to his patient (failure to perform a legal duty), and that he engaged in repeated incompetent and unskilled acts (acting in a criminally or grossly negligent manner). The prosecutor argued that there are different levels of deviation from the standard of care: a minor deviation, a serious deviation, or an egregious/extreme deviation. It was those acts that were extreme deviations from the standard of care that were evidence of gross negligence by Dr. Murray and supported a conviction of involuntary manslaughter.

He then laid out several facts that established this extreme deviation from the standard of care in this case. The first and foremost was the use of propofol under these circumstances. Propofol is intended for use in a highly monitored setting, such as the operating room of a hospital. Using it in someone's

[17] *The People v. Stanley Burroughs*, 35 Cal. 3d 824 (1984).

[18] *The People v. Stanley Burroughs, supra* at 833.

[19] Ibid.

[20] *Conrad Murray Trial—Judge's Instructions to Jury.*

private home, in their bedroom, was an extreme violation of the standard of care and, he argued, an act that constituted criminal negligence. The following arguments and evidence presented at trial established other allegations of extreme violations of the standard of care that were, individually and in combination, criminal negligence:

- Leaving Jackson alone without continuous monitoring while administering propofol, which the prosecutor argued amounted to abandonment of the patient
- Using propofol to treat insomnia, or to put someone to sleep, instead of using it for the induction and maintenance of general anesthesia and for procedural sedation
- Failing to have standard resuscitation equipment and drugs available while administering propofol
- Using propofol combined with benzodiazepines in this particular setting and under these conditions

It should be noted that there was an argument made in this case that, as evidenced by the contract that was signed by Murray, this was not a doctor–patient relationship but an employee–employer relationship and that Dr. Murray did not act as a medical professional using sound medical judgment. Instead, the physician used his medical training and license to give Jackson access to unlimited supplies of propofol, which were then administered without regard for Jackson's safety or his life. As stated by the prosecutor at trial, Dr. Murray had a legal duty of care to use his best medical judgment and to "do no harm" to his patient. Instead, he administered "massive amounts" of propofol and had regards only for the contract and not for the patient (see Fig. 36.7).

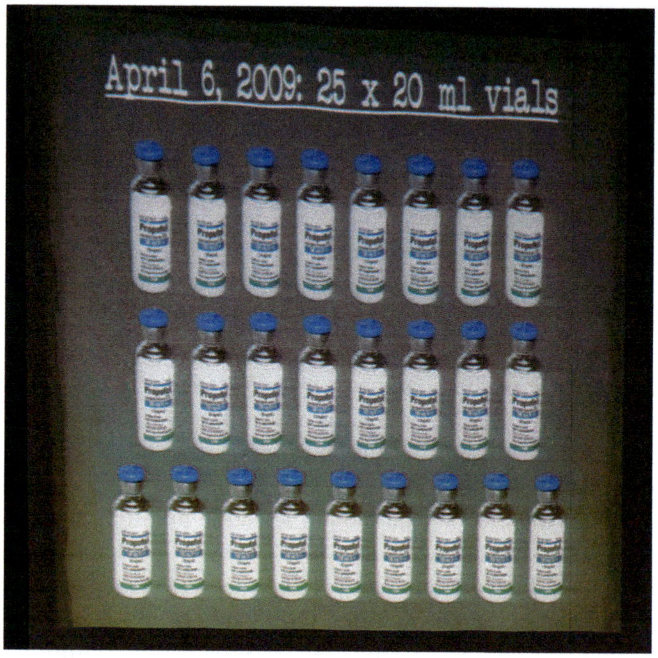

Fig. 36.7 In this photo from Al Seib, Associated Press, you see a slide projection shown in the courtroom displaying a single order of propofol made by Dr. Conrad Murray (used with permission from the Associated Press)

It should also be noted that the *defense*[21] attorney at this trial did not defend much of Dr. Murray's conduct. He did not claim that Dr. Murray was a trained anesthesiologist, or that he should have administered propofol for this purpose or in this setting. Instead, the defense took the position that the doctor's acts did not cause Jackson's death. The defense argued that Murray gave Jackson such a small dose of propofol, which would dissipate rather quickly, that Jackson had to have self-administered more of the narcotic while Dr. Murray was not in the room in order for him to have died from propofol poisoning. Therefore, although Dr. Murray may have acted with criminal negligence, his actions did not result in the death.[22] However, the prosecution was able to show that Dr. Murray gave Jackson more than the 25 mg of propofol that he admitted to administering, and the jury rejected this defense completely.

An examination of the facts and arguments show not only how easily the conduct of Dr. Murray fits within the definition of involuntary manslaughter, but also how extreme his conduct was compared with conventional medical treatment and with conventional use of anesthetics. Going back to the legal definition of criminal negligence, the question for the jury was whether the facts of the case and the facts that they found concerning the treatment given by Dr. Murray were such a departure from what would be the conduct of an ordinarily prudent man (doctor) under the same circumstances as to be incompatible with a proper regard for human life. The trial judge defined criminal negligence to the jury in his charge, telling them that it is acting recklessly in such a way that creates a high risk of death or great bodily injury, and that a reasonable person would have known that acting in such a manner created that type of risk. He also specifically told the jury that criminal negligence involves more than ordinary carelessness, inattention, or mistake in judgment. In other words, the doctor's conduct needed not only to be reckless, but it had to be knowingly reckless.

The Death of Michael Jackson: Professionalism and Medical Ethics

The definition of what is legal is reasonably straightforward: that which violates criminal law. But what is professionalism? "Professionalism" encompasses the conduct, qualities, and aims that characterize *a person* engaged in doing certain types of work. In the medical profession, that conduct involves not only the competent completion of technical tasks and treatments, but the requirement that they are done within the generally recognized goals of the profession, namely to improve the lives of patients in medically meaningful

[21] Please refer to glossary for definition.

[22] *Conrad Murray Trial—Opening and Closing Arguments of Ed Chernoff.*

ways, and to relieve suffering. Furthermore, the accomplishment of these tasks must occur within the professional and ethical boundaries of the practice of medicine. It might be possible, for example, to relieve the suffering of another human being by killing him, but it would only be considered consistent with medical professionalism and ethical conduct under very narrow circumstances, only in a few select countries, or (in the view of many) never consistent with ethical medical conduct at all. Thus, professionalism and ethics reach beyond the mere technical performance of specific tasks, and additionally consider the context in which such tasks are performed. The reason for such standards of conduct rests in the "social contract" that physicians hold. The practice of medicine involves an expectation by society of special service in return for special privileges such as prestige, financial advancement, and social status.

The term "professional" has come to refer in common language to almost any work for which a person gets paid—a "professional" is the opposite of an "amateur." But in this discussion the terms "professional" and "professionalism" carry a different meaning. In the not-too-distant past, there were only three "true" professions recognized in Western society: physicians, clergy, and practitioners of the legal profession [1]. These three occupations have in common the characteristics that the practitioners possess information and/or skills that have the power to profoundly affect the lives of persons upon whom they practice: the physician holds the keys to health, the clergy to salvation, and the legal profession to freedom. Each requires the practitioner to use utmost discretion for the sake of the persons served. Each assumes a dedication to competently practicing the skills taught within the profession. Each profession requires the active participation of the practitioners of its arts in the development of future members of the profession. Entry into each of these professions involves indoctrination into a "universal" philosophy of practice, subjugation of personal interests in pursuit of the profession's values and goals, and the commitment via "vows" to the philosophy, fraternity, and values and standards of the profession.

Violation of the standards of conduct in each of these professions risks dire consequences for the people who are being served: of depriving a patient of their health, a parishioner of their salvation, a legal client of their freedom. Breaches of confidence in each of these professions may have serious social consequences for these people as well. It is no coincidence that each of these professions is afforded special privileges under the law regarding confidentiality: doctors, clergy, and lawyers are generally not required to disclose their clients' secrets, even under oath, outside of extreme and explicit exceptions. Maintaining standards of professionalism and ethics is in the interest not only of the clients the professions serve but is in the interest of the members of the profession itself: Failure to perform their duties with the competence and confidentiality that society expects puts the practitioners at risk of losing their special social privileges, both individually and as a class. Failure to meet professional standards is unlikely to result in legal sanctions in most cases, but can often lead to limitations of practice, loss of licensure, loss of hospital privileges, and expulsion from the profession or professional societies.

In examining the events leading to Michael Jackson's death, a number of questions concerning professionalism and ethical standards arise. Were Dr. Murray's treatments in fact even the practice of medicine, or were they a corruption or caricature of the physician's privileges and skills applied to serve some other purpose? Did a legitimate physician–patient relationship even exist between Michael Jackson and Dr. Murray? If so, did Dr. Murray adhere to principles of professionalism in his relationship to his patient? If his treatments were in fact medical therapy, were they carried out competently and within the standards of medical practice, or were they managed incompetently or perhaps even negligently?

Was Dr. Murray Practicing Medicine?

The question of whether Dr. Murray's actions even constituted the practice of medicine is not an insignificant one. Many actions can seem like medical practice when they involve procedures that are also commonly carried out by physicians, but are not consistent within the goals and values of the profession and are therefore not actually the practice of medicine. It is not merely the action itself, but the *context* in which an action takes place that determines if it is the practice of medicine. Placing a needle or catheter into a vein in order to administer antibiotics for an infection is the practice of medicine. Placing the same needle or catheter in order to inject heroin for recreational purposes is not. The practice of medicine has certain required elements: The action must serve some beneficial medical purpose, involving the diagnosis and assessment of health issues. Treatment must be based on sound knowledge of the condition at hand, and be backed by theoretical, clinical, or experimental evidence that leads to a reasonable conclusion that the treatment has a significant chance of altering the course of the disorder in a positive way. In extreme cases such as terminal illness, medical care may be solely comfort based, but it is generally not sufficient to treat symptoms alone if there are also effective treatments for the condition underlying the symptoms. Simply giving a drug addict another "hit" of their favorite drug to alleviate the suffering of withdrawal without also attending to the underlying affliction (addiction) is not the practice of medicine—it is drug trafficking.

What can we say with regard to the treatments Dr. Murray administered to Michael Jackson? It is known that Jackson had a chronic history of insomnia and of improper and chronic use of benzodiazepine medication as a sleep aid, apparently escalating his use to extraordinary doses of medication that at times were unsuccessful in inducing sleep. His affliction and behavior bear the typical hallmarks of drug addiction, abuse, or at the very least significant misuse. When self-medication was not effective and he was engaged in stressful preparations for a concert tour, he contracted with Dr. Murray to manage his requirement for sleep drugs. Nominally at least, Dr. Murray was also to provide other emergency and routine medical care—although it is not clear from the public record that he did so to any significant degree. For that service, Jackson offered what can only be described as an exorbitant price of $150,000 per month. Dr. Murray, who allegedly was in significant financial debt, abandoned his medical practice to be available to perform this service exclusively to Jackson.

Insomnia is a legitimate medical condition with well-described diagnostic procedures and standard treatments, none of which appear to have been followed in Dr. Murray's "care" of Jackson. Murray did not have specialty training in sleep disorders or neurology, nor did he consult with or refer Jackson to specialists in these fields. In fact, it appears that it was Jackson himself who first requested and then demanded propofol by name, and that Murray complied by stockpiling extraordinary supplies of the drug and administering it to Jackson in an unmonitored setting in a bedroom at the singer's home.

Propofol is known to be an addictive drug that increasingly is being used as a drug of choice by abusers, particularly health care workers. The most common reason given for propofol use that leads to addiction was to treat insomnia [2]. Propofol infusion exposes the user to significant risks of respiratory depression—particularly when simultaneously administered, as it was in this case, with high doses of benzodiazepines. Only one small study investigates the use of propofol to treat insomnia—and that in a highly structured and monitored setting as a short series of infusions, and not as chronic repeated treatments [3].

Given these considerations, it is reasonable to conclude that Dr. Murray was not engaged in the practice of medicine with Jackson, because he did not attempt to diagnose and assess the singer's problem in any standard way, and he rendered contraindicated "therapy." Murray appears to have been placed under contract to use his prescriptive privileges for the purpose of accessing a restricted drug for a third party's abuse, and to use his technical skills to administer the drug in a nonmedical setting. A physician who uses the privileges and skills afforded to him or her by the profession to pursue nonmedical activities is guilty of a very serious breach of professionalism and ethics.

Did a Legitimate Physician–Patient Relationship Exist?

The physician–patient relationship is one of unequal power. The physician owns specialized skills and knowledge with which to guide medical care. The patient is at the mercy of the physician to practice these skills competently and effectively. Each member of the relationship has both rights and responsibilities. The patient is expected to be truthful with the physician about aspects of his or her medical condition, because without accurate information, the physician's conclusions regarding diagnosis and treatment are illegitimized. Because such truthfulness may expose extreme patient vulnerabilities, the physician is expected to keep such information in strict confidence. Patients and physicians are expected to work together to agree on legitimate medical goals that incorporate the patient's needs and the physician's (competent) clinical judgment. In the position of power, the physician is vulnerable to corruption. In the position of dependence, the patient is vulnerable to coercion. Therefore, a physician's fees are required to be usual and customary. They cannot be so great as to prevent a patient from seeking help or to corrupt the physician into acting unprofessionally. They also cannot be "unusual"—a physician cannot require sex or the patient's enslavement, for example, in return for services.

In the Murray–Jackson relationship, it is difficult to decisively conclude that a true doctor–patient relationship ever existed. In this case, the patient, rather than the physician "prescribed" the treatment and paid what is potentially a corrupting amount of money to induce the physician to carry out a treatment to order that had no basis in medical theory. Dr. Murray was vulnerable to corruption because of the extraordinary fee being offered in the face of his personal debt, and perhaps also out of a desire for notoriety and social privilege by being associated with a famous star.

Ethical Principles in Medical Care

Presuming that, contrary to the aforementioned arguments, there was a genuine doctor–patient relationship, and Dr. Murray was practicing medicine when he administered propofol to Michael Jackson, we are still left with determining whether such practice met the minimum standards of medical ethics. While there are many possible ethical constructs in medicine, in Western medicine, the predominant ethical theory surrounding the physician–patient relationship consists of several core principles: respect for patient autonomy, beneficence (doing good), and nonmaleficence (avoiding harm).[23]

Respect for Autonomy

Of all of the principles to consider in the Jackson case, respect for patient autonomy is likely to cause the most confusion, because some might interpret it to say that the doctor is obliged to do what the patient wants. If Jackson desired to sleep and to have propofol, then does respect for patient autonomy require the doctor to provide it? The answer, of

[23]For further reading on basic principles in medical ethics, see Beauchamp T, Childress JF. *Principles of Biomedical Ethics, 7th Ed.* Oxford University Press, Oxford, UK. 2012.

course, is no. Professionalism limits the physician to practice within the values and boundaries of conduct that defines the profession. Jackson cannot require his physician to provide procedures and therapies not contained within those boundaries. Physicians are not required to, nor should they provide futile or grotesque care, and they should not provide care that falls below professional standards of competency. They are not required to provide procedures or medications that serve no medically sanctioned purpose. Within those parameters, the principle of respect for patient autonomy requires that the physician try to understand and honor the patient's values and to provide care that takes into account as far as possible the patient's preferences. Jackson could request whatever treatments he desired, but his physician was obliged to adhere only to those that were within the scope of professional and competent care. Not only is propofol administration contraindicated in the chronic treatment of insomnia, administration of propofol in an unmonitored, nonmedical setting as a common sleep aid is far below professional standards.

Beneficence

Interestingly, the principle of beneficence (doing good) was not necessarily violated simply because Dr. Murray's actions resulted in Mr. Jackson's death. While certainly a great harm resulted to Jackson, medical care is fraught with unintended and unanticipated complications, and outcomes are not always what we expect or wish them to be. The principle of beneficence applies first and foremost to what the physician *desired and intended* the results to be and how he went about trying to produce the desired results, and only modestly to what the results actually were. Why is that? In ethics, a predominant theory is *deontology,* or "rules-based" ethics. In deontologic ethical theory, the determination of whether "good" was done is based on the intentions and actions of the doer, and not necessarily on the outcomes. Good intentions require competency; in other words, the physician cannot simply commit a random act while hoping that it turns out well in order to meet the principle of beneficence. Rather, he or she must *do their best* to make it turn out well, and doing their best means having appropriate knowledge, choosing a course of action or treatment that has a reasonable chance of success, and carrying out that treatment in the safest and most competent manner. Deontologic ethical theory recognizes that even if the physician does all of those things, outside influences and circumstances that are beyond the physician's control may yet lead to a poor outcome. A physician might appropriately administer penicillin to treat a dental abscess, with neither the patient nor physician knowing that the patient suffers from a fatal allergy to penicillin. The patient dies. This is a bad outcome, but the physician was intending to perform a beneficent act, had appropriate knowledge to enable her to do so, chose an appropriate treatment, and administered the drug in a competent manner. An underlying and previously unknown condition resulted in a bad outcome despite the physician's actions, yet the physician was acting appropriately under the principle of beneficence.

In Dr. Murray's treatment of Michael Jackson, however, we see several violations of the principle of beneficence. As mentioned before, the "treatment" Dr. Murray undertook ignored the underlying problem (insomnia that might have been due to addiction or some underlying neurological condition requiring treatment), was contraindicated, and posed an extreme and well-recognized risk to Jackson.

Administration of propofol is governed by numerous standards: It is advised that only a physician or practitioner who is learned in the administration of general anesthesia use propofol outside of a closely monitored setting, such as an intensive care unit, and/or in an intubated patient. Use of propofol for sedation is discouraged by any physician or practitioner not qualified and trained in the "the administration of general anesthesia" and the US Food and Drug Administration (FDA) warns users of this advisory and of the risk of airway obstruction [4]. The literature is replete with reports of respiratory depression and death when this particular drug is used in conjunction with benzodiazepines, or administered without continuous monitoring of vital signs and respiratory effectiveness. Murray was not a professionally trained anesthesiologist or nurse anesthetist. He was either unaware of, or chose to ignore, basic principles of monitoring and safety while administering propofol. He left his "patient" unattended after administering the drug for some unknown period of time, which however brief or long, was nevertheless of sufficient duration to lead to Michael Jackson's death. It is difficult to find a single aspect of Dr. Murray's care that meets the medical principle of beneficence.

Nonmaleficence

The principle of avoiding harm is the flip-side of the beneficence coin. Not only are physicians obligated to try to produce good, but they must use their knowledge and expertise, choices, and skills in such a way as to minimize the potential harms to patients. In our previous hypothetical example, if the physician knew the patient had a history of penicillin allergy and simply ignored that history, did not pretreat the patient for possible reactions and/or did not choose a different, appropriate drug for treatment, then logically we would say they violated the principle of nonmaleficence, since they had the knowledge and wherewithal to avoid the penicillin reaction, knew about the allergy, and yet chose recklessly to proceed with dangerous therapy.

Even though Dr. Murray chose to administer an unsafe drug that was contraindicated for Jackson's condition, he still had an opportunity to avoid further mischief by adhering to safe practices. In an appropriate setting, such as a medically

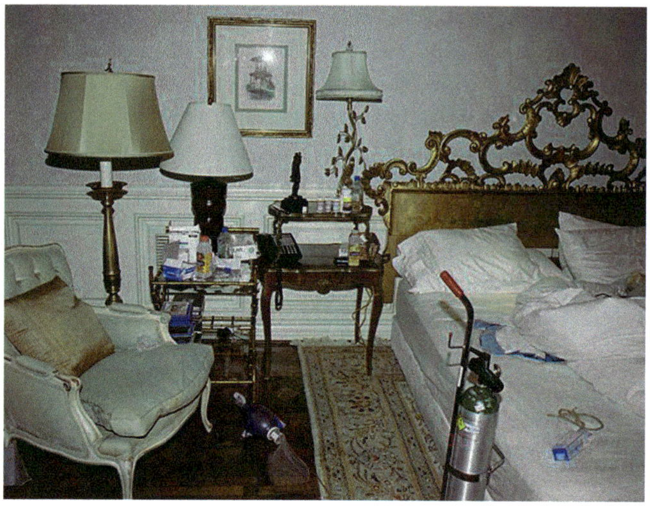

Fig. 36.8 This photo from the Los Angeles Police Department was taken in the master bedroom at the home of Michael Jackson, also known as the Carolwood residence

equipped sedation suite, with appropriate heart, blood pressure, blood oxygen and respiration monitoring, and with the continuous presence of a qualified anesthesia practitioner, it is actually unlikely that Jackson would have died from the propofol administration (see Fig. 36.8). Murray would still have been guilty of egregious incompetence or willfully disregarding standard medical practice in administering the drug for a condition in which it was contraindicated, but Jackson would perhaps not have paid the ultimate price for his actions).

An important question remains to be asked: if Dr. Murray was not practicing medicine when he committed willful acts that led to the death of Michael Jackson, and if he did not have a legitimate doctor–patient relationship with Jackson, then how should his conduct be examined and possible penalties for that conduct be assessed? In which court should his actions be tried? Since so much of what Murray did appears to fall *outside* of the practice, values, ethical principles, and context of the medical profession, then criminal prosecution indeed appears to be a more appropriate venue for examining the details of the case than a civil case for medical malpractice.

Outcome of the Case

The jury in the Jackson case convicted Dr. Murray of one count of involuntary manslaughter. On November 29, 2011, Dr. Conrad Murray was sentenced to 4 years incarceration by Judge Michael Pastor, the trial judge in the case. This was the maximum sentence that could be imposed under the statutory scheme for involuntary manslaughter in California. Judge Pastor spoke at length about the reasons he imposed that sentence, some of which reflected the evidence and arguments that were presented at the trial. He stated that Dr. Murray abandoned his patient, Mr. Jackson, and that the doctor violated the trust of the medical community and of his patient by his conduct when treating Jackson. The judge also focused on Murray's conduct after Jackson's death, stating that Dr. Murray repeatedly lied and engaged in deceitful conduct and that Murray had no sense of remorse or fault. Judge Pastor also noted that Dr. Murray remained dangerous if allowed to remain at large and practice medicine.

The judge did not address Dr. Murray's medical license, since that was not within the purview of the court. However, Murray's license to practice medicine in California was suspended on December 29, 2011, 1 month after he was sentenced. That board has yet to render a decision on revocation. His Texas medical license was suspended in February of 2012 and revoked on August 30, 2013. Murray's attorneys have filed to have his Texas license reinstated.

On October 28, 2013, Dr. Murray was released from jail after serving 2 years of his 4 year sentence. His shortened sentence was the result of prison overcrowding and the fact that he was convicted as a nonviolent felon. His attorneys have appealed his conviction for involuntary manslaughter to the California Appellate Court.

Another Sedation Case

The analysis of the Michael Jackson case from legal and professional perspectives is instructive, but represents a grotesque caricature of medical care. How do these principles apply in cases that are more mainstream, but when the outcome for the patient is nevertheless catastrophic? Let us consider another case involving death following a procedure with "sedation."

The Case[24]

In a state that requires medical direction of nurse anesthetists, a 58-year-old man presents to a gastroenterologist for a routine screening colonoscopy. The gastroenterologist schedules him for the procedure at a free-standing endoscopy center in which he has a controlling financial interest, with sedation provided by a nurse anesthetist that he employs and medically directs. The patient has a history of morbid obesity, hypertension, and symptoms and signs highly predictive of sleep apnea (male gender, snoring loudly enough

[24] Some details in this case have been altered from the actual case to protect patient privacy. The analyses provided here are based only on the facts presented in this text, and do not represent actual legal rulings.

to be heard through a closed door, daytime somnolence, body mass index 60, increased neck circumference, hypertension, and age over 50). The nurse anesthetist proceeds to provide "sedation" under monitored conditions for sedation in an operating suite with the patient receiving supplemental mask oxygen. Blood pressure, pulse, and arterial oxygen saturation are observed throughout. The patient receives fentanyl 100 μg and midazolam 2 mg IV, after which he falls asleep and begins snoring loudly. When the procedure begins, the patient moans and starts to move and the gastroenterologist asks for more sedation. Administration of three separate boluses of 50 mg of intravenous propofol silence the snoring and keep the patient completely still during the rest of the procedure. Arterial oxygen saturation remains above 92 % throughout. In the recovery room, the patient does not wake up, and is noted to have snoring and sometimes "gasping" respirations. The oxygen saturation monitor is intermittently unable to read oxygen saturation, but at times show oxygen saturation of >92 %. Approximately 1 h later, he has still not awakened and does not respond purposefully to painful stimulation. The patient is transported unintubated to a hospital approximately 20 min away, where upon arrival he is still unresponsive and snoring. The emergency physician intubates the patient without obtaining an initial arterial blood gas, although blood gases 1 h after intubation are essentially normal. The patient does not regain consciousness, and dies approximately 4 weeks later. Thirty days after his death, the family files a malpractice lawsuit against the physician and nurse anesthetist.

Legal Analysis

This case can be analyzed in relation to potential criminal charges according to typical state statutory schemes relating to involuntary manslaughter/negligent homicide. The two questions that should be asked are whether the conduct of the nurse anesthetist somehow violated the law and, if not, whether that conduct was still so far beyond the standard of care that it constitutes criminal or gross negligence.

The answer to the first question is a simple "no," there is no underlying criminal conduct in this case. In contrast with the *Burroughs* case cited previously, there is no allegation of practicing medicine without a license or anything that remotely approaches a violation of the law in connection with this treatment.[25]

The second question is a bit more complicated but is still clear. Although this conduct might be found to violate the standard of care that is established for a civil negligence claim, it is nowhere near the type of violation that gives rise to criminal negligence. One can apply the standard from *Burroughs* and determine whether there is evidence of conduct incompatible with a proper regard for human life or of indifference to consequences. One could apply the charge on the law given in the Jackson case by the court and determine whether this was a case of ordinary carelessness, inattention or mistake in judgment, or a case where the conduct was so egregious that it created a high risk of death or serious bodily injury. Or one could analyze the conduct in the same manner the prosecution did in the Jackson case and determine whether there are repeated, extreme violations of the standard of care that give rise to gross negligence.

The answer in each case is the same. This is treatment by licensed, trained professionals acting within their area of expertise and experience in a medical facility, albeit not a hospital. This is an acceptable type of treatment that is common in this setting. If there is a breach of the standard of care here, it is not so egregious, nor of the type to constitute repeated, extreme violations of the standard of care, or reckless behavior under the law that would lead to criminal charges being brought. Criminal charges brought in the context of medical treatment against doctors or nurses is extraordinarily rare, and for good reason. This type of conduct will be examined at most under civil law in a potential malpractice litigation, not in a criminal context.

Professionalism and Ethics

When we compare this case to the Michael Jackson case from the perspective of professionalism and medical ethics, several stark differences are immediately apparent. The basic elements of professional medical care were present and observed in this case. A true provider/patient relationship appears to exist; one in which the nurse anesthetist was prescribing and monitoring treatment for which he or she was professionally qualified by virtue of having completed specific training in the administration of anesthesia-related medications, including propofol. The care was within the scope of professionalism of the practice, and according to accepted medical theory. The provider "prescribed" the therapy, rather than simply providing drugs on demand, and the therapy was appropriate for the procedure being performed. There was an obvious attempt to adhere to medical standards. Appropriate drug selection and dosing was used, and most monitoring was according to standards set by several professional bodies.

But other important elements of medical professionalism and ethics nevertheless fell short. It is well recognized that certain patients—either those who are seriously ill, or some who suffer from specific conditions—are of sufficient risk

[25] A more difficult analysis could exist in cases when there is a legal requirement that a licensed physician be present during the procedure, that requirement is violated and a patient dies due to administration of anesthesia that is below the standard of care. In the context of criminal charges, difficult questions would arise concerning the quality of the care, the extent to which the administration of anesthesia violated the standard of care, and whether there is evidence that the absence of a licensed physician was a contributing cause of the death.

for surgery and anesthesia that they should not undergo invasive procedures in anything other than a hospital setting. Guidelines have been established for the selection of patients to undergo care in free-standing procedural centers [5]. This patient suffered from not one, but several conditions that should have alerted his care providers that he was a poor candidate for this procedure in that type of setting, and that he should have the colonoscopy done in a hospital. Those included his morbid obesity, and the fact that he had multiple risk factors suggesting that he might have moderate to severe obstructive sleep apnea—a condition that generally requires extended observation following sedation for procedures, may require emergency airway intervention, and is notorious for being associated with difficult airway management [6]. Under established guidelines, he should have undergone this procedure in a hospital environment, where more resources would be available if airway issues arose.

Established national standards state that when a medically directed nurse anesthetist or other practitioner is supervised by a non-anesthesiologist, that physician must nevertheless be "qualified and trained in the recognition of and rescue from general anesthesia" [7]. From the review of the case, it is apparent that this standard was not followed. While there is nothing about the standard that would prohibit a gastroenterologist from supervising the nurse anesthetist in administering the sedation, it is clear from review of the case that, in fact, a general anesthetic was administered. The definition of general anesthesia is that it produces unconsciousness, lack of pain, and lack of purposeful movement in response to procedural stimulus [8]. The nurse anesthetist documented administering enough medication such that movement and response to stimulation did not occur. This was beyond the scope of the gastroenterologist's practice, who was not trained in the administration of general anesthesia. Because of this critical issue, the patient was not "rescued" from general anesthesia, and this first problem opened the door for what followed.

In the administration of general anesthesia, several standards also were not met. Whenever general anesthesia is administered, oxygenation and ventilation must be monitored throughout [9]. While oxygen saturation was monitored in this case, end-tidal CO_2 was not, nor were any other quantitative assessments of ventilation recorded. This is particularly disturbing because obvious clinical signs of airway obstruction were present (snoring, gasping respiratory movements).

The competency and judgment of the medical providers can be called into question in that they appeared not to recognize, nor did they appropriately treat, airway obstruction for which obvious signs were present. This led to a sequence of events (hypercarbia, somnolence, probable systemic acidosis) that are at the very least not within the expected standards of care, and at the worst may have actually caused the patient's demise.

A possible contributing factor in this situation may have been a financial conflict of interest: The anesthetist may have been reluctant to refuse the case since doing so may have had the potential to cost her employment. The gastroenterologist may have ignored important evidence that the procedure should not be performed at a free-standing procedural center because of the financial impact involved.

Ethically, the principles of beneficence and nonmaleficence were violated by either willful disregard of published standards, or more likely failure through ignorance or incompetence to meet well-published standards of care in delivering sedation in this clinical setting, as well as inadequate training and knowledge on the part of the supervising gastroenterologist. The providers failed in both a professional and ethical sense regardless of the patient's ultimate outcome.

Conclusion

Violations of legal, ethical, and professional standards can sometimes accompany or even be the root causes of misadventures in anesthesia and sedation care. (Refer to Chap. 29.) While legal, ethical, and professional standards are not synonymous, they often parallel one another. Legal actions are generally taken because of adverse outcomes in medical cases, and may be civil or criminal in nature. The differentiation between civil and criminal liability takes into account whether there were violations in medical, ethical, and professional standards, whether such violations were intentional or unintentional, and whether such actions were extreme enough to demonstrate disregard for human life. Whether a violation of professionalism and/or medical ethics has taken place on the other hand, is not based in the medical outcome, although such violations may come to our attention because of an adverse outcome. Rather, ethics and professionalism establish the required quality and character of the practitioner involved, the principles within which a physician acts, and the context that defines medical practice.

Glossary

The following are general lay definitions of terms common to the practice of criminal and civil law. Some of the precise definitions vary from state to state according to that state's laws and practice.

Civil lawsuit A legal case brought on behalf of an individual (plaintiff) against another individual or entity (defendant) who acted negligently (below some standard of care) and thereby caused them harm. This case is brought for a monetary recovery for damages sustained by the plaintiff. The plaintiff's burden of proof in a civil lawsuit is typically by a preponderance of the evidence, a lesser burden of proof than in a criminal prosecution. A successful civil lawsuit usually results in the payment of money for the losses sustained by the plaintiff.

Criminal negligence Acting in a grossly negligent manner. Typically, this involves the conscious disregard of a known risk of death or serious injury.

Defense Those responsible for representing a defendant in a criminal case or a civil lawsuit. The defense does not have the burden of proving innocence or lack of fault.

Homicide The unlawful taking of another's life. Homicide ranges from first-degree murder (the taking of a life with specific intent to kill and with malice) to involuntary manslaughter (an accidental killing where the defendant acts unintentionally and without malice but with criminal negligence).

Informed consent The consent given by a patient to a doctor that allows the doctor to perform a certain procedure or render particular treatment. The consent is "informed" because the doctor has explained the specifics of the procedure or treatment to the patient, including the risks and alternatives, who has then made a knowing, informed decision about whether they want to proceed.

Involuntary manslaughter The unlawful taking of another's life without intent to kill or to harm and without malice, but the act is committed with criminal negligence.

Malpractice Professional negligence. This is an act of negligence committed by a professional such as a doctor, a lawyer, and an engineer while acting within their profession. The negligent conduct is measured by the standard of care in that profession and in that specialty in which the professional practices. A doctor who commits malpractice is said to have breached the standard of care in their area of specialty.

Negligence Failing to act in a reasonably prudent manner.

Prosecution Charging an individual (defendant) with a violation of criminal law, marshaling the evidence against that individual, presenting the evidence to a court or jury and, if a conviction is obtained, proceeding to sentencing against the individual. The prosecutor represents the people of the state where the crime occurred and technically not the victim of the crime, although the prosecutor often speaks on behalf of the victim. The prosecutor bears the burden of proving guilt beyond a reasonable doubt. If a conviction is obtained, the defendant faces incarceration.

References

1. Perks RW. Accounting and society. London: Chapman & Hall; 1993. p. 2.
2. Early PH, Finver T. Addiction to propofol; a study of 22 treatment cases. J Addict Med. 2013;7(3):169–76.
3. Xu Z, Jiang X, Li W, Gao D, Li X, Liu J. Propofol-induced sleep: efficacy and safety in patients with refractory chronic primary insomnia. Cell Biochem Biophys. 2011;60(3):161–6.
4. http://www.drugs.com/monograph/propofol.html. Accessed 13 May 2013.
5. American Society of Anesthesiologists Task Force on Perioperative Management of patients with obstructive sleep apnea. Practice guidelines for the perioperative management of patients with obstructive sleep apnea: an updated report by the American Society of Anesthesiologists Task Force on Perioperative Management of Patients with Obstructive Sleep Apnea. Anesthesiology. 2014;120(2):268–86. Also available at http://www.asahq.org/For-Members/Practice-Management/Practice-Parameters.aspx.
6. Enterlein G, Byhahn C. Practice guidelines for management of the difficult airway: update by the American Society of Anesthesiologists task force. Anaesthesist. 2013;62(10):832–5. Also available at http://www.asahq.org/For-Members/Practice-Management/Practice-Parameters.aspx.
7. Statement on granting privileges to nonanesthesiologist physicians for personally administering or supervising deep sedation. American Society of Anesthesiologists, Park Ridge, IL. 2012. https://www.asahq.org/For-Members/Standards-Guidelines-and-Statements.aspx
8. Continuum of depth of sedation: definition of general anesthesia and levels of sedation/analgesia. American Society of Anesthesiologists, Park Ridge, IL. https://www.asahq.org/For-Members/Standards-Guidelines-and-Statements.aspx. Amended Oct 2009.
9. Standards for basic anesthetic monitoring. American Society of Anesthesiologists, Park, IL. https://www.asahq.org/For-Members/Standards-Guidelines-and-Statements.aspx. Effective 1 July 2011.

Ethics and Clinical Aspects of Palliative Sedation in the Terminally Ill Child

37

Gail A. Van Norman

Abstract

More than 50,000 children in the United States die every year. Causes of death in children differ significantly from causes of death in adults—and palliative care guidelines and practices that may be appropriate for adults may not be appropriate in children. For children suffering terminal illness, the end-of-life period—defined as the average period between the realization by parents that their child cannot be cured and the child's death—lasts an average of 9 weeks. Physician realization that a child cannot be cured precedes the parental realization by an average of 100 days. During the final 63 days, health care decisions evolve from those with goals of treatment and cure to those with goals of comfort and palliation. Grief experienced after the death of a child has been shown to have profound adverse effects on mental and physical health of the parents for more than 9 years after the death of a child, and parental perceptions of child distress at end of life are correlated with longer duration of parental distress. Evidence shows that effective palliative care has an important role to play not only in the relief of distress of the child, but in the future well-being of the parents.

Keywords

Sedation • Palliative care • End-of-life care • Terminal illness • Anxiolysis • Deep continuous sedation (DCS) • Euthanasia • Pain • Hydration • Nutrition • Physician-assisted suicide (PAS) • Suffering • Principle of double effect • Richmond Agitation Sedation Scale (RASS) • Guide for Sedation of the Royal Dutch Medical Association (KNMG)

Introduction

More than 50,000 children in the United States die every year. Causes of death in children differ significantly from causes of death in adults—and palliative care guidelines and practices that may be appropriate for adults may not be appropriate in children.

For children suffering terminal illness, the end-of-life period—defined as the average period between the realization by parents that their child cannot be cured and the child's death—lasts an average of 9 weeks [1]. Physician realization that a child cannot be cured precedes the parental realization by an average of 100 days [2]. During the final 63 days, health care decisions evolve from those with goals of treatment and cure to those with goals of comfort and palliation. Grief experienced after the death of a child has been shown to have profound adverse effects on mental and physical health of the parents for more than 9 years after the death of a child [3], and parental perceptions of child distress at end of life are correlated with longer duration of parental distress [4]. Evidence shows that effective palliative care has an important role to play not only in the relief of distress of the child, but in the future well-being of the parents. (Refer to Chap. 16.)

G.A. Van Norman, M.D. (✉)
Department of Anesthesiology and Pain Medicine, University of Washington, 1959 Pacific Street, Seattle, WA 98195, USA

Department of Biomedical Ethics, University of Washington Medical Center, Seattle, WA, USA
e-mail: gvn@uw.edu

K.P. Mason (ed.), *Pediatric Sedation Outside of the Operating Room: A Multispecialty International Collaboration*, DOI 10.1007/978-1-4939-1390-9_37, © Springer Science+Business Media New York 2015

Palliative treatments focus on the relief of physical symptoms (pain, dyspnea, nausea, anorexia) and existential conditions (loneliness, hopelessness, feelings of meaninglessness, despair, fear) that prevent the child from experiencing and enjoying a good quality of life.

Inadequate management of terminal symptoms is disturbingly common in both adults and children. Costantini et al. [5] reported up to 82.3 % of adult terminal cancer patients experienced pain at end of life, and 61 % had very distressing pain. Only 59.5 % of patients received opioid analgesia for moderate to severe pain. In 54 % of patients with very distressing or severe pain, pain was "only partially" or "not at all" relieved. The end-of-life landscape does not look much better for children. Symptoms in children that are reported as "most distressing" by parents (pain, nausea, and fatigue) are extremely common, occurring in about two-thirds of dying children in one study [6]. And in approximately one-third of cases in which such physical symptoms occur, treatment was rated as unsuccessful. Psychological and spiritual distress is addressed much less often, with parents reporting that psychological symptoms at end of life were addressed in fewer than half of children, and in only 25 % of children were such symptoms adequately managed [7].

When suffering becomes intractable to "conventional" therapies and the end of life nears, physicians are increasingly turning to sedation practices to reduce or eliminate the patient's perceptions of unpleasant physical, psychological, and spiritual symptoms. There is widespread physician acceptance of "palliative sedation" or "terminal sedation" as an appropriate adjunct in end-of-life care in adults. Widespread practice, however, is not in fact sufficient evidence that such a process is ethical, and historical examples abound of social philosophies and practices (e.g., racism and slavery) that are now condemned as being immoral despite at one time being widely accepted. Far from being a settled issue, palliative sedation practice is still ethically controversial.

Sedation practices at end of life are plagued by vague and nonstandardized terminology, a lack of outcomes research, a queasy association with physician-assisted suicide (PAS) and euthanasia, misunderstanding of the ethical principle of double effect, poorly understood concepts of human suffering, and unsettled and culturally diverse philosophies about the role suffering and transcendence plays in the meaning of human life. Some authors suggest that deep continuous sedation (DCS), a form of palliative sedation, is merely euthanasia in disguise, camouflaged to circumvent legal sanctions and moral objections. When the patient is a terminally ill *child*, we are further faced with questionable assumptions about suffering among persons who may or may not be cognitively and/or emotionally fully developed, who may be incapable of understanding and contextualizing suffering, and who are utterly dependent upon surrogate decision-makers for their health care and well-being.

Any physician considering palliative sedation as an adjunct to end-of-life care, whether for adult or pediatric patients, should not only be well trained in the clinical aspects of these therapies, but the moral dimensions as well. Recipes for palliative sedation are readily available in the medical literature and can be found in references provided at the end of this chapter. The main thrust of this discussion, however, is not to provide instruction on the pharmacologic practice of palliative sedation, but to consider the ethical dimensions of palliative sedation in general and in the end-of-life care of children in particular.

Palliative Sedation: What *Exactly* Are We Talking About?

While it may seem strange to say that outcomes for sedation in end-of-life care have not been "well studied"—since the main eventual clinical "endpoint" is the patient's death—nevertheless it is true that important outcomes remain underexamined, even in adult patients. These outcomes include validation of objective measurements of patient suffering, family perceptions of patient comfort, family satisfaction with the sedation process, and family knowledge and expectations about sedation and how well these expectations were met. Sedation at end of life in children is even less understood than the processes in adults. A major barrier to formulating clinical guidelines and measuring these outcomes is a lack of unifying terminology for a range of sedation practices in end-of-life care. Authors often apply their own definitions to a variety of terms, or use disparate terms interchangeably, making it difficult to draw unifying conclusions from what little research has been done.

Common terms used in describing sedation at end of life include palliative sedation (a currently preferred, but imprecise term that can refer to a host of different sedation practices), terminal sedation (which has fallen out of favor because of a perceived connection with euthanasia), "total" sedation, DCS, sedation for refractory symptoms, sedation for intractable distress in the dying patient, and (inappropriately) "slow euthanasia."

Sedation at end of life clinically runs on a spectrum between, on the one end, the administration of anxiolytics to reduce anxiety while having minimal effects on consciousness, to "deep continuous sedation" in which the goal is to keep the patient completely unconscious permanently until death occurs. The ethical nuances of these practices are different and deserve different approaches. Simple anxiolysis without intent to significantly alter the patient's consciousness, competence, or ability to interact with others may have some ethical implications with regard to the patient's ability to participate in ongoing health care decisions, but is far less ethically perplexing than intentionally rendering a patient deeply unconscious for the remainder of his or her life. As Sinclair and Stephenson state, "The common practice of prescribing sedatives (i.e., benzodiazepines, barbiturates) or medicines that may cause sedation (i.e., tricyclic antidepressants, antipsychotics, anticonvulsants, opioids) for basic symptom control is *not* palliative sedation, but instead basic end-of-life care" [8].

This chapter will concentrate on ethical issues surrounding the practice of rendering a patient unconscious until death for the control of intractable suffering. The author prefers the term *deep continuous sedation* (DCS) for this practice, as it accurately describes both the intention and the result of the clinical treatment and accurately distinguishes it from all other palliative sedation practices.

Deep Continuous Sedation

Regardless of what name it is called, DCS is uniformly described in the medical literature as the use of sedating medications to deliberately induce and maintain a deep sleep until death—*without the intention of producing death itself* [9, 10]. Death supposedly occurs as a natural consequence of the patient's disease process and not as a result of efforts to hasten its arrival. DCS is NOT routine end-of-life care, and in fact constitutes "a radical medical procedure, since it lowers the patient's level of consciousness until the moment of death" [11].

While the definition of DCS appears simple on the surface, it is nevertheless problematic on several levels. For one, the controversy over DCS has resurrected debates regarding the definitions and implications of death and loss of personhood—some authors have suggested that DCS permanently deprives the individual of "personhood" and therefore is a form of killing. For another, it is difficult to assure that DCS does not hasten biological death, when it places the patient at significant risks, such as starvation, dehydration, and aspiration—all of which *can and do* kill under the right circumstances. The principle of "double effect," which is used by many authors to justify such risks may not ethically apply to this practice at all, as we will see. And while the physician, at least in theory, should not intend to hasten death by instituting DCS, studies of physicians employing DCS show that in fact that many actually *do* explicitly intend to hasten death [12, 13].

Epidemiology of DCS

When symptoms of suffering are not adequately relieved in a terminally ill patient, physicians are increasingly instituting DCS. In one recent study DCS was reportedly involved in 15 % of all deaths in Belgium, 17 % of all deaths in the United Kingdom, and 8 % of all deaths in the Netherlands [13, 14]. Between 3 % and 52 % of terminally ill patients in the United States are believed to have received DCS for a variety of refractory physical symptoms [15, 16] (Tables 37.1 and 37.2). The *exact* prevalence of DCS practice, however, is not precisely known, due to the lack of consensus of definitions and terminology for palliative sedation.

While the use of DCS for the relief of refractory physical symptoms and even some psychological symptoms (e.g., anxiety, agitation) appears to be widely accepted by physicians and other health care workers, the same professionals are less convinced that it is appropriate to use DCS to relieve spiritual anguish and/or existential suffering [16, 17]. In fact, although these latter symptoms are common (Table 37.3) and can be even more distressing to patients than physical ones, many health care workers hold beliefs that patients

Table 37.1 Common distressing physical symptoms at end of life [15, 16]

Symptom	Prevalence
Fatigue	83 %
Dyspnea	50–63 %
Malaise/restlessness	40 %
Pain	25–48 %
Confusion	36 %
Anxiety	31 %
Depression	28 %
Agitation	21 %
Nausea/vomiting	6–25 %
More than one symptoms	54 %

Table 37.2 Frequency of physical symptoms in pediatric cancer patients in palliative phase of care [7]

Symptom	Frequency
Pain	75 %
Anorexia	75 %
Fatigue	72 %
Lack of mobility	66 %
Vomiting	53 %
Dyspnea	41 %

Table 37.3 Frequency of psychological symptoms of children (mean age 10.9 years) in the palliative phase of cancer care [7]

Symptom	Frequency
Sadness	65 %
Difficulty in talking about their feelings	41 %
Fear of being alone	37 %
Loss of perspective	36 %
Loss of independence	32 %
Anger	30 %
Fear of death	16 %
Feelings of guilt	12 %
Depression	3 %

achieve transcendence and spiritual growth by experiencing them and are reluctant to use pharmacologic means to reduce the patient's awareness of these forms of suffering [8].

What is Suffering?

The experience of suffering is to be distinguished from the occurrence of physical stress or responses to unpleasant stimuli. "Suffering" is the conscious processing of unpleasant physical or other experiences. "Suffering" implies that the victim on some level perceives and/or anticipates the discomfort—whether physical, mental, or spiritual—and that such perception and/or anticipation is extremely unpleasant. Every anesthesiologist knows that even under general anesthesia, the body may physically respond to painful stimuli and manifest the physical stress response it induces through tearing, sweating, rises in blood pressure or pulse, or increasing respirations. Physiologically, even under general anesthesia, painful stimulation causes the release of "stress hormones," such as cortisol and epinephrine. But while the body responds to pain, most anesthesiologists would not describe the patient's experience under general anesthesia as "suffering" unless the patient at some point becomes consciously aware of the stimulation.

The primary justification for DCS at end of life rests in the assertion that it is used to prevent suffering in patients for whom the symptoms are intractable and cannot otherwise be relieved, by reducing the patient's awareness of them [18]. As such, DCS is not justified, for example, for use in patients who are already unconscious of their surroundings or physical experiences. Even if physical manifestations of terminal symptoms can still be observed, unless the patient is aware of them, there is no ethical justification for using DCS to relieve the suffering of the patient, since "suffering" in that case does not exist. And yet many studies show that DCS is requested and employed, even in minimally aware or even unconscious patients, and at times with the physician's explicit intention to hasten death [12], in some cases even to facilitate the death of nonterminal patients [13].

Existential Suffering and Transcendence

While it may seem out of place to discuss the concept of transcendence in a medical textbook, transcendence nevertheless plays a key role in controversies concerning DCS. Not only have physicians been historically slow to accept that spiritual and psychological aspects of end of life impact the physical process of dying, but many even deny that it is the role of physicians to incorporate such thinking and understanding in the care of the dying patient. Little research is available to teach us about the impact of spirituality and religiosity on adult dying patients, and none at all is available regarding the dying child. Yet it is reasonable to assume that, at the very least, what little we do know about adult patients will apply to many older children—and may apply to younger children as well.

What do we mean by *transcendence*? While there are many different definitions offered, one way to consider transcendence in the dying patient is as the opportunity and potential for the patient to find comfort in understanding their own death in a broader context than simply the physical one. For the dying patient, psychological, spiritual, and religious resolution and comfort may assume much greater importance than physical comfort. Denying patients the opportunity to seek and achieve such an understanding at the end of life may deny them an important path toward relief of their overall suffering. Transcendence, ultimately, is surpassing what we have already become, through our experiences and understanding of those experiences.

Although many physicians and family members worry that knowing that death is imminent may cause patients to despair, lose hope, and even seek to hasten their own deaths, research in adult patients confirms exactly the opposite: that achieving transcendent understanding of their own death can be profoundly comforting to patients.

Kellehear, in a theoretical model of spiritual needs in palliative care, defined a framework for understanding spirituality and religiosity in the dying patient [19]. "Spirituality" refers to a feeling of connectedness to the universe and the search for the meaning of life that may or may not be connected to any religious figure. "Religiosity" is an organized set of beliefs and rituals that are carried out with the goal of connecting to a higher power, such as a god [20, 21]. In Kellehear's model, spiritual meaning arises from three types of needs: situational, moral, and biographical [19]. Situational needs arise from individual personal and social experiences played out in the context of the individual patient's illness. Patients seek meaning, purpose, and hope within their own experience of their illness. Moral and biographical needs are met by finding reconciliation of past dilemmas, reunion with others, forgiveness, and closure. The patient may seek moral and social analysis of their life and dying process. Religious needs are met through seeking divine reconciliation and forgiveness, through the experience of religious rites, visitation and literature, and through discussion of eternal life and hope. In this model, research with adult patients to determine the effect of spiritual and/or religious well-being at end of life demonstrates that patients who are informed and aware of the imminence of death generally have significantly *higher* scores on a spiritual well-being scale than those from whom explicit information is withheld [22]. Patients who are aware of their terminal condition may use remaining time to redirect and re-evaluate their lives, and focus on resolving their spiritual needs.

As de Benedetto et al. commented about listening to patients at end of life:

> We allow them to transform their chaos stories into quest stories, in which their illnesses become teaching tools for all involved. Quest stories are stories of transcendence [23].

Many doctors are uncomfortable with spiritual and experiential discussions with dying patients, and may justify ignoring or curtailing such conversations as a means of reducing patient suffering—when exactly the opposite may in fact be true. Premature institution of DCS, ostensibly to relieve the "anxiety" that causes patients to seek spiritual comfort may prevent patients from being able to fulfill critical spiritual needs at end of life.

Spiritual experiences are common among dying patients. Renz et al. [24] reported on 251 patients in whom 135 described experiences of peace, freedom, transformed perception or consciousness, experiences of God within and outside of the experience of suffering, and experiences of spirit and energy—a sort of divine light. All patients in the Renz study reported reduced pain, less anxiety, and better body awareness, as well as a different attitude toward illness, life, death, and the divine shortly before they died. Other studies also demonstrate that significant proportions of terminally ill patients experience spiritual and transcendent phenomenon [25], with many, but not all, of these experiences occurring very shortly before death. As one patient stated of their experience, "Simple. Elegant. Beautiful. And I hang on to that with everything I've got" [25]. A significant shift toward peace and contentment is one hallmark of these experiences, and they appear to permanently eradicate a patient's fear, dread, and anxiety as death approaches.

It is understandable that some health care providers question the use of DCS toward end of life, since even minimal studies seem to indicate that these are important, comforting, and transforming experiences that mitigate suffering for both the patient and family, and since many of these experiences happen when the patient is close to death and consideration of DCS might be in play. But are such "transcendent experiences" of real value to patients, particularly to children?

The impact of transcendent experiences on dying children is entirely unstudied, but spirituality is known to play an important positive role in the comfort and well-being of dying children [26, 27]. And while terminal spiritual experiences in younger children are not extensively described, they certainly exist based on reports of near-death experiences in children—one type of terminal spiritual event [28]. DCS in even young children may therefore deprive them of important experiences with regard to meaning in life and spiritual comfort. This may be especially true when DCS is employed to treat "anxiety" rather than to mitigate intractable physical pain, or worse, to relieve the anxiety of others around the child, such as parents, family, and caregivers—for it may then not best serve the child. At the very least, the reasons and goals for employing DCS should be carefully explored, and consideration given to the important experiences DCS may obliterate as well as ameliorate.

DCS and Euthanasia: Is Permanent Loss of Consciousness a Form of Death?

One concern regarding the practice of DCS is whether it ethically amounts to a subtle form of euthanasia—one that simply serves to camouflage the true nature of the physician's actions and skirt legal sanctions and professional oaths against killing patients. To examine this concern, we need to consider what determines if an act is euthanasia, what defines death, and the role of intention and the principle of double effect in DCS practice.

What is Euthanasia?

Euthanasia is a general term that is derived from Greek roots *eu*, meaning good or well, and *thanatos*, meaning death. In modern usage, euthanasia always refers to an act of killing, but one that must meet certain conditions. Not every act of killing is euthanasia, but every act of euthanasia is a killing, for every act of euthanasia ends in death. Furthermore, the term "euthanasia" itself has no intrinsic or independent ethical or legal value: Various acts of euthanasia can be ethical, unethical, legal, or illegal.

Intentions, foresights, and motives are crucial determinants of euthanasia. Euthanasia is above all a *deliberate* act and requires the explicit intention that the object of the act will be killed. It is neither an accidental side effect nor even a recognized but acceptable risk of an action that is intended primarily to produce results other than death. Thus, administration of pain medication with the explicit intention only of relieving pain, but which causes a possible, but not necessarily wished-for side effect of respiratory depression and death, is not euthanasia. If this was not so, then any physician who attempts to treat a critically ill patient by administering an intravenous antibiotic that unintentionally results in immediate anaphylaxis and death—a known albeit small risk of such action—commits euthanasia. Because personal intentions can be difficult to independently verify, it may be difficult to determine with certainty whether some acts of killing are really euthanasia or merely unintended side effects of other well-intentioned actions.

Intention and foresight are important concepts in both the legal and medical concepts of euthanasia, and they are not synonymous. *Intention* refers to the specific goals and desired results of an action. *Foresight* is conceiving of outcomes that we may or may not intend. We might consider the risks of many "secondary outcomes" as significant, without primarily desiring them. In a recent news article, a hunter accidentally killed his hunting partner with a gunshot, while trying to kill the bear that was attacking him. Certainly the hunter may have *foreseen* a risk, even a significant one, that since both bear and human were in his sights, he might actually shoot the human. But his *intention* was to kill the bear. Foreseeing a possible outcome does not mean that it is our intention.

Finally, for an act to be euthanasia it must have at its heart a special type of *motive*. Motive differs from intention in that motive refers to the reasons *behind* our intentions. Motive is an incitement to action, whereas intention is the intended outcome of the action that is incited. Euthanasia has *mercy* at the heart of its incitement and *altruism* as its core virtue. In these ways it shares common roots with DCS, whose intention is also merciful and virtue is altruistic. Harold Shipman, a British physician who administered lethal drugs to patients because he stood to inherit large sums of money from their estates, committed murder and not euthanasia *even* if many of the deaths he caused were swift and painless and *even* if as a "side effect" they sometimes ended the life of someone who was suffering and actually wanted to die. That is because his primary motive was based neither in mercy nor altruism, but rather in self-enrichment [29].

The term "euthanasia" does not require nor even imply that the subject is always able to understand, consent to, or request a "good death." This becomes most obvious when we speak of the euthanasia of nonhuman animals, which *always* occurs without consent. Euthanasia recipients can include incompetent and never-competent humans, such as infants. Whether it is legal, ethical, or desirable to subject such individuals to euthanasia is a complex topic beyond the scope of this chapter. However, because "mercy" is a core requirement in order for a killing to be considered euthanasia, it follows that in the case of competent persons of any age who are capable of deciding whether euthanasia represents a merciful death for them, consent by the patient is required.

Why do we worry about physicians performing euthanasia? Ancient oaths have emphasized the physician's role as healer; indeed proscribing practices that, intentionally or otherwise, hasten death. Such prohibitions have rested in the traditional role of physicians as healers and not killers, and the "societal contract" physicians owe to protect lives in return for being pulled into their patients' privacy and confidences, and for being given unprecedented power in affecting the quality and duration of patients' lives. Physicians have been prohibited by their oaths since ancient times from participating in the killing of human beings. But the changing physical and moral landscapes of end of life in the last century have led to serious reconsideration of the appropriate role of the physician when death is inevitable. And even in the face of intense debate, PAS and euthanasia is still permitted in only a handful of places in the world. It is important, therefore, to consider whether DCS is, as some suggest, a disguised form of euthanasia.

Defining Death

Proponents of deep conscious sedation (DCS) argue that DCS can be differentiated from euthanasia because DCS is reversible, while death (due to euthanasia) is not.

Death, however, has been a difficult concept for human beings to strictly define. In 1968 when the ad hoc Committee of the Harvard Medical School defined "brain death" [30], they considered whether "death of personhood" was another way of defining death. The Committee defined brain death as irreversible cessation of the function of the whole brain. Lesser, but still permanent brain dysfunctions were also considered, such as permanent coma, in which various degrees of dysfunction of the cortex were present, but brainstem function remained essentially intact. Proponents of a "personhood" definition of death argued that once a human being reached some threshold level of cognitive dysfunction, their inability to participate in a social context in their lives essentially rendered them "dead," and that therefore certain comatose patients could be declared dead [31]. Some authors have discussed the ethics of using such comatose patients for unconsented vital organ donation, for example [32].

In whatever way death is defined, however, one common requirement is that death is a permanent state of affairs. Even in patients whose hearts have stopped and then been restored to beating, we do not say medically that they were biologically dead. We say we have "resuscitated" them, not "resurrected" them. To be sure, death hovered close by—prolonged cardiac arrest would have progressed quickly from "resuscitatible" to "nonresuscitatible" and therefore permanent. Loss of brain function would have progressed from "reversible" to "irreversible." The attainment of a permanent loss of these functions is a key element to declaring death.

Because DCS can be reversed (i.e., the medications can be stopped and the person presumably restored to higher levels of awareness), it is argued by many physicians that it cannot be considered "death," and therefore instituting it is not a form of "euthanasia" [33]. Anesthesiologists regularly produce a state of profound unconsciousness in their patients, for example, but no one equates that state with death, nor the practitioner of anesthesia with having committed an act of killing. However, others point out that the *intention and practice* of DCS produces *permanent* loss of consciousness, and therefore permanent loss of "personhood." If death can be defined as an intended permanent loss of social participation and awareness, then DCS certainly produces a type of death [34].

Defining the nature of such a "social death" proved elusive for the ad hoc committee, due to the spectrum of cognitive dysfunction that could be considered "dead" under such a definition, together with the potential temporary nature of loss of personhood. There were concerns that a "slippery slope" may then allow physicians and families to kill vulnerable persons who have been disabled by varying levels of cognitive dysfunction. Furthermore, subsequent research indicated that many human beings considered to be permanently "comatose" and therefore having "lost personhood," in fact have high levels of awareness and are merely prevented from demonstrating awareness and interacting with others due to other disabilities imposed on them by their brain injuries [35]. For these and other reasons, loss of personhood has never been accepted legally or ethically as a definition of death in the United States, and ethical arguments that DCS constitutes euthanasia are somewhat weak.

DCS and Hastening Death

The Principle of Double Effect and DCS

Many argue that DCS, even if it causes or hastens death, is ethically permissible under the ethical principle of "double effect." Double effect is the concept that an action can have a combination of beneficial and harmful results, but is still ethical if the intent is *only* to produce the beneficial ones. The principle of double effect is rooted in Catholic theology and was first mentioned in the writings of St. Thomas Aquinas regarding self-defense as a "duality of the results of single human actions" [36]. In the process of defending oneself, the defender might kill the aggressor without intending to kill but merely to fend off an attack. The defender would then be held less culpable for the outcome (although it is important to note that they would not necessarily be *entirely* inculpable).

The principle of double effect can be asserted only if several assertions are true: (1) the action has both potential "good" and "bad" results, (2) the action is not in and of itself immoral, (3) the action is undertaken solely with the purpose of producing the good effect and not that bad one—even though the bad effect may be foreseen, (4) the good effect is not achieved by means of the bad effect, and (5) the action is undertaken for a "proportionally grave" reason [37].

To invoke the principle of double effect to justify DCS, we have to suppose that DCS may hasten death in some cases. If we accept for the moment that supposition, and if we review the five assertions of double effect in the context of DCS, we can accept the assertions that (1) DCS has both potentially good and bad results as it may hasten death, and (5) DCS is (or at least should be) undertaken for a proportionally "grave" reason—the relief of intractable suffering in a dying patient when relief cannot otherwise be achieved. But with the second, third, and fourth assertions we run into problems.

Is DCS morally neutral, as required in the second assertion? In the case of patients who stop eating and drinking *because of DCS*, the treatment is not neutral, but directly, necessarily, and predictably could lead to harm, unless nutrition and hydration are then artificially administered. The combination of DCS with withdrawal of hydration and nutrition therefore presents particular problems with the concept of the moral neutrality of DCS. The institution of DCS increases the risk of complications that may hasten death (such as aspiration) and *requires* that the patient be put into a state of enhanced risk. This raises questions about the validity of the fourth assertion.

Is the third assertion, that the action is undertaken only to produce the good effect, upheld in DCS? Many authors suggest that DCS carries as its underlying motive a fundamental harm: the wish to hasten death [37, 38]. Studies demonstrate that in a significant portion of cases physicians actually *intend* to hasten death. Surveys of Dutch physicians, where euthanasia is legal, demonstrate that hastening death is actually an explicit *intention* in 17 % of cases of DCS, and it is cited as partly the intention in 47 % of cases [39]. A study of United Kingdom doctors also indicated that DCS was somewhat intended to hasten death in a significant proportion of cases [40]. A recent survey carried out by the Association of American Physicians and Surgeons found that 16 % of American physicians said that they had "first-hand knowledge of patients who were placed on 'terminal sedation' with denial of fluids and nutrition in United States hospitals, when in [their] opinion they might recover with aggressive treatment" [41]. It is almost certain therefore that in some cases, in the perception of the physician and/or family, a "good effect" is achieved through the intended death of the patient, which also violates the fourth assertion of double effect.

Studies show that the situation is not much better when the terminally ill patient is a child. A significant percentage (13 %) of parents report that they considered requesting hastening the death of their terminally ill child, and in 9 % of cases, actually discussed this possibility [42]. This intention increased if the child's primary symptoms were related to pain. Retrospectively, about 34 % of parents indicated that they would have considered hastening their child's death if the child had experienced uncontrolled pain, and 15 % for intractable psychological suffering. When a child is unable to communicate during the terminal stages of illness, mothers are more likely to believe that death is better for their child, and when a child faces six or more years of illness, fathers are more likely to consider death to be preferable for the child [43].

Table 37.4 Time to death after institution of deep conscious sedation (DCS) [11]

Time to death after institution of DCS	% of patients
≤24 h	47
1–7 days	47
2 weeks	4
>2 weeks	2

DCS and Withdrawal of Hydration and Nutrition

Is it ethical to withdraw nutrition and hydration when DCS is initiated? Or is it, as some assert, a form of "slow euthanasia"?

On the one hand, adult patients and their surrogates in the United States have rights under federal law and the Constitution to refuse even life-saving medical care [44]. The courts have repeatedly determined that withdrawal of nutrition and hydration is no different than withdrawing other medically initiated life-sustaining care, and may be withheld at the request of a competent patient or a patient's surrogate decision-makers [45, 46]. However, the issues concerning withdrawal/withholding of treatments in children are less clear—particularly in very young children who may not completely understand the issues and may not be able to express preferences or to have true decisional autonomy. Court-ordered cancer treatment for minor children that overrides parental and child religious objections, for example, is not all that unusual.

Studies indicate that palliative sedation does not appear by itself to shorten life—largely because it is initiated in the final phases of terminal illness [47] (Table 37.4). Dehydration associated with withholding of artificial fluids and/or nutrition at the time of initiation of palliative sedation typically results in death within 2 weeks [48]. The practice of withdrawing/withholding artificial nutrition and hydration at the time of initiation of DCS is widespread [49] and occurred in up to 64 % of patients who received DCS according to a European survey [50].

Since the indication for DCS is to treat intractable symptoms by rendering the patient permanently unconscious and *not* to deliberately hasten death, caution is indicated when these two ethically diverse decisions are combined in one event.

The decision to withdraw hydration and nutrition should be made separately and distinctly from the decision to initiate DCS, and the intent of each action made clear to the patient, to family members, and to health care workers involved. Some authors point out that the patient's (or parents') preferences regarding the use of artificial hydration and nutrition should be clearly established *separately and before* any decision to initiate DCS [51]. If death from the underlying cause is expected within 2 weeks, the decision to withhold nutrition and hydration may not be morally significant.

Legal Precedents and Physician Attitudes Regarding DCS

Although some argue that DCS and euthanasia, or PAS, are ethically similar, legal precedent and physician opinion nevertheless clearly distinguish between the two.

In 1997, in the case of Washington et al. v. Gucksberg et al., the United States Supreme Court held that the (then) ban in Washington State[1] on PAS was not unconstitutional [52]. Justice Sandra Day O'Connor, in her concurring opinion, not only distinguished the practice of DCS from euthanasia, but stated that "a patient who is suffering from a terminal illness and who is experiencing great pain has no legal barriers to obtaining medication from qualified physicians to alleviate that suffering, even to the point of causing unconsciousness *and hastening death*" (author's italics). There is no doubt that DCS constitutes legal end-of-life care in the United States.

About 78 % of physicians in one survey supported the use of DCS in end-of-life care, but almost half of those who supported DCS were opposed to PAS and euthanasia [53]. This could indicate either that physicians are unaware of ethical arguments that place these actions in the same moral boat or that they use perceived differences in these actions to justify DCS and alleviate themselves of culpability *even when hastening death is their intention.* In one survey of Dutch physicians, many indicated that, unlike with PAS or euthanasia, the physician experienced a patient's death following DCS as a "natural death," with an entirely different emotional context than if actively assisting a death [53, 54]. This feeling was by no means universal however, with some physicians in the survey reporting that they experienced the "social death" of the patient and their final goodbyes at the initiation of DCS similarly to deaths from PAS or euthanasia.

Professional Societies and Opinions Regarding DCS

The American Medical Association has released an opinion by the Council for Ethical and Judicial Affairs that endorses DCS in terminally ill patients who suffer from intractable physical symptoms (pain, nausea and vomiting, shortness of breath, and agitated delirium) as well as severe psychological distress [55]. They exclude purely existential suffering as an indication for DCS, stating, for example, that loneliness

[1] In 2008, Washington State passed a law allowing physician-assisted suicide.

Table 37.5 Recommendations of the American Medical Association regarding palliative sedation [55]

The patient must be in the final stages of terminal illness, and the rationale for palliative care must be documented in the chart
DCS may be considered when symptoms do not respond to aggressive, symptom-specific treatments
Informed consent should be obtained from the patient and/or the patient's surrogate for DCS
Physicians should consult with a multidisciplinary team, including experts in palliative care to assure that symptom-specific treatments have been sufficiently employed and DCS is now the most appropriate course
Physicians should discuss with patients considering DCS the care plan, including degree and length, intermittent or constant, and specific expectations for continuing, withdrawing, or withholding future life-sustaining treatments
Once palliative sedation is begun, measures to monitor treatment must be in place
Palliative sedation is not appropriate for purely existential suffering
Palliative sedation must never be used to intentionally cause a patient's death

and isolation should be treated by broader social and spiritual support. This exclusion is interesting in that is presupposes that such interventions are actually effective for intractable existential suffering, when no such efficacy has ever been shown. They caution that proportionality of treatment is key in DCS—sedation should be used only to the level necessary to relieve distressing symptoms. In the report, they present clinical guidelines for practicing palliative sedation (Table 37.5).

Guidelines

There are a few authoritative statements and guidelines for the use of DCS. Essentially all indicate that the patient must be in a terminal condition, and DCS can be instituted only if symptoms are intolerable and refractory. All endorse that expected survival should be very short—from days up to about 2 weeks. Most professional societies approach the issue of palliative sedation similarly to the American Medical Association, whose recommendations are summarized in Table 37.5.

The aspect in which guidelines and statements often differ significantly is on the issue of whether DCS is permissible to treat existential suffering (Table 37.6) [11, 55–59].

Initiating DCS: Goals, Monitoring, and Evaluation of Efficacy

Common sedatives used in DCS include midazolam, lorazepam, haloperidol, pentobarbital, phenobarbital, and propofol. Most are administered intravenously or subcutaneously in a continuous regimen, with the goal being to reach a dose that achieves sedation of sufficient depth to achieve the endpoint of alleviation of the patient's distressing symptoms. Typical dosing can be found in many sources [8], but the range of dosing is wide and ultimately based on achieving the desired result of diminished or absent awareness of terminal symptoms. For midazolam, for example, usual maintenance dosing for an intravenous infusion is anywhere from 20 to 120 mg/day in adult patients [8].

Commonly, opioids are erroneously discontinued at the time that DCS is initiated, under the mistaken understanding that sedation is all that is needed. Medications targeted for the patient's source of suffering (e.g., opioids for pain) should be continued and sedation used to augment those treatments to achieve the goal of diminished or absent awareness of residual discomfort [8]. Reducing pain medication while initiating sedation can lead to opioid withdrawal and increased suffering, or increasing pain with diminished ability of the patient to communicate about symptoms.

Monitoring of symptoms should include clinical observation, periodic vital signs, conversations with family and other observers about their impressions of the patient's comfort level, and, if complete unconsciousness is not intended or achieved, conversations with the patient. Usual measures to assess depth of sedation, such as the application of painful physical stimuli to gauge arousal, are contraindicated in DCS.

Recommendations for Initiating DCS in Pediatric Patients [60]

The initiation of DCS should follow certain prescribed steps:

Step 1: Once it is determined that a patient is terminally ill, establishment of general palliative therapy should include discussion of the patient's (or their surrogates') goals, given the terminal prognosis. Desires regarding resuscitation and treatments such as artificial hydration and nutrition should be discussed prior to and separately from discussion of DCS.

Step 2: Symptom-specific therapy should be optimized prior to consideration of DCS. Palliative sedation therapy should only then be considered if intractable suffering is still present despite optimization of symptom-directed therapy. The patient and/or their parents should be informed of the expected results of treatments, including the fact that simultaneously withdrawing hydration and nutrition with initiation of DCS does not appear to hasten

Table 37.6 Guidelines statements regarding use of DCS for treatment of existential suffering [11, 55–59]

Society	Is DCS permissible for existential suffering?
American Academy of Hospice and Palliative Medicine [56]	Not specified
American College of Physicians – American Society of Internal Medicine Consensus Panel [57]	Not specified, although only physical symptoms are addressed
AMA Council on Ethical and Judicial Affairs [55]	No
Royal Dutch Medical Association [11]	Yes
Harvard University Community Ethics Committee (CEC) [58]	Yes
Veterans Health Administration [59]	Did not specifically exclude it in their final recommendations, but weighed against it in their discussion

Table 37.7 The KNMG Sedation Scale [11]

Sedation	Description
Level 1	(a) Awake and oriented (b) Drowsy (c) Eyes closed, responds to verbal commands (d) Eyes closed, responds only to physical stimulation
Level 2	Not arousable by physical stimulation
Level 3	Not arousable, basic brain function affected (e.g., depressed respiration)

Table 37.8 The Richmond Agitation-Sedation Scale [62]

Score	Observation
+4	Combative: violent, danger to staff
+3	Very agitated: pulls at tubes, aggressive toward staff
+2	Agitated: frequent nonpurposeful movement or ventilatory dyssynchrony
+1	Restless: anxious, but movements nonvigorous
0	Alert and calm
−1	Drowsy: not fully alert, but eye contact >10 s to voice
−2	Light sedation: eye contact, but <10 s to voice
−3	Moderate sedation: any movement (no eye contact) to voice
−4	Deep sedation: no response to voice, but movement with physical stimulation
−5	Unarousable: no response to voice or physical stimulation

death. Pediatric patients should be included in discussion of these measures to the level of their ability to do so.

Step 3: The patient, family members, and health care workers should have a clear idea of treatment goals, and clear indicators should be established that will be used to assess patient comfort and the need to further titrate sedation. These matters should include the observation points and times, and who does what and when. The overall process should be evaluated personally by the physician a *minimum* of once a day. New symptoms can arise that require attention.

Step 4: Palliative sedation therapy should start with a trial of sedation titrated to provide adequate symptom control. If lesser degrees of sedation than DCS provide adequate symptom relief, then permanent unconsciousness need not be pursued, and generally should not be. *The treating physician should always be present at the initiation of DCS* [11]. It is an "emotionally charged" event and may feel/appear to the family emotionally comparable to the death of the patient. Use of opioids for the sole purpose of DCS is specifically contraindicated and under some guidelines is specifically called out as "bad practice" [11]. Opioids, such as morphine, do not reliably reduce awareness, but do have side effects that can increase patient suffering, such as delirium and myoclonus. If opioids are being used to treat pain or dyspnea, for example, they should be continued.

Two validated scales to assess sedation were found in one study to be the most reliable for use in palliative sedation [61]: the Guide for Sedation of the Royal Dutch Medical Association (KNMG) (Table 37.7) and the Richmond Agitation-Sedation Scale (RASS) (Table 37.8) [62].

Conclusion

Palliative care involves a turn from goals of cure to those of comfort and terminal symptom control. When suffering at end of life becomes intractable, many physicians are turning to the use of DCS to control problematic symptoms. In cases where the terminally ill patient is a child, the quality of palliative care has been shown to have effects on parental well-being for many years following the child's death.

Sedation that is aimed at producing drowsiness and reduced agitation may have ethical implications regarding patient participation in end-of-life decisions, but DCS is ethically much more controversial, and in all cases is considered a "radical medical treatment." While there appears to be widespread agreement that DCS should be used to treat intractable physical symptoms, there is significant disagreement about the use of DCS to treat existential suffering, even though such symptoms can be more problematic to patients than physical ones. The nature of existential suffering in terminally ill patients is poorly studied and remains virtually unknown in children, particularly young children.

Significant controversy regarding DCS centers on whether DCS constitutes a form of euthanasia that circumvents normal legal and moral sanctions against killing. These concerns have resurrected debates about whether "loss of personhood" at end of life represents another legitimate definition of death.

Justification of DCS by the principle of double effect may not be appropriate application of ethical theory, and the very assertion that DCS hastens physical death appears to have been substantially refuted by medical studies.

The clinical practice of DCS is poorly studied overall and remains virtually unstudied in pediatric patients. Poor clinical practices, such as discontinuing opioids with initiation of DCS, or using opioids as a primary agent to produce DCS, are common. More research and better training in the clinical and ethical aspects of DCS is needed for physician caring for patients of all ages.

Acknowledgment The author wishes to sincerely thank the Brocher Foundation, Hermance Switzerland, for the opportunity to study the ethics of end-of-life decision-making, including palliative sedation, physician-assisted suicide, and euthanasia. While no monetary contribution was made toward the writing of this chapter, the scholarly work that residency at the foundation permitted was an invaluable asset.

References

1. Hechler T, Blankenburg M, Friedrichsdorf SJ, et al. Parents' perspective on symptoms, quality of life, characteristics of death and end-of-life decisions for children dying from cancer. Klin Padiatr. 2008;220(3):166–74.
2. Valdimarsdottir U, Kreicbergs U, Hauksdottir A, et al. Parents' intellectual and emotional awareness of their child's impending death to cancer: a population-based long-term follow-up study. Lancet Oncol. 2007;8:706–14.
3. Lannen PK, Wolfe J, Prigerson HG, et al. Unresolved grief in a national sample of bereaved parents: impaired mental and physical health 4 to 9 years later. J Clin Oncol. 2008;26(36):5870–6.
4. Kreicbergs U, Valdimarsdottir U, Onelov E, et al. Care-related distress: a nationwide study of parents who lost their child to cancer. J Clin Oncol. 2005;23(36):9162–71.
5. Costantini M, Ripamonti C, Beccaro M, et al. Prevalence, distress, management, and relief of pain during the last 3 months of cancer patients' life. Results of an Italian mortality follow-back survey. Ann Oncol. 2009;20(4):729–35.
6. Lutzau P, Otto M, Hechler G, et al. Children dying of cancer; parents' perspectives on symptoms, quality of life, characteristics of death, and end-of-life decisions. J Palliat Care. 2012;28(4):274–81.
7. Theunissen JMJ, Hoogerbrugge PM, van Achterberg T, et al. Symptoms in the palliative phase of children with cancer. Pediatr Blood Cancer. 2007;49(2):160–5.
8. Sinclair CT, Stephenson RC. Palliative sedation: assessment, management, and ethics. Hosp Physician. 2006;42:33–8.
9. Hahn MP. Review of palliative sedation and its distinction from euthanasia and lethal injection. J Pain Palliat Care Pharmacother. 2012;26:30–9.
10. Broeckaert B. Palliative sedation, physician assisted suicide, and euthanasia: "same, same but different"? Am J Bioeth. 2011;11(6):62–4.
11. Guideline for Palliative Sedation. Utrecht: Royal Dutch Medical Association (KNMG). 2009. http://knmg.artsennet.nl/web/file?uuid=d57c9dec-49d3-43a2-9c4d-1b15005c615c&owner=a8a9ce0e-f42b-47a5-960e-be08025b7b04&contentid=66977. Accessed 2 Feb 2014.
12. Sercu M, Pype P, Christiaens T, et al. Belgian general practitioners' perspectives on the use of palliative sedation in end-of-life home care: a qualitative study. J Pain Symptom Manage. 2014;47(6):1054–63.
13. Anquinet L, Rietjens JA, Vandervoort A, et al. Continuous deep sedation until death in nursing home residents with dementia: a case series. J Am Geriatr Soc. 2013;61(10):1768–76.
14. Anquinet L, Rietjens JAC, Seale C, et al. The practice of continuous deep sedation until death in Flanders (Belgium), the Netherlands, and the U.K.: a comparative study. J Pain Symptom Manage. 2012;44(1):33–43.
15. Kohara H, Ueoka H, Takeyama H, et al. Sedation for terminally ill patients with cancer with uncontrollable physical distress. J Palliat Med. 2005;8(1):20–5.
16. Klinkenberg M, Willems DL, van der Wal G, Deeg DJH. Symptom burden in the last week of life. J Pain Symptom Manage. 2004;27:5–13.
17. Beauverd M, Bernard M, Currat T, et al. French Swiss physician's attitude toward palliative sedation: influence of prognosis and type of suffering. Palliat Support Care. 2013;17:1–6.
18. Tsu PSH. Elimination of pain versus elimination of suffering: why CDS is ethically preferable to PAS. Am J Bioeth. 2011;11(6):45–6.
19. Kellehear A. Spirituality and palliative care: a model of needs. Palliat Med. 2000;14:149–55.
20. Bryson KA. Spirituality, meaning and transcendence. Palliat Support Care. 2004;2:3321–8.
21. Vachon M, Fillion L, Archille M. A conceptual analysis of spirituality at the end of life. J Palliat Med. 2009;12(1):53–9.
22. Leung KK, Chiu TY, Chen CY. The influence of awareness of terminal condition on spiritual well-being in terminal cancer patients. J Pain Symptom Manage. 2006;31(5):449–56.
23. De Benedetto MAC, de Castro AG, de Carvalho E, et al. From suffering to transcendence. Can Fam Physician. 2007;53:1277–9.
24. Renz M, Mao SM, Omlin A, et al. Spiritual experiences of transcendence in patients with advanced cancer. Am J Hosp Palliat Care. 2013;2(1):17–26.
25. Arnold BL, Lloyd LS. Harnessing complex emergent metaphors for effective communication in palliative care: a multimodal perceptual analysis of hospice patients' reports of transcendence experiences. Am J Hosp Palliat Care. 2014;31(3):292–9.
26. Lima NN, Nscimento VB, Carvalho SM, et al. Spirituality in childhood cancer care. Neuropsychiatr Dis Treat. 2013;9:1539–44.
27. Petersen CL. Spiritual care of the child with cancer at the end of life: a concept analysis. J Adv Nurs. 2014;70(6):1243–53.
28. Atwater P. Our tiniest near-death experiencers: startling evidence suggestive of a brain shift. J Relig Psych Res. 2003;26(2):86–97.
29. BBC News. Harold Shipman, the killer doctor. http://news.bbc.co.uk/2/hi/uk_news/3391897.stm. Accessed 2 Feb 2014.
30. A definition of irreversible coma. A report of the Ad Hoc Committee of the Harvard Medical School to Examine the Definition of Brain Death. JAMA. 1968;206(6):337–40.
31. Schonberger RB, Rosenbaum SH. Brain death. In: Van Norman GA, Jackson S, Rosenbaum SH, Palmer S, editors. Clinical ethics in anesthesiology: a case-based textbook. Cambridge: Cambridge University Press; 2010. p. 108–13.
32. Koppelman ER. The dead donor rule and the concept of death: severing the ties that bind them. Am J Bioeth. 2003;3(1):1–9.
33. LiPuma SH. The lacking of moral equivalency for continuous sedation and PAS. Am J Bioeth. 2011;11(6):48–9.
34. Lipuma S. Continuous sedation until death as physician-assisted suicide/euthanasia, a conceptual analysis. J Med Philos. 2013;38:190–204.
35. Owen AM, Coleman MR. Detecting awareness in the vegetative state. Ann N Y Acad Sci. 2008;1129:130–8.
36. Aquinas ST. Summa Theologica I–II; 1947.
37. Dudzinski DM. The principle of double effect in palliative care: euthanasia by another name? In: Van Norman GA, Jackson S, Rosenbaum SH, Palmer S, editors. Clinical ethics in anesthesiology:

a case-based textbook. Cambridge: Cambridge University Press; 2010. p. 85–91.
38. Carvalho TB, Rady MY, Verheijde JL, Robert JS. Continuous deep sedation in end-of-life care: disentangling palliation form physician-assisted suicide. Am J Bioeth. 2011;11(6):60–2.
39. Rietjens JA, van der Heide A, Vrakking AM, et al. Physician reports of terminal sedation without hydration or nutrition for patients nearing death in The Netherlands. Ann Intern Med. 2004;141: 178–85.
40. Seale C. Continuous deep sedation in medical practice: a descriptive study. J Pain Symptom Manage. 2010;39(1):44–53.
41. Association of American Physicians and Surgeons. https://aaps.wufoo.com/reports/terminal-sedation-survey-results/. Accessed 24 Jan 2014.
42. Dussel V, Joffe S, Hilden JM, et al. Considerations about hastening death among parents of children who die of cancer. Arch Pediatr Adolesc Med. 2010;164(3):231–7.
43. Hunt H, Valdimarsdottir U, Mucci L, et al. When death appears best for the child with severe malignancy: a nationwide parental follow up. Palliat Med. 2006;20(6):567–77.
44. H.R. 5067—101st Congress: Patient Self Determination Act of 1990 (1990).
45. Cruzan v. Director, Missouri Department of Health, 497 U.S. 261 (1990)
46. Altenbernd CW. (for The Court) (2001-01-24). "In re Guardianship of Theresa Marie Schiavo, Incapacitated. Robert Schindler and Mary Schindler, Appellants, v. Michael Schiavo, as Guardian of the person of Theresa Marie Schiavo, Appellee, Case Number: 2D00-1269".
47. Rietjens JA, van Zuylen L, van Veluw H, et al. Palliative sedation in a specialized unit for acute palliative care in a cancer hospital: comparing patients dying with and without palliative sedation. J Pain Symptom Manage. 2008;36(3):228–34.
48. Berger JT. Rethinking guidelines for the use of palliative sedation. Hastings Cent Rep. 2010;40:32–8.
49. Raus K, Sterckz S, Mortier F. Is continuous sedation at the end of life an ethically preferable alternative to physician -assisted suicide? Am J Bioeth. 2011;11(6):32–40.
50. Miccinesi GJ, Rietjens L, Deliens L, et al. Continuous deep sedation: physician's experiences in six European countries. J Pain Symptom Manage. 2006;331(2):122–9.
51. Schildmann J, Schildmann E. Clinical and ethical challenges of palliative sedation therapy. The need for clear guidance and professional competencies. Int J Clin Pract. 2013;11:1086–8.
52. Washington et al v Gluckberg et al, 521 U.S. 702 (S.C., 1997, 736-737)
53. Kaldjian LC, Jekel JF, Bernene JL, et al. Internists' attitudes towards terminal sedation in the end of life care. J Med Ethics. 2004;30(5):499–503.
54. van de Vathorst S, Schermer M. Additional reasons for not viewing continuous sedation as preferable alternative for physician-assisted suicide. Am J Bioeth. 2011;11(6):43–4.
55. Levine M. Report of the Council on Ethical and Judicial Affairs of the American Medical Association. Sedation to unconsciousness in end-of-life care. 2008. 5-A-08. http://www.ama-assn.org/resources/doc/code-medical-ethics/2201a.pdf
56. American Academy of Hospice and Palliative Sedation Position Statement on Palliative Sedation; approved by the board of directors. 2006. http://www.aahpm.org/positions/default/sedation.html Accessed 1 Feb 2014.
57. Quill TE, Byock IR, American College of Physicians-American Society of Internal Medicine. Responding to intractable terminal suffering: the role of terminal sedation and voluntary refusal of food and fluids. End of life Consensus Panel. http://www.acponline.org/clinical_information/resources/end_of_life_care/intractable_suffering.pdf Accessed 1 Feb 2014.
58. Powers CL, McLean PC, Harvard Community Ethics Committee. The community speaks: continuous deep sedation as caregiving versus physician-assisted suicide as killing. Am J Bioeth. 2011;11(6):65–6.
59. National Ethics Committee Veterans Health Administration. The ethics of palliative sedation as a therapy of last resort. Am J Hosp Palliat Care. 2007;23(6):483–91.
60. Anghlelescu DL, Hamilton H, Faughnan LG, et al. Pediatric palliative sedation therapy with propofol: recommendations based on experience in children with terminal cancer. J Palliat Med. 2012; 15(10):1082–90.
61. Arevalo JJ, Brinkkemper T, van der Heide A, et al. Palliative sedation: reliability and validity of sedation scales. J Pain Symptom Manage. 2012;44(5):704–14.
62. Sessler CN, Gosnell MS, Grap MJ, et al. The Richmond Agitation-Sedation Scale: validity and reliability in adult intensive care unit patients. Am J Respir Crit Care Med. 2002;166:1338–44.

Future of Pediatric Sedation

38

James R. Miner

Abstract

This concluding chapter will summarize the progress that has already been made and reflect on the opportunities and ongoing needs for advancing the field of pediatric sedation. The future of pediatric sedation will benefit from our ability to more accurately target and achieve the optimal level of sedation, analgesia, and amnesia needed for a given procedure. Advances in sedation will require that we improve our ability to proactively identify, anticipate, prepare for, and treat adverse events. The important areas that remain to be explored and advanced will be reviewed.

Keywords

Sedation • Depth of sedation • Consciousness monitoring • Pulse oximetry • Capnography • Risk assessment • Analgesia • Prophylaxis • Training • Credentialing • Simulations • Safety • Guidelines • Computerized provider order entry (CPOE) • Checklists • Adverse event reporting • Targeted controlled infusion (TCI) • Computer-assisted personalized sedation device (CAPS) • Remimazolam • Objective Risk Assessment Tool for Sedation (ORATS) • SEDASYS • Center for Medicaid and Medicare (CMS) • Word Society of Intravenous Anesthesia (World SIVA) • International Sedation Task Force (ISTF)

Introduction

Over the past two decades, pediatric sedation outside of the operating room has evolved rapidly and is an important part of the care of children. It is now an area of interest, research, and clinical practice that encompasses multiple specialties. Policies, procedures, and guidelines have been created worldwide by specialty organizations and even governmental agencies, all designed to maximize safety and outcome. Clinical research continues in efforts to further our knowledge of sedation practice, predictors of adverse outcome, and improve safety. However, there still remains to be many opportunities to optimize the safe practice of pediatric sedation, as well as improve the efficiency and efficacy of its implementation [1].

Often, when we look for advances in sedation, we look to new agents to improve our practice. The perfect sedation agent would allow the physician to provide adequate analgesia and amnesia of the painful sedation, have a precisely controllable duration of action, and then quickly have complete recovery without any adverse events. Unfortunately, such an agent does not currently exist, and we are left to adjust the protocols that we have to come as close as possible to this goal.

This concluding chapter will summarize the progress that has already been made and reflect on the opportunities and ongoing needs for advancing the field of pediatric sedation. The future of pediatric sedation will benefit from our ability to more accurately target and achieve the optimal level of sedation, analgesia, and amnesia needed for a given procedure. Advances in sedation will require that we improve our

J.R. Miner, M.D. (✉)
Department of Emergency Medicine, Hennepin County Medical Center, 701 Park Avenue S. Mail Code R2, Minneapolis, MN 55415, USA
e-mail: miner015@umn.edu

K.P. Mason (ed.), *Pediatric Sedation Outside of the Operating Room: A Multispecialty International Collaboration*, DOI 10.1007/978-1-4939-1390-9_38, © Springer Science+Business Media New York 2015

ability to proactively identify, anticipate, prepare for, and treat adverse events. The important areas that remain to be explored and advanced will be reviewed.

The Optimal Level of Sedation

Outcome Assessment and Standardization of Adverse Event Identification and Documentation

From the patient's perspective, a swift return to preprocedure mental status after having achieved adequate amnesia and analgesia represents a good outcome measure of a successful sedation. To achieve this outcome, the sedation provider would need to achieve a level of sedation adequate to induce amnesia in order to avoid the procedural recall associated with lighter levels [2–4]. Balancing patient comfort and satisfaction with safety requires that the provider anticipates that the deepest levels of sedation place patients at the highest risk for complications. These risks are most prone to occur within 3–20 min of receiving intravenous (IV) sedatives and when noxious stimuli are removed (immediately after the procedure) [3].

In terms of an assessment of the risk to the patient, the presence and nature of any adverse events that occurred during the sedation procedure are a good measure of the procedure's outcome. Adverse event rates for procedural sedation outside of the operating room (OR) have been described to range from 2.5 to 7.7 % [5–10], but the actual rate depends on what is considered to constitute an adverse event and it has varied among studies. Indicators of adverse events during procedural sedation that have been reported include sedation to a deeper level than intended, hypoxia, the need for assisted ventilations, clinically significant hypotension, aspiration, and endotracheal intubation.

The indicators that we use to compare and assess sedation outcomes, however, are not always clearly defined or accepted. For example, the occurrences of hypoxia and hypotension are identifiers that have no standardized definition. A review of the published sedation literature indicates that the definitions of hypoxia range from a 5 to 20 % drop in oxygen saturation and hypotension is defined as a 0–30 % deviation from either the patient's presedation vital signs or from established normal values [11]. Without clearly defined, standardized, and objective identifiers of adverse events, it is difficult to evaluate and compare sedation outcomes in the literature.

A recent set of recommendations [12] has advocated for the adoption of objective, standardized definers that could be applied not only to clinical studies, but also to quality assurance programs. These recommendations advocate that the need to "intervene" is an easily identifiable and objective identifier of the occurrence of an adverse or noteworthy event. Physician interventions are robust to clinically insignificant events and sensitive to events that are not necessarily captured with physiologic monitors and would identify events that require physician intervention in order to avoid, treat, or resolve complicated events during the procedure. This advance in research may help identify risk factors associated with the need for intervention and may ultimately highlight factors, predictors, and protocols that may be associated with significant adverse events. Identifying risk factors for the need for physician intervention may allow us to refine our pediatric sedation techniques and guide our training and credentialing process using clinically significant events, rather than using unclear changes in vital signs or rare outcomes.

Defining the Depth of Sedation

The Sedation Continuum is another topic of interest and advancement [13, 14]. Clinical outcomes, policies, guidelines, and recommendations are usually founded on the target depth of sedation for a procedure and risks associated with that depth. For example, the qualifications necessary to administer deep sedation is a controversial topic. Specialty societies worldwide, the Center for Medicaid and Medicare Services in the United States as well as the government sponsored health services abroad, have all weighed in with different opinions and guidelines [10, 15–25]. The basic tenet of this controversy, however, is founded on a relatively subjective scoring system: The assessment of a patient's response to verbal, tactile, and painful stimulation is used to define the depth of sedation on the sedation continuum. The tenet of the sedation continuum is that the depth of sedation is fluid and a patient can fluctuate between levels. There are limitations to this scoring system: It is subjective and not always a feasible method of assessment usually performed by the same provider administering the sedative. Accurate, continuous monitoring is not always possible, appropriate, or safe, particularly when the sedated patient is far removed from the sedation provider (magnetic resonance imaging (MRI) studies) or undergoing a procedure that discourages patient response (angiography) [26].

Sedation scales have been proposed in efforts to minimize the subjective component of the scoring process [27]. (Refer to Chap. 5.) None, however, have eliminated the subjective contribution. Rather, these markers are associated with increasing levels of sedation and respiratory depression and are not accurate identifiers of procedural success, patient recall, and the incidence of adverse events [28]. In order to advance our ability to detect adequate sedation, more precise measures of the depth of sedation must be developed [14, 26].

Table 38.1 Objective risk assessment tool for sedation (ORATS)

New levels (as yet unnamed)	Escalating risk of serious adverse event	Physiological monitoring parameters (singular or combination)[a]	Recommended sedationist skill set	Recommended resources[b]
1	≤1:10,000	Consistent with normal awake pattern and frequency	Ability to observe and interpret the agreed-upon physiological monitoring parameters	Appropriate for risk level
2	1:1,000	← Objective monitoring predicts this level of risk	Skills appropriate for maintaining sedation at this risk level and for rescuing from the subsequent level	Appropriate for risk level
3	1:100	← Objective monitoring predicts this level of risk	Skills appropriate for maintaining sedation at this risk level and for rescuing from the subsequent level	Appropriate for risk level
4	≥1:10	← Objective monitoring predicts this level of risk	Skills appropriate for maintaining a patient at this risk level	Appropriate for risk level

Preliminary sample schematic: The choice of four levels here is arbitrary and for illustration purposes only; the final tool would contain the minimum number of discrete levels with independent predictive value [14]

[a]Focused research would be required to validate the specific variables, parameters, and thresholds that predict the progressive levels of serious adverse event risk. Evaluation of capnography, for example, could include but not be limited to evaluation of waveform, frequency, pattern, and/or numerical value on inspiration or expiration

[b]To be determined at each level by consensus panel and would include but not be limited to recommendations on adjuvant personnel, intravenous access, availability of rescue medications, and airway equipment

Green and Mason have advocated a reformulation of the sedation continuum. Instead of basing the scale on subjective or semiobjective criteria, scales based on objective physiologic monitoring would be devised. The reformulated sedation continuum would be based on an objective means of assessing and stratifying sedation risk. The tool would be identified as the Objective Risk Assessment Tool for Sedation (ORATS) [14] (Table 38.1). The ORATS tool would be used in conjunction with a Comfort Assessment Tool for Sedation (CATS), which reconfigures the existing sedation continuum to reflect and follow the degree of comfort [14]. Focused research will be required to validate the specific variables, thresholds, and parameters to define such a system, but the standardization of adverse events, using this "intervention-based" approach and the application of a new tool to assess depth of sedation, will be an important step to supplement our assessment of the depth of sedation and associated risks at each level [12].

"Consciousness" Monitoring as an Indication of Sedation Depth

Amnesia and analgesia are important to our patients. Without an "amnesia" monitor, we tend to target a deep level of sedation in order to minimize the risk of recall. The deeper the level of sedation achieved during procedural sedation, however, the higher the rate of respiratory depression, and therefore the higher the risk of adverse events [2]. Ideally, the optimal sedation encounter would ensure amnesia and analgesia with minimal risk of respiratory depression and other adverse events.

To date, there is no means of ensuring amnesia during sedation [29]. Currently, a patient's level of sedation is mainly determined through interactive, subjective assessments, which integrate the physiological vital signs with a patient's response to verbal or painful stimulation. Factors such as eye opening, response to voice, and response to pain are often used to extrapolate depth of sedation and likelihood of amnesia. These factors, although likely to be associated with the progression toward deeper levels of sedation and associated adverse events, do not predict recall or analgesia. Patients who appear alert may actually have no recall following a painful procedure with propofol [28], and patients who appear to have a much decreased level of consciousness may have recall of a procedure with an opioid [30]. As we advance our knowledge of sedation, it will be important to determine the presence of procedural amnesia in order to guide us in our titration of sedation while minimizing the risk of adverse outcome.

The future of sedation would benefit from a physiological monitor that accurately follows "depth" of sedation and likelihood of amnesia. The Bispectral Index (BIS) is a monitor that was originally introduced to monitor the depth of anesthesia. It is a noninvasive monitor that monitors electroencephalogram (EEG) activity from adhesive leads that are placed on the forehead. Using a 1–100 analog score, BIS denotes a number that is intended to reflect brain activity and provide an objective monitor of depth of anesthesia [2, 3, 28, 31]. Although initially hoped to be a monitor that could follow depth of sedation and provide a surrogate marker for risk of patient recall, BIS is neither accurate nor reliable for most sedation [31–33]. It often defaults to high values in sedated patients when there is motion artifact, limiting its utility for pediatric sedation. Currently, its practical application as a monitor for depth of sedation is controversial, and its use remains investigational. Mid-latency auditory-evoked potentials (MLAEPs) have also been described as demonstrating the depth of sedation in a dose-dependent fashion and may also represent a potential depth of sedation measurement [34]. The development of an objective monitor that would quantify the level of consciousness and improve the precision in achieving adequate sedation and amnesia without progressing to a deeper level of sedation will be an important step forward in the advancement of procedural sedation [2].

Assessment of Oxygenation, Respiration, and Identification of Hypoxia

Pulse Oximetry

A patient's oxygen saturation is typically monitored during procedural sedation using pulse oximetry and is a standard of care for most specialties who provide sedation [1, 3, 10, 22, 35–37]. There is, however, a limitation to its utility: There is a variable lag time between the onset of hypoventilation or apnea and a change in oxygen saturation, especially in patients who receive supplemental oxygen, that can delay the recognition of changes in the patient's ventilation [11, 38, 39].

Pulse oximetry measures oxygenation and not ventilation. A patient breathing supplemental oxygen may not exhibit changes in their oxygen saturation until several minutes after the onset of hypoventilation, making it a late sign of hypoventilation [40, 41]. It is possible that in the future pulse oximetry may be replaced or supplemented with newer technologies that use near-infrared spectroscopy to monitor nonpulsatile signals of arterioles, capillaries, and venules, indication of tissue or cerebral oxygenation. Unlike conventional pulse oximetry, which monitors the pulsatile signal component reflecting arterial circulation, tissue perfusion monitoring can be reliable in low perfusion states, shock, and cardiac arrest situations. Changes in peripheral tissue perfusion were recently shown to correlate with the need for supportive airway maneuvers during procedural sedation [42]. The effectiveness of peripheral tissue monitoring relative to pulse oximetry or capnography has yet to be determined, and further work will be required to determine its utility in sedation monitoring.

Similarly, the role of cerebral oximetry has yet to be validated for use in procedural sedation: A recent procedural sedation study demonstrated poor correlation between cerebral oximetry, pulse oximetry, and capnography [43]. In this study, 100 children ages 9 months to 18 years were sedated with various agents (ketamine, fentanyl, pentobarbital, dexmedetomidine, or propofol). Changes in rSO_2 occurred in 2.1 % of patients and were associated with changes in SpO_2 23 % of the time and changes in end-tidal CO_2 29 % of the time. Only a minority of hypoxic episodes resulted in a decrease in rSO_2, while of the majority of the changes in rSO_2 occurred in the absence of changes in cardiorespiratory parameters. Although rSO_2 appears to be a more sensitive measure of cerebral oxygenation than pulse oximetry, there is no clear rSO_2 threshold under which clinically significant brain hypoxia occurs [44]. Improvements in the ability to detect changes in oxygenation and perfusion will likely aid in the detection of impending over-sedation and the need for intervention.

Capnography

Capnographic monitoring measures expired carbon dioxide, allowing it to follow changes in ventilation. Changes in the shape of the waveform of the capnograms display can demonstrate changes in ventilation, while changes in end-tidal CO_2, the maximum CO_2 concentration at the end of each tidal breath, can be used to estimate the severity of these changes, the response to interventions, and to quantify the degree of respiratory depression [45]. Large changes in the end-tidal CO_2 values and in the waveform shapes have been associated with respiratory depression in sedated patients and may allow earlier identification of possible hypoventilation than oximetry [38, 39, 46]. (Refer to Chap. 6.)

Capnography can rapidly detect apnea, upper airway obstruction, laryngospasm, bronchospasm, and respiratory failure [15, 47]. Capnography is more sensitive than pulse oximetry in identifying impending hypoxia in patients who are receiving supplemental oxygen [11, 38, 39, 46, 47]. A recent study by Deitch et al. demonstrated a decrease in hypoxic events among patients who were monitored using capnography in addition to standard monitoring during sedation [46].

There has been a great deal of research in capnography during sedation. Currently, these findings are made through gross visual examination of the waveform and trends in the end-tidal carbon dioxide value. As research and experience in this area continues, it is likely that these monitors will be used to detect subtle changes in respiratory effort and ventilator capacity that will be associated with both the depth of sedation and the need for airway interventions prior to the onset of an adverse event. There is sufficient evidence available, however, to recommend the routine use of capnography in procedural sedation [48, 49].

A recent study by Yu et al. of the entropy of tracheal sounds developed a novel method to assess for apnea in sedated patients. This study analyzed sounds recorded by a microphone over the trachea and was able to accurately detect apnea of 15 s or longer with a sensitivity of 95 % and a specificity of 92 % [50]. This may represent the potential for an apnea monitor more robust than pulse oximetry and more accurate in terms of false-positive detection than capnography. Hopefully further work will lead to the development of this monitor for regular use.

Risk Assessment in Balancing the Urgency for the Procedure with the Associated Risk of Sedation

The urgency of the patient's requirement for procedural sedation and the patient's current medical condition play an important role in determining the level of risk for adverse events that can be accepted for a procedure. A common tool used to assess the severity of a patient's underlying illness is the American Society of Anesthesiologists (ASA) physical status classification system [51]. Most research in the area of pediatric sedation outside of the operating room has focused on physical status class 1 and 2 patients, and the risk of an adverse event in these patients is well known. The risk of adverse effects of procedural sedation is likely higher in patients who have physical status scores of 3 or 4 [52]. The urgency of a patient's need for the procedure for which one is being sedated is based on the nature of the problem that requires sedation. Emergent indications for procedures may include cardioversion for life-threatening arrhythmias, reduction of fractures or dislocations with soft tissue or vascular compromise, or intractable pain or suffering. Not all procedures are emergent, however, and the remainder must be triaged to urgent, semiurgent, or elective/nonurgent. The degree of urgency often guides the acceptable level of risk for adverse events for procedural sedation. Patients with an emergent need for sedation are unlikely to benefit from a delay in the procedure if they have eaten food prior to the procedure [53], whereas a patient with a nonurgent need for sedation is much more likely to benefit from such a delay.

Other than the ASA physical status score, the patient's current medical condition, NPO status, and the assessment of the patient's airway and respiratory status, there has not been a great deal of investigation into the risk factors for adverse events that can be identified before the procedure has begun. As our knowledge of procedural sedation increases, the risk of adverse events subsequent to specific procedures and in patients with a variety of medical conditions needs to be established. Once these data are available, this information, along with the risk of adverse events associated with various depths of sedation, can be used to decide on the best level and timing for procedural sedation for each given procedure and can allow us to better tailor sedation to a given circumstance for a patient's specific medical situation and sedation needs.

Analgesia, Prophylaxis, and Avoiding Conditioned Behaviors

Patients who present in pain would benefit from analgesics prior to initiating the sedation. The combination of sedatives and analgesics, however, may increase the likelihood of adverse outcomes [6, 54–57]. The optimal method to treat procedural pain during sedation, and the degree to which it should be relieved, has not been determined. It is likely that patients who receive more preprocedural analgesia are more prone to respiratory depression during the sedation [48]. Recent work has demonstrated that during brief procedures, the physiologic stress of respiratory depression may be more pronounced than the stress of unrecalled pain [57].

The determination of the optimal balance between pain management and safety is difficult and requires close assessment of the patient's ongoing pain. Future work should focus on improving our ability to provide analgesia without increasing the risk of adverse events. In those situations in which the procedure is successfully completed albeit with some pain, it will be important to determine whether the inability to recall this painful experience, because of the amnestic effects of the medication, could have enduring, subversive, psychological effects.

Since pain is a subjective experience, our knowledge of a child's pain is achieved by patient report. Due to the limitations of communication with children, especially in younger children, the assessment of pain is often done simply by observation, and many methods of assessing exist [58–67]. Numerous studies have found that healthcare providers consistently underestimate a child's pain, as do the child's parents (although the parents are usually closer to the child's rating than the healthcare providers) [68]. Furthermore, it has been recently shown that sedatives may increase pain perception, at least in terms of how it is reported [69]. It is often difficult to distinguish a child's pain and agitation from distress due to the situation surrounding the pain.

The physiologic measurement of pain remains beyond current capabilities, and there is no blood test or physical sign that can accurately predict how much pain a patient experiences, leaving the situation more difficult in children than it is in adults. In the setting of repeated painful experiences, children will begin to recognize the activities of the event and develop conditioned behaviors related to upcoming painful events. The determination of which aspects of the pain response are most associated with changes in future pain behavior will guide us in modifying our sedation technique to reduce the risk of sensitizing the child to future painful procedures.

Training and Credentialing of Sedation Providers

Most of the data on procedural sedation are drawn from large academic centers with high sedation volumes. Sedation data from lower volume settings suggest that their outcomes are similar to that of busy nonacademic centers [70], but it is difficult to make conclusive comparisons regarding these two settings. Since many aspects of safe and effective procedural sedation rely on the interactive monitoring, experience, and the judgment of the operator, such as the ability to accurately recognize the depth of sedation and adequacy of ventilatory effort, it seems likely that less experienced providers would experience a comparatively higher rate of adverse events. There is likely a minimal amount of experience required in order to bring a provider to the point where he can balance the sedation depth with the adverse event risk effectively. Determining the point at which a provider can safely perform these tasks will be important in the determination of appropriate training for procedural sedation. At a national, state, and professional society level, there has been evolving interest and commitment to setting guidelines and standards for sedation delivery among healthcare professionals.

At a national level, the Joint Commission does not mandate specific credentialing for moderate sedation, but leaves it to the organizations to determine the necessary training and skills. In an update on July 7, 2010, the Joint Commission reiterated that "the individuals who are 'permitted' to administer sedation are able to rescue patients at whatever level of sedation or anesthesia is achieved either intentionally or unintentionally, e.g., when the patient slips from moderate into deep sedation or from deep sedation into full anesthesia. Each organization is free to define how it will determine that the individuals are able to perform the required types of rescue. Acceptable examples include, but are not limited to, ACLS certification, a satisfactory score on a written examination developed in concert with the department of anesthesiology, or a mock rescue exercise evaluated by an anesthesiologist" [71].

In the United States, some specialty organizations such as the American Dental Association (ADA) have released policy statements that put the onus of credentialing on the dental boards of each state. In their October 2007 Policy Statement on the Use of Sedation and General Anesthesia by Dentists, the ADA leaves the responsibility for credentialing in the hands of the individual states: "Appropriate permitting of dentists utilizing moderate sedation, deep sedation and general anesthesia is highly recommended. State dental boards have the responsibility to ensure that only qualified dentists use sedation and general anesthesia. State boards set acceptable standards for safe and appropriate delivery of sedation and anesthesia care, as outlined in this policy and in the ADA Guidelines for the Use of Sedation and General Anesthesia by Dentists" [23]. (Refer to Chap. 20.) The ASA has been much more specific in making recommendations for training and credentialing. They issued a Statement on "Granting Privileges For Deep Sedation To Non-Anesthesiologist Sedation Practitioners" on October 20, 2010 [22]. It recommends that the nonanesthesiologist be able to bag-valve-mask ventilate, insert an oro/pharyngeal airway and laryngeal mask airway, and perform an endotracheal intubation. This should include a minimum of 35 patients, inclusive of simulator experience. Practitioners should also be familiar with the use and interpretation of capnography. Deep sedation of children requires PALS and ACLS certification as well as separate education training and credentialing [72]. The ASA statement recommends that nonanesthesiologists be proficient in advanced airway management for rescue when they deliver deep sedation. This proficiency and competency would be determined by the Director of Anesthesia Services of the facility in which the sedation is delivered [17, 22]. In addition, the ASA specified that performance evaluation and a performance improvement program would be required for privileging—both of which would be developed with and reviewed by the Director of Anesthesia Services [22].

The topic of training, credentialing, and privileging process of nonanesthesia specialists has become an area of debate. In response to the aforementioned ASA statement, in July 2011 the American College of Emergency Physicians released a policy statement entitled "Procedural Sedation and Analgesia in the Emergency Department: Recommendations for Physician Credentialing, Privileging, and Practice" [72]. This policy iterated that the chief of the Emergency Medicine Service at each institution will be responsible for establishing criteria for credentialing and recommending emergency physicians for sedation privileges. Sedation training should "focus on the unique ED environment." (Refer to Chaps. 2, 6 and 19.)

The federal government has also issued guidelines via the Center for Medicaid and Medicare Services (CMS), and as recently as May 2010 and February 2011, updated the Hospital Anesthesia Services Condition of Participation 42 CFR 482.52 (a) [24]. The ASA recognizes the Center for Medicare and Medicaid Services (CMS) as defining those qualified to administer deep sedation. The 2010 CMS guidelines limited deep sedation to be delivered only by an anesthesiologist, nonanesthesiologist MD or DO, dentist, oral surgeon, podiatrist, Certified Registered Nurse Anesthetist (CRNA), or Anesthesia Assistant (AA) [24]. These CMS guidelines toward nonanesthesia providers of sedation were revised in January 2011 in the PUB 100–07 State Operations Provider Certification, which revises Appendix A for various provisions of 42 CFR 482.52 concerning anesthesia services [24]. (Refer to Chap. 12.) These revisions were made in response to feedback from practitioners and allow the individual hospitals to establish their own policies and procedures with respect to the qualifications of analgesia providers and the clinical situations that distinguish anesthesia from analgesia. The policies must follow nationally recognized guidelines and can include guidelines of one or more specialty societies.

In response to the January 2011 update to the CMS guidelines [24], the American College of Emergency Physicians used their policy statement of July 2011, entitled "Procedural Sedation and Analgesia in the Emergency Department: Recommendations for Physician Credentialing, Privileging, and Practice" to delineate who would be appropriate to deliver deep sedation [72]. (Refer to Chap. 2.) The emergency medicine physicians, physician assistants, and nurse practitioners could be credentialed to deliver sedation. Furthermore, the policy acknowledges that the emergency medicine physician may commonly administer general anesthesia for specific situations in the emergency department (intubation, postintubation, procedures on intubated patients). It expands the role of the emergency physicians as well as emergency medicine nurses by condoning the capability of qualified ED nurses to "administer propofol, ketamine, and other sedatives under the direct supervision of a privileged emergency physician." The policy also recognizes that there may be occasions whereby the emergency medicine environment may not lend itself to having a separate physician administer the sedative and another to perform the procedure: For these situations, the policy states "Deep sedation may be accomplished by the same emergency physician both administering sedation and performing the procedure" [72].

California has taken the initiative to credential sedation care providers. Specifically, the California Board of Medicine recently sponsored and passed legislation (AB2637.Eng, Chap. 499) allowing the dental board to issue a dental sedation assistant permit after a minimum of 12 months of work experience. The permit allows the assistant to monitor conscious sedation or general anesthesia from noninvasive instrumentation. They may also add drugs, medications, and fluids to intravenous lines using a syringe [73].

At a state level, the New York State Department of Health has already recognized the importance of safe delivery of sedation in the office-based setting. In 2007, the state required that office-based surgery (OBS) be performed in an accredited setting. Expounding on this, on July 14, 2009, the state became more specific: any physician performing "office-based surgery" (OBS) must do so either in an Article 28 licensed hospital, ambulatory surgery center, diagnostic and treatment center, or in a private physician's office that is accredited [74]. Accreditation may come from one of three organizations: The Joint Commission, Accreditation Association for Ambulatory Health Care (AAAHC), or American Association for Accreditation of Ambulatory Surgery Facilities (AAAASF).

In the future, it is very likely that other states will follow New York's lead and increase the vigilance and scrutiny of OBS, which requires moderate to deep sedation. We anticipate that there will be increased requirements for accrediting outpatient facilities to perform moderate or deep sedation and to credential practitioners in those settings. Outpatient clinics and providers will likely be held to the same standards as hospital-based centers. This will further increase the need for standardized and effective practitioner training and assessment.

In general, all sedation care providers agree that sedation training, credentialing, and privileging are important. There is a lack of consensus among the different specialties as to who should be responsible for developing the sedation training programs as well as for credentialing the provider. One skill set required for the safe delivery of sedation, however, remains universally accepted: the ability to recognize and manage a compromised airway. This skill set will remain a critical and integral component of the training and credentialing process and would benefit from a standardized approach among all providers.

A possible approach to facilitate and standardize the credentialing process would be to develop simulation training as an added tool to the didactic and hands-on experience. (Refer to Chap. 35.) These simulators could develop scenarios that are specific for the specialty, patient population, and type of facility (office versus hospital-based setting). They could also be used as a research tool to evaluate adverse events: By artificially creating an adverse event model, one could develop techniques to identify the contributing factors as well as ways in which to monitor, detect, and manage these occurrences. Such a model was recently described by Tobin et al., who developed a sedation simulation course, and found participants preferred it to standard didactic training [75]. Further research in the impact of such training and the validity of such models for determining sedation competency are needed, but the goal of developing sedation simulation for training appears at hand. A recent study of pediatric residents described a sedation simulation model that was able to differentiate the skills and identify the educational needs of residents, highlighting the potential use of simulation as an assessment and credentialing tool [76]. This model of training has long been in existence in the airline industry. Flight simulation dates back to before World War I and has been used to train pilots and subsequently crew and air traffic controllers [77]. The roots of *Crew Resource Management* training in the United States are usually traced back to a workshop, *Resource Management on the Flight Deck*, sponsored by the National Aeronautics and Space Administration (NASA) in 1979. This conference was the outgrowth of NASA research into the causes of air transport accidents. The research presented at this meeting identified human error aspects of the majority of air crashes as failures of interpersonal communications, decision making, and leadership. At this meeting, the label Cockpit Resource Management (CRM) was applied to the process of training crews to reduce "pilot error" by making better use of the human resources on the flight deck [78].

The Federal Aviation Authority (FAA) as well as NASA have incorporated and mandated simulation training for credentialing, licensing, and continued education. The enactment of incidences that occur with low incidence, potentially so low that a pilot may never actually even experience the real-life scenario, offers the pilot the advantage to rehearse for such an occasion. These "rehearsals" could be as important to ensuring the safety of the passengers on an airplane as they are to the children that we sedate. Simulation models and training have already been implemented throughout the specialties for training purposes [79–82]. The importance of adopting sedation-directed simulation scenarios into the training and credentialing process has been recently explored by Babl et al., who found an improvement in sedation safety 3 years after the implementation of a simulation-based sedation training curriculum [83].

Educating the Public

With recent publicity over the sedation-related deaths of celebrities (Anna Nicole Smith, Heath Ledger, Michael Jackson), the public awareness of sedation, the sedation agents (propofol, in particular), and the risk of mixing multiple sedatives is in the spotlight. (Refer to Chap. 36.) The National Institute of Health has even published a three-page patient education brochure entitled "Conscious (Moderate) Sedation for Adults" [84] in order to educate the layperson. In New York, as of 14 July 2009, patients can refer to www.nyhealth.gov to determine whether the OBS center that is using more than minimal sedation to perform a surgical or invasive procedure is accredited. Any practices that perform such procedures with more than minimal sedation and no accreditation are hence guilty of professional misconduct and disciplinary action. Patient awareness and scrutiny of sedation practice, including the agents, qualifications, and experience of providers, emergency preparedness, and outcome data should drive the field of pediatric sedation forward.

Developing the "Safety Culture" of Sedation: Implementing Safety Measures

Establishing a "safe culture" around sedation practice is important. (Refer to Chap. 30.) Credentialing, standardizing the definition of adverse events, improving sedation delivery methods and techniques, introducing new sedatives, incorporating simulation into provider training, and using more objective means of identifying the depth of sedation and associated risks are all important first steps. There are also new methods that could be adopted. Once again, the airline industry has been on the forefront of adopting and exploring new methods at ensuring safety. The industry has adopted the use of checklists. The airline industry, National Aeronautics and Space Administration (NASA), and FAA have been developing checklists since before World War II. Checklists have begun to be adopted in the medical community as a means to foster active discussions and teamwork [85–88]. In 2009, a multi-institutional, international group of eight hospitals published prospectively collected data on a total of 7,688 consecutive patients, before and after the adoption of a 19-item Surgical Safety Checklist. This was an initiative of the World Health Organization's (WHO) Safe Surgery Saves Lives Program. The mortality rate (at 30 days) decreased from 1.5 to 0.8 % following implementation [88]. A global commitment by the sedation community to develop checklists to foster teamwork and the "safety culture" may ultimately improve patient outcomes [86, 89].

A method of increasing procedural safety may also be the use of computerized provider order entry (CPOE). A recent study of the effect on error reduction in hospitals that have introduced CPOE shows a moderate improvement [90]. It is likely the CPOE will improve sedation safety, especially in terms of dosing errors and adjuvant medications. Electronic systems have the added benefit of the potential to facilitate the use of safety checklists before, during, and after the procedure.

Collecting Outcome Data to Guide Safety and Practice Parameters: Adoption of Standardized Definitions of Sedation-Related Adverse Events

As described previously, the works of the Pediatric Sedation Research Consortium and the ketamine individual patient data meta-analysis are important first steps toward generating the data required to carefully assess sedation practice in children outside the OR. Recently, the World Society of Intravenous Anesthesia (World SIVA) established an International Sedation Task Force (ISTF) represented by 26 members from multispecialties, both adult and pediatric, from 11 countries. The ISTF has proposed an Adverse Event Reporting Tool designed to standardize the collection of sedation outcome data worldwide [91]. This tool is an open-access web-based tool, available to providers globally.[1] The data collected will be available to individual and institutional users and will, in addition, populate the global ISTF sedation

[1] www.AESedationReporting.com or www.InternationalSedationTaskForce.com

database. (Refer to Chap. 28.) The collection of large data from multispecialists globally will be an important first step to identify and carefully evaluate the range of variables that effect sedation-related adverse event rates. Such studies must be broad reaching in scope yet flexible enough to consider new developments in sedation techniques and monitoring as well as the use of the ever-emerging new sedation drugs that become available.

Compiling standardized data sets allowing for the aggregation of data will only be possible through the rigorous adherence to the use of standardized adverse events definitions and reporting structures such as described in the Quebec Guidelines and by the ISTF. Such an advancement will allow for the meaningful comparison of studies and the analysis of uncommon but important adverse events such as the need for endotracheal intubation [92]. National and international multispecialty collaboration will be required to develop such databases with sufficient patient numbers and the clinical data required to develop and evaluate sedation practice based on patient populations and providers, procedures performed, and drugs administered. The feasibility of such a collaborative endeavor requires not only cooperation of multiple specialties using cutting-edge data collection technology, but also a level of funding that to date has not been realized.

Sedatives: Exploring New Agents and Alternative Methods and Modes of Delivery

The ideal agent for procedural sedation would provide analgesia, anxiolysis, amnesia, and somnolence rapidly and predictably with no adverse effects. Ideally, this drug would be devoid of respiratory side effects and ensure hemodynamic stability. To date, such a drug does not exist. Currently, there are still a limited number of sedatives with pediatric labeling and Food and Drug Administration (FDA) approval. Labeling with pediatric information is in less than 50 % of drug products [93]. The Best Pharmaceuticals for Children Act of 2002 and the Pediatric Research Equity Act of 2003 advocated for expanding the number of drugs with pediatric labeling [94, 95]. In March, 2014 the American Academy of Pediatrics and its Committee on Drugs published a policy statement on off-label drugs in children. The policy concluded that "evidence, not label indication, remains the gold standard from which practitioners should draw when making therapeutic decisions for their patients." The statement made recommendations for off-label drug administration and the advocating of off-label drug research and publication. Finally, the policy statement recommended, "institutions and payers should not use labeling status as the sole criterion that determines the availability on formulary or reimbursement status for medications in children. Similarly, less expensive therapeutic alternatives considered appropriate for adults should not automatically be considered appropriate first-line treatment in children. Finally, off-label uses of drugs should be considered when addressing various drug-related concerns, such as drug shortages." [96] (Refer to Chap. 26.)

It is highly unlikely that a perfect sedative will ever be developed. Alternatives could include the introduction of sedatives that are reversible, shorter action, or that use new delivery methods. In addition, evidence now suggests that pharmacogenetics has a role in the effect of analgesic, sedative, and local anesthetic medications [97]. Variants in the μ opioid receptor gene change the analgesic effect of opioid medications, ibuprofen clearance varies between individuals based on genotype, as does midazolam metabolism, and the efficacy of lidocaine [98–101]. It is possible that in the future, pharmacogenetic approaches may facilitate personalized sedation. (Refer to Chap. 11.)

Fospropofol is a water-soluble prodrug of propofol that was originally intended to be offered as a sedative that confers the same advantages of propofol (relatively rapid onset of sedation, brief time to recovery) with the added benefit of having less associated risk of respiratory depression [102]. It did not receive FDA approval as a sedative and instead has the same "anesthetic agent" labeling as propofol. Its slow onset and long duration of action, however, made it appear unsuitable for procedural sedation. Furthermore, the metabolism of fospropofol produces formaldehyde, which has not been found to be in toxic levels but is not ideal. Further studies are needed to determine the efficacy and safety profile of fospropofol, as currently the published studies are largely limited to adults undergoing gastrointestinal endoscopy procedures [102]. A similar propofol prodrug (HX0969w) that releases propofol and gamma hydroxyl butyrate rather than formaldehyde has been recently described and will likely undergo trials in the near future [103]. This change in metabolite may be a key advantage, given the sedative properties of gamma hydroxyl butyrate. This property, however, may complicate the determination of the duration of effect or the progression of sedative effects with cumulative dosing and will require detailed work to determine its safety, efficacy, and optimal uses. The combination of a more gradual onset and offset could diminish complications during the start of the procedure, and decrease the need for further sedative dosing late in the procedure, and these may be qualities that will result in a larger therapeutic window than is currently available with standard propofol.

Alfentanil [30], remifentanil [104], and sufentanil [105] have all been recently described in procedural sedation protocols with some success. These short-acting opioids may prove to have some uses in procedural sedation as isolated agents rather than as the supplemental opioids for which they have been studied, but further work is required to determine the relative efficacy to other agents and the spectrum of situations in which they would prove a useful alternative. Recent trials comparing dexmedetomidine to short-acting opioids have found them inferior for sedation for awake intubation [105, 106]. Opioids are not typically amnestic at doses not associated with respiratory depression, and often result in procedural recall at doses sufficient for procedural compliance when used as sole sedative agents. The relative importance of procedural amnesia versus recall of a compliant state in children, however, remains to be determined. The determination of the effect of recall and the state of the child's comfort will be an important area of research in the future to determine the utility of short-acting opioids for procedural sedation.

Another agent in development is remimazolam. This is an ultra-short acting benzodiazepine that is currently undergoing trials as a procedural sedation agent. It appears from initial studies to have a similar achieved sedation depth and a shorter recovery time than midazolam [107–109]. This agent will likely have a future role in pediatric sedation outside of the operating room, depending on its associated rates of respiratory depression, onset and offset, and effects on procedural recall.

Given the few new sedative drugs in development, it has also been beneficial to explore alternate routes to deliver sedatives and analgesics that are currently available. As different routes (intramuscular, sublingual, intranasal, buccal, rectal, oral, intravenous, subcutaneous) of delivery have different uptake and onset of action, their efficacy, outcome, and adverse event profiles differ. The development of non-parenterally administered sedatives would offer alternatives to establishing intravenous access. This model already exists for some opiates. Fentanyl has been well described for transmucosal administration, but has not been developed for use in procedural sedation [110]. Sufentanil is being developed for sublingual administration and is demonstrating an onset of action comparable to parenteral opioids [111]. Intramuscular ketamine has been well described in children and is currently a widely used option for those children who do not require intravenous access [15, 112, 113]. Intranasal ketamine as well as intranasal dexmedetomidine have been recently described and compared, and both were found to be effective premedications for children undergoing MRI [114]. Sedation for radiologic procedures is common, and the intranasal route has many advantages, making these advances in the route of administration promising.

Nitrous oxide offers the advantages of an inhalational delivery method and has been used for procedural sedation for almost a century, especially in dentistry and oral surgery, and will likely continue to play a large role in the sedation of children [113, 115]. Current advances in nitrous delivery have included improved scavenger systems, breath-actuated gas delivery, and dynamic gas mixing. Advances in nitrous oxide delivery systems may someday enable children to assist in the self-administration of nitrous oxide via a patient-controlled delivery system, which only delivers when triggered by inspiratory pressure, has a built-in scavenging system, and guarantees that a hypoxic mixture will never be delivered.

In addition to exploring outcomes with different routes of sedation, the future of sedation could rely on our ability to incorporate and validate new delivery methods. Targeted controlled infusions (TCI) are another option for more precise drug delivery. (Refer to Chap. 31.) TCI infusion devices deliver a medication to a target blood concentration (brain) using validated pharmacokinetic models to achieve the targeted end point. TCI is already being used worldwide by the anesthesia community as a method to titrate the intravenous anesthetic to the patient's physiological vital signs and predicted plasma serum levels. Adult TCI models for many medications (ketamine, remifentanil, propofol, fentanyl) have been incorporated into specialized TCI infusion pumps, which are widely used in Europe but are not available in the United States (Alaris PK Syringe Pump, Cardinal Health, Switzerland; Master TCI, Fresenius Kabi, Germany; Perfusor Space, Braun, Germany). Advances in patient-controlled infusions or TCI and more importantly, the development of pediatric models for TCI delivery, may allow currently used sedatives, analgesics, and anesthetics to be administered to children in a more precise and safe manner.

A recent study by Guen et al. compared a manual sedation algorithm to an automated system for the titration of a propofol/remifentanil infusion for sedated patients in ICU. This study used the BIS monitor to determine adequate sedation and drive the algorithm and the automated system, and found the automated system to be superior to the manual algorithm for maintaining deep sedation [116]. Such automated systems hold great promise for improving sedation, both in terms of decreasing adverse events and in maintaining stable sedation levels through procedures.

Currently, a computer-assisted personalized sedation device (CAPS) has been developed for adult use. SEDASYS (Ethicon Endo Surgery Inc., Cincinnati, OH) is a CAPS device that recently completed a multicenter Phase III trial delivering propofol for gastrointestinal endoscopy [106]. (Refer to Chap. 31.) CAPS is designed to integrate patient data into computerized programs in order to guide drug delivery. The goal of CAPS is to provide moderate sedation, with patients still able to respond to verbal or tactile instructions by squeezing a hand held switch. Initial CAPS outcome data in adult patients undergoing gastrointestinal endoscopy appear promising [117]. In June 2009, the FDA Advisory Committee for Anesthesiology and Respiratory Therapy Devices recommended that the FDA approve the SEDASYS device, with a few caveats; the agency should require special training on the device for physicians and should require teams of at least three clinicians, including one doctor or nurse. The advisory committee also recommended that the system be limited to adults aged 70 or younger and that additional studies were needed. In May of 2013, the FDA granted premarket approval for the SEDASYS system, and it is expected to be introduced on a limited basis in 2014.

The future of pediatric sedation may well rest in the development and introduction of TCI and CAPS (for those children who are developmentally and cognitively able). A collaboration between the pharmaceutical and device industry as well as the clinical investigators will be essential not only to trial the CAPS, but also to create TCI models for children. The potential application of CAPS for pediatric use could offer cognitively able children the ability to control the delivery of their own sedation and analgesia. The future of CAPS and TCI for the pediatric population in the United States and abroad depends on pediatric trials, industry initiative, financial support, and the FDA's commitment to approach this new technique with an open mind.

Conclusion

There are a variety of advances currently underway likely to improve the safety and effectiveness of sedation. Future advances in pediatric procedural sedation will rely as much on the standardization and refinement of existing technology and resources as the development of new monitoring techniques, sedation protocols, sedation medications, administration routes, and methods of sedative delivery.

References

1. Miner JR, Krauss B. Procedural sedation and analgesia research: state of the art. Acad Emerg Med. 2007;14(2):170–8 [Review].
2. Miner JR, Biros MH, Heegaard W, Plummer D. Bispectral electroencephalographic analysis of patients undergoing procedural sedation in the emergency department. Acad Emerg Med. 2003;10(6):638–43 [Clinical Trial Comparative Study].
3. Miner JR, Biros MH, Seigel T, Ross K. The utility of the bispectral index in procedural sedation with propofol in the emergency department. Acad Emerg Med. 2005;12(3):190–6.
4. Miner JR, Huber D, Nichols S, Biros M. The effect of the assignment of a pre-sedation target level on procedural sedation using propofol. J Emerg Med. 2007;32(3):249–55.
5. Burton JH, Miner JR, Shipley ER, Strout TD, Becker C, Thode Jr HC. Propofol for emergency department procedural sedation and analgesia: a tale of three centers. Acad Emerg Med. 2006;13(1): 24–30.
6. Cote CJ, Karl HW, Notterman DA, Weinberg JA, McCloskey C. Adverse sedation events in pediatrics: analysis of medications used for sedation. Pediatrics. 2000;106(4):633–44 [Research Support, Non-U.S. Gov't].
7. Cravero JP, Blike GT. Pediatric sedation. Curr Opin Anaesthesiol. 2004;17(3):247–51.
8. Pena BM, Krauss B. Adverse events of procedural sedation and analgesia in a pediatric emergency department. Ann Emerg Med. 1999;34(4 Pt 1):483–91.
9. Rex DK, Deenadayalu VP, Eid E, Imperiale TF, Walker JA, Sandhu K, et al. Endoscopist-directed administration of propofol: a worldwide safety experience. Gastroenterology. 2009;137(4): 1229–37; quiz 1518–9 [Research Support, Non-U.S. Gov't Review].
10. Vargo JJ, Cohen LB, Rex DK, Kwo PY. Position statement: non-anesthesiologist administration of propofol for GI endoscopy. Gastroenterology. 2009;137(6):2161–7 [Practice Guideline].
11. Deitch K, Chudnofsky CR, Dominici P. The utility of supplemental oxygen during emergency department procedural sedation and analgesia with midazolam and fentanyl: a randomized, controlled trial. Ann Emerg Med. 2007;49(1):1–8 [Randomized Controlled Trial].
12. Bhatt M, Kennedy RM, Osmond MH, Krauss B, McAllister JD, Ansermino JM, et al. Consensus-based recommendations for standardizing terminology and reporting adverse events for emergency department procedural sedation and analgesia in children. Ann Emerg Med. 2009;53(4):426–35.e4 [Consensus Development Conference Research Support, Non-U.S. Gov't].
13. American Society of Anesthesiologists. Continuum of depth of sedation: definition of general anesthesia and levels of sedation/analgesia. http://www.asahqorg/For-Members/Clinical-Information/Standards-Guidelines-and-Statements.aspx. Amended on 21 October 2009; Accessed June 2013.
14. Green SM, Mason KP. Stratification of sedation risk—a challenge to the sedation continuum. Paediatr Anaesth. 2011;21(9):924–31 [Research Support, Non-U.S. Gov't Review].
15. Green SM, Krauss B. Clinical practice guideline for emergency department ketamine dissociative sedation in children. Ann Emerg Med. 2004;44(5):460–71.
16. Miner JR, Burton JH. Clinical practice advisory: emergency department procedural sedation with propofol. Ann Emerg Med. 2007;50(2):182–7, 187.e1.
17. Dumonceau JM, Riphaus A, Aparicio JR, Beilenhoff U, Knape JT, Ortmann M, et al. European Society of Gastrointestinal Endoscopy, European Society of Gastroenterology and Endoscopy Nurses and associates, and the European Society of Anaesthesiology Guideline: non-anesthesiologist administration of propofol for GI endoscopy. Endoscopy. 2010;42(11):960–74 [Practice Guideline].
18. Reed A TJ, Roelofse JA, Gray R. de Kock M, Peircy J. Paediatric procedural sedation and analgesia (PSA) guidelines. South African Society of Anaesthesiologists. 2011. Accessed at http://sasaweb.com.
19. Peiry J, Roelofse J. SASA sedation guidelines 2010. South Afr J Anaesth Analg. 2010;16(4):1612.
20. CBO. Summary of draft guidelines on sedation and/or analgesia (PSA) at locations outside the operating theatre. Part III: in children. Netherlands Society of Anesthesiologists and Dutch Society of Pediatrics. Utrecht: DIfHICAO; 2011.
21. SIGN. Safe sedation of children undergoing diagnostic and therapeutic procedures. A national clinical guideline. Edinburgh: Scottish Intercollegiate Guidelines Network; 2004.
22. American Society of Anesthesiologists. Granting privileges for deep sedation to non-anesthesiologist sedation providers. Approved by ASA House of Delegates October 2010. 2010
23. American Dental Association. Guidelines for the use of sedation and general anesthesia by dentists. ADA House of Delegates adopted October 2007. 2007.
24. Department of Health & Human Services, CfMMS. Revised hospital anesthesia services interpretive guidelines-state operations manual (SOM) appendix A; 2011. Accessed at http://cms.gov.
25. Anonymous. Sedation in children and young people (CG112). National Institute for Health and Care Excellence (NICE). 2013. http://guidance.nice.org.uk/cg112
26. Green SM, Mason KP. Reformulation of the sedation continuum. JAMA. 2010;303(9):876–7.

27. Avramov MN, White PF. Methods for monitoring the level of sedation. Crit Care Clin. 1995;11(4):803–26.
28. Miner JR, Bachman A, Kosman L, Teng B, Heegaard W, Biros MH. Assessment of the onset and persistence of amnesia during procedural sedation with propofol. Acad Emerg Med. 2005;12(6):491–6 [Clinical Trial Research Support, Non-U.S. Gov't].
29. Atkins JH, Mandel JE. Recent advances in patient-controlled sedation. Curr Opin Anaesthesiol. 2008;21(6):759–65.
30. Miner JR, Gray R, Delavari P, Patel S, Patel R, Plummer D. Alfentanil for procedural sedation in the emergency department. Ann Emerg Med. 2011;57(2):117–21.
31. Gill M, Green SM, Krauss B. A study of the bispectral index monitor during procedural sedation and analgesia in the emergency department. Ann Emerg Med. 2003;41(2):234–41.
32. Mason KP, Michna E, Zurakowski D, Burrows PE, Pirich MA, Carrier M, et al. Value of bispectral index monitor in differentiating between moderate and deep Ramsay Sedation Scores in children. Paediatr Anaesth. 2006;16(12):1226–31.
33. Malviya S, Voepel-Lewis T, Tait AR, Watcha MF, Sadhasivam S, Friesen RH. Effect of age and sedative agent on the accuracy of bispectral index in detecting depth of sedation in children. Pediatrics. 2007;120(3):e461–70 [Meta-Analysis Research Support, Non-U.S. Gov't].
34. Kuhnle GE, Hornuss C, Lenk M, Salam AP, Wiepcke D, Edelman-Gahr V, Flake G, Daunderer M, Oberhauser M, Muller HH, Feuerecker M. Impact of propofol on mid-latency auditory-evoked potentials in children. Br J Anaesth. 2013;110(6):1001–9.
35. Cote CJ, Wilson S. Guidelines for monitoring and management of pediatric patients during and after sedation for diagnostic and therapeutic procedures: an update. Paediatr Anaesth. 2008;18(1): 9–10 [Guideline].
36. Godwin SA, Caro DA, Wolf SJ, Jagoda AS, Charles R, Marett BE, et al. Clinical policy: procedural sedation and analgesia in the emergency department. Ann Emerg Med. 2005;45(2):177–96.
37. Miner JR, Danahy M, Moch A, Biros M. Randomized clinical trial of etomidate versus propofol for procedural sedation in the emergency department. Ann Emerg Med. 2007;49(1):15–22.
38. Burton JH, Harrah JD, Germann CA, Dillon DC. Does end-tidal carbon dioxide monitoring detect respiratory events prior to current sedation monitoring practices? Acad Emerg Med. 2006;13(5): 500–4 [Evaluation Studies].
39. Miner JR, Heegaard W, Plummer D. End-tidal carbon dioxide monitoring during procedural sedation. Acad Emerg Med. 2002; 9(4):275–80.
40. Keidan I, Gravenstein D, Berkenstadt H, Ziv A, Shavit I, Sidi A. Supplemental oxygen compromises the use of pulse oximetry for detection of apnea and hypoventilation during sedation in simulated pediatric patients. Pediatrics. 2008;122(2):293–8 [Comparative Study].
41. Lightdale JR, Goldmann DA, Feldman HA, Newburg AR, DiNardo JA, Fox VL. Microstream capnography improves patient monitoring during moderate sedation: a randomized, controlled trial. Pediatrics. 2006;117(6):e1170–8 [Randomized Controlled Trial Research Support, N.I.H., Extramural Research Support, Non-U.S. Gov't Research Support, U.S. Gov't, P.H.S.].
42. Miner JR, Plummer D. Using near infrared spectroscopy for tissue oxygenation monitoring during procedural sedation: the association of Sto_2 changes with supportive airway measures. Ann Emerg Med. 2012;60(4):s152.
43. Padmanabhan P, Berkenbosch JW, Lorenz D, Pierce MC. Evaluation of cerebral oxygenation during procedural sedation in children using near infrared spectroscopy. Ann Emerg Med. 2009;54(2):205–13.
44. Carlin RE, McGraw DJ, Calimlim JR, Mascia MF. The use of near-infrared cerebral oximetry in awake carotid endarterectomy. J Clin Anesth. 1998;10(2):109–13 [Clinical Trial].
45. Krauss B, Hess DR. Capnography for procedural sedation and analgesia in the emergency department. Ann Emerg Med. 2007;50(2):172–81.
46. Deitch K, Miner J, Chudnofsky CR, Dominici P, Latta D. Does end tidal CO2 monitoring during emergency department procedural sedation and analgesia with propofol decrease the incidence of hypoxic events? A randomized, controlled trial. Ann Emerg Med. 2010;55(3):258–64 [Randomized Controlled Trial].
47. Green SM, Krauss B. Pulmonary aspiration risk during emergency department procedural sedation—an examination of the role of fasting and sedation depth. Acad Emerg Med. 2002;9(1):35–42 [Review].
48. Mohr NM, Wessman B. Continuous capnography should be used for every emergency department procedural sedation. Ann Emerg Med. 2013;61(6):697–8.
49. Waugh JB, Epps CA, Khodneva YA. Capnography enhances surveillance of respiratory events during procedural sedation: a meta-analysis. J Clin Anesth. 2011;23(3):189–96 [Meta-Analysis].
50. Yu L, Ting CK, Hill B, Orr J, Brewer L, Johnson K, Egan T, Westenkow D. Using entropy of tracheal sounds to detect apnea during sedation in healthy nonobese volunteers. Anesthesiology. 2013;118(6):1341–9.
51. American Society of Anesthesiologists. Physical status classification system. 2004. www.asahq.org/clinical/physicalstatus.htm. Accessed 30 Mar 2004.
52. Green SM, Roback MG, Kennedy RM, Krauss B. Clinical practice guideline for emergency department ketamine dissociative sedation: 2011 update. Ann Emerg Med. 2011;57(5):449–61.
53. Green SM, Roback MG, Miner JR, Burton JH, Krauss B. Fasting and emergency department procedural sedation and analgesia: a consensus-based clinical practice advisory. Ann Emerg Med. 2007;49(4):454–61.
54. American Society of Anesthesiologists. Statement on the safe use of propofol. 2004. www.asahq.org. Accessed June 2005
55. Messenger DW, Murray HE, Dungey PE, van Vlymen J, Sivilotti ML. Subdissociative-dose ketamine versus fentanyl for analgesia during propofol procedural sedation: a randomized clinical trial. Acad Emerg Med. 2008;15(10):877–86.
56. Miner JR, Gray RO, Stephens D, Biros MH. Randomized clinical trial of propofol with and without alfentanil for deep procedural sedation in the emergency department. Acad Emerg Med. 2009;16(9):825–34 [Comparative Study Randomized Controlled Trial].
57. Miner JR, Moore JC, Plummer D, Gray RO, Patel S, Ho JD. Randomized clinical trial of the effect of supplemental opioids in procedural sedation with propofol on serum catecholamines. Acad Emerg Med. 2013;20(4):330–7.
58. Bailey B, Daoust R, Doyon-Trottier E, Dauphin-Pierre S, Gravel J. Validation and properties of the verbal numeric scale in children with acute pain. Pain. 2010;149(2):216–21 [Research Support, Non-U.S. Gov't Validation Studies].
59. Hicks CL, von Baeyer CL, Spafford PA, van Korlaar I, Goodenough B. The faces pain scale-revised: toward a common metric in pediatric pain measurement. Pain. 2001;93(2):173–83.
60. Lynch-Jordan AM, Kashikar-Zuck S, Goldschneider KR. Parent perceptions of adolescent pain expression: the adolescent pain behavior questionnaire. Pain. 2010;151(3):834–42 [Validation Studies].
61. Palermo TM, Lewandowski AS, Long AC, Burant CJ. Validation of a self-report questionnaire version of the child activity limitations interview (CALI): the CALI-21. Pain. 2008;139(3):644–52 [Research Support, Non-U.S. Gov't Validation Studies].
62. Solodiuk JC, Scott-Sutherland J, Meyers M, Myette B, Shusterman C, Karian VE, et al. Validation of the Individualized Numeric Rating Scale (INRS): a pain assessment tool for nonverbal children with intellectual disability. Pain. 2010;150(2):231–6 [Validation Studies].

63. Spafford PA, von Baeyer CL, Hicks CL. Expected and reported pain in children undergoing ear piercing: a randomized trial of preparation by parents. Behav Res Ther. 2002;40(3):253–66 [Clinical Trial Comparative Study Randomized Controlled Trial].
64. Spagrud LJ, von Baeyer CL, Ali K, Mpofu C, Fennell LP, Friesen K, et al. Pain, distress, and adult-child interaction during venipuncture in pediatric oncology: an examination of three types of venous access. J Pain Symptom Manage. 2008;36(2):173–84 [Controlled Clinical Trial Research Support, Non-U.S. Gov't].
65. Tomlinson D, von Baeyer CL, Stinson JN, Sung L. A systematic review of faces scales for the self-report of pain intensity in children. Pediatrics. 2010;126(5):e1168–98 [Research Support, Non--U.S. Gov't Review].
66. von Baeyer CL, Forsyth SJ, Stanford EA, Watson M, Chambers CT. Response biases in preschool children's ratings of pain in hypothetical situations. Eur J Pain. 2009;13(2):209–13 [Research Support, Non-U.S. Gov't].
67. von Baeyer CL, Spagrud LJ, McCormick JC, Choo E, Neville K, Connelly MA. Three new datasets supporting use of the Numerical Rating Scale (NRS-11) for children's self-reports of pain intensity. Pain. 2009;143(3):223–7 [Validation Studies].
68. Singer AJ, Gulla J, Thode Jr HC. Parents and practitioners are poor judges of young children's pain severity. Acad Emerg Med. 2002;9(6):609–12 [Comparative Study Validation Studies].
69. Frolich MA, Kui Z, Ness TJ. Effects of sedation on pain perception. Anesthesiology. 2013;118(3):611–21.
70. Sacchetti A, Senula G, Strickland J, Dubin R. Procedural sedation in the community emergency department: initial results of the ProSCED registry. Acad Emerg Med. 2007;14(1):41–6.
71. Anonymous. Permission to administer moderate sedation. The Joint Commission. 2010. http://www.jointcommission.org/mobile/standards_information/jcfaqdetails.aspx?StandardsFAQId=457&StandardsFAQChapterId=66. Accessed 26 Dec 2013.
72. O'Connor RE, Sama A, Burton JH, Callaham ML, House HR, Jaquis WP, et al. Procedural sedation and analgesia in the emergency department: recommendations for physician credentialing, privileging, and practice. Ann Emerg Med. 2011;58(4):365–70 [Practice Guideline].
73. Newsletter MBoC. Newsletter. 2009:109.
74. Anonymous. Office based surgery laws: New York State Department of Health. http://www.health.ny.gov/professionals/office-based_surgery/obs_faq.htm. Accessed 26 Dec 2013.
75. Tobin C, Clark CA, McEvoy MD, Reves JG, Schaefer JJ, Wolf BJ, Reeves ST. An approach to moderate sedation simulation training. Simul Healthc. 2013;8(2):114–23.
76. Schinasi DA, Nadel FM, Hales R, Boswinkel JP. Assessing pediatric residents' clinical performance in procedural sedation. Pediatr Emerg Care. 2013;29(4):447–52.
77. Nikolic MI, Sarter NB. Flight deck disturbance management: a simulator study of diagnosis and recovery from breakdowns in pilot-automation coordination. Hum Factors. 2007;49(4):553–63 [Research Support, U.S. Gov't, Non-P.H.S.].
78. Anonymous. Mercado da Aviacao. 2012. http://www.mercadodaaviacao.com.br/cursos-apostilas/visualizar/crm-evolution-faa-ingles/. Accessed 26 Dec 2013.
79. Gaba DM. The future vision of simulation in healthcare. Simul Healthc. 2007;2(2):126–35.
80. Gaba DM. Adapting space science methods for describing and planning research in simulation in healthcare: science traceability and decadal surveys. Simul Healthc. 2012;7(1):27–31.
81. Shavit I, Keidan I, Hoffmann Y, Mishuk L, Rubin O, Ziv A, et al. Enhancing patient safety during pediatric sedation: the impact of simulation-based training of nonanesthesiologists. Arch Pediatr Adolesc Med. 2007;161(8):740–3 [Clinical Trial].
82. Siu LW, Boet S, Borges BC, Bruppacher HR, LeBlanc V, Naik VN, et al. High-fidelity simulation demonstrates the influence of anesthesiologists' age and years from residency on emergency cricothyroidotomy skills. Anesth Analg. 2010;111(4):955–60 [Comparative Study Research Support, Non-U.S. Gov't].
83. Babl FE, Krieser D, Belousoff J, Theophilos T. Evaluation of a paediatric procedural sedation training and credentialing programme: sustainability of change. Emerg Med J. 2010;27: 577–81.
84. National Institutes of Health. Conscious (moderate) sedation for adults. 2013.
85. Koppel R, Metlay JP, Cohen A, Abaluck B, Localio AR, Kimmel SE, et al. Role of computerized physician order entry systems in facilitating medication errors. JAMA. 2005;293(10):1197–203 [Evaluation Studies Research Support, U.S. Gov't, Non-P.H.S. Research Support, U.S. Gov't, P.H.S.].
86. Verdaasdonk EG, Stassen LP, Hoffmann WF, van der Elst M, Dankelman J. Can a structured checklist prevent problems with laparoscopic equipment? Surg Endosc. 2008;22(10):2238–43.
87. Weiser TG, Haynes AB, Lashoher A, Dziekan G, Boorman DJ, Berry WR, et al. Perspectives in quality: designing the who surgical safety checklist. International J Qual Health Care. 2010;22(5):365–70 [Research Support, Non-U.S. Gov't].
88. Haynes AB, Weiser TG, Berry WR, Lipsitz SR, Breizat AH, Dellinger EP, et al. A surgical safety checklist to reduce morbidity and mortality in a global population. N Engl J Med. 2009;360(5):491–9 [Multicenter Study Research Support, Non-U.S. Gov't].
89. Eslami S, de Keizer NF, Abu-Hanna A. The impact of computerized physician medication order entry in hospitalized patients—a systematic review. Int J Med Inform. 2008;77(6):365–76 [Meta-Analysis Review].
90. Radley DC, Wasserman MR, Olsho LE, Shoemaker SJ, Spranca MD, Bradshaw B. Reduction in medication errors in hospitals due to adoption of computerized provider order entry systems. JAMIA. 2013;20(3):470–6 [Research Support, U.S. Gov't, P.H.S.].
91. Mason KP, Green SM, Piacevoli Q. Adverse event reporting tool to standardize the reporting and tracking of adverse events during procedural sedation: a consensus document from the World SIVA International Sedation Task Force. Br J Anaesth. 2012; 108(1):13–20.
92. Chassin MR, Loeb JM, Schmaltz SP, Wachter RM. Accountability measures—using measurement to promote quality improvement. N Engl J Med. 2010;363(7):683–8.
93. Sachs AN, Avant D, Lee CS, Rodriguez W, Murphy MD. Pediatric information in drug product labeling. JAMA. 2012;307(18): 1914–5.
94. Best Pharmaceuticals for Children Act. Public Law No. 107-109. 2002. http://www.fda.gov/Drugs/DevelopmentApprovalProcess/DevelopmentResources/ucm049876.htm. Accessed 8 Apr 2014.
95. Pediatric Research Equity Act. Public Law No. 108-155. 2003. http://www.gpo.gov/fdsys/pkg/PLAW-108publ155/content-detail.html. Accessed 8 Apr 2014.
96. American Academy of Pediatrics Committee on Drugs. Policy statement: off-label use of drugs in children. Pediatrics. 2014; 133(3):563–7.
97. Cohen M, Sadhasivam S, Vinks AA. Pharmacogenetics in perioperative medicine. Curr Opin Anaesthesiol. 2012;25(4):419–27 [Review].
98. Hajj A, Khabbaz L, Laplanche JL, Peoc'h K. Pharmacogenetics of opiates in clinical practice: the visible tip of the iceberg. Pharmacogenomics. 2013;14(5):575–85 [Research Support, Non-U.S. Gov't].
99. Sadhasivam S, Chidambaran V. Pharmacogenomics of opioids and perioperative pain management. Pharmacogenomics. 2012;13(15): 1719–40 [Research Support, Non-U.S. Gov't Review].
100. Ashenhurst JR, Bujarski S, Ray LA. Delta and kappa opioid receptor polymorphisms influence the effects of naltrexone on

subjective responses to alcohol. Pharmacol Biochem Behav. 2012;103(2):253–9 [Research Support, N.I.H., Extramural].

101. Saruwatari J, Matsunaga M, Ikeda K, Nakao M, Oniki K, Seo T, et al. Impact of CYP2D6*10 on H1-antihistamine-induced hypersomnia. Eur J Clin Pharmacol. 2006;62(12):995–1001 [Research Support, Non-U.S. Gov't].
102. Cohen LB, Cattau E, Goetsch A, Shah A, Weber JR, Rex DK, et al. A randomized, double-blind, phase 3 study of fospropofol disodium for sedation during colonoscopy. J Clin Gastroenterol. 2010;44(5):345–53 [Clinical Trial, Phase III Comparative Study Multicenter Study Randomized Controlled Trial Research Support, Non-U.S. Gov't].
103. Zhou Y, Yang J, Liu J, Wang Y, Zhang WS. Efficacy comparison of the novel water-soluble propofol prodrug HX0969w and fospropofol in mice and rats. Br J Anaesth. 2013;111(5):825–32.
104. Sacchetti A, Jachowski J, Heisler J, Cortese T. Remifentanil use in emergency department patients: initial experience. Emerg Med J. 2012;29(11):928–9.
105. Shen SL, Xie YH, Wang WY, Hu SF, Zhang YL. Comparison of dexmedetomidine and sufentanil for conscious sedation in patients undergoing awake fibreoptic nasotracheal intubation: a prospective, randomized and controlled clinical trial. Clin Respir J. 2014;8(1):100–7.
106. Zhang JQ, Meng FM, Xue FS. Is dexmedetomidine or remifentanil alone an optimal sedation scheme for awake intubation? J Anesth. 2013;27(4):627–8.
107. Antonik LJ, Goldwater DR, Kilpatrick GJ, Tilbrook GS, Borkett KM. A placebo- and midazolam-controlled phase I single ascending-dose study evaluating the safety, pharmacokinetics, and pharmacodynamics of remimazolam (CNS 7056): part I. Safety, efficacy, and basic pharmacokinetics. Anesth Analg. 2012;115(2):274–83 [Clinical Trial, Phase I Randomized Controlled Trial Webcasts].
108. Rogers WK, McDowell TS. Remimazolam, a short-acting GABA(A) receptor agonist for intravenous sedation and/or anesthesia in day-case surgical and non-surgical procedures. IDrugs. 2010;13(12):929–37 [Review].
109. Wiltshire HR, Kilpatrick GJ, Tilbrook GS, Borkett KM. A placebo- and midazolam-controlled phase I single ascending-dose study evaluating the safety, pharmacokinetics, and pharmacodynamics of remimazolam (CNS 7056): part II. Population pharmacokinetic and pharmacodynamic modeling and simulation. Anesth Analg. 2012;115(2):284–96 [Clinical Trial, Phase I Randomized Controlled Trial Research Support, Non-U.S. Gov't Webcasts].
110. Klein EJ, Diekema DS, Paris CA, Quan L, Cohen M, Seidel KD. A randomized, clinical trial of oral midazolam plus placebo versus oral midazolam plus oral transmucosal fentanyl for sedation during laceration repair. Pediatrics. 2002;109(5):894–7.
111. Minkowitz HS, Singla NK, Evashenk MA, Hwang SS, Chiang YK, Hamel LG, et al. Pharmacokinetics of sublingual sufentanil tablets and efficacy and safety in the management of postoperative pain. Reg Anesth Pain Med. 2013;38(2):131–9 [Clinical Trial, Phase I Clinical Trial, Phase II Comparative Study Randomized Controlled Trial Research Support, Non-U.S. Gov't].
112. Green SM, Roback MG, Krauss B. Laryngospasm during emergency department ketamine sedation: a case-control study. Pediatr Emerg Care. 2010;26(11):798–802 [Review].
113. Babl FE, Belousoff J, Deasy C, Hopper S, Theophilos T. Paediatric procedural sedation based on nitrous oxide and ketamine: sedation registry data from Australia. Emerg Med J. 2010;27(8):607–12 [Research Support, Non-U.S. Gov't].
114. Gyanesh P, Haldar R, Srivastava D, Agrawal PM, Tiwari AK, Singh PK. Comparison between intranasal dexmedetomidine and intranasal ketamine as premedication for procedural sedation in children undergoing MRI: a double-blind, randomized, placebo-controlled trial. J Anesth. 2014;28(1):12–8.
115. Kennedy RM, Luhmann JD, Luhmann SJ. Emergency department management of pain and anxiety related to orthopedic fracture care: a guide to analgesic techniques and procedural sedation in children. Paediatr Drugs. 2004;6(1):11–31.
116. Le Guen M, Liu N, Bourgeois E, Chazot T, Sessler DI, Rouby JJ, et al. Automated sedation outperforms manual administration of propofol and remifentanil in critically ill patients with deep sedation: a randomized phase II trial. Intensive Care Med. 2013;39(3):454–62 [Research Support, Non-U.S. Gov't].
117. Pambianco DJ, Vargo JJ, Pruitt RE, Hardi R, Martin JF. Computer-assisted personalized sedation for upper endoscopy and colonoscopy: a comparative, multicenter randomized study. Gastrointest Endosc. 2011;73(4):765–72 [Comparative Study Multicenter Study Randomized Controlled Trial].

Epilogue

Anthony R. Absalom, M.B.Ch.B., F.R.C.A., F.H.E.A., M.D.
Professor of Anesthesia
Department of Anesthesiology
University Medical Center Groningen
Groningen, The Netherlands

Karel Allegaert, M.D., Ph.D.
Associate Professor of Anesthesia
Department of Growth and Regeneration
KU Leuven and Neonatal Intensive Care Unit
University Hospitals Leuven
Leuven, Belgium

Brian J. Anderson, M.B.Ch.B., Ph.D., F.A.N.Z.C.A., F.J.F.I.C.M.
Adjunct Professor of Anesthesiology
Department of Anesthesiology
University of Auckland School of Medicine
Pediatric Intensive Care Unit
Auckland Children's Hospital
Auckland, New Zealand

Dean B. Andropoulos, M.D., M.H.C.M.
Chief of Anesthesiology
Texas Children's Hospital
Professor of Anesthesiology and Pediatrics
Baylor College of Medicine
Houston, TX, USA

Franz E. Babl, M.D., M.P.H.
Associate Professor of Anesthesia
University of Melbourne
Emergency Department
Royal Children's Hospital
Melbourne, VIC, Australia

Douglas W. Carlson, M.D.
Professor of Pediatrics
Director, Division of Pediatric Hospitalist Medicine
Division of Pediatric Hospitalist Medicine
Department of Pediatrics
St. Louis Children's Hospital
Washington University
St. Louis, MO, USA

Xuan Chen, M.Med.
Department of Anesthesia
Hong Kong University
Shenzhen, Guangdong, China

Vincent W. Chiang, M.D.
Associate Professor of Pediatrics
Harvard Medical School
Chief of Inpatient Services
Boston Children's Hospital
Associate Program Director
Boston Combined Residency
Boston, MA, USA

Stewart L. Cohen, Esq.
Partner/Shareholder
Cohen, Placitella & Roth, P.C.
Philadelphia, PA, USA

Luciane Ribeiro de Rezende Sucasas da Costa, D.D.S., M.S., Ph.D.
Professor of Pediatric Dentistry
Faculty of Dentistry
Division of Pediatric Dentistry
Federal University of Goiás
Goiania, Goias, Brazil

Paulo Sérgio Sucasas da Costa, M.S., Ph.D.
Associate Professor of Pediatrics
Department of Pediatrics
Federal University of Goiás
Goiania, Goias, Brazil

Joseph P. Cravero, M.D.
Associate Professor of Anesthesia
Harvard Medical School
Department of Anesthesiology, Perioperative, and Pain Medicine
Boston Children's Hospital
Boston, MA, USA

Stuart R. Dalziel, M.B.Ch.B., F.R.A.C.P., Ph.D.
Pediatric Emergency Medicine Specialist
Children's Emergency Department

K.P. Mason (ed.), *Pediatric Sedation Outside of the Operating Room: A Multispecialty International Collaboration*, DOI 10.1007/978-1-4939-1390-9, © Springer Science+Business Media New York 2015

Director of Emergency Medicine Research
Starship Children's Hospital
Auckland District Health Board
Auckland, New Zealand

Andrew J. Davidson, M.B.B.S., M.D., F.A.N.Z.C.A.
Associate Professor
Department of Pediatrics
Senior Staff Anesthetist
Director of Clinical Research
Department of Anaesthesia and Pain Management
The Royal Children's Hospital Melbourne
Murdoch Children's Research Institute
University of Melbourne
Melbourne, VIC, Australia

James J. Fehr, M.D.
Associate Professor of Anesthesia
Department of Anesthesiology and Pediatrics
St. Louis Children's Hospital
St. Louis, MO, USA

Lynne R. Ferrari, M.D.
Associate Professor of Anesthesia
Harvard Medical School
Medical Director and Chief, Perioperative Anesthesia
Departments of Anesthesiology, Perioperative
and Pain Medicine
Boston Children's Hospital
Boston, MA, USA

Daniela Hearst, B.Sc. (Hons.), M.Phil.
Consultant Clinical Psychologist and Joint Head
of Pediatric Psychology
Department of Pediatric Psychology, Psychosocial
and Family Services
Great Ormond Street Hospital for Children NHS
Foundation Trust
London, UK

Robert S. Holzman, M.D., M.A. (Hon.), F.A.A.P.
Professor of Anaesthesia
Harvard Medical School
Department of Anesthesiology, Perioperative
and Pain Medicine
Boston Children's Hospital
Boston, MA, USA

Timothy Horeczko, M.D., M.S.C.R.
Assistant Professor of Emergency Medicine
Department of Emergency Medicine
Harbor – UCLA Medical Center
Torrance, CA, USA

Marie Therese Hosey, D.D.S., M.Sc. (Med. Sci.), B.D.S., F.D.S.R.C.P.S. (Glas.)
Head of Pediatric Dentistry
Department of Pediatric Dentistry
Professor of Dentistry
King's College London, Dental Institute
London, UK

Michael G. Irwin, M.B.Ch.B., M.D., F.H.K.C.A., F.A.N.Z.C.A., F.R.C.A., F.H.K.A.M.
Professor and Head
Department of Anesthesiology
The University of Hong Kong
Chief of Service in Anesthesia
Queen Mary Hospital, China
Chief of Service in Anesthesia
HKU Shenzen Hospital, China
President, Society of Anesthetists, Hong Kong
President, International Federation of Intravenous
Anesthesia Society
President, Organizing Committee for World Congress
of Anaesthesia 2016

Ian A. Jenkins, M.B.B.S., F.R.C.A., F.R.C.P.E., F.F.I.C.M.
Consultant in Pediatric Intensive Care & Anaesthesia
Bristol Royal Hospital for Children
Bristol, UK
Past President of the Pediatric Intensive Care Society
Past Chair of the Pediatric Intensive Care Society
Sedation Group

Robert M. Kennedy, M.D.
Professor of Pediatrics
Associate Director, Education Affairs
Emergency Services
Washington University School of Medicine
Department of Pediatrics
St. Louis Children's Hospital
St. Louis, MO, USA

Baruch S. Krauss, M.D., Ed.M.
Associate Professor of Pediatrics
Harvard Medical School
Director, Inpatient Sedation Service
Division of Emergency Medicine
Boston Children's Hospital
Boston, MA, USA

Piet L.J.M. Leroy, M.D., Ph.D.
Associate Professor of Pediatrics
Department of Pediatrics
Division of Pediatric Critical Care
Pediatric Procedural Sedation Unit
Maastricht University Medical Centre
Maastricht, The Netherlands

Bi-lian Li, M.D.
Department of Anesthesiology
Guangzhou Women and Children's Medical Centre
Guangzhou, Guangdong, China

Jenifer R. Lightdale, M.D., M.P.H.
Professor of Pediatrics, University of Massachusetts Medical School
Division Chief, Pediatric Gastroenterology, Hepatology and Nutrition
Chief Quality Officer UMass Memorial Children's Medical Center
Division of Pediatric Gastroenterology, Hepatology and Nutrition
UMass Memorial Children's Medical Center
Department of Pediatrics
University of Massachusetts Medical School
Worcester, MA, USA

Yuan-Chi Lin, M.D., M.P.H.
Director, Medical Acupuncture Service
Department of Anesthesiology, Perioperative and Pain Medicine
Boston Children's Hospital
Associate Professor of Anesthesia (Pediatrics)
Harvard Medical School

Mohamed Mahmoud, M.D.
Associate Professor of Pediatrics and Anesthesiology
Director, Radiology Anesthesia and Sedation
Department of Anesthesia
Cincinnati Children's Hospital Medical Center
Cincinnati, OH, USA

Keira P. Mason, M.D.
Associate Professor of Anesthesia
Harvard Medical School
Director of Radiology Anesthesia and Sedation
Department of Anesthesiology, Perioperative and Pain Medicine
Boston Children's Hospital
Boston, MA, USA
Vice President, World Society of Intravenous Anesthesia (SIVA)
Chairman, International Sedation Task Force (ISTF) and Pediatric Committee, World SIVA

Lisa L. Mathis, M.D.
Executive Medical Director
Department of Global Regulatory Affairs and Safety
Maternal and Pediatric Safety and Regulatory
Amgen Inc.
Thousand Oaks, CA, USA

Ian McKenzie, M.B.B.S., Dip. R.A.C.O.G., F.A.N.Z.C.A.
Assistant Professor
University of Queensland, Brisbane, Australia
Director, Department of Anesthesia and Pain Management
The Royal Children's Hospital
Parkville, VIC, Australia

Suzanne Swanson Mendez, M.D.
Pediatric Hospitalist
Department of Pediatrics
Santa Clara Valley Medical Center
San Jose, CA, USA

Alan F. Merry, O.N.Z.M., M.B.Ch.B., F.A.N.Z.C.A., F.P.M.A.N.Z.C.A., F.R.C.A.
Professor and Head of School of Medicine
University of Auckland
Department of Anesthesiology
Auckland City Hospital
Auckland, New Zealand
Chairman, Board of the New Zealand Health Quality and Safety Commission

James R. Miner, M.D.
Professor of Emergency Medicine
University of Minnesota Medical School
Department of Emergency Medicine
Hennepin County Medical Center
Minneapolis, MN, USA

Itai M. Pessach, M.D., Ph.D.
Israel Center for Medical Simulation (MSR)
Sheba Medical Center
Tel-Hashomer, Israel

Randy P. Prescilla, M.D.
Instructor in Anesthesia
Harvard Medical School
Department of Anesthesiology, Perioperative and Pain Medicine
Children's Hospital Boston
Boston, MA, USA

Mark G. Roback, M.D.
Professor of Pediatrics and Emergency Medicine
University of Minnesota Medical School
Co-Director, Pediatric Emergency Medicine
Department of Pediatrics
University of Minnesota Amplatz Children's Hospital
Minneapolis, MN, USA

James A. Roelofse, M.B.Ch.B., M.Med. (Anes.)
Professor of Anesthesiology
Head of Sedation and Pain Control
University of the Western Cape
Department of Anesthesiology
Tygerberg Hospital
Bellville, Cape Province, South Africa
Visiting Professor of Anesthesiology
Director, Post-Graduate Certificate in Sedation and Pain Management
University College London
Visiting Professor of Anesthesiology

Khan University, Nairobi, Kenya
President, Society of Sedation Practitioners of South Africa (SOSPOSA)

Joel S. Rosen, Esq.
Partner
Cohen, Placitella & Roth, P.C.
Philadelphia, PA, USA

Cyril Sahyoun, M.D.
Assistant Professor of Clinical Pediatrics
Department of Pediatric Emergency Medicine
Morgan Stanley Children's Hospital of New York
Columbia University Medical Center
New York, NY, USA

Steven M. Selbst, M.D.
Professor of Pediatrics
Thomas Jefferson University Hospital
Department of Pediatrics
Nemours/Alfred I. duPont Hospital for Children and Jefferson Medical College
Wilmington, DE, USA

Wang Ning ShangGuan, M.D., Ph.D.
Associate Professor
Department of Anesthesiology
The 2nd Affiliated Hospital
Wenzhou Medical University
Wenzhou, Zhejiang, China

Devona J. Slater, C.H.A., C.H.C., C.M.C.P.
President and Compliance Auditor
Auditing for Compliance and Education, Inc. (ACE)
Overland Park, KS, USA

Sulpicio G. Soriano, M.D.
Professor and BCH Endowed Chair in Pediatric Neuroanesthesia
Harvard Medical School
Department of Anesthesiology, Perioperative and Pain Medicine
Boston Children's Hospital
Boston, MA, USA

Michael J. Stabile, M.D., M.B.A.
Chief, Department of Anesthesia
Centennial Medical Center
Nashville, TN, USA
Cheif of Anesthesia, Operation Smile

Michael R.J. Sury, M.B.B.S., F.R.C.A., Ph.D.
Consultant Pediatric Anesthetist
Great Ormond Street Hospital for Children
Honorary Senior Lecturer in Anaesthesia
PORTEX Unit of Pediatric Anesthesia
Institute of Child Health
University College of London
London, England

Joss J. Thomas, M.B.B.S., M.P.H., F.C.C.P.
Clinical Associate Professor of Anesthesia
Department of Anesthesia
University of Iowa Hospitals and Clinics
Iowa City, IA, USA

Joseph D. Tobias, M.D.
Chief, Department of Anesthesiology & Pain Medicine
Department of Anesthesiology & Pain Medicine
Nationwide Children's Hospital
Columbus, OH, USA

Johannes van den Anker, M.D., Ph.D.
Professor, Department of Pediatrics, Pharmacology and Physiology
Department of Pediatrics, Pharmacology and Physiology
Children's National Medical Center, Washington, DC, USA
Intensive Care, Erasmus Medical Center-Sophia Children's Hospital, Rotterdam, The Netherlands
Department of Pediatric Pharmacology, University Children's Hospital Basel, Switzerland

Gail A. Van Norman, M.D.
Professor Anesthesiology and Pain Medicine
Adjunct Professor Biomedical Ethics
Department of Anesthesiology and Pain Medicine
Department of Biomedical Ethics
University of Washington Medical Center
Seattle, WA, USA

Robert A. Veselis, M.D.
Professor of Anesthesiology
Weill Cornell Medical College
Director, Neuroanesthesiology Research Laboratory
Department of Anesthesiology/CCM
Memorial Sloan Kettering Cancer Center
New York, NY, USA

Pablo O. Sepúlveda Voullième, Dr. Med.
Professor of Anesthesia
Servicio de Anestesia
Clinica Alemana Santiago Chile
Santiago, Chile

Laszlo Vutskits, M.D., Ph.D.
Staff Anesthesiologist and Senior Lecturer
Department of Anesthesiology, Pharmacology and Intensive Care
Department of Fundamental Neuroscience
Geneva Neuroscience Center
University of Geneva
Geneva, Switzerland

Chunyan Wang, M.Med.
Department of Anesthesiology
Hong Kong University Shenzhen Hospital
Shenzhen, Guangdong, China

Craig S. Webster, B.Sc., M.Sc. (Hon.), Ph.D.
Senior Lecturer
Centre for Medical and Health Sciences Education
School of Medicine
University of Auckland
Auckland, New Zealand

Graeme S. Wilson
Senior Specialist
Department of Anaesthesia
University of Cape Town, Red Cross War Memorial Children's Hospital
Rondebosch, Western Cape, South Africa

Stephen Wilson, D.M.D., M.A., Ph.D.
Professor, University of Cincinnati Department of Pediatrics
Medical Director, Division of Pediatric Dentistry
Division of Pediatric Dentistry
Cincinnati Children's Hospital Medical Center
Cincinnati, OH, USA

Ying Xu, Ph.D., M.D.
Associate Professor
Department of Anesthesiology
Children's Hospital of Chongqing Medical University
Chongqing, Chongqing, China

Lynne P. Yao, M.D.
Associate Director
Office of New Drugs
Pediatric and Maternal Health Staff
Center for Drug Evaluation and Research
United States Food and Drug Administration (FDA)
Silver Spring, MD, USA

Vivian Man-ying Yuen, M.B.B.S., F.A.N.Z.C.A., F.H.K.C.A., F.H.K.A.M.
Consultant of University of Hong Kong Shenzhen Hospital
Honorary Clinical Associate Professor
Department of Anesthesiology
University of Hong Kong
Honorary Consultant
Department of Anesthesiology
Queen Mary Hospital
Shenzhen, Guangdong, China

Index

K.P. Mason (ed.), *Pediatric Sedation Outside of the Operating Room: A Multispecialty International Collaboration*, DOI 10.1007/978-1-4939-1390-9, © Springer Science+Business Media New York 2015

E

F

G

O

S

T

U

PGMO 05/23/2018